D1449964

CONSUMER HEALTH USA
Essential Information from the
Federal Health Network

Edited by Alan M. Rees

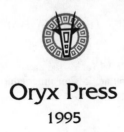

Oryx Press
1995

The rare Arabian Oryx is believed to have inspired the myth of the unicorn. This desert antelope became virtually extinct in the early 1960s. At that time several groups of international conservationists arranged to have 9 animals sent to the Phoenix Zoo to be the nucleus of a captive breeding herd. Today the Oryx population is over 800 and nearly 400 have been returned to reserves in the Middle East.

Library of Congress Cataloging-in-Publication Data

Consumer health USA / edited by Alan M. Rees.
    p.   cm.
    Includes index.
    ISBN 0-89774-889-1 (acid-free paper)
    1. Medicine, Popular. 2. Consumer education. I. Rees, Alan M.
RC81.C725 1994   94-37594
616—dc20   CIP

CONTENTS

■ ■ ■

PREFACE

■ ■ ■

The Need for Medical Information

Consumers demand concise, accurate, up-to-date, meaningful, and understandable information about the many and diverse medical problems they experience in their daily lives. Medical consumerism is driven by the desire to acquire, understand, and process information in order to make intelligent health decisions. This need propels people to consult libraries, toll-free hotlines, patient educators, magazines, information clearinghouses, Ask-a-Nurse, or any other convenient information source to amplify, explain, verify, or deny what they have learned from their health care providers.

Health Publications from the Government

One of the most valuable sources of authoritative, concise and current information is the United States federal government. The National Institutes of Health and the Public Health Service in particular produce a vast quantity of information of interest to consumers. This information, in effect, represents a condensation and digest of the findings of the national medical research investment. In this manner, the National Cancer Institute offers information to consumers concerning most types of cancer, current treatments, clinical trials, and research, while the Agency for Health Care Policy and Research translates the current state of the art in many areas of clinical practice into patient versions of practice guidelines. Patient versions of clinical practice guidelines are now available on topics such as treatment of unstable angina, depression, acute pain management, prostate enlargement, sickle cell disease, heart failure, cataracts, urinary incontinence, and early HIV infection. The High Blood Pressure Education Program and the National Cholesterol Education Program produce pamphlets and booklets with the specific intention of educating the general public.

The publications are carefully edited and screened by government researchers for scientific accuracy. Many contain helpful charts and diagrams. Often, they include lists of resources, phone numbers, and addresses of support groups. Few would argue with either the quality or value of these publications.

Access Problems

The major problem confronting the consumer is how to *access* this body of literature. It is most difficult to identify, locate, order, and obtain copies of health-related consumer publications. There is no established and integrated announcement mechanism, with the result that consumers must ask to be added to the mailing list of each publishing agency. Frequent purging of mailing lists results in consumers being denied receipt of further newsletters. The *NIH Publications List* is not always current and accurate, and some agencies are not represented. Most of the announced publications are not available from the U.S. Government Printing Office and must be ordered from each agency. A telephone or mail order may take up to six weeks for fulfillment. To save money, fourth-class mail, the slowest delivery method, is frequently used to fill orders. Often a number of follow-up calls must be made to check the status of an order and to determine why requested items have not been received. Unfortunately, the publication of this large corpus of valuable information has outstripped the federal announcement and distribution system.

Several agencies have initiated fax-based services to shorten document delivery time. Fax messages now exist on a wide variety of topics such as cancer, tetanus, chronic fatigue syndrome, measles, Lyme disease, chicken pox, and shingles. In many instances, there is no print equivalent. The availability of fax machines is, however, still limited so that many individuals do not have this type of access.

The Purpose of This Publication

The purpose of *Consumer Health USA* is to bring together in one convenient location 151 consumer health information documents currently available on topics of most concern to the general public. The publication is designed to facilitate easy identification and to provide materials for photocopying, thereby eliminating the considerable time and effort involved in physically locating and acquiring elusive documents. Moreover, this volume will make it easier for libraries to maintain a complete collection with minimum risk of vandalism and loss.

Immediate and convenient access is provided to a vast store of current, authoritative, concise, and readily understandable health information produced by the federal government for consumer use. The information has been assembled from key agencies of the U.S. government such as the National Institutes of Health; Food and Drug Administration; National Institute on Aging; National Institute of Arthritis and Musculoskeletal and Skin Diseases; National Eye Institute; National Heart, Blood, and Lung Institute; National Institute of Neurological Diseases and Stroke; and the National Institute of Mental Health. Both print and fax-based messages are included. Most of the fax documents are those made available by the National Cancer Institute through CancerFax and the Centers for Disease Control through the CDC Fax Information Service.

Text of these documents is reproduced in this volume unedited. In order to make *Consumer Health USA* as compact as possible, only those illustrations essential to the text have been reproduced. Publisher information is located at the end of each document under the heading "Document Source."

Arrangement

Documents are arranged according to body system, thereby bringing together publications related, for example, to Heart Disease and Blood Vessel Disorders, Skin Diseases and Disorders, Gastrointestinal System Disorders, and Women's Health. Documents concerning cancer in general are contained in the Cancer, General section, while those related to a particular body system are printed under the relevant sections. Consequently, lung cancer is to be found in the Lung and Respiratory Disorders section, and cervical cancer in Women's Health. Within body system sections, documents are arranged alphabetically by title. Cross references to related documents in this book are located at the end of each entry, and a subject index assists the reader further in locating information.

I would like to acknowledge the creative and skilled efforts of Janet Woolum and Susan Slesinger of Oryx Press in transforming a vast array of diverse and complex textual material into a finished book.

Alan M. Rees
Cleveland, Ohio
October 1994

AIDS AND SEXUALLY TRANSMITTED DISEASES

■ ■ ■

CARING FOR SOMEONE WITH AIDS

Information for Friends, Relatives, Household Members, and Others Who Care for a Person with AIDS at Home

One of the best places for a person with AIDS to receive care is at home, surrounded by those who can provide love and care.

Most people with AIDS can lead an active life for long periods of time. In fact, most of the time a person with AIDS does not need to be in a hospital. A person with AIDS often recovers from AIDS-related illnesses more quickly and comfortably at home with the support of friends and loved ones. Also, home care can help reduce the stress and cost of hospitalization.

Each person with AIDS is different, and is affected by the disease in different ways, and to different degrees. The person's doctor or nurse will keep you updated on the amount and kind of care that is needed. Often, one of the hardest things for a person with AIDS to do is to keep up with the everyday routines of shopping, getting and answering the mail, paying bills, and tidying up. These are the types of roles in which you can play a major part.

What Will You Need to Do?

If you are planning to provide home care for a person with AIDS, you should consider taking a home care course. Contact your local Red Cross chapter, Visiting Nurse Association, or AIDS service agency to find out about home care training offered in your area.

While it's not always possible, it's nice if you can get to know the person's doctor, or at least the nurse, social worker, and other care providers. Work with them to create a plan for home care. Ask them to provide you with clear written instructions regarding medications and procedures. Make sure you know about any adverse reactions to drugs that may occur. Learn whom to call or what to do in the event of an emergency.

Be prepared to keep the doctor or nurse posted of changes if they occur in the person's health or behavior. For example, a cough, fever, diarrhea, or confusion may indicate an infection or complication that requires special treatment or hospitalization. The doctor or nurse will also let you know about changes in the person's condition which may indicate that home care is not the best option for the person with AIDS.

Providing Emotional Support for the Person with AIDS

It is important to think about the emotional well-being of the person you are caring for. Since every person's emotional needs are different, no single approach is best for everybody.

Here are some suggestions for giving emotional support to people with AIDS.

- Encourage the person with AIDS to become involved in his or her own care, set a schedule, and make decisions whenever possible. These actions will provide a sense of control and independence.
- Don't avoid the person with AIDS. Include him or her in activities whenever possible. You don't always have to talk. Your company can be more important than your words. Just having you there while reading or watching television may be appreciated. Allow for quiet time. Like anyone else, he or she may feel anger, frustration, depression, and all other emotions.
- Don't be afraid to discuss the disease. Often, people with AIDS need to talk about it to work out what is happening in their own mind. Offer to help find professional counseling if it is desired. Let the doctors, nurses, and social workers understand your relationship to the person with AIDS, and your role as a caregiver.
- Don't be afraid to touch a person with AIDS. Holding a hand, giving a hug, or giving a back rub can greatly raise the person's spirits. However, be sensitive to people who do not wish to accept physical closeness.

The virus that causes AIDS can damage the brain and cause psychological problems. These problems can include difficulty in thinking clearly and changes in feelings and moods. A common problem for a person with AIDS is dementia. It can result in forgetfulness and poor concentration; slowing down of movements, speech, and thinking; decreased alertness; loss of interest and pleasure in work, and most other activities; and unpredictable or exaggerated changes in mood.

These problems can be very disturbing to the person with AIDS and to others in the home. They can also make it difficult to follow the routines for home care and for protecting the person with AIDS from infection. If these or other psychological problems develop, they should be discussed with the doctor, nurse, social worker, or mental health professional.

Protecting Yourself from Infection with the Virus That Causes AIDS

The virus that causes AIDS is the *human immunodeficiency virus.* You will hear it called by its initials—HIV. Studies indicate that HIV is present in blood, semen, and vaginal fluids of infected persons, and is usually transmitted by

♦ having sex with a person infected with HIV; or
♦ using, sharing, or sticking yourself with a needle or syringe that has previously been used by or for a person infected with HIV.

In addition, women infected with HIV can pass the virus to their babies during pregnancy or during birth. In some cases they can also pass it on when breast-feeding. Some people have been infected by receiving blood transfusions, although the risk of infection has been virtually eliminated since careful screening and laboratory testing of the blood supply began in 1985.

You won't get the AIDS virus through everyday contact. You won't get the disease from the air, food, water, insects, animals, dishes, or toilet seats. Because the virus which causes AIDS is found in the blood of infected persons, you should consider blood or other body fluids which contain visible blood (for example, bloody stool) as a potential source of infection. However, in the many instances when health care providers have come in contact with HIV-infected blood, only a small number of HIV infections have resulted. These have all taken place because of needle stick injuries or when blood was splashed on skin that had sores or breaks, or on mucous membranes (mouth, nose, or eyes). *In the absence of sores or breaks, no HIV infections are known to have occurred at all.* The risk of becoming infected with HIV through needle stick injury or blood coming in contact with your skin is very low. Simple precautions can virtually eliminate this already very small risk. Wear gloves if you may have contact with blood or blood-tinged body fluids. Also, if you have any cuts, sores, or breaks on exposed skin, cover them with a bandage. You will want to wear gloves to clean up articles soiled with urine, feces, or vomit to avoid other germs, even though infections with HIV have not been observed following such contact.

Two types of gloves can be used, depending upon the task. You can use disposable hospital-type gloves to prevent contact with blood when you provide nursing care to a person with AIDS. These gloves should be used once and thrown away. For household chores that involve contact with blood, you may also use household rubber gloves. These gloves can be cleaned, disinfected, and reused. Just make sure they are in good condition. Don't use gloves that are peeling, cracked, or have holes in them.

Always wash your hands with soap and water after any hand contact with blood, even if gloves are worn. In addition to wearing gloves, if large amounts of blood are present, you may want to wear an apron or smock to prevent your clothing from being soiled. If the person with AIDS is bleeding frequently or heavily, contact the doctor or nurse, as home care may no longer be adequate. Remove blood from surfaces and containers with soap and water or a household cleaning solution, then disinfect the area with a solution made by mixing household bleach and water.

The same precautions you take when blood is present need to be taken in the presence of vaginal secretions and semen.

Medication needles may be present if the person with AIDS is diabetic, has hemophilia, or is having other special treatment at home. Handle needles carefully to avoid sticking yourself.

A Handy Disinfecting Solution

A solution of one part bleach freshly diluted with 100 parts water (for example, one tablespoon in one quart of water) can be used on floors, showers, tubs, sinks, and other items, such as mops and sponges. Wear gloves while cleaning up blood, and wash your hands with soap and water after removing gloves. Discard the bleach solution after 24 hours, since it is less effective when it is old. Keep the solution out of the reach of children.

♦ Do not put caps back on needles by hand, do not remove needles from the syringes, and do not break, bend, or otherwise handle needles, because you might stick yourself in the process.
♦ When you handle a used needle and syringe, pick it up by the barrel of the syringe and carefully drop it into a puncture-proof container. The doctor, nurse, or AIDS service organization can provide you with a container especially made for this purpose. If a special container is not available, you can use any puncture-proof container that has a plastic top, such as a coffee can.
♦ Keep the disposal container in a room where needles and syringes are used, but well out of the reach of children and visitors.
♦ Be sure to dispose of the container before it is overflowing with needles. Ask your doctor or nurse about further instructions for disposal of the container.
♦ If you stick yourself with a used needle, wash the site of exposure thoroughly with soap and water. Then, contact your doctor as soon as possible to get further evaluation, advice, and, perhaps, treatment.

You can wash clothing and linens used by a person with AIDS as you ordinarily would. When using an automatic washing machine, use soap or detergent and either hot or cold washing cycles. Follow the instructions on the soap or detergent package.

If stains due to blood, semen, or vaginal secretions are present, soaking the clothes in cold water and using bleach may help to remove the stains. However, it is not necessary to add bleach to washing machines to kill the virus. Clothes may also be dry-cleaned or hand-washed.

A person with AIDS does not require separate dishes or eating utensils, and dishes used by a person with AIDS do not require special methods of cleaning. They should be washed as you ordinarily would, with soap or detergent and hot water.

A person with AIDS can prepare food for others, provided that he/she does not have diarrhea due to a germ that can be spread by food. It is a good idea for anyone preparing food—including a person with AIDS—to wash his or her hands before beginning.

A person with AIDS should not share razors or toothbrushes because these items sometimes draw blood.

Flush all liquid waste containing blood down the toilet. Be careful to avoid splashing blood when you are pouring liquids into the toilet. Tissues, or other flushable items with blood, semen, or vaginal fluid on them, may also be flushed.

Paper towels, sanitary pads and tampons, wound dressings, and other items soiled with blood, semen, or vaginal fluid that are not flushable should be placed in a plastic bag. Close the bag securely before placing in a trash container. Check with your doctor, nurse, or local health department to be sure you are following trash disposal regulations for your area.

Protecting the Person with AIDS from Infection

A person with AIDS or AIDS-related illnesses has a difficult time fighting off certain infections. A person with AIDS should avoid close contact with people with contagious illnesses until symptoms have disappeared. That includes diseases such as colds, the flu, or stomach flu (gastroenteritis).

If you have a cold or flu and nobody else is available to provide care, you should wear a surgical-type mask and wash your hands before touching the person with AIDS.

If you have skin infections such as boils, cold sores or fever blisters (*herpes simplex*), or shingles (zoster), you should avoid close contact with a person with AIDS. If such contact is unavoidable, you should keep skin sores covered and wash hands before contact. Wear gloves if you have a rash or sores on your hands.

If there are pets in the house, the person with AIDS should wash his or her hands with soap and water after handling them and especially after cleaning their litter or living areas (such as cages and tanks). This is to protect against infections the animals may carry. Litter boxes should be emptied (not sifted) daily. Pet birds should be checked by a veterinarian for psittacosis, a disease which may be harmful to a person with AIDS. Sick pets should be checked promptly by a veterinarian. Neither sick pets nor their litter should be handled by the person with AIDS.

Everyone caring for or living with a person with AIDS should consider getting a flu (influenza) shot to reduce the chance of getting the flu and passing the disease on to the person with AIDS. To be effective, flu shots must be taken *every year*.

Everyone caring for or living with a person with AIDS should be up-to-date on all of their "childhood" shots, not only for their own protection, but also to avoid getting any of these diseases outside the home and then transmitting the disease to the person with AIDS.

Even if you believe that you and everybody living with the person with AIDS have had all the recommended childhood shots, ask your doctor if you need any boosters or shots for measles, mumps, or rubella, since these shots may not have been available when you were a child. If the person with AIDS is exposed to measles, contact the person's doctor within 24 hours. There is a special medicine which, if given promptly, may help to prevent measles in a person with AIDS.

Children or adults who live with a person with AIDS and who need a polio shot should get a special form of polio shot known as "inactivated virus" vaccine. The oral polio vaccine (drops on the tongue or "sugar cube vaccine") can be dangerous to a person with AIDS.

Chicken pox can make a person with AIDS very sick, and can even be deadly. If the person with AIDS has had chicken pox in the past, he or she will probably not get it again. However, the following precautions should be taken in any case.

♦ *Under no circumstances* should someone with chicken pox be in the same room with the person with AIDS until all of the chicken pox have completely crusted over.

♦ Anyone who has recently been *exposed* to chicken pox and who has not yet had chicken pox should not be in the same room as the person with AIDS from the 10th through 21st day after exposure. If it is not possible to stay out of the room, keep the exposure time to a minimum. The exposed person should wear a surgical-type mask and wash hands before providing care.

♦ Most adults have already had chicken pox, but persons giving care should be especially alert to check whether children who are visiting or living with the person with AIDS and who have not had chicken pox have been recently exposed.

♦ If you have shingles (zoster), you should not care for the person with AIDS until all the shingles have healed over. This is because contact with shingles can cause chicken pox in a person who has not had chicken pox. If no one else is available to care for the person with AIDS, you should keep the shingles completely covered and wash your hands carefully before providing care.

♦ If the person with AIDS is exposed to chicken pox or shingles, contact the person's doctor within 24 hours. There is a special medicine which, if given promptly, may help to prevent serious complications from chicken pox in the person with AIDS.

The handling of food for the person with AIDS requires some special care (though these rules actually apply to anyone).

The person with AIDS can eat virtually any food that might seem appealing (the healthier the appetite the better). However, there are some guidelines that need to be followed to protect the person with AIDS from diseases and infections to which they may be susceptible.

♦ Avoid raw (unpasteurized) milk.
♦ Never serve raw eggs. Remember that they may be present in homemade mayonnaise, hollandaise sauce, homemade ice cream, fruit "smoothies," as well as other foods that might seem healthful.
♦ Meats and poultry should be well-cooked, not pink in the middle. Raw fish or shellfish, as well as raw or undercooked meats and poultry, can also cause problems.

As you can see, it is important that foods are fully cooked. There are also some other precautions you can take during preparation to avoid cross-contamination. This is especially important when you are handling uncooked poultry and meats.

♦ Wash your hands before handling any food, and between handling different food items.
♦ Wash all utensils before reusing with other foods.
♦ Keep uncooked food juices (such as blood from meats, water from shrimp or other seafood) from coming in contact with other foods.
♦ Use a plastic cutting board rather than a wooden one, because a plastic board is easier to clean.
♦ Scrub fresh vegetables thoroughly.

Protecting Yourself from Other Infections

A person with AIDS may sometimes have other infections that you and persons who live or visit in the home need to take precautions to avoid catching. Stay in touch with the person's doctor or nurse to find out if he or she develops any other infections and what this means for you and others in the home. This is especially important if you have HIV infection yourself.

For example, diarrhea in a person with AIDS may be caused by an infection (gastroenteritis). You should wear gloves during contact with diarrheal discharge from a person with AIDS and wash your hands carefully afterward. A person with AIDS (or anybody else) who has diarrhea due to an infection should not prepare food for others.

If the person with AIDS has a cough lasting more than a week or two, he or she should see a doctor to be checked for tuberculosis (TB). If the person with AIDS has TB, then you and others who live or visit in the home should be checked several times, even if you are not coughing. Discuss this and other precautions with your doctor, nurse, or local health department.

If the person with AIDS develops acute hepatitis (yellow jaundice) or is a carrier of the *hepatitis B virus*, then you, and any children and adults living with the person, and especially any current or recent sexual partners of the person with AIDS should ask their doctor about receiving treatment and/or a vaccine to prevent hepatitis.

If the person with AIDS has either chicken pox or shingles (zoster), anyone who has never had chicken pox should not be in the same room. If being in the same room is unavoidable, then you should wear a surgical-type mask, and gloves, and wash your hands before and after providing care. These precautions should be taken until the chicken pox or shingles are completely crusted over. You should also consult your physician. There is a special medicine which may protect you from serious complications that can result from chicken pox.

If a person with AIDS has fever blisters or cold sores (*herpes simplex*) around the mouth or nose, you should avoid kissing or touching these sores. If you must touch these sores with your hands, wear gloves and wash hands carefully afterward. This is particularly important if you have eczema (allergic skin), since the *herpes simplex virus* can cause severe skin disease in persons with eczema.

Many people with AIDS are infected with a virus called *cytomegalovirus* (CMV) which may be present in urine and saliva. You should wash hands carefully after touching saliva and urine. This is particularly important for someone who may be pregnant, since a pregnant woman who becomes infected with CMV may sometimes transmit this virus to the baby that she is carrying.

Help for the Caregiver

Providing home care can be a stressful and emotional experience. You may feel very frustrated watching a person become sicker despite your efforts. To help cope with feelings of frustration, share your feelings with others, including other caregivers, counselors, clergy, or health professionals. Call your local AIDS service organization for support.

Be sure to arrange for some backup help so you can have some free time occasionally. This is especially important during times when the person with AIDS is very ill. You may need to be relieved of your responsibilities periodically so you can also maintain your energy level.

When caring for a loved one who is very sick, it is important not to ignore your own needs. Unless you take care of yourself, you will not have the inner resources to care for the person with AIDS.

Remember that you are not alone. There are others like you who have gone through this experience before. You can gain knowledge and strength from what they can tell you.

Would You Like More Information?

If you'd like more information about caring for a person with AIDS, if you would like to volunteer, or if you would just like more information about AIDS, contact a doctor, your local health department, your local AIDS volunteer health group, or call 1-800-342 AIDS. The Spanish hotline is 1-800-344-7432. The deaf access hotline is 1-800-AIDS-TTY.

■ **Document Source:**
  U.S. Department of Health and Human Services, Public Health Service
  Centers for Disease Control and Prevention

CONDOMS AND SEXUALLY TRANSMITTED DISEASES . . . ESPECIALLY AIDS

A Condom Could Save Your Life!

This booklet is to help you understand why it's important to use condoms (rubbers, prophylactics) to help reduce the spread of sexually transmitted diseases. These diseases include AIDS, chlamydia, genital herpes, genital warts, gonorrhea, hepatitis B and syphilis. You can get them through having sex—vaginal, anal or oral.

The surest way to avoid these diseases is to not have sex altogether (abstinence). Another way is to limit sex to one partner who also limits his or her sex in the same way (monogamy). Condoms are not 100% safe, but if used properly, will reduce the risk of sexually transmitted diseases, including AIDS. **Protecting yourself against the AIDS virus is of special concern because this disease is fatal and has no cure**.

About two-thirds of the people with AIDS in the United States got the disease during sexual intercourse with an infected partner. **Experts believe that many of these people could have avoided the disease by using condoms**.

Condoms are used for both birth control and reducing the risk of disease. That's why some people think that other forms of birth control—such as the IUD, diaphragm, cervical cap or pill—will protect them against diseases, too. But that's not true. **So if you use any other form of birth control, you still need a condom in addition to reduce the risk of getting sexually transmitted diseases**.

A condom is especially important when an uninfected pregnant woman has sex, because it can also help protect her and her unborn child from a sexually transmitted disease.

This booklet will answer many of your questions about condoms. You will learn:

- Who should use a condom;
- What the Federal Government and condom manufacturers are doing to help ensure that the condoms you buy are of high quality;
- What you need to know to choose, store, and use condoms the right way.

Keep this booklet handy and refer to it when you have questions about condoms. Note well: Condoms are not 100% safe, but if used properly, will reduce the risk of sexually transmitted diseases, including AIDS.

Facts About Sexually Transmitted Diseases

- Sexually transmitted diseases (STDs) affect 12 million men and women in the United States each year.
- Anyone can become infected through sexual intercourse with an infected person.
- Many of those infected are teenagers or young adults.
- Changing sexual partners adds to the risk of becoming infected.

- Sometimes, early in the infection, there may be no symptoms, or symptoms may be easily confused with other illnesses.

Sexually transmitted diseases can cause:

- Tubal pregnancies, sometimes fatal to the mother and always fatal to the unborn child
- Death or severe damage to a baby born to an infected woman
- Sterility (loss of ability to get pregnant)
- Cancer of the cervix in women
- Damage to other parts of the body, including the heart, kidneys and brain
- Death to infected individuals

See a doctor if you have any of these symptoms of STDs:

- Discharge from the vagina, penis and/or rectum
- Pain or burning during urination and/or intercourse
- Pain in the abdomen (women), testicles (men), and buttocks and legs (both)
- Blisters, open sores, warts, rash, and/or swelling in the genital area, sex organs, and/or mouth
- Flu-like symptoms, including fever, headache, aching muscles, and/or swollen glands

You can get more information about preventing sexually transmitted diseases by calling the National AIDS Hotline, the National Sexually Transmitted Diseases Hotline, or your state or local hotlines.

Answers to Your Questions

1. Who should use a condom?

A person who takes part in risky sexual behavior should always use a condom.

The **highest** risk comes from having intercourse—vaginal, anal or oral—with a person who has a sexually transmitted disease. If you have sex with an infected person, you're taking a big chance. **If you know your partner is infected, the best rule is to avoid intercourse (including oral sex).** If you do decide to have sex with an infected partner, you should **always** be sure a condom is used from start to finish, every time.

And it's risky to have sex with someone who has shared needles with an infected person.

It's also risky to have sex with someone who had sex with an infected person in the past. If your partner had intercourse with a person infected with HIV (the AIDS virus), he or she could pass it on to you. That can happen even if the intercourse was a long time ago and even if your partner seems perfectly healthy.

With sexually transmitted diseases, you often can't tell whether your partner has been infected. If you're not sure about yourself or your partner, you should choose to **not** have sex at all. **But if you do have sex, be sure to use a condom that covers the entire penis to reduce your risk of being infected**. This includes oral sex where the penis is in contact with the mouth.

If you think you and your partner should be using condoms but your partner refuses, then you should say **NO** to sex with that person.

2. Will a condom guarantee I won't get a sexually transmitted disease?

No. There's no absolute guarantee even when you use a condom. But most experts believe that the risk of getting AIDS and other sexually transmitted diseases can be greatly reduced if a condom is used **properly**.

In other words, sex with condoms **isn't** totally "safe sex," but it **is** "less risky" sex.

3. How can I get the most protection from condoms?

♦ Choose the right kind of condoms to prevent disease.
♦ Store them properly.
♦ Remember to use a **new** condom **every time** you have sex.
♦ Use the condom the right way, from start to finish.

4. How does a condom protect against sexually transmitted diseases?

A condom acts as a barrier or wall to keep blood, or semen, or vaginal fluids from passing from one person to the other during intercourse.

These fluids can harbor germs such as HIV (the AIDS virus). If no condom is used, the germs can pass from the infected partner to the uninfected partner.

5. How do I choose the right kind of condoms to prevent disease?

Always read the label. Look for two things:

♦ **The condoms should be made of latex (rubber)**. Tests have shown that latex condoms can prevent the passage of the AIDS, hepatitis and herpes viruses. But natural (lambskin) condoms may not do this.

In the future, manufacturers may offer condoms of other materials and designs for disease prevention. As with all new products that make medical claims, such as "prevention of sexually transmitted diseases," these new condoms would have to be reviewed by the U.S. Food and Drug Administration (FDA) before they are allowed to be sold.

♦ **The package should say that the condoms are to prevent disease**. If the package doesn't say anything about preventing disease, the condoms may not provide the protection you want, even though they may be the most expensive ones you can buy.

Novelty condoms will not say anything about either disease prevention or pregnancy prevention on the package. They are intended only for sexual stimulation, not protection.

Condoms which do not cover the entire penis are not labeled for disease prevention and should not be used for this purpose. For proper protection, a condom **must** unroll to cover the entire penis. This is another good reason to read the label carefully.

6. What is the government doing about condom quality?

The FDA is working with condom manufacturers to help ensure that the latex condoms you buy are not damaged.

Manufacturers "spot check" their condoms using a "water-leak" test. FDA inspectors do a similar test on sample condoms they take from warehouses. The condoms are filled with water and checked for leaks. An average of 996 of 1000 condoms must pass this test.

(Don't try the water-leak test on condoms you plan to use, because this kind of testing weakens condoms.)

Government testing can **not** guarantee that condoms will always prevent the spread of sexually transmitted diseases. **How well you are protected will also depend a great deal on which condoms you choose and how you store, handle and use them**.

7. Are condoms strong enough for anal intercourse?

The Surgeon General has said, "Condoms provide some protection, but anal intercourse is simply too dangerous a practice."

Condoms may be more likely to break during anal intercourse than during other types of sex because of the greater amount of friction and other stresses involved.

Even if the condom doesn't break, anal intercourse is very risky because it can cause tissue in the rectum to tear and bleed. These tears allow disease germs to pass more easily from one partner to the other.

8. Should spermicides be used with condoms?

In test tubes, a spermicide called nonoxynol-9 (a chemical used to kill the man's sperm for birth control) has been shown to kill the germs that cause sexually transmitted diseases. Some experts believe nonoxynol-9 may kill the AIDS virus during intercourse, too. **So you might want to use a spermicide along with a latex condom as an added precaution in case the condom breaks during intercourse**.

Condoms with spermicides have an expiration date. Pay attention to that date.

9. How do I buy spermicides and how should they be used?

Spermicides generally come in the form of jellies, creams or foams. You can buy them in pharmacies and some grocery stores.

You can also buy condoms with a small amount of spermicide already applied. But some experts believe it's a good idea to add more spermicide to the amount that comes on the condom.

If you do add a spermicide, place a small amount inside the condom at its tip. After the condom is on the penis, put more on the outside. Spermicides can also be put inside the woman's vagina. Follow the directions for use.

If you have oral sex, use a condom without a spermicide. Although swallowing small amounts of spermicide has not proven harmful in animal tests, we don't know if this is always true for people.

Spermicide products and condoms with spermicides have expiration dates. Don't buy or use a package that is outdated.

10. Should I use a lubricant with a condom?

Some condoms are already lubricated with dry silicone, jellies or creams. **If you buy condoms not already lubricated, it's a good idea to apply some yourself**. Lubricants may help prevent condoms from breaking during use and may prevent irritation, which might increase the chance of infection.

If you use a separate lubricant, be sure to use one that's **water-based** and made for this purpose. If you're not sure which to choose, ask your pharmacist.

Never use a lubricant that contains oils, fats, or greases such as petroleum-based jelly (like Vaseline® brand), baby oil or lotion, hand or body lotions, cooking shortenings or oily cosmetics like cold cream. They can seriously weaken latex, causing a condom to tear easily.

11. Does it matter which styles of condoms I use?

It's most important to choose latex condoms that say "disease prevention" on the package. Other features are a matter of personal choice.

12. What do the dates mean on the package?

Some packages show "DATE MFG." This tells you when the condoms were made. It is **not** an expiration date.

Other packages may show an expiration date. The condoms should not be purchased or used after that date.

13. Are condoms from vending machines any good?

It depends. Vending machine condoms **may** be OK:

♦ If you know you are getting a latex condom,
♦ If they are labeled for disease prevention,
♦ If you know the spermicide (if any) is not outdated, and
♦ If the machine is not exposed to extreme temperatures and direct sunlight.

14. How should condoms be stored?

You should store condoms in a cool, dry place out of direct sunlight, perhaps in a drawer or closet. If you want to keep one with you, put it in a loose pocket, wallet or purse for no more than a few hours at a time.

Extreme temperatures—especially heat—can make latex brittle or gummy (like an old balloon). So, don't keep these latex products in a hot place like a glove compartment.

15. How should condoms be handled?

Gently! When opening the packet, don't use your teeth, scissors or sharp nails. Make sure you can see what you're doing.

16. What defects should I look for?

If the condom material sticks to itself or is gummy, the condom is no good. Also, check the condom tip for other damage that is obvious (brittleness, tears, and holes). Don't

unroll the condom to check it because this could cause damage.

Never use a damaged condom.

17. How should I use a condom?

Follow these guidelines:

♦ Use a new condom for every act of intercourse.
♦ If the penis is uncircumcised, pull the foreskin back before putting the condom on.
♦ Put the condom on after the penis is erect (hard) and before **any** contact is made between the penis and any part of the partner's body.
♦ If using a spermicide, put some inside the condom tip.
♦ If the condom does not have a reservoir tip, pinch the tip enough to leave a half-inch space for semen to collect.
♦ While pinching the half-inch tip, place the condom against the penis and unroll it all the way to the base. Put more spermicide or lubricant on the outside.
♦ If you feel a condom break while you are having sex, stop immediately and pull out. Do not continue until you have put on a new condom and used more spermicide.
♦ After ejaculation and before the penis gets soft, grip the rim of the condom and carefully withdraw from your partner.
♦ To remove the condom from the penis, pull it off gently, being careful semen doesn't spill out.
♦ Wrap the used condom in a tissue and throw it in the trash where others won't handle it. Because condoms may cause problems in sewers, don't flush them down the toilet. Afterwards, wash your hands with soap and water.
♦ Finally, beware of drugs and alcohol! They can affect your judgment, so you may forget to use a condom. They may even affect your ability to use a condom properly.

Sexually Transmitted Diseases, including AIDS, Can Be Prevented!

Learn the facts so that you can protect yourself and others from getting infected. Condoms are not 100% safe, but if used properly, will reduce the risk of sexually transmitted diseases, including AIDS. If you have unprotected sex now, you can contract sexually transmitted diseases. Later, if you decide to have children, you might pass the diseases on to them.

If you would like more information about condoms and how to prevent sexually transmitted diseases, talk with your doctor or call:

The National AIDS Hotline. It's open 24 hours a day. Trained operators will answer your questions and can send you more information.

For AIDS information in English, **1-800-342-AIDS**

For AIDS information in Spanish, **1-800-344-SIDA**

Deaf Access, **1-800-AIDS-TTY**

The National STD Hotline, 1-800-227-8922.

Condom Shopping Guide

Use this handy shopping guide as a reminder of what to look for when buying condoms, lubricants and spermicides.

Be sure to choose:

- **Latex**
- **Disease prevention claim on package label**

Also consider:

- With spermicide
- Separate spermicide
  - Gel
  - Cream
  - Foam
- With lubricant
- Separate lubricant (Select only *water-based* lubricants made for this purpose.)

■ **Document Source:**
U.S. Department of Health and Human Services, Public Health Service
Center for Devices and Radiological Health
Food and Drug Administration
DHHS Publication FDA 90-4239

HIV AND YOUR CHILD

Purpose of This Booklet

Even before HIV causes AIDS, it can cause health problems. Learning about how the virus can affect your child's body and getting care early, before health problems worsen, can help your child live a longer and healthier life.

This booklet is a guide to understanding HIV and getting the right care for your child. It gives you questions to ask your doctor, nurse, or other medical care provider. What you learn about HIV and AIDS will help you become more involved in your child's health care.

HIV affects everyone in a family, whether only one or several family members are infected. Babies with HIV and their infected parents need to be followed very closely by a medical care provider such as a doctor, nurse, or other medical professional.

Babies who may have HIV infection should be tested for HIV as soon as possible after birth and have regular followup exams. This is very important to help your baby stay as healthy as possible.

The Immune System and HIV

The body's health is defended by its immune system. White blood cells called lymphocytes (B cells and T cells) protect the body from "germs" such as viruses, bacteria, parasites, and fungi. When germs are detected, B cells and T cells are activated to defend the body.

This process is hindered in the case of the acquired immunodeficiency syndrome (AIDS). AIDS is a disease in which the body's immune system breaks down. AIDS is caused by the human immunodeficiency virus (HIV).

When HIV enters the body, it infects special T cells, where the virus grows. The virus kills these cells slowly. As more and more of the T cells die, the body's ability to fight infection weakens.

A person with HIV infection may remain healthy for many years. People with HIV infection are said to have AIDS when they are sick with serious illnesses and infections that can occur with HIV. The illnesses tend to occur late in HIV infection, when few T cells remain.

Where Did HIV and AIDS Come From?

We may never know where or how HIV and AIDS began. Many experts believe that AIDS was present in the United States, Europe, and Africa for several decades or longer before the earliest cases appeared in 1980 and 1981.

HIV was first identified in 1984 by French and American scientists, but the human immunodeficiency virus did not get its name until 1986.

Facts About HIV in Babies and Children

- HIV can be passed to a baby during pregnancy or delivery.
- An HIV-infected woman's chances of having a baby with HIV are one in four (25 percent) for each pregnancy.
- HIV can be passed to a baby through breast milk from an HIV-infected mother.
- Like adults, children and adolescents can get HIV from contact with blood or body fluids or through sex.
- Bathing, kissing, feeding, and playing with your child are not risky and do not cause the spread of HIV.
- In the past, some babies and children became infected through blood transfusions. Today the blood from all donors is screened for the virus, and HIV infection from this source is unlikely.
- Special blood tests can show whether your infant is infected with HIV.
- Your child needs to see a health care provider who has experience treating HIV-infected babies and children.
- Early immunizations (shots) can help protect your child from other HIV-related diseases.

How Will I Know If My Baby Has HIV?

Before a baby is born, it shares its mother's blood supply. If you are infected with HIV, you can transmit HIV to your child through your blood before birth. The baby also can become infected during delivery.

For the first few months your baby may test positive for HIV infection because it still has some parts of your blood, so early tests are not accurate. After several months, the child's own system takes over. Test results then become accurate for your child and can indicate HIV infection.

When your child is less than 2 years old, his or her blood should be tested every 2 to 3 months until the system matures.

After age 2, a single blood test can show if your child is infected with HIV.

What Will Happen to My Baby?

Some babies who have HIV infection may become ill in the first year of life. Others remain healthy for many years.

Regular medical checkups and blood tests will help your doctor keep track of how your child is doing and decide whether special medicines are needed. Ask your health care provider how you can help protect your child.

How Can I Help My Child Stay Healthy?

It is very important to seek medical care as soon as you know that your child has HIV. Although there is no cure as yet for HIV, there are things you can do to help your child stay as healthy as possible.

Because your child has HIV infection, you will want to learn as much as you can about the virus. You can prevent many illnesses by:

♦ Keeping your home safe and clean.
♦ Observing and listening to your child.
♦ Telling your health care provider right away about unusual behavior or symptoms.
♦ Working with the doctor, nurse, or other health care provider to plan your child's care.
♦ Making sure your child gets all recommended baby shots and booster shots.
♦ Try to keep a positive outlook. Hope is very important. Every day, there are new drugs and treatments for HIV that may help your child. Each time you take your child for health care, be sure to ask about new treatments or clinical trials that might be right for your child.

Prevent Illness

Immunize against infection

With HIV infection, your child is more likely to get common childhood illnesses, and these may be more serious. You can protect your child by making sure all the baby shots are given on time. These shots include:

♦ Diptheria, pertussis (whooping cough), and tetanus (DPT).
♦ Polio (IPV).
♦ Mumps, measles, rubella (MMR).

Your health care provider may recommend other immunizations, depending on the results of medical tests. These include:

♦ *Haemophilus influenzae* type B (HIb)
♦ Hepatitis B (HepB)
♦ Pneumococcal infection (after 2 years of age)
♦ Influenza (yearly)

Avoid common illnesses

Some infections cannot be prevented by shots. Infections from the bacteria and viruses that cause sores, colds, and influenza (flu) can weaken your child and make it harder to resist more serious HIV-related diseases. Keep your child away from people who are sick, and tell the doctor or nurse if you think your child has been near someone with tuberculosis (TB) or other infections.

Provide a Healthy Home Life

As the parent or guardian of a child who has HIV infection, you will want to take special care of yourself so that you can care for your child. The advice that follows can help both you and your child stay as healthy as possible.

Teach personal care. Wash your hands often, and teach your child to do the same as soon as he or she is able. Keep your child away from human or animal waste.

Brush the child's teeth until he or she is able. Your child will need to visit the dentist twice a year. Ask the dentist to help you teach your child proper mouth care. The first sign of your child's HIV infection may be sores in the mouth. At each visit, the doctor or nurse will examine your child's mouth.

Eat healthy foods. Your child needs healthy foods in order to grow and to help fight infections. A proper diet will also help you and your child have strength and energy. Your child's health care provider can help you decide which foods are best. Ask how to help a "picky eater" learn to enjoy healthy foods.

Get regular exercise. Most children with HIV infection are active; however, some need encouragement to get physical exercise (in fresh air and sunshine if possible). Regular exercise is important to help you and your child keep up your strength.

Get plenty of sleep. HIV-infected children need rest. Sleep will renew your child's energy for the next day, especially for going to day care or school, where there may be little time for rest during the day.

Play with, talk to, and hug your child often. Spending time together will help you spot problems that should be reported to your child's health care provider.

Give medication correctly and on time. Your child needs medicines to slow the HIV infection and prevent other infections, such as pneumonia, that can occur when the immune system is weak.

Your doctor or nurse will tell you exactly what medicine your child should have. Giving your child the right amount of medicine, and giving it on time, can mean the difference between staying healthy and becoming severely ill.

Do not allow your child to take any other medicines, alcohol, or illegal (street) drugs.

See the end of this booklet for some helpful hints on giving medicine to a young child. Your child's health care provider can show you how to hold the baby and use medicine droppers or syringes correctly.

Help your child lead a normal life. Playing with other children in your home and in the neighborhood is good for your child. It is not dangerous for your child or for the other children. HIV infection is not spread by touching or being in close contact with a friend.

Report Symptoms Promptly

Watch your child carefully. Report any of the following to your health care provider right away:

- ♦ Fever.
- ♦ Cough.
- ♦ Fast or difficult breathing.
- ♦ Loss of appetite and poor weight gain.
- ♦ White patches or sores in the mouth.
- ♦ Diaper rash that won't go away.
- ♦ Blood in the diaper or bowel movements.
- ♦ Diarrhea (frequent loose, watery, bowel movements).
- ♦ Vomiting.
- ♦ Contact with a person who has chicken pox, measles, TB, or other diseases that can spread.

Be Sure Your Child Gets Medical Treatment

Your child may stay strong and healthy for a long time, but to be sure, regular blood tests will be needed to show how well the immune system is working.

Special T cells, called CD4 cells, in the blood help the body defend itself from attackers, such as viruses. But CD4 cells can be destroyed as your child's HIV infection worsens, leaving your child unable to fight off other infections and illnesses.

Your child's health care provider will do a CD4 cell count every few months. This test shows the number of CD4 cells in your child's blood and lets the doctor know when special medicine is needed.

The doctor will probably prescribe medicine, such as AZT (now called ZDV, for zidovudine), didanosine (ddI), or dideoxycytidine (ddC) to help slow your child's HIV infection.

Another drug, trimethoprim-sulfamethoxazole or TMP-SMX (Bactrim®, Septra®, and generic products), may be given to prevent *Pneumocystis carinii* pneumonia (PCP). PCP is the most common serious pneumonia in children with HIV. Your child may need other medicines to prevent "opportunistic" infections that can take advantage of a weakened immune system.

These treatments are strong and can cause problems. Watch for and report side effects such as problems in sleeping, headaches, vomiting, muscle or belly pain, numbness in hands or feet, or hyperactivity.

Your health care provider will take blood tests regularly to see how well your child can resist infections. Be sure to ask your doctor about other tests and treatments your child may need, including:

- ♦ New HIV drugs or vaccines. New medicines are tested on people to see if they are safe or helpful. This is called a clinical trial. Usually, new HIV medicines must be tested in a clinical trial before a doctor can give them to patients who are not part of the clinical trial.
- ♦ Special x-rays and other tests for growth, development, and nervous system function.
- ♦ Special feedings or formulas.
- ♦ Physical, occupational, or speech therapy.

Telling Others About Your Child's HIV Infection

When you learn about your child's HIV infection, you may have mixed feelings, including fear, anger, sadness, or guilt. Telling people that your child has the virus may be hard. You will need to think about many things when deciding whom to tell about your child's HIV infection.

Signs and Symptoms of HIV Infection in Babies

- ♦ Swelling in the lymph glands in the neck, under the arms, and in the diaper area
- ♦ Swollen belly, sometimes with diarrhea (frequent loose, watery, bowel movements)
- ♦ Itchy skin rashes
- ♦ Frequent lung infections (pneumonia)
- ♦ Frequent ear and sinus infections
- ♦ Problems with gaining weight or growth
- ♦ Inability to do the kinds of things healthy babies do (such as sitting alone, crawling, walking)
- ♦ Crankiness, irritability, and constant crying

Most important, talk with your health care provider right away about anything you notice that seems unusual for your baby.

Although it is risky, sharing information about your child's HIV infection can be helpful in a number of ways. Telling others may help you seek the medical care your child needs and apply for other kinds of help. You can begin actively planning for your child's care and your family's future.

Talking About Your Child's HIV Infection

Possible Benefits

- ♦ More support from family and friends
- ♦ In some states, better health and welfare benefits
- ♦ More acceptance of the child's infection

Possible Risks

- ♦ Rejection by family, friends, or day care, school, or social programs
- ♦ Changes in health benefits

Your doctor, nurse, social worker, or other members of the health care team can help you plan how and when to share information about your child's HIV infection. They can help you tell others. Your list of people to tell may include:

- ♦ Your child, if he or she is old enough to understand.
- ♦ Family members.
- ♦ Day care workers or babysitters.
- ♦ Teachers, classmates, and other people at school.
- ♦ Health professionals who work with your child or your family, including your family doctor and dentist, nurses, social workers, nutrition counselors, and pharmacists.

Your doctor may be required by law to report your child's HIV infection to the state or local health department. Ask about the laws, confidentiality, and anonymous HIV testing in your state.

Talking with Your Child About HIV Infection

Consider your child's age. Talk with your child about HIV when he or she seems ready, possibly around age 5. How you talk with an older child about HIV infection depends on whether the child has had HIV since infancy or is newly diagnosed.

Young children. Children born with the virus have learned a lot about living with HIV infection by the time they reach the age when they can understand what it means to have HIV. Your child will have had regular visits to doctors and other health care providers and will have experienced blood drawing and shots. Taking medicines may be routine. Perhaps your child knows or can say the name of the infection, too.

Young children are usually content with knowing only a little bit about HIV. You can give short, simple answers to most of the questions your young child asks.

School-age children. Older children can understand much more. It is very important to give your child correct information and honest answers about your feelings. Otherwise the child may get the wrong information from someone else.

A child who has HIV infection that is kept secret may suffer silently because of shame or fear. An older child who is having trouble coping with HIV infection may:

♦ Have problems sleeping.
♦ Pull away from friends and family.
♦ Be depressed or sad.
♦ Have problems at school.

Even a young child may have many of the same problems as an adult when dealing with HIV infection. Counselors and health care providers who work with children who have HIV can help you recognize changes in your child's behavior. They can help the child, and you, find ways to talk about these problems.

Older children. The older child—from 12 to 21 years of age—who has recently become infected with HIV may feel and express many of the same emotions as an adult in the same situation: disbelief, fear, sadness, depression, shame. At the same time, the child may behave in some of the same ways as a younger child.

Learning as much as possible about HIV and AIDS will help you talk with your child. For example, your child may ask (or might like to ask):

♦ Am I going to get sick? When?
♦ What will happen to me?
♦ Will I have to go to the hospital or see the doctor more often?
♦ How will HIV affect my family, friends, and people at school?
♦ How can I prevent giving HIV to others?

It is important to talk with older children who have HIV about using condoms for safe sex, as well as the dangers of needle-sharing. It may be very hard to stay calm and neutral

when talking with your older child about HIV infection. You may want to arrange for your child to meet privately with an HIV/AIDS health counselor who knows how to interact with teenagers. Ask your child's health care provider to help you find a counselor who can meet with your child.

Talking with your older child in an open and friendly way will do much to ease fears about rejection by other family members and friends. You may decide together whom to tell about the HIV infection and when.

How Can We Get the Support Our Family Needs?

A person or family with HIV may need many kinds of support. Your child's health care provider and your local health and social services departments can assist you in finding the help you need. Help may include someone to:

♦ Answer your questions about HIV and AIDS.
♦ Help you find health care providers and make health care decisions.
♦ Provide transportation to and from health care appointments.
♦ Assist in planning ways to meet financial and daily needs.
♦ Arrange home nursing care or rehabilitation services.
♦ Refer you and your loved ones to support groups.
♦ Represent your family in legal matters.

Sometimes it helps to talk with others who also have HIV or a child with HIV. Here are some ways of finding them:

♦ Read HIV newsletters.
♦ Join a support group for friends and family.
♦ Volunteer to help others.
♦ Attend social events to meet other families living with HIV.

Additional Resources

There are many ways to get information about living with HIV. You may find it helpful to read about HIV and learn how others have cared for themselves or their family members.

♦ You can get information from your local health department about HIV, including where to get tested for the virus and the kinds of services available to your child and your family.
♦ Your local or state medical society can help you find a doctor.
♦ Your library may have information that you can share with your child. Ask your librarian if there is a special directory that lists groups for families whose children have HIV.
♦ Some hospitals and churches offer programs and sponsor support groups.

National hotlines and information clearinghouses can send you free publications and give you the latest news about drug-testing and clinical trials. Here are some telephone numbers to help you get the information you need:

General Information

National AIDS Hotline
English (800) 342-AIDS (2437)
Spanish (800) 344-SIDA (7432)

TDD Service for the Deaf
(800) 243-7889

National AIDS Clearinghouse
(800) 458-5231

National Pediatric HIV Resource Center
(800) 362-0071

HIV/AIDS Treatment Information

American Foundation for AIDS Research
(800) 39AMFAR (392-6327)

AIDS Treatment Data Network
(212) 268-4196

Project Inform
(800) 822-7422

Clinical Trials Conducted by the National Institutes of Health or Food and Drug Administration-Approved Trials:

AIDS Clinical Trials Information Service
800-TRIALS-A (874-2572)

Social Security Disability Benefits

For confidential assistance in applying for social security disability benefits, call the Social Security Administration at (800) 772-1213. You may request a personal earnings and benefit estimate statement (PEBES) to help you estimate the retirement, disability, and survivor benefits payable on your social security record.

Hints for Giving Medicine to Babies and Toddlers

Giving medicine to your baby or young child does not have to be a chore for either of you. Just follow these steps:

1. Prepare the medicine and place it and other things you will need on a table within reach of the hand you will feed with.
2. Hold the baby on your lap. If you are right handed, hold the baby on your left (if left handed, on your right).
3. With your left hand, hold baby's left arm: baby's right arm should go under your left arm, around your back.
4. Support baby's head and shoulder firmly between your left arm and chest, and tilt the head back a little bit.
5. Squirt small amounts of medicine into the side of the baby's mouth alongside the back of the tongue on the side closest to your body (baby will have a hard time spitting and will not choke).
6. Keep baby's mouth closed and hold baby's body upright until the medicine is swallowed.

Helpful Hints:

♦ For liquids, use a soft plastic dropper or syringe.
♦ Try mixing medicine in food for spoon-feeding.
♦ Sit in a firm, comfortable chair.
♦ Put a bib or towel on baby.
♦ Stay calm and use a soft voice.
♦ Reward baby with juice or water to rinse the mouth.

■ **Document Source:**
U.S. Department of Health and Human Services, Public Health Service
Agency for Health Care Policy and Research
Executive Office Center, Suite 501, 2101 East Jefferson Street, Rockville, MD 20852
AHCPR Publication No. 94-0576
January 1994

HIV INFECTION AND AIDS: ARE YOU AT RISK?

While it's almost certain that you've heard quite a bit about AIDS in the past few years, the term HIV might be new to you.

HIV and AIDS are closely related, and if you understand HIV infection, you can better understand AIDS.

What is AIDS?

AIDS stands for *acquired immunodeficiency syndrome*, a disease in which the body's immune system breaks down. Normally, the immune system fights off infections and certain other diseases. When the system fails, a person with AIDS can develop a variety of life-threatening illnesses.

AIDS is caused by HIV

AIDS is caused by the virus called the *human immunodeficiency virus*, or HIV. A virus is one of the smallest "germs" that can cause disease.

If you have sex or share needles or syringes with an infected person, you may become infected with HIV. Specific blood tests can show evidence of HIV infection. You can be infected with HIV and have no symptoms at all. You might feel perfectly healthy, but if you're infected, you can pass the virus to anyone with whom you have sex or share needles or syringes.

Will you get AIDS if you are infected with HIV?

About half of the people with HIV develop AIDS within 10 years, but the time between infection with HIV and the onset of AIDS can vary greatly. The severity of the HIV-related illness or illnesses will differ from person to person, according to many factors, including the overall health of the individual.

Today there are promising new medical treatments that can postpone many of the illnesses associated with AIDS. This is a step in the right direction, and scientists are becoming optimistic that HIV infection will someday be controllable. In the meantime, people who get medical care to monitor and treat their HIV infection can carry on with their lives, including their jobs, for longer than ever before.

How can you become infected with HIV?

You can become infected with HIV in two main ways:

♦ Having sexual intercourse—anal, vaginal, or oral—with an infected person.
♦ Sharing drug needles or syringes with an infected person.

Also, women infected with HIV can pass the virus to their babies during pregnancy or during birth. They can also pass it on when breast-feeding. Some people have become infected by receiving blood transfusions. Since 1985, however, when careful screening and laboratory testing of all blood donations began, this possibility has been greatly reduced.

You cannot be infected by giving blood at a blood bank.

HIV can be spread through sexual intercourse, from male to male, male to female, female to male, and, in theory, from female to female.

You can get HIV from sexual intercourse

HIV is sexually transmitted, and HIV is not the only infection that is passed through intimate sexual contact. Other sexually transmitted diseases, such as gonorrhea, syphilis, herpes, and chlamydia, can also be contracted through anal, vaginal, and oral intercourse. If you have one of these infections and engage in sexual behaviors that can transmit the virus, you are at greater risk of getting HIV.

HIV may be in an infected person's blood, semen, or vaginal secretions. HIV can enter the body through cuts or sores in the skin or the moist lining of the vagina, penis, rectum, or even the mouth. Some of these cuts or sores are so small you don't even know they're there. Anal intercourse with an infected person is one of the ways HIV has been most frequently transmitted. Other forms of sexual intercourse, including oral sex, can spread it as well. During oral sex, a person who takes semen, blood, or vaginal secretions into their mouth is at risk of becoming infected.

Many infected people have no symptoms and have not been tested. If you have sex with one of them, you unknowingly put yourself in danger. Also, the more sexual partners you have, the greater your chances of encountering one or more who are infected and of becoming infected yourself. The only sure way to avoid infection through sex is to abstain from sexual intercourse or engage in sexual intercourse only with someone who is not infected and only has sex with you. Latex condoms have been shown to help prevent HIV infection and other sexually transmitted diseases. But they are not foolproof. You have to use condoms properly. And you have to use them every time you have sex—vaginal, anal, or oral.

You can get HIV from sharing needles

Sharing needles or syringes, even once, is a very likely way to become infected with HIV and other germs. HIV from an infected person can remain in a needle or syringe and then be injected directly into the bloodstream of the next person who uses it. Sharing needles to inject IV drugs is the most dangerous form of needle sharing.

Sharing needles for other purposes may also transmit HIV and other germs. These types of needles include those used to inject steroids and those used for tattooing or ear-piercing.

If you plan to have your ears pierced or get a tattoo, make sure you go to a qualified person who uses brand-new or sterile equipment. Don't be shy about asking questions. Responsible technicians will explain the safety measures they follow.

HIV and babies

A woman infected with HIV can pass the virus on to her baby during pregnancy, while giving birth, or when breast-feeding. If a woman is infected before or during pregnancy, her child has about one chance in three of being born with HIV infection. There is no known way to prevent this transmission.

Any woman who is considering having a baby and who thinks she might have done something that could have caused her to become infected with HIV—even if this occurred years ago—should seek counseling and testing for HIV infection to help her make an informed choice about becoming pregnant. To find out where to go in your area for counseling and testing, call your local health department or the CDC National AIDS Hotline (1-800-342-AIDS).

Blood transfusions and HIV

In the past some people became infected with HIV from receiving blood transfusions. This risk has been practically eliminated. Since 1985, potential blood donors at highest risk of HIV infection have been asked not to donate blood. All donated blood has been tested for evidence of HIV. All blood found to contain evidence of HIV infection is discarded. Currently in the United States, there is only a very small chance of infection with HIV through a blood transfusion.

You cannot get HIV from giving blood at a blood bank or other blood collection center. The needles used for blood donations are sterile. They are used once, then destroyed.

How you *cannot* get HIV

HIV infection doesn't "just happen." You can't "catch" it like a cold or flu. Unlike cold or flu viruses, HIV is not spread by coughs or sneezes. Again, you get HIV by receiving infected blood, semen, or vaginal fluids from another person.

♦ You won't get HIV through everyday contact with infected people at school, work, home, or anywhere else.
♦ You won't get HIV from clothes, phones, or toilet seats. It can't be passed on by things like forks, cups, or other objects that someone who is infected with the virus has used.
♦ You cannot get HIV from eating food prepared by an infected person.
♦ You won't get HIV from a mosquito bite. HIV does not live in a mosquito, and it is not transmitted through a mosquito's bite like other germs, such as the ones that cause malaria. You won't get it from bedbugs, lice, flies, or other insects, either.
♦ You won't get HIV from sweat or tears.

Not all of the answers are in

You won't get HIV from a simple kiss. Experts are not completely certain about HIV transmission through deep, prolonged, or "french" kissing. Most scientists agree that although transmission of HIV through deep or prolonged kissing may be possible, it would be unlikely.

Who is really at risk for HIV infection?

There is evidence that HIV, the virus that causes AIDS, has been in the U.S. at least since 1978. The following are known risk factors for HIV. You may be at increased risk of infection if any of the following have applied to you since 1978.

♦ Have you shared needles or syringes to inject drugs or steroids?
♦ If you are a male, have you had sex with other males?
♦ Have you had sex with someone who you believe may have been infected with HIV?
♦ Have you had a sexually transmitted disease (STD)?
♦ Have you received blood transfusions or blood products between 1978 and 1985?
♦ Have you had sex with someone who would answer yes to any of the above questions?

If you answered yes to any of the above questions, you should discuss your need for testing with a trained counselor. If you are a woman in any of the above categories and you plan to become pregnant, counseling and testing are even more important.

If you have had sex with someone and you didn't know their risk behavior, or you have had many sexual partners in the last 10 years, then you have increased the chances that you might be HIV-infected.

What about the HIV test?

The only way to tell if you have been infected with HIV is by taking an HIV-antibody blood test. This test should be done through a testing site, doctor's office, or clinic familiar with the test. It is important that you discuss what the test may mean with a qualified health professional, *both before and after the test is done.*

Do you need more information about HIV or HIV counseling and testing?

You can receive free publications from the Centers for Disease Control and Prevention. To receive brochures, or to ask any questions about HIV infection or AIDS, call the CDC National AIDS Hotline at 1-800-342-AIDS. (Spanish: 1-800-344-7432; deaf access: 1-800-243-7889 [TDD]). The Hotline is staffed with information specialists who can offer a wide variety of written materials or answer your questions about HIV infection and AIDS in a prompt, confidential manner. There are also local groups that can help you find the information you need. Contact your state or local health department, AIDS service organization, or other community-based organization dealing with HIV and AIDS. The National AIDS Hotline can tell you how to contact all of these.

■ Document Source:
U.S. Department of Health and Human Services, Public Health Service
Centers for Disease Control and Prevention
NAIEP 9/93

See also: HIV and Your Child (page 8)

ALLERGIES

■■■

ALLERGIC DISEASES

Who gets allergies?

Allergies are incredibly common. More than 50 million Americans—1 out of 5—suffer from allergic diseases. One out of every 11 office visits to the doctor is for an allergic disease.

Inheritance has a major influence on allergy. If one parent has allergies, the odds are that one in three of the children will have allergies. If both parents have allergies, then all the children will probably have allergies.

Aside from inheritance, it is not known why some people get allergies and others do not. Some believe that hormonal influences, viral infections, smoking, and a number of other influences affect whether one develops allergies. No one knows all the reasons why people with equal likelihood to develop allergies become allergic to different things, or why some have hay fever and others have asthma.

Second, a person has to be exposed to an allergen, a foreign protein that causes allergy. Ragweed pollen is the major cause of allergy in the United States. It is an unusual allergen that is found in high concentrations only in this country. Most people who move to the United States are exposed to ragweed for the first time. Many have never had allergies previously in their families for centuries, yet they develop allergies within two or three years of living in the United States. A large part of why they develop allergies is exposure to ragweed, which is an incredibly potent allergy-producing plant.

Each ragweed plant produces about one billion pollen grains during an average allergy season. Those pollen grains are very small—microscopic. They float in the air and may be carried out to sea as many as 300 or 400 miles. So it does not matter if people do not have ragweed plants in their backyards; they are clearly exposed to ragweed every place in the United States except for the arid southwest and southern California, where ragweed does not grow.

Other major allergens include grass pollens, tree pollens, dust, molds, and animal dander. Worldwide, however, the major allergen is the dust mite. All temperate climate areas in the world have dust mites, which live in carpeting, mattresses, and upholstery. They have to have temperatures above 60

degrees to reproduce. Most people keep the temperature in their homes above 60 degrees all year. Dust mites also need a relative humidity above 50 percent.

People are not actually allergic to the dust mite; they are allergic to its feces. The fecal balls are sticky, heavy materials that bind to carpeting or upholstery. One of the worst ways to bring dust mite allergens into the air is to vacuum the floor; this blows the dust up into the air, where it floats for a couple of hours and makes up the moats in a beam of sunlight.

How do allergies work?

There are three components to allergies: mast cells, which contain chemicals like histamine; antibodies, a specific type of protein made by the immune system, known as IgE; and allergens, which trigger the reaction. Mast cells are the allergy-causing cells and are found in every tissue throughout the body, though they are most heavily concentrated in those tissues that are exposed to the outside world—the skin, linings of the nose and lungs, gastrointestinal tract, and reproductive system.

The IgE antibody, which actually causes allergy, sits on the surface of these mast cells. A mast cell has about 1,000 histamine-containing granules in its cytoplasm, and on its surface are between 100,000 and 1 million receptors for IgE. When the IgE encounters the allergen, it triggers the mast cell to release granules from its cytoplasm. Those granules contain histamine and other chemicals. These mediators that are released then interact with the tissues, causing the allergic symptoms.

With ragweed, for example, the pollen grains from the plant are male gametes equivalent to sperm. They carry the male genetic code from a male ragweed plant to a female ragweed plant. Since the pollen grains are wind borne and do not have a particular way of finding a female plant, many excess pollen grains are produced in the hopes that one or another will find a female plant and fertilize it.

On the surface of a pollen grain are enzymes that help the pollen grain enter female plants. Unfortunately, people breathe in pollen grains that are floating in the air. When a pollen grain gets on the skin that lines the inside of the nose, those enzymes are released from the pollen grain and work their way through the mucus in the nose. The enzymes sensitize the person by initiating the production of IgE antibodies, which then sensitize mast cells that are in the nose. It generally takes about two to five seasons of allergen exposure before a person makes enough IgE to result in allergy symptoms.

Everyone makes some IgE. Only people with genetic predispositions toward allergies make large quantities. IgE, like other antibodies that the body produces, is part of the body's defense mechanism. Some antibodies, like IgG, get rid of Streptococcus and help cure those infected with a strep throat. Other antibodies get rid of cold viruses. The IgE antibody is directed against parasites. Its function is to protect the body against parasitic infections. There are few parasites in the United States, but the IgE antibody system reacts against the enzymes from the surface of pollen grains as if they were parasites and elicits an allergic response. The body is misdirecting an extremely important immune response at pollens, dust, dander, and molds.

Most antibodies last in the body about three weeks, but IgE may sit on its receptor on mast cells and sensitize the mast cells for years. For example, someone who had an adverse allergic reaction to penicillin as a child could still be allergic to the drug as an adult. The IgE antibody the person made as a 6-year-old child would still be present in the 40-year-old adult. It is sitting on the mast cells, which are long-lived cells, and it conveys incredibly long-lived sensitivity to allergens.

In one research study, we looked at mast cell histamine release under the electron microscope. We sensitized a mast cell to IgE, making it allergic to grass, trees, ragweed, and certain breeds of cats and dogs. We then took this mast cell and exposed it to an extract of ragweed. Over a 15-minute period, many of the granules in its cytoplasm disappeared. Fifteen minutes later, the granules were all gone.

Although the mast cell had no visible secretory granules in its cytoplasm, it was alive and well; over the next 6 to 24 hours it would reconstitute all the granules that had disappeared. After releasing histamine from its granules, a mast cell can once again do damage to the person the next day when he or she breathes in ragweed.

The chemicals that are released from mast cells are the mediators that cause allergies. At last count, there were 28 separate chemicals released by mast cells that orchestrate allergic responses. The allergic symptoms a person experiences depend on the tissue in which the mediators are released. For example, if these chemicals are released in the nose, the person will get hay fever, allergic rhinitis. If they are released in the chest, the person will get asthma or coughing. Chemicals released in the skin will produce hives or eczema, in the intestine will produce food allergy or diarrhea, and in the brain may result in a migraine. There is a whole spectrum of problems that these mediators can cause.

Allergic reactions often take place very quickly. Those who experience allergy may go outside on a bright, sunny, windy morning during the ragweed season and within 15 minutes begin to have allergic reactions. This reaction is referred to as immediate hypersensitivity. When mast cells release their chemicals, they cause immediate reactions.

Some people also experience late-phase reactions. When mast cells release their chemicals, they cause an inflammatory response. The site of the allergic reaction gets red, swollen, hot, and tender, causing a more prolonged response. A person may go out at 8 a.m. and experience a late reaction at 4 p.m. Such reactions may last one day, two days, one week, or one month from a single allergen exposure. They are part of the underlying problem for chronic asthma, rhinitis, eczema, hives, and other allergic diseases.

How are allergies diagnosed?

Allergy is diagnosed through skin testing, which shows an immediate reaction to allergens. The procedure traditionally involves introducing a minute amount of allergen into the skin. The tip of the needle is used to puncture the skin, causing an interaction between the allergen and a mast cell.

When doctors administer skin tests, they are introducing allergen into the skin and causing the same reaction that the patients experience in their noses or lungs during the allergy season. In the past, doctors used to take small needles and inject them under the skin surface and put a minute amount of allergen in the skin. Within 15 minutes a welt formed, like a mosquito bite, if the patient had a positive reaction. That was minimally uncomfortable, but it was still uncomfortable.

Today, doctors use a needle to put a drop of allergen on the skin without breaking the skin surface. They "tent" the skin by putting the needle through the droplet and lifting up the skin without breaking the skin surface. It is essentially painless, yet it is very sensitive and specific.

Diagnosis, preferentially, is done by skin testing. Skin tests are fast; they take about 5 minutes to administer and can be read within 15 minutes. They are very sensitive, relatively cheap, cause minimal discomfort, but require some medical expertise.

A second way to diagnosis allergy is with a blood test that looks for IgE antibodies. This test is relatively expensive, slightly less sensitive, requires a blood drawing, and does not require expertise. It is done frequently by non-allergists who want to see if the patient has allergies. In proper hands, both tests are equally informative.

Allergic rhinitis

Allergic rhinitis (hay fever) is a disease of incredible proportion. Thirty-five million Americans—17 percent of the population—experience allergic rhinitis. It is the single most common chronic disease experienced by human beings. As a single entity, 1 out of every 40 doctor office visits (2.5 percent) are due to allergic rhinitis.

Allergic rhinitis is caused by exposure to airborne allergens. The process of allergic rhinitis takes place in the nose. Pollen grains, dust, and dander are trapped by hairs in the nose and are trapped in the mucus that lines the inside of the nose. The allergens release soluble proteins that reach the mucous membranes, causing allergic rhinitis.

The skin that lines the inside of the nose is a succulent tissue full of glands and blood vessels. The submucous glands in this living tissue produce the mucus in the nose. In fact, that is why the lining is called a mucous membrane—it specifically makes mucus. Although many people think of mucus as a bother, mucus is quite helpful.

Mucus is important because it humidifies and protects the mucous membrane. It contains antimicrobial factors that protect people from both bacterial and viral infections. When people get colds, it is despite the fact that they have mucus; if they did not have that mucus, they would have infections all the time.

What about nasal congestion? The body has cavities in the lining of the nose where blood can pool. The nose can become swollen with blood pooling in these sinusoids. When blood is diverted into these sinusoids, this tissue gets markedly enlarged and the person cannot breathe through his or her nose. Everyone experiences nasal congestion; every 45 minutes to 2 hours, one side of the nose congests and the other side constricts. People breathe preferentially through one side, resting the other side, and then alternating sides. One never breathes evenly through both sides of the nose because of this process of congestion. Of course, during allergic rhinitis it gets much worse and the allergy sufferer experiences more severe, chronic nasal congestion.

What can the mucous membrane do? It can congest by pooling blood in these sinusoids; it can become itchy or sneezy by stimulating some of the sensory nerves in the nose; and it can produce secretions. These are the processes that people experience when they have rhinitis—allergic rhinitis, vasomotor rhinitis, rhinitis from colds, or from eating hot and spicy foods.

The most common features of allergic rhinitis are sneezing attacks and itching of the nose, eyes, pharynx, and palate. Clicking the tongue on the top of the mouth is the way one scratches the soft palate, and the soft palate itches if one has allergic rhinitis. One also gets a runny nose or congestion of the nose.

To confirm a diagnosis of allergic rhinitis, the doctor performs a nasal examination and looks for changes in the mucous membrane. If the patient has allergic rhinitis, the mucous membrane becomes very pale because it is swollen. In fact, it takes on a whitish-blue tint. It is very wet with a watery secretion. A smear of the mucus would be loaded with a type of white blood cell known as an eosinophil, which is very characteristic of allergic diseases, and the patient would have an increase of eosinophils in his or her blood. If the doctor does a skin test or a blood test, called a RAST test, which measures an increase in the patient's IgE antibody, both would be positive.

There are two kinds of allergic rhinitis—seasonal and perennial. Seasonal allergic rhinitis characteristically occurs as spring-fall allergies. Springtime begins with tree allergies. Grass is another major springtime allergen.

In the eastern United States, there are few allergens in July and early August, and individuals with allergic rhinitis get better. Pollen from plants that bloom in the summer is spread by the insects, not by the wind, so that is a good time for most people unless they are allergic to molds. Seasonal allergies begin again when ragweed pollinates, starting from mid-August and lasting until the first frost.

Some people also have seasonal allergies to dust during the winter months when the house is closed up and the dust mite feces are richest in the air. But most people with dust allergy have year-round—perennial—symptoms.

Other things that cause year-round allergies are molds. Many people who live in humid areas have damp cellars in which molds form. These molds cause major problems for people with mold allergies.

The other common cause of year-round allergies is allergens from pets. Cats are the worst source of pet allergens, much worse than dogs. The source of allergen from cats is not their fur or skin; it is their saliva, or the proteins in their saliva. And what do cats do all day? They preen. They put saliva on their fur, the saliva dries, aerosolizes, and is the source for the allergen. Dogs—sloppy, friendly little animals that they are—only preen selected parts of their body and are much less likely to expose humans to salivary allergens.

Dogs are still a major source of allergy, especially if they slobber, but if one had to choose between the two, one would choose a dog over a cat. Ideally, allergy sufferers would not have any furred animals in the house because they all cause allergy. Cockroaches also are a major source of year-round allergens.

How is allergic rhinitis treated?

Seasonal allergic rhinitis generally has a better prognosis because it is not a year-round exposure. It is easier to treat and tends to be much less severe. By contrast, perennial disease tends to be much more difficult to treat and is harder to control.

When treating patients with allergic rhinitis, doctors try specifically to take away the causes of the disease. By using allergy avoidance, they get rid of the allergen and the patient is better. Other common treatments include antihistamines, allergy immmunotherapy (allergy shots), a drug called cromolyn sodium, and topical corticosteroids.

To avoid pollen allergens, one must know when the pollen counts are highest. They are generally highest early in the morning, about 6 a.m., on a bright, sunny, breezy day. That is the time allergy sufferers should try to stay inside. If they ride in a car, they should use the car air conditioner. Allergy sufferers should use their house air conditioner, too. Air conditioning filters the air very well, taking out more than 99 percent of all the pollen- and allergen-producing material in the air. If people who are very sensitive during the ragweed, grass, or tree season must go outside in the yard, they should wear nuisance masks, which are like surgical masks and available in drug stores. They are comfortable and will reduce the likelihood of inhaling allergens.

Those with dust allergy should design their bedrooms accordingly. The worst things to have in the bedroom of an allergic person are venetian blinds, which are dust traps; down-filled blankets; feather pillows; heating vents with forced hot air; carpeting; dogs; cats; and closets full of clothing.

Instead of venetian blinds, people should have shades over the windows because they cannot trap dust. If curtains are used, they should be washable curtains that are cleaned periodically in hot water to kill the dust mites. A hardwood or linoleum floor is best, but a washable throw rug is acceptable if it is cleaned in hot water regularly. The bedding should be encased within allergen-proof encasements that are airtight to keep in dust mites, along with their feces. Pillows should be hypoallergenic and replaced every one to two years because when people sleep, they sweat and the sweat makes the pillows moldy over time. Blankets and bedding should be hypoallergenic—definitely not down filled. If at all possible, clothing should be kept in another room. Ideally, the closets would be empty in order to remain dust free. Heat registers should be covered with a filter. New products are appearing in the market that can kill dust mites in carpeting and may prove to be a boon to allergy sufferers.

Allergy shots are extremely effective. Eighty-five percent of the people who receive allergy shots to treat hay fever due to grass, ragweed, trees, and dust get better. It usually takes one to two years. Many people get better for years, and some even permanently. Allergy shots, which are the only known way to turn off allergic disease, reduce the production of IgE and cause the body to make another class of antibody called IgG, which actually protects people from allergic diseases. Shots are the only method available for long-lasting protection from allergies.

Patients with problems only two to four weeks of the year usually are treated with medications. Those with perennial disease are more likely to be put on allergy shots unless their condition can be controlled completely with allergy medications.

There are several medications available to treat allergic rhinitis. One is cromolyn sodium administered in the nose, which prevents allergic reactions from taking place. This drug actually stops the release of chemical mediators like histamine from the mast cell. It is often a very effective therapy. Unfortunately, it must be used about four times a day as a nasal spray.

A second major improvement in therapy of allergic rhinitis has been the use of topical nasal steroids. These steroids are not anabolic steroids. They are anti-inflammatory steroids that stop the late phase reaction. They reduce the number of mast cells in the nose, reduce mucus secretion and swelling, and have other beneficial actions. Because they are given topically, they have no effects elsewhere in the body—only in the nose.

The other major medication used is antihistamines. Over the last five or six years, nonsedating antihistamines have become available. These antihistamines are just as effective as older antihistamines, but they do not cause sleepiness. However, they are considerably more expensive than some of the over-the-counter antihistamines.

Antihistamines work beautifully for immediate hypersensitivity. They reduce sneezing, itching, runny nose, and partially reduce the congestion of allergic rhinitis. Unfortunately, they have no effect on late phase reactions. Antihistamines and nasal steroids are effective combinations to treat allergic rhinitis.

Asthma

Fifteen million people—seven percent of those who live in the United States—have asthma. It is the number one cause for school absenteeism among all chronic diseases. It is the number six cause for hospitalization of all diseases and the number one cause for hospitalization of children.

It is estimated that $4.5 billion is spent every year on medically related charges for the treatment of asthma. That includes hospital and doctor visits. This is an extremely important disease that kills as many as 4,000 Americans a year.

Asthma is a disease of the airways, the tubes through which people breathe. The causes of airflow obstruction in asthma are swelling of the airways, excessive mucus production, inflammation of the airways with eosinophils and neutrophils, and airway smooth muscle contraction. Asthmatic airways are full of secretions, mucus containing eosinophils

and neutrophils—white blood cells—that reflect the underlying inflammation. The epithelial cells that line the airways have been lifted off and the airways are denuded. The muscles contract, closing the airways, and the glands are very reactive and produce large quantities of mucus.

Asthma is an inability to breathe out. Normally when people breathe in, they lower their diaphragms, raise their ribs, and breathe in. It is an active process. To breathe out, they stop breathing in. Breathing out is passive. They breathe out because the lungs are made of elastic tissue, like a rubber band. When a person stops breathing in, the lungs try to assume their relaxed size and do so by letting the air out—if there is no obstruction.

Asthmatic airways have excess mucus, are swollen and inflamed, and have their muscles contracted. As people with asthmatic airways breathe in, they open up their chests and their lungs get bigger. As a result, the airways get bigger and they can move air around these obstructions. They have opened up the airways. When they stop breathing in to breathe out, these obstructions close, there by trapping the air in the lungs.

Take a deep breath to the maximum and do not let it out for the next minute. Breathe at the top of your lungs and do not let out any air. That is what it feels like to have asthma. Asthmatics trap 2 liters of air in their chests, which is the amount of air in a basketball. They have to breathe at the top of their lungs. It is exhausting and feels terrible.

What causes asthma?

The most common cause of asthma is allergy. Of the children under 16 years old who have asthma, 90 percent are allergic. Of the people under 30 who have asthma, 70 percent are allergic. Of the people over 30, 50 percent have allergies.

Asthma also may be caused by infections such as bronchitis, which is a wheezing disease that effects children less than 2 years old and is caused by a viral infection of the airways. This disease leads to asthma; more than half the children who get bronchiolitis have asthma until they are at least 7 years old.

Adults with asthma also get infections that make their asthma worse. They will have colds that commonly develop into bronchitis. Because their lungs are inflamed, the lungs get irritated by a cold very readily and go into an asthmatic attack.

Drugs like aspirin cause asthma in 10 percent of asthmatics. Aspirin and aspirinlike drugs specifically cause asthma in a population of patients that have recurring sinusitis, or infections of the sinuses, and have nasal polyps.

Other drugs that may cause asthma or make it worse are beta-adrenergic blocking agents, which are used for treatment of such conditions as migraine, too rapid a heart rate, congestive heart failure, tremor, and glaucoma.

A third type of agent that may cause asthma is sulfiting agents, which are chemicals that are added to processed foods to keep them from turning brown. If a food should ordinarily turn brown and has not, it has sulfiting agents in it. This includes dried fruits, fruit juices, vegetables, and wines. As sulfites are eaten, they mix with acids in the stomach and become sulfuric acid, which is a gas. The gas travels up through the esophagus, is breathed in, and provokes asthma.

Industrial and occupational exposures also have a bad effect on asthma. On smoggy days, the air is loaded with exhaust from motor vehicles. This is a major source of pollutants, and people with asthma experience increased asthmatic symptoms as a result.

How is asthma diagnosed?

An allergist will do spirometry to measure the patient's ability to blow air out of the chest. The patient takes a deep breath and blows into a machine called a spirometer. The doctor then measures how much and how quickly air was blown out. Most people blow all the air in their chest out within 3 seconds; 75 percent of the air is exhaled within 1 second. The point of maximum expiration is called the "peak flow."

Asthmatics have trouble blowing out the air. That is because of airflow obstruction during breathing out. As a result, they have a very hard time blowing out air and it takes much longer.

Over the past few years, the availability of inexpensive and accurate peak flow meters has made life easier for doctors. Patients can measure their own peak flow in the morning and evening. The patient blows into the flow meter and it measures the peak expiratory flow rate.

For home use it is reliable and inexpensive. A patient can use it before and after taking bronchodilators. It tells the doctor how much airflow increased with the use of bronchodilators and can be used to regulate medications. It also tells the doctor when the patient is doing well, and warns when trouble is coming.

Airway hyperresponsiveness is increased reactivity of the airways, a "twitchiness" of the airways. Asthmatics have nonspecific airway responsiveness. They react when breathing in certain chemicals, including irritants and chemical mediators, or under certain physical conditions like exercise. The importance of airway hyperreactivity is that it clearly separates those who do not have hyperreactivity from asthmatics. Airway hyperreactivity actually predicts who will develop asthma. Patients who have abnormal hyperreactivity are very likely to be predisposed to developing asthma under the right conditions.

There is a range of abnormal airway hyperreactivity among people with asthma, ranging from mild to severe, and doctors can use that range of near normal to very abnormal to determine which medications are required.

Airway hyperreactivity gets worse with allergic reactions that cause late phase reactions. But airway hyperreactivity can get better if the patient avoids allergens, goes on allergy shots, and uses inhaled cromolyn or corticosteroids. Recently, it has been recognized that one of the major targets for the treatment of asthma is airway reactivity.

How is asthma treated?

In order to treat asthma and airway reactivity, doctors recommend that asthma patients avoid the allergens to which they are sensitive whenever possible. They put the patients on allergy shots if they have allergic asthma in hopes of reducing the allergic contribution to the asthma. They use inhaled cromolyn, which stops allergic reactions, and often use in-haled corticosteroids, which stop inflammation of the airways and reduce airway hyperreactivity.

With all patients, doctors also use symptomatic treatment of asthma involving agents that relax the airways. These agents include beta-adrenergic agonists, theophylline, anti-cholinergics, and occasionally expectorants and mucolytics. These medications are employed to try to reverse the airflow obstruction, but they do not have any effect on the underlying causes of asthma.

Until recently, the therapy of asthma was based on the drug theophylline. This drug is an excellent, time-proven, time-tested, and very reliable bronchodilator that opens up asthmatic airways. It was the foundation of asthma therapy from 1970 to 1990.

In the 1980's beta-adrenergic agents became available. These medications relax the airways and make many people better. They became very important in asthma therapy, and have become the predominant drug used to relax airways.

In 1990, asthma therapy shifted so that all asthmatics are now treated with specific therapy aimed at the underlying causes of the disease—allergy avoidance, inhaled corticosteroids, perhaps allergy shots, and perhaps inhaled cromolyn. Nearly all patients use inhaled corticosteroids or cromolyn for the treatment of their airway inflammation. For control of airway obstruction, patients use beta-adrenergic agonists, as well as theophylline and ipratropium, which is an anti-cholinergic agent. Theophylline, however, has gone from being the foundation of treatment to a second-line therapy. It is added later and taken away sooner.

What about general treatments? It is recommended that all asthmatics exercise. Some patients have exercise-induced asthma, so it sounds contradictory, but with the proper medications every asthmatic—particularly children—can and should exercise. Swimming is the preferred form of exercise; biking is the second preferred; and running is the least preferred. It is recommended that asthmatics do not smoke, and that people with asthmatic children stop smoking. Patients are advised to monitor their pulmonary function with a home peak flow meter and learn as much as possible about asthma.

Questions and answers

Q. Nobel Laureate Linus Pauling made mention of the fact that vitamin C has some effect on allergic reactions. What is the latest on that?
A. Scientifically it has not been proven that vitamin C has any effect, beneficial or detrimental, on allergies. It is not harmful, at least in reasonable doses, but it will not help the disease.

Q. How are food allergies effectively identified and then treated?
A. Dr. Dean Metcalfe, here at the National Institute of Allergy and Infectious Diseases, screened adults for food allergy, and he found that when people came in and said, "I'm allergic to strawberries," they were likely to be allergic to strawberries. If people came in and said, "I'm allergic to food," they were almost never allergic to food. When people come in and can identify the food to which they are sensitive, we can confirm that by skin testing. In the case of a specific allergen, the skin tests are positive almost all the time. And, if we do a double-blind food challenge, it is frequently positive.

We have many examples where people have said, "I haven't been able to eat eggs for 25 years," and we skin tested them and the tests were negative. We did a provocation challenge, and the only response was they did not care for the taste of eggs. So, the skin test plus a good history is how we screen for food allergies.

Q. Have you ever observed any ophthalmological effects from allergies such as double vision?
A. The eye is always involved in allergy, but the symptoms are generally itching, swelling, and redness. Eye movement and visual acuity are not affected.

Q. What advice would you give to parents, both of whom suffer from allergies, regarding the introduction of foods for their infant children?
A. Our instructions are very simple. We would recommend, especially if you have two allergic parents, that solids not be introduced until the children are at least 6 months of age. We recommend exclusive breast-feeding through at least the first 6 months. There is some suggestion that very allergenic foods, like cow's milk and peanuts, should be avoided by the mother during breast-feeding because she can transfer some allergens in breast milk. But the opportunity for a child to become allergic to allergens in breast milk is very limited versus drinking cow's milk. Thus, breast-feeding is highly recommended.

Q. I have two questions. First, what are the possible side effects of allergy medications and how often do they occur? Second, I read that in some cases either asthma or hay fever, or some combination, can be due to emotional problems. Is there any information about that?
A. It has often been claimed that asthma is a psychological disease. That is not the case. Asthma is a real, very important disease that can kill you. It may be worsened by psychological stresses, but it is not caused by stress. It is not psychological. The parents of asthmatics often feel very guilty that their child has asthma, and they wonder if it is their fault in some way that influenced their child's asthma. That is not the case.

The side effects for drugs is a very broad question, very hard to answer, but I can tell you that the agents that we use today have been selected from many others because of their efficacy versus their very limited side effects. And the reason that theophylline is being used less today is because it has some side effects we wish to avoid.

Q. I would like your comment on sinusitis. Is it associated with allergies?
A. Sinusitis is an infection of the sinus areas of the skull, which are between the eyes, on either side of the cheeks, in the forehead, and center of the head. They are frequently associated with allergies and the development of sinus congestion; sinus infections are frequent accompaniments of allergy.

Q. What about the long-term effects of corticosteroids? Did I understand you to say that that was no problem?
A. Corticosteroids have major complications associated with them. In the past, we balanced the use of oral corticosteroids, which have systemic side effects, with the effects of the disease. When the disease was bad enough, we gave oral steroids and accepted the side effects if we had to. Now, with topical, inhaled steroids we have little or no systemic effects,

so we get all the beneficial capabilities of steroids with none of the unwanted side effects.

Q. Why do some medications like Benadryl, which you might give a child for hives, say, "Do not give to a child with asthma"? Is it dangerous to give a child Benadryl when he or she has hives and not asthma?
A. That is an interesting and good question. The classical (older) antihistamines, like Benadryl, if you read the label, are not supposed to be used in asthma. Testing in the early 1950's suggested that antihistamines made asthma worse. So there is a label insert that says they should not be used in asthma. We do not use any of the classical or older antihistamines for the treatment of asthma because they do not work very well. Despite the labeling, however, we do not believe they have any danger for people with asthma.

Some of the new, nonsedating antihistamines do have some efficacy in asthma, and they are being used cautiously for asthma treatment. These new antihistamines have no limitations on their use in asthma and may, indeed, be useful.

Q. I wondered if there has ever been a program to eradicate ragweed.
A. Yes, there has been. A woman in the Pennsylvania area and her family had terrible ragweed allergies and she organized the community to eradicate ragweed. It did not make any difference because ragweed moves through the air for such a long distance.

Q. Many of the over-the-counter antihistamines say, "Do not take it for more than seven days." If I want to take them longer, should I get a prescription from a doctor?
A. Antihistamines have been available since the 1940's and many people have taken antihistamines for more than 30 years. They have been among the world's safest drugs. That does not mean that you should use an over-the-counter antihistamine without caution. By and large, we would recommend that everyone would benefit from an appropriate diagnosis and proper therapy, which might include over-the-counter drugs, but might also include prescription drugs, which are really quite a bit more potent and maybe more specific.

■ Document Source:
  National Institutes of Health
  Clinical Center Communications
  NIH Publication No. 91-3221
  April 1991

See also: Facts About Asthma (page 258)

SOMETHING IN THE AIR: AIRBORNE ALLERGENS

Introduction

When is sneezing not a symptom of a cold? Very often, when it represents an allergic reaction to something in the air. It is estimated that 35 million Americans suffer from upper respiratory allergic reactions to airborne pollen. Pollen allergy, commonly called hay fever, is one of the most common chronic diseases in the United States. Worldwide, airborne dust causes the most problems for people with allergies. The respiratory symptoms of asthma, which affects approximately 15 million Americans, are often provoked by airborne allergens (substances that cause an allergic reaction).

Allergic diseases are among the major causes of illness and disability in the United States, affecting as many as 40 to 50 million Americans. The National Institute of Allergy and Infectious Diseases, a component of the National Institutes of Health, conducts and supports research on allergic diseases. The goals of this research are to provide a better understanding of the cause of allergy, to improve the methods for diagnosing and treating allergic reactions, and eventually to prevent allergies. This booklet summarizes what is known about the causes and symptoms of allergic reactions to airborne allergens, how these reactions are diagnosed and treated, and what medical researchers are doing to help people who suffer from these allergies.

What is an allergy?

An allergy is a specific immunologic reaction to a normally harmless substance, one that does not bother most people. Allergic people often are sensitive to more than one substance. Types of allergens that cause allergic reactions include food, dust particles, medicines, insect venom, mold spores, or pollen.

Why are some people allergic to these substances while others are not?

Scientists think that people inherit a tendency to be allergic, although not to any specific allergen. Children are much more likely to develop allergies if their parents have allergies. Even if only one parent is allergic, a child has a one in four chance of developing allergies. Exposure to allergens at certain times when the body's defenses are lowered or weakened, such as after a viral infection, during puberty, or during pregnancy, seems to contribute to the development of allergies.

What is an allergic reaction?

Normally, the immune system functions as the body's defense against invading agents such as bacteria and viruses. In most allergic reactions, however, the immune system is responding to a false alarm. When allergic persons first come into contact with an allergen, their immune systems treat the allergen as an invader and mobilize to attack. The immune system does this by generating large amounts of a type of antibody (a disease-fighting protein) called immunoglobulin E, or IgE. Only small amounts of IgE are produced in nonallergic people. Each IgE antibody is specific for one particular allergenic (allergy-producing) substance. In the case of pollen allergy, the antibody is specific for each type of pollen: one antibody may be produced to react against oak pollen and another against ragweed pollen, for example.

These IgE molecules attach themselves to the body's mast cells, which are tissue cells, and to basophils, which are blood cells. When the allergen next encounters the IgE, it attaches to the antibody like a key fitting into a lock, signalling the cell to which the IgE is attached to release (and in some cases to produce) powerful inflammatory chemicals like histamine, prostaglandins, and leukotrienes. These chemicals move into various parts of the body, such as the respiratory system, and cause the symptoms of allergy.

Some people with allergy develop asthma. The symptoms of asthma include coughing, wheezing, and shortness of breath due to a narrowing of the bronchial passages (airways) in the lungs and to excess mucus production. Asthma can be disabling and sometimes can be fatal. If wheezing and shortness of breath accompany allergy symptoms, it is a signal that the bronchial tubes also have become involved, indicating the need for medical attention.

Symptoms of Allergies to Airborne Substances

The signs and symptoms are familiar to many:

- Sneezing often accompanied by a runny or clogged nose
- Coughing and postnasal drip
- Itching eyes, nose, and throat
- Allergic shiners (dark circles under the eyes caused by increased blood flow near the sinuses)
- The "allergic salute" (in a child, persistent upward rubbing of the nose that causes a crease mark on the nose)
- Watering eyes
- Conjunctivitis (an inflammation of the membrane that lines the eyelids, causing red-rimmed, swollen eyes and crusting of the eyelids).

In people who are not allergic, the mucus in the nasal passages simply moves foreign particles to the throat, where they are swallowed or coughed out. But something different happens to a person who is sensitive to airborne allergens.

As soon as the allergen lands on the mucous membranes lining the inside of the nose, a chain reaction occurs that leads the mast cells in these tissues to release histamine. This powerful chemical enlarges the many small blood vessels in the nose. Fluids escape through these expanded vessel walls, which causes the nasal passages to swell, resulting in nasal congestion.

Histamine can also cause sneezing, itching, irritation, and excess mucus production, which can result in allergic rhinitis (runny nose). Other chemicals made and released by mast cells, including prostaglandins and leukotrienes, also contribute to allergic symptoms.

Pollen Allergy

Each spring, summer, and fall tiny particles are released from trees, weeds, and grasses. These particles, known as pollen, hitch rides on currents of air. Although their mission is to fertilize parts of other plants, many never reach their targets. Instead, they enter human noses and throats, triggering a type of seasonal allergic rhinitis called pollen allergy, which many people know as hay fever or rose fever (depending on the season in which the symptoms occur).

Of all the things that can cause an allergy, pollen is one of the most widespread. Many of the foods, drugs, or animals that cause allergies can be avoided to a great extent; even insects and household dust are escapable. Short of staying indoors when the pollen count is high—and even that may not help—there is no easy way to evade windborne pollen.

People with pollen allergies often develop sensitivities to other troublemakers that are present all year, such as dust. For these allergy sufferers, the "sneezin' season" has no limit. Year-round airborne allergens cause perennial allergic rhinitis, as distinguished from seasonal allergic rhinitis.

What is pollen?

Plants produce microscopic round or oval pollen grains to reproduce. In some species, the plant uses the pollen from its own flowers to fertilize itself. Other types must be cross-pollinated; that is, in order for fertilization to take place and seeds to form, pollen must be transferred from the flower of one plant to that of another plant of the same species. Insects do this job for certain flowering plants, while other plants rely on wind transport.

The types of pollen that most commonly cause allergic reactions are produced by the plain-looking plants (trees, grasses, and weeds) that do not have showy flowers. These plants manufacture small, light, dry pollen granules that are custom-made for wind transport. Samples of ragweed pollen have been collected 400 miles out at sea and 2 miles high in the air. Because airborne pollen is carried for long distances, it does little good to rid an area to an offending plant—the pollen can drift in from many miles away. In addition, most allergenic pollen comes from plants that produce it in huge quantities. A single ragweed plant can generate a million grains of pollen a day.

The chemical makeup of pollen is the basic factor that determines whether it is likely to cause hay fever. For example, pine tree pollen is produced in large amounts by a common tree, which would make it a good candidate for causing allergy. The chemical composition of pine pollen, however, appears to make it less allergenic than other types. Because pine pollen is heavy, it tends to fall straight down and does not scatter. Therefore, it rarely reaches human noses.

Among North American plants, weeds are the most prolific producers of allergenic pollen. Ragweed is the major culprit, but others of importance are sagebrush, redroot pigweed, lamb's quarters, Russian thistle (tumbleweed), and English plantain.

Grasses and trees, too, are important sources of allergenic pollens. Although more than 1,000 species of grass grow in North America, only a few produce highly allergenic pollen. These include timothy, Johnson, Bermuda, redtop, orchard, sweet vernal, and Kentucky bluegrass. Trees that produce allergenic pollen include oak, ash, elm, hickory, pecan, box elder, and mountain cedar.

It is common to hear people say that they are allergic to colorful or scented flowers like roses. In fact, only florists, gardeners, and others who have prolonged, close contact with flowers are likely to become sensitized to pollen from these plants. Most people have little contact with the large, heavy, waxy pollen grains of many flowering plants because this type of pollen is not carried by wind but by insects such as butterflies and bees.

When do plants make pollen?

One of the most obvious features of pollen allergy is its seasonal nature—people experience its symptoms only when the pollen grains to which they are allergic are in the air. Each plant has a pollinating period that is more or less the same from year to year. Exactly when a plant starts to pollinate seems to depend on the relative length of night and day—and therefore on geographical location — rather than on the weather. (On the other hand, weather conditions during pollination can affect the amount of pollen produced and distributed in a specific year.) Thus, the farther north you go, the later the pollinating period and the later the allergy season.

A pollen count, which is familiar to many people from local weather reports, is a measure of how much pollen is in the air. This count represents the concentration of all the pollen (or of one particular type, like ragweed) in the air in a certain area at a specific time. It is expressed in grains of pollen per square meter of air collected over 24 hours. Pollen counts tend to be highest early in the morning on warm, dry, breezy days and lowest during chilly, wet periods. Although a pollen count is an approximate and fluctuating measure, it is useful as a general guide for when it is advisable to stay indoors and avoid contact with the pollen.

Mold Allergy

Along with pollens from trees, grasses, and weeds, molds are an important cause of seasonal allergic rhinitis. People allergic to molds may have symptoms from spring to late fall. The mold season often peaks from July to late summer. Unlike pollens, molds may persist after the first killing frost. Some can grow at subfreezing temperatures, but most become dormant. Snow cover lowers the outdoor mold count drastically but does not kill molds. After the spring thaw, molds thrive on the vegetation that has been killed by the winter cold.

In the warmest areas of the United States, however, molds thrive all year and can cause year-round (perennial) allergic problems. In addition, molds growing indoors can cause perennial allergic rhinitis even in the coldest climates.

What is mold?

There are thousands of types of molds and yeast, the two groups of plants in the fungus family. Yeasts are single cells that divide to form clusters. Molds consist of many cells that grow as branching threads called hyphae. Although both groups can probably cause allergic reactions, only a small number of molds are widely recognized offenders.

The seeds or reproductive particles of fungi are called spores. They differ in size, shape, and color among species. Each spore that germinates can give rise to new mold growth, which in turn can produce millions of spores.

What is mold allergy?

When inhaled, microscopic fungal spores or, sometimes, fragments of fungi may cause allergic rhinitis. Because they are so small, mold spores may evade the protective mechanisms of the nose and upper respiratory tract to reach the lungs and bring on asthma symptoms. Build-up of mucus, wheezing, and difficulty in breathing are the result. Less frequently, exposure to spores or fragments may lead to a lung disease known as hypersensitivity pneumonitis, which will be discussed later.

In a small number of people, symptoms of mold allergy may be brought on or worsened by eating certain foods, such as cheeses, processed with fungi. Occasionally, mushrooms, dried fruits, and foods containing yeast, soy sauce, or vinegar will produce allergic symptoms. There is no known relationship, however, between a respiratory allergy to the mold *Penicillium* and an allergy to the drug penicillin, made from the mold.

Where do molds grow?

Molds can be found wherever there is moisture, oxygen, and a source of the few other chemicals they need. In the fall they grow on rotting logs and fallen leaves, especially in moist, shady areas. In gardens, they can be found in compost piles and on certain grasses and weeds. Some molds attach to grains such as wheat, oats, barley, and corn, making farms, grain bins, and silos likely places to find mold.

Hot spots of mold growth in the home include damp basements and closets, bathrooms (especially shower stalls), places where fresh food is stored, refrigerator drip trays, house plants, air conditioners, humidifiers, garbage pails, mattresses, upholstered furniture, and old foam rubber pillows.

Bakeries, breweries, barns, dairies, and greenhouses are favorite places for molds to grow. Loggers, mill workers, carpenters, furniture repairers, and upholsterers often work in moldy environments.

Which molds are allergenic?

Like pollens, mold spores are important airborne allergens only if they are abundant, easily carried by air currents, and allergenic in their chemical makeup. Found almost everywhere, mold spores in some areas are so numerous they often outnumber the pollens in the air. Fortunately, however, only a few dozen different types are significant allergens.

In general, *Alternaria* and *Cladosporium (Hormodendrum)* are the molds most commonly found both indoors and outdoors throughout the United States. *Aspergillus, Penicillium, Helminthosporium, Epicoccum, Fusarium, Mucor, Rhizopus,* and *Aureobasidium (Pullularia)* are also common.

Are mold counts helpful?

Similar to pollen counts, mold counts may suggest the types and relative quantities of fungi present at a certain time and place. For several reasons, however, these counts probably cannot be used as a constant guide for daily activities. One reason is that the number and types of spores actually present in the mold count may have changed considerably in 24 hours because weather and spore dispersal are directly related. Many of the common allergenic molds are of the dry spore type— they release their spores during dry, windy weather. Other fungi need high humidity, fog, or dew to release their spores. Although rain washes many larger spores out of the air, it also causes some smaller spores to be shot into the air.

In addition to the effect of day-to-day weather changes on mold counts, spore populations may also differ between day and night. Day favors dispersal by dry spore types and night favors wet spore types.

Are there other mold-related disorders?

Fungi or microorganisms related to them may cause other health problems similar to allergy. Some kinds of *Aspergillus* especially may cause several different illnesses, including both infections and allergy. These fungi may lodge in the airways or a distant part of the lung and grow until they form a compact sphere known as a "fungus ball." In people with lung damage or serious underlying illnesses, *Aspergillus* may grasp the opportunity to invade and actually infect the lungs or the whole body.

In some individuals, exposure to these fungi can also lead to asthma or to an illness known as "allergic bronchopulmonary aspergillosis." This latter condition, which occurs occasionally in people with asthma, is characterized by wheezing, low-grade fever, and coughing up of brown-flecked masses or mucous plugs. Skin testing, blood tests, x-rays, and examination of the sputum for fungi can help establish the diagnosis. Corticosteroid drugs are usually effective in treating this reaction; immunotherapy (allergy shots) is not helpful. The occurrence of allergic aspergillosis suggests that other fungi might cause similar respiratory conditions.

Inhalation of spores from fungus-like bacteria, called actinomycetes, and from molds can cause a lung disease called hypersensitivity pneumonitis. This condition is often associated with specific occupations. For example, farmer's lung disease results from inhaling spores growing in moldy hay and grains in silos. Occasionally, hypersensitivity pneumonitis develops in people who live or work where an air conditioning or a humidifying unit is contaminated with and emits these spores.

The symptoms of hypersensitivity pneumonitis may resemble those of a bacterial or viral infection such as the flu. Bouts of chills, fever, weakness, muscle pains, cough, and shortness of breath develop 4 to 8 hours after exposure to the offending organism. The symptoms gradually disappear when the source of exposure is removed. If this is not possible, such as in occupational settings, it may be necessary to increase the ventilation of the workplace, wear a mask with a filter capable of removing spores, or change jobs. If hypersensitivity pneumonitis is allowed to progress, it can lead to serious heart and lung problems.

Dust Allergy

An allergy to dust found in houses is perhaps the most common cause of perennial allergic rhinitis. House dust allergy usually produces symptoms similar to pollen allergy.

What is house dust?

Rather than a single substance, house dust is a varied mixture of potentially allergenic materials. It may contain fibers from different types of fabrics; cotton lint, feathers, and other stuffing materials; bacteria; mold and fungus spores (especially in damp areas); food particles; bits of plants and insects; and other allergens peculiar to an individual home.

Dust also may contain microscopic mites. These mites, which also live in bedding, upholstered furniture, and carpets, thrive in summer and die in winter. However, in a warm, humid house, they continue to thrive even in the coldest months. The particles seen floating in a shaft of sunlight are dead dust mites and their waste-products. These waste-products, which are proteins, actually provoke the allergic reaction. House dust mite allergy is the major year-round allergy in the world, though ragweed allergy is more prevalent in the United States.

Waste-products of cockroaches are also an important cause of allergy symptoms from household allergens, particularly in some urban areas of the United States.

Animal Allergy

Household pets are the main culprits in causing allergic reactions to animals. It was once thought that pet allergy was provoked by dander or fur from cats and dogs. Now, however, the allergen is known to be proteins in the saliva that is present on the dander or fur. Cats win the prize for causing the most allergic reactions. One reason may be that cats preen themselves more than other furry pets. This preening coats the hairs with saliva containing allergens, which become airborne when the saliva dries. Also, it may because cats are held more and often spend more time in the house, close to humans, than do dogs.

Some rodents, such as guinea pigs and gerbils, have become increasingly popular as household pets. They, too, can cause allergic reactions in some people. Urine is the major source of allergens from these animals.

Allergies to animals can take 2 years or more to develop and may not subside until 6 months or more after ending contact with the animal. Carpet and furniture are a reservoir for pet allergens, and the allergens can remain in them for 4 to 6 weeks. In addition, these allergens can stay in household air for months after the animal has been removed. Therefore, it is wise for people with an animal allergy to check with the landlord or previous owner to find out if furry pets had lived previously on the premises.

Chemical Sensitivity

"Allergic to the twentieth century" is a phrase that has been used to describe people who seem to react to everything in their environment—indoors and outdoors. These allergy-like reactions can result from exposure to man-made substances, such as those found in paints or carpeting, or to natural substances, such as odors emitted by plants and flowers. Although the symptoms may resemble some of the manifestations of true allergies, sensitivity to chemicals does not represent a true allergic reaction.

Diagnosing Allergic Diseases

People with allergy symptoms, such as allergic rhinitis, may at first suspect they have a cold — but the "cold" lingers on. It is important to see a doctor about any respiratory illness that lasts longer than a week or two. When it appears that the symptoms are caused by an allergy, the patient should see a physician who understands the diagnosis and treatment of allergies. If the patient's medical history indicates that the symptoms recur at the same time each year, the physician will work under the theory that a seasonal allergen (like pollen) is involved. Properly trained specialists recognize the patterns of the local seasons and the association between these and patterns and symptoms. The medical history suggests which allergens are the likely culprits. The doctor will also examine the mucous membranes, which often appear swollen and pale or bluish in persons with allergic conditions.

Skin tests

To confirm which allergen is responsible, skin testing may be recommended using extracts from allergens such as dust, pollens, or molds commonly found in the local area. A diluted extract of each kind of allergen is injected under the patient's skin or is applied to a scratch or puncture made on the patient's arm or back.

With a positive reaction, a small, raised, reddened area with a surrounding flush (called a wheal and flare) will appear at the test site. The size of the wheal can provide the physician with an important diagnostic clue, but a positive reaction does not prove that a particular pollen is the cause of a patient's symptoms. Although such a reaction indicates that IgE antibody to a specific allergen is present in the skin, respiratory symptoms do not necessarily result.

Blood tests

Skin testing is not advisable in some people such as those with widespread skin conditions like eczema. Diagnostic tests can be done using a blood sample from the patient to detect levels of IgE antibody to a particular allergen. One such blood test is called the RAST (radioallergosorbent test), which can be performed when eczema is present or if a patient has taken medications that interfere with skin testing.

It is expensive to perform, takes several weeks to yield results, and is somewhat less sensitive than skin testing. Overall, skin testing is the most sensitive and least costly diagnostic tool.

Treating Allergic Diseases

There are three general approaches to the treatment of these allergies: avoidance of the allergen, medication to relieve symptoms, and allergy shots. Although no cure for allergies has yet been found, one of these strategies or a combination of them can provide varying degrees of relief from allergy symptoms.

Avoidance

Complete avoidance of allergenic pollen or mold means moving to a place where the offending substance does not grow and where it is not present in the air. But even this extreme solution may offer only temporary relief since a person who is sensitive to a specific pollen or mold may subsequently develop allergies to new allergens after repeated exposure. For example, people allergic to ragweed may leave their ragweed-ridden communities and relocate to areas where ragweed does not grow, only to develop allergies to other weeds or even to grasses or trees in their new surroundings. Because relocating is not a reliable solution, allergy specialists do not encourage this approach.

There are other ways to evade the offending pollen: remaining indoors in the morning, for example, when the outdoor pollen levels are highest. Sunny, windy days can be especially troublesome. If persons with pollen allergy must work outdoors, they can wear face masks designed to filter pollen out of the air and keep it from reaching their nasal passages. As another approach, some people take their vacations at the height of the expected pollinating period and choose a location where such exposure would be minimal. The seashore, for example, may be an effective retreat for many with pollen allergies.

Mold allergens can be difficult to avoid, but some steps can be taken to at least reduce exposure to them. First, the allergy sufferer should avoid those hot spots mentioned earlier where molds tend to be concentrated. The lawn should be mowed and leaves should be raked up, but someone other than the allergic person should do these chores. If such work cannot be delegated, wearing a tightly fitting dust mask can greatly reduce exposure and resulting symptoms. Travel in the country, especially on dry, windy days or while crops are being harvested, should be avoided as should walks through tall vegetation. A summer cabin closed up all winter is probably full of molds and should be aired out and cleaned before a mold-sensitive person stays there.

Around the home, a dehumidifier will help dry out the basement, but the water extracted from the air must be removed frequently to prevent mold growth in the machine.

Those with dust allergy should pay careful attention to dust-proofing their bedroom. The worst things to have in the bedroom are wall-to-wall carpets, venetian blinds, down-filled blankets, feather pillows, heating vents with forced hot air, dogs, cats, and closets full of clothing. Shades are preferred over venetian blinds because they do not trap dust. Curtains can be used if they are washed periodically in hot water to kill the dust mites. Bedding should be encased in a zippered, plastic, airtight, and dust-proof cover.

Although shag carpets are the worst type for the dust-sensitive person, all carpets trap dust and make dust control impossible. In addition, vacuuming can contribute to the amount of dust, unless the vacuum is equipped with a special high-efficiency particulate air (HEPA) filter. Wall-to-wall carpets should be replaced with washable throw rugs over hardwood, tile, or linoleum floors.

Reducing the amount of dust in a home may require new cleaning techniques as well as some changes in furnishings to eliminate dust collectors. Water is often the secret to effective dust removal. Washable items should be washed often using water hotter than 130° Fahrenheit. Dusting with a damp cloth or oiled mop should be done frequently.

The best way for a person allergic to pets, especially cats, to avoid allergic reactions is to find another home for the animal. There are, however, some suggestions that help keep cat allergens out of the air: bathe the cat weekly and brush it more frequently, remove carpets and soft furnishing, and use a vacuum cleaner with a high-efficiency filter and a room air cleaner (see section below). Wearing a face mask while house and cat cleaning and keeping the cat out of the bedroom are other methods that allow many people to live more happily with their pets.

Irritants such as chemicals can worsen airborne allergy symptoms and should be avoided as much as possible. For example, during periods of high pollen levels, people with pollen allergy should try to avoid unnecessary exposure to irritants such as dust, insect sprays, tobacco smoke, air pollution, and fresh tar or paint.

Air conditioners and filters

Use of air conditioners inside the home or in a car can help prevent pollen and mold allergens from entering. Various types of air-filtering devices made with fiberglass or electrically charged plates may help reduce allergens produced in the home. These can be added to the heating and cooling systems. In addition, portable devices that can be used in individual rooms are especially helpful in reducing animal allergens.

An allergy specialist can suggest which kind of filter is best for the home of a particular patient. Before buying a filtering device, it is wise to rent one and use it in a closed room (the bedroom, for instance) for a month or two to see whether allergy symptoms diminish. The air-flow should be sufficient to exchange the air in the room five or six times per hour; therefore, the size and efficiency of the filtering device should be determined in part by the size of the room.

Persons with allergies should be wary of exaggerated claims for appliances that cannot really clean the air. Very small air cleaners cannot remove dust and pollen—and no air purifier can prevent viral or bacterial diseases such as influenza, pneumonia, or tuberculosis. Buyers of electrostatic precipitators should compare the machine's ozone output with Federal standards. Ozone can irritate the nose and airways of persons with allergies, especially those with asthma, and can increase the allergy symptoms. Other kinds of air filters such as HEPA filters do not release ozone into the air.

Medication

For people who find they cannot adequately avoid the allergens, the symptoms often can be controlled with medications. Effective medications that can be prescribed by a physician include antihistamines, topical nasal steroids, and cromolyn sodium—any of which can be used alone or in combination. Many effective antihistamines and decongestants also are available without a prescription.

Antihistamines. As the name indicates, an antihistamine counters the effects of histamine, which is released by the mast cells in the body's tissues and contributes to allergy symptoms. For many years, antihistamines have proven useful in relieving sneezing and itching in the nose, throat, and eyes and in reducing nasal swelling and drainage.

Many people who take antihistamines experience some distressing side effects: drowsiness and loss of alertness and coordination. In children, such reactions can be misinterpreted as behavior problems. During the last few years, however, antihistamines that cause fewer of these side effects have become available by prescription. These new nonsedating antihistamines are as effective as other antihistamines in preventing histamine-induced symptoms, but do so without causing sleepiness.

Topical nasal steroids. This medication should not be confused with anabolic steroids that have serious side effects. Topical nasal steroids are anti-inflammatory drugs that stop the allergic reaction. In addition to other beneficial actions, they reduce the number of mast cells in the nose and reduce mucus secretion and nasal swelling. The combination of anti-histamines and nasal steroids is a very effective way to treat allergic rhinitis.

Cromolyn sodium. Cromolyn sodium stops allergic reactions from starting. It is administered as a nasal spray, and it can prevent the release of chemicals like histamine from the mast cell.

Immunotherapy

Immunotherapy, or a series of allergy shots, is the only available treatment that has a chance of reducing the allergy symptoms over the long haul. Patients receive injections of increasing concentrations of the allergen(s) to which they are sensitive. These injections reduce the amount of IgE antibodies in the blood and cause the body to make a protective antibody called IgG. About 85 percent of patients with allergic rhinitis will have a significant reduction in their hay fever symptoms and in their need for medication within 24 months of starting immunotherapy. Many patients are able to stop the injections with good, long-term results. As better allergens for immunotherapy are produced, this technique will become an even more effective treatment.

Allergy Research

The National Institute of Allergy and Infectious Diseases (NIAID) conducts and supports research on allergies focused on understanding what happens to the body during the allergic process—the sequence of events leading to the allergic response and the factors responsible for allergic diseases. This understanding will lead to better methods of preventing and treating allergies.

NIAID supports a network of Asthma, Allergic and Immunologic Diseases Cooperative Research Centers throughout the United States. The centers encourage close coordination among scientists studying the immune system, genes, biochemistry, and pharmacology. This interdisciplinary approach helps move research knowledge as quickly as possible from research scientists to physicians and their allergy patients.

Educating patients and health care workers is an important tool in controlling allergic diseases. All of these research centers conduct and evaluate educational programs focused on methods to control allergic diseases.

NIAID's National Cooperative Inner-City Asthma Study Centers are examining ways to prevent asthma in minority children in inner-city environments. Asthma, a major cause of illness and death among these children, is provoked by a number of possible factors, including allergies to airborne substances.

Although several factors provoke allergic responses, scientists know that heredity is a major influence on who will develop an allergy. Therefore, researchers are trying to identify and describe the genes that make a person susceptible to allergic diseases.

Other studies are aimed at seeking better ways to diagnose and treat people with allergic diseases and to better understand the factors that regulate IgE production in order to reduce the allergic response in patients. Several research institutions are focusing on ways to influence the cells that participate in the allergic response.

These studies offer the promise of improving treatment and control of allergic diseases and the hope that one day allergic diseases will be preventable as well.

Information Resources

American Academy of Allergy and Immunology
611 East Wells Street
Milwaukee, WI 53202
1-800-822-ASMA

Asthma and Allergy Foundation of America
1125 15th Street, NW, Suite 502
Washington, DC 20005
1-800-7-ASTHMA

Allergy and Asthma Network
3554 Chain Bridge Road, Suite 200
Fairfax, VA 22030
1-800-878-4403

For information on air-cleaning devices:

Environmental Protection Agency
Public Information Service
401 M Street, SW
Washington, DC 20460
1-800-438-4318

■ Document Source:
   U.S. Department of Health and Human Services, Public Health Service
   National Institutes of Health
   National Institute of Allergy and Infectious Diseases
   NIH Publication No. 93-493
   March 1993

See also: Facts About Asthma (page 258)

BLOOD DISEASES AND DISORDERS

◼ ▨ ◼

CancerFax from the National Cancer Institute

ADULT ACUTE LYMPHOCYTIC LEUKEMIA

Description

What Is Adult Acute Lymphocytic Leukemia?

Adult acute lymphocytic leukemia (also called acute lymphoblastic leukemia or ALL) is a disease in which too many infection-fighting white blood cells called lymphocytes are found in your blood and bone marrow. Lymphocytes are made by the bone marrow and by other organs of the lymph system. Your bone marrow is the spongy tissue inside the large bones in your body. The bone marrow makes red blood cells (which carry oxygen and other materials to all tissues of the body), white blood cells (which fight infection), and platelets (which make your blood clot). Normally, the bone marrow makes cells called blasts that develop (mature) into several different types of blood cells that have specific jobs to do in the body.

The lymph system is made up of thin tubes that branch, like blood cells, into all parts of the body. Lymph vessels carry lymph, a colorless, watery fluid that contains lymphocytes. Along the network of vessels are groups of small, bean-shaped organs called lymph nodes. Clusters of lymph nodes are found in the underarm, pelvis, neck, and abdomen. The spleen (an organ in the upper abdomen that makes lymphocytes and filters old blood cells from the blood), the thymus (a small organ beneath the breastbone), and the tonsils (an organ in your throat) are also part of the lymph system.

Lymphocytes fight infection by making substances called antibodies, which attack germs and other harmful bacteria in your body. In ALL, the developing lymphocytes do not mature and become too numerous. These immature lymphocytes are then found in the blood and bone marrow. They also collect in the lymph tissues and make them swell. Lymphocytes may crowd out other blood cells in the blood and bone marrow. If your bone marrow cannot make enough platelets to make your blood clot normally, you may bleed or bruise easily. The cancerous lymphocytes can also invade other organs, the spinal cord, and the brain.

Leukemia can be acute (progressing quickly with many immature cancer cells) or chronic (progressing slowly with more mature-looking leukemia cells). Acute lymphocytic leukemia progresses quickly. ALL can occur in children and adults. Treatment is different for children than it is for adults. If you want information on childhood ALL, refer to the PDQ patient information statement on childhood acute lymphocytic leukemia. Separate PDQ patient information statements are also available for chronic lymphocytic leukemia, chronic myelogenous leukemia, adult or childhood acute myeloid leukemia, and hairy cell leukemia.

Like most cancers, acute lymphocytic leukemia is best treated when it is found (diagnosed) early. It is often difficult to diagnose ALL. The early signs may be similar to the flu or other common diseases. You should see your doctor if you have a fever that won't go away, you feel weak or tired all the time, your bones or joints ache, or your lymph nodes swell.

If you have symptoms, your doctor may order blood tests to count the number of each of the different kind of blood cells. If the results of the blood test are not normal, your doctor may do a bone marrow biopsy. During this test, a needle is inserted into a bone and a small amount of bone marrow is taken out and looked at under the microscope. Your doctor can then tell what kind of leukemia you have and plan the best treatment.

Your doctor may also do a spinal tap in which a needle is inserted through your back to take a sample of the fluid that surrounds your brain and spine. The fluid is then looked at under a microscope to see if leukemia cells are present.

Your chance of recovery (prognosis) depends on how the leukemia cells look under a microscope, how far the leukemia has spread, your age, and your general health.

Stage Explanation

Stages of Adult Acute Lymphocytic Leukemia

There is no staging for adult acute lymphocytic leukemia. Your choice of treatment depends on whether you have been treated or not.

Untreated
Untreated ALL means no treatment has been given except to treat symptoms. There are too many white blood cells in the blood and bone marrow, and there may be other signs and symptoms of leukemia.

In remission

Treatment has been given and the number of white blood cells and other blood cells in the blood and bone marrow is normal. There are no signs or symptoms of leukemia.

Relapsed/refractory

Relapsed disease means the leukemia has come back (recurred) after going into remission. Refractory disease means the leukemia has failed to go into remission following treatment.

Treatment Options Overview

How Adult Acute Lymphocytic Leukemia Is Treated

There are treatments for all patients with adult ALL. The primary treatment for ALL is chemotherapy. Radiation therapy may be used in certain cases. Bone marrow transplantation is being studied in clinical trials.

Chemotherapy uses drugs to kill cancer cells. Chemotherapy may be taken by pill, or it may be put into the body by a needle in a vein or muscle. Chemotherapy is called a systemic treatment because the drug enters the bloodstream, travels through the body, and can kill cancer cells throughout the body. Chemotherapy may sometimes be put into the fluid that surrounds the brain through a needle in the brain or back (intrathecal chemotherapy).

Radiation therapy uses x-rays or other high-energy rays to kill cancer cells and shrink tumors. Radiation for ALL usually comes from a machine outside the body (external radiation therapy).

There are two phases of treatment for ALL. The first stage is called induction therapy. The purpose of induction therapy is to kill as many of the leukemia cells as possible and make you go into remission. Once you go into remission and there are no signs of leukemia, a second phase of treatment is given (called continuation therapy), which tries to kill any remaining leukemia cells. You may receive chemotherapy for up to several years to keep you in remission.

If the leukemia cells have spread to the brain, you will receive radiation or chemotherapy to the brain. During induction and remission, you may also receive therapy to prevent leukemia cells from growing in the brain. This is called central nervous system (CNS) prophylaxis.

Bone marrow transplantation is used to replace your bone marrow with healthy bone marrow. First, all of the bone marrow in your body is destroyed with high doses of chemotherapy with or without radiation therapy. Healthy marrow is then taken from another person (a donor) whose tissue is the same as or almost the same as yours. The donor may be a twin (the best match), a brother or sister, or another person not related. The healthy marrow from the donor is given to you through a needle in the vein, and the marrow replaces the marrow that was destroyed. A bone marrow transplant using marrow from a relative or person not related to you is called an allogeneic bone marrow transplant.

Another type of bone marrow transplant, called autologous bone marrow transplant, is being studied in clinical trials. To do this type of transplant, bone marrow is taken from you and treated with drugs to kill any cancer cells. The marrow is frozen to save it. Next, you are given high-dose chemotherapy with or without radiation therapy to destroy all of your remaining marrow. The frozen marrow that was saved for you is then thawed and given to you through a needle in a vein to replace the marrow that was destroyed.

A greater chance for recovery occurs if your doctor chooses a hospital which does more than 5 bone marrow transplantations per year.

Treatment by Stage

Treatment for adult acute lymphocytic leukemia depends on the type of your disease, your age, and your overall condition.

You may receive treatment that is considered standard based on its effectiveness in a number of patients in past studies, or you may choose to go into a clinical trial. Not all patients are cured with standard therapy and some standard treatments may have more side effects than are desired. For these reasons, clinical trials are designed to find better ways to treat cancer patients and are based on the most up-to-date information. Clinical trials are going on in most parts of the country for most stages of ALL. If you want more information, call the Cancer Information Service at 1-800-4-CANCER (1-800-422-6237).

Treatment options: Untreated adult acute lymphocytic leukemia

Your treatment will probably be systemic chemotherapy. You may also receive intrathecal chemotherapy alone or plus either radiation therapy to the brain or high doses of systemic chemotherapy to treat or prevent leukemia in the brain. Your treatment may also include blood transfusions, antibiotics, and instructions to keep your body and teeth especially clean. Clinical trials are testing new drugs.

Treatment options: Adult acute lymphocytic leukemia in remission

Your treatment may be one of the following:
1. Systemic chemotherapy. Intrathecal chemotherapy plus either radiation to the brain or high doses of systemic chemotherapy is also given to prevent leukemia cells from growing in the brain.
2. Clinical trials of bone marrow transplantation.
3. Clinical trials of new chemotherapy drugs.

Treatment options: Relapsed adult acute lymphocytic leukemia

You may choose to take part in a clinical trial of new chemotherapy drugs or bone marrow transplantation.

To learn more about adult acute lymphocytic leukemia, call the National Cancer Institute's Cancer Information Service at 1-800-4-CANCER (1-800-422-6237). By dialing this toll-free number, you can speak with someone who can answer your questions.

■ **Document Source:**
National Cancer Institute
  Building 31, Room 10A24, 9000 Rockville Pike, Bethesda, MD
    20892
  PDQ 208/01024
  02/01/94

See also: Chemotherapy and You: A Guide to Self-Help During Treatment (page 40); Radiation Therapy and You: A Guide to Self-Help During Treatment (page 56)

CancerFax from the National Cancer Institute

ADULT ACUTE MYELOID LEUKEMIA

Description

What Is Adult Acute Myeloid Leukemia?

Adult acute myeloid leukemia (AML) is a disease in which cancer (malignant) cells are found in your blood and bone marrow. AML is also called acute nonlymphocytic leukemia or ANLL. Your bone marrow is the spongy tissue inside the large bones in your body. The bone marrow makes red blood cells (which carry oxygen and other materials to all tissues of the body), white blood cells (which fight infection), and platelets (which make your blood clot).

Normally, the bone marrow makes cells called blasts that develop (mature) into several different types of blood cells that have specific jobs to do in the body. AML affects the blasts that are developing into white blood cells called granulocytes. In AML, the blasts do not mature and become too numerous. These immature blast cells are then found in the blood and the bone marrow.

Leukemia can be acute (progressing quickly with many immature blasts) or chronic (progressing slowly with more mature-looking cancer cells). Acute myeloid leukemia progresses quickly. AML can occur in children or adults. If you want information on the treatment of childhood AML, refer to the PDQ patient information statement on childhood acute myeloid leukemia. Separate PDQ statements are also available for chronic lymphocytic leukemia, chronic myelogenous leukemia, adult acute lymphocytic leukemia, and hairy cell leukemia.

Like most cancers, adult acute myeloid leukemia is best treated when it is found (diagnosed) early. It is often difficult to diagnose AML. The early signs may be similar to the flu or other common diseases. You should see your doctor if you have a fever that won't go away, you feel weak or tired all the time, or your bones or joints ache.

If you have symptoms, your doctor may order blood tests to count the number of each of the different kind of blood cells. If the results of the blood test are not normal, your doctor may do a bone marrow biopsy. During this test, a needle is inserted into a bone and a small amount of bone marrow is taken out and looked at under the microscope. Your doctor can then tell what kind of leukemia you have and plan the best treatment.

Your chance of recovery (prognosis) depends on the type of AML you have, your age, and your general health.

Stage Explanation

Stages of Adult Acute Myeloid Leukemia

There is no staging for acute myeloid leukemia. Your choice of treatment depends on whether you have been treated or not.

Untreated

Untreated adult acute myeloid leukemia means no treatment has been given except to treat symptoms. There are too many white blood cells in the blood and bone marrow and there may be other signs and symptoms of leukemia.

In remission

Treatment has been given and the number of white blood cells and other blood cells in the blood and bone marrow is normal. There are no signs or symptoms of leukemia.

Relapsed/refractory

Relapsed disease means the leukemia has come back (recurred) after going into remission. Refractory disease means the leukemia has not gone into remission following treatment.

Treatment Options Overview

How Adult Acute Myeloid Leukemia Is Treated

There are treatments for all patients with adult acute myeloid leukemia. The primary treatment for AML is chemotherapy. Radiation therapy may be used in certain cases. Bone marrow transplantation and biological therapy are being studied in clinical trials.

Chemotherapy uses drugs to kill cancer cells. Drugs may be given by mouth or they may be put into the body by a needle in a vein or muscle. Chemotherapy is called a systemic treatment because the drug enters the bloodstream, travels through the body, and can kill cancer cells throughout the body. Chemotherapy may sometimes be put into the fluid that surrounds the brain through a needle in the brain or back (intrathecal chemotherapy).

Radiation therapy uses x-rays or other high-energy rays to kill cancer cells and shrink tumors. Radiation for AML usually comes from a machine outside the body (external radiation therapy).

If the leukemia cells have spread to the brain you will receive radiation therapy to the brain or intrathecal chemotherapy.

There are two phases of treatment for AML. The first stage is called induction therapy. The purpose of induction therapy is to kill as many of the leukemia cells as possible and make you go into remission. Once you go into remission and there are no signs of leukemia, a second phase of treatment is given (called continuation therapy), which tries to kill any remaining leukemia cells. You may receive chemotherapy for several years to keep you in remission.

Bone marrow transplantation is used to replace your bone marrow with healthy bone marrow. First, all of the bone marrow in your body is destroyed with high doses of chemotherapy with or without radiation therapy. Healthy marrow is then taken from another person (a donor) whose tissue is the same as or almost the same as yours. The donor may be a twin (the best match), a brother or sister, or another person not related. The healthy marrow from the donor is given to you through a needle in the vein, and the marrow replaces the marrow that was destroyed. A bone marrow transplant using marrow from a relative or person not related to you is called an allogeneic bone marrow transplant.

Another type of bone marrow transplant, called autologous bone marrow transplant, is being studied in clinical trials. To do this type of transplant, bone marrow is taken from you and treated with drugs to kill any cancer cells. The marrow is then frozen to save it. Next, you are given high-dose chemotherapy with or without radiation therapy to destroy all of your remaining marrow. The frozen marrow that was saved for you is then thawed and given to you through a needle in a vein to replace the marrow that was destroyed. Cells for the transplant may be taken from your own blood for a procedure called peripheral stem cell transplantation.

A greater chance for recovery occurs if your doctor chooses a hospital which does more than 5 bone marrow transplantations per year.

Biological therapy tries to get your own body to fight cancer. It uses materials made by your own body or made in a laboratory to boost, direct, or restore your body's natural defenses against disease. Biological therapy is sometimes called biological response modifier (BRM) therapy or immunotherapy.

Treatment by Stage

Treatment for adult AML depends on the type of your disease, your age, and your overall health.

You may receive treatment that is considered standard based on its effectiveness in a number of patients in past studies, or you may choose to go into a clinical trial. Not all patients are cured with standard therapy and some standard treatments may have more side effects than are desired. For these reasons, clinical trials are designed to find better ways to treat cancer patients and are based on the most up-to-date information. Clinical trials are going on in most parts of the country for most stages of adult acute myeloid leukemia. If you want more information, call the Cancer Information Service at 1-800-4-CANCER (1-800-422-6237).

Treatment options: Untreated adult acute myeloid leukemia

Your treatment will probably be systemic chemotherapy. If leukemia cells are found in the brain, you may receive intrathecal chemotherapy. Clinical trials are testing new drugs.

Treatment options: Adult acute myeloid leukemia in remission

Your treatment may be one of the following:
1. Systemic chemotherapy. Clinical trials are testing new chemotherapy drugs and new ways of giving the drugs.
2. Clinical trials of bone marrow or peripheral stem cell transplantation.

Treatment options: Relapsed adult acute myeloid leukemia

You may choose to take part in clinical trials of new chemotherapy drugs or bone marrow transplantation.

To learn more about adult acute myeloid leukemia, call the National Cancer Institute's Cancer Information Service at 1-800-4-CANCER (1-800-422-6237). By dialing this toll-free number, you can speak with someone who can answer your questions.

■ Document Source:
National Cancer Institute
Building 31, Room 10A24, 9000 Rockville Pike, Bethesda, MD 20892
PDQ 208/01029
02/01/94

See also: Chemotherapy and You: A Guide to Self-Help During Treatment (page 40); Radiation Therapy and You: A Guide to Self-Help During Treatment (page 56)

CancerFax from the National Cancer Institute
CHRONIC MYELOGENOUS LEUKEMIA

Description

What Is Chronic Myelogenous Leukemia?

Chronic myelogenous leukemia (also called CML or chronic granulocytic leukemia) is a disease in which too many white blood cells are made in the bone marrow. Your bone marrow is the spongy tissue inside the large bones in your body. The bone marrow makes red blood cells (which carry oxygen and other materials to all tissues of the body), white blood cells (which fight infection), and platelets (which make your blood clot).

Normally, bone marrow cells called blasts develop (mature) into several different types of blood cells that have specific jobs to do in the body. CML affects the blasts that are developing into white blood cells called granulocytes. The blasts do not mature and become too numerous. These immature blast cells are then found in the blood and the bone marrow. In most people with CML, the genetic materials (chromosomes) in the leukemia cells have a feature that is not normal called a Philadelphia chromosome. This chromosome usually doesn't go away, even after treatment.

Leukemia can be acute (progressing quickly with many immature blasts) or chronic (progressing slowly with more mature-looking cancer cells). Chronic myelogenous leukemia progresses slowly and usually occurs in people who are middle-aged or older, although it also can occur in children. In the first stages of CML, most people don't have any symptoms of cancer. You should see your doctor if you have any of the following: tiredness that won't go away, a feeling of no energy, fever, not feeling hungry, or night sweats. The spleen (the organ in the upper abdomen that makes other types of white blood cells and filters old blood cells from the blood) may be swollen.

If you have symptoms, your doctor may order blood tests to count the number of each of the different kinds of blood cells. If the results of the blood test are not normal, your doctor may order more blood tests. A bone marrow biopsy also may be done. During this test, a needle is inserted into a bone and a small amount of bone marrow is taken out and looked at under the microscope. Your doctor can then tell what kind of leukemia you have and plan the best treatment.

There are separate PDQ patient information statements on acute lymphocytic leukemia (adult and childhood), acute myeloid leukemia (adult and childhood), chronic myelogenous leukemia, and hairy cell leukemia.

Stage Explanation

Stages of Chronic Myelogenous Leukemia

Once chronic myelogenous leukemia (CML) has been found (diagnosed), more tests may be done to find out if leukemia cells have spread into other parts of the body such as the brain. This is called staging. CML progresses through different phases and these phases are the stages used to plan treatment. The following stages are used for chronic myelogenous leukemia:

Chronic phase
There are few blast cells in the blood and bone marrow and there may be no symptoms of leukemia. This phase may last from several months to several years.

Accelerated phase
There are more blast cells in the blood and bone marrow, and fewer normal cells.

Blastic phase
More than 30% of the cells in the blood or bone marrow are blast cells. The blast phase of CML is sometimes called "blast crisis." Sometimes blast cells will form tumors outside of the bone marrow in places such as the bone or lymph nodes. Lymph nodes are small bean-shaped structures that are found throughout the body. They produce and store infection-fighting cells.

Meningeal
Leukemia cells are found in the fluid that surrounds the brain and/or spinal cord. Meningeal CML can occur during the accelerated phase or the blastic phase.

Refractory
Leukemia cells do not decrease even though treatment is given.

Treatment Options Overview

How Chronic Myelogenous Leukemia Is Treated

There are treatments for all patients with chronic myelogenous leukemia. Three kinds of treatment are used:

chemotherapy (using drugs to kill cancer cells)
radiation therapy (using high-dose x-rays or other high-energy rays to kill cancer cells)
bone marrow transplantation (killing the bone marrow and replacing it with healthy marrow).

The use of biological therapy (using your body's immune system to fight cancer) is being tested in clinical trials. Surgery may be used in certain cases to relieve symptoms.

Chemotherapy uses drugs to kill cancer cells. Chemotherapy may be taken by pill, or it may be put into the body by a needle in the vein or muscle. Chemotherapy is called a systemic treatment because the drug enters the bloodstream, travels through the body, and can kill cancer cells throughout the body. Chemotherapy also can be put directly into the fluid around the brain and spinal cord through a tube inserted into the brain or back. This is called intrathecal chemotherapy.

Radiation therapy uses x-rays or other high-energy rays to kill cancer cells and shrink tumors. Radiation for CML usually comes from a machine outside the body (external radiation therapy) and is sometimes used to relieve symptoms or as part of therapy given before a bone marrow transplant.

Bone marrow transplantation is used to replace your bone marrow with healthy bone marrow. First, all of the bone marrow in your body is destroyed with high doses of chemotherapy with or without radiation therapy. Healthy marrow is then taken from another person (a donor) whose tissue is the same as or almost the same as yours. The donor may be a twin (the best match), a brother or sister, or another person not related. The healthy marrow from the donor is given to you through a needle in the vein, and the marrow replaces the marrow that was destroyed. A bone marrow transplant using marrow from a relative or person not related to you is called an allogeneic bone marrow transplant.

Another type of bone marrow transplant, called autologous bone marrow transplant, is being tested in clinical trials. To do this type of transplant, bone marrow is taken from you and treated with drugs to kill any cancer cells. The marrow is then frozen to save it. You are given high-dose chemotherapy with or without radiation therapy to destroy all of your remaining marrow. The frozen marrow that was saved for you is then thawed and given to you through a needle in a vein to replace the marrow that was destroyed.

A greater chance for recovery occurs if your doctor chooses a hospital which does more than 5 bone marrow transplantations per year.

Biological therapy tries to get your own body to fight cancer. It uses materials made by your own body or made in a laboratory to boost, direct, or restore your body's natural defenses against disease. Biological therapy is sometimes called biological response modifier (BRM) therapy or immunotherapy.

If the spleen is swollen, your doctor may take out the spleen in an operation called a splenectomy.

Treatment by Stage

You may receive treatment that is considered standard based on its effectiveness in a number of patients in past studies, or you may choose to go into a clinical trial. Most patients are not cured with standard therapy and some standard treatments may have more side effects than are desired. For these reasons, clinical trials are designed to find better ways to treat cancer patients and are based on the most up-to-date information. Clinical trials are going on in most parts of the country for patients with CML of any phase. If you wish to know more about clinical trials, call the Cancer Information Service at 1-800-4-CANCER (1-800-422-6237).

Treatment options: Chronic phase chronic myelogenous leukemia
Your treatment may be one of the following:
1. No treatment if blood counts are nearly normal.
   Your doctor will follow you carefully to see if the

disease is progressing so that treatment can be given.

2. Chemotherapy to lower the number of white blood cells.
3. Bone marrow transplantation.
4. Surgery to remove the spleen (splenectomy).
5. Clinical trials of biological therapy with and without chemotherapy or after bone marrow transplantation.

Treatment options: Accelerated phase chronic myelogenous leukemia

Your treatment may be one of the following:

1. Chemotherapy to lower the number of white blood cells.
2. Transfusions of blood or blood products to relieve symptoms.
3. Clinical trials of bone marrow transplantation.

Treatment options: Blastic phase chronic myelogenous leukemia

Your treatment may be one of the following:

1. Chemotherapy. Clinical trials are testing new chemotherapy drugs and new combinations of drugs.
2. Radiation therapy to relieve symptoms caused by tumors formed in the bone.
3. Clinical trials of bone marrow transplantation.

Treatment options: Meningeal chronic myelogenous leukemia

Your treatment may be one of the following:

1. Intrathecal chemotherapy.
2. Radiation therapy to the brain.

Treatment options: Refractory chronic myelogenous leukemia

Your treatment depends on many factors. You may wish to consider entering a clinical trial.

To learn more about chronic myelogenous leukemia, call the National Cancer Institute's Cancer Information Service at 1-800-4-CANCER (1-800-422-6237). By dialing this toll-free number, you can speak with someone who can answer your questions.

■ **Document Source:**
National Cancer Institute
Building 31, Room 10A24, 9000 Rockville Pike, Bethesda, MD
20892
PDQ 208/01031
Current as of: 02/01/94

See also: Chemotherapy and You: A Guide to Self-Help During Treatment (page 40); Radiation Therapy and You: A Guide to Self-Help During Treatment (page 56)

SICKLE CELL DISEASE IN NEWBORNS AND INFANTS: A GUIDE FOR PARENTS

Purpose of this booklet

This booklet can help you understand sickle cell disease and how it can affect your child.

The best way to help your baby is to learn as much as you can about the disease, the problems it can cause, and what you can do to care for your baby. Talk about this booklet and your baby's health care choices with your doctor and others who know about sickle cell disease. Working together, you can give your child the best possible care.

You will find a description of the kinds of problems a baby with sickle cell disease may have on the next page of this booklet. Remember when you read it that not all babies will have all of these problems. At the back of this booklet, you will find a list of terms often used by doctors and nurses when they talk about sickle cell disease.

What is sickle cell disease?

Sickle cell disease is an inherited disorder of the red blood cells. Red blood cells carry oxygen to all parts of the body by using a protein called hemoglobin. Normal red blood cells contain only normal hemoglobin and are shaped like doughnuts. These cells are very flexible and move easily through small blood vessels.

But in sickle cell disease, the red blood cells contain sickle hemoglobin, which causes them to change to a curved shape (sickle shape) after oxygen is released. Sickled cells become stuck and form plugs in small blood vessels. This blockage of blood flow can damage the tissue. Because there are blood vessels in all parts of the body, damage can occur anywhere in the body.

The most common types of sickle cell disease are:
Sickle cell anemia
Hemoglobin SC disease
Sickle beta-thalassemia

Types of sickle cell disease

There are several forms of sickle cell disease. The most common is sickle cell anemia. Your doctor or nurse will tell you what kind of sickle cell disease your baby has. Be sure to write down the name so that you can refer to it if your baby has to go to a new doctor or clinic.

How are babies affected?

Babies with sickle cell disease may have:

◆ **Anemia** (a low number of red blood cells). People with anemia may tire easily.

♦ **Aplastic crisis**. Babies with sickle cell disease may stop making red blood cells for a short time. Signs include paleness, less activity than normal, fast breathing, and fast heartbeat. A baby with these signs must be seen quickly by the doctor.

♦ **Hand-and-foot syndrome**. Babies with sickle cell disease may have pain and swelling in their hands or feet.

♦ **Painful episodes** (mostly in the arms, hands, legs, feet, or abdomen). This happens when sickle cells plug blood vessels and block the flow of blood. Doctors call this a painful episode, event, or crisis.

♦ **Severe infections**. The child with sickle cell anemia is at great risk for serious infections—such as sepsis (a blood stream infection), meningitis, and pneumonia. The risk of infection is increased because the spleen does not function normally.

♦ **Splenic sequestration crisis**. The spleen is the organ that filters blood. In children with sickle cell disease, the spleen can enlarge rapidly from trapped red blood cells. This condition is called splenic sequestration crisis and can be life-threatening.

♦ **Stroke**. This happens when blood vessels in the brain are blocked by sickled red blood cells. Signs include seizure, weakness of the arms and legs, speech problems, and loss of consciousness. A baby with any of these signs must be seen quickly by a doctor.

Who is affected?

In the United States, most people who have sickle cell disease are African Americans. About 1 in 375 African-American children has sickle cell disease. Hispanic Americans from the Caribbean, Central America, and parts of South America may also have the disease. Sickle cell disease is also found in individuals from Turkey, Greece, Italy, the Middle East, or East India.

What causes sickle cell disease?

All forms of sickle cell disease are inherited. Children inherit genes for the disease from their parents.

Genes are substances within the father's sperm and the mother's egg that determine all of the physical characteristics of a baby. Children inherit the genes for hemoglobin from their parents. Persons who inherit both normal and sickle hemoglobin have sickle cell trait. Sickle cell trait is not a disease and does not change to disease. The individual sperm or egg from a person with sickle cell trait may contain either a gene for normal hemoglobin or a gene for sickle hemoglobin.

When both parents have sickle cell trait, for each pregnancy, the chances are:

♦ 1 in 4 that the baby will have only normal hemoglobin.

♦ 2 in 4 that the baby will have both normal and sickle hemoglobin (sickle cell trait).

♦ 1 in 4 that the baby will have only sickle hemoglobin (sickle cell anemia).

The inheritance of other forms of sickle cell disease can be explained by your doctor.

How do I know if my baby has sickle cell disease?

All newborn babies should be tested for sickle cell disease. Many states have screening programs that test babies born in the hospital within a few days of birth. A blood sample is taken from the baby's heel for the sickle cell test, as well as screening tests for several other medical conditions.

If the test shows your baby might have sickle cell disease, the doctor will do the test again to make sure. The doctor may ask one or both parents for blood samples to test. If your baby has sickle cell disease, the doctor will tell you as soon as possible.

What if my baby has sickle cell disease?

If your baby has sickle cell disease, the doctor will help you find the best medical care for your child. This care could be provided by your family doctor, a pediatrician (children's doctor), or a pediatric hematologist (children's blood specialist), or a special sickle cell clinic. You also may want to see a counselor who can talk with you about your chances of having another baby with sickle cell disease.

Sickle cell disease is not just a medical problem. You may have many concerns about your baby and your family—for example, how to cope with your feelings and how to pay the medical bills. Your doctor or nurse can talk with you about your concerns. They also can help you find a local social service agency to assist you. In many areas there are sickle cell support groups, as well as community organizations that offer testing, education, and support to families affected by sickle cell disease.

How can I help my baby?

The best way to help your baby is to learn as much as you can about the disease and to make sure your baby gets the best health care possible. The child with sickle cell disease has special needs and must have regular medical care to stay as healthy as possible. The doctor or nurse will explain how often to bring your baby for medical care and what you can do if your baby becomes ill.

By 2 months of age, your baby should start taking penicillin by mouth twice each day. *It is very important to give the medicine exactly as the doctor tells you*. This will help prevent life-threatening infections. Penicillin should be continued until at least 5 years of age.

Also by 2 months of age, your baby will get a shot to protect against *H. influenzae*, a type of bacteria that causes an infection which can be dangerous to people with sickle cell disease. The baby also will need a shot to protect against hepatitis B, a liver disease. At age 2, your child should receive pneumococcal vaccine. Your child should have all the other shots that children normally receive.

Here are some of the most important things you need to know about caring for a baby with sickle cell disease:

♦ *If your baby has a fever (over 101 degrees), you must get medical help right away*. A fever in a child with sickle cell disease can be a sign of serious medical problems. Always take your baby's temperature when your baby appears sick. Your doctor will tell you what to do if your baby has a fever.

♦ If any new doctor or health care provider sees your baby for any reason, explain that your baby has sickle cell disease.

♦ A good diet is very important for all babies. Ask your doctor or other health care provider about the right foods and liquids for your baby. Make sure your baby drinks plenty of liquids. Find out if your baby also should have vitamins or iron.

♦ Make sure your baby does not become overheated or chilly. Keep your baby warm. Cold baths or cold air can slow the baby's blood flow and cause problems.

If your baby is sick, you must get medical help right away. Any sign of illness in a child with sickle cell disease can be serious. Your baby needs to see the doctor quickly if the baby:

♦ Is breathing fast or having a problem with breathing
♦ Coughs frequently
♦ Is cranky and cries more than usually
♦ Screams when touched
♦ Is very tired or has little energy
♦ Is very weak
♦ Vomits
♦ Does not want to eat
♦ Has diarrhea
♦ Has fewer wet diapers
♦ Has pain or swelling in the abdomen
♦ Has swollen hands or feet
♦ Has pale blue or grey lips or skin

Questions to ask

You should always feel free to ask any questions about sickle cell disease and how it affects you and your family. Here are some questions you may want to ask the doctor, nurse, counselor, or social worker.

♦ What does my baby have? How did he or she get it?
♦ What do I have? How did I get it? How will it affect me and my family?
♦ How often does my baby need to see you?
♦ What medicine does my baby need? What do I need to know about giving it?
♦ What should my baby eat and drink?
♦ Is there anything my baby should not do?
♦ How can I tell if my baby gets sick?
♦ What should I do, and who should I call, if my baby gets sick?
♦ What other help is available to my family?

Additional resources

To learn more about sickle cell disease and how to cope with it, contact:

National Association for Sickle Cell Disease
3345 Wilshire Boulevard, Suite 1106
Los Angeles, CA 90010-1880
Telephone: 1-800-421-8453

Additional organizations that can provide help include:

California State Department of Health
Childrens Medical Services Branch
Sacramento, CA 95814
Telephone: 916-654-0499

Cincinnati Comprehensive Sickle Cell Center
Children's Hospital Medical Center
Cincinnati, OH 45229
Telephone: 513-559-4200

Clinical Center Communications
9000 Rockville Pike
Building 10, Room 1C255
Bethesda, MD 20892
Telephone: 301-496-2563

Education Programs Associates
1 West Campbell Ave, Building D
Campbell, CA 95008
Telephone: 408-374-1210

Howard University
Comprehensive Sickle Cell Center
2121 Georgia Ave
Washington, DC 20059
Telephone: 202-806-7930

March of Dimes
Birth Defects Foundation
1275 Mamaroneck Ave
White Plains, NY 10605
For faster service, look in the telephone book for a local March of Dimes chapter in your area.

Mid-South Sickle Cell Center
Le Bonheur Children's Medical Center
Memphis, TN 38103
Telephone: 901-522-6792

Mississippi State Department of Health
Genetics Division
PO Box 1700
Jackson, MS
Telephone: 601-960-7619

National Maternal and Child Health Clearinghouse
8201 Greensboro Dr, Suite 600
McLean, VA 22102
Telephone: 703-821-8955

New York State Department of Health
Newborn Screening Program
Wadsworth Center for Laboratories and Research
PO Box 509
Albany, NY 12201-0509
Telephone: 518-473-7552

Northern California Comprehensive Sickle Cell Center
San Francisco, CA 94110
Telephone: 510-428-3651

Texas Department of Health
Newborn Screening Program
1100 West 49th St
Austin, TX 78756-3199
Telephone: 512-458-7111

This is not a complete list. Check with your state or local health department or sickle cell agency for more information.

Common sickle cell terms

Your doctor, nurse, or other caregiver may use these terms in talking with you about sickle cell disease and your child.

Acute chest syndrome. A serious condition caused by infection or trapped red blood cells in the lungs. Fast or difficult breathing, chest pain, and coughing are signs of acute chest syndrome in the child with sickle cell disease. A child with acute chest syndrome usually will have to go to the hospital for treatment.

Anemia. A reduced number of red blood cells. Anemia occurs in persons with sickle cell disease because sickled red blood cells do not live as long as normal red blood cells. A child with sickle cell disease cannot make red blood cells fast enough to keep up with the rapid breakdown, so the person with sickle cell disease has fewer red blood cells than normal and is anemic.

Aplastic crisis. Occurs when a child's bone marrow temporarily stops producing red blood cells. A child with aplastic crisis may appear pale and be tired and less active than usual.

Capillaries. Tiny blood vessels where sickle-shaped blood cells may get trapped and cause problems.

Gene. The biological units that are passed from both parents to a child. Genes determine all of the child's characteristics—for example, hair, eye, and skin color, foot size, height—and whether the child will have sickle cell disease or another inherited disease.

Haemophilus influenzae. A type of bacteria that causes infection and can lead to serious problems in the child with sickle cell disease. Babies must receive a special vaccine beginning at 2 months of age to protect them from this condition.

Hand-and-foot syndrome. Pain and swelling of the hands and feet caused by sickle-shaped red blood cells that plug blood vessels in the hands and feet. Often this will be the baby's first problem caused by sickle cell disease.

Hemoglobin. A molecule found in red blood cells that carries oxygen from the lungs to other parts of the body.

Pain event or painful episode. Pain caused by plugging of blood vessels by sickled blood cells. Pain is most often felt in the arms, legs, back, and abdomen. The pain may last only a few hours or as long as a week or two. The pain may be mild or so severe that pain medicine is needed. The number of pain events a person has may vary greatly.

Sepsis. The presence of infection in the blood stream.

Sickle cell anemia. The most common form of sickle cell disease. Other types of sickle cell disease include hemoglobin SC disease and sickle beta-thalassemia; there are also other, less common types of sickle cell disease.

Sickle cell disease. A group of inherited disorders in which anemia is present and sickle hemoglobin is produced.

Sickle cell trait. The condition in which a person has both normal and sickle hemoglobin in the red cells as a result of inheriting a normal hemoglobin gene and a gene for sickle hemoglobin. Sickle cell trait is not a disease and does not change to sickle cell disease. Persons with sickle cell trait may pass the sickle gene to their children.

Sickled cells. In children with sickle cell disease, hemoglobin molecules in red blood cells stick to one another and cause the red cells to become crescent or sickle shaped. Sickled cells cannot pass easily through tiny blood vessels.

Splenic sequestration crisis. Occurs when a large portion of the child's blood becomes trapped in the spleen. Early signs include paleness, an enlarged spleen, and pain in the abdomen.

Streptococcus pneumoniae. A bacteria that causes a very serious type of pneumonia in children with sickle cell disease. Twice daily doses of penicillin by mouth, starting at about 2 months of age, can help to prevent this life-threatening infection in children with sickle cell anemia and sickle beta-thalassemia.

For more information

The information in this booklet was taken from the *Clinical Practice Guideline on Sickle Cell Disease: Screening, Diagnosis, Management, and Counseling in Newborns and Infants*. The guideline was written by a panel of experts sponsored by the Agency for Health Care Policy and Research. Other guidelines on common health problems also are being developed.

For more information about guidelines, or to order extra copies of this booklet, contact:

Agency for Health Care Policy and Research
Publications Clearinghouse
PO Box 8547
Silver Spring, MD 20907
Or call 1-800-358-9295 (for callers outside the US, only: 301-495-3453) weekdays, 9 am to 5 pm, Eastern time.

■ Document Source:
   U.S. Department of Health and Human Services, Public Health Service
   Agency for Health Care Policy and Research
   Executive Office Center, Suite 501, 2101 East Jefferson Street, Rockville, MD 20852
   AHCPR Publication No. AHCPR 93-0564
   April 1993

WHAT YOU NEED TO KNOW ABOUT HODGKIN'S DISEASE

The National Cancer Institute (NCI) has prepared this booklet to help patients and their families better understand and deal with Hodgkin's disease. We also hope it will encourage all readers to learn more about this type of cancer. The information presented here—on the symptoms, diagnosis, and treatment of Hodgkin's disease and on living with the disease—is intended to add to talks with doctors, nurses, and other members of the medical team.

Our knowledge about Hodgkin's disease is increasing. Research sponsored by NCI and other groups has led to improved treatment of Hodgkin's disease. Presently, well over half of all Hodgkin's patients can be cured. For up-to-date information, call the NCI-supported Cancer Information Service (CIS) toll-free at 1-800-4-CANCER.

Throughout this booklet, words that may be new to readers are printed in *italics*. Definitions of these and other terms related to Hodgkin's disease are listed in the "Medical Terms" section. For some words, a "sounds-like" spelling is also given.

Other NCI publications about cancer, its treatment, and coping with the disease, and the CIS are described at the end of this booklet.

What Is Hodgkin's disease?

Hodgkin's disease is a type of *lymphoma*. Lymphomas are cancers that develop in the *lymphatic system*, part of the body's circulatory system. The job of the lymphatic system is to help fight diseases and infection.

The lymphatic system includes a network of thin tubes that branch, like blood vessels, into the tissues throughout the body. Lymphatic vessels carry *lymph*, a colorless, watery fluid that contains infection-fighting cells called *lymphocytes*. Along this network of vessels are groups of small, bean-shaped organs called *lymph nodes* that filter the lymph as it passes through the nodes. Clusters of lymph nodes are found in the underarm, *groin*, neck, and abdomen.

Other parts of the lymphatic system are the *spleen, thymus*, tonsils, and *bone marrow*.

Like all types of cancer, Hodgkin's disease affects the body's cells. Healthy cells grow, divide, and replace themselves in an orderly manner. This process keeps the body in good repair. In Hodgkin's disease, cells in the lymphatic system grow abnormally and can spread to other organs. As the disease progresses, the body is less able to fight infection.

Hodgkin's disease is rare. It accounts for less than 1 percent of all cases of cancer in this country. It is most often seen in young people aged 15 to 34 and in people over the age of 55. Other cancers of the lymphatic system, called non-Hodgkin's lymphomas, are discussed in the booklet *What You Need To Know About Non-Hodgkin's Lymphomas*.

Symptoms of Hodgkin's Disease

The most common symptom of Hodgkin's disease is a painless swelling in the lymph nodes in the neck, underarm, or groin. Other symptoms may include fevers, night sweats, tiredness, weight loss, or itching skin. However, these symptoms are not sure signs of cancer. They may also be caused by many common illnesses, such as the flu or other infections. But it is important to see a doctor if any of these symptoms lasts longer than 2 weeks. Any illness should be diagnosed and treated as early as possible, and this is especially true of Hodgkin's disease.

Diagnosing Hodgkin's Disease

If Hodgkin's disease is suspected, the doctor will ask about the patient's medical history and will do a thorough physical exam. Blood tests and x-rays of the chest, bones, liver, and spleen will also be done.

Tissue from an enlarged lymph node will be removed. This is known as a *biopsy*. It is the only sure way to tell if cancer is present. A *pathologist* will look at the tissue under the microscope for *Reed-Sternberg cells*, abnormal cells that are usually found with Hodgkin's disease.

When Hodgkin's disease is diagnosed, the doctor needs to know the *stage*, or extent, of the disease. Knowing the stage

is very important for planning treatment. The stage indicates where the disease has spread and how much tissue is affected. In staging, the doctor checks:

♦ The number and location of affected lymph nodes;
♦ Whether the affected lymph nodes are above, below, or on both sides of the *diaphragm* (the thin muscle under the lungs and heart that separates the chest from the abdomen); and
♦ Whether the disease has spread to the bone marrow or to places outside the lymphatic system, such as the liver.

In staging, the doctor usually orders several tests, including biopsies of the lymph nodes, liver, and bone marrow. Many patients have *lymphangiograms*, x-rays of the lymphatic system using a special dye to outline the lymph nodes and vessels. Another test is *computed tomography* (also called CT or CAT scan), a series of x-rays of cross-sections of the body.

Treating Hodgkin's Disease

Treatment decisions for Hodgkin's disease are complex. Before starting treatment, the patient might want a second doctor to review the diagnosis and treatment plan. There are a number of ways to find a doctor for a second opinion:

♦ The patient's doctor may be able to suggest a doctor who has a special interest in Hodgkin's disease.
♦ The Cancer Information Service, at 1-800-4-CANCER, can tell callers about cancer centers and other NCI-supported programs in their area.
♦ Patients can get the names of doctors from the local medical society, a nearby hospital, or a medical school.
♦ The *Directory of Medical Specialists* lists doctors' names and gives their background. It is in most public libraries.

Methods of Treatment

Treatment for Hodgkin's disease usually includes *radiation therapy* or *chemotherapy*. Sometimes, both are given. Treatment decisions depend on the stage of disease, its location in the body, which symptoms are present, and the general health and age of the patient. (Treatment for children with Hodgkin's disease is more complex and is not discussed here.)

Often, patients are referred to doctors or medical centers that specialize in the different treatments of Hodgkin's disease. Also, patients may want to talk with their doctor about taking part in a research study of new treatment methods. Such studies are called *clinical trials*.

Radiation therapy uses high-energy rays to damage cancer cells and stop their growth. Radiation therapy is generally given in a hospital or clinic. Most often, patients receive radiation therapy 5 days a week for several weeks as outpatients. Weekend rest periods allow time for healthy tissue to recover.

Chemotherapy is the use of drugs to kill cancer cells. To treat Hodgkin's disease, the doctor prescribes a combination of drugs that work together. The drugs may be given in different ways: some are given by mouth; others are injected into an artery, vein, or muscle. The drugs travel through the bloodstream to almost every part of the body. Chemotherapy is usually given in cycles: a treatment period followed by a rest period, then another treatment period, and so on.

Side Effects of Treatment

The methods used to treat Hodgkin's disease are very powerful. That's why the treatment often causes side effects—both short-term and permanent. Side effects depend on the type of treatment and on the part of the body being treated. Also, each patient may respond differently.

During radiation therapy, patients may become unusually tired as therapy continues. Resting as much as possible is important. Skin reactions (redness or dryness) in the area being treated are also common. Patients should be gentle with the treated area of skin. Lotions and creams should not be used without the doctor's advice. When the chest is treated, patients may have a dry, sore throat and may have trouble swallowing. Sometimes, they have shortness of breath or a dry cough. Radiation treatment to the lower abdomen may cause nausea, vomiting, or diarrhea. Some patients have tingling or numbness in their arms, legs, and lower back. These side effects gradually disappear when treatment is over.

The side effects of chemotherapy depend mainly on the drugs that are given. In general, anticancer drugs affect rapidly growing cells, such as blood cells that fight infection, cells that line the digestive tract, and cells in hair follicles. As a result, patients may have side effects such as lower resistance to infection, nausea, vomiting, or mouth sores. They may also have less energy and may lose their hair.

Loss of appetite can be a problem for patients receiving radiation therapy or chemotherapy. Researchers are learning that patients who eat well may be better able to tolerate the side effects of their treatment. Therefore, nutrition is an important part of the treatment plan. Eating well means getting enough calories to prevent weight loss and having enough protein in the diet to build and repair skin, hair, muscles, and organs. Many patients find that eating several small meals and snacks throughout the day is easier than trying to have three large meals.

Treatment for Hodgkin's disease can cause fertility problems. Women's menstrual periods may stop. Periods are more likely to return in younger women. In men, both Hodgkin's disease and its treatment can affect fertility. Younger men are more likely to regain their fertility. Sperm banking before treatment may be an option for some men.

The side effects that patients have during cancer therapy vary from person to person and may even be different from one treatment to the next. Doctors try to plan treatment to keep problems to a minimum. Doctors, nurses, and dietitians can explain the side effects of cancer treatment and can suggest ways to deal with them. Helpful information about cancer treatment and coping with the side effects is given in the NCI publications *Radiation Therapy and You, Chemotherapy and You,* and *Eating Hints.*

Followup Care

Regular followup exams are very important for anyone who has been treated for Hodgkin's disease. The doctor will continue to watch the patient closely for several years. Gener-

ally, checkups include a careful physical exam, x-rays, blood tests, and other laboratory tests.

Patients treated for Hodgkin's disease have an increased risk of developing other types of cancer later in life, especially leukemia. Patients should follow their doctor's recommendations on health care and checkups. Having regular checkups allows problems to be detected and treated promptly if they should arise.

Adjusting to the Disease

When people have cancer, life can change for them and for the people who care about them. These changes in daily life can be difficult to handle. It's natural for a person with Hodgkin's disease to have many different and sometimes confusing emotions.

At times, patients and family members may be depressed, angry, or frightened. At other times, feelings may vary from hope to despair or from courage to fear. Patients usually are better able to cope with their emotions if they can talk openly about their illness and their feelings with family members and friends.

Concerns about the future—as well as about medical tests, treatments, a hospital stay, and medical bills—are common. Talking to doctors, nurses, or other members of the health care team may help to ease fear and confusion. Patients can take an active part in decisions about their medical care by asking questions about their treatment. Patients and family members often find it helpful to write down questions for the doctor as they think of them. Taking notes during visits to the doctor can help them remember what was said. Patients should ask the doctor to explain anything that is not clear.

Patients have many important questions to ask about their disease, and their doctor is the best person to provide answers. Most people want to learn how Hodgkin's disease can be treated, how successful the treatment is likely to be, and how much the treatment is expected to cost. The following are some other questions that patients might want to ask the doctor:

♦ What are the expected benefits of treatment?
♦ Would a clinical trial be appropriate for me?
♦ What are the risks and possible side effects of treatment?
♦ Will treatment affect my fertility?
♦ Can I keep working during treatment?
♦ Will I have to change my normal activities?
♦ How often will I need checkups?

The patient's doctor is the best person to give advice about working or limiting other activities, but it may be hard for some people to talk to the doctor about their feelings and other very personal matters. Many patients find it helpful to talk with others who are facing similar problems. This kind of help is available through cancer-related support groups. It also may be helpful to talk with a nurse, social worker, counselor, or member of the clergy.

Living with any serious disease can be a difficult challenge. The public library is a good source of books and articles on adjusting to cancer. Also, cancer patients and their families can find helpful suggestions in the NCI booklet called *Taking Time.*

Support for Cancer Patients

Adapting to the changes brought about by having cancer is easier for both patients and their families when they have helpful information and support services. Often, the social service office at the hospital or clinic can suggest local and national agencies that will help with emotional support, financial aid, transportation, home care, or rehabilitation. The American Cancer Society and the Leukemia Society of America are two nonprofit organizations that offer a variety of services to patients and their families. Their local offices may be listed in the telephone book.

Information about other resources and services is available through the Cancer Information Service toll free at 1-800-4-CANCER.

What the Future Holds

More than 7 million Americans living today have had some type of cancer. Thirty years ago, few patients with Hodgkin's disease recovered from their illness. Now, because of modern radiation therapy and combination chemotherapy, more than 75 percent of all newly diagnosed Hodgkin's disease patients are curable. The chances for recovery continue to improve as scientists find new and more effective treatments.

Doctors often talk about "surviving" cancer, or they may use the word "remission" rather than "cure." Even though many patients recover completely, doctors use these terms because Hodgkin's disease can show up again. Patients are naturally concerned about their future and may try to use statistics they have read or heard about to try to figure out their own chances of being cured. It is important to remember, however, that statistics are averages based on the experiences of large numbers of people, and no two cancer patients are alike. Only the doctor who takes care of a patient knows enough about that person to discuss the *prognosis*.

The Promise of Cancer Research

Scientists at hospitals and medical centers throughout the country are studying Hodgkin's disease. They are trying to learn more about the possible causes of the disease and how it might be prevented.

In addition, scientists are exploring new methods of treatment, including new drugs, drug combinations, and combinations of radiation therapy and chemotherapy. Other methods, such as *bone marrow transplantation* and *biological therapy*, are being studied with some Hodgkin's disease patients in clinical trials. These trials are designed to answer scientific questions and to find out whether a promising new treatment is both safe and effective. Patients who take part in clinical trials make an important contribution to medical science and may have the first chance to benefit from improved treatment methods.

Hodgkin's disease patients may consider participating in a trial and should discuss this possibility with their doctors. *What Are Clinical Trials All About?* is an NCI publication for patients who may be interested in taking part in clinical research.

The NCI's PDQ database helps doctors across the country learn about clinical trials. A doctor can obtain information from PDQ by using an office computer or the services of a medical library. Most Cancer Information Service offices provide PDQ searches and can tell doctors how to obtain regular access to the database. Information about current research is also available to patients and the public through the Cancer Information Service toll free at 1-800-4-CANCER.

Medical Terms

Benign tumor (bee-NINE). A noncancerous growth that does not spread to other parts of the body.

Biological therapy (by-o-LOJ-i-kal). Treatment with substances that can stimulate the immune system to fight disease more effectively. Also called immunotherapy.

Biopsy (BY-op-see). The removal of a sample of tissue followed by microscopic examination to see whether cancer cells are present.

Bone marrow. The soft, spongy tissue in the center of large bones that produces white blood cells, red blood cells, and platelets.

Bone marrow transplantation. Treatment in which healthy bone marrow replaces bone marrow that has been affected by a disease or by treatment for a disease.

Cancer. A general term for more than 100 diseases that are characterized by uncontrolled, abnormal growth of cells. Cancer cells can spread through the bloodstream and lymphatic system to other parts of the body.

Chemotherapy (kee-mo-THER-a-pee). Treatment with anticancer drugs.

Clinical trial. Research conducted with cancer patients, usually to evaluate a new treatment. Each trial is designed to answer scientific questions and to find better ways to treat patients.

Computed tomography (tom-OG-rah-fee). An x-ray procedure that uses a computer to produce a detailed picture of a cross section of the body; also called CAT or CT scan.

Diaphragm (DY-a-fram). The thin muscle below the lungs and heart that separates the chest from the abdomen.

Fertility. The ability to have children.

Groin. The area where the thigh meets the hip.

Lymph (limf). The almost colorless fluid that bathes body tissues and carries cells that help fight infection.

Lymph nodes. Small, bean-shaped organs located along the lymphatic system. Nodes filter out bacteria or cancer cells that may travel through the lymphatic system; also called lymph glands.

Lymphangiogram (limf-AN-jee-o-gram). An x-ray of the lymphatic system. A dye is injected to outline the lymphatic vessels and organs.

Lymphatic system (lim-FAT-ik). The tissues and organs (including the bone marrow, spleen, thymus, and lymph nodes) that produce and store cells that fight infection and the network of vessels that carry lymph.

Lymphocytes (LIMF-o-sites). White blood cells that fight infection and disease.

Malignant (ma-LIG-nant). Cancerous (see *Cancer*).

Oncologist (on-KOL-o-jist). A doctor who specializes in treating cancer.

Pathologist (path-OL-o-jist). A doctor who specializes in identifying diseases by studying cells and tissues under a microscope.

Prognosis (prog-NO-sis). The probable outcome of a disease; the prospect of recovery.

Radiation therapy (ray-dee-AY-shun THER-a-pee). Treatment with high-energy radiation from x-rays or other sources of radiation.

Reed-Sternberg cell. A type of cell that appears in patients with Hodgkin's disease. The number of these cells increases as the disease advances.

Sperm banking. Freezing sperm for future use. This procedure can allow men to father children after loss of fertility.

Spleen. An organ that produces lymphocytes, filters the blood, stores blood cells, and destroys those that are aging. It is located on the left side of the abdomen near the stomach.

Stage. The extent to which cancer has spread from its original site to other parts of the body.

Tumor. An abnormal mass of tissue that results from excessive cell division. Tumors perform no useful body function. They may be either benign (not cancer) or malignant (cancer).

Thymus. An organ in which lymphocytes mature and multiply. It lies behind the breastbone.

Resources

Information about cancer is available from many sources. Three are listed below. You also may wish to check your local library or contact support groups in your community.

Cancer Information Service (CIS)
1-800-4-CANCER

The Cancer Information Service, a program of the National Cancer Institute, includes a telephone service for cancer patients and their families and friends, the public, and health professionals. The staff can answer questions and can send booklets about cancer. They also may know about local resources and services. One toll-free number, 1-800-4-CANCER, connects callers all over the country to the office that serves their area. Spanish-speaking staff members are available.

American Cancer Society (ACS)
1599 Clifton Road, N.E.
Atlanta, GA 30329
1-800-ACS-2345

The American Cancer Society is a voluntary organization with a national office (at the above address) and local units all over the country. It supports research, conducts educational programs, and offers many services to patients and their families. To obtain information about services and activities in local areas, call the Society's toll-free number, 1-800-ACS-2345, or the number listed under American Cancer Society in the white pages of the telephone book.

Leukemia Society of America (LSA)
733 Third Avenue
New York, NY 10017
1-800-955-4LSA
(212) 573-8484

Another voluntary organization, the Leukemia Society of America is concerned with leukemia, non-Hodgkin's lymphoma, and Hodgkin's disease. It provides information about these diseases and offers many services, including physician referrals, financial assistance, and support for families. Further information about these services is available by contacting the national headquarters or a local chapter, which may be listed in the telephone book.

For Further Information

The printed materials listed below may be helpful to cancer patients, their families, and others. They are available free of charge by calling 1-800-4-CANCER or writing:

Office of Cancer Communications
National Cancer Institute
Building 31, Room 10A24
Bethesda, MD 20892

♦ *Chemotherapy and You: A Guide to Self-Help During Treatment*
♦ *Eating Hints: Tips and Recipes for Better Nutrition During Cancer Treatment*
♦ *Facing Forward: A Guide for Cancer Survivors*
♦ *Radiation Therapy and You: A Guide to Self-Help During Treatment*
♦ *Taking Time: Support for People With Cancer and the People Who Care About Them*
♦ *What Are Clinical Trials All About?*
♦ *When Someone in Your Family Has Cancer*

■ **Document Source:**
U.S. Department of Health and Human Services, Public Health Service
National Institutes of Health
NIH Publication No. 92-1555
Revised August 1991. Printed December 1991

See also: Chemotherapy and You: A Guide to Self-Help During Treatment (page 40); Radiation Therapy and You: A Guide to Self-Help During Treatment (page 56); What Are Clinical Trials All About? A Booklet for Patients with Cancer (page 68)

CANCER, GENERAL*

■ ▦ ▦

CHEMOTHERAPY AND YOU: A GUIDE TO SELF-HELP DURING TREATMENT

About This Booklet

This booklet will help you, your family, and your friends understand **chemotherapy,** the use of drugs to treat cancer. It will answer many of the questions you may have about this method of cancer treatment. It will also show you how you can help yourself during chemotherapy.

Taking care of yourself during chemotherapy is important for several reasons. For one thing, it can lessen some of the physical side effects you may have from your treatment. As you will see, some simple tips can make a big difference in how you feel. But the benefits of self-help aren't just physical; they're psychological, too. Knowing some ways to take care of yourself can give your emotions a boost at a time when you may be feeling that much of what's happening to you is out of your control. This feeling can be easier to deal with when you discover how much you can contribute to your own well-being, in partnership with your doctors and nurses.

Chemotherapy and You will help you become an informed partner in your care. Remember, though, it is only a guide. Self-help is never a substitute for professional medical care. Be sure to ask your doctor and nurse any questions you may have about chemotherapy, and tell them about any side effects you may have.

You will find several helpful sections at the back of this booklet. The section called "Resources for Patients and Their Families" tells you how to get more information about cancer and how to find many services available to cancer patients and their families. The section on "Paying for Chemotherapy" gives you information about insurance and other payment methods. The glossary explains many terms related to cancer and chemotherapy.

This edition of *Chemotherapy and You* does not include the tear-out cards for drug information that were in previous versions. A series of fact sheets on anticancer drugs is available from the National Cancer Institute (See "Resources for Patients and Their Families.")

Understanding Chemotherapy

What is chemotherapy?

Chemotherapy is the use of drugs to treat cancer. The drugs are often called "anticancer" drugs.

How does chemotherapy work?

Normal cells grow and die in a controlled way. But cancer cells keep growing and reproducing and take a long time to die. Anticancer drugs destroy cancer cells by stopping them from growing or multiplying at one or more points in their life cycle. Because some drugs work better together than alone, chemotherapy may consist of more than one drug. This is called **combination chemotherapy.** In addition to chemotherapy, other methods are sometimes used to treat cancer. For example, certain drugs can block the effect of hormones—natural substances, made by the body, that help some cancers grow. Doctors may also use biological response modifiers to boost the body's natural defenses against cancer.

What can chemotherapy achieve?

Depending on the type of cancer and its stage of development, chemotherapy can be used:

- ◆ To cure cancer.
- ◆ To keep the cancer from spreading.
- ◆ To slow the cancer's growth.
- ◆ To relieve symptoms that may be caused by the cancer.

Chemotherapy is a very effective cancer treatment. Even when chemotherapy cannot cure the disease, it can help people live longer and more comfortably.

* Information on specific types of cancer are located in the relevant body system chapter. (For example, gallbladder cancer is covered in the chapter on Liver and Gallbladder Disorders.) Check the table of contents or index to find the right publication for you.

Will chemotherapy be my only treatment for cancer?

Sometimes chemotherapy is the only therapy a patient receives. More often, however, chemotherapy is used in addition to surgery and/or radiation therapy. There are several reasons why chemotherapy may be given in addition to other treatment methods. For instance, chemotherapy may be used to shrink a tumor before surgery or radiation therapy. It may also be used after surgery and/or radiation therapy to help destroy any microscopic collections of cancer cells that may remain. When it is used for this purpose it is called **adjuvant therapy.**

Which drugs will I get?

Your doctor decides which drug or drugs will work best for you. The decision depends on what kind of cancer you have, where it is, the extent of its growth, how it is affecting your normal body functions, and your general health.

Your doctor may also suggest that you join a clinical trial for chemotherapy, or you may want to bring up this option with your doctor. Clinical trials are carefully designed research studies that test promising new cancer treatments. Patients who take part in research may be the first to benefit from improved treatment methods. These patients also can make an important contribution to medical care because the results of the studies may help many people. Patients participate in clinical trials only if they choose to and are free to leave at any time.

To learn more about clinical trials, call the National Cancer Institute's Cancer Information Service and ask for the booklet *What Are Clinical Trials All About?* You also may want to ask about the video "Patient to Patient: Cancer Clinical Trials and You." This videotape can put to rest fears you may have about being part of clinical trials. The Cancer Information Service can be reached by dialing 1-800-4-CANCER (1-800-422-6237).

Where will I get chemotherapy?

You may get your chemotherapy at home, in your doctor's office, in a clinic, in your hospital's outpatient department, or in a hospital. The choice of where you get chemotherapy depends on which drug or drugs you are getting, your hospital's policies, and your doctor's preferences. When you first start chemotherapy, you may need to stay at the hospital for a short time so that your doctor can watch the medicine's effects closely and make any adjustments that are needed.

How often will I get chemotherapy, and how long will I get it?

How often—and for how long—you get chemotherapy depends on the kind of cancer you have, the goals of the treatment, the drugs that are used, and how your body responds to them. You may get chemotherapy every day, every week, or every month. Chemotherapy is often given in on-and-off cycles that include rest periods so that your body has a chance to build healthy new cells and regain its strength. In most cases, the treatments continue for at least 3 months up to about 3 years. Your doctor should be able to estimate how long you will be getting chemotherapy.

Whatever schedule your doctor prescribes, it is very important to stay with it. Otherwise, the anticancer drugs might not have their desired effect. If you miss a treatment session or skip a dose of medication, contact your doctor at once for instructions about what to do.

How will I get chemotherapy?

Depending on the type of cancer you have and the drug or drugs you are getting, your chemotherapy may be given in one or more of the following ways:

- By mouth (**orally**, or **PO**) in pill, capsule, or liquid form. You will swallow the drug, just as you do many other medications.
- Topically. The medication will be applied onto the skin.
- Into a muscle (**intramuscularly**, or **IM**), under the skin (**subcutaneously**, or **SC**), or directly into a cancerous area in the skin (**intralesionally**, or **IL**). You will get an injection with a needle.
- Into a vein (**intravenously**, or **IV**). You will get the drug through a thin needle inserted into a vein, usually on your hand or lower arm. Another way to get IV chemotherapy is by means of a **catheter**, a thin tube that is placed into a large vein in your body and remains there as long as it is needed.

Chemotherapy may also be delivered to specific areas of the body using a catheter. Catheters may be placed into the spinal fluid, abdominal cavity, bladder, or liver.

Two kinds of pumps—external and internal—may be used to control the rate of delivery of chemotherapy. External pumps remain outside of the body. Some are portable and allow a person to move around while the pump is in use. Other external pumps are not portable and may restrict activity. Internal pumps are surgically placed inside the body, usually right under the skin. They contain a small reservoir (storage area) that delivers the drugs into the catheter. Internal pumps allow people to go about most of their daily activities.

Does chemotherapy hurt?

Getting chemotherapy by mouth, on the skin, or by injection generally feels the same as taking other medications by these methods. Getting chemotherapy intravenously usually feels like having blood drawn for a lab test, although the needle remains in place for a longer period of time. Some people feel a coolness or other unusual sensation in the area of the injection when the IV is started. Report these feelings to your doctor or nurse. Be sure that you also report any pain, burning, or discomfort that occurs during or after an IV treatment.

Many people have little or no trouble having the IV needle in their hand or lower arm. However, if a person has a hard time for any reason, or if it becomes difficult to insert the needle into a vein for each treatment, it may be possible to place a catheter in a large vein and leave it there for as long as it is needed. This avoids repeated insertion of the needle into the vein.

Catheters cause no pain or discomfort if they are properly placed and cared for, although a person usually remains aware that they are there. It is important to report any pain or discomfort with a catheter to your doctor or nurse.

Can I take other medicines while I am getting chemotherapy?

Some medicines may interfere with the effects of your chemotherapy. That is why you should take a list of all your medications to your doctor before you start chemotherapy. Your list should include the name of each drug, how often you take it, the reason you take it, and the dose. Remember to include over-the-counter drugs such as laxatives, cold pills, pain relievers, and vitamins. Your doctor will tell you if you should stop taking any of these medications before you start chemotherapy. After your treatments begin, be sure to check with your doctor before taking any new medicines or stopping the ones you are already taking.

Will I be able to work during chemotherapy?

Most people are able to continue working while they are being treated with anticancer drugs. It may be possible to schedule your treatments late in the day or right before the weekend, so they interfere with work as little as possible.

If your chemotherapy makes you very tired, you might want to think about adjusting your work schedule for a while. Speak frankly with your employer about your needs and wishes at this time. You may be able to agree on a part-time schedule, or perhaps you can do some of your work at home.

Under Federal and state laws, some employers may actually be required to allow you to work a flexible schedule to meet your treatment needs. To find out about your on-the-job protections, check with your local American Cancer Society, a social worker, or your congressional or state representative. The National Cancer Institute's publication *Facing Forward: A Guide for Cancer Survivors* also has information on work-related concerns.

How will I know if my chemotherapy is working?

Your doctor and nurse will use several methods to measure how well your treatments are working. You will have frequent physical exams, blood tests, scans, and x-rays. Don't hesitate to ask the doctor about the test results and what they show about your progress.

While tests and exams can tell a lot about how chemotherapy is working, side effects tell very little. (Side effects—such as nausea or hair loss—occur because chemotherapy harms some normal cells as well as cancer cells.) Sometimes people think that if they don't have side effects, the drugs aren't working or that if they do have side effects, the drugs are working well. But side effects vary so much from person to person, and from drug to drug, that having them or not having them usually isn't a sign of whether the treatment is effective.

If you **do** have side effects, there is much you can do to help relieve them. The next section of this booklet describes some of the most common side effects of chemotherapy and gives you some hints for coping with them.

Coping with Side Effects

If you have questions about side effects, you are not alone. Before chemotherapy starts, most people are concerned about whether they will have side effects and, if so, what they will be like. Once treatments begin, people who do have side effects want to know the best ways to cope with them. This section will answer some of your questions about side effects.

If you are reading this section before you start chemotherapy, you may feel overwhelmed by the wide range of side effects it describes. But remember: Every person doesn't get every side effect, and some people get few, if any. In addition, the severity of side effects varies greatly from person to person. Whether you have a particular side effect, and how severe it will be, depends on the kind and dose of chemotherapy you get and how your body reacts. Be sure to talk to your doctor and nurse about which side effects are most likely to occur with your chemotherapy, how long they might last, how serious they might be, and when you should seek medical attention for them.

What causes side effects?

Because cancer cells grow and divide rapidly, anticancer drugs are made to kill fast-growing cells. But certain normal, healthy cells also multiply quickly, and chemotherapy can affect these cells, too. When it does, side effects may result. The fast growing, normal cells most likely to be affected are blood cells forming in the bone marrow and cells in the digestive tract, reproductive system, and hair follicles. Anticancer drugs can also damage cells of the heart, kidney, bladder, lungs, and nervous system. The most common side effects of chemotherapy include nausea and vomiting, hair loss, and fatigue.

How long do side effects last?

Most normal cells recover quickly when chemotherapy is over, so most side effects gradually disappear after treatment ends and the healthy cells have a chance to grow normally. The time it takes to get over some side effects and regain energy varies from person to person. How soon you will feel better depends on many factors, including your overall health and the kinds of drugs you have been taking.

While many side effects go away fairly rapidly, certain ones may take months or years to disappear completely. Sometimes, the side effects can last a lifetime, as when chemotherapy causes permanent damage to the heart, lungs, kidneys, or reproductive organs. And certain types of chemotherapy may occasionally cause delayed effects, such as a second cancer, that show up many years later.

It is important to remember that many people have no long-term problems due to chemotherapy. It is also reassuring to know that doctors are making great progress in preventing some of chemotherapy's more serious side effects. For instance, they are using many new drugs and techniques that increase chemotherapy's powerful effects on cancer cells while decreasing its harmful effects on the body's healthy cells.

The side effects of chemotherapy can be unpleasant, but they must be measured against the treatment's ability to destroy cancer. People getting chemotherapy sometimes become discouraged about the length of time their treatment is taking or the side effects they are having. If that happens to you, talk to your doctor. It may be that your medication or the treatment schedule can be changed. Or, your doctor may be able to suggest ways to reduce side effects or make them easier to live with. Remember, though, your doctor will not ask you to continue treatments unless the expected benefits outweigh any problems you might have.

On the pages that follow, you will find suggestions for dealing with some of the more common side effects of chemotherapy.

Nausea and vomiting

Chemotherapy can cause nausea and vomiting by affecting the stomach, the area of the brain that controls vomiting, or both. Some people who have this side effect feel mildly nauseated most of the time. Others become severely nauseated for a limited time after a treatment. Their symptoms may start soon after a treatment or 8 to 12 hours later. They may feel sick for just a few hours or for 12 to 24 hours. Some even begin to feel nauseated or to vomit before their treatment begins. This is called **anticipatory nausea.** Be sure to tell your doctor or nurse if you are very nauseated and/or have vomited for more than a day or if your nausea is so bad that you cannot even keep liquids down.

Nausea and vomiting can often be controlled or at least lessened. If you experience this side effect, your doctor can choose from a wide and ever-growing range of drugs that help curb nausea and vomiting. Different drugs work for different people, and it may be necessary to use more than one drug to get relief. Don't give up. Continue to work with your doctor and nurse to find the drug or drugs that work best for you.

You can also try the following ideas:

♦ Avoid big meals so your stomach won't feel too full. Eat small meals throughout the day.
♦ Drink liquids at least an hour before or after mealtime, instead of with your meals.
♦ Eat and drink slowly.
♦ Stay away from sweet, fried, or fatty foods.
♦ Eat foods cold or at room temperature so you won't be bothered by strong smells.
♦ Chew your food well for easier digestion.
♦ If nausea is a problem in the morning, try eating dry foods like cereal, toast, or crackers before getting up. (Don't try this if you have mouth or throat sores or if you are troubled by a lack of saliva.)
♦ Drink cool, clear, unsweetened fruit juices, such as apple or grape juice, or light-colored sodas, such as ginger ale, that have lost their fizz.
♦ Suck on ice cubes, mints, or tart candies. (Don't use tart candies if you have mouth or throat sores.)
♦ Try to avoid odors that bother you, such as cooking smells, smoke, or perfume.
♦ Prepare and freeze meals in advance for days when you don't feel like cooking.
♦ Rest in a chair after eating, but don't lie flat for at least 2 hours.
♦ Wear loose-fitting clothes.

♦ Breathe deeply and slowly when you feel nauseated.
♦ Distract yourself by chatting with friends or family members, listening to music, or watching a movie or TV show.
♦ Use relaxation techniques to help prevent anticipatory nausea.
♦ Avoid eating for at least a few hours before treatment if nausea usually occurs during chemotherapy.

Hair loss

Hair loss is a common side effect of chemotherapy, but it doesn't always happen. Your doctor can tell you whether hair loss is likely to occur with the drug or drugs you are taking. When hair loss does occur, the hair may become thinner or may fall out entirely. The hair usually grows back after the treatments are over. Some people even start to get their hair back while they are still having treatments.

Hair loss can occur on all parts of the body, not just the head. Facial hair, arm and leg hair, underarm hair, and public hair may all be affected.

Hair loss usually doesn't happen right away; more often, it begins after a few treatments. At that point, hair may fall out gradually or in clumps. It breaks at or near the skin, and the scalp may become tender. Any hair that is still growing may become dull and dry.

To care for your scalp and hair during chemotherapy:

♦ Use mild shampoos.
♦ Use soft hair brushes.
♦ Use low heat when drying your hair.
♦ Don't use brush rollers to set your hair.
♦ Don't dye your hair or get a permanent.
♦ Have your hair cut short. A shorter style will make your hair look thicker and fuller. It will also make hair loss easier to manage if it occurs.

Some people who lose all or most of their hair choose to wear turbans, scarves, caps, wigs, or hairpieces. Others leave their head uncovered. Still others switch back and forth, depending on whether they are in public or at home with friends and family members. There are no "right" or "wrong" choices; do whatever feels comfortable for you.

Here are some tips if you choose to cover your head:

♦ Get your wig or hairpiece before you lose a lot of hair. That way, you can match your natural color and current hair style if you wish.
♦ Consider borrowing a wig or hairpiece, rather than buying one. Check with the local chapter of the American Cancer Society or with the social work department at your hospital.
♦ Remember that a hairpiece needed because of cancer treatment is a tax-deductible expense and may be at least partially covered by your health insurance. Be sure to check your policy.

Losing hair from your head, face, or body can be hard to accept. It's common—and perfectly all right—to feel angry or depressed about this loss. Talking about your feelings can help. So can remembering that the hair lost during chemotherapy may grow back even thicker than ever.

Fatigue/anemia

Chemotherapy can reduce the bone marrow's ability to make red blood cells, which carry oxygen to all parts of your body. When there are too few red blood cells, body tissues don't get enough oxygen to do their work. This condition is called **anemia**.

Anemia can make you feel very weak and tired. Other symptoms of anemia include dizziness, chills, or shortness of breath. Be sure to report any of these symptoms to your doctor.

Your doctor will check your red blood cell count often during your treatment. If your red count falls too low, you may need a blood transfusion to increase the number of red blood cells in your body.

Here are some things you can do to help yourself feel better if you develop anemia:

♦ Get plenty of rest. Sleep more at night and take naps during the day if you can.
♦ Limit your activities: Do only the things that are most important to you.
♦ Don't be afraid to get help when you need it. Ask family and friends to pitch in with things like child care, shopping, housework, or driving.
♦ Eat well, and be sure to include plenty of iron-rich foods. Add more green, leafy vegetables and red meats, especially liver, to your diet.
♦ When sitting or lying down, get up slowly. This will help prevent dizziness.

Infection

Chemotherapy can make you more likely to get infections. This happens because most anticancer drugs affect the bone marrow and decrease its ability to produce white blood cells, the cells that fight infections. Almost any part of your body can get an infection, including your mouth, skin, lungs, urinary tract, rectum, and reproductive tract.

Your doctor will check your blood cell count often while you are getting chemotherapy. If your white cell count falls too low, your doctor may postpone your next treatment or give you a lower dose of drugs for a while.

When your white count is lower than normal, it is very important to try to prevent infections by taking the following steps:

♦ Wash your hands often during the day. Be sure to wash them extra well before you eat and before and after you use the bathroom.
♦ Clean your rectal area gently but thoroughly after each bowel movement. Ask your doctor or nurse for advice if the area becomes irritated or if you have hemorrhoids.
♦ Stay away from people who have diseases you can catch, such as a cold, the flu, measles, or chickenpox. Also try to avoid crowds.
♦ Don't cut or tear the cuticles of your nails. Use cuticle cream and remover instead.
♦ Be careful not to cut or nick yourself when using scissors, needles, or knives.
♦ Use an electric shaver instead of a razor to prevent breaks or cuts in your skin.

♦ Use a soft toothbrush that won't hurt your gums.
♦ Don't squeeze or scratch pimples.
♦ Take a warm (not hot) bath, shower, or sponge bath every day. Pat your skin dry using a light touch. Don't rub.
♦ Use lotion or oil to soften and heal your skin if it becomes dry and cracked.
♦ Clean cuts and scrapes right away with warm water, soap, and an antiseptic.
♦ Wear protective gloves when gardening or cleaning up after animals.
♦ Do not get any immunization shots without checking first with your doctor to see if it's all right.

Even if you take extra care, you may still get an infection. Be alert to the signs that you might have an infection and check your body regularly for its signs, paying special attention to your eyes, nose, mouth, and genital and rectal areas. The symptoms of infection include:

♦ Fever over 100 degrees F.
♦ Chills.
♦ Sweating.
♦ Loose bowels (this can also be a side effect of chemotherapy).
♦ A burning feeling when you urinate.
♦ A severe cough or sore throat.
♦ Unusual vaginal discharge or itching.
♦ Redness or swelling, especially around a wound, sore, pimple, or boil.

Report any signs of infection to your doctor right away. If you have a fever, don't use aspirin or any other medicine to bring your temperature down without first checking with your doctor.

Blood clotting problems

Anticancer drugs can affect the bone marrow's ability to make platelets, the blood cells that help stop bleeding by making your blood clot. If your blood does not have enough platelets, you may bleed or bruise more easily than usual, even from a minor injury.

Be sure to let your doctor know if you have unexpected bruising, small red spots under the skin, reddish or pinkish urine, or black or bloody bowel movements. Also report any bleeding from your gums or nose. Your doctor will check your platelet count often while you are having chemotherapy. If your platelet count falls too low, the doctor may give you a transfusion to build the count up.

Here are some ways to avoid problems if your platelet count is low:

♦ Don't take any medicine without first checking with your doctor or nurse. This includes aspirin or aspirin-free pain relievers.
♦ Don't drink any alcoholic beverages unless your doctor says it's all right.
♦ Use a very soft toothbrush to clean your teeth.
♦ Clean your nose by blowing gently; never use your fingers.
♦ Take care when using knives or tools.

- Be careful not to burn yourself when ironing or cooking. Use a padded glove when you reach into the oven.
- Avoid contact sports and other activities that might result in injury.
- Wear heavy gloves for digging in the garden or working near plants with thorns.

Mouth, gum, and throat problems

Anticancer drugs can cause sores in the mouth and throat. They can also make these tissues dry and irritated or cause them to bleed. In addition to being painful, mouth sores can become infected by the many germs that live in the mouth. Because infections can be hard to fight during chemotherapy and can lead to serious problems, it's important to take every possible step to prevent them.

Here are some suggestions for keeping your mouth, gums, and throat healthy:

- If possible, see your dentist before you start chemotherapy to have your teeth cleaned and to take care of any problems such as cavities, abscesses, gum disease, or poorly fitting dentures. Ask your dentist to show you the best ways to brush and floss your teeth during chemotherapy. Chemotherapy can make you more likely to get cavities, so your dentist may suggest using a fluoride rinse or gel each day to help prevent decay.
- Brush your teeth after every meal. Use a soft toothbrush and a gentle touch; brushing too hard can damage soft mouth tissues. If your gums are too sensitive for even a soft toothbrush, use a cotton swab or gauze. Use a nonabrasive toothpaste or a paste of baking soda and water.
- Rinse your toothbrush well after each use and store it in a dry place.
- Avoid commercial mouthwashes that contain a large amount of salt or alcohol. Ask your doctor or nurse about a mild mouthwash that you might use.

If you develop sores in your mouth, be sure to contact your doctor or nurse because you may need medical treatment for the sores. If the sores are painful or keep you from eating, you can also try these ideas:

- Ask your doctor if you may apply Maalox® or milk of magnesia to the sores with a swab. The doctor may also prescribe a medicine you can use to ease the pain.
- Eat foods cold or at room temperature. Hot and warm foods can irritate a tender mouth and throat.
- Choose soft, soothing foods such as ice cream, milkshakes, baby food, soft fruits such as bananas and applesauce, mashed potatoes, cooked cereals, soft-boiled or scrambled eggs, cottage cheese, macaroni and cheese, custards, puddings, and gelatin. You can also puree cooked foods in the blender to make them smoother and easier to eat.
- Avoid irritating, acidic foods such as tomatoes, citrus fruit and fruit juice (orange, grapefruit, and lemon); spicy or salty foods; and rough, coarse, or dry foods such as raw vegetables, granola, and toast.

If mouth dryness bothers you or makes it hard for you to eat, try these tips:

- Ask your doctor if you should use an artificial saliva product to moisten your mouth.
- Drink plenty of liquids.
- Suck on ice chips, popsicles, or sugarless hard candy. You can also chew sugarless gum.
- Moisten dry foods with butter, margarine, gravy, sauces, or broth.
- Dunk crisp, dry foods in mild liquids.
- Eat soft and pureed foods like those listed above.
- Use lip balm if your lips become dry.

Diarrhea

When chemotherapy affects the cells lining the intestine, the result can be diarrhea (loose stools). If you have diarrhea that continues for more than 24 hours, or if you have pain and cramping along with the diarrhea, call your doctor. In severe cases, the doctor may prescribe an antidiarrhea medicine.

You can also try these ideas to help control diarrhea:

- Eat smaller amounts of food, but eat more often.
- Avoid high-fiber foods, which can lead to diarrhea and cramping. High-fiber foods include whole-grain breads and cereals, raw vegetables, beans, nuts, seeds, popcorn, and fresh and dried fruit. Eat low-fiber foods instead. Low-fiber foods include white bread, white rice or noodles, creamed cereals, ripe bananas, canned or cooked fruit without skins, cottage cheese, yogurt, eggs, mashed or baked potatoes without the skin, pureed vegetables, chicken or turkey without the skin, and fish.
- Avoid coffee, tea, alcohol, and sweets. Stay away from fried, greasy, or highly spiced foods, too. They are all irritating and can cause diarrhea and cramping.
- Unless your doctor has told you otherwise, eat more high-potassium foods because diarrhea can cause you to lose this important mineral. Bananas, oranges, potatoes, and peach and apricot nectars are good sources of potassium.
- Drink plenty of fluids to replace those you have lost through diarrhea. Mild, clear liquids such as apple juice, water, weak tea, clear broth, or ginger ale are best. Drink them slowly, and make sure they are at room temperature. Let carbonated drinks lose their fizz before you drink them.
- If your diarrhea is severe, ask your doctor if you should try a clear liquid diet to give your bowels time to rest. As you feel better, you can gradually add the low-fiber foods listed above. A clear liquid diet doesn't provide all the nutrients you need, so don't follow one for more than 3 to 5 days.
- Avoid milk and milk products if they make your diarrhea worse.

Constipation

Some people who get chemotherapy become constipated because of the drugs they are taking. Others may become constipated because they are less active or less well-nourished than usual. Tell your doctor if you have not had a bowel movement for more than a day or two. You may need to take a laxative or stool softener or use an enema, but **don't** use these remedies unless you have checked with your doctor.

You can also try these ideas to deal with constipation:

♦ Drink plenty of fluids to help loosen the bowels. Warm and hot fluids work especially well.

♦ Eat a lot of high-fiber foods. High-fiber foods include bran, whole-wheat breads and cereals, raw or cooked vegetables, fresh and dried fruit, nuts, and popcorn.

♦ Get some exercise. Simply getting out for a walk can help, as can a more structured exercise program. Be sure to check with your doctor before becoming more active.

Nerve and muscle effects

Your nervous system affects just about all your body's organs and tissues. So it's not surprising that when chemotherapy affects the cells of the nervous system—as the drugs sometimes do—a wide range of side effects can result. For example, certain drugs can cause **peripheral neuropathy**, a condition that may make you feel a tingling, burning, weakness, or numbness in the hands and/or feet. Other nerve-related symptoms include loss of balance, clumsiness, difficulty picking up objects, walking problems, jaw pain, hearing loss, stomach pain, and constipation. In addition to affecting the nerves, certain anticancer drugs can also affect the muscles and make them weak, tired, or sore.

In some cases, nerve and muscle effects—though annoying—may not be serious. In other cases, nerve and muscle symptoms may indicate serious problems that need medical attention. Be sure to report any suspected nerve or muscle symptoms to your doctor.

Caution and common sense can help you deal with nerve and muscle problems. For example, if your fingers become numb, be very careful when grasping objects that are sharp, hot, or otherwise dangerous. If your sense of balance or muscle strength is affected, avoid falls by moving carefully, using handrails when going up or down stairs and using bathmats in the bathtub or shower. Do not wear slippery shoes.

Effects on skin and nails

You may have minor skin problems while you are having chemotherapy. Possible side effects include redness, itching, peeling, dryness, and acne. Your nails may become brittle or cracked or develop vertical lines or bands.

You will be able to take care of most of these problems yourself. If you develop acne, try to keep your face clean and dry and use over-the-counter medicated creams or soaps. For itching, apply cornstarch as you would a dusting powder. To help avoid dryness, take quick showers or sponge baths rather than long, hot baths. Apply cream and lotion while your skin is still moist and avoid perfume, cologne, or aftershave lotion that contains alcohol. You can strengthen your nails with the remedies sold for this purpose, but be alert to signs of a worsening problem because these products can be irritating to some people. Protect your nails by wearing gloves when washing dishes, gardening, or performing other work around the house. Get further advice from your doctor if these skin and nail problems don't respond to your efforts.

Certain anticancer drugs, when given intravenously, may produce a fairly dramatic darkening of the skin all along the vein. Some people use makeup to cover the area, but this can become difficult and time-consuming if several veins are affected, which sometimes happens. The darkened areas will usually fade on their own a few months after treatment ends.

Exposure to the sun may increase the effects some anticancer drugs have on your skin. Check with your doctor or nurse about using a sunscreen lotion with a skin protection factor of 15 to protect against the sun's effects. They may even suggest that you avoid being in direct sunlight or that you use a product, such as zinc oxide, that blocks the sun's rays completely.

Some people who have had radiation therapy develop "radiation recall" during their chemotherapy. During or shortly after the treatment is given, the skin over the area that was treated with radiation turns red—a shade anywhere from light to very bright—and may itch or burn. This reaction may last hours or even days. You can soothe the itching and burning by putting a cool, wet compress over the affected area. Radiation recall reactions should be reported to your doctor or nurse.

Most skin problems are not serious, but a few demand immediate attention. For example, certain drugs given intravenously can cause serious and permanent tissue damage if they leak out of the vein. Tell your doctor or nurse **right away** if you feel any burning or pain when you are getting IV drugs. These symptoms don't always mean there's a problem, but they always must be checked out at once.

You should also let your doctor or nurse know **right away** if you develop sudden or severe itching, if your skin breaks out in a rash or hives, or if you have wheezing or any other trouble breathing. These symptoms may mean you are having an allergic reaction that may need to be treated at once.

Kidney and bladder effects

Some anticancer drugs can irritate the bladder or cause temporary or permanent damage to the kidneys. Be sure to ask your doctor if your anticancer drugs are among the ones that have this effect, and notify the doctor if you have any symptoms that might indicate a problem. Signs to watch for include:

♦ Pain or burning when you urinate.
♦ Frequent urination.
♦ A feeling that you must urinate right away ("urgency").
♦ Reddish or bloody urine.
♦ Fever.
♦ Chills.

In general, it's a good idea to drink plenty of fluids to ensure good urine flow and help prevent problems; this is especially important if your drugs are among those that affect the kidney and bladder. Water, juice, coffee, tea, soup, soft drinks, broth, ice cream, soup, popsicles, and gelatin are all considered fluids. Your doctor will let you know if you must increase your fluid intake.

You should also be aware that some anticancer drugs cause the urine to change color (orange, red, or yellow) or to take on a strong or medicine-like odor. The color and odor of semen may be affected, as well. Check with your doctor to see if the drugs you are taking have this effect.

Flu-like syndrome

Some people report feeling as though they have the flu a few hours to a few days after chemotherapy. Flu-like symptoms—muscle aches, headache, tiredness, nausea, slight fever, chills, and poor appetite—may last from 1 to 3 days. These symptoms can also be caused by an infection or by the cancer itself, so it's important to check with your doctor if you have flu-like symptoms.

Fluid retention

Your body may retain fluid when you are having chemotherapy. This may be due to hormonal changes from your therapy, to the effect of the drugs themselves, or to your cancer. Check with your doctor or nurse if you notice swelling or puffiness in your face, hands, feet, or abdomen. You may need to avoid table salt and foods with a high sodium content. If the problem is severe, your doctor may prescribe medicine to help your body get rid of excess fluids.

Sexual effects: physical and psychological

Chemotherapy may—but does not always—affect sexual organs and functioning in both men and women. The side effects that might occur depend on the drugs used and the person's age and general health.

Men

Chemotherapy drugs may lower the number of sperm cells, reduce their ability to move, or cause other abnormalities. These changes can result in infertility, which may be temporary or permanent. Infertility affects a man's ability to father a child but does **not** affect his ability to have sexual intercourse.

Because permanent sterility may occur, it's important to discuss this issue with your doctor before you begin chemotherapy. If you wish, you might consider sperm banking, a procedure that freezes sperm for future use..

Men undergoing chemotherapy should use an effective means of birth control with their partners during treatment because of the harmful effects of the drugs on chromosomes. Ask your doctor when you can stop using birth control for this purpose.

Women

Anticancer drugs can damage the ovaries and reduce the amount of hormones they produce. As a result, some somen find that their menstrual periods become irregular or stop completely while they are having chemotherapy.

Damage to the ovaries may result in infertility, the inability to become pregnant. In some cases, the infertility is a temporary condition; in other cases, it may be permanent. Whether infertility occurs, and how long it lasts, depends on many factors, including the type of drug, the dosage given, and the woman's age.

Although pregnancy may be possible during chemotherapy, it is still not advisable because some anticancer drugs may cause birth defects. Women of childbearing age—from the teens through the end of menopause—are urged to use birth control throughout their treatment.

If a woman is pregnant when her cancer is discovered, it may be possible to delay chemotherapy until after the baby is born. For a woman who needs treatment sooner, the doctor may suggest starting chemotherapy after the 12th week of pregnancy, when the fetus is beyond the stage of greatest risk. In some cases, termination of the pregnancy may be considered.

The hormonal effects of chemotherapy may also cause menopause-like symptoms such as hot flashes and itching, burning, or dryness of vaginal tissues. These tissue changes can make intercourse uncomfortable, but the symptoms can often be relieved by using a water-based vaginal lubricant. The tissue changes can also make a woman more likely to get vaginal infections. To help prevent infection, avoid oil-based lubricants such as Vaseline, wear cotton underwear and pantyhose with a ventilated cotton lining, and don't wear tight slacks or shorts. Your doctor may also prescribe a vaginal cream or suppository to reduce the chances of infection. If infection does occur, it should be treated right away. (For more information, see "Infection.")

Sexuality

Sexual feelings and attitudes vary among people during chemotherapy. Some people find that they feel closer than ever to their partners and have an increased desire for sexual activity. Others experience little or no change in their sexual desire and energy level. Still others find that their sexual interest declines because of the physical and emotional stresses of having cancer and getting chemotherapy. These stresses may include worries about changes in appearance; anxiety about health, family, or finances; or side effects, including fatigue and hormonal changes. All of these can lessen the desire for sexual activity.

A partner's concerns or fears can also affect the sexual relationship. Some may worry that physical intimacy will harm the person who has cancer; others may fear that they might "catch" the cancer or be affected by the drugs. Many of these issues can be cleared up by talking about misunderstandings. Both you and your partner should feel free to discuss sexual concerns with your doctor, nurse, or other counselor who can give you the information and the reassurance you need.

You and your partner should also try to share your feelings with one another. If it's difficult for you to talk to each other about sex, or cancer, or both, you may want to speak to a counselor who can help you communicate more openly. People who can help include psychiatrists, ecologists, social workers, marriage counselors, sex therapists, and members of the clergy.

If you were comfortable with and enjoyed sexual relations before starting therapy, chances are you will still find pleasure in physical intimacy during your treatment. You may discover, however, that intimacy takes on a new meaning and character. Hugging, touching, holding, and cuddling may become more important, while sexual intercourse may become less so. Remember that what was true before you started chemotherapy remains true now: There is no one "right" way to express your sexuality. It's up to you and your partner to determine together what is pleasurable and satisfying to you both.

The American Cancer Society has two booklets on sexuality that may be helpful—one for women and one for men. Contact your local unit or the national office for copies.

Eating Well During Chemotherapy

It is very important to eat as well as you can while you are undergoing treatment. People who eat well can cope with side effects better and are able to fight infection more easily. In addition, their bodies can rebuild healthy tissues faster.

Eating well during chemotherapy means choosing a well-balanced diet that contains all the nutrients the body needs. A good way to do this is to eat foods from each of the four major food groups: fruits and vegetables; poultry, fish, and meat; cereals and breads; and dairy products. Eating well also means having a diet high enough in calories to keep your weight up and, most important, high enough in protein to build and repair skin, hair, muscles, and organs.

You may also need to drink extra amounts of fluid to protect your bladder and kidneys during your treatment. (For more information, see "Kidney and Bladder Effects.")

What if I don't feel like eating?

Even when you know it's important to eat well, there may be days when you feel you just can't. This may happen because side effects such as nausea or mouth and throat problems make it difficult or painful to eat. If this is the case, be sure to read the sections in this booklet on your particular discomforts. They will give you tips that can make it easier for you to eat. You can also lose your appetite if you feel depressed or tired.

When a poor appetite is the problem, try these hints:

♦ Eat small meals or snacks whenever you want. You don't have to eat three regular meals each day.
♦ Vary your diet and try new foods and recipes.
♦ When possible, take a walk before meals to make you feel hungrier.
♦ Try changing your mealtime routine. For example, eat by candlelight or in a different location.
♦ Eat with friends or family members. When eating alone, listen to the radio or watch TV.
♦ If you live alone, you might want to arrange for "Meals on Wheels" or a similar program to bring food to you. Ask your doctor, nurse, local American Cancer Society office, or the Cancer Information Service about these programs, which are provided in most large communities.

The National Cancer Institute's booklet *Eating Hints* provides more tips about how to make eating easier and more enjoyable. It also gives many ideas about how to eat well and increase your protein and calorie intake during cancer treatment. For a free copy of *Eating Hints,* call the Cancer Information Service at 1-800-4-CANCER or write to the National Cancer Institute. (See "Resources for Patients and Their Families," for more information.)

Can I drink alcoholic beverages?

Small amounts of alcohol can help you relax and increase your appetite. On the other hand, alcohol may interact with some drugs to reduce their effectiveness or worsen their side effects. For this reason, some people must drink less alcohol or avoid alcohol completely during chemotherapy. Be sure to ask your doctor if it's okay for you to drink beer, wine, or other alcoholic beverages.

Should I take vitamin or mineral supplements?

There is no single answer to this question, but one thing is clear. No diet or nutritional plan can "cure" cancer, and taking vitamin and mineral supplements should **never** be considered a substitute for medical care. Some people may benefit from taking extra vitamins and minerals during their treatments. Other people may not benefit, or may even be harmed. You should not take any supplements without your doctor's knowledge and consent.

Talking with Your Doctor and Nurse

Some people with cancer want to know every detail about their condition and their treatment. Others prefer only general information. The choice of how much information to seek is yours, but there are questions that every person getting chemotherapy should ask. These include:

♦ Why do I need chemotherapy?
♦ What are the benefits of chemotherapy?
♦ What are the risks of chemotherapy?
♦ What drug or drugs will I be taking?
♦ How will the drugs be given?
♦ Where will I get my treatments?
♦ How long will my treatment last?
♦ What are the possible side effects?
♦ Are there any side effects that I should report right away?
♦ Are there any other possible treatment methods for my type of cancer?

This list is just a start. You should always feel free to ask your doctor and nurse as many questions as you want. If you don't understand their answers, keep asking until you do. Remember, when it comes to cancer and cancer treatment there is no such thing as a "stupid" question. To make sure you get all the answers you want, you may find it helpful to draw up a list of questions before your appointment. Some people even keep a "running list" and jot down each new question as it occurs to them.

To help remember your doctor's answers, you may want to take notes during your appointment. Don't feel shy about asking your doctor to slow down when you need more time to write. You might also ask if you can use a tape recorder during your visit. That way, you can review your conversation later as many times as you wish. Some doctors like this idea and others don't, so be sure to check before you try it. Another way to help you remember is to bring a friend or family member to sit with you while you talk to your doctor. This person can help you understand what your doctor says during your visit and help refresh your memory afterward.

Chemotherapy and Your Emotions

Chemotherapy can bring major changes to a person's life. It can affect overall health, threaten a sense of well-being, disrupt day-to-day schedules, and put a strain on personal relationships. No wonder, then, that many people feel fearful, anxious, angry, or depressed at some point during their chemotherapy.

These emotions are perfectly normal and understandable, but they can also be disturbing. Fortunately, there are ways to cope with these emotional "side effects," just as there are ways to cope with the physical side effects of chemotherapy.

How can I get the support I need?

There are many sources of support you can draw on. Here are some of the most important:

♦ *Doctors and nurses.* If you have questions or worries about your cancer treatment, talk with members of your health care team. See "Talking With Your Doctor and Nurse," for some communication tips.

♦ *Counseling professionals.* There are many kinds of counselors who can help you express, understand, and cope with the emotions cancer treatment can cause. Depending on your preferences and needs, you might want to talk with a psychiatrist, psychologist, social worker, sex therapist, or member of the clergy.

♦ *Friends and family members.* Talking with friends or family members can help you feel a lot better. Often, they can comfort and reassure you in ways that no one else can. You may find, though, that you'll need to help them help you. At a time when you might expect that others will rush to your aid, you may have to make the first move.

Many people do not understand cancer, and they may withdraw from you because they're afraid of your illness. Others may worry that they will upset you by saying "the wrong thing."

You can help relieve these fears by being open in talking with others about your illness, your treatment, your needs, and your feelings. By talking openly, you can correct mistaken ideas about cancer. You can also let people know that there's no single "right" thing to say, so long as their caring comes through loud and clear. Once people know they can talk with you honestly, they may be more willing and able to open up and lend their support.

The National Cancer Institute's booklet *Taking Time* offers useful advice to help cancer patients and their families and friends communicate with one another. For more information about this booklet, see "Resources for Patients and Their Families."

♦ *Support groups.* Support groups are made up of people who are going through the same kinds of experiences as you. Many people with cancer find they can share thoughts and feelings with group members that they don't feel comfortable sharing with anyone else. Support groups can also serve as an important source of practical information about living with cancer.

Support can also be found in one-to-one programs that put you in touch with another person very similar to you in terms of age, sex, type of cancer, and so forth. In some programs, this person comes to visit you. In others, a "hotline" puts you in touch with someone you can talk with on the telephone.

Sources for information about support programs include your hospital's social work department, the local office of your American Cancer Society, and the National Cancer Institute's Cancer Information Service.

How can I make my daily life easier?

Here are some tips to help yourself while you are getting chemotherapy:

♦ Try to keep your treatment goals in mind. This will help you keep a positive attitude on days when the going gets rough.

♦ Remember that eating well is very important. Your body needs food to rebuild tissues and regain strength.

♦ Learn as much as you want to know about your disease and its treatment. This can lessen your fear of the unknown and increase your feeling of control.

♦ Keep a journal or diary while you're in treatment. A record of your activities and thoughts can help you understand the feelings you have as you go through treatment, and highlight questions you need to ask your doctor or nurse. You can also use your journal to record the steps you take to cope with side effects, and how well those steps work. That way, you'll know which methods worked best for you in case you have the same side effects again.

♦ Set realistic goals and don't be too hard on yourself. You may not have as much energy as usual, so try to get as much rest as you can, let the "small stuff" slide, and only do the things that are most important to you.

Try new hobbies and learn new skills. Exercise if you can. Using your body can make you feel better about yourself, help you get rid of tension or anger, and build your appetite. Ask your doctor or nurse about a safe and practical exercise program.

How can I relieve stress?

You can use a number of methods to cope with the stresses of cancer and its treatment. The techniques described here can help you relax. They can also help relieve the nausea and vomiting that may occur before a treatment. Try some of these methods to find the one (or ones) that work best for you. If you have lung problems, check with your doctor before trying any method that involves deep breathing.

♦ *Muscle tension and release.* Lie down in a quiet room. Take a slow, deep breath. As you breathe in, tense a particular muscle or group of muscles. For example, you can squeeze your eyes shut, frown, clench your teeth, make a fist, or stiffen your arms or legs. Hold your breath and keep your muscles tense for a second or two. Then breathe out, release the tension, and let your body relax completely. Repeat the process with another muscle or muscle group.

You can also try a variation of this method, called "progressive relaxation." Start with the toes of one foot and, working upward, progressively tense and relax all the muscles of one leg. Next, do the same with the other leg. Then tense and relax the rest of the muscle groups in your body, including those in your scalp. Remember to hold your breath while tensing your muscles and to breathe out when releasing the tension.

♦ **Rhythmic breathing.** Get into a comfortable position and relax all your muscles. If you keep your eyes open, focus on a distant object. If you close your eyes, imagine a peaceful scene or simply clear your mind and focus on your breathing.

Breathe in and out slowly and comfortably through your nose. If you like, you can keep the rhythm steady by saying to yourself, "In, one two; Out, one two." Feel yourself relax and go limp each time you breathe out.

You can do this technique for just a few seconds or for up to 10 minutes. End your rhythmic breathing by counting slowly and silently from one to three.

♦ **Biofeedback.** With training in biofeedback, you can control body functions such as heart rate, blood pressure, and muscle tension. A machine will sense when your body shows signs of tension and will let you know in some way such as making a sound or flashing a light. The machine will also give you feedback when you relax your body. Eventually, you will be able to control your relaxation responses without having to depend on feedback from the machine. Your doctor or nurse can refer you to someone trained in teaching biofeedback.

♦ **Imagery.** Imagery is a way of daydreaming that uses all your senses. It is usually done with your eyes closed. To begin, breathe slowly and feel yourself relax. Imagine a ball of healing energy—perhaps a white light—forming somewhere in your body. When you can "see" the ball of energy, imagine that as you breathe in you can blow the ball to any part of the body where you feel pain, tension, or discomfort such as nausea. When you breathe out, picture the air moving the ball away from your body, taking with it and painful or uncomfortable feelings. (Be sure to breathe naturally; don't blow.) Continue to picture the ball moving toward you and away from you each time you breathe in and out. You may see the ball getting bigger and bigger as it takes away more and more tension and discomfort.

To end the imagery, count slowly to three, breathe in deeply, open your eyes, and say to yourself, "I feel alert and relaxed."

If you choose to use imagery as a relaxation technique, please be sure to read the caution in the following section.

♦ **Visualization.** Visualization is a method that is similar to imagery. With visualization, you create an inner picture that represents your fight against cancer. Some people getting chemotherapy use images of rockets blasting away their cancer cells or of knights in armor battling their cancer cells. Others create an image of their white blood cells or their drugs attacking the cancer cells.

Visualization and imagery are excellent ways to relieve stress and to increase your sense of self-control. But it is very important to remember that they can never take the place of the medical care your doctor prescribes to treat your cancer.

♦ **Hypnosis.** Hypnosis puts you in a trance-like state that can reduce discomfort and anxiety. You can be hypnotized by a qualified person, or you can learn how to hypnotize yourself. If you are interested in learning more, ask your doctor or nurse to refer you to someone trained in the technique.

♦ **Distraction.** You use distraction any time an activity takes your mind off your worries or discomforts. Try watching TV, listening to the radio, reading, going to the movies, or working with your hands by doing needlework or puzzles, building models, or painting. You may be surprised how comfortably the time goes by.

Paying for Chemotherapy

The cost of chemotherapy varies with the kinds and dose of drugs used, how long and how often they are given, and whether you get them at home, in a clinic or office, or in the hospital. Most health insurance policies (including Medicare Part B, which helps pay for doctors' bills and many other medical services) cover at least part of the cost of many kinds of chemotherapy.

Sometimes, however, an insurer may not pay for the use of certain drugs for certain kinds of cancers—at least not at first. If your insurer denies payment for your treatment, don't give up. Most people do get payment eventually.

Teamwork with your doctor and the office staff is important. Be sure to let them know if you have been denied payment. They can consult with your insurer and help answer any questions your insurer may have. They can also consult with the company that makes the drug or drugs you are taking. Often, these companies can provide information or other services that will help you get payment.

In some states, Medicaid (which makes health care services available for people with financial need) may help pay for certain treatments. Contact the office that handles social services in your city or county to find out whether you are eligible for Medicaid and whether your chemotherapy is a covered expense.

If you need help paying for treatments, contact your hospital's social service office, the Cancer Information Service, or the local office of the American Cancer Society. They may be able to direct you to other sources of help. Another possibility is the Leukemia Society of America. You may also be eligible for special assistance programs run by the company or companies that make the drugs your doctor prescribes. (See "Patient Drug Assistance Programs.")

A Final Word

The National Cancer Institute hopes *Chemotherapy and You* help you and your family, whether you are waiting to begin chemotherapy or have already begun your treatment. Discuss the information in this booklet with your doctor and nurse, and take good care of yourself during your chemotherapy. By working together, you, your family, and your health care providers will make the strongest possible team in your fight against cancer. We wish you success.

Resources for Patients and Their Families

National Cancer Institute, Cancer Information Service

The Cancer Information Service (CIS), supported by the National Cancer Institute, is a nationwide telephone service that answers questions from cancer patients and their families, health care professionals, and the public. Information specialists are not doctors, but they can provide information and publications on all aspects of cancer. They also may know about cancer-related services in your local area.

By dialing 1-800-4-CANCER (1-800-422-6237), you will be connected to a CIS office serving your area, where a trained staff member can answer your questions and listen to your concerns. Spanish-speaking staff members are available.

PDQ

People who have cancer, those who care about them, and doctors need up-to-date and accurate information about cancer treatment. To meet these needs, the National Cancer Institute developed PDQ (Physician Data Query), a computer database that gives quick and easy access to:

♦ State-of-the-art treatment information.
♦ Information about current clinical trials (research studies) that are testing new and promising cancer treatments.
♦ Names of organizations and doctors involved in caring for people with cancer.

To use PDQ, doctors may use an office computer or the services of a medical library. Doctors and patients can get PDQ information by calling the CIS at 1-800-4-CANCER.

Publications

You may want to read some other National Cancer Institute booklets that discuss various aspects of cancer, cancer treatment, and patient concerns. The following publications are available free of charge and may be ordered by calling the Cancer Information Service at 1-800-4-CANCER or by writing to the National Cancer Institute, Building 31, Room 10A24, Bethesda, MD 20892.

♦ *Answers to Your Questions About Metastatic Cancer.*
♦ *Eating Hints: Recipes and Tips for Better Nutrition During Cancer Treatment.*
♦ *Facing Forward: A Guide for Cancer Survivors.*
♦ *Questions and Answers About Pain Control.*
♦ *Radiation Therapy and You: A Guide to Self-Help During Treatment.*
♦ *Research Reports.* A series of in-depth booklets about different types of cancer.
♦ *Taking Time: Support for People With Cancer and the People Who Care About Them.*
♦ *What You Need To Know About Cancer.* A series of booklets about different types of cancer; ask for the booklet about the type of cancer you have.
♦ *Anticancer Drug Information Sheets.* A series of fact sheets on 59 common anticancer drugs, available in Spanish as well as English. Ask for the information sheet about the drug or drugs you need.

American Cancer Society

The American Cancer Society is a nonprofit organization that offers a variety of services to patients and their families. Local American Cancer Society units offer such programs as information, counseling, and guidance; referral to community health services and resources; equipment loans for care of the homebound patient; and transportation to and from treatment. Many local units also sponsor group and individual support programs. To find a chapter near you, check your local telephone book or contact the national headquarters at:

American Cancer Society
National Headquarters
1599 Clifton Road, NE
Atlanta, GA 30329
1-800-ACS-2345

Patient drug assistance programs

Many drug companies have drug assistance programs for patients who cannot afford the drugs in any other way. For the most current information on these programs, contact the Cancer Information Service at 1-800-4-CANCER.

Glossary

This glossary reviews the meaning of some words used in *Chemotherapy and You.* It also explains some words related to chemotherapy that are not mentioned in this booklet but that you may hear from your doctor or nurse.

Adjuvant therapy. Anticancer drugs or hormones given after surgery and/or radiation to help prevent the cancer from coming back.

Alopecia. Hair loss.

Anemia. Having too few red blood cells. Symptoms of anemia include feeling tired, weak, and short of breath.

Anorexia. Poor appetite.

Antiemetic. A medicine that prevents or controls vomiting.

Benign. A term used to describe a tumor that is not cancerous.

Biological response modifiers (BRMs). Natural and man-made substances that help control the immune system in its fight against cancer.

Blood count. The number of red blood cells, white blood cells, and platelets in a sample of blood. This is also called the complete blood count (CBC).

Bone marrow. The inner, spongy tissue of large bones where red blood cells, white blood cells, and platelets and made.

Cancer. A general name for more than 100 diseases in which abnormal cells grow out of control; a malignant tumor.

Catheter. A tube used to inject or withdraw fluids.

Chemotherapy. The use of drugs to treat cancer.

Combination chemotherapy. The use of more than one drug to treat cancer.

Gastrointestinal. Having to do with the digestive tract, which includes the mouth, esophagus, stomach, and intestines.

Hormones. Natural substances released by one organ that can influence the function of other organs in the body.

Infusion. Slow and/or prolonged intravenous delivery of a drug or fluids.

Injection. Using a syringe and needle to push fluids or drugs into the body; often called a "shot."

Intra-arterial (IA). Into an artery.

Intracavitary (IC). Into a cavity or space, specifically the abdomen, pelvis, or the pleural cavity of the chest.

Intralesional (IL). Into the cancerous area in the skin.

Intramuscular (IM). Into a muscle.

Intrathecal (IT). Into the spinal fluid.

Intravenous (IV). Into a vein.

Malignant. Used to describe a cancerous tumor.

Metastasis. When cancer cells break away from their original site and spread through the body.

Platelets. Special blood cells that help stop bleeding.

Radiation therapy. Cancer treatment with radiation (high-energy rays).

Red blood cells. Cells that supply oxygen to tissues throughout the body.

Remission. The disappearance of signs and symptoms of disease.

Stomatitis. Sores on the inside lining of the mouth.

Subcutaneous. Under the skin.

Tumor. An abnormal growth of cells or tissues. Tumors may be benign (noncancerous) or malignant (cancerous).

White blood cells. The blood cells that fight infection.

■ **Document Source:**
U.S. Department of Health and Human Services, Public Health Service
National Institutes of Health
National Cancer Institute
NIH Publication No. 92-1136
Third Edition. December 1991

See also: What Are Clinical Trials All About? A Booklet for Patients with Cancer (page 68); When Cancer Recurs: Meeting the Challenge Again (page 74)

MANAGING CANCER PAIN

Purpose of This Booklet

This booklet is about cancer pain and how it can be controlled. Not everyone with cancer has pain. But those who do can feel better with proper pain treatment.

Reading this booklet should help you to:

♦ Learn why pain control is important to you.
♦ Work with your doctors and nurses to find the best method to control your pain.
♦ Talk to your doctors and nurses about your pain and how well the treatment is working for you.

Facts About Cancer Pain Treatment

If you are being treated for cancer pain, you may have concerns about your medicine or other treatments. Here are some common concerns people have and the facts about them.

Concern: I can only take medicine or other treatments when I have pain.

Fact: You should not wait until the pain becomes severe to take your medicine. Pain is easier to control when it is mild than when it is severe. You should take your pain medicine regularly and as your doctor or nurse tells you. This may mean taking it on a regular schedule and around-the-clock. You can also use the other treatments, such as relaxation and breathing exercises, hot and cold packs, as often as you want to.

Concern: I will become "hooked" or "addicted" to pain medicine.

Fact: Studies show that getting "hooked" or "addicted" to pain medicine is very rare. Remember, it is important to take pain medicine regularly to keep the pain under control.

Concern: If I take too much medicine, it will stop working.

Fact: The medicine will not stop working. But sometimes your body will get used to the medicine. This is called tolerance. Tolerance is not usually a problem with cancer pain treatment because the amount of medicine can be changed or other medicines can be added. Cancer pain can be relieved, so don't deny yourself pain relief now.

Concern: If I complain too much, I am not being a good patient.

Fact: Controlling your pain is an important part of your care. Tell your doctor or nurse if you have pain, if your pain is getting worse, or if you are taking pain medicine and it is not working. They can help you to get relief from your pain.

You may have concerns about your treatment that were not discussed here. Talk to your doctor or nurse about your concerns.

Why Pain Should Be Treated

Pain can affect you in many ways. It can keep you from being active, from sleeping well, from enjoying family and friends, and from eating. Pain can also make you feel afraid or depressed.

When you are in pain or uncomfortable, your family and friends may worry about you.

With treatment, most cancer pain can be controlled. When there is less pain, you will probably feel more active and interested in doing things you enjoy.

If you have cancer and you are feeling pain, you need to tell your doctor or nurse right away. Getting help for your pain early on can make pain treatment more effective.

What Causes Cancer Pain?

There are many causes of cancer pain. Most of the pain of cancer comes when a tumor presses on bone, nerves, or body organs. Cancer treatment can cause pain, too.

You may also have pain that had nothing to do with your illness or its treatment. Like everyone else, you can get headaches, muscle strains, and other aches and pains. Because you may be taking medicine for cancer treatment or pain, check with your doctor or nurse on what to take for these everyday aches and pains.

Other conditions, such as arthritis, can cause pain, too. Pain from these other conditions can be treated along with cancer pain. Again, talk to your doctor or nurse about your medical history. They will be able to tell you how each condition can be treated and what is best for you.

Treating Cancer Pain

Cancer pain is usually treated with medicine. But surgery, radiation therapy, and other treatments can be used along with medicine to give even more pain relief. Ask your doctor or nurse how the other treatments can help you.

Choosing the Right Medicine

Pain treatments work differently for different people. Even when a doctor or nurse uses the right medicines and treatments in the right way, you may not get the pain relief you need. While you are being treated for your pain, tell your doctor or nurse how you feel and if the treatments help. The information you give them will help them to help you get the best pain relief.

Your doctor and nurse will work to find the right pain medicine and treatments for you. You can help by talking with them about:

- Pain medicines you have taken in the past and how well they have worked for you.
- Medicines and other treatments (including health foods, vitamins, and other "nonmedical" treatments) you are taking now. Your doctor or nurse needs to know about other treatments you are trying and other medicines you take. This is important because some treatments and medicines do not work well together. **Your doctor or nurse can find medicines that can be taken together**.
- Allergies that you have, including allergies to medicines.
- Fears and concerns that you have about the medicine or the treatment. Talk to your doctor or nurse about your fears and concerns. They can answer your questions and help you to understand your pain treatment.

Types of Pain Medicine

Many medicines are used to treat cancer pain, and your doctor may give you one or more of them to take. The list below describes the different types of medicine that you may be taking and the kind of pain they work on. Ask your doctor or nurse to tell you more about the medicine you are taking.

Do not start to take a new medicine without checking with your doctor or nurse first. Even aspirin can be a problem in some people who are taking other medicines or having cancer treatment.

- For mild to moderate pain—
  Nonopioids: Acetaminophen and nonsteroidal anti-inflammatory drugs (NSAIDs), such as aspirin and ibuprofen. You can buy many of these over-the-counter (without a prescription). Others need a prescription.
- For moderate to severe pain—
  Opioids: Morphine, hydromorphone, oxycodone, and codeine. A prescription is needed for these medicines. Nonopioids may be used along with opioids for moderate to severe pain.
- For tingling and burning pain—
  Antidepressants: Amitriptyline, imipramine, doxepin, trazodone. A prescription is needed for these medicines. Taking an antidepressant does not mean that you are depressed or have a mental illness.
  Anticonvulsants: Carbamazepine and phenytoin. A prescription is needed for these medicines. Taking an anticonvulsant does not mean that you are going to have convulsions.
- For pain caused by swelling—
  Steroids: Prednisone, dexamethasone. A prescription is needed for these medicines.

About Side Effects

All medicines can have some side effects, but not all people get them. Some people have different side effects than others. Most side effects happen in the first few hours of treatment and gradually go away. Some of the most common side effects of pain medicines are:

- **Constipation** (not being able to have a bowel movement). The best way to prevent constipation is to drink lots of water, juice, and other liquids, and to eat more fruits and vegetables. Exercise also helps to prevent constipation. Your doctor or nurse may also be able to give you a stool softener or a laxative.
- **Nausea and vomiting.** When this happens, it usually only lasts for the first day or two after starting a medicine. Tell your doctor or nurse about any nausea or vomiting. They can give you medicine to stop these side effects.
- **Sleepiness.** Some people who take opioids feel drowsy or sleepy when they first take the medicine. This usually does not last too long. Talk to your doctor or nurse if this is a problem for you.
- **Slowed breathing.** This sometimes happens when the dose of medicine is increased. Your doctor or nurse can tell you what to watch for and when to report slowed breathing.

Most serious side effects of pain medicines are rare. As with the more common side effects, they usually happen in the first few hours of treatment. They include trouble breathing, dizziness, and rashes. If you have any of these side effects, you should call your doctor or nurse right away.

How Pain Medicine Is Taken

Most pain medicine is taken by mouth (orally). Oral medicines are easy to take and usually cost less than other kinds of medicine. Most oral medicines are in tablet form, but sometimes they are liquids that you drink. If it is hard for you to swallow and you cannot take in tablet or liquid for some other reason, there are other ways to get these medicines. These include:

- **Rectal suppositories** (medicine that dissolves in the rectum and is absorbed by the body).
- **Patches that are filled with medicine and placed on the skin** (transdermal patches).
- **Injections.** There are many kinds of injections to give pain relief. Most injections use a tube or needle to place medicine directly into the body. These include:

  Subcutaneous injection—medicine is placed just under the skin using a small needle.

  Intravenous injection—medicine is placed directly into the vein through a needle that stays in the vein.

  Epidural or intrathecal injections—medicine is placed directly into the back using a small tube. Most of these injections give pain relief that lasts for many hours.

  Subdermal and intramuscular injections—commonly known as "shots," are injections that are placed more deeply into the skin or muscle using a needle. These injections are not recommended for long-term cancer pain treatment. Constantly having shots into the skin and muscle can be painful. Also, shots take longer to work, and you have to wait for them.

When to Take Your Pain Medicine

To help your pain medicine work best:

- Take your medicine on a regular schedule (by the clock). Taking medicine regularly and as your doctor tells you will help to keep pain under control. Do not skip a dose of medicine or wait for the pain to get worse before taking your medicine.
- Ask your doctor or nurse how and when to take extra medicine. If some activities make your pain worse (for example, riding in a car), you may need to take extra doses of pain medicines before these activities. The goal is to PREVENT the pain. Once you feel the pain, it is harder to get it under control.

Treating pain is important, and there are many medicines and treatments that can be used. If one medicine or treatment does not work, there is another one that can be tried. Also, if a schedule or way that you are taking the medicine does not work for you, changes can be made. Talk to your doctor or nurse because they can work with you to find the pain medicine that will help you the most.

It may be helpful for you to keep a record of how the medicine is working. Keeping a record and sharing it with your doctor or nurse will help to make your treatment more effective.

Other Treatments

Your doctor or nurse may recommend that you try other treatments along with your medicine to give you even more pain relief. Relaxation exercises help reduce pain. Many people find that cold packs, heating pads, massage, and rest help to relieve pain. Music or television may distract you from the pain. Your family members may want to help you to use these treatments. These treatments will help to make your medicines work better and relieve other symptoms, but they should not be used instead of your medicine.

Nondrug Treatments of Pain

Here are a few examples of treatments that can help to relieve your pain. You may use these treatments along with your regular medicine:

- Biofeedback.
- Breathing and relaxation.
- Imagery.
- Massage, pressure, vibration.
- Transcutaneous electrical nerve stimulation (TENS).
- Distraction.
- Hot or cold packs.
- Rest.

Talk to your doctor or nurse about these treatments. They will be able to give you more information. Also, the counseling and support groups listed below may be able to tell you more.

When Medicine Is Not Enough

Some patients have pain that is not relieved by medicine. In these cases other treatments can be used to reduce pain:

- **Radiation therapy.** This treatment reduces pain by shrinking a tumor. A single dose of radiation may be effective for some people.
- **Nerve blocks.** Pain medicine is injected directly around a nerve or into the spine to block the pain.
- **Neurosurgery.** In this treatment pain nerves (usually in the spinal cord) are cut to relieve the pain.
- **Surgery.** When a tumor is pressing on nerves or other body parts, operations to remove all or part of the tumor can relieve pain.

Talk to your doctor about other pain treatments that will work for you.

The First Step

The key to getting the best pain relief is talking with your doctor or nurse about your pain. They will want to know how much pain you feel, where it is, and what it feels like. Answering the questions below may help you describe your pain.

- **Where is the pain?** You may have pain in more than one place. Be sure to list all of the painful areas.
- **What does the pain feel like?** Does it ache? Throb? Burn? Tingle? You may wish to use other words to describe your pain.
- **How bad is the pain?** You can also use a number scale and rate your pain from 0 to 10: 0 means no pain and 10 means the worst pain. You may want to use a pain intensity scale to put a number to your pain. You can also describe your pain with words like none, mild, moderate, severe, or worst possible pain.

♦ **What makes the pain better or worse?** You may have already found ways to make your pain feel better. For example, using heat or cold, or taking certain medicines. You may have also found that sitting or lying in certain positions or doing some activities affects the pain.

♦ **If you are being treated for pain now, how well is the treatment working?** You may want to describe how well the treatment is working by saying how much of the pain is relieved—all, almost all, none, etc.

♦ **Has the pain changed?** You may notice that your pain changes over time. It may get better or worse or it can feel different. For example, the pain may have been a dull ache at first and has changed to a tingle. It is important to report changes in your pain. Changes in pain do not always mean that the cancer has come back or grown. Describe how the pain was before and how it is now.

After talking with you about your pain, your doctor or nurse may want to examine you or order x-rays or other tests.

These tests will help the doctor or nurse find the cause of your pain.

Having a Plan

You can work with your doctor or nurse to write a pain control plan to meet your needs. In a pain control plan, you and your doctor or nurse plan your pain control activities. This will include when to take your medicine, how and when to take extra medicine, and other things you can do to ease and prevent your pain. Your doctor or nurse may also list the medicines and other treatments you can use to help you with any side effects or other aches and pains, such as headaches.

Making the Plan Work

Some people find that the first pain control plan does not work for them. You and your doctor or nurse can change your pain control plan at any time. Here are some questions to ask yourself about the pain plan:

♦ Is the pain plan hard to follow?
♦ Is there any part of the plan that is hard to understand?
♦ Are you pleased with the pain control?
♦ Are you having trouble getting the medicine?
♦ Are you having trouble taking the medicine?
♦ Are you having side effects from the medicine?
♦ Is the medicine or the treatment causing a problem for you or your family?
♦ Are the nondrug treatments working for you?

Benefits and Risks of Treatment

This booklet talks about many different treatments for cancer pain. It also talks about side effects of medicines. Information about benefits and risks (side effects) of medicines may also be important to you. The list below describes the benefits and risks of the different types of medicines.

Nonopioids:

Benefits: Control mild to moderate pain. Some can be bought without a prescription.

Risks: Some of these medicines can cause stomach upset. They can also cause bleeding in the stomach, slow blood clotting, and cause kidney problems. Acetaminophen does not cause these side effects, but high doses of it can hurt the liver.

Opioids:

Benefits: These medicines control moderate to severe pain and do not cause bleeding.

Risks: May cause constipation, sleepiness, nausea and vomiting. Opioids sometimes cause problems with urination or itching. They may also slow breathing, especially when they are first given, but this is unusual in people who take opioids on a regular basis for pain.

Antidepressants:

Benefits: Antidepressants help to control tingling or burning pain from damaged nerves. They also improve sleep.

Risks: These medicines may cause dry mouth, sleepiness, and constipation. Some cause dizziness and lightheadedness when standing up suddenly.

Anticonvulsants:

Benefits: Help to control tingling or burning from nerve injury.

Risks: May hurt the liver and lower the number of red and white cells in the blood. It is important to have regular blood tests to check for these effects.

Steroids:

Benefits: Help relieve bone pain, pain caused by spinal cord and brain tumors, and pain caused by inflammation. Steroids also increase appetite.

Risks: May cause fluid to build up in the body. May also cause bleeding and irritation to the stomach. Confusion is a problem for some patients when taking steroids.

Counseling and Peer Support

Pain can make you feel many emotions. You may feel sad, helpless, vulnerable, angry, depressed, lonely, isolated, or other emotions. Lots of people feel these things when they are in pain. Often, when the pain is successfully treated, these feelings lift. Many people who have had cancer feel that counseling, religious, and other support groups have helped them to get back a sense of control and well being.

To find out more about support groups and to receive books and pamphlets about cancer pain, call or write to:

National Cancer Institute
Cancer Information Service
800-4-CANCER
Ask for the booklet *Questions and Answers About Pain Control.*

American Cancer Society
800-ACS02345
The booklet *Questions and Answers About Pain Control* is also available from this group.

Wisconsin Cancer Pain Initiative
Medical Science Center, Room 3675
University of Wisconsin Medical School
1300 University Avenue
Madison, WI 53706
608-262-0978
For adults, ask for *Cancer Pain Can Be Relieved.* For children with cancer pain, ask for *Children's Cancer Pain Can Be Relieved.* For adolescents with cancer pain, ask for *Jeff Asks About Cancer Pain.*

Slow Rhythmic Breathing for Relaxation

Deep breathing exercises can help relax you. These exercises may work along with your medicine to lessen or relieve your pain.

1. Breathe in slowly and deeply.
2. As you breathe out slowly, feel yourself beginning to relax; feel the tension leaving your body.
3. Now breathe in and out slowly and regularly, at whatever rate is comfortable for you.
4. To help you focus on your breathing and breathe slowly and rhythmically: (a) breathe in as you say silently to yourself, "in, two, three"; (b) breathe out as you say silently to yourself, "out, two, three," or each time you breathe out, say silently to yourself a word such as "peace" or "relax."
5. Do steps 1 through 4 only once or repeat steps 3 and 4 for up to 20 minutes.
6.   End with a slow deep breath. As you breathe out say to yourself "I feel alert and relaxed."

Document Source: McCaffery and Beebe, *Pain: Clinical manual for nursing practice*, 1989. Adapted and reprinted with permission.

■ **Document Source:**
   U.S. Department of Health and Human Services, Public Health Service
   Agency for Health Care Policy and Research
   Executive Office Center, Suite 501, 2101 East Jefferson Street,
      Rockville, MD 20852
   AHCPR Publication No. 94-0595
   March 1994

RADIATION THERAPY AND YOU: A GUIDE TO SELF-HELP DURING TREATMENT

Introduction

This booklet is for you if you are receiving radiation therapy for cancer. Its main purpose is to help you know what to expect and how to care for yourself during your treatment. It describes external radiation therapy and brachytherapy using radiation implants, the two most common types of radiation therapy. Information is included on radiation therapy methods

and the general effects of treatment. There are also some self-help "pointers" for specific side effects.

You may not want to read this whole booklet at one time. Flip through it, read the sections that are of interest to you right now, and look at the others as needed. Because your treatment will be planned specially for you and the type of cancer you have, some sections of the booklet will not apply to you.

Radiation therapy can vary among different doctors and hospitals. Therefore, your treatment program or the advice of your doctor (the radiation oncologist) may differ from what you read here. Be sure to ask questions and discuss your concerns with your doctor, nurse, or radiation therapist. Ask whether they have other booklets that also might help you.

You will find some helpful sections at the back of this booklet. Words that relate to radiation therapy and other aspects of cancer care appear in bold throughout this booklet; these words are defined in the "Glossary." Knowing the meanings of words can help you understand more about your illness and the roles of the people involved in your care. The "Resources" section tells you how to get more information about cancer and services for cancer patients from the National Cancer Institute and the American Cancer Society.

Radiation in Cancer Treatment

What is radiation therapy?

Radiation is a special kind of energy carried by waves or a stream of particles. It can come from special machines or from radioactive substances. Many years ago doctors learned how to use this energy to see inside the body and find disease. You've probably seen a chest x-ray or x-ray pictures of your teeth or your bones. When radiation is used at high doses (many times those used for x-ray exams), it can be used to treat cancer and other illnesses. Special equipment is used to aim the radiation at tumors or areas of the body where there is disease. The use of high-energy rays or particles to treat disease is called radiation therapy. Sometimes it's called **radiotherapy,** x-ray therapy, cobalt therapy, electron beam therapy, or irradiation.

How does radiation therapy work?

High doses of radiation can kill cells or keep them from growing and dividing. Radiation therapy is a useful tool for treating cancer because cancer cells grow and divide more rapidly than many of the normal cells around them. Although some normal cells are affected by radiation, most normal cells appear to recover more fully from the effects of radiation than do cancer cells. Doctors carefully limit the intensity of treatments and the area being treated so that the cancer will be affected more than normal tissue.

What are the benefits and goals of radiation therapy?

Radiation therapy is an effective way to treat many kinds of cancer in almost any part of the body. Half of all people with cancer are treated with radiation, and the number of cancer patients who have been cured is rising every day. For many patients, radiation is the only kind of treatment needed. Thousands of people are free of cancer after having radiation treatments alone or in combination with surgery, **chemotherapy,** or **biological therapy.**

Doctors can use radiation before surgery to shrink a **tumor.** After surgery, radiation therapy may be used to stop the growth of any cancer cells that remain. Your doctor may choose to use radiation therapy and surgery at the same time. This procedure, known as **intraoperative radiation,** is explained more fully later in this booklet. In some cases, doctors use radiation along with anticancer drugs to destroy the cancer, instead of surgery.

Even when curing the cancer is not possible, radiation therapy still can bring relief. Many patients find the quality of their lives improved when radiation therapy is used to shrink tumors and reduce pressure, bleeding, pain or other symptoms of cancer. This is called **palliative care.**

Are there risks involved?

Like many other treatments for disease, there are risks for patients who are receiving radiation therapy. The brief high doses of radiation that damage or destroy cancer cells also can hurt normal cells. When this happens, the patient has side effects. These side effects and what to do about them are discussed later in this booklet. The risk of side effects is usually less than the benefits of killing cancer cells.

Your doctor will not advise you to have any treatment unless the benefits—control of disease and relief from symptoms—are greater than the known risks. Although it will be many years before scientists know all of the possible risks of radiation therapy, they *now* know that it can control cancer.

How is radiation therapy given?

Radiation therapy can be in either of two forms: external or internal. Some patients have both forms, one after the other.

Most people who receive radiation therapy for cancer have the external type. It is usually given during outpatient visits to a hospital or treatment center. In external therapy, a machine directs the high-energy rays or particles at the cancer and the normal tissue surrounding it.

One type of machine that is used for radiation therapy is called a **linear accelerator.** High-energy rays may also come from a machine that contains a radioactive substance such as **cobalt-60.**

The various machines used for external radiation work in slightly different ways. Some are better for treating cancers near the skin surface; others work best on cancers deeper in the body. Your doctor decides which machine is best for you.

When **internal radiation** therapy is used, a radioactive substance, or source, is sealed in small containers such as thin wires or tubes called implants. The implant is placed directly into a tumor or inserted into a body cavity. Sometimes, after a tumor has been removed by surgery, implants are put into the area around the incision to kill any tumor cells that may remain.

Another type of internal radiation therapy uses unsealed radioactive sources. The source is either taken by mouth or is injected into the body. If you have this type of treatment, you will probably need to stay in the hospital for several days.

Who gives radiation treatments?

A doctor who has had special training in using radiation to treat disease—a **radiation oncologist**—will prescribe the type and amount of treatment that best suits your needs. The radiation oncologist is the person referred to as "your doctor" throughout this booklet.

The radiation oncologist works closely with other doctors involved in your care and also heads a highly trained health care team. Your radiation therapy team may include:

- The **radiation physicist,** who makes sure that the equipment is working properly and ensures that the machines deliver the right dose of radiation.
- The **dosimetrist,** who helps carry out your treatment plan by calculating the number of treatments and how long each treatment should last.
- The radiation therapy nurse, who provides nursing care and helps you learn about treatment and how to manage side effects.
- The **radiation therapist,** who sets you up for your treatments and runs the equipment that delivers the radiation.

You also may use the services of a **dietitian,** a **physical therapist,** a social worker, and other health care professionals.

Is radiation therapy expensive?

Treatment of cancer with radiation can be costly. It requires very complex equipment and the services of many health care professionals. The exact cost of your radiation therapy will depend on the type and number of treatments you need.

Most health insurance policies, including Part B of Medicare, cover charges for radiation therapy. It's a good idea to talk with your doctor's office staff or the hospital business office about your policy and how expected costs will be paid.

In some states, the Medicaid program may help you pay for treatments. You can find out from the office that handles social services in your city or county whether you are eligible for Medicaid and whether your radiation therapy is a covered expense.

If you need financial aid, contact the hospital social service office, the Cancer Information Service, or the local office of the American Cancer Society. They may be able to direct you to sources of help. These organizations are listed in the "Resources" section.

External Radiation Therapy: What to Expect

How does the doctor plan the treatment?

The radiation used in radiation therapy can come from a variety of sources. Your doctor may choose to use **x-rays,** an **electron beam,** or cobalt-60 **gamma rays.** Choosing which type of radiation to use depends on what type of cancer you have and on how deep into your body the doctor wants the radiation to penetrate. High-energy radiation is used to treat many types of cancer. Low-energy x-rays are used to treat some kinds of skin diseases.

After a physical exam and a review of your medical history, the radiation oncologist may need to do some special planning to pinpoint the treatment area. In a process called **simulation,** you will be asked to lie very still on a table while the radiation therapist uses a special x-ray machine to define your **treatment port** or **field.** This is the exact place on your body where the treatment will be aimed. You may have more than one treatment port. Simulation may take from a half hour to about 2 hours.

The radiation therapist often will mark the treatment port on your skin with tiny dots of colored, semipermanent ink to outline the treatment area. Be careful when you bathe because the marks must not be washed off until all of your treatment is over. If they start to fade, tell the therapist who will darken them so that they can be seen easily. Do not try to draw over faded lines at home unless they will be completely gone before your next visit. If you do replace the marks, be sure to tell the therapist at your next visit.

Using the information from the simulation, other tests, and your medical background, your doctor will meet with the radiation physicist and the dosimetrist. Your doctor then decides how much radiation is needed, how it will be delivered, and how many treatments you should have. This process often takes several days.

After you have started the treatments, your doctor will follow your progress, checking your response to treatment and your overall well-being at least once a week. The treatment plan may be revised by your doctor, if needed. It's very important that you have all of your scheduled treatments to get the most benefit from your therapy. Unnecessary delays can lessen the effectiveness of your radiation treatment.

How long does the treatment take?

Radiation therapy usually is given 5 days a week for 6 or 7 weeks. When radiation is used for palliative care, the course of treatment lasts for 2 to 3 weeks. These types of schedules, which use small amounts of daily radiation, rather than a few large doses, help protect normal body tissues in the treatment area. Weekend rest breaks allow normal cells to recover. The total dose of radiation and the number of treatments you need will depend on the size and location of your cancer, type of tumor, your general health, and any other treatments you're receiving.

What happens during each treatment visit?

Before your treatment is given, you may need to change into a hospital gown or robe. It's best to wear clothing that is easy to take off and put on again.

In the treatment room, the radiation therapist will use the marks on your skin to locate the treatment area. You will sit in a special chair or lie down on a treatment table. For each external radiation therapy session, you will be in the treatment room about 15 to 30 minutes, but you will be getting your dose of radiation for only about 1 to 5 minutes of that time. Receiving external radiation treatments is painless, just like having an x-ray taken.

The radiation therapist may put special shields (or blocks) between the machine and certain parts of your body to help protect normal tissues and organs. There might also be plastic or plaster forms to help you stay in exactly the right place. *You will need to remain very still during the treatment so that the radiation reaches only the area where it's needed and the same area is treated each time.* You don't have to hold your breath—just breathe normally.

The radiation therapist will leave the treatment room before the machine is turned on. The machine is controlled from a small area that is nearby. You will be watched on a television screen or through a window in the control room. Although you may feel alone, keep in mind that you can be seen and heard at all times by the therapist who can talk with you through a speaker.

The machines used for radiation treatments are very large, and they make noises as they move around to aim at the treatment area from different angles. Their size and motion may be frightening at first. Remember that the machines are being moved and controlled by your radiation therapist. They are checked constantly to be sure they're working right. If you are concerned about anything that happens in the treatment room, ask your therapist to explain.

You will not see or hear the radiation, and, most likely, you won't feel anything. If you do feel ill or very uncomfortable during the treatment, tell your therapist at once. The machine can be stopped at any time.

What is hyperfractionated radiation therapy?

Radiation is usually given once a day in a dose that is based on the type and location of the tumor. In **hyperfractionated radiation** therapy, the daily dose is divided into smaller doses that are given more than once a day. If more than one treatment is given per day to an area, the treatments usually are separated by 4 to 6 hours. Doctors are studying hyperfractionated therapy to see if it is equally or even more effective than once-a-day therapy. Early results in certain tumors are encouraging, and hyperfractionated therapy is becoming a more common way to give radiation treatments.

What is intraoperative radiation?

Intraoperative radiation combines surgery and radiation therapy at the same time. The surgeon removes as much as possible of the tumor; then a large dose of radiation is given directly to the tumor bed and nearby areas where cancer cells might have spread. In some hospitals, there is an operating room right in the radiation therapy department; in others, the patient is treated in the radiation therapy department and then returned to the operating room for surgery. Sometimes high-dose intraoperative radiation is used in addition to external radiation therapy to give the cancer cells a larger amount of radiation than would be safe with external radiation alone.

What are the effects of treatment?

External radiation therapy does not cause your body to become radioactive. There is no need to avoid being with other people because of your treatment. Even hugging, kissing, or having sexual relations with others poses no risk to them of radiation exposure.

Side effects of radiation therapy most often are related to the area that is being treated. Your doctor and nurse will tell you about the possible side effects and how you should deal with them. You should contact your doctor or nurse if you have any unusual symptoms during your treatment, such as coughing, sweating, fever, or unusual pain. Most side effects that occur during radiation therapy, although unpleasant, are not serious and can be controlled with medication or diet. They usually go away within a few weeks after treatment ends. However, some side effects can last longer. Many patients have no side effects at all. In another section of this booklet, "Managing Side Effects," you will find advice on how to cope with the side effects that might occur during and after your therapy.

Throughout your treatment, your radiation oncologist will regularly check on the effects of the treatment. You may not be aware of changes in the cancer, but you probably will notice decreases in pain, bleeding, or other discomforts you may have had, especially after your treatment is completed. You may continue to notice more improvements with time. Your doctor probably will recommend some tests to be sure that the radiation is causing as little damage to normal cells as possible. You may have routine blood tests to check the levels of **white blood cells** and **platelets,** which may be lower than normal during treatment.

What can I do to take care of myself during therapy?

Each patient's body responds to radiation therapy in its own way. That's why the doctor must plan, and sometimes adjust, your treatment just for you. In addition, your doctor or nurse will give you advice for caring for yourself at home that is specific for your treatment and the side effects that might result.

Nearly all cancer patients receiving radiation therapy need to take special care of themselves to protect their health and help the treatment succeed. Some guidelines to remember are given below:

- Be sure to get plenty of rest. Sleep as often as you feel the need. Your body will use a lot of extra energy over the course of your treatment, and you may feel very tired. In fact, fatigue may last for 4 to 6 weeks after your treatment is finished.
- Good nutrition is a must. Try to eat a balanced diet that will prevent weight loss. For patients who have problems with eating or diet planning, the section titled "Managing Side Effects" offers practical tips.
- Avoid wearing tight clothes such as girdles or close-fitting collars over the treatment area. It's best to wear older garments that feel comfortable and that you can wash or throw away if the ink marks rub off on them.
- Be *extra* kind to the skin in the treatment area.
  - *Do not use any soaps, lotions, deodorants, medicines, perfumes, cosmetics, talcum powder, or other substances in the treated area without talking with your doctor.*
  - Wear loose, soft cotton clothing over the treated area.
  - Do not starch your clothes.
  - Do not rub or scrub treated skin.
  - Do not use adhesive tape on treated skin. If bandaging is necessary, use paper tape. Try to apply the tape outside of the treatment area.

- Do not apply heat or cold (heating pad, ice pack, etc.) to the treatment area. Even hot water can hurt your skin, so use only lukewarm water for bathing the treated area.
- Use an electric shaver if you must shave the area—but only after checking with your doctor or nurse. Do not use a preshave lotion or hair remover products.
- Protect the area from the sun. If possible, cover treated skin (with light clothing) before going outside. Ask your doctor if you should use a lotion that contains a sunblock. If so, use a PABA sunscreen or a sunblocking product with a protection factor of at least 15. Reapply the sunscreen often, even after your skin has healed following your treatment. Continue to protect your skin from sunlight for at least 1 year after radiation therapy.
- Be sure your doctor knows about any medicines you are taking before starting treatment. If you need to start taking any medicines, even aspirin, let your doctor know before you start.
- Ask your doctor, nurse, or radiation therapist any questions you have. They are the only ones who can properly advise you about your treatment, side effects, at-home care, and any other medical concerns you may have.

Internal Radiation Therapy: What to Expect

When is internal radiation therapy used?

Your doctor may decide that very intense radiation given to a small area of your body is the best way to treat your cancer. Internal radiation therapy places the source of the high-energy rays as close as possible to the cancer cells so that fewer normal cells are exposed to radiation. By using internal radiation therapy, the doctor can give a higher total dose of radiation in a shorter time than is possible with external treatment. Instead of using a large radiation machine, the radioactive material is placed directly into (or as close as possible to) the affected area. Some of the radioactive substances used for internal radiation treatment include radium, cesium, iridium, iodine, phosphorus, and palladium.

Internal radiation therapy often is used for cancers of the head and neck, breast, uterus, thyroid, cervix, and prostate. Your doctor may recommend a combination of internal and external radiation therapy.

Implant radiation as used in this booklet means internal radiation treatment. You also may hear the terms **interstitial radiation, intracavitary radiation,** or **brachytherapy**; each is a form of internal radiation therapy. Some people use the term "brachytherapy" whenever they are talking about any form of internal radiation therapy.

When interstitial radiation is given, the radiation source is placed right in the affected tissue, usually in small tubes or containers. These **implants** may be temporary or permanent. When intracavitary radiation is used, a container of radioactive material is placed in a cavity of the body such as the uterus. In brachytherapy, the radioactive source, which is sealed in a small container, is placed on the surface of the body near the tumor or a short distance from the affected area. The radioactive source also may be delivered to the tumor through tubes; this is called **remote brachytherapy.** Internal radiation also may be given by injecting a solution of radioactive substance into the bloodstream or a body cavity. When the substance is injected, it is not sealed in a container and may be called **unsealed internal radiation therapy.**

How is the implant placed in the body?

For most types of implants, you will need to be in the hospital and have general or local **anesthesia** while the doctor places the container for the radioactive material in your body. In many hospitals, the radioactive material is placed in the container after you return to your room so that others are not exposed to radiation.

To get the radiation as close as possible to the cancer, doctors may use implants of radioactive material sealed in wires, seeds, capsules, or needles. The type of implant and the method of placing it depend on the size and location of the cancer. Implants may be put right into the tumor, in special applicators inside a body cavity, on the surface of a tumor, or in the area from which the tumor has been taken.

Does the implant spread radiation to others?

The radioactive substance in your implant may transmit rays outside your body. While you're receiving implant therapy, the hospital may require you to stay in a private room. Although the nurses and other people caring for you will not be able to spend a long time in your room, they will give you all of the care you need. You should call for a nurse when you need one, but keep in mind that the nurse will work quickly and speak to you from the doorway more often than from your bedside. In most cases, your urine and stool will contain no radioactivity. However, either one may contain some radioactive material if you have unsealed internal radiation therapy.

There also will be limits on visitors while your implant is in place. Most hospitals do not let children younger than 18 or pregnant women visit patients who have an implant. Visitors should sit at least 6 feet from your bed and stay for only a short time each day (10 to 30 minutes). Have visitors ask your nurse for specific instructions before thay enter your room.

Are there any side effects?

You are not likely to have severe pain or feel ill during implant therapy. However, if an applicator is holding your implant in place, it may be somewhat uncomfortable. If you need it, the doctor will order medicine to help you relax or to relieve pain. Some patients feel drowsy, weak, or nauseated after having the anesthesia to place the implant, but these effects do not last long.

Be sure to tell the nurse if you have any side effects such as burning, sweating, or other unusual symptoms. In the section of this booklet called "Managing Side Effects," you will find tips on skin care and what you can do about problems that might occur after implant therapy.

How long does the implant stay in place?

The total amount of time that an implant is left in place depends on the dose (amount) of radioactivity with which the patient is treated. The implant may be low dose rate and left in place for several days, or it may be high dose rate and removed after a few minutes. Generally, low dose rate implants are left in place from 1 to 7 days. Your treatment schedule will depend on the type of cancer, where it is, your general health, and other cancer treatments you have had. Depending on where the implant is placed, you may have to stay in bed and lie fairly still to keep the implant from shifting.

For some cancer sites, the implant may be left in place permanently. If your implant is permanent, you may need to stay in your room away from other people in the hospital for a few days while the radiation is most active. The implant will lose energy each day, so by the time you are ready to go home, the radiation in your body will be much weaker. Your doctor will advise you if there are any special precautions you need to use at home.

High dose rate remote brachytherapy allows a person to be treated within a few minutes in inpatient or outpatient clinics. With remote brachytherapy, a very powerful radioactive source travels by remote control through tubes, or **catheters,** to the tumor. The radioactivity remains at the tumor for only a few minutes. This procedure is done by the brachytherapy team, who will watch you on a closed-circuit television. They will talk to you through an intercom. In some cases, several remote treatments may be required. Sometimes, the catheter stays in place between treatments and sometimes it is removed, depending on your condition.

High dose rate treatments are short (usually a few minutes) and result in less discomfort than other types of radiation therapy. Because radioactive materials are not left in your body, you can return home soon after you recover. Remote brachytherapy has been used to treat cancers of the cervix, breast, lung, pancreas, prostate, and esophagus.

What happens after the implant is removed?

Usually there is no need to have an anesthetic to take out the implant. Most can be taken out right in the patient's hospital room. If you had to stay in bed during implant therapy, you might have to remain in the hospital an extra day or so after the implant is removed. Once the implant is removed, there is no radioactivity in your body. The nurses and your visitors no longer will have to observe any special rules.

Your doctor will tell you if you should limit your activities after leaving the hospital. Most patients are allowed to do as much as they feel like doing. You may need some extra sleep or rest breaks during your first days at home, but you will feel stronger quickly.

The area that has been treated with an implant may be sore or sensitive for some time after therapy. Your doctor may advise you to limit sports and sexual activity for a while if they cause irritation in the treatment area.

Managing Side Effects

Are side effects the same for everyone?

The side effects of radiation treatment vary from patient to patient. You may have no side effects or only a few mild ones through your course of treatment. Or you may have more serious side effects. The side effects that you have depend mostly on the treatment dose and the part of your body that is treated. Your general health also can affect how your body reacts to radiation therapy and whether you have side effects. Before beginning your treatment, ask your doctor and nurse about the side effects you might experience, how long they might last, and how serious they might be.

There are two main types of side effects: acute and chronic. Acute, or short-term, side effects occur close to the time of the treatment and usually are gone completely within a few weeks of finishing therapy. Chronic, or long-term, side effects may take months or years to develop and usually are permanent.

The most common side effects are fatigue, skin changes, and loss of appetite. They can result from radiation to any treatment site. Other side effects are related to treatment of specific areas. For example, temporary or permanent hair loss may be a side effect of radiation treatment to the head. This chapter discusses common side effects first. Then side effects involving specific body parts are described.

Fortunately, most side effects will go away in time. In the meantime, there are ways to reduce the discomfort they cause. If you have a side effect that is particularly severe, the doctor may prescribe a break in your treatments or change the kind of treatment you're receiving.

Be sure to tell your doctor, nurse, or radiation therapist about any side effects that you notice. They can help you treat the problems and tell you how to lessen the chances that the side effects will come back. The information in this booklet can serve as a guide to handling some side effects, but it cannot replace talking with your health care team.

Will side effects limit my activity?

Not necessarily. It will depend on what side effects you have and how severe they are. Many patients are able to go to work, keep house, and enjoy leisure activities while they are receiving radiation therapy. Others find that they need more rest than usual and therefore cannot do as much. You should try to do the things you enjoy as long as you don't become too tired.

Your doctor may suggest that you limit activities that might irritate the area being treated. In most cases, you can have sexual relations if you wish. Your desire for physical intimacy may be lower because radiation therapy may cause you to feel more tired than usual. For most patients, these feelings are temporary.

What causes fatigue?

During radiation therapy, the body uses a lot of energy healing itself. Stress related to your illness, daily trips for treatment, and the effects of radiation on normal cells all may contribute to fatigue. Most people begin to feel tired after a few weeks of radiation therapy. Feelings of weakness or weariness will go away gradually after your treatment is finished.

You can help yourself during radiation therapy by not trying to do too much. If you feel tired, limit your activities and use your leisure time in a restful way. Do not feel that you have to do all the things you normally do. Try to get more sleep at night, and rest during the day if you can.

If you have been working a full-time job, you may want to continue. Although treatment visits are time-consuming, you can ask your doctor's office or the radiation therapy department to help by trying to schedule treatments with your workday in mind.

Some patients prefer to take a few weeks off from work while they're receiving radiation therapy; others work a reduced number of hours. You may want to speak frankly with your employer about your needs and wishes during this time. You may be able to agree on a part-time schedule, or perhaps you can do some work at home.

Whether you're going to work or not, it's a good idea to ask family members or friends to help with daily chores, shopping, child care, housework, or driving. Neighbors may be able to help by picking up groceries for you when they do their own shopping. You also could ask someone to drive you to and from your treatment visits to help conserve your energy.

How are skin problems treated?

You may notice that your skin in the treatment area may begin to look reddened, irritated, sunburned, or tanned. After a few weeks you may have very dry skin from the therapy. Ask your doctor or nurse for advice on relieving itching or discomfort. With some kinds of radiation therapy, treated skin may develop a "moist reaction," especially in areas where there are skin folds. When this happens, the skin is wet and it may become very sore. It's important to notify your doctor or nurse if your skin develops a moist reaction. They can give you some suggestions on how you can keep these areas dry. Other helpful tips can be found below.

During radiation therapy you will need to be very gentle with the skin in the treatment area. Avoid irritating treated skin. When you wash, use only luke-warm water and mild soap. Don't wear tight clothing over the area. It's important not to rub, scrub, or scratch any sensitive spots. Also avoid putting anything that is very hot or very cold, such as heating pads or ice packs, on your treated skin. Don't use any powders, creams, perfumes, deodorants, body oils, ointments, lotions, or home remedies in the treatment area while you're being treated or for several weeks afterward (unless approved by your doctor or nurse). Many skin products can leave a coating on the skin that can interfere with radiation therapy or healing.

Avoid exposing the area to the sun during treatment and for at least 1 year after your treatment is completed. If you expect to be in the sun for more than a few minutes you will need to be very careful. Wear protective clothing (such as a hat with a broad brim and a shirt with long sleeves) and use a sunscreen. Ask your doctor or nurse about using sunblocking lotions.

The majority of skin reactions to radiation therapy should go away a few weeks after treatment is finished. In some cases, though, the treated skin will remain darker than it was before.

What can be done about hair loss?

Radiation therapy can cause hair loss, also known as **alopecia**, but only in the area being treated. For example, if you are receiving treatment to your hip, you will not lose the hair from your head. However, radiation to your head may cause you to lose some or all of the hair on your scalp. Many patients find that their hair grows back again after the treatments are finished, but accepting the loss of hair—whether from scalp, face, or body—can be a hard adjustment. The amount of hair that grows back will depend on how much radiation you receive and the type of radiation treatment your doctor recommends. Other types of treatment, such as chemotherapy, also can affect how your hair grows back. For example, if your radiation therapy is for palliative care, your hair probably will grow back slowly. However, if the goal of your radiation therapy is to cure rather than to relieve the symptoms of your cancer, then your hair may not grow back, and if it does, it probably will be very fine.

Although your scalp may be tender after the hair is lost, you may want to cover your head with a hat, turban, or scarf while you're in treatment. Also, you should wear a protective cap or scarf when you're in the sun. If you prefer a wig or toupee, be sure the lining does not irritate your scalp. A hairpiece that you need because of cancer treatment is a tax-deductible expense and may be covered in part by your health insurance. If you plan to buy a wig, it's a good idea to select it early in your treatment so that you can match the color and style to your own hair.

What about side effects on the blood?

Sometimes radiation therapy can cause low white blood cell counts or low levels of platelets. These blood cells help your body fight infection and prevent bleeding. If your blood tests show this side effect, your treatment might be delayed for about a week to allow your blood counts to increase.

What if there are eating problems?

Many side effects can cause problems with eating and digesting food, but you always should try to eat enough to help damaged tissues rebuild themselves. It's very important not to lose weight during radiation therapy. Try to eat small meals often and eat a variety of different foods. Your doctor or nurse can tell you whether your treatment calls for a special diet, and a dietitian will have a lot of ideas to help you maintain your weight.

Coping with short-term diet problems may be easier than you expect. There are a number of diet guides and recipe booklets for patients who need help with eating problems. Another NCI booklet, *Eating Hints,* tells how to get more calories and protein without eating more food and provides further tips to help you enjoy eating. The recipes it contains can be used for the whole family and are marked for people with special concerns, such as low-salt diets.

If you have pain when you chew and swallow, your doctor may advise you to use a powdered or liquid diet supplement. Many of these products, available at the drugstore without prescription, are made in a variety of flavors. They are tasty when used alone, or they can be combined with other foods, such as pureed fruit, or added to milkshakes. Some of the companies that make diet supplements have produced recipe booklets to help you increase your nutrient intake. Ask your dietitian or pharmacist for further information.

You may lose interest in food during your treatment. Loss of appetite can happen when changes occur in normal cells. Some people just don't feel like eating because of stress from their illness and treatment or because the treatment changes the way foods taste. Even if you're not very hungry, it's important that you make every effort to keep your protein and calorie intake high. Doctors have found that patients who eat well can better handle both their cancer and the side effects of treatment.

The list below suggests ways to perk up your appetite when it's poor and to make the most of it when you do feel like eating.

- ♦ Eat when you are hungry, even if it is not mealtime.
- ♦ Eat several small meals during the day rather than three large ones.
- ♦ Use soft lighting, quiet music, brightly colored table settings, or whatever helps you feel good while eating.
- ♦ Vary your diet and try new recipes.
- ♦ If you enjoy company while eating, try to have meals with family or friends, or turn on the radio or television.
- ♦ Ask your doctor or nurse whether you can have a glass of wine or beer with your meal to increase your appetite. Keep in mind that in some cases, alcohol may not be allowed because of the chance that it will worsen the side effects of treatment. This may be especially true if you are receiving radiation therapy for cancer of the head or neck.
- ♦ When you feel up to it, make some simple meals in batches and freeze them to use later.
- ♦ Keep healthy snacks close by for nibbling when you get the urge.
- ♦ If other people offer to cook for you, let them. And don't be shy about telling them what you'd like to eat.
- ♦ If you live alone, you might want to arrange for "Meals on Wheels" to bring food to you. Ask your doctor, nurse, local American Cancer Society office, or Cancer Information Service about "Meals on Wheels." This service is active in most large communities.

If you are able to eat only small amounts of food, you can increase the calories per serving by trying the following ideas:

- ♦ Add butter or margarine if you like the flavor.
- ♦ Mix canned cream soups with milk or half-and-half rather than water.
- ♦ Drink eggnogs, milkshakes, or prepared liquid supplements between meals.
- ♦ Add cream sauce or melted cheese to your favorite vegetables.

Some people find they can handle large amounts of liquids even when they don't feel like eating solid foods. If this is the case for you, try to get the most from each glassful by having drinks enriched with powdered milk, yogurt, honey, or prepared liquid supplements.

Does radiation therapy affect the emotions?

Nearly all patients who receive treatment for cancer feel some degree of emotional upset. It's not unusual to feel depressed, afraid, angry, frustrated, alone, or helpless. Radiation therapy may affect the emotions indirectly through fatigue or changes in hormone balance, but the treatment itself is not a direct cause of mental distress.

Many patients help themselves by talking about their feelings with a close friend, family member, chaplain, nurse, social worker, or psychologist with whom they feel at ease. You may want to ask your doctor or nurse about meditation or relaxation exercises that could help you unwind and feel better.

American Cancer Society nationwide programs can provide support. Groups such as the United Ostomy Association and the Lost Chord Club offer opportunities to meet with others who share the same problems and concerns. Some medical centers have formed peer support groups so that patients can meet to discuss their feelings and inspire each other.

There are several helpful books and other materials on this subject. The Cancer Information Service can direct you to reading matter and other resources in your area.

What side effects occur with radiation therapy to the head and neck area?

Some people who are having radiation to the head and neck have redness and irritation in the mouth, a dry mouth, difficulty in swallowing, changes in taste, or nausea. Try not to let these symptoms keep you from eating.

Other problems that may occur during treatment to the head and neck are a loss of your sense of taste, earaches (caused by hardening of ear wax), and swelling or drooping of skin under the chin. There may be changes in your skin texture. You also may notice that your jaw feels stiff and that you cannot open your mouth as wide as before your treatment. Jaw exercises may help this problem. Report any side effects to your doctor or nurse and ask what you should do about them.

If you are receiving radiation therapy to the head or neck, you need to take especially good care of your teeth, gums, mouth, and throat. Side effects from treatment to these areas most often involve the mouth, which may be sore and dry.

Here are a few tips that may help you manage mouth problems:

- Avoid spices and coarse foods such as raw vegetables, dry crackers, and nuts.
- Don't smoke, chew tobacco, or drink alcohol.
- Stay away from sugary snacks that promote tooth decay.
- Clean your mouth and teeth often, using the method your dentist or doctor recommends.
- Do not use a commercial mouthwash; the alcohol content has a drying effect on mouth tissues.

Dental care

Radiation treatment for head and neck cancer can increase your chances of getting cavities. Mouth care designed to prevent problems will be a very important part of your treatment. Before starting radiation therapy, notify your dentist and arrange for a complete dental/oral checkup. *Ask your dentist to consult with your radiation oncologist about any dental work you need before your radiation treatments begin.*

Your dentist probably will want to see you often over the course of your radiation therapy. Your dentist can give you very detailed instructions about caring for your mouth and teeth to reduce the risk of tooth decay and will help you deal with possible problems such as soreness of the tissues in your mouth. It is important to your total well-being that you follow the dentist's advice while you're receiving radiation therapy. Most likely, you will be advised to:

- Clean teeth and gums thoroughly with a soft brush after meals and at least once more each day.
- Use a fluoride toothpaste that contains no abrasives.
- Floss gently between teeth daily, especially if you flossed regularly before your illness.
- Use a disclosing solution or tablet after brushing to reveal plaque that you've missed.
- Rinse your mouth well with a salt and baking soda solution after you brush. Use 1/2 teaspoon of salt and 1/2 teaspoon of baking soda in 1 quart of water.
- Apply **fluoride** regularly as prescribed by your dentist.

Your dentist can explain how to use disclosing tablets, how to mix the salt and baking soda mouthwash, and how to use the fluoride treatment method that best suits your needs. Most likely you can get printed instructions for proper dental care at the dentist's office.

Handling mouth or throat problems

Soreness in your mouth or throat may appear in the second or third week of external radiation therapy. It is likely to decrease from the fifth week on and end a month or so after your treatment ends. You may have trouble swallowing during this time because your mouth feels dry. Your doctor or dentist can prescribe medicine for mouth discomfort and advise your about methods to relieve other mouth problems.

If you wear dentures you may notice that they no longer fit well. This may happen if the radiation causes swelling in your gums. It's important not to let your dentures cause gum sores that may become infected. You may need to stop wearing your dentures until your radiation therapy is over.

Your glands may produce less saliva than usual, making your mouth feel dry. It's helpful to sip cool drinks often throughout the day. Water probably is your best choice. In the morning, fill up a large cup or glass with ice, add water, and carry it with you so you have something to drink during the day. Keep a glass of cool water at your bedside at night, too. Many radiation therapy patients say that drinking carbonated beverages helps relieve dry mouth. Sugar-free candy or gum also may help. Avoid tobacco and alcoholic drinks because they will dry and irritate your mouth tissues even more. Moisten food with gravies and sauces to make eating easier. If these measures are not enough, ask your dentist about artificial saliva. Dry mouth may continue to be a problem even after treatment is over.

Tips on eating

If you are having radiation therapy to the chest, you may find swallowing difficult or painful. Some patients say that it feels like something is stuck in their throat.

Soreness or dryness in your mouth or throat can make it hard to eat. However, there are several ways to ease your discomfort:

- Choose foods that taste good to you and are easy to eat.
- Try changing the consistency of foods by adding fluids and using sauces and gravies to make them softer.

♦ Avoid highly spiced foods and textures that are dry and rough, such as crackers.

♦ Eat small meals, and eat more frequently than usual.

♦ Cut your food into small, bite-sized pieces.

♦ Ask your doctor for special liquid medicines that can help you eat and swallow more easily by reducing the pain in your throat.

♦ Ask your doctor about liquid food supplements. These can help you meet your energy needs.

♦ If you are being treated for lung cancer, and you get your doctor's okay, try to drink extra fluids. This will help keep mucus and other secretions thin and manageable.

♦ If your sense of taste changes during radiation therapy, try different methods of food preparation.

Also, many helpful suggestions can be found in the NCI booklet, *Eating Hints*.

What side effects occur with radiation therapy to the breast and chest?

Radiation treatment to the chest may cause several changes. You will notice some of these changes yourself, and your treatment team will keep an eye on these and others. For example, you may find that it is hard to swallow or that swallowing hurts. Your may develop a cough. Or you may develop a fever, notice a change in the color or amount of mucus when you cough, or feel short of breath. It is important to let your treatment team know right away if you have any of these symptoms. Your doctor also may check your blood counts regularly, especially if the radiation treatment area on your body is large. Just keep in mind that your doctor and nurse will be alert for these changes and will help you deal with them.

If you are receiving radiation therapy after a lumpectomy or mastectomy, it's a good idea to go without wearing a bra whenever possible. If this is not possible, wear a soft cotton bra without underwires. This will help reduce the irritation to your skin in the treatment area. You may have several other side effects if you are receiving radiation therapy for breast cancer. For example, you may notice a lump in your throat or develop a dry cough. Or, your shoulder may feel stiff; if so, ask your doctor or nurse about exercises to keep your arm moving freely. Other side effects that may appear are breast soreness and swelling from fluid build up in the treated area. These side effects, as well as skin reddening or tanning, most likely will disappear in 4 to 6 weeks. If fluid buildup continues to be a problem, your doctor will tell you what steps to take.

Women who have radiation therapy after a lumpectomy may notice other changes in the breast after the therapy. These long-term side effects may continue for a year or longer after treatment. The redness of the skin will fade, and you may notice that your skin is slightly darker, just as when a sunburn fades to a suntan. The pores may be enlarged and more noticeable. Some women report increased sensitivity of the skin on the breast; others have decreased feeling. The skin and the fatty tissue of the breast may feel thicker, and you may notice that your breast is firmer than it was before your radiation treatment. Sometimes the size of your breast changes—it may become larger because of fluid buildup or smaller because of the development of fibrous tissue. Many women have little or no change in size.

Your radiation therapy plan may include implants of radioactive material a week or two after external treatment is completed. You may have some breast tenderness or a feeling of tightness while the implants are in your breast. After they are removed, you are likely to notice some of the same effects that occur with external treatment. If so, follow the advice given above and let your doctor know about any problems that persist.

After 10 to 12 months, no further changes are likely to be caused by the radiation therapy. If you see new changes in breast size, shape, appearance, or texture after this time, report them to your doctor at once.

What side effects occur with radiation therapy to the stomach and abdomen?

If you are having radiation treatment to the stomach or some portion of the abdomen, you may have to deal with an upset stomach, nausea, or diarrhea. Your doctor can prescribe medicines to relieve these problems. Do not take any home remedies during your treatment unless you first check with your doctor or nurse.

Managing nausea

Some patients report feeling queasy for a few hours right after radiation therapy to the stomach or abdomen. If you have this problem, do not eat for several hours before your treatment time. You may be able to handle the treatment better on an empty stomach. After your treatment, you may find it helpful to wait 1 to 2 hours before eating again. If the problem persists, ask your doctor to prescribe a medicine (an **antiemetic**) to prevent nausea. If antiemetics are prescribed, try to take them when your doctor suggests, even if you sometimes feel that they are not needed.

If your stomach feels upset just before your treatment, try a bland snack such as toast or crackers and apple juice before your appointment. This type of side effect may be related to your emotions and concerns about treatment. Try to unwind a bit before you have your treatment. If you have to spend time in a waiting room, reading a book, writing letters, or working a crossword puzzle may help you relax.

Here are some tips to help an unsettled stomach:

♦ Stick to any special diet that your doctor or dietitian gives you.

♦ Eat small meals.

♦ Eat often and try to eat and drink slowly.

♦ Avoid foods that are fried or are high in fat.

♦ Drink cool liquids between meals.

♦ Eat foods that have only a mild aroma and those that can be served cool or at room temperature.

♦ For a severe upset stomach, try a clear liquid diet (broth and juices) or bland foods that are easy to digest, such as dry toast and gelatin.

How to handle diarrhea

Diarrhea most often begins in the third or fourth week of radiation therapy. Your doctor may suggest you change your diet, prescribe medicine for you, or give you special instructions to help with the problem. Tell the doctor or nurse if these changes are not controlling your diarrhea.

The following changes in your diet also may help:

♦ Try a clear liquid diet (water, weak tea, apple juice, clear broth, plain gelatin) as soon as diarrhea starts or when you feel that it's going to start.

♦ Ask your doctor or nurse to advise you about liquids that won't make your diarrhea worse. Apple juice, peach nectar, weak tea, and clear broth are frequent suggestions.

♦ Avoid foods that are high in fiber or can cause cramps or a gassy feeling such as raw fruits and vegetables, coffee, beans, cabbage, whole grain breads and cereals, sweets, and spicy foods.

♦ Eat frequent small meals.

♦ Avoid milk and milk products if they irritate your bowels.

♦ When the diarrhea starts to improve, try eating small amounts of low-fiber foods such as rice, bananas, apple-sauce, mashed potatoes, low-fat cottage cheese, and dry toast.

♦ Be sure your diet includes foods that are high in potassium (bananas, potatoes, apricots), an important mineral that you may lose through diarrhea.

Diet planning is a very important part of radiation treatment of the stomach and abdomen. Keep in mind that these problems will be reduced greatly when treatment is over. In the meantime, try to pack the highest possible food value into even small meals so that you will have enough calories and vital nutrients.

What side effects occur with radiation therapy to the pelvis?

If you are having radiation therapy to any part of the pelvis (the area between your hips), you might have one or more of the digestive problems already described. You also may have some irritation to your bladder. This can cause discomfort or frequent urination. Drinking fluids can help relieve some of your discomfort. Your doctor can prescribe some medicine to deal with these problems.

There are also certain side effects that occur only in the reproductive organs. The effects of radiation therapy on sexual and reproductive functions depend on which organs are treated. Some of the more common side effects for both men and women do not last long after treatment. Others may be long-term or permanent. Before your treatment begins, ask your doctor about possible side effects and how long they might last.

Effects on fertility

Scientists are still studying how radiation treatment affects fertility. If you are a women in your childbearing years, you should discuss birth control measures with your doctor. It is not a good idea to become pregnant during radiation therapy. Radiation may injure the fetus. In addition, pregnancy, childbirth, and caring for a very young child can add to the physical and emotional stress of having cancer. If you are pregnant before beginning radiation therapy, special steps should be taken to protect the fetus from radiation.

Depending on the radiation dose, women having radiation therapy in the pelvic area may stop menstruating and may have other symptoms of menopause. Treatment also can result in vaginal itching, burning, and dryness. You should report these symptoms to your doctor or nurse, who can suggest treatment.

For men, radiation therapy to an area that includes the testes can reduce both the number of sperm and their effectiveness. This does not mean that conception cannot occur, however. If you're having this type of treatment, discuss your concerns and your birth control measures with your doctor. If you want to father a child and are concerned about reduced fertility, you can look into the option of banking your sperm before treatment.

Sexual relations

During treatment to the pelvis, some women are advised not to have intercourse. Others may find that intercourse is painful. You most likely will be able to resume having sex within a few weeks after your treatment ends.

Some shrinking of vaginal tissues occurs during radiation therapy. After your radiation therapy is finished your doctor will advise you about sexual intercourse and how to use a dilator, a device that gently stretches the tissues of the vagina.

With most types of radiation therapy, neither men nor women are likely to suffer any change in their ability to enjoy sex. Both sexes, however, may notice a decrease in their level of desire. This is more likely to be due to the stress of having cancer than to the effects of radiation therapy. This effect most likely will go away when the treatment ends, so it should not become a major concern. A booklet on sexuality and cancer is available without charge from your local American Cancer Society office. There are different versions for male and female patients.

Followup Care

What does "followup" mean?

Once your course of radiation therapy is finished, it is important to have regular exams to check the results of your treatment. No matter what type of cancer you've had, you will need regular checkups and perhaps lab tests and x-rays. The radiation oncologist will want to see you at least once after your treatment ends. The doctor who referred you for radiation therapy will schedule followup visits as needed. Followup care, in addition to checking the results of your treatment, might also include more cancer treatment, rehabilitation, and counseling. Taking good care of yourself is also a part of following through after radiation treatments.

Who provides care after therapy?

Most patients return to the radiation oncologist for regular followup visits. Others are referred back to their original doctor, to a surgeon, or to a **medical oncologist**, a doctor who is trained to give chemotherapy (treatment with anticancer drugs). Your followup care will depend on the kind of cancer you have and on other treatments that you had or may need.

What other care might be needed?

Just as every patient is different, followup care varies. Your doctor will prescribe and schedule the followup care that you need. Don't hesitate to ask about the tests or treatments that your doctor orders. Try to learn all the things you should do to take good care of yourself.

Following are some of the questions that you may want to ask your doctor after you have finished your radiation therapy:

- How often do I need to return for checkups?
- Why do I need more x-rays, scans, blood tests, and so on? What will these tests tell us?
- Will I need chemotherapy, surgery, or other treatments?
- How will you know if I'm cured of cancer? What are the chances that it will come back?
- How soon can I go back to my regular activities?
  - Work?
  - Sexual activity?
  - Sports?
- Do I need to take any special precautions?
- Do I need a special diet?
- Should I exercise?
- Can I wear a prosthesis?
- How soon can I have reconstructive surgery?

You may want to write down other questions and take the list with you to your doctor's office.

What if pain is a problem?

A few patients need help to manage pain if it continues after radiation therapy. You should not use a heating pad or warm compress to relieve pain in any area treated with radiation. Mild pain medicine may be enough for some people. If you have severe pain, ask the doctor about prescription drugs or other methods of relief. Be as specific as possible when telling the doctor about your pain so you can get the best treatment for it. If you are unable to get relief from pain, you may want to talk with a doctor who is a pain specialist.

Because pain can be worse when you are afraid or worried, it may help to try relaxation exercises. Other methods such as hypnosis, biofeedback, and acupuncture may be useful for some cancer patients. *Questions and Answers About Pain Control* is a free booklet that may help you understand more about cancer pain.

How can I help myself after radiation therapy?

Patients who have had radiation therapy need to continue some of the special care used during treatment at least for a short while. For instance, you may have skin problems for several weeks after your treatments end. You should continue to be gentle with skin in the treatment area until all signs of irritation are gone. Don't try to scrub off the marks in your treatment area. They will fade and wear away.

You may find that you still need extra rest while your healthy tissues are rebuilding. Keep taking naps as needed and try to get more sleep at night. You may need some time to test your strength, little by little, so you may not want to resume a full schedule of activities right away.

When should I call the doctor?

After treatment for cancer, you're likely to be more aware of your body and to notice even slight changes in how you feel from day to day. The doctor will want you to report any unusual symptoms. If you have any of the problems listed below, tell your doctor at once:

- A pain that doesn't go away, especially if it's always in the same place.
- Lumps, bumps, or swelling.
- Nausea, vomiting, diarrhea, or loss of appetite.
- Unexplained weight loss.
- A fever or cough that doesn't go away.
- Unusual rashes, bruises, or bleeding.
- Any other signs mentioned by your doctor or nurse.

What about returning to work?

Many people continue to work during radiation therapy, but if you have stopped working, you can return to your job as soon as you feel up to it, even while your radiation therapy is continuing. If your job requires lifting or heavy physical activity, you may need to change your activities until you have regained your strength.

When you are ready to return to work, it is important to learn about your rights regarding your job and health insurance. If you have any questions about employment issues, contact the Cancer Information Service or the American Cancer Society. They can help you find local agencies that respond to problems cancer survivors sometimes face regarding employment and insurance rights. These organizations are listed in the "Resources" section at the end of this booklet.

Conclusion

We hope the information in this booklet will help you understand how radiation therapy is used to treat cancer. Knowing what to expect when you go for your treatments should lessen the anxiety you may be feeling. Don't forget to call on your health care team whenever you need more information.

Glossary

These are words that appear in this booklet or that you may hear your health team use.

Adjuvant therapy. A treatment method used in addition to the primary therapy. Radiation therapy often is used as an adjuvant to surgery.

Alopecia (al-oh-PEE-she-ah). Hair loss.

Anesthesia. Loss of feeling or sensation resulting from the use of certain drugs or gases.

Antiemetic (an-tee-eh-MET-ik). A medicine to prevent or relieve nausea or vomiting.

Benign tumor. A growth that is not a cancer and does not spread to other parts of the body.

Biological therapy. Treatment by stimulation of the body's immune defense system.

Biopsy. The removal of a sample of tissue to see whether cancer cells are present.

Brachytherapy (BRAK-ee-THER-ah-pee). Internal radiation treatment achieved by implanting radioactive material directly into the tumor or very close to it. Sometimes called "internal radiation therapy."

Cancer. A general term for more than 100 diseases that have uncontrolled, abnormal growth of cells that can invade and destroy healthy tissues.

Catheter. A thin, flexible tube through which fluids enter or leave the body.

Chemotherapy. Treatment with anticancer drugs.

Cobalt 60. A radioactive substance used as a radiation source to treat cancer.

Dietitian (also registered dietitian). A professional who plans diet programs for proper nutrition.

Dosimetrist (do-SIM-uh-trist). A person who plans and calculates the proper radiation dose for treatment.

Electron beam. A stream of particles that produces high-energy radiation to treat cancer.

External radiation. Radiation therapy that uses a machine located outside of the body to aim high-energy rays at cancer cells.

Fluoride. A chemical applied to the teeth to prevent tooth decay.

Gamma rays. High-energy rays that come from a radioactive source such as cobalt-60.

Gray. A measurement of absorbed radiation dose; 1 Gray = 100 rads.

High dose rate remote brachytherapy. A type of internal radiation in which each treatment is given in a few minutes while the radioactive source is in place. The source of radioactivity is removed between treatments. Also known as high dose rate remote radiation therapy.

Hyperfractionated radiation. Division of the total dose of radiation into smaller doses that are given more than once a day.

Implant. A small container of radioactive material placed in or near a cancer.

Internal radiation. A type of therapy in which a radioactive substance is implanted into or close to the area needing treatment.

Interstitial radiation. A radioactive source (implant) placed directly into the tissue (not in a body cavity).

Intracavitary radiation. A radioactive source (implant) placed in a body cavity such as the chest cavity or the vagina.

Intraoperative radiation. A type of external radiation used to deliver a large dose of radiation therapy to the tumor bed and surrounding tissue at the time of surgery.

Linear accelerator. A machine that creates high-energy radiation to treat cancers, using electricity to form a stream of fast-moving subatomic particles. Also called megavoltage (MeV) linear accelerator or a linac.

Malignant. Cancerous (see *Cancer*).

Medical oncologist. A doctor who specializes in using chemotherapy to treat cancer.

Metastasis. The spread of a cancer from one part of the body to another. Cells in the second tumor are like those in the original tumor.

Oncologist. A doctor who specializes in treating cancer.

Palliative care. Treatment to relieve, rather than cure, symptoms caused by cancer. Palliative care can help people live more comfortably.

Physical therapist. A health professional trained in the use of treatments such as exercise and massage.

Platelets. Special blood cells that help stop bleeding.

Prosthesis. An artificial replacement of a part of the body.

Rad. Short form for "radiation absorbed dose;" a measurement of the amount of radiation absorbed by tissues (100 rads = 1 Gray).

Radiation. Energy carried by waves or a stream of particles.

Radiation oncologist. A doctor who specializes in using radiation to treat cancer.

Radiation physicist. A person trained to ensure that the radiation machine delivers the right amount of radiation to the treatment site.

Radiation therapist. A person with special training who runs the equipment that delivers the radiation.

Radiation therapy. The use of high-energy penetrating rays or subatomic particles to treat disease. Types of radiation include x-ray, electron beam, alpha and beta particles, and gamma rays. Radioactive substances include cobalt, radium, iridium, and cesium. (See also *gamma rays, brachytherapy, teletherapy, and x-ray.*)

Radiologist. A physician with special training in reading diagnostic x-rays and performing specialized x-ray procedures.

Radiotherapy. See radiation therapy.

Remote brachytherapy. See high dose rate remote brachytherapy.

Simulation. A process involving special x-ray pictures that are used to plan radiation treatment so that the area to be treated is precisely located and marked for treatment.

Teletherapy. Treatment in which the radiation source is at a distance from the body. Linear accelerators and cobalt machines are used in teletherapy.

Treatment port or field. The place on the body at which the radiation beam is aimed.

Tumor. An abnormal mass of tissue. Tumors are either **benign** or **malignant.**

Unsealed internal radiation therapy. Internal radiation therapy given by injecting a radioactive substance into the bloodstream or a body cavity. This substance is not sealed in a container.

White blood cells. The blood cells that fight infection.

X-ray. High-energy radiation that can be used at low levels to diagnose disease or at high levels to treat cancer.

Resources

Information about cancer is available from the sources listed below. You may wish to check for additional information at your local library or bookstore and from support groups in your community.

Cancer Information Service (CIS)

The Cancer Information Service, a program of the National Cancer Institute, is a nationwide telephone service for cancer patients and their families and friends, the public, and health care professionals. The staff can answer questions and can send booklets about cancer. They also may know about local resources and services. One toll-free number, 1-800-4-CANCER (1-800-422-6237), connects callers with the office that serves their area. Spanish-speaking staff members are available.

PDQ

People who have cancer, those who care about them, and doctors need up-to-date and accurate information about cancer treatment. To meet these needs, PDQ was developed by NCI. PDQ contains an up-to-date list of trials all over the country. The Cancer Information Service, at 1-800-4-CANCER, can provide PDQ information to doctors, patients, and the public.

Publications

Cancer patients, their families and friends, and others may find the following books useful. They are available free of charge by calling 1-800-4-CANCER.

- ♦ *Chemotherapy and You: A Guide to Self-Help During Treatment.*
- ♦ *Eating Hints: Recipes and Tips for Better Nutrition During Cancer Treatment.*
- ♦ *Questions and Answers About Pain Control.*
- ♦ *Taking Time: Support for People With Cancer and the People Who Care About Them.*
- ♦ *What You Need To Know About Cancer.* A series of booklets about different types of cancer; ask for the type of cancer you have.

American Cancer Society (ACS)

The American Cancer Society is a voluntary organization with a national office and local units all over the country. It supports research, conducts educational programs, and offers many services to patients and their families. To obtain information about services and activities in local areas, call the Society's toll-free number, 1-800-ACS-2345 (1-800-227-2345), or the number listed under "American Cancer Society" in the white pages of the telephone book.

American Cancer Society
1599 Clifton Road, N.E.
Atlanta, GA 30329
1-800-ACS-2345

■ Document Source:
   National Institutes of Health
   National Cancer Institute
   NIH Publication No. 94-2227
   Revised October 1993

See also: Managing Cancer Pain (page 52); Radiation Therapy: A Treatment for Early Stage Breast Cancer (page 438)

WHAT ARE CLINICAL TRIALS ALL ABOUT? A BOOKLET FOR PATIENTS WITH CANCER

Foreword

Research studies conducted with patients are called clinical trials. As a cancer patient, you may take part in a clinical trial. This booklet is written for you, your family and friends, to explain what clinical trials are and to help you make a decision about entering a trial.

The time when cancer is diagnosed or when treatment decisions are being made is very difficult. It is often hard to understand or remember complex medical explanations. The information in this booklet is meant to supplement what your doctors tell you. It provides answers to questions asked most often about clinical trials. (You may not want to read the whole book at one time. It is broken down into questions and answers that you can read now or later.)

You may wish to write down questions to ask your doctor or nurse. There is a glossary of words that relate to clinical trials and cancer care. This is a quick way to look up terms that you may hear or read. More information on many cancer-related topics is available at no cost in other publications from the National Cancer Institute.

We hope this booklet will help to explain how clinical studies are designed and carried out. Of course, there are good treatments and good care for cancer patients if they take part in clinical trials or if they receive standard treatments. You may decide not to take part in a trial, and you can still receive good medical care. The decision to enter a clinical trial or not is always up to you.

What is a clinical trial?

In cancer research, a clinical trial is a study conducted with cancer patients, usually to evaluate a new treatment. Each study is designed to answer scientific questions and to find new and better ways to help cancer patients.

The search for good cancer treatments begins with basic research in laboratory and animal studies. The best results of that research are tried in patient studies, hopefully leading to findings that may help many people.

Before a new treatment is tried with patients, it is carefully studied in the laboratory. This research points out the new methods most likely to succeed, and, as much as possible, shows how to use them safely and effectively. But this early research cannot predict exactly how a new treatment will work with patients. With any new treatment there may be risks as well as possible benefits. There may also be some risks that are not yet known. Clinical trials help us find out if a promising new treatment is safe and effective for patients. During a trial, more and more information is gained about a new treatment, its risks, and how well it may or may not work.

Standard treatments, the ones now being used, are often the base for building new, hopefully better treatments. Many new treatments are designed on the basis of what has worked in the past, in efforts to improve on this.

Only patients who wish to, take part in a clinical trial. You may be interested in or asked to enter a trial. Learn as much as you can about the trial, before you make up your mind.

Why are clinical trials important?

Advances in medicine and science are the results of new ideas and approaches developed through research. New cancer treatments must prove to be safe and effective in scientific studies with a certain number of patients before they can be made widely available.

Through clinical trials, researchers learn which approaches are more effective than others. This is the best way to test a new treatment. A number of standard treatments were first shown to be effective in clinical trials. These trials help us find new and better treatments.

Why would a patient be interested in a clinical trial?

Patients take part in clinical trials for many reasons. Usually, they hope for benefits for themselves. They may hope for a cure of disease, a longer time to live, a way to feel better. Often they want to contribute to a research effort that may help others.

Based on what researchers learn from laboratory studies, and sometimes earlier clinical studies and standard treatments as well, they design a trial to see if a new treatment will improve on current treatments. The hope is that it will. Often researchers use standard treatments as the building blocks to try to design better treatments.

Many trials have turned out to be better than standard treatments; others have either been not as good as or no better than the treatments already being used. Although there is always a chance that a new treatment will be disappointing, the researchers involved in a study have reason to believe that it will be as good as, or better than, current treatments.

The patients in a clinical trial are among the first to receive new research treatments before they are widely available. How a treatment will work for a patient in a trial can't be known ahead of time. Even standard treatments, although effective in many patients, do not carry sure benefits for everyone. But, patients should choose if they want to take part in a study or not, only after they understand both the possible risks and benefits.

The patients who take part in clinical trials that do prove to be better treatments, have the first chance to benefit from them. All patients in clinical trials are carefully monitored during a trial and followed up afterwards. They become part of a network of clinical trials carried out around the country. In this network, doctors and researchers pool their ideas and experience to design and monitor clinical studies. They share their knowledge from many specialties about cancer treatment and care. Patients in these studies receive the benefit of their expertise. At cancer centers, patients receive care from a special research team. Through new programs, community hospitals and doctors are also coming more and more into the research network.

Are there risks or side effects in clinical trials?

Yes. The treatments used in clinical trials can cause side effects and risks depending on the type of treatment and the patient's condition. Side effects vary from patient to patient.

Because clinical trials are research into new areas of treatment, the risks involved are not always known ahead of time, though efforts have been made to find out what they might be. For this reason, trials can carry unknown dangers and side effects as well as hoped-for benefits. Patients need to know what is involved in a study—what side effects may be expected—and, as much as possible, what "unknowns" or uncertainties they may be facing.

You will be told about the treatments being tested and will be given a form to read that discusses the risks and hoped-for benefits. If you agree to take part, you will be asked to sign a form, called the informed consent form. Before you sign, be sure you understand what risks you face. Ask the doctor or nurse to explain any parts of the form or the trial that are not clear. If you do not want to be in the trial, you may refuse. Even if you sign the form, you are free to leave the trial at any time and can receive other available medical care.

In clinical trials, most side effects are temporary and will gradually go away once treatment is stopped. For example, some anticancer drugs cause hair loss and nausea and some do not. They can also affect the bone marrow which produces blood cells. During treatment, the number of blood cells, called blood counts, may fall too low. Since this could lead to possible infection or other problems, patients have their blood counts checked often. Luckily, bone marrow has a great ability to replace blood cells, so that blood counts can usually return to normal.

Some side effects in clinical trials can be permanent and serious, even life-threatening. Also, certain side effects may not appear until later, after the treatment itself is over. (These "late" effects may include damage to a major organ like the heart, lungs, or kidneys; sterility; or a second cancer.) Many cancer patients are now living longer, largely because of better treatments. Researchers are concerned and trying to prevent late complications of treatments.

As a patient, it can be hard to decide about your treatment. There are a number of things to consider. Cancer is a life-threatening disease which causes symptoms of its own that are not related to treatment. In each case, the unavoidable risks of the cancer itself, and your condition, should be weighed against the potential risks and benefits of a new research treatment.

Standard treatments, as well as treatments in clinical trials, can also cause side effects and risks.

Why does cancer treatment have side effects?

Any medical treatment can carry the potential for side effects in some patients. Cancer treatment is particularly powerful, because it is designed to destroy constantly dividing cancer cells. It can also affect healthy dividing cells and this can cause side effects. The challenge to researchers has been to develop treatments that destroy cancer cells but do not harm healthy cells.

What is being done to lessen side effects of treatment?

Cancer researchers are trying to make cancer treatment more effective and lessen its side effects for the cancer patient. Results of such efforts include:

♦ new anticancer drugs with less side effects;
♦ better antinausea medicine;
♦ some shorter periods of time on anticancer drugs;
♦ special ways to protect normal tissues during radiation therapy;
♦ new methods of surgery that are less extensive and less damaging to the body; and
♦ psychological support programs and information on ways to cope during difficult times. How patients feel during and after treatment is important.

If you are thinking of entering a clinical trial . . . are you eligible for a clinical trial?

Every clinical trial is designed to answer a set of research questions. If you fit the guidelines for a trial, you may be eligible to take part. Each study enrolls patients with certain types and stages of cancer and certain health status. A study that involves two or more treatments can yield reliable answers only if all the patient cases are the same so they can be compared with each other.

Before a decision is made about your treatment (whether it is in a clinical trial or not), your type of cancer will be diagnosed and "staged." Staging tells how far the disease has spread. Deciding on treatment depends on many things, including the stage of the disease and your general condition. You would most likely be referred to a trial by your own doctor or by a doctor who knows your case. Some patients find out about trials from other sources. In any case, you must have a reasonable understanding of your role in a research study and be freely willing to take part in it. Ask what you can expect if you take part in a trial.

What trials are available for your type of cancer?

There are many ways to find out what your treatment choices are. Talk with your doctors and get the opinion of cancer specialists (oncologists). You should not be afraid to ask for a second opinion. A helpful, new computer information system called PDQ, is supported by the National Cancer Institute. PDQ can give your doctor the latest information on clinical trials being offered around the country for each type and stage of cancer. This ready reference is kept up to date. Your doctor can check it from a library or personal computer.

The Cancer Information Service (CIS) is another source of information. This program, also sponsored by the National Cancer Institute, answers cancer-related questions from the public, cancer patients and their families, and health professionals. If you have questions, call the toll-free number: 1-800-4-CANCER, and you will be connected to the CIS office serving your area.

What is best for you?

This is a big question. Finding answers and making decisions are often hard for a cancer patient. The diagnosis of cancer and deciding what to do about it can be overwhelming, and you may be confused and upset. It is important to discuss your options with medical experts—including your own doctor—and with those close to you. Your personal doctor, who may be your family doctor, and cancer specialists can counsel you about your choices for standard treatment or clinical trials.

Talk to them and ask questions about the problems you are facing. If you understand what is going on, you can help your doctor work with you more effectively. You may want to take a friend or relative along with you when you talk to your doctor about your case.

Take time to ask your questions and to discuss what you want to know. It may help you and your doctor if you plan what to ask and write questions down ahead of time. No question is foolish. Learn what is available to you. Find out your choices and the risks and benefits of each. Each patient is different. You are an individual with individual needs, and your health is important. If you are a parent of a child with cancer, of course, you have great concerns about making the best decision for your child's care.

As you decide about treatment, if it is in a clinical trial or not, remember that you are not alone. There are many people to help you—doctors, nurses, social workers, clergy, your family, friends, and other patients. Although it is YOUR decision, they can help you think about it and decide what is best for you.

What are important questions to ask about a clinical trial?

If you are thinking about taking part in a clinical trial, here are some important questions to ask:

♦ What is the purpose of the study?
♦ What does the study involve? What kinds of tests and treatments? (Find out what is done and how it is done.)
♦ What is likely to happen in my case with, or without, this new research treatment? (What may the cancer do and what may this treatment do?)
♦ What are other choices and their advantages and disadvantages? (Are there standard treatments for my case and how does the study compare with them?)
♦ How could the study affect my daily life?
♦ What side effects could I expect from the study? (There can also be side effects from standard treatments and from the disease itself.)
♦ How long will the study last? (Will it require an extra time commitment on my part?)
♦ Will I have to be hospitalized? If so, how often and for how long?
♦ Will I have any costs? Will any of the treatment be free?*
♦ If I am harmed as a result of the research, what treatment would I be entitled to?
♦ What type of long-term followup care is part of the study?

What is informed consent?

Informed consent, a key part of a good trial, is required in studies that are federally regulated or funded as well as by many state laws. Informed consent means that as a patient, you are given information so you can understand what is involved

---

* Costs are a major concern of patients and families. Different arrangements and policies exist at different institutions and, of course, insurance coverage varies. Patients should freely discuss what costs are involved in their cases ahead of time. If you need financial aid, contact the hospital social services office, the Cancer Information Service, or the local American Cancer Society chapter. They may be able to direct you to a source of help.

in a trial, including its potential benefits and risks, and then decide freely to take part in it or not. The nature of the treatment is explained by the doctors and nurses in the trial. You are given an informed consent form to read and consider carefully. Ask any questions you may have. Then, if you agree to take part, you can sign the form. Of course, you may also refuse.

The informed consent process is an ongoing process. If you enter a trial, you will continue to receive any new information about your treatment that may affect your willingness to stay in the trial. Signing a consent form does not bind you to the study. You can still leave at any time.

What is it like to be a patient in a clinical trial?

Whether cancer patients are in a research study or not, they face a new world of medical terms and procedures. For some people, myths and fears of "experimentation" or of being a "guinea pig" come with the idea of clinical trials. And, surely, there are fears of the unknown. Understanding what is involved can ease some of your anxieties. Patients in a clinical trial, for example, receive their care in the same places that standard treatments are given—at cancer centers, hospitals, clinics, or doctors' offices.

Because a growing number of cancer specialists are now in private practice in the community, most cancer care can be given in an area near your home. Doctors, nurses, social workers and other health professionals from many different specialties may help care for you. They are working together for your good. There is consideration for your privacy and well-being.

If you join a research study, you will be watched closely and data on your case will be carefully recorded. You may receive more examinations and tests than are usually given. (These are to follow your progress as well as to collect study data.) Of course, tests can carry certain risks and benefits or discomforts of their own. Although they can be inconvenient, these tests can assure an extra ounce of observation along the way.

During the course of a study, if it is clear that a treatment is not in your best interest, you will be removed from the study and you can discuss other options.

Can you leave a trial at any time?

Yes. Just as you can refuse to join a study, you may leave a study at any time. Your rights as an individual do not change because you are a patient in a clinical trial. You may choose to take part or not, and you can always change your mind later, even after you enter a trial.

You may also refuse to take part in any aspect of the research. If you have questions at any time about any part of the study, be sure to ask your doctors. If you are not satisfied with the answers, you may consider leaving the study. If you decide to leave, it will not be held against you. Don't be afraid that you will receive no further care. You can freely discuss other possible treatments and care with your doctors and nurses.

What protection do you have as a patient in a clinical trial?

The ethical and legal codes that govern medical practice apply to clinical trials. In addition, most clinical research is federally regulated or federally funded (at least in part), with built-in safeguards to protect patients. These safeguards include regular review of the protocol (the study plans) and the progress of each study by researchers at other places.

For example, federally funded and federally regulated clinical trials must first be approved by an Institutional Review Board (IRB) located at the institution where the study is to take place. IRBs, designed to protect patients, are made up of scientists, doctors, clergy and other people from the local community. An IRB reviews a study to see that it is well designed with safeguards for patients, and that the risks are reasonable in relation to the potential benefits.

Federally supported or regulated studies also go through reviews by a government agency, such as the National Cancer Institute, which sponsors and monitors many trials around the country.

Any well-run clinical trial, whether federally supported or not, is carefully reviewed for medical ethics, patient safety, and scientific merit by the research institution. Every study should provide for monitoring the data and the safety of patients on an ongoing basis.

As discussed earlier, informed consent is also an important process that helps to protect patients.

After patients join a clinical trial and it progresses, the doctors report the results of the trial to scientific meetings, to medical journals whose articles are approved by experts, and to various government agencies.

What can help you learn if a trial is sound and well run?

Things that make a sound, well-run trial to safeguard patients include the items discussed in the previous section of this booklet. Keeping these items in mind, here are some important questions for you to ask to find out if a study is well run:

♦ What is its purpose?
♦ Who has reviewed and approved the study?
♦ Who is sponsoring the study?
♦ How are the study data and patient safety being checked?
♦ Where will information from the study go? (In government-related research, for example, reports might go to the National Cancer Institute and/or the Food and Drug Administration.)

For your own protection, be sure to get satisfactory answers to these questions before you agree to take part.

What kinds of clinical trials are there?

There are many kinds of clinical trials. They range from studies of ways to prevent, detect and diagnose, control and treat cancer, to studies of the psychological impact of the disease and ways to improve the patient's comfort and quality of life (including pain control).

Most cancer clinical trials deal with new treatments. These treatments often involve surgery, radiation therapy (the use of x-rays, neutrons or other types of cell-destroying radiation), and chemotherapy (the use of anticancer drugs). Alone, or in combination, these types of treatments can cure many cancer patients and prolong the lives of many others. A fairly new area of cancer treatment is biological therapy—the use of biologicals (substances produced by the body's own cells) and biological response modifiers (substances that affect the body's natural defense systems against disease).

How are trials divided into phases?

Clinical trials are carried out in phases, each designed to find out certain information. Patients may be eligible for studies in different phases depending on their general condition and the type and stage of their cancer. More patients take part in the later phases of studies than in the earlier ones.

In a Phase I study, a new research treatment is given to a small number of patients. The researchers must find the best way to give a new treatment and how much of it can be given safely. They watch carefully for any harmful side effects. The research treatment has been well tested in laboratory and animal studies but no one knows how patients will react. Phase I studies may involve significant risks for this reason. They are offered only to patients whose cancer has spread and who would not be helped by other known treatments. Phase I treatments may produce anticancer effects, and some patients have been helped by these treatments.

Phase II studies determine the effect of a research treatment on various types of cancer. Each new phase of a clinical trial depends on and builds on information from an earlier phase. If a treatment has shown activity against cancer in Phase II, it moves to Phase III. Here it is compared with standard treatment to see which is more effective. Often researchers use standard therapy as the base to design new, hopefully better treatments. Then in Phase III, the new treatment is directly compared to the old one. In Phase IV studies, the new research treatment becomes part of standard treatment in patient care. For example, a new drug that has been found effective in a clinical trial may then be used together with other effective drugs, or with surgery, and/or radiation therapy.

How are clinical trials conducted?

The doctors who conduct a clinical trial follow a carefully designed treatment plan called a "protocol." This spells out what will be done and why. Studies are planned to safeguard the medical and psychological health of patients as well as to answer research questions.

Some clinical trials test one research treatment in one group of patients. Other trials compare two or more treatments in separate groups of patients who are similar in certain ways, such as the extent of their disease. This way, the treatment groups are alike and the results from each can validly be compared.

One of the groups may receive standard (the most accepted) treatment so the new treatments can be directly compared to it. The group receiving the standard treatment is called the "control" group. For example, one group of patients (the control group) may receive the usual surgical treatment for a certain cancer, while another patient group with the same type of cancer may receive surgery plus radiation therapy to see if this improves disease control.

Sometimes, no standard treatment yet exists for certain cancer patients. In drug studies for such cases, one group of patients might receive a new drug and the control group, none. But no patient is placed in a control group without treatment if there is any known treatment that would benefit that patient. The control group is followed as often and carefully as the "treatment" group.

One of the ways to prevent the bias of a patient or doctor from influencing study results is "randomization." If a patient agrees to be randomized, this means he or she is selected by chance to be in one group or another. The researchers do not know which treatment is best. From what is known at the time, any one of the treatments chosen could be of equal benefit to the patient.

If the treatment in a trial is not helping the patient, the patient's doctor can decide to take him or her out of the study. Of course, the patient can decide to leave, as well, and still receive other available care. There are regular reviews of the results of a trial and the information is shared. This is important, because if a treatment is found to be too harmful or not effective, it is stopped. Also, when there is firm evidence that one method is better than the others in a study, the trial is stopped and all patients in the trial are given the benefit of the new information. Such information may help present and future patients.

Throughout a clinical study, a patient's personal doctor will be kept informed of the patient's progress. Patients are encouraged to maintain contact with their referring doctors.

The National Cancer Program and clinical trials

A nationwide effort to conquer cancer intensified with the National Cancer Act of 1971. As a result of the National Cancer Program, created by that legislation, more cancer patients are being cured today than ever before, and many others are living longer with improved quality of life.

The National Cancer Program brings together a network of researchers at many public and private institutions around the country. These include the National Cancer Institute, cancer centers, universities, community hospitals and private industry. Groups involving hundreds of researchers are working to discover and put to use new knowledge to benefit the cancer patients of today and tomorrow.

Knowledge gained from research studies with patients—clinical trials—has been essential to overall progress. Such studies have led to increased survival for childhood cancers, Hodgkin's disease, breast, uterine, testicular and bladder cancers, as well as others. These studies continue to play a key role in progress against cancer.

Today, major scientific discoveries in the laboratory are part of a revolution in biology. New tools to unravel the process of cancer are leading to exciting new approaches against cancer. Clinical trials continue to be the link between such basic research and patients. The goal is to translate the best of that research into findings that directly help people.

Glossary

Adjuvant Chemotherapy (ad'ju-vant kee-mother'a-pee). One or more anticancer drugs used in combination with surgery or radiation therapy as part of the treatment of cancer. Adjuvant usually means "in addition to" initial treatment.

Antibody (an'ti-bod-ee). A protein produced by a plasma cell in the lymphatic system or bone marrow. An antibody binds to the specific antigen that has stimulated the immune system. Once bound, the antigen can be destroyed by other cells of the immune system. See **Immune System.**

Antigen (an'ti-jen). A substance, foreign to the body, that stimulated the production of antibodies by the immune system. Antigens include foreign proteins, bacteria, viruses, pollen and other materials.

Biological Therapy. Use of biologicals (substances produced by our own cells) or biological response modifiers (substances that affect the patient's defense systems) in the treatment of cancer.

Blood Count. Measurement of the number of red cells, white cells, and platelets in a sample of blood.

Bone Marrow (mair'oh). The inner, spongy core of bone that produces blood cells.

Cancer (kan'ser). A general term for more than 100 diseases characterized by abnormal and uncontrolled growth of cells. The resulting mass, or tumor, can invade and destroy surrounding normal tissues. Cancer cells from the tumor can spread through the blood or lymph to start new cancers in other parts of the body.

CCOP (Community Clinical Oncology Program). This new program links community physicians with NCI clinical research programs, so that more cancer patients can participate in clinical trials in their own communities.

Chemotherapy (kee-mo-ther'a-pee). Treatment with anticancer drugs.

Clinical Trial. The systematic investigation of the effects of materials or methods, according to a formal study plan and generally in a human population with a particular disease or class of diseases. In cancer research, a clinical trial generally refers to the evaluation of treatment methods such as surgery, drugs or radiation techniques, although methods of prevention, detection or diagnosis also may be the subject of such studies.

Combination Chemotherapy (kee-mo-ther'a-pee). Use of two or more anticancer drugs.

Combination Therapy (ther'a-pee). The use of two or more modes of treatment—surgery, radiotherapy, chemotherapy, immunotherapy—in combination, alternately or together, to achieve optimum results against cancer.

Control Group. In clinical studies this is a group of patients which receives *standard treatment,* a treatment or intervention currently being used and considered to be of proved effectiveness on the basis of past studies. Results in patients receiving newly developed treatments may then be compared to the control group. In cases where no standard treatment yet exists for a particular condition, the control group would receive no treatment. No patient is placed in a control group without treatment if there is any beneficial treatment known for that patient.

Double-blind. Characteristic of a controlled experiment in which neither the patient nor the attending physician knows whether the patient is getting one or another drug or dose. In *single-blind* studies, patients do not know which of several treatments they are receiving, thus preventing personal bias from influencing their reactions and study results. In either case, the treatment can be quickly identified, if necessary, by a special code.

Hormone. Chemical product of the endocrine glands of the body, which, when secreted into body fluids, has a specific effect on other organs.

Immune System. A complex network of organs, cells and specialized substances distributed throughout the body and defending it from foreign invaders that cause infection or disease.

Immunotherapy (im-mew-no-ther'a-pee). A form of biological therapy. An experimental method of treating cancer, using substances which stimulate the body's immune defense system.

Informed Consent. The process in which a patient learns about and understands the purpose and aspects of a clinical trial and then agrees to participate. Of course, a patient may decline to participate. This process includes a document defining how much a patient must know about the potential benefits and risks of therapy before being able to agree to undergo it knowledgeably. (Informed consent is required in federally conducted, funded or regulated studies as well as by many state laws.) If a patient signs an informed consent form and enters a trial, he or she is still free to leave the trial at any time, and can receive other available medical care.

Interferon (in-tur-feer'on). A protein substance produced by white blood cells and other types of cells that have been exposed to certain viruses. In test animals, interferon has shown some activity against tumors. Studies of its usefulness in treating some types of human cancer are under way. One of a number of new agents available as biological therapy.

Investigational New Drug. A drug allowed by the Food and Drug Administration (FDA) to be used in clinical trials but not approved by the FDA for commercial marketing.

Investigator. An investigator is the experienced clinical researcher who prepares a protocol or treatment plan and implements it with patients.

Metastasis (me-tas'ta-sis). The transfer of disease from one part of the body to another. In cancer, metastasis is the migration of cancer cells from the original tumor site through the blood and lymph vessels to produce cancers in other tissues. Metastasis also is the term used for a secondary cancer growing at a distant site.

Metastatic Cancer (met-a-stat'ik). Cancer that has spread from its original site to one or more additional body sites.

Monoclonal Antibodies (mon-o-klone'al an'ti-bod-eez). One of several new substances used in biological therapy. These antibodies, all exactly alike, are mass-produced and designed to home in on target cancer cells. Monoclonal antibodies are products of new scientific techniques and may prove useful in both cancer diagnosis and treatment.

Multimodality Therapy (mul'ti-mo-dal'i-tee ther'a-pee). The combined use of more than one method of treatment, for example, surgery and chemotherapy.

Oncologist (on-kol'o-jist). A physician who is a cancer specialist.

PDQ. PDQ, supported by NCI, is a computerized database available to physicians nationwide. Geographically matrixed, it offers the latest information on standard treatments and ongoing clinical trials for each type and stage of cancer. The information is easily accessible for physicians via libraries and personal computers.

Placebo (pla-see'bo). An inactive substance resembling a medication, given for psychological effect or as a control in evaluating a medicine believed to be active. It is usually a tablet, capsule, or injection that contains a harmless substance but appears to be the same as the medicine being tested. A placebo may be compared with a new drug when no one knows if any drug or treatment will be effective.

Protocol (pro'to-kol). The outline or plan for use of an experimental procedure or experimental treatment.

Radiation Therapy, also called Radiotherapy. Treatment using x-rays, cobalt-60, radium, neutrons, or other types of cell-destroying radiation.

Radiosensitizers (ray'dee-o-sen-si-ty'zers). Drugs being studied to try to boost the effect of radiation therapy.

Randomized Clinical Trials (ran-duh'mized). A study in which patients with similar traits, such as extent of disease, are chosen or selected by chance to be placed in separate groups that are comparing different treatments. Because irrelevant factors or preferences do not influence the distribution of patients, the treatment groups can be considered comparable and results of the different treatments used in different groups can be compared. (There is no way at the time for the researchers to know which of the treatments is best.) See also **Clinical Trials.** (It is the patient's choice to be in a randomized trial or not.)

Regression (ree-gresh'un). The state of growing smaller or disappearing; used to describe the shrinkage or disappearance of a cancer.

Remission (ree-mish'un). The decrease or disappearance of evidence of a disease; also the period during which this occurs.

Risk/Benefit Ratio. The relation between the risks and benefits of a given treatment or procedure. Institutional Review Boards (IRBs) (located where the study is to take place) determine that the risks in a study are reasonable with respect to the potential benefits. It is also up to the patient to decide if it is reasonable for him or her to take part in a study.

Side Effect. A secondary and usually adverse effect, as from a drug or other treatment. For example, nausea is a side effect of some anticancer drugs.

Single Blind. (See **Double Blind**)

Staging. Methods used to establish the extent of a patient's disease.

Standard Treatment. A treatment or other intervention currently being used and considered to be of proved effectiveness on the basis of past studies.

Study Arm. Patients in clinical trials are assigned to one part or segment of a study—a study "arm." One arm receives a different treatment from another.

Therapeutic (ther'a-pew'tik). Pertaining to treatment.

For additional information on this subject, write to the Office of Cancer Communications, National Cancer Institute, Bethesda, MD 20892, or call the toll-free telephone number of the Cancer Information Service at **1-800-4-CANCER**

In Hawaii, on Oahu call 524-1234 (neighbor islands call collect).

Spanish-speaking staff members are available to callers from the following areas (daytime hours only): California, Florida, Georgia, Illinois, New Jersey (area code 201), New York and Texas.

The National Cancer Institute has developed PDQ (Physician Data Query), a computerized database designed to give doctors quick and easy access to:

♦ The latest treatment information for most types of cancer;
♦ Descriptions of clinical trials that are open for patient entry; and
♦ Names of organizations and physicians involved in cancer care.

To get access to PDQ, a doctor may use an office computer with a telephone hookup and a PDQ access code or the services of a medical library with online searching capability. Most Cancer Information Service offices (1-800-4-CANCER) provide a physician with one free PDQ search, and can tell doctors how to get regular access to the database. Patients may ask their doctor to use PDQ or may call 1-800-4-CANCER themselves. Information specialists at this toll-free number use a variety of sources, including PDQ, to answer questions about cancer prevention, diagnosis, and treatment.

■ **Document Source:**
U.S. Department of Health and Human Services, Public Health Service
National Institutes of Health
National Cancer Institute
NIH Publication No. 90-2706
Reprinted December 1989

WHEN CANCER RECURS: MEETING THE CHALLENGE AGAIN

Introduction

In the back of every cancer patient's mind is the possibility that the disease may return. And yet when it does, most patients think, "How can this be happening to me again?"

The shock is back. The fears are back—of telling your family and friends, of more treatment, and possibly of death. The anger is there too—after all you've been through, it should have been enough. And the unanswered question is, "Will the treatment work this time?"

Even though you may feel some of the same things you felt when you first were diagnosed, now there's a difference. You've been through this before. You've faced cancer and its treatment and the changes that came to your life. You know that medical and emotional support is available to you. Facing cancer again is difficult, but it is a challenge you can handle.

This booklet is about cancer that has returned—its diagnosis and treatment, suggestions for coping, and where to get help. The glossary at the end of the booklet explains some of the terms that you will read or that you may hear in talking with your treatment team.

As you read this booklet, remember that there are more than 100 different types of **cancer.** Each is different, and each person responds to treatment differently. No booklet can cover every situation for every person. For this reason, the information given here is general, and some of it may not apply to you.

Still, a lot of people have found ways to handle recurring cancer in similar ways, and their experiences may help you.

Many people who have faced the return of cancer will tell you that learning more about your illness and its treatment helps you take part in your care. Having a positive attitude toward treatment may help you control some of your emotional and physical reactions to it. Drawing on your own strengths and the support from the people and resources around you can help you meet this challenge again.

You can call the Cancer Information Service (CIS) at 1-800-4-CANCER to get the most up-to-date information about treatment for your type of cancer and to talk with someone who can offer suggestions on how to cope. Spanish-speaking CIS staff members are also available.

Why Cancer Can Recur

Recurrence means "the reappearance." When cancer recurs, it means that the disease that was thought to be cured, or at least to be inactive (in **remission**), has become active again. Cancer may recur after several months, a few years, or many years.

Cancer that has recurred is very much like the first cancer in the way that it starts: Abnormal cells begin to grow and multiply quickly. If not stopped, cancer cells can destroy normal tissues and organs.

Recurrent cancer starts from cells that were not killed by the original therapy. Your previous treatment was meant to destroy the original cancer and the cells that may have broken away from it. However, a small number of cancer cells may have survived and only now have grown into large enough tumors to be detected.

The cancer that recurs is the same type as the original cancer, no matter where it is found. For example, if colon cancer recurs in the liver, it is not liver cancer; it is colon cancer that has spread to the liver.

Where Cancers Can Recur

Not every cancer cell that breaks away from a **tumor** is able to grow elsewhere. Most are stopped by the body's natural defenses or destroyed by treatment. Cancers differ in their ability to recur and in the places where they may recur. For this reason, recurrent cancers are classified by location: local, regional, or metastatic.

Local recurrence means that the cancer has come back in the same place as the original cancer. The term "local" also means that there is no sign of cancer in nearby lymph nodes or other tissues. For instance, a woman who has had a mastectomy could later have a local recurrence of breast cancer in or around the area of the surgery.

A *regional* recurrence involves growth of a new tumor in **lymph nodes** or tissues near the original site but with no evidence of cancer at distant places in the body. A man who has had a melanoma removed from his arm, for instance, might have a regional recurrence in the lymph nodes under his arm.

In *metastatic* recurrence, cancer has spread to organs or other tissues far from the original site. For example, a man with prostate cancer could have **metastasis** to his bones.

Diagnosing Recurrent Cancer

Over the past several months or years, you may have had a number of tests and checkups. Most likely, your doctor told you to watch for changes in your body and to report any unusual symptoms.

You may have noticed a weight change, bleeding, or constant pain, or your doctor may have found signs of further illness while examining you. In either case, tests are used to find the exact cause of the problem and decide on the best treatment.

Specific procedures and tests help your doctor answer these questions:

♦ Are the signs and symptoms caused by cancer or by some other medical problem?
♦ If cancer is present, is it a recurrence or is it a new type of cancer?
♦ Has the cancer spread to more than one place?

Because certain types of cancer tend to recur in certain parts of the body, your doctor is likely to check those places first. Information from physical exams and tests helps the doctor make an accurate diagnosis and choose the treatment that is best for you.

Physical Exams

In addition to your routine physical exam, besides feeling for lumps and swelling, your doctor may need to look at your colon, stomach, bladder, breathing passages, or other organs. A number of instruments are used for viewing different parts of the body. The names of most of the instruments end in "scope." For example, a bronchoscope is used to view the air passages of a lung. In some cases, the doctor may even take a tissue sample (biopsy) through the scope and look at the sample under a microscope.

Laboratory Tests

A number of lab tests are used to help diagnose recurrent cancer. For example, blood samples can be tested to check the levels of certain tumor markers that may change when cancer recurs. The carcinoembryonic antigen (CEA) test is a blood test that detects changes in this **tumor marker** that often accompany some cancers.

Other tests, such as the examination of a stool smear, can detect internal bleeding that may be too slight for you to notice. If blood is found, a series of x-rays or another type of test is done to learn if the bleeding is caused by cancer or by some other problem.

These are only a few examples of lab tests used to diagnose cancer and other health problems. Your doctor will select those that may be helpful in your case.

X-Rays and Scans

To learn the location and size of suspected cancer, the doctor can use x-rays, computed tomography (CT) scans, nuclear scanning, ultrasound, or magnetic resonance imaging (MRI).

These tests use radiation, computers, magnets, and other sophisticated equipment. If you have questions about how they are used, their risks or benefits, or what you should expect during the procedure, be sure to talk with your doctor, nurse, or technician about your concerns.

X-Rays

Tumors that cause a change in density of a normal structure can often be seen with a standard **x-ray:** for example, decreased bone density from breast cancer that has spread or increased density of lung cancer that has grown into the air spaces of the lung. Other tests combine x-rays with a barium solution, dye, or air to give sharp pictures of organs such as the stomach, kidney, and colon that cannot be seen clearly with x-rays alone. An example of this kind of study is the "lower GI series" (barium enema followed by an x-ray of the **gastrointestinal tract**).

CT Scan

In a **CT scan,** a series of x-rays are taken from many directions and combined into one cross-sectional picture with the aid of a computer. The CT scan gives more detailed pictures than standard x-rays for certain body parts and often is used for tissues such as the liver and brain.

Nuclear Scanning

Nuclear scans often are used to see many parts of the body. A substance that is very slightly radioactive is swallowed or injected into the bloodstream. A machine called a scanner then takes pictures of the areas of the body where the substance is taken up. A cancer can show up in the pictures as an area of more or less radioactivity than the tissue around it.

Ultrasound

An ultrasound test uses a microphone-like device that sends sound waves that bounce off internal organs. The sound echoes made by the sound waves are converted into a picture by computer.

MRI

Instead of x-rays, **MRI** uses radio waves and a powerful magnet to create images of internal organs. Like a CT scan, MRI uses a computer to combine many images into a single picture. That picture may include organs, muscles, blood vessels, and other parts of the body that are hard to see with other kinds of scanners.

Biopsy

A **biopsy** is often the best way to tell if cancer is present. While an abnormal area may be seen through scopes or on x-ray films, a biopsy shows whether it is made of cancer cells.

For some cancers, the doctor uses a needle to withdraw fluid (aspirate) or remove small tissue samples (needle biopsy). A surgical biopsy, done under local or general anesthesia, removes the entire tumor or a piece of it. The sample of cells or tissues that is removed is examined under a microscope.

If your cancer has recurred, an accurate diagnosis is the first step in determining the best course of treatment and getting the disease under control again.

Treatment Methods

In planning your treatment for recurrent cancer, many of the same factors that affected treatment decisions for the original cancer will be taken into account. How your cancer is treated depends on the type of cancer, its size and location, your general health, and other treatments you've had.

Your doctor may recommend surgery, radiation, anticancer drugs (chemotherapy), or a combination of these treatments. For certain cancers, such as those in the reproductive organs, the doctor may suggest hormone therapy. In other cases, biological therapy may be considered.

It is important that you take an active part in your treatment by asking questions and expressing your feelings. Talk to your doctor about treatment goals, methods, and side effects to help determine which treatment will be best for you.

The following paragraphs describe the most common treatments, some of the newer methods now under study, and "unproven" treatments about which you may have heard. You also will find a list of questions that patients often ask about the various treatments.

Surgery

Surgery often is used to treat cancer when it is first diagnosed, but it is used less often in recurrent disease. Your doctor may recommend an operation to remove a recurrence if it seems to be limited to a single spot on the skin or in the lung, liver, bone, brain, or lymph nodes. For many sites of recurrence, other methods such as radiation, chemotherapy, or biological therapy have been shown to be more effective.

When cancer recurs in a weight-bearing bone (such as in the leg), there may be a threat of fracture caused by the growing tumor. In such a case, the doctor may suggest an operation to support the bone and prevent a break. This procedure can help relieve pain and keep the patient active while waiting for other forms of treatment to take effect and control the cancer.

Radiation Therapy

Radiation treatment directs high levels of radiation (tens of thousands of times the amount used to produce a chest x-ray) at a cancerous tumor to destroy the cancer cells. Both normal and cancer cells are affected by radiation, so special equipment is used to aim the radiation at tumors or areas of the body where there is disease. Because cancer cells are growing and dividing more rapidly than many of the normal cells around them, most normal cells appear to recover more fully from radiation effects than cancer cells.

Doctors use radiation to treat cancer in almost every part of the body. Sometimes **radiation therapy** is used before surgery to shrink a cancerous tumor. After surgery, it may be used to stop the growth of any cancer cells that remain in a certain part of the body. In some cases, doctors use radiation and anticancer drugs, rather than surgery, to destroy a cancer and prevent it from returning.

The type of cancer, location, stage (extent of disease), and other factors will determine whether radiation therapy is right for a patient. Sites that may be treated with radiation include the brain, lung, and bone.

Although radiation treatment can cause side effects, most are not serious. They usually disappear within a few weeks after treatment ends, although some last longer. The type of side effects often will depend on the part of the body that is being treated and the amount of radiation received. Fatigue and skin irritation are common side effects among patients receiving radiation therapy. Many patients have no side effects at all. If radiation therapy is prescribed for you, ask your doctor to explain the side effects that might occur and how your can best manage them. *Radiation Therapy and You,* a booklet available from the National Cancer Institute (NCI), answers many questions about this type of treatment.

Chemotherapy

Chemotherapy is the use of drugs to treat cancer. These drugs may be used alone or in combination with radiation therapy, surgery, or biological therapy.

Chemotherapy may be given by mouth or by injection into the veins or muscles. The drugs reach and destroy cancer cells in nearly every part of the body. Treatment may consist of a single drug or a combination of drugs.

Because anticancer drugs can reach sites that are far away from the original cancer and can destroy cancer cells throughout the body, chemotherapy is the primary treatment for many kinds of recurrent cancers that have spread beyond a single site or region.

Chemotherapy can affect any rapidly growing cells in the body, normal as well as cancer cells. The normal cells most likely to be affected are the blood-producing cells in the bone, cells lining the digestive tract and reproductive organs, and hair follicles. Again, many normal cells are able to replace themselves.

Every person reacts differently to chemotherapy. Some people have few or no side effects; others say their side effects are less severe than they expected; still others have a more difficult time. Ask your doctor, nurse, or pharmacist about side effects that could occur with the specific anticancer drugs prescribed for you. They can give you suggestions to help manage problems that may occur during treatment. Most side effects gradually begin to stop after treatment ends. However, the fatigue that some patients experience during chemotherapy sometimes lingers for a while.

The NCI booklet *Chemotherapy and You* provides further information about this type of cancer treatment.

Hormone Therapy

Some cancers are sensitive to changes in **hormone** levels. By adding, removing, or limiting the activity of a certain hormone, doctors can slow the growth or activity of cells affected by that hormone. **Hormone** therapy is often used to treat cancers of the breast and prostate.

Sometimes surgery or radiation treatment is used to stop the body from producing hormones that cancer cells need to grow. Hormone therapy can cause a number of side effects, depending on the type of drug or surgical procedures. Patients may have nausea, swelling, or weight gain. In some cases, the treatment interferes with the body's production or use of hormones. For example, breast cancer patients taking tamoxifen may have some symptoms of menopause, such as hot flashes.

Biological Therapy

Biological therapy—sometimes called immunotherapy—is a promising new area of cancer treatment. It uses both natural and manmade substances to boost the body's own immune (defense) system against cancer. Called "biological response modifiers" (BRMs), they help the body's immune system fight the growth of cancer cells. Researchers are studying biological therapies in clinical trials to learn how BRMs work best and against which cancers.

Supportive Therapy

When you were first treated for cancer, you may have had physical therapy or used the services of a psychological counselor or social worker. You may want to consider seeking those kinds of help again. Two other types of supportive therapy that also could be important to you are nutritional support and pain management.

Nutrition

Eating well during cancer therapy is very important. Studies have shown that patients who eat well may be able to cope better with the cancer and its treatment.

Eating well means choosing foods that have the protein, calories, and other elements needed to keep the body working normally. Dieting during treatment is not advised because it deprives the body of needed calories and nutrients.

You could have problems with eating and digesting food because of treatment side effects. There are ways to ease some of these side effects, however. The NCI publication *Eating Hints* has many suggestions for healthy ways to eat during treatment, as do the booklets *Chemotherapy and You* and *Radiation Therapy and You,* which discuss specific nutrition problems associated with those treatments.

If eating enough to stay at your normal weight continues to be a problem in spite of your efforts, ask a dietitian at the hospital where you had your treatment to help plan a diet for you. For severe nutrition problems, special treatments can be given at home or in the hospital.

Pain Control

Having cancer does not always mean having pain. But if pain does occur, there are many ways to relieve or reduce it. Cancer pain almost always can be relieved or controlled. You have a right to ask those caring for you to help you control your pain as much as possible. The best way to manage pain is to treat its cause. Whenever possible, the cause of pain is treated by removing the tumor or decreasing its size. To do this your doctor may recommend surgery, radiation therapy, or chemotherapy. When none of these procedures can be done, or when the cause of pain is unknown, pain-relief methods are used. Most pain can be controlled by using oral pain medicines. Your doctor may recommend nonprescription or over-the-counter pain medicines for mild to moderate pain, or your doctor may give you a prescription pain reliever for more severe pain.

Many patients try to avoid using pain medicine on a regular basis. Bear in mind, though, that the medicine works best if taken before the pain becomes severe. Talk with your doctor if you are concerned about how often to take the medicine or if it doesn't seem to be working. If you're having radiation therapy or chemotherapy, be sure to check with your doctor before taking any medicines.

When describing pain to your doctor, be as specific as you can. To recommend the best pain treatment for you, your doctor will want to know the following things:

- Where exactly is your pain? Does it ever move from one spot to another?
- How does the pain feel (dull, sharp, burning, etc.)?
- How often does it occur?
- How long does it last?
- Does it start at a specific time (before or after meals, after certain activities, etc.)?
- Does anything (lying down, sitting, eating, etc.) seem to relieve the pain?

Because pain can be worse when you are frightened or worried, you may find some relief by using relaxation exercises or meditation. These activities, which usually involve deep, rhythmic breathing and quiet concentration, can be done almost anywhere.

A number of nonmedical ways to reduce pain have been gaining attention in recent years. Hypnosis and biofeedback have been helpful for some people with serious illness. If you want to learn about them, ask your doctor or nurse to refer you to a health professional who is trained to teach these methods. A booklet on handling pain, *Questions and Answers About Pain Control,* is available from the Cancer Information Service (CIS) of the NCI or from the American Cancer Society (ACS). To obtain a copy, call the CIS at 1-800-4-CANCER or contact your local ACS office listed in the telephone directory.

Investigational and Unproven Treatments

The words "investigational" and "unproven" may be similar in meaning, but there are important differences when they are used to describe cancer treatments. Understanding the difference can help you when discussing and choosing among you treatment options.

Investigational Treatments

Investigational treatments are new methods of treating disease that are given under strict scientific controls. These methods have been tested on animals and have shown promise for treating humans. Doctors test the value of new treatments with the help of cancer patients who take part in studies called clinical trials.

Patients who take part in clinical trials may be the first to benefit from improved treatment methods. They also can make an important contribution to medical care because the results of the studies may help many people. Patients participate in clinical trials only if they so choose and are free to leave the trial at any time. More information about these studies is provided in NCI's booklet *What Are Clinical Trials All About?*

Examples of investigational treatments of cancer being studied in clinical trials at this time include new combinations of drugs, biological therapies, and bone marrow transplants. If proven effective, the investigational treatments of today could become standard treatments in the future.

Unproven Methods

A treatment method described as "unproven" is one for which the substance used (a vitamin, food, etc.) or the way it is given has not been shown to be effective by accepted scientific methods. **Unproven methods** you may have heard about use various diets, vitamins, and herb mixtures.

The ACS has developed a list of clues to help you know whether a new treatment is "investigational" or "unproven." One way is to look at how results of the treatment are reported. Findings from clinical trials usually are reported first in medical and scientific journals and later may be reported in newspapers and magazines directed to the general public. Unproven methods usually are reported only in newspapers and magazines. They generally rely on first-person accounts by patients and do not discuss scientific data. Using these unproven treatments actually may be harmful because they may cause dangerous reactions or may delay or interfere with treatments proven to be effective.

Call the CIS if you want to learn more about unproven methods. The booklet *Unproven Methods of Cancer Management,* available from the ACS, provides information about many of these treatments. Be sure to consider carefully the list of suggested questions below as you think about your treatment options.

Questions to Ask the Doctor

Before you and your doctor agree on a treatment plan, you should understand why one treatment is recommended over others. Evaluate the possible benefits, risks, side effects, and impact on the quality of your life of the recommended treatment when compared with other treatments.

The questions listed below are examples of what patients often want to know about their treatment. You may want to add your own questions to the list to discuss with your doctor, nurse, or social worker. Family members or others close to you may have questions, too.

Questions to ask about any recommended treatment:

- What is the goal of this treatment? Is it a cure, will it shrink the tumor and relieve the symptoms, or is it for comfort only?
- Why do you think this treatment is the best one for me?
- Is this the standard treatment for my type of cancer?
- Are there other treatments? What are they?
- Am I eligible for any clinical trials?
- What benefits can I expect from the treatment?
- Are there side effects with this treatment? Are they temporary or permanent?
- Is there any way to prevent or relieve the side effects?
- How safe is this treatment? What are the risks?
- How will I know if the treatment is working?
- Will I need to be in the hospital?
- What will happen if I don't have the treatment?

♦ What does my family need to know about the treatment? Can they help?
♦ How long will I be on this treatment?
♦ How much will the treatment cost?

About radiation therapy:

♦ What benefits can I expect from this therapy?
♦ What type of radiation treatment will I be getting?
♦ How long do the treatments take? How many will I need? How often?
♦ Can I schedule treatments at a certain time of day?
♦ What if I have to miss a treatment?
♦ What risks are involved?
♦ What side effects should I expect? What can I do about them?
♦ Who will give me the treatments? Where are they given?
♦ Will I need a special diet?
♦ Will my activities be limited?

About chemotherapy and hormone therapy:

♦ What do you expect the drugs to do for me?
♦ Which drugs will I be getting? How is each one given?
♦ Where are the treatments given?
♦ How long do the treatments take? How many will I need?
♦ What happens if I miss a dose?
♦ What risks are involved?
♦ What side effects should I expect? What can I do about them?
♦ Will I need a special diet or other restrictions?
♦ Can I take other medicines during treatment?
♦ Can I drink alcoholic beverages during treatment?

About biological therapy:

♦ Exactly what kind of therapy will I receive? How is it given?
♦ Has this type of therapy already been shown to work against my kind of cancer?
♦ What side effects should I expect? What can be done about them?
♦ Where will I have to go for treatment?
♦ Who will be the doctor responsible for my care?
♦ How long will the treatment last, and how long will I be in the hospital?
♦ How much will the treatment cost? Will my insurance pay for it?

About investigational treatments or unproven methods:

♦ What benefits can I expect from the treatment?
♦ What can I learn from it?
♦ Is there scientific evidence that the treatment can help?
♦ What are the known or potential risks? Possible side effects?
♦ Will I have to get the new treatment from a different doctor?
♦ Will my insurance cover the costs of treatment?
♦ Will I have to travel to get the treatment? How often?

Helping Yourself

You may remember that much of the fear and anxiety that you felt the first time cancer appeared in your life was "fear of the unknown." You can help yourself again by gathering information, taking part in your treatment as actively as possible, and finding the support you need to deal with your feelings about the recurrence of your cancer.

Gathering Information

If you know how your illness can affect your body and if you stay informed about the progress of your treatment, you have a better chance to take part in your care.

Learn as much as you can about what is happening to you. If you have questions, ask your doctor and other members of your treatment team. Your pharmacist is a good person to talk to if you have questions about your medicines. If you don't understand the answer to a question, ask it again.

Some patients hesitate to ask their doctors about their treatment options. They may think that doctors do not like to have their recommendations questioned. Most doctors, however, believe that the best patient is an informed patient. They understand that coping with treatment is easier when patients understand as much as possible, and they encourage patients to discuss their concerns.

When you see your doctor to talk about possible treatments or to get help for problems that come up during treatment, take your list of questions and ask a friend or relative to go with you. You'll get the most useful advice if you and your companion speak openly with the doctor about your needs, expectations, wishes, and concerns.

Taking Part in Your Treatment

Taking an active part in your care can help you have a sense of control and well-being. You can be involved in many ways. One is to follow your doctor's recommendations about caring for yourself such as staying on a special diet or avoiding alcohol.

Another way you can help is to keep your doctor informed. Report honestly how you feel, and if problems arise, be as specific as possible when describing them. Don't ever hesitate to report symptoms to your doctor or to ask advice about what to do about them. Although many health-related signs and symptoms may not seem important to you, they could provide valuable information to your doctor. Know what signs you should look for, and if any of them appear, tell your doctor as soon as possible.

Remember the difference between "doing" and "overdoing." Rest is very important to you now both physically and emotionally. Some things you can do to keep up your strength are to:

♦ *Eat well.* This may be one of the most important things you can do to improve your body's response to treatment.
♦ *Get extra rest.* Your body will use a lot of extra energy during treatment. Get more sleep at night, and take naps whenever you feel the need.
♦ *Adjust activities.* Try not to demand too much of yourself. Ask other people to take over some of your tasks if

necessary. If your energy level is low, do the things that are most important to you and cut back on the others.

Managing Your Emotions

The diagnosis of cancer, whether for the first time or when it recurs, can threaten anyone's sense of wellbeing. Some people, when they first find out that cancer has returned, feel shock and denial. Many had put their experiences with cancer completely behind them, and the new diagnosis hits them as hard as—or even harder than—it did the first time. Others are not surprised, as if they had been expecting it all along.

There may be times when you'll feel overcome by fear, anxiety, depression, or anger. These emotions are natural. They are common ways to cope with a difficult situation, and many people with recurrent cancer experience them. Feel free to express these feelings if they occur. None of these is a "wrong" reaction, and letting them out will help you deal with them.

Starting cancer treatment again can place demands on your spirits as well as your body. Your attitudes and actions really can make a difference. Remember that you have coped with this situation before. Keeping your treatment goals in mind may help you keep your spirits up during therapy and see you through "down" spells that may occur.

As you go through treatment, you're bound to feel better about yourself on some days than on others. The uncertainty of living with recurrent cancer can sometimes contribute to ups and downs. When a bad day comes along, try to remember that there have been good days, and there will be more. Feeling low today does not mean you will feel that way tomorrow or that you are giving up. At these times, try distracting yourself with a book, a hobby, or plans for a new garden. Many people say it helps to have something to look forward to—even simple things like a drive, a visit from a friend, or a telephone call. Sometimes, however, you may just want to cry, and that's okay too.

You may need to rely more on the people closest to you to help during your treatment, but this may be difficult at first. You may not want to accept help, and some people may have trouble giving it. Many people do not understand cancer, and they may avoid you because they are afraid of your illness. Others may worry that they will upset you by saying the wrong thing.

At a time when you might expect others to rush to your aid, you may have to make the first move. Try to be open in talking with others about your illness, your treatment, your needs, and your feelings. Once people know that you can discuss these things, they may be more willing to open up and help.

By sharing your feelings, you and your loved ones will be better able to help each other through a difficult time. Another booklet from the NCI, *Taking Time,* offers useful advice for cancer patients and their families.

Sometimes it is easier to talk to someone outside your family or your friends. Try talking to health professionals such as your doctor, nurse, psychologist, social worker, or a clergyman with whom you feel comfortable. These professionals care about your emotional as well as physical well-being. When they know about your personal concerns, how your home life or lifestyle has been affected, and what changes in your situation you'd like to see, they will be better able to support you emotionally.

At times you are likely to feel stressed by the continuing changes in your life. Some stress can help because it may push you to take action. Too much stress, though, can harm your health and make you feel like you are losing control. You may not be able to remove all the stress around you, but you can try to limit it. Relaxation techniques can be used to reduce stress and help you cope better with your illness. Rhythmic breathing, imagery, and distraction are among the techniques that are easy to learn and use whenever you need them. If you are interested, ask your doctor or nurse to refer you to someone trained to teach these techniques. The local library also has useful books on relieving stress.

There are many reasons for cancer patients to feel sad, worried, or depressed. You probably can manage some of these problems on your own or with the help of family, friends, or clergy, but for others you may want professional help. A counselor trained to help cancer patients deal with their feelings can offer the support you may need. These counselors understand the special problems that go along with serious illness as well as the various ways of coping that others have found useful. If you think this kind of professional support could help you, ask your doctor or nurse for the name of an appropriate counselor.

Employment and Insurance Issues

If you have a job, you may want to return to work as soon as you can. You even may find it possible to continue to work during the time you are receiving treatment. This depends on the kind of treatment you are getting, what side effects you have, and how you feel about working.

Sometimes cancer patients find that they are treated differently on the job because of their medical condition. If this happens to you, be aware of your rights. Your employer may be violating laws that protect you from such unfair practices.

Although as many as 1 million cancer patients in the United States experience some form of employment discrimination, this practice is illegal. The Americans with Disabilities Act, which went into effect in 1992, bans discrimination by both private and public employers against qualified workers who have disabilities or histories of disability. The Federal Rehabilitation Act of 1973 states that Federal employers or companies receiving Federal funds cannot discriminate against handicapped workers, including cancer patients. In addition to Federal protection, you may be eligible for protection under state laws. Find out the legal facts on equal opportunity by contacting your local department of employment services.

You need to understand fully your insurance rights, not only as a cancer patient but also as an employee of your company. Carefully read the health insurance policy provided by your employer. If you have any questions, contact your state insurance commission or department. This agency determines what types of insurance policies must be offered and when rates may be raised.

If you have trouble learning what your rights are, or if you have any questions about employment issues, contact the National Coalition for Cancer Survivorship at (301) 585-2616.

They can help you find local agencies that respond to problems cancer survivors face regarding their rights.

Glossary

Biological therapy. Treatment with substances called biological response modifiers that can help the immune system fight disease more effectively. Also called immunotherapy.

Biopsy. The removal of a sample of tissue for examination under a microscope to check for cancer cells.

Cancer. A term for the more than 100 diseases in which abnormal cells multiply out of control. Cancer cells can spread through the bloodstream and lymphatic system to other parts of the body.

Chemotherapy. Treatment with anticancer drugs.

CT or CAT scan. A series of detailed pictures of areas inside the body created by a computer linked to an x-ray machine. Also called compound tomography scan or computed axial tomography scan.

Gastrointestinal tract. The digestive tract, where the body processes and uses food. It includes the esophagus, stomach, liver, small and large intestines, and rectum.

Hormones. Chemicals produced by certain glands in the body. Hormones control the way certain cells or organs act.

Hormone therapy. Treatment of cancer by adding or blocking the production of hormones.

Investigational treatments. Treatments that use new substances or methods of treating disease and are given under strict scientific controls.

Lymph nodes. Small, bean-shaped structures in the lymphatic system. The lymph nodes store special cells that can trap cancer cells or bacteria traveling through the body in lymph.

Metastasis. The spread of cancer from one part of the body to another. Cells in the metastatic (secondary) tumor are like those in the original (primary) tumor.

MRI. A procedure that uses a magnet linked to a computer to create pictures of areas inside the body. Also called magnetic resonance imaging.

Nuclear scans. Pictures of the inside of the body taken after slightly radioactive material is swallowed or injected into the bloodstream.

Radiation therapy. Treatment with high-energy rays from x-rays or other sources to kill cancer cells.

Recurrence. The reappearance of the signs and symptoms of cancer.

Remission. Disappearance of the signs and symptoms of cancer. When this happens, the disease is said to be "in remission." A remission can be temporary or permanent.

Surgery. An operation.

Tumor. An abnormal mass of tissue.

Tumor marker. A substance in blood or other body fluids that may suggest that a person has cancer.

Ultrasound. A test that bounces sound waves off tissues and changes the echoes into pictures (sonograms). These pictures are shown on a monitor like a TV screen. Different types of tissue reflect sound waves differently. This makes it possible to find abnormal growths.

Unproven methods. Treatments that use substances or methods of treating disease that have not been shown effective by accepted scientific methods.

X-ray. High-energy radiation. It is used in low doses to diagnose diseases and in high doses to treat cancer.

Resources

Information about cancer is available from the sources listed below. You may wish to check for additional information at your local library or bookstore and from support groups in your community.

Additional Reading

Cancer patients, their families and friends, and others may find the following books useful. They are available free of charge by calling 1-800-4-CANCER or writing:

Office of Cancer Communications
National Cancer Institute
Building 31, Room 10A24
Bethesda, MD 20892

Chemotherapy and You: A Guide to Self-Help During Treatment. Explains chemotherapy and addresses problems and concerns of patients undergoing this treatment.

Datos sobre el tratamiento de quimioterapia contra el c ncer. Introduces chemotherapy to Spanish-speaking persons.

Eating Hints: Recipes and Tips for Better Nutrition During Cancer Treatment. Provides recipes that help patients meet their needs for good nutrition during treatment.

El tratamiento de radioterapia: gu¡a para el paciente durante el tratamiento. Provides an explanation of radiation therapy for Spanish-speaking persons.

Questions and Answers About Metastatic Cancer. Presents information on detection, treatment methods, and common areas of recurrence.

Questions and Answers About Pain Control. Discusses pain control using both medical and non-medical methods. This is also available from the American Cancer Society.

Radiation Therapy and You: A Guide to Self-Help During Treatment. Explains radiation therapy and addresses concerns of patients receiving radiation treatment.

Taking Time: Support for People With Cancer and the People Who Care About Them. Discusses the emotional side of cancer—how to deal with the disease and learn to talk with friends, family members, and others about cancer.

What Are Clinical Trials All About? Explains clinical trials (studies of new cancer treatments) to help patients decide if they want to take part in a trial.

What You Need To Know About... This is a series of booklets. Each provides information about a specific type of cancer. These booklets discuss symptoms, diagnosis, treatment, emotional issues, and questions to ask the doctor about a number of types of cancer. Some are available in Spanish.

Additional Resources

Cancer Information Service (CIS)
The Cancer Information Service, a program of the National Cancer Institute, provides a nationwide telephone service for cancer patients and their families and friends, the public, and health care professionals. The staff can answer questions and can send booklets about cancer. They also may know about local resources and services. One toll-free number, 1-800-4-CANCER (1-800-422-6237), connects callers with the office that serves their area. Spanish-speaking staff members are available.

PDQ

People who have cancer, those who care about them, and doctors need up-to-date and accurate information about cancer treatment. To meet these needs, PDQ was developed by NCI. PDQ contains an up-to-date list of trials all over the country. Doctors can obtain an access code and use a personal computer to get PDQ information. Also, the Cancer Information Service, at 1-800-4-CANCER, can provide PDQ information to doctors, patients, and the public.

American Cancer Society (ACS)

The American Cancer Society is a voluntary organization with a national office and local units all over the country. It supports research, conducts educational programs, and offers many services to patients and their families. To obtain information about services and activities in local areas, call the Society's toll-free number, 1-800-ACS-2345 (1-800-227-2345), or the number listed under "American Cancer Society" in the white pages of the telephone book.

American Cancer Society
1599 Clifton Road, N.E.
Atlanta, GA 30329
1-800-ACS-2345

■ **Document Source:**
National Institutes of Health
National Cancer Institute
NIH Publication No. 93-2709
Revised November 1989. Reprinted October 1992

See also: Chemotherapy and You: A Guide to Self-Help During Treatment (page 40); Radiation Therapy and You: A Guide to Self-Help During Treatment (page 56); What Are Clinical Trials All About? A Booklet for Patients with Cancer (page 68)

CONTRACEPTION AND REPRODUCTION

■ ■ ■

DEPO-PROVERA: THE QUARTERLY CONTRACEPTIVE

by Dori Stehlin

It may be the birth control compromise many woman have been looking for. Falling in between the daily effort of remembering the pill and the once-every-five-years appointment for the implant, one injection of Depo-Provera in the muscle of the arm or buttocks protects against pregnancy for three months.

The Food and Drug Administration approved Depo-Provera, manufactured by The Upjohn Co., Kalamazoo, Mich., for contraception last October. The active ingredient in Depo-Provera is a synthetic hormone similar to the natural hormone progesterone.

"I was not happy with other methods," says Becky Schroder, of Jacksonville, Fla. "I was a poor pill taker. I forgot. And I thought that barrier methods were inconvenient and messy."

Schroder, 31, started on Depo-Provera three years ago, when its use as a contraceptive was still investigational. (FDA had previously approved the drug for treating endometrial and renal cancers.)

Depo-Provera inhibits the production of another hormone, gonadotropin, which, in turn, prevents ovulation. Depo-Provera also causes changes in the lining of the uterus that make pregnancy less likely to occur.

Depo-Provera's estimated effectiveness in preventing pregnancy is 99 percent, on a par with Norplant, the contraceptive implant. Norplant contains another synthetic progestin hormone, levonorgestrel. (See "Norplant: Birth Control at Arm's Reach" in the May 1991 *FDA Consumer.*)

Mark Your Calendar

The amount of Depo-Provera in the bloodstream is at the highest level just after injection. Over time, the level drops and after three months, the level may no longer offer enough protection against conception.

"Go back on time for the next injection," says Ridgely Bennett, M.D., the FDA medical officer responsible for reviewing the new drug application for Depo-Provera. "That should be made abundantly clear."

He adds that if the time between injections is greater than 14 weeks, the physician should make sure the woman isn't pregnant before giving her the next injection.

Getting Started

A woman should get her first injection of Depo-Provera within five days after the start of her menstrual period. The drug is effective immediately, so no other birth control is necessary.

Because Depo-Provera is not a barrier contraceptive, however, it offers no protection against sexually transmitted diseases such as AIDS, herpes, chlamydia, and gonorrhea. For optimum protection from both disease and pregnancy, couples may choose to use both Depo-Provera and a condom.

A woman who has just had a baby—and wants to wait before having another—should get her shot within five days after the birth if she is not breast-feeding, and six weeks after the baby is born, if she is.

Although numerous studies by the World Health Organization have shown that Depo-Provera does not have any adverse effects on breast milk production or composition, or on the health of the nursing infant, it's best not to expose a newborn to the drug in the first six weeks, according to Philip Corfman, M.D., a supervisory medical officer in FDA's division of metabolism and endocrine drug products. "It's just a precaution," he says.

If a woman decides at the end of three months that she wants to get pregnant, she simply doesn't get the next injection. But, because the length of time between the last injection and becoming pregnant varies widely, any woman starting Depo-Provera should be sure she doesn't want to become pregnant for the next year or two, says Susan Wysocki, executive director of the National Association of Nurse Practitioners in Reproductive Health.

According to the approved physician's label, "the median time to conception for those who do conceive is 10 months following the last injection with a range of four to 31 months." Since Depo-Provera does not accumulate in the body, the return to fertility is independent of the number of injections received, but may be affected by a woman's age or weight.

A woman should not take Depo-Provera if she has acute liver disease, unexplained vaginal bleeding, breast cancer, or blood clots in the legs, lungs or eyes.

"She also shouldn't have a fear of injections," Wysocki says.

Side Effects

Change in the menstrual cycle is the most common side effect of Depo-Provera. At first there may be irregular bleeding or spotting, but that usually diminishes and eventually disappears after several injections. After a year on Depo-Provera, menstruation will stop completely in approximately half of the women.

Normal menstruation will usually return within a few months once the injections stop.

Women who continue to menstruate while on Depo-Provera may have decreased blood flow, which, in turn, reduces the chance of anemia. There may also be a decrease in menstrual cramps and pain, as well as ovulatory pain.

Schroder, who had very painful premenstrual symptoms before starting Depo-Provera, says she thinks of these side effects as benefits.

After menstrual changes, the most common side effect is weight gain. "It's not clear whether the weight gain is due to water retention or a metabolic effect that increases appetite and body fat," says David Grimes, M.D., a professor with the department of obstetrics and gynecology at the University of Southern California School of Medicine. "But it is real, and women should know about it."

In addition, some patients may experience headache, nervousness, abdominal pain, dizziness, weakness, or fatigue.

Breast Cancer Concerns

The possibility of a link between Depo-Provera and breast cancer was first considered in the early 1970s, after breast cancers were found in beagles treated for more than three years with a dose of Depo-Provera equivalent to 25 times that of the human contraceptive dose. However, those studies were eventually discounted at an October 1981 meeting of the World Health Organization. Experts at that meeting concluded, and FDA later agreed, that beagles were not appropriate animal models for determining what the potential effects of Depo-Provera would be on women.

Ten years later, WHO presented the results of a study of over 11,000 women who used Depo-Provera, mainly in Thailand and New Zealand. (The drug has been approved for contraception in about 90 countries.) Based on the study, published in the Oct. 5, 1991, issue of *The Lancet*, WHO concluded that, overall, women on Depo-Provera are not at increased risk of breast cancer. In addition, breast cancer risk did not increase the longer a woman stayed on the injectable contraceptive.

The study did find a slight increase in the risk of breast cancer during the first four years of use, primarily in women under 35. That increase, however, is statistically weak and comparable to the risk associated with oral contraceptives, according to the researchers.

But the National Women's Health Network disagrees with the researchers' conclusion. In testimony presented to FDA's Fertility and Maternal Health Drugs Advisory Committee last June, Cindy Pearson, a representative of the National Women's Health Network, said that the WHO studies were conducted in countries with breast cancer rates less than half that of the United States and therefore can't be accurately applied to women in this country.

She adds that comparing the breast cancer risk to that associated with oral contraceptives is also misleading. "These disturbing data are emerging from much smaller groups of women than was the case with oral contraceptives," she said. "Only three epidemiologic studies have been done on Depo-Provera and breast cancer, and all three raise a red flag."

However, to Grimes, that increased risk in younger women isn't a link to Depo-Provera. Instead, "It suggests to me that women who start taking Depo-Provera may be coming into the health-care system for the first time and having preexisting tumors discovered."

"It should be noted," says FDA's Bennett, "that more data on breast cancer risk is now available for Depo-Provera than has been required for any other drug prior to marketing."

The results of the WHO study also indicated that Depo-Provera use did not increase the overall risk of cancer of the liver, ovaries, endometrium, or cervix.

Osteoporosis Risk?

A study by Tim Cundy and colleagues, published in the July 6, 1991, issue of the British Medical Journal found that the bone density in 30 women who had been using Depo-Provera for at least five years was less than the bone density of other women of similar age. Cundy recommends "that women with more than one risk factor for osteoporosis [family history, underweight, cigarette smoking, European or Asian origin] should have bone mineral density measurements undertaken if they are considering Depo-Provera use on a continuing basis, and those in the lower third of the normal range are advised to consider other contraceptive methods."

While FDA's Corfman agrees that a woman considering Depo-Provera needs to discuss the possibility of bone thinning with her doctor, he adds, "[the risk of] osteoporosis is just part of the calculation. There are many other issues involved."

FDA is requiring Upjohn to conduct additional research on the effects of Depo-Provera on bone density.

Best Candidates

"[Depo-Provera] has been a godsend for women who've been unable or unwilling to use other methods," says Grimes.

Becky Schroder's plans to have a baby in the next two or three years made her decide against Norplant. Although the implant can be removed at any time, "it isn't cost effective if it's taken out early," she says.

But Pearson, of the National Women's Health Network, is concerned that Depo-Provera will be forced on poor women. She told FDA's advisory committee that "the women's health movement has already documented many cases of coercion even while Depo-Provera was not approved as a contraceptive."

Wysocki acknowledges Pearson's concern. "That concern stems from some very real things that happened back in the 60s, particularly with sterilization, but there's no reason to believe that because the technology is available that it will be abused. The problem itself should be addressed, not the drug."

Wysocki adds that Depo-Provera is a safe, low-cost method of contraception that requires little attention. "No one method of contraception is perfect for all women at all times during their reproductive years," she says. "However, additional options increase the likelihood that a method of contraception that matches each woman's need will be found."

(For more information on all methods of contraception, see the *FDA Consumer* reprint "Comparing Contraceptives." Write to FDA, HFE-88, 5600 Fishers Lane, Rockville, MD 20857, for single copies.)

Dori Stehlin is a staff writer for FDA Consumer.

■ Document Source:
U.S. Department of Health and Human Services, Public Health Service
Food and Drug Administration
FDA Consumer
March 1993

FACTS ABOUT ORAL CONTRACEPTIVES

When oral contraceptives were introduced in the United States in 1960, many women believed they had found the answer to the need for convenient, safe and reliable birth control. By 1965, "the pill" was America's leading contraceptive.

With the 1970's came disillusionment: The pill was not perfect. While it was highly effective and convenient, it had many minor side effects and a few serious ones. Though severe complications were rare, "pill scare" reports created an aura of danger. Pill use dropped in the mid-70's.

Today the pill has been put into perspective. It is not for everyone, but recent studies show it to be safe for most young, healthy, nonsmoking users. Despite widespread publicity on the pill's drawbacks, its benefits must be substantial. It is still the most popular reversible birth control method in America, with more than seven million women taking it daily.

Two Decades of Research. Oral contraceptives are probably the most extensively studied medication in history, yet they are not fully understood. Twenty years of research has, however, brought much safer pills and a long list of guidelines to help doctors screen out women most likely to develop serious complications.

The most important outcome of recent research is that groups of women with a high risk of developing pill complications have been identified. These include smokers, older women (the risks start to rise at 30), and those with a history of certain illnesses. While current knowledge is not precise enough to predict exactly which individuals will suffer serious pill complications, it is continually improving.

New studies also show benefits of pill use, besides contraception, such as protection from pelvic inflammatory disease and other conditions. Many doctors today stress that women should be made aware of these benefits, as well as the possible problems, so they can make informed decisions about the pill.

Research on oral contraceptives continues. Each year the National Institute of Child Health and Human Development (NICHD), a part of the National Institutes of Health, spends millions of dollars to evaluate current pills and develop better ones. This brochure, prepared by staff of the NICHD, describes the latest news on oral contraceptives.

Today's Pills

The most popular oral contraceptives are "combined" pills. These contain two synthetic hormones (an estrogen and a progestogen) similar to the hormones the ovary normally produces.

When studies linked the amount of estrogen in birth control pills with serious side effects—including blood clots, heart attacks, and strokes—researchers developed new pill formulas with less estrogen. They also developed a progestogen-only pill known as the "minipill."

Ten years ago, doctors often prescribed combined pills with 100 to 150 micrograms of estrogen. Today the Food and Drug Administration urges physicians to start patients on combined pills with no more than 50 micrograms of estrogen and, if possible, one of the newer "low dose" combined pills with only 30 or 35 micrograms of estrogen.

Major studies have concluded that switching from higher doses to pills with 50 micrograms of estrogen cuts the blood clot risk substantially. Recent research suggests that pills with less than 50 micrograms of estrogen cut the risk even further.

Progestogen levels in pills have also dropped over the years. Minipills contain even less progestogen than low-dose combined pills, which may make the minipill the safest oral contraceptive known.

How they work. Combined birth-control pills, including the newer low-dose forms, work by suppressing ovulation, the release of an egg from the ovary. Without a released egg, pregnancy cannot occur. Though rare, it is possible for women using combined pills to ovulate. Then other mechanisms work to prevent pregnancy.

Both kinds of pills make the cervical mucus thick and "inhospitable" to sperm, discouraging entry to the uterus. In addition, they make it difficult for a fertilized egg to implant, by causing changes in fallopian tube contractions and in the uterine lining. These actions explain why the minipill works, as it generally does not suppress ovulation.

Effectiveness. Taken properly, the combined pills are better than 99 percent effective. Some formulas with less estrogen may be slightly less effective, about 98 to 99 percent.

Minipills are comparable in effectiveness to the IUD, at around 98 percent. But they must be taken without fail every day—ideally at the same time. Missing just one minipill can undo the contraceptive protection. Also, because minipills do not generally suppress ovulation, many doctors recommend a backup method, such as a diaphragm or condoms, at midcycle.

Why Pills Fail

If you take oral contraceptives, you should be prepared to use an additional form of birth control, because there are times the pill's effectiveness can be diminished.

Skipping pills. This is probably the main reason for reduced effectiveness. Directions for what to do after missing a dose vary with the pill formula and are included in the package insert that comes with all pills. Using a backup method for the rest of the cycle (while continuing to take the pill) will increase protection from pregnancy.

Illness. If you become sick with vomiting or diarrhea, your oral contraceptives may not be fully absorbed. It is safest to use an additional method for the rest of the cycle.

Drug interaction. Some medications can diminish the pill's effectiveness, including certain antibiotics (rifampin, and perhaps ampicillin and tetracycline); epilepsy drugs (Dilantin); anti-inflammatory or antiarthritic drugs (phenylbutazone); and barbiturates (phenobarbital). If you are treated for any ailment, even one that seems totally unrelated to pill use, be sure to inform your physician if you take birth control pills.

Should You Take the Pill?

Many women are attracted by the advantages of the pill but are also concerned by the list of possible complications. Keep in mind that the process of weighing the benefits and risks is a highly individual one. No two women have exactly the same medical history or birth control needs. A doctor will help you make the best decision for *you.*

For some women the pill is ruled out altogether. Using pills with estrogen is too risky for women who have had blood clots, heart attack, or stroke; chest pain caused by angina pectoris; known or suspected breast cancer or cancer of the uterine lining; undiagnosed abnormal vaginal bleeding (which may indicate cancer and must be checked out); liver tumors; or jaundice during pregnancy.

Other health problems may also forbid pill use. These include fibroid uterine growths, diabetes, high cholesterol levels, high blood pressure, obesity, depression, gall bladder disease, and exposure to DES before birth.

In addition, because the pill tends to cause the body to retain water, women with a history of migraine headaches, asthma, epilepsy, or kidney and heart diseases may find the pill worsens their condition. If they choose to take it, they must be monitored closely by their doctors. Cigarette smoking and age also add to the chances of a woman developing serious pill-related complications.

But what about a woman without any of these risk factors? Once a woman's doctor has found that she has no detectable physical reason for avoiding the pill, the decision is in her hands. The pill carries a relatively small risk of serious complications even to the safest group of users—young, healthy nonsmokers. Therefore it is important that the decision be an informed one.

Understanding the risks. The "patient leaflet" that comes with all pills contains a complete list of potential complications. Women should remember, though:

♦ The pill affects all body cells, so the potential complications linked with it are many. But the chances of most young, healthy, nonsmoking women developing a particular complication are slim.

♦ The most serious side effects are also the most rare.

♦ Many of the risks known today were estimated through studies of *older* women using the *higher* dose pills. Therefore some experts believe that these studies may overstate the likelihood of complications in *younger* women using the newer *low-dose* pills or minipills.

♦ Knowledge of the health risks associated with childbirth can help to place in perspective the problems associated with pill use. The chances of dying from a childbirth complication exceed the chances of dying from a pill complication, *except* for smoking pill users aged 35 and over. As shown in the chart below, in either event, death is very rare. (Many women die each year for other reasons, including accidents and other health problems, as shown by the overall death rate included below for comparison.)

Estimated Annual Deaths per 100,000 Women

Cause of Death	Ages 15-19	20-24	25-29	30-34	35-39	40-44
Childbirth	5	6	7	13	21	22
Pill complications, smokers	2	4	6	12	31	61
Pill complications, nonsmokers	1	1	2	3	9	18
All causes, including accidents	54	67	74	98	146	237

Other considerations: minor side effects. The pill also causes many minor side effects. Although they are not life threatening, they are nuisances and many women stop taking the pill because of them.

A minority of women on the pill experience nausea or vomiting (usually only in the first few cycles), weight changes, breast tenderness, abdominal cramps, or skin discoloration. Bladder and vaginal infections may also occur more frequently with pill use. In addition, some women report changes in sex drive (either increased or decreased), a loss of scalp hair, or an intolerance to contact lenses (because of water retention).

Many of these complaints disappear after the first few cycles of pill use. They may occur less often with low-dose pills and minipills. The newer formulas, however, are more likely to cause menstrual irregularities, such as spotting, breakthrough bleeding (which should be reported to a doctor), or, rarely, a lack of periods altogether. Menstrual irregularities are much more common with minipills than with combined pills, but cycles often become regular with time.

Knowing the benefits, too. The combined pill, when taken properly, is unmatched in effectiveness. And the pill in general allows more spontaneity in sexual relations than barrier methods that must be applied at the time of intercourse.

These benefits have long been known. But we are now learning that the pill protects women from some relatively common and potentially serious disorders that have nothing to do with its use as a contraceptive. According to recent estimates, each year, the pill prevents:

- 51,000 cases of pelvic inflammatory disease, 13,300 of which would have required hospitalization,
- 20,000 hospitalizations for certain types of noncancerous breast disease,
- 9,900 hospitalizations for ectopic pregnancy,
- 3,000 hospitalizations for ovarian cysts,
- 27,000 cases of iron deficiency anemia, and
- 2,700 cases of rheumatoid arthritis.

The protection against pelvic inflammatory disease (PID) may be the most important noncontraceptive benefit of the pill. PID—a bacterial infection of the uterus, fallopian tubes, or ovaries—affects an estimated 850,000 U.S. women yearly. It can lead to infertility or, in rare cases, death. Studies have shown that women on the pill have half the chance of developing PID compared to women using no form of birth control. (Women using barrier devices also have half the chance.)

Other advantages of the pill include less menstrual cramping, lighter blood flow, and for those using combined pills, very regular periods. Some women using oral contraceptives also have diminished premenstrual tension. And women with acne often find the pill improves their complexion.

The Major Risk

The most serious side effect of oral contraceptive use is an increased risk of cardiovascular disease—specifically blood clots, heart attacks, and strokes. But even these complications are occurring less frequently, according to Bruce Stadel, M.D. (NICHD), as a result of lower hormone content in pills, better screening of women who might be at high risk, and, perhaps most importantly, the recent drop in pill use among women over 35.

What are the odds? Pill-related heart attacks are very rare. They occur in an estimated one in 14,000 users between the ages of 30 and 39. Between the ages of 40 and 44 the risk rises to about one case in 1,500 women on the pill.

Strokes occur five times more frequently among women taking oral contraceptives. But they are a rare event, too, affecting about one in 2,700 women on the pill.

Although clots in the veins occur more often than heart attacks or strokes, they are still uncommon, affecting about one in 500 previously healthy women on the pill. Hormone changes in pregnancy cause clots far more frequently than pills do.

Who are the high-risk women? The vast majority of heart attacks and strokes among pill users occur in women who smoke, women over 35, and women with other health conditions, such as high blood pressure, that ordinarily contribute to cardiovascular risk. Women with a combination of two or more of these factors carry the greatest risk of all. (See "Compounding the Risks.")

Some research shows that the length of pill use can affect the chances of having a cardiovascular complication. A recent study found that women aged 40 to 49 who had taken the pill for five or more years had twice the average heart attack risk—even years after they stopped taking the pill. Heavy

smoking adds far more to the chances of having a heart attack, however.

Perhaps surprisingly, age and smoking habits do not seem to increase the chances of developing blood clots in the veins. But women with certain blood types—A, B, or AB—are twice as likely to develop clots as women with type O. This is true whether a woman is on the pill or not.

NICHD-funded research has shown that women who experience clotting disorders may lack the ability to produce extra amounts of a certain anticlotting blood protein that women on the pill need. Unfortunately it is not yet possible to predict who will have this problem. But researchers have found evidence suggesting that women may counteract it through regular exercise, which may spur the body to produce more of the anticlotting protein.

Because oral contraceptives double the chances of developing blood clots after surgery, doctors advise women taking the pill to stop, if possible, at least four weeks before any scheduled operation. And all women on the pill should know the symptoms that indicate a possible blood clot—sharp pain in the chest, coughing blood, or sudden shortness of breath; pain in the calf; or sudden partial or complete loss of vision—and notify their doctors immediately if they experience any of them.

High blood pressure. Although many women experience a mild elevation in blood pressure when they are taking oral contraceptives, it usually remains within the normal range and returns to "prepill" levels when they stop. Studies several years ago found that pill users have three to six times the average risk of developing high blood pressure. It has been estimated to occur in one to four percent of women who take the pill and is usually confined to those over 35. Newer studies show that high blood pressure is not a common problem for today's younger pill takers. But *all* women on the pill should have their blood pressure checked every six to 12 months.

Compounding the Risks

Factors such as smoking, increasing age, or high blood pressure add to the chances of developing cardiovascular disorders—problems in the heart or blood vessels. Combine any of these factors with oral contraceptive use, and the risks multiply. And when a woman has more than one risk factor, her chances of a serious pill complication skyrocket.

Smoking. Most of the women who have a heart attack or stroke while using the pill are smokers. The mechanism is not understood, but the pill somehow intensifies the adverse effects of smoking on the circulatory system.

To illustrate: One study found that either using oral contraceptives or smoking increased the odds of having a stroke by about six times. In women who both smoked *and* took the pill, the risks did not just add together. Instead, they jumped to 22 times the risk of stroke in women who neither smoked nor took the pill.

All smokers using the pill are at greater risk than nonsmokers. The likelihood of heart attack or stroke rises sharply for those who smoke more than 15 cigarettes per day. From the standpoint of safety, doctors now advise pill users not to just cut back, but to quit smoking altogether.

Age. The natural aging process also increases the chances of developing cardiovascular disorders, and birth control pills accentuate the risk. An example: In women who *don't* use the pill, those aged 40 to 44 are about five times as likely to have a heart attack as those aged 30 to 39. But in pill users, the older age group is about nine times as likely to have a heart attack.

The cardiovascular risks of the pill begin to rise substantially around age 30, particularly in smokers. However, there is no definite cutoff age for pill use. Some doctors believe that regardless of smoking habits, women should consider other forms of contraception starting at age 30. Others feel that at age 30, women *who smoke* and take the pill should choose between the two, while *nonsmokers* are relatively safe until age 35. Still others hold that the new low-dose pills and minipills may be safe options for women over 35 who do not smoke or have other unfavorable health conditions.

Obviously, the final word is not yet in. Over the next few years, NICHD-supported studies should help clarify the pill's risks to women over 30.

Health conditions. Women at any age with health problems that ordinarily increase the chances of cardiovascular disease are even more at risk when using the pill. The conditions include:

♦ high blood pressure,
♦ a history of high blood pressure in pregnancy,
♦ obesity,
♦ diabetes mellitus, and
♦ elevated cholesterol.

Combined risk factors. When more than one of the above risk factors are present, the chances of a serious pill complication increase dramatically. A recent study found that the odds of having a heart attack are increased by:

♦ 3 times among pill users,
♦ 5 times among smokers,
♦ 8 times among people with high blood pressure, and
♦ 170 times among pill users with high blood pressure who smoke.

An expert on oral contraceptives at the Centers for Disease Control (CDC), Dr. Howard Ory, stresses that "the most serious adverse effect of pill use—death from cardiovascular disease—is also the *most preventable.*"

"If women who use the pill would not smoke," he states, "at least *half* of all deaths associated with pill use could be avoided. If in addition, women with other predisposing factors for cardiovascular disease, such as high blood pressure, high cholesterol, and diabetes mellitus would not use the pill, deaths could be further reduced."

The Pill and Cancer

Probably the question women ask most frequently about oral contraceptives is, "Does the pill cause cancer?"

Because most kinds of cancer take so long to develop, the answer must still be tentative, but it is reassuring: There is no firm evidence that the pill causes cancer.

The NICHD and the CDC are currently cosponsoring a long-term project to analyze the pill's relationship to breast cancer and cancer of the reproductive tract. Although final results will not be available until the mid-1980's, the preliminary results are encouraging, showing no association between the pill and breast cancer. Early results also suggest that women who have used the pill for at least one year have *half* the average risk of developing cancer of the ovary and of the endometrium (the lining of the uterus).

No clear cause-and-effect relationship has been established between the pill and cancer of the cervix, but most doctors still feel it is very important for women on the pill to have yearly Pap smears.

One kind of potentially life-threatening cell growth that is linked with the pill is an extremely rare liver tumor known as hepatic adenoma. Although it is not cancerous, it can cause internal bleeding. It occurs in about one in 33,000 pill users per year, mostly women who have taken the pill for about five years or more. Early detection of the condition can make a difference. Make sure that your checkups include a physical exam of the abdomen.

The Pill and Body Chemistry

Studies of women taking combined pills with at least 50 micrograms of estrogen show changes in the levels of sugars, fats and proteins in the blood, and alterations in the way the body uses certain nutrients. These and other metabolic changes can cause slightly altered thyroid, liver and blood tests, though results usually remain within the normal range.

While it appears that metabolic changes are lessened with the newer formulas, the long-range effects of even small changes in body chemistry in pill users are unknown. Current studies supported by the NICHD are expected to define these changes more precisely and to determine whether they affect the risk of cardiovascular disease in pill users.

Nutritional changes. Oral contraceptives can affect nutritional status, but studies of this topic often have conflicting results. This is because many variables, such as hormone shifts throughout a menstrual cycle, can also change the body's nutritional needs.

In women taking the combined pill, studies have found increased levels of vitamin A and iron; decreased levels of vitamins B-6, B-12, C, and riboflavin; and both increases and decreases in levels of folic acid and zinc.

A lowered level of vitamin B-6 is the most consistently reported nutritional change in pill users. One NICHD-funded study found that lowered levels of B-6 during pregnancy and location were more common in women who used the pill for a long time (more than 30 months), and became pregnant within four months after stopping the pill. Nevertheless, it is uncertain whether pill use is a cause of true vitamin B-6 deficiency, which is linked with depression (see next page). Other symptoms of vitamin deficiency include weakness, lethargy, dizziness, skin and gum irritations, and an increased susceptibility to infection.

Next to vitamin B-6, folic acid is the nutrient most significantly affected by the pill. Changes in folic acid metabolism have been reported in connection with two conditions in pill users. A few women using oral contraceptives have developed a rare but serious anemia which responds to treatment with folic acid supplements. In addition, the pill is linked with changes in folic acid metabolism in cells around the cervix, which may be related to a kind of abnormal cell growth called cervical dysplasia. An NICHD-supported study found that cervical dysplasia sometimes improves with folic acid supplements.

For pill users, a balanced diet is often recommended over routine vitamin and mineral supplements for two reasons. First, overdosing on supplements can be toxic, and second, people taking supplements often do not try as hard to get a balanced diet. Vitamin supplements cannot take the place of a balanced diet; in fact, they need to have proper foods present to work right. But when medical tests show a vitamin deficiency, vitamin supplement therapy may be in order.

Recent studies on oral contraceptives and metabolism found that pill users do not eliminate caffeine or valium as efficiently as nonusers. This means that either substance can accumulate in the body. As a result, women using the pill may be more prone to caffeine side effects such as nervousness and insomnia. Those using valium could become oversedated if the dosage is not carefully watched.

Depression

Oral contraceptives alleviate depression in some women and worsen it in others. Symptoms of depression related to pill use include pessimism, dissatisfaction, listlessness, tension, crying, and perhaps anxiety or a loss of sex drive. Although many of the reports of pill-related depression came when higher doses of estrogen were widely used, it is not clear whether depression is less common with the newer low-dose pills or minipills.

Depression can be a symptom of vitamin B-6 deficiency. The pill can affect the body's use of B-6 and other vitamins and minerals, and studies have found that some depressed pill users are B-6 deficient. These women may respond to vitamin B-6 therapy. Women who become seriously depressed while on the pill should discuss it with their physicians, and consider switching to another form of birth control.

The Pill and Childbearing

Many women taking birth control pills are planning to have children at some time. For them the news is good: There appears to be little risk that use of the pill leads to sterility. In fact, because the pill protects many women from pelvic inflammatory disease, which can damage the fallopian tubes, it guards against a leading cause of infertility.

Fertility. Former pill users may take a few months longer to conceive than other women, but an estimated 80 percent of women resume normal reproductive functions within three months after stopping the pill and more than 95 percent are ovulating within a year.

Women who do not regain normal periods within six months should see a doctor for a complete evaluation. Most women who have menstrual problems after stopping the pill had irregular periods before they started taking it. But some studies suggest that there is a very slim chance that the pill itself causes a condition known as "post-pill amenorrhea"—a lack of periods. Though the cause of the problem is a matter

of much debate among researchers, infertility after stopping the pill generally is temporary and responds to treatment.

Pregnancy. Many doctors recommend that women who wish to become pregnant use traditional barrier contraceptives for at least three months after stopping the pill. Usually, a woman's menstrual cycle will become regular during this time, which permits the doctor to accurately date the start of the pregnancy. When former pill users do become pregnant, they have no greater risk of complications than other women.

Although it happens extremely rarely, oral contraceptives can fail even when a woman has been conscientious about taking them every day. In addition to causing an unplanned pregnancy, pill failure can lead to inadvertent exposure of a developing fetus to extra hormones. Some studies show a slight increased risk of birth defects in infants exposed before birth to oral contraceptive hormones; other studies have found no risk. Experts generally agree that the risks, if they exist at all, are very small.

But for absolute safety, if you even suspect you might be pregnant, immediately stop taking the pill, switch to another form of contraception, and have a pregnancy test as soon as possible. Studies have shown no added risk of birth defects when conception occurs one month after stopping the pill.

Breastfeeding. Physicians often recommend methods other than the pill for women who are nursing babies. For one thing, the estrogen in combined pills can suppress milk production. Also, very small quantities of hormones pass from the mother to her nursing infant. Although no long-term effects of this ingestion have been reported, the possibility of risk to the baby has not been extensively studied. For women who want to breastfeed and use an oral contraceptive, doctors frequently suggest the minipill, since it does not suppress lactation.

How to Minimize the Risks

Both doctors and the women for whom they prescribe birth control pills have a role in reducing the chances of pill-related complications. Doctors must screen patients carefully, follow up conscientiously, and prescribe the lowest possible dose that is compatible with an individual woman's needs. Yet as recently as 1978, one-fourth of the women taking the pill in the United States were still using formulas with more than 50 micrograms of estrogen. Check your prescription: If it contains more than 50 micrograms, you might ask your physician if you can try a lower dose.

Women must be open with their doctors, informing them of any health problems. They must also know the signs that indicate a possibly serious complication of pill use and call their doctors immediately (see next page). In addition, women on the pill should exercise regularly. Above all, they should have medical checkups at least yearly (more frequently if their doctors advise).

Twenty years ago there was hope that the pill would prove to be the perfect form of birth control: effective, convenient, and safe for all women. Ten years ago reports of side effects brought disillusionment. Today we know that the pill, though imperfect, is an option many women can use safely. We now have better formulas, better screening of women, and a better informed public. And as these trends continue we can look forward to even safer use of the pill.

Warning Signals

Women taking oral contraceptives should be alert to any physical or mental change that may warrant a visit to the doctor. If you experience any of the following symptoms, notify your physician at once and remind him or her that you are on the pill.

- ♦ Severe abdominal pain
- ♦ Chest pain, coughing, shortness of breath
- ♦ Pain or tenderness in calf or thigh
- ♦ Severe headache, dizziness, or faintness
- ♦ Muscle weakness or numbness
- ♦ Speech disturbance
- ♦ Eye problems: blurred vision, flashing lights, blindness
- ♦ Breast lump
- ♦ Severe depression
- ♦ Yellowing of skin

"Facts About Oral Contraceptives" was written by Maureen B. Gardner, Office of Research Reporting, National Institute of Child Health and Human Development (NICHD). It is reprinted from the June 1983 issue of *Good Housekeeping* magazine with permission of the publisher.

The NICHD, part of the Federal Government's National Institutes of Health, conducts and supports research on the various processes that determine the health of children, adults, families and populations. For more copies of this fact sheet or others in this series, write to NICHD, P.O. Box 29111, Washington, D.C. 20040.

Other Publications in This Series:

- ♦ *Facts About Anorexia Nervosa*
- ♦ *Facts About Cesarean Childbirth*
- ♦ *Facts About Childhood Hyperactivity*
- ♦ *Facts About Down Syndrome*
- ♦ *Facts About Dyslexia*
- ♦ *Facts About Dysmenorrhea and Premenstrual Syndrome*
- ♦ *Facts About Precocious Puberty*
- ♦ *Facts About Pregnancy and Smoking*
- ♦ *Facts About Premature Birth*
- ♦ *Facts About Vasectomy Safety*

■ Document Source:
   U.S. Department of Health and Human Services, Public Health Service
   National Institutes of Health
   National Institute of Child Health and Human Development

FACTS ABOUT VASECTOMY SAFETY

Until recent years, few people questioned the long-term safety of vasectomy. A couple considering vasectomy was more likely to ask a doctor about the operation itself, its effectiveness, or how it might change their sexual relationship.

Things have changed. Men considering vasectomy and their partners now want to know about long-term side effects. Their biggest concern is hardening of the arteries or heart disease—issues raised by animal studies in the late 1970s. Researchers speculated then that sperm antibodies, produced

by many men following vasectomy, could be responsible for these and other health risks.

This concern prompted the National Institute of Child Health and Human Development (NICHD), the nation's largest supporter of research on birth control methods, to start a multimillion dollar program of vasectomy research. Fortunately for the millions of men with vasectomies and their families, the latest news about its long-term safety is good.

Almost 40,000 men took part in four studies completed in recent years under contracts with the Institute. The findings are reassuringly similar: None show an increased risk of hardening of the arteries or other forms of cardiovascular disease in men with vasectomies. In fact, one study found that, for unknown reasons, men who have had vasectomies are healthier in some ways than those who have not.

While this is good news for men with vasectomies, those who are considering it should still give the decision serious thought, because vasectomy is generally permanent. Although new techniques for reversing vasectomies may increase the odds that fertility will return, there are no guarantees. Realizing this, and being up-to-date on news about long-term safety, can help couples today to make informed decisions about vasectomy.

After Decline, Vasectomy Popularity Jumps

Sterilization—including both vasectomy and female sterilization—is now the most popular form of birth control in the United States, chosen by four out of 10 couples who use contraception.

Vasectomy is far simpler and less expensive than sterilization for women. Yet today, fewer men than women undergo sterilization procedures. Just a short while ago, this was not the case.

In the mid-1970s, men and women had sterilizations in nearly equal numbers. Gradually, however, more and more couples opted for female sterilization, until these procedures outnumbered vasectomies by 2 to 1 in 1982.

Fears about the long-term safety of vasectomy were at least partly responsible for a decline in vasectomies, experts believe, along with easier and safer sterilization operations for women.

But now that trend seems to be reversing. The Association for Voluntary Sterilization (AVS) noted a 50 percent jump in vasectomies performed between 1982 and 1983. The AVS credits this increase to "evidence from scientific studies that has dispelled lingering doubts about the safety of vasectomy."

Long-Term Safety: The Antibody Question

Concern over the long-term safety of vasectomy first arose several years ago when researchers discovered that many men produce antibodies to sperm following the operation. Fortunately, investigators have since found no evidence that this immune response causes health problems in men.

Antibodies are disease-fighting substances that circulate in the bloodstream. Normally they protect the body from invaders such as viruses, bacteria, and foreign cells. In the case of many vasectomized men, however, the body's immune system mistakes sperm for foreign cells and forms antibodies against them.

This happens because early in infancy, the immune system learns what is native to the body and what is foreign. Sperm cells are not produced until years later, at puberty. But at that time, they are essentially hidden from the immune system by barriers in the reproductive tract, so antibodies are not formed.

After vasectomy, however, the protective barriers can be broken. The testicles still produce sperm, which the body absorbs. In the process, antibodies often form.

One-half to two-thirds of men who have had vasectomies develop antibodies to sperm after the procedure. It is not known why some men produce more or fewer antibodies than other, and some none at all. A very small percent of men without vasectomies also develop sperm antibodies because of surgery, infection, or inborn abnormalities of the reproductive tract.

Counseling—A Must

Before a man has a vasectomy, it is very important that he and his partner receive thorough counseling that permits them to ask questions and express any fears they may have. This forces a couple to become sure of their decision; without it, some anxieties are likely to remain. Vasectomy counselors are urged to explain all other methods of birth control, in addition to giving full details on the benefits and possible drawbacks of vasectomy.

In men with vasectomies, the antibodies may persist for 10 years or more after surgery. Doctors became concerned about this immune response because they felt that, in theory, it might have adverse consequences.

The most serious side effect that was suggested by studies in monkeys is a worsening of hardening of the arteries. When these studies were reported in the late 1970s, the investigators thought the antibodies might play a part in damaging inner walls of arteries. Nevertheless, research to date has not demonstrated that these findings apply to men.

As an example, one study showed that the level of sperm antibodies in a man's bloodstream does not affect his risk of developing coronary heart disease. At the Battelle Human Affairs Research Centers in Seattle, WA, a group of scientists found that high levels of sperm antibodies were equally common in men with and without heart disease. There was no evidence, moreover, that the antibody levels increase over time.

Largest Study on Vasectomy: Healthier Men

Even before the findings from the monkey studies were reported, the NICHD started a project that became the largest study on vasectomy performed to date. The study, involving more than 20,000 men in four U.S. cities, was designed to find out if the immune reaction following vasectomy could lead to any health problems.

In announcing the study, health officials stated that because it is the most comprehensive assessment ever performed on this topic, the results are especially encouraging. In almost every category of illness, the men with vasectomies were either

no more prone to disease than the other men, or even less likely to become ill.

In this study, based at the University of California at Los Angeles, scientists compared the rates of more than 100 diseases in 10,590 men who had vasectomies and an equal number who had not. When the study began in 1976, they were mainly interested in diseases that might be related to an immune response, such as rheumatoid arthritis. But when early results from the monkey studies appeared the next year, they added a special focus on cardiovascular disease.

The study's results, reported widely in 1983, showed that men with vasectomies have no more health problems than other men—including diseases involving the immune system, cardiovascular disease, cancer, and impotence. This held true for specific diseases that had been cited as possible complications of vasectomy, including hardening of the arteries, rheumatoid arthritis, blood clotting disorders, gout, and multiple sclerosis.

The only condition seen markedly more often in the vasectomized men was epididymitis, a local inflammation near the site of the operation. This complication, which was previously known, occurs mostly within the first year after vasectomy. Treated with heat, it usually clears up in a week.

Otherwise, men with vasectomies were just as healthy as other men, if not more so. Besides having fewer cases of cancer and heart disease, the men with vasectomies also had one-third fewer deaths. The lower death rate was found for all causes of death except accidents and violence, which killed the same number of men with and without vasectomies. The researchers do not know why men with vasectomies had better survival rates overall.

Quick Operation, Rapid Recovery

The vasectomy operation is quick, safe, and inexpensive. Usually it is performed in a doctor's office or clinic and takes only 10 to 15 minutes.

After giving the patient a local anesthetic, a doctor generally makes two small incisions, one on either side of the scrotum, then locates the two thin tubes that carry sperm, seals them off, and closes the incisions. The patient rests for an hour or two before going home.

The cost for vasectomy averaged $240 in 1982, a price one-fifth that of female sterilization.

Recovery from the vasectomy operation is rapid, and serious complications are rare. Swelling, bruising, and pain—the most common complaints—occur in about half of men after vasectomy. The discomfort subsides within a week or two and usually responds to treatment with ice packs, mild pain killers, scrotal support and rest. Men are generally advised to avoid strenuous work or exercise for about 2 days after the operation.

A minority of men develop a small lump of inflammatory tissue called a granuloma near the incision site. Granulomas, caused by sperm leaking into surrounding tissues, usually stay so small that they don't cause symptoms. If they do cause pain, it is generally treated with bed rest and mild pain killers.

Fewer than 3 in 100 men develop complications such as infection, hematoma (bleeding under the skin), or epididymitis (inflammation of the tube that collects sperm from the testes). All can be treated, and no deaths from vasectomy have been reported in the United States.

Delayed Effectiveness

Vasectomy is one of the most effective means of birth control, with a less than 1 to 100 chance of failure. It does not offer immediate protection from unwanted pregnancy, however.

The reproductive tract is not clear of sperm for several weeks, and other forms of birth control must be used until a semen sample, generally checked at 6 to 8 weeks, shows no sperm. The most common reason for vasectomy failure is probably unprotected intercourse before all sperm have cleared the reproductive tract.

Other Major Studies: Consistent Findings

While the UCLA project looked at the rates of all possible diseases in men, other studies in the NICHD's program of vasectomy research have taken a more specialized approach. Three large studies in men have focused on the question raised in animal studies about hardening of the arteries and heart disease. Again, the findings for men with vasectomies are favorable.

One study involved more than 7,000 men who had hardening of the coronary arteries, which supply the heart muscle with blood. Researchers at the Medical College of Wisconsin looked for factors that might influence the severity of coronary blockage. They found no connection between vasectomy and the disease, but they did confirm that age, smoking, and high blood pressure all make coronary blockage more severe.

The question of long-term safety was tackled in another study—this one involving 5,000 men—based at the Battelle Human Affairs Research Centers in Seattle, WA. Many men in the study had had vasectomies for more than 25 years, while the average time since vasectomy was 15 years, the longest in any study to date.

Regardless of the length of time since the procedure, the men with vasectomies did not have a greater risk of heart disease. The researchers reported that "this finding strengthens the results of all previous studies in humans," which also found no relation between vasectomy and heart disease.

Similarly reassuring findings have come from the latest study, a Boston University project involving about 6,000 men. Results show no higher risk of heart attack in men with vasectomies.

In all, the NICHD and other organizations have sponsored more than a dozen large studies on vasectomy involving more than 100,000 men. None show a greater risk of any serious illness in men with vasectomies. And contrary to the findings in monkeys, none demonstrate an increased risk of hardening of the arteries or heart disease.

When Permanence Is a Problem

While safety is a major consideration in choosing a birth control method, another important factor is convenience. Vasectomy's permanence makes it convenient; within a few weeks after the operation, no other steps must be taken to prevent pregnancy.

Although this is an advantage to most men who have the operation, it is a drawback for a very small percent of them.

Approximately 2 in 1000 men who have vasectomies regret it later and wish to have the operation reversed.

The main reasons for requesting a reversal are remarriage, death of a child, or an improvement in finances followed by a wish for another child. Fewer than 10 percent of men who request reversals do so because of physical or psychological problems following vasectomy.

Sex After Vasectomy: No Difference

After vasectomy, a man can safely resume having sex (using another form of birth control until his semen is free of sperm) as soon as he feels comfortable. Because the sperm and fluids from the area sealed off by vasectomy make up only a small fraction of the total fluid ejaculated, he should notice no difference in the amount of fluid nor in its appearance. The size of the testicles remains unchanged as well.

Two common worries about vasectomy are that it will reduce a man's sex hormone levels or take away his ability to have sex. These myths have no biological basis, however, because vasectomy only prevents the escape of sperm from the reproductive system, not the release of testosterone, the male sex hormone, into the bloodstream.

Both sperm and testosterone are produced in the testicles, but they leave by different routes. Sperm move through a series of ducts that channel through the reproductive organs to the outside of the body, while tiny veins in the testicles transport testosterone into the bloodstream.

So when vasectomy seals the tubes that carry sperm, it doesn't affect the transfer of testosterone into the bloodstream. Therefore there is no physical reason for a loss of sex drive or other sexual characteristics. A small percentage of men—less than 1 to 5 percent—have psychological problems after vasectomy that can include a drop in sex drive. But according to a report from the Johns Hopkins University Population Information Program, reactions like these can be reduced with careful counseling before the operation.

Serious marital, psychological, or sexual instability should be treated as possible reasons for not having a vasectomy, according to the report. It also states that "vasectomized men and their wives usually report either no change or an improvement in marital happiness and sexual satisfaction."

Reversal Operations: No Guarantees

In contrast to the original operation, the vasectomy reversal is a complicated, delicate and expensive procedure that is not covered by medical insurance. The difficulty lies in trying to reconnect the sperm-carrying tube's inner canal, which is the size of a pinpoint. And although new surgical techniques are improving the chances of success, no doctor can guarantee that a reversal operation will result in both the reappearance of sperm in the semen and, ultimately, the achievement of pregnancy.

Pregnancy rates following vasectomy reversal range from 16 to 85 percent. Success depends on several factors, including the ability of the surgeon performing the reversal, the way in which the original operation was performed, and the time lapsed since vasectomy.

Some reports show that when reversal is performed within 2 years of the original operation, men can expect sperm counts eventually to return to normal. If it is done between 2 and 10 years later, they have about a 90 percent chance, and if it is more than 10 years they have only a 35 percent chance of regaining normal sperm counts.

But returning sperm counts to normal is only half the battle; the other half is achieving pregnancy. Here, the fertility of the woman must be considered as well. Another factor in question is whether men with high levels of antibodies to sperm are less likely to regain fertility following a reversal operation.

Physicians are often asked about the possibility of storing frozen semen in sperm banks before vasectomy, as a safety measure. Few men follow up on this, however. While it is possible to bank sperm and later establish pregnancy, it works an estimated one time out of four. Some experts believe that individuals who want to bank sperm probably shouldn't have a vasectomy, because they most likely have doubts about giving up their ability to father a child.

Peace of Mind

For most men with vasectomies, though, the permanence is a benefit; it frees them from worries of unwanted pregnancies and the hassles of other forms of birth control. And now they can also take reassurance from findings of current research on vasectomy's long-term safety.

More information on vasectomy is available from the following sources:

Association for Voluntary Sterilization
122 East 42nd Street
New York, NY 10168
(Brochures for men and women interested in sterilization)

Population Information Program
Johns Hopkins University
Hampton House
624 North Broadway
Baltimore, MD 21205
(In-depth reports on vasectomy and other forms of birth control)

National Clearinghouse for Family Planning Information
P.O. Box 12921
Arlington, VA 22209
(Bibliography on male and female sterilization; other birth control information)

Planned Parenthood
Publications Department
810 7th Avenue
New York, NY 10019
(Send 50¢ for brochure called "All About Vasectomy")

"Facts About Vasectomy Safety" was written by Maureen B. Gardner, Office of Research Reporting, National Institute of Child Health and Human Development (NICHD).

The NICHD, part of the Federal Government's National Institutes of Health, conducts and supports research on the processes that determine the health of children and adults. For copies of this fact sheet or others in this series, write to the National Institute of Child Health and Human Development, P.O. Box 29111, Washington, D.C., 20040.

Other Publications in This Series:

- ◆ Facts About Anorexia Nervosa
- ◆ Facts About Cesarean Childbirth
- ◆ Facts About Childhood Hyperactivity
- ◆ Facts About Dyslexia
- ◆ Facts About Premenstrual Syndrome
- ◆ Facts About Oral Contraceptives
- ◆ Facts About Precocious Puberty
- ◆ Facts About Pregnancy and Smoking
- ◆ Facts About Premature Birth

■ **Document Source:**
U.S. Department of Health and Human Services, Public Health Service
National Institutes of Health
National Institute of Child Health and Human Development

INFERTILITY SERVICES

About one in six U.S. couples is infertile. If you are among them, you may have considered contacting a health care provider that offers advanced infertility services.

Most infertility service providers will tell you what their record has been in helping couples. But in talking with or writing to different providers, you may find that success rates are calculated differently—making it confusing to select among the more than 200 programs offering these advanced services.

In addition, a particular infertility service may have a lower success rate than others, but specialize in more difficult cases. Or, a service may have a very good overall success rate, but not be the best one to treat your particular problem. Infertility experts emphasize that your chances for success depend on many factors, such as age and cause of infertility.

The staff at the Federal Trade Commission has reviewed how success-rate claims are calculated by infertility services. The following information may help in evaluating these claims and selecting the best program for your specific needs.

How Success Rates Are Advertised

As you contact infertility service providers, consider carefully how success rates are calculated. Make sure to ask for the success rate for people who fit your particular patient profile, such as your age and cause of infertility.

Ask which specific procedures are included or omitted in the figures. This information can be difficult to understand, so ask for it in "plain English."

Included here are explanations of some frequently used success-rate calculations. For help in understanding these definitions, please refer to "Terms You Need to Know."

Live Birth Rate per Egg Stimulation

This figure tells how many births occurred in relation to the number of egg-stimulation procedures performed. Experts say this figure is the most meaningful overall success-rate statistic, because it includes live births as well as all procedures performed, including those that failed.

Live Birth Rate per Embryo Transfer

This figure refers to the percentage of births from all embryo transfer procedures. Although this number reflects live births—which may be the most meaningful figure—it does not include those instances where the attempt at egg stimulation, egg retrieval, and fertilization did not succeed.

Terms You Need to Know

In vitro fertilization (IVF): In this procedure, a woman's eggs are retrieved and combined with sperm to fertilize in the laboratory. Any fertilized eggs, called embryos, are returned to the uterus.

The steps involved in IVF are:

Step 1   Egg Stimulation
Step 2   Egg Retrieval
Step 3   Fertilization
Step 4   Embryo Transfer

If all goes well, the next two steps are:

Step 5   Clinical Pregnancy
Step 6   Live Birth

Gamete intrafallopian transfer (GIFT): This procedure differs from IVF in that retrieved eggs and sperm are injected into a woman's fallopian tubes where fertilization can take place.

Because fertilization does not take place outside the body, there is no embryo transfer step in GIFT.

Egg Stimulation: This refers to the administration of fertility drugs to a woman to "stimulate" and increase egg production.

Egg Retrieval: This process involves the removal of an egg or eggs from the ovaries and follicles for subsequent fertilization through IVF or GIFT.

Fertilization: The retrieved egg is mixed with sperm, after which the egg becomes fertilized and forms what then becomes an embryo.

Embryo Transfer: After an egg and sperm fertilize in the laboratory, the newly formed embryo is transferred to the uterus.

Clinical Pregnancy: This is a pregnancy which has been confirmed by ultrasound or other clinical means. Prior to this point, a blood test or a urinary pregnancy test may indicate a pregnancy. Such tests look for human chorionic gonadotropin or hCG. If the blood or urinary tests indicate a positive reading, then the pregnancy is referred to as a "chemical pregnancy." Infertility service providers generally do not accept chemical pregnancies as anything more than an indicator because conditions other than pregnancy can account for a positive reading.

Live Birth: This refers to the actual live birth of one or more babies. In determining success-rate data using live births, the industry standard is to count a "live birth" as a single delivery, regardless of how many babies were born.

Pregnancy Rate per Attempted Egg Stimulation

This rate refers to the number of clinical pregnancies resulting from all egg-stimulation attempts. This figure does not tell you whether these pregnancies resulted in live births, but does include the women who received multiple treatments.

Pregnancy Rate per Woman in the Program

This rate refers to how many clinical pregnancies occurred per woman in the program. Excluded from this figure are the number of births and the number of times an individual woman may have undergone the procedure prior to achieving a pregnancy.

Pregnancy Rate per Attempted Egg Retrieval

This rate reflects the number of clinical pregnancies resulting from all egg-retrieval attempts. This statistic does not tell whether these pregnancies resulted in live births and does not include instances where egg stimulation did not produce an egg to retrieve.

Pregnancy Rate per Embryo Transfer

This usually refers to how many clinical pregnancies occurred in relation to the number of embryo-transfer procedures performed. This figure does not say how many births occurred or how successful the program was in stimulating egg production, in obtaining egg retrieval, and in fertilizing eggs retrieved.

It takes time for new infertility service providers to establish success rates based on live births. For this reason, some providers cite only national statistics in discussing success rates. Be wary of any claims not based on a provider's own experience. Experts say it is fair for new providers to report anticipated births by including those pregnancies that have progressed beyond 26 weeks—at which point the pregnancy is highly likely to continue to term.

Some providers also favor reporting "cumulative" pregnancy and birth rate claims. Cumulative rates suggest the overall probability of a pregnancy or birth occurring based on women undergoing several successive procedures. You may want to ask how such calculations are made and what percentage of patients were able to go through multiple treatments. Evaluate all claims of success carefully.

How to Select an Infertility Service

You may want to begin your search for fertility specialists by asking your gynecologist, obstetrician, family doctor, or friends and relatives for recommendations. Ask your local hospital or medical society for names. In addition, you may want to contact local infertility support groups, which can provide you with both information and emotional support.

Plan to talk with several providers of infertility services before taking any particular course of action. By doing so, you can compare programs, gain more information about the field, and learn about different treatments applicable to your situation.

You may want to contact infertility programs first by telephone, study any literature sent to you and, then, visit those that most interest you. Try to select an infertility provider that you feel comfortable with and is convenient for you. Here are some questions to ask providers.

1. What is your infertility service's success rate and how is it calculated? *For established programs:* What is your live birth rate per egg stimulation attempted? *For new programs:* What is your live birth rate plus ongoing pregnancies past 26 weeks per egg stimulation?

You will want to examine how each infertility service tabulates its success rate and consider how meaningful these figures are.

2. What is your success rate with couples who have problems similar to ours?

Most importantly, find out how successful an infertility service has been in helping couples with your specific problems. Tell the staff your individual circumstances. Then ask: "Given our particular medical history, what are our chances of having a baby after undergoing a single egg-stimulation procedure?"

3. How long has your infertility service been in existence? How many patients have you treated? What is the specific training of your medical personnel?

You probably will want to select a program that is well-established, has worked with many patients, and has a highly-trained medical staff.

4. Is your infertility service associated with a medical board specializing in infertility?

You may wish to determine whether the infertility service has a doctor who is board-certified by the American Board of Obstetrics and Gynecology in the subspecialty of Reproductive Endocrinology. This board certification provides recognition of tested expertise in IVF and GIFT procedures.

5. Can you send me written material about the particular procedure you are recommending?

It is helpful to get written information about any medical procedures you may undergo. IVF and GIFT treatments should be explained to you in detail so that you fully understand the nature of these procedures.

6. What are the fees for these procedures? How much will drugs cost? What is typically covered by insurance?

Costs for infertility procedures are relatively expensive, and coverage by health insurance plans varies. Ask the cost of each step in the IVF or GIFT procedure. Most infertility services charge you as you advance through each step of the procedure rather than require a payment-in-full prior to the start of a treatment. You should review your health insurance to see which parts, if any, of the IVF or GIFT procedures are covered and discuss the matter with the provider of your choice.

7. Can we talk with several former or current patients who have had problems similar to ours?

Talking with a provider's patients can help in confirming your impressions of an infertility program, particularly the way in which patients are treated. You frequently can get an idea of a program's strengths and weaknesses from those who have participated in it.

Where to Go for More Information

For help in researching or checking possible complaints about particular infertility programs, you may want to contact the state medical board or county medical society. For more information about infertility, write to the American Fertility Society (2140 Eleventh Avenue South, Suite 200, Birmingham, Alabama 35205-2800). In addition, an infertility support group such as RESOLVE, with national headquarters in Arlington, Massachusetts and numerous local chapters, may be of immediate help to you. If you have further questions or want to discuss possible problems about this issue, contact the

FTC at (202) 326-3123 or write to the Division of Service Industry Practices, Federal Trade Commission, Washington, D.C. 20580. Although the FTC does not usually intervene in individual cases, the information you provide may indicate a pattern of possible law violations requiring action by the Commission.

■ Document Source:
Office of Consumer/Business Education
Bureau of Consumer Protection

A Reprint from FDA Consumer Magazine

NORPLANT: BIRTH CONTROL AT ARM'S REACH

by Marian Segal

The newest birth control option for women is literally at arm's reach. The Norplant contraceptive, approved by the Food and Drug Administration last December and marketed since February, is implanted just under the skin of the inner arm, right above the elbow. Developed by the Population Council of New York, this birth control alternative is distinctly different form methods previously available.

New Form, Old Content

Norplant consists of a familiar ingredient in a new package. Six silicone rubber capsules about the size of matchsticks contain a synthetic progestin hormone long used in birth control pills. The flexible tubes are inserted in a fan-like arrangement and can be felt but not easily seen.

Once in place, they steadily release a low dose of hormone into the bloodstream. Effective within 24 hours after insertion, Norplant can continue to prevent pregnancy for up to five years.

The hormone usually inhibits ovulation so that eggs are not produced regularly, and causes the mucus of the cervix to thicken, making it more difficult for sperm to reach the egg. Other ways that Norplant may provide contraceptive effects have been proposed but not proven.

Experimental Attitude

Jennifer Collier, a 28-year-old New York law student, entered a study of Norplant at the Robert Wood Johnson Institute in New Brunswick, N.J., in the spring of 1984 and is now on her second implant, inserted last June.

It sounded like a really neat invention, so I decided to try it," says Collier. She had been dissatisfied with the weight gain and irritability she experienced using oral contraceptives. With Norplant, she says, she isn't troubled with either of those side effects. Collier describes the implant as visible, "but not terribly obvious. No one has noticed it unless they were looking for it, probably partly because of where it's inserted."

Each Norplant capsule is 2.4 millimeters (about one-tenth of an inch) in diameter and 34 millimeters (just under one-and-a-half inches) long, and holds 36 milligrams of powdered crystals of the progestin levonorgestrel. The tubes are made of Silastic, a silicone material long used in surgical implants such as heart valves and hip joints.

The hormone seeps through the permeable tubes into the bloodstream, initially at a rate of about 85 micrograms a day. The amount declines gradually to about 50 micrograms by nine months, 35 by 18 months, and about 30 micrograms at the end of five years. In comparison, birth control pills that contain levonorgestrel provide about 50 to 150 micrograms of the progestin a day, plus estrogen. (The only progestin-only contraceptive available in the United States contains 75 micrograms of norgestrel, a progestin similar to levonorgestrel.)

When the hormone supply dwindles, usually in about five years, a new implant can be inserted if desired. On the other hand, if a woman wishes to become pregnant earlier, she can have the implants removed at any time, and fertility is restored very soon. Blood levels of the progestin are undetectable within 5 to 14 days.

Population Council Project

Norplant has been marketed in other countries for several years. According to the Population Council, more than half a million women in 46 countries have used the implant since it was first approved in Finland—where it is manufactured—in 1983. It now has regulatory approval in 17 other countries as well, including Sweden, Indonesia, the Dominican Republic, Thailand, China, Peru, and the United States. Norplant's U.S. distributor is the Philadelphia-based pharmaceutical firm Wyeth-Ayerst Laboratories.

"The first implants were tested in 1968," says Population Council vice president Wayne Bardin, M.D., "and then the council began to develop and test implants that released a whole variety of progestins. By 1974, we came up with what is now the Norplant implant, using levonorgestrel. The first clinical trial of that was begun in 1975."

FDA approval of the implant was based on the results of clinical studies involving 2,400 women in the United States, Finland, Sweden, Denmark, Jamaica, Brazil, Chile, and the Dominican Republic.

In the studies, the contraceptive's effectiveness approached that of sterilization in the first year.

Pregnancy rates were slightly higher in heavier women, increasing after the third year of use in those who weighed more than 69 kilograms (153 pounds). Nevertheless, the protection is still quite good. For example, among 100 women of all weights using the implant for five years, it is expected that four would become pregnant during that time. By contrast, of 100 women using the pill for the same time, at least 15 might be expected to become pregnant.

Norplant's effectiveness does not depend on patient compliance—a feature shared by only one other type of reversible contraceptive—the intrauterine device, or IUD. This particularly appeals to Collier for the convenience it affords. "Unlike the pill, you don't have to remember to take it every day, and, unlike the diaphragm, there's no problem with spontaneity," she says.

Effectiveness Rates of Contraceptive Methods

(Shown are the number of pregnancies for every 100 women during the first year of use)

Method	Lowest Expected	Typical
Male sterilization	0.1	0.15
Norplant	0.2	0.2
Female sterilization	0.2	0.4
Oral contraceptives		3
Combined	0.1	*
Progestin only	0.5	*
IUD	<1	3
Condom without spermicide	2	12
Cervical cap	6	18
Diaphragm with spermicide cream or jelly	6	18
Vaginal sponge		
women who haven't borne children	6	18
women who have borne children	9	28
Spermicides alone (foams, creams, jellies, and vaginal suppositories)	3	21
Periodic abstinence (all methods)	1-9	20
No contraception (planned pregnancy)	85	85

* = not available
(Document Source: Adapted from Table 1 in Studies in Family Planning, 1990, by J. Trussell et al.)

Because Norplant is not a barrier contraceptive, however, it offers no protection against sexually transmitted diseases such as AIDS, herpes, chlamydia, and gonorrhea. For optimum protection from both disease and pregnancy, couples may choose to use both Norplant and a condom.

The Drawbacks

As with virtually any drug or medical device, Norplant isn't entirely troublefree. Side effects that women have reported with the implant during the first year include irregular menstrual bleeding, headache, nervousness, depression, nausea, dizziness, skin rash, acne, change of appetite, breast tenderness, weight gain, enlargement of the ovaries, and excessive growth of body or facial hair.

Some Norplant users have also reported breast discharge, vaginal discharge, inflammation of the cervix, abdominal discomfort, and muscle and skeletal pain. These effects, however, cannot be linked to use of the implant because the complaints are common among the general population and could stem from many other causes. There is no known biological reason to link the complaints specifically to use of the contraceptive.

By far, the most common side effect is menstrual cycle irregularity. "To give the percentage of women with menstrual irregularities is complex," says Bardin, "because it changes with time." He says that over a five-year period of use, about 45 percent of women will have irregular periods and another 45 percent will have normal periods. The remaining 10 percent will have long periods of time—three to four months—with no bleeding. "That's an average," says Bardin. "Basically what happens is you have more women with irregular periods in the first year and that tends to diminish with continuing use."

The bleeding irregularities result from the continuous hormone release. "With the oral contraceptive pills, estrogen and progestin are taken for three weeks and withdrawn for one week, causing regular bleeding," explains Lisa Rarick, M.D., a medical officer in FDA's division of endocrine and metabolism drug products. "Norplant, on the other hand," says Rarick, "provides no cyclic withdrawal, and thus each individual creates her own bleeding pattern."

In the multi-center trials, more women had increases in their hemoglobin concentrations than decreases, indicating that they lost less menstrual blood when using Norplant. (Hemoglobin is the oxygen-carrying pigment of red blood cells that gives them their red color and serves to transport oxygen to tissues.) Bardin says that this is because, on average, even if the number of bleeding days increases in the first year of use, the total amount of blood lost may be less than would be lost without hormonal contraception.

He says that most women who use Norplant don't perceive bleeding as a problem. "To illustrate," he says, "if you say, 'What is the biggest complaint that women have about Norplant,' it's bleeding irregularities. But if you ask all women if bleeding irregularities bother them, something like 60 percent say 'no.'"

Collier says she has spotting and a lighter flow with Norplant. "Sometimes, I have no discernible cycle at all," she says, but maintains that "although of course I'd rather have regular periods, the effects are not that bad."

Nevertheless, the major reason women give for discontinuing Norplant is bleeding problems, accounting for about 9 percent of those who stop in the first year, according to FDA's Rarick. Another 5 percent stop for other medical reasons, from headaches to dizziness, and perhaps another 5 percent stop for other reasons, including to have a baby. She estimates that about 60 to 65 percent of women continue with the implant longer than two years.

Not for Everyone

More serious complications are possible as well, and Norplant is not recommended for everyone. As with oral contraceptives, women with acute liver disease or liver tumors—whether malignant or benign—unexplained vaginal bleeding, breast cancer, or blood clots in the legs, lungs or eyes should not use the implant.

Norplant contains only progestin, whereas most oral contraceptives contain both progestin and estrogen. Some side effects of the pill, such as eye disorders and increased risk of cardiovascular problems among women who smoke, are believed to be related to the estrogen component. Nevertheless, FDA advises physicians to "consider the possible increased risks associated with oral contraceptives, including elevated blood pressure, thromboembolic disorders [blood clots obstructing blood vessels], and other vascular problems that might occur with use of the contraceptive implant."

Bardin suggests that Norplant will be most attractive to women who:
◆ wish to use highly effective low-dose hormone contraception
◆ want long-term contraception after completing their family, but don't want sterilization
◆ want to delay childbearing for an extended period of time
◆ cannot use estrogens
◆ are unhappy with other forms of contraception.

On the flip side, Bardin expects the implant to be less popular among women who:
◆ are happy with their present form of contraception
◆ cannot or do not want to pay the upfront cost of Norplant
◆ will not tolerate irregular menstrual bleeding if it should occur
◆ do not want to use a method that requires a visit to a health-care professional to discontinue. ("Some women feel that puts them at the mercy of the clinic and they want to be able to stop it any time they want," says Bardin. "That's why they like pills and barrier methods—it's under their control," he says.)

Surgical Insertion

Successful use of the Norplant system depends on careful insertion of the capsules. Wyeth-Ayerst markets the implant as a kit with detailed instructions for insertion and removal, and, through the Association of Reproductive Health Professionals, offers physician training programs as well.

The firm describes the insertion as a minor, outpatient surgical procedure requiring only 10 to 15 minutes. The area is numbed with a local anesthetic, and a small incision, less than an eighth of an inch long, is made. Using a special instrument called a trocar, the physician places the six capsules just under the skin. The incision is then covered with protective gauze and a small adhesive bandage. Stitches are not required.

When the anesthetic wears off, there may be some tenderness or itching, and perhaps some temporary discoloration, bruising and swelling. Infection at the site of insertion has also been reported.

It takes a bit longer to remove the implant than to insert it—usually from 15 to 20 minutes, according to the distributor. As with insertion, a small incision is made under a local anesthetic. Then the physician removes the capsules and, again, the incision is covered with an adhesive bandage. Sometimes, some capsules may be more difficult to remove than others. When this happens, the woman may have to return a second time, after the area has healed, for removal of the remaining capsules.

The reason for suggesting the second visit, Bardin says, is to let the physician know that "if you have trouble removing, don't cut a big hole in the woman's arm and go fishing around looking for it [the capsule]." If the anesthetic has caused the area to puff up, for example, it may be difficult to feel the implant. "Wait until the next week or whenever she can come in again," says Bardin, "and you'll be able to see it and take it out with minimal trauma."

If desired, a new set of implants can be inserted at the same time the old set is removed, either in the same arm and through the same incision, or in the other arm.

The price to the medical professional for a single Norplant system, which includes all the necessary apparatus for insertion and removal as well as the set of six capsules, has been set at $350. Fees for insertion and related costs, such as counseling and removal, vary, depending on the physician.

Collier says that this will probably be the last Norplant she'll have, at least for a while, as she plans to get pregnant eventually. She's not sure if she would come back to the implant later. "Hormone therapy and the risks associated with it—more with the pill and estrogen than with Norplant—concern me," she says. "I'll just have to see what else might be available when that time comes." For now, Collier is pleased with Norplant and would recommend it to any woman, "espe-

cially," she says, "if they're going to be on hormone therapy anyway."

Marian Segal is a member of FDA's public affairs staff.

■ **Document Source:**
   U.S. Department of Health and Human Services, Public Health Services
   Food and Drug Administration
   DHHS Publication No. (FDA) 92-3194
   Reprinted May 1991

DENTAL CARE AND ORAL HEALTH

■ ■ ■

DRY MOUTH (XEROSTOMIA)

Do you feel the need to moisten your mouth frequently? Does your mouth feel dry at mealtime? Do you have less saliva than you once did? Do you have difficulty swallowing? Do you have trouble eating dry foods such as crackers or toast?

If you answer "yes" to these questions, you may be one of the many people who suffer from dry mouth, or xerostomia (pronounced "zero-stoh'-me-a").

Although xerostomia is not a disease in itself, it is a symptom of certain diseases. Dry mouth also is a common side effect of some medications and medical treatments. Most cases of dry mouth are caused by failure of the salivary glands to function properly. But in some people, the sensation of a dry mouth occurs even though their salivary glands are normal.

Dry mouth is a significant health problem because it can affect nutrition and psychological well-being, while also contributing to tooth decay and other mouth infections. Dry mouth also may signal more serious problems in the body. If you have a dry mouth, you should be seen by a dentist or physician to determine the cause of the symptom.

Why is saliva important?

Saliva has many important functions in the body. Each person needs adequate amounts of healthy saliva to:

♦ Limit the growth of bacteria that cause tooth decay and other oral infections
♦ Preserve teeth by bathing them with protective minerals that allow early cavities to remineralize and heal
♦ Lubricate the soft tissues lining the mouth to keep them pliable and make speaking and chewing easier
♦ Dissolve foods and allow us to experience their sweet, sour, salty, and bitter tastes
♦ Assist digestion by providing enzymes that break down food
♦ Lubricate food so it can be swallowed easily
♦ Cleanse the teeth and mouth of food particles

What causes dry mouth?

Changes in salivary gland function, brought on by:

Medications. Over 400 commonly used drugs can cause the sensation of dry mouth. The main culprits are the antihypertensives (for high blood pressure) and antidepressants. Both are prescribed for millions of Americans. Painkillers, tranquilizers, diuretics, and over-the-counter antihistamines can also decrease saliva.

Cancer treatment. Radiation therapy can permanently damage salivary glands if they are in the field of radiation. Chemotherapy can change the composition of saliva, creating a sensation of dry mouth.

Diseases. Siogren's syndrome is an autoimmune disorder whose symptoms include dry mouth and dry eyes. Some Siogren's patients also have a connective tissue disorder, most commonly rheumatoid arthritis or systemic lupus erythematosus.

Other conditions. Bone marrow transplants, endocrine disorders, nutritional deficiencies, anxiety, mental stress, and depression can cause a dry mouth.

Changes not related to salivary glands, such as:

Nerve damage. Trauma to the head and neck area from surgery or wounds can damage the nerves that supply sensation to the mouth. While the salivary glands may be left intact, they cannot function normally without the nerves that signal them to produce saliva.

Altered perception. Conditions like Alzheimer's disease or stroke may change the ability to perceive oral sensations.

Does aging cause dry mouth?

Until recently dry mouth was regarded as a normal part of aging. Researchers now know that healthy older adults do not produce less saliva. When older people do experience dry mouth, it is because they suffer from diseases that cause the condition or they take medications that produce dry mouth as a side effect.

What happens when you have dry mouth?

Dry mouth caused by malfunctioning salivary glands is associated with changes in saliva. The flow of saliva can decrease. Or the composition of saliva can change.

Patients with dry mouth have varying degrees of discomfort. Some people feel a dry or burning sensation in their mouths. A dry mouth may affect their ability to chew, taste, swallow, and speak. Changes in saliva also can affect oral and dental health. Severe cases of dry mouth can result in cracking of the lips, slits at the corners of the mouth, changes in the surface of the tongue, rampant tooth decay, ulceration of the mouth's linings, and infection.

Is relief available?

Although there is no single way to treat dry mouth, there are a number of steps you can follow to keep teeth in good health and relieve the sense of dryness. These suggestions will not correct the underlying cause of xerostomia, but may help you feel more comfortable.

To preserve your teeth:

♦ Brush your teeth at least twice a day.
♦ Use dental floss daily.
♦ Use a toothpaste that contains fluoride. Ask your dentist about using a topical fluoride.
♦ Avoid sticky, sugary foods or brush immediately after eating them.
♦ See your dentist at least three times a year for cleanings and early treatment of cavities.
♦ Ask your dentist if you should use a remineralizing solution or prescription-strength fluoride.

To relieve dryness and preserve the soft tissues:

♦ Take frequent sips of water or drinks without sugar. Pause often while speaking to sip some liquid. Avoid caffeine-containing coffee, tea, and soft drinks.
♦ Drink frequently while eating. This will make chewing and swallowing easier and may increase the taste of foods.
♦ Keep a glass of water by your bed for dryness during the night or upon awakening.
♦ Chew sugarless gum. The chewing may produce more saliva.
♦ Eat sugarless mints or hard sugarless candies, but let them dissolve in your mouth. Cinnamon and mint are often most effective.
♦ Place a small piece of lemon rind or a cherry pit in your mouth. The sucking action helps stimulate saliva.
♦ Avoid tobacco and alcohol.
♦ Avoid spicy, salty, and highly acidic foods that may irritate the mouth.
♦ Ask your dentist about using artificial salivas to help lubricate the mouth.
♦ Use a humidifier, particularly at night.

What is being done about dry mouth?

At the National Institute of Dental Research (NIDR), one of the National Institutes of Health in Bethesda, MD, scientists study the causes of dry mouth and possible treatments for this condition. In 1983, they opened a Dry Mouth Clinic to evaluate, diagnose, and treat patients with salivary gland dysfunction.

Researchers at the NIDR Dry Mouth Clinic have developed better methods of diagnosing salivary gland dysfunction. A complete evaluation of a patient with dry mouth includes measurement of both "stimulated" salivary flow—found when a person actively chews, sips, or tastes sour substances—and "unstimulated" flow—found when a person is at rest or sleeping. Researchers also analyze saliva composition and look at other aspects of saliva secretion to distinguish between salivary gland dysfunction and other causes of dry mouth.

The investigators are now testing a drug—pilocarpine— to treat dry mouth in patients with minimally functioning salivary glands. Their studies show that pilocarpine can stimulate saliva production and relieve a patient's sense of oral dryness without causing untoward side effects. The increased output of saliva might also help prevent tooth decay, ulcerations, and infections. Further studies are needed, however, before the drug will be available to the public. NIDR investigators are also looking into other possible treatments for dry mouth. Several research studies focus on the cause of Siogren's syndrome and treatment for the dry mouth associated with this condition.

Patient volunteers

The NIDR Dry Mouth Clinic seeks patients with dry mouth caused by head and neck radiation therapy and Siogren's syndrome. A number of research studies are underway to examine the causes of salivary dysfunction in these patients, the long-term consequences of salivary changes, and new methods of treatment.

For further information about the NIDR Dry Mouth Clinic, write to:

Dr. Philip C. Fox
The Dry Mouth Clinic
National Institute of Dental Research
Building 10, Room 1N-113
National Institutes of Health
Bethesda, MD 20892

Support groups

As many as two million Americans may suffer from Siogren's syndrome. Two voluntary organizations have chapters in major cities around the country that offer support for these patients.

For further information, contact:

Siogren's Syndrome Foundation, Inc.
382 Main Street
Port Washington, NY 11050

National Siogren's Syndrome Association
3201 West Evans Drive
Phoenix, AZ 85023

■ Document Source:
   U.S. Department of Health and Human Services, Public Health Service
   National Institutes of Health
   National Institute of Dental Research
   Bethesda, MD 20892
   NIH Publication No. 91-3174

TMD: TEMPOROMANDIBULAR DISORDERS

You may have read articles in newspapers and magazines about "TMD"—temporomandibular (jaw) disorders, also called "TMJ syndrome." Perhaps you have even felt pain sometimes in your jaw area, or maybe your dentist or physician has told you that you have TMD.

If you have questions about TMD, you are not alone. Researchers, too, are looking for answers to what causes TMD, what are the best treatments, and how we can prevent these disorders. The National Institute of Dental Research has written this pamphlet to share with you what we have learned about TMD.

TMD is not just one disorder, but a group of conditions, often painful, that affect the jaw joint (temporomandibular joint or TMJ) and the muscles that control chewing. Although we don't know how many people actually have TMD, the disorders appear to affect about twice as many women as men.

The good news is that for most people, pain in the area of the jaw joint or muscles is not a signal that a serious problem is developing. Generally, discomfort from TMD is occasional and temporary, often occurring in cycles. The pain eventually goes away with little or no treatment. Only a small percentage of people with TMD pain develop significant, long-term symptoms.

What is the temporomandibular joint?

The temporomandibular joint connects the lower jaw, called the mandible, to the temporal bone at the side of the head. If you place your fingers just in front of your ears and open your mouth, you can feel the joint on each side of your head. Because these joints are flexible, the jaw can move smoothly up and down and side to side, enabling us to talk, chew and yawn. Muscles attached to and surrounding the jaw joint control its position and movement.

When we open our mouths, the rounded ends of the lower jaw, called condyles, glide along the joint socket of the temporal bone. The condyles slide back to their original position when we close our mouths. To keep this motion smooth, a soft disc lies between the condyle and the temporal bone. This disc absorbs shocks to the TMJ from chewing and other movements.

What are temporomandibular disorders?

Today, researchers generally agree that temporomandibular disorders fall into three main categories:

- myofascial pain, the most common form of TMD, which is discomfort or pain in the muscles that control jaw function and the neck and shoulder muscles;
- internal derangement of the joint, meaning a dislocated jaw or displaced disc, or injury to the condyle;
- degenerative joint disease, such as osteoarthritis or rheumatoid arthritis in the jaw joint.

A person may have one or more of these conditions at the same time.

What causes TMD?

We know that severe injury to the jaw or temporomandibular joint can cause TMD. A heavy blow, for example, can fracture the bones of the joint or damage the disc, disrupting the smooth motion of the jaw and causing pain or locking. Arthritis in the jaw joint may also result from injury.

Other causes of TMD are less clear. Some suggest, for example, that a bad bite (malocclusion) can trigger TMD, but recent research disputes that view. Orthodontic treatment, such as braces and the use of headgear, has also been blamed for some forms of TMD, but studies now show that this is unlikely.

And there is no scientific proof that gum chewing causes clicking sounds in the jaw joint, or that jaw clicking leads to serious TMJ problems. In fact, jaw clicking is fairly common in the general population. If there are no other symptoms, such as pain or locking, jaw clicking usually does not need treatment.

Researchers believe that most people with clicking or popping in the jaw joint likely have a displaced disc—the soft, shock-absorbing disc is not in a normal position. As long as the displaced disc causes no pain or problems with jaw movement, no treatment is needed.

Some experts suggest that stress, either mental or physical, may cause or aggravate TMD. People with TMD often clench or grind their teeth at night, which can tire the jaw muscles and lead to pain. It is not clear, however, whether stress is the cause of the clenching/grinding and subsequent jaw pain, or the result of dealing with chronic jaw pain or dysfunction. Scientists are exploring how behavioral, psychological and physical factors may combine to cause TMD.

TMD signs and symptoms

A variety of symptoms may be linked to TMD. Pain, particularly in the chewing muscles and/or jaw joint, is the most common symptom. Other likely symptoms include:

- limited movement or locking of the jaw,
- radiating pain in the face, neck or shoulders,
- painful clicking, popping or grating sounds in the jaw joint when opening or closing the mouth.
- a sudden, major change in the way the upper and lower teeth fit together.

Symptoms such as headaches, earaches, dizziness and hearing problems may sometimes be related to TMD. It is important to keep in mind, however, that occasional discomfort in the jaw joint or chewing muscles is quite common and is generally not a cause for concern. Researchers are working to clarify TMD symptoms, with the goal of developing easier and better methods of diagnosis and improved treatment.

Diagnosis

Because the exact causes and symptoms of TMD are not clear, diagnosing these disorders can be confusing. At present, there is no widely accepted, standard test to correctly identify TMD. In about 90 percent of cases, however, the patient's description of symptoms, combined with a simple physical examination of the face and jaw, provides information useful for diagnosing these disorders.

The examination includes feeling the jaw joints and chewing muscles for pain or tenderness; listening for clicking, popping or grating sounds during jaw movement; and examining for limited motion or locking of the jaw while opening or closing the mouth. Checking the patient's dental and medical history is very important. In most cases, this evaluation provides enough information to locate the pain or jaw problem, to make a diagnosis, and to start treatment to relieve pain or jaw locking.

Regular dental x-rays and TMJ x-rays (transcranial radiographs) are not generally useful in diagnosing TMD. Other x-ray techniques, such as arthrography (joint x-rays using dye); magnetic resonance imaging (MRI), which pictures the soft tissues; and tomography (a special type of x-ray), are usually needed only when the practitioner strongly suspects a condition such as arthritis or when significant pain persists over time and symptoms do not improve with treatment. Before undergoing any expensive diagnostic test, it is always wise to get another independent opinion.

One of the most important areas of TMD research is developing clear guidelines for diagnosing these disorders. Once scientists agree on what these guidelines should be, it will be easier for practitioners to correctly identify temporomandibular disorders and to decide what treatment, if any, is needed.

Treatment

The key words to keep in mind about TMD treatment are "conservative" and "reversible." Conservative treatments are as simple as possible and are used most often because most patients do not have severe, degenerative TMD. Conservative treatments do not invade the tissues of the face, jaw or joint. Reversible treatments do not cause permanent, or irreversible, changes in the structure or position of the jaw or teeth.

Because most TMD problems are temporary and do not get worse, simple treatment is all that is usually needed to relieve discomfort. Self-care practices, for example, eating soft foods, applying heat or ice packs, and avoiding extreme jaw movements (such as wide yawning, loud singing and gum chewing) are useful in easing TMD symptoms. Learning special techniques for relaxing and reducing stress may also help patients deal with pain that often comes with TMD problems.

Other conservative, reversible treatments include physical therapy you can do at home, which focuses on gentle muscle stretching and relaxing exercises, and short-term use of muscle-relaxing and anti-inflammatory drugs.

The health care provider may recommend an oral appliance, also called a splint or bite plate, which is a plastic guard that fits over the upper or lower teeth. The splint can help reduce clenching or grinding, which eases muscle tension. An oral splint should be used only for a short time and should not cause permanent changes in the bite. If a splint causes or increases pain, stop using it and see your practitioner.

The conservative, reversible treatments described are useful for temporary relief of pain and muscle spasm—they are not "cures" for TMD. If symptoms continue over time or come back often, check with your doctor.

There are other types of TMD treatment, such as surgery or injections, that invade the tissues. Some involve injecting pain relieving medications into painful muscle sites, often called "trigger points." Researchers are studying this type of treatment to see if these injections are helpful over time.

Surgical treatments are often irreversible and should be avoided where possible. When such treatment is necessary, be sure to have the doctor explain to you, in words you can understand, the reason for the treatment, the risks involved, and other types of treatment that may be available.

Scientists have learned that certain irreversible treatments, such as surgical replacement of jaw joints with artificial implants, may cause severe pain and permanent jaw damage. Some of these devices may fail to function properly or may break apart in the jaw over time. *Before undergoing any surgery on the jaw joint, it is very important to get other independent opinions.*

> The Food and Drug Administration has recalled artificial jaw joint implants made by Vitek, Inc., which may break down and damage surrounding bone. If you have these implants, see your oral surgeon or dentist. If there are problems with your implants, the devices may need to be removed. Persons who have Vitek implants should call Medic Alert at 1-800-554-5297 for more information.

Other irreversible treatments that are of little value—and may make the problem worse—include orthodontics to change the bite; restorative dentistry, which uses crown and bridge work to balance the bite; and occlusal adjustment, grinding down teeth to bring the bite into balance.

Although more studies are needed on the safety and effectiveness of most TMD treatments, scientists strongly recommend using the most conservative, reversible treatments possible before considering invasive treatments. Even when the TMD problem has become chronic, most patients still do not need aggressive types of treatment.

If you think you have TMD . . .

Keep in mind that for most people, discomfort from TMD will eventually go away whether treated or not. Simple self-care practices are often effective in easing TMD symptoms. If more treatment is needed, it should be conservative and reversible. Avoid, if at all possible, treatments that cause permanent changes in the bite or jaw. If irreversible treatments are recommended, be sure to get a reliable second opinion.

Many practitioners, especially dentists, are familiar with the conservative treatment of TMD. Because TMD is usually painful, pain clinics in hospitals and universities are also a good source of advice and second opinions for these disorders. Specially trained facial pain experts can often be helpful in diagnosing and treating TMD.

Research

The National Institute of Dental Research supports an active research program on TMD. Developing reliable guidelines for diagnosing these disorders is a top priority. Studies are also under way on the causes, treatments, and prevention of TMD.

Through continued research, pieces of the TMD puzzle are falling slowly but steadily into place.

■ Document Source:
National Institutes of Health
National Institute of Dental Research
NIH Publication No. 94-3487

DIABETES AND OTHER ENDOCRINE DISORDERS

■ ■ ■

NIDDK Fact Sheet

ADDISON'S DISEASE

Addison's disease is a rare endocrine, or hormonal, disorder that affects about 1 in 100,000 people. It occurs in all age groups and afflicts men and women equally. The disease is characterized by weight loss, muscle weakness, fatigue, low blood pressure, and sometimes darkening of the skin in both exposed and nonexposed parts of the body.

Addison's disease occurs when the adrenal glands do not produce enough of the hormone cortisol and in some cases, the hormone aldosterone. For this reason, the disease is sometimes called chronic adrenal insufficiency, or hypocortisolism.

Cortisol is normally produced by the adrenal glands, located just above the kidneys. It belongs to a class of hormones called glucocorticoids, which affect almost every organ and tissue in the body. Scientists think that cortisol has possibly hundreds of effects in the body. Cortisol's most important job is to help the body respond to stress. Among its other vital tasks, cortisol:

- helps maintain blood pressure and cardiovascular function;
- helps slow the immune system's inflammatory response;
- helps balance the effects of insulin in breaking down sugar for energy; and
- helps regulate the metabolism of proteins, carbohydrates, and fats.

Because cortisol is so vital to health, the amount of cortisol produced by the adrenals is precisely balanced. Like many other hormones, cortisol is regulated by the brain's hypothalamus and the pituitary gland, a bean-sized organ at the base of the brain. First, the hypothalamus sends "releasing hormones" to the pituitary gland. The pituitary responds by secreting other hormones that regulate growth, thyroid and adrenal function, and sex hormones such as estrogen and testosterone. One of the pituitary's main functions is to secrete ACTH (adrenocorticotropin), a hormone that stimulates the adrenal glands. When the adrenals receive the pituitary's signal in the form of ACTH, they respond by producing cortisol. Completing the cycle, cortisol then signals the pituitary to lower secretion of ACTH.

Aldosterone belongs to a class of hormones called mineralocorticoids, also produced by the adrenal glands. It helps maintain blood pressure and water and salt balance in the body by helping the kidney retain sodium and excrete potassium. When aldosterone production falls too low, the kidneys are not able to regulate salt and water balance, causing blood volume and blood pressure to drop.

Causes

Failure to produce adequate levels of cortisol, or adrenal insufficiency, can occur for different reasons. The problem may be due to a disorder of the adrenal glands themselves (primary adrenal insufficiency) or to inadequate secretion of ACTH by the pituitary gland (secondary adrenal insufficiency).

Primary Adrenal Insufficiency

Most cases of Addison's disease are caused by the gradual destruction of the adrenal cortex, the outer layer of the adrenal glands, by the body's own immune system. About 70 percent of reported cases of Addison's disease are due to autoimmune disorders, in which the immune system makes antibodies that attack the body's own tissues or organs and slowly destroy them. Adrenal insufficiency occurs when at least 90 percent of the adrenal cortex has been destroyed. As a result, often both glucocorticoid and mineralocorticoid hormones are lacking. Sometimes only the adrenal gland is affected, as in idiopathic adrenal insufficiency; sometimes other glands also are affected, as in the polyendocrine deficiency syndrome.

The polyendocrine deficiency syndrome is classified into two separate forms, referred to as type I and type II. Type I occurs in children, and adrenal insufficiency may be accompanied by underactive parathyroid glands, slow sexual development, pernicious anemia, chronic candida infections, chronic active hepatitis, and, in very rare cases, hair loss. Type II, often called Schmidt's syndrome, usually afflicts young adults. Features of type II may include an underactive thyroid gland, slow sexual development, and diabetes mellitus. About

10 percent of patients with type II have vitiligo, or loss of pigment, on areas of the skin. Scientists think that the polyendocrine deficiency syndrome is inherited because frequently more than one family member tends to have one or more endocrine deficiencies.

Tuberculosis (TB) accounts for about 20 percent of cases of primary adrenal insufficiency in developed countries. When adrenal insufficiency was first identified by Dr. Thomas Addison in 1849, TB was found at autopsy in 70 to 90 percent of cases. As the treatment for TB improved, however, the incidence of adrenal insufficiency due to TB of the adrenal glands has greatly decreased.

Less common causes of primary adrenal insufficiency are chronic infections, mainly fungal infections; cancer cells spreading from other parts of the body to the adrenal glands; amyloidosis; and surgical removal of the adrenal glands. Each of these causes is discussed in more detail below.

Secondary Adrenal Insufficiency

This form of Addison's disease can be traced to a lack of ACTH, which causes a drop in the adrenal glands' production of cortisol but not aldosterone. A temporary form of secondary adrenal insufficiency may occur when a person who has been receiving a glucocorticoid hormone such as prednisone for a long time abruptly stops or interrupts taking the medication. Glucocorticoid hormones, which are often used to treat inflammatory illnesses like rheumatoid arthritis, asthma, or ulcerative colitis, block the release of both corticotropin- releasing hormone (CRH) and ACTH. Normally, CRH instructs the pituitary gland to release ACTH. If CRH levels drop, the pituitary is not stimulated to release ACTH, and the adrenals then fail to secrete sufficient levels of cortisol.

Another cause of secondary adrenal insufficiency is the surgical removal of benign, or noncancerous, ACTH-producing tumors of the pituitary gland (Cushing's disease). In this case, the source of ACTH is suddenly removed, and replacement hormone must be taken until normal ACTH and cortisol production resumes.

Less commonly, adrenal insufficiency occurs when the pituitary gland either decreases in size or stops producing ACTH. This can result from tumors or infections of the area, loss of blood flow to the pituitary, radiation for the treatment of pituitary tumors, or surgical removal of parts of the hypothalamus or the pituitary gland during neurosurgery of these areas.

Symptoms

The symptoms of adrenal insufficiency usually begin gradually. Chronic, worsening fatigue and muscle weakness, loss of appetite, and weight loss are characteristic of the disease. Nausea, vomiting, and diarrhea occur in about 50 percent of cases. Blood pressure is low and falls further when standing, causing dizziness or fainting. Skin changes also are common in Addison's disease, with areas of hyperpigmentation, or dark tanning, covering exposed and nonexposed part of the body. This darkening of the skin is most visible on scars; skin folds; pressure points such as the elbows, knees, knuckles, and toes; lips; and mucous membranes.

Addison's disease can cause irritability and depression. Because of salt loss, craving of salty foods also is common. Hypoglycemia, or low blood sugar, is more severe in children than in adults. In women, menstrual periods may become irregular or stop.

Because the symptoms progress slowly, they are usually ignored until a stressful event like an illness or an accident causes them to become worse. This is called an addisonian crisis, or acute adrenal insufficiency. In most patients, symptoms are severe enough to seek medical treatment before a crisis occurs. However, in about 25 percent of patients, symptoms first appear during an addisonian crisis.

Symptoms of an addisonian crisis include sudden penetrating pain in the lower back, abdomen, or legs; severe vomiting and diarrhea, followed by dehydration; low blood pressure; and loss of consciousness. Left untreated, an addisonian crisis can be fatal.

Diagnosis

In its early stages, adrenal insufficiency can be difficult to diagnose. A review of a patient's medical history based on the symptoms, especially the dark tanning of the skin, will lead a doctor to suspect Addison's disease.

A diagnosis of Addison's disease is made by biochemical laboratory tests. The aim of these tests is first to determine whether there are insufficient levels of cortisol and then to establish the cause. X-ray exams of the adrenal and pituitary glands also are useful in helping to establish the cause.

ACTH Stimulation Test

This is the most specific test for diagnosing Addison's disease. In this test, blood and/or urine cortisol levels are measured before and after a synthetic form of ACTH is given by injection. In the so-called short, or rapid, ACTH test, cortisol measurement in blood is repeated 30 to 60 minutes after an intravenous ACTH injection. The normal response after an injection of ACTH is a rise in blood and urine cortisol levels. Patients with either form of adrenal insufficiency respond poorly or do not respond at all.

When the response to the short ACTH test is abnormal, a "long" ACTH stimulation test is required to determine the cause of adrenal insufficiency. In this test, synthetic ACTH is injected either intravenously or intramuscularly over a 48- to 72-hour period, and blood and/or urine cortisol are measured the day before and during the 2 to 3 days of the injection. Patients with primary adrenal insufficiency do not produce cortisol during the 48- to 72-hour period; however, patients with secondary adrenal insufficiency have adequate responses to the test on the second or third day.

In patients suspected of having an addisonian crisis, the doctor must begin treatment with injections of salt, fluids, and glucocorticoid hormones immediately. Although a reliable diagnosis is not possible while the patient is being treated, measurement of blood ACTH and cortisol during the crisis and before glucocorticoids are given is sufficient to make the diagnosis. Once the crisis is controlled and medication has been stopped, the doctor will delay further testing for up to 1 month to obtain an accurate diagnosis.

Insulin-Induced Hypoglycemia Test

A reliable test to determine how the hypothalamus and pituitary and adrenal glands respond to stress is the insulin-induced hypoglycemia test. In this test, blood is drawn to measure the blood glucose and cortisol levels, followed by an injection of fast-acting insulin. Blood glucose and cortisol levels are measured again at 30, 45, and 90 minutes after the insulin injection. The normal response is for blood glucose levels to fall and cortisol levels to rise.

Other Tests

Once a diagnosis of primary adrenal insufficiency has been made, x-ray exams of the abdomen may be taken to see if the adrenals have any signs of calcium deposits. Calcium deposits may indicate TB. A tuberculin skin test also may be used.

If secondary adrenal insufficiency is the cause, doctors may use different imaging tools to reveal the size and shape of the pituitary gland. The most common is the CT scan, which produces a series of x-ray pictures giving a cross-sectional image of a body part. The function of the pituitary and its ability to produce other hormones also are tested.

Treatment

Treatment of Addison's disease involves replacing, or substituting, the hormones that the adrenal glands are not making. Cortisol is replaced orally with hydrocortisone tablets, a synthetic glucocorticoid, taken once or twice a day. If aldosterone is also deficient, it is replaced with oral doses of a mineralocorticoid, called fludrocortisone acetate (Florinef), which is taken once a day. Patients receiving aldosterone replacement therapy are usually advised by a doctor to increase their salt intake. Because patients with secondary adrenal insufficiency normally maintain aldosterone production, they do not require aldosterone replacement therapy. The doses of each of these medications are adjusted to meet the needs of individual patients.

During an addisonian crisis, low blood pressure, low blood sugar, and high levels of potassium can be life threatening. Standard therapy involves intravenous injections of hydrocortisone, saline (salt water), and dextrose (sugar). This treatment usually brings rapid improvement. When the patient can take fluids and medications by mouth, the amount of hydrocortisone is decreased until a maintenance dose is achieved. If aldosterone is deficient, maintenance therapy also includes oral doses of fludrocortisone acetate.

Special Problems

Surgery

Patients with chronic adrenal insufficiency who need surgery with general anesthesia are treated with injections of hydrocortisone and saline. Injections begin on the evening before surgery and continue until the patient is fully awake and able to take medication by mouth. The dosage is adjusted until the maintenance dosage given before surgery is reached.

Pregnancy

Women with primary adrenal insufficiency who become pregnant are treated with standard replacement therapy. If nausea and vomiting in early pregnancy interfere with oral medication, injections of the hormone may be necessary. During delivery, treatment is similar to that of patients needing surgery; following delivery, the dose is gradually tapered and the usual maintenance doses of hydrocortisone and fludrocortisone acetate by mouth are not reached until about 10 days after childbirth.

Patient Education

A person who has adrenal insufficiency should always carry identification stating his or her condition in case of an emergency. The card should alert emergency personnel about the need to inject 100 mg of cortisol if its bearer is found severely injured or unable to answer questions. The card should also include the doctor's name and telephone number and the name and telephone number of the nearest relative to be notified. When traveling, it is important to have a needle, syringe, and an injectable form of cortisol for emergencies. A person with Addison's disease also should know how to increase medication during periods of stress or mild upper respiratory infections. *Immediate medical attention is needed when severe infections or vomiting or diarrhea occur.* These conditions can precipitate an addisonian crisis. A patient who is vomiting may require injections of hydrocortisone.

It is very helpful for persons with medical problems to wear a descriptive warning bracelet or neck chain to alert emergency personnel. Bracelets and neck chains can be obtained from:

Medic Alert Foundation International
2323 Colorado
Turlock, California 95381
(209) 668-3333

Suggested Reading

The following materials can be found in medical libraries, many college and university libraries, and through interlibrary loan in most public libraries.

Wingert, Terence D. and Mulrow, Patric J., "Chronic Adrenal Insufficiency," in *Current Diagnosis,* edited by Rex B. Conn. Philadelphia, W.B. Saunders Company, 1985, pp 860-863.

Bravo, Emmanuel L., "Adrenocortical Insufficiency," in *Conn's Current Therapy,* edited by Robert E. Rakel. Philadelphia, W.B. Saunders Company, 1987, pp 493-495.

Bondy, Philip K., "Disorders of the Adrenal Cortex," in *Williams Textbook of Endocrinology,* seventh edition, edited by Jean D. Wilson and Daniel W. Foster. Philadelphia, W.B. Saunders Company, 1985, pp 844-858.

Loriaux, D. Lynn and Cutler, Gordon B., "Diseases of the Adrenal Glands," in *Clinical Endocrinology,* edited by Peter O. Kohler. New York, John Wiley & Sons, 1986, pp 208-215.

Williams Gordon H. and Dluhy, Robert G., "Diseases of the Adrenal Cortex," in *Harrison's Principles of Internal Medicine,* 11th edition, edited by Eugene Braunwald, Kurt J. Isselbacher, Robert G. Petersdorf, Jean D. Wilson, Joseph B. Martin, and Anthony S. Fauci. New York, McGraw-Hill Book Company, 1987, pp 1769-1772.

Baxter, John D. and Tyrrell, J. Blake, "The Adrenal Cortex," in *Endocrinology and Metabolism*, second edition, edited by Phillip Felig, John D. Baxter, Arthur E. Broadus, and Lawrence A. Frohman. New York, McGraw-Hill Book Company, 1987, pp 581-599.

Other Resources

National Addison's Disease Foundation
505 Northern Boulevard, Suite 200
Great Neck, New York 11021
(516) 487-4992

This fact sheet was written by Eileen K. Corrigan of NIDDK's Office of Health Research Reports. The draft was reviewed by Dr. George P. Chrousos, National Institute of Child Health and Human Development, Dr. Judith Fradkin, National Institute of Diabetes and Digestive and Kidney Diseases, and by Dr. Richard Horton, University of Southern California Medical Center.

■ **Document Source:**
   U.S. Department of Health and Human Services, Public Health Service
   National Institutes of Health
   National Institute of Diabetes, and Digestive and Kidney Diseases
   NIH Publication No. 90-3054
   November 1989

NIDDK Fact Sheet

CUSHING'S SYNDROME

Cushing's syndrome is an endocrine, or hormonal, disorder. Although symptoms vary from person to person, most patients have upper-body obesity, severe fatigue and muscle weakness, high blood pressure, backache, elevated blood sugar, easy bruising, and bluish-red stretch marks on the skin. In women, there may be increased growth of facial and body hair, and menstrual periods may become irregular or stop completely.

Cushing's syndrome is caused by prolonged exposure of the body's tissues to high levels of the hormone cortisol. For this reason, the disorder is sometimes called "hypercortisolism."

Cortisol is normally produced by the adrenal glands, located just above the kidneys. It belongs to a class of hormones called glucocorticoids, which affect almost every organ and tissue in the body. Scientists think that cortisol has possibly hundreds of effects in the body. Among its vital tasks, cortisol:

- helps maintain blood pressure and cardiovascular function;
- helps slow the immune system's inflammatory response;
- helps balance the effects of insulin in breaking down sugar for energy; and
- helps regulate the metabolism of proteins, carbohydrates, and fats.

One of cortisol's most important jobs is to help the body respond to stress. In fact, the adrenal glands naturally produce more cortisol during stress. High levels of the hormone normally occur in women during the last 3 months of pregnancy and in highly trained athletes. Increased cortisol levels also are found in people suffering from depression, alcoholism, malnutrition, and panic disorders.

To understand the different ways that cortisol production can go wrong, it helps to look at how hormones normally do their work. Endocrine glands differ from other organs in the body because they release hormones into the bloodstream. Hormones travel through the blood, instructing cells in other parts of the body to release another hormone or to perform a specific function. Among the major endocrine glands are the thyroid, parathyroid, thymus, pituitary, and adrenals. Together, they play a major role in growth, metabolism, reproduction, and overall health.

The leaders in this carefully balanced performance are the brain's hypothalamus and the pituitary gland, a bean-sized organ at the base of the brain. First, the hypothalamus sends "releasing hormones" to the pituitary gland. The pituitary responds by secreting other hormones that regulate growth, thyroid function, and sex hormones such as estrogen and testosterone. One of the pituitary's main duties is to secrete ACTH (adrenocorticotropin), a hormone that stimulates the adrenal glands. When the adrenals receive the pituitary's signal in the form of ACTH, they respond by producing cortisol. Completing the cycle, cortisol then signals the pituitary to lower secretion of ACTH.

Normally, the amount of cortisol released by the adrenals is precisely balanced to meet the body's daily needs. If something goes wrong during this process—for example, with the adrenals, or their regulating switches in the brain (the pituitary gland or the hypothalamus)—cortisol production can go awry.

Causes

Exposure to too much cortisol can occur for different reasons. A common cause of elevated cortisol is the long-term use of glucocorticoid hormones such as prednisone for the treatment of inflammatory illnesses like rheumatoid arthritis. People who have taken these hormones for a long time may develop the symptoms of Cushing's syndrome, for example, the rounded or "moon face" and muscle weakness.

Elevated levels of cortisol also can be traced to abnormalities of the pituitary gland or the adrenal glands. High cortisol production also can be caused by tumor cells that release ACTH, in turn signaling the adrenals to overproduce cortisol. Each of these causes is discussed in more detail below.

Pituitary Adenomas

Most cases of Cushing's syndrome are caused by benign, or noncancerous tumors of the pituitary gland called adenomas, which secrete increased amounts of ACTH. Most patients have a single adenoma. This form of the syndrome, known as "Cushing's disease," afflicts more women than men. Adenomas are unlikely to spread; rarely, however, some pituitary tumors have the features of cancer, including the ability to spread.

Ectopic ACTH Syndrome

About 17 percent of Cushing's syndrome cases are due to the production of ACTH by various types of potentially malignant tumors that arise in different parts of the body. By far, the most common form of ACTH-producing tumor is oat cell, or small cell, lung cancer, which accounts for about 25 percent of all lung cancer cases. Other, less common types of cancer that can produce ACTH are thymomas, carcinoid tumors, pancreatic islet cell tumors, and medullary carcinomas of the thyroid.

Adrenal Tumors

In about 15 percent of patients with Cushing's syndrome, the cause can be traced to an abnormality of the adrenal glands, most often an adrenal tumor. In about one-half of these cases, the tumors are noncancerous growths of adrenal tissue, called adrenal adenomas, which release excess cortisol into the blood.

Adrenocortical carcinomas, or adrenal cancers, are the least common cause of Cushing's syndrome, accounting for about 7 percent of cases. They tend to occur in children. Cancer cells secrete excess levels of several adrenal cortical hormones, causing cortisol and adrenal androgen levels to remain elevated. Adrenal carcinomas also can be marked by very high hormone levels and rapid development of symptoms.

Incidence

Cushing's syndrome is relatively rare. It affects about 10 people per million population every year, or approximately 1 in 5,000 hospital admissions, with most cases occurring between the ages of 20 and 50 years.

About 70 percent of reported cases are diagnosed with pituitary adenomas that overproduce ACTH (Cushing's disease). This form of the syndrome affects more women than men at a ratio of 5:1.

The ectopic ACTH syndrome, caused by ACTH-producing tumors, is responsible for about 17 percent of the cases of Cushing's syndrome. Of these, over 50 percent are due to lung tumors, with a 3:1 ratio of males to females.

Adrenal tumors account for the remainder of cases, occurring in about two per million population annually. The average age of onset is about 40 years.

Symptoms

There is no single symptom shared by all patients with Cushing's syndrome, although some features of the disorder occur more often than others.

Obesity

The most common symptom is weight gain, with rounding of the face and increased fat in the neck and above the collar bone, while the arms and legs tend to stay thin. Obesity associated with poor growth is most common in children.

Skin

Skin changes also are common in Cushing's syndrome. The cheeks redden as the skin becomes thin, making the blood vessels more visible. The thin, fragile skin breaks easily, and ulcers may arise from minor injury. The ulcers may persist for a long time because of poor wound healing. Easy bruising and

bluish-red stretch marks, which often appear on the abdomen, thighs, buttocks, arms, armpits, and breasts, result from weakened connective tissue. Connective tissue not only provides the supportive framework of the body and its internal organs, but it is a major structural component of arteries and veins as well as the skin.

Excess Hair Growth

In women, excess hair growth, or hirsutism, often appears on the face, neck, chest, abdomen, and thighs. It occurs in about 80 percent of women with Cushing's syndrome.

Menstrual Disorders

Menstrual disorders are common. Periods become irregular and often stop. In men, there is decreased fertility with diminished or absent libido.

High Blood Pressure

Blood pressure above the normal range, or hypertension, occurs in 85 percent of Cushing's patients. More than 50 percent of patients have elevated diastolic pressure, and practically all patients have elevated systolic pressure. High blood pressure is associated with increased atherosclerosis, a buildup of fat in the arteries.

Muscle and Bone Weakness

Severe fatigue and weak, fragile muscles are characteristic of Cushing's syndrome. Backache is common due to osteoporosis, a weakening of the bones resulting from decreased bone mass. In Cushing's syndrome, rib fractures are frequent, and vertebral (spinal column) compression fractures may occur during routine activities such as bending, lifting, or rising from a chair.

High Blood Sugar

High blood sugar, or hyperglycemia, is seen in 80 percent of patients with Cushing's syndrome following the oral glucose tolerance test. However, diabetes mellitus occurs in less than 20 percent of people with Cushing's syndrome, and usually only in those with a family history of the disorder.

Diagnosis

The diagnosis of Cushing's syndrome is based on a review of the patient's medical history, physical examination, laboratory tests, and often x-ray exams of the adrenal or pituitary glands. The aim of these tests is first to determine whether excess levels of cortisol are present and then to establish the cause.

24-Hour Urinary Free Cortisol Level

This is the most specific test for diagnosing Cushing's syndrome. The patient's urine is collected over a 24-hour period and then tested for the amount of cortisol. Levels higher than 100 micrograms a day for an adult suggest Cushing's syndrome. (Persons suffering from depression or alcoholism, who tend to produce higher than normal levels of cortisol, may need further testing to confirm a diagnosis of Cushing's syndrome.)

Once Cushing's syndrome has been diagnosed, it is important to determine its cause. Various other tests are used to find the abnormality that leads to excess cortisol production. The choice of test depends in part on the preference of the endocrinologist or the center where the test is performed. Two very specialized tests that may be used are described below.

Dexamethasone Suppression Test

In this test, dexamethasone, a synthetic cortisol, is given by mouth every 6 hours for a period of 4 days. For the first 2 days, low doses of dexamethasone are given, and for the last 2 days, higher doses are given. The normal response after taking dexamethasone is a drop in blood and urine cortisol levels. Depending on the cause of Cushing's syndrome, different responses of cortisol to dexamethasone are obtained. The dexamethasone suppression test helps to distinguish patients with pituitary adenomas from those with ACTH-or cortisol-producing tumors.

The dexamethasone test can produce false-positive results in response to depression, alcohol abuse, high estrogen levels, acute illness, and stress. Conversely, drugs such as phenytoin and phenobarbital may cause false results in response to dexamethasone suppression. For this reason, patients should stop taking these drugs for at least 1 week before the test is performed.

CRH Stimulation Test

The corticotropin-releasing hormone (CRH) stimulation test is a relatively new diagnostic tool that also may be used to identify the cause of Cushing's syndrome. Patients with pituitary adenomas, after receiving an injection of CRH, usually have a rise in blood levels of ACTH and cortisol. This response is rarely seen in patients with ectopic ACTH syndrome and practically never in patients with cortisol-secreting adrenal tumors.

Direct Visualization of Endocrine Glands

Doctors use different imaging tools to reveal the size and shape of the pituitary and adrenal glands. The most common are the CT (computerized tomography) scan and MRI (magnetic resonance imaging). A CT scan produces a series of x-ray pictures giving a cross-sectional image of a body part. MRI also produces images of the internal organs of the body but without exposing the patient to ionizing radiation. A CT scan or MRI of the pituitary gland may help determine if a tumor is present, causing an overproduction of ACTH. Occasionally, doctors use a special radioisotope procedure, known as the iodocholesterol scan, to view the adrenal glands. If these tests do not establish the source of ACTH, some centers are experienced in performing catheterization procedures that sample the blood leaving the pituitary gland to determine if the pituitary is the source of high ACTH.

Treatment

Treatment of Cushing's syndrome depends on the specific reason for cortisol overproduction. If the cause is long-term use of glucocorticoid hormones to treat another disorder, the doctor will gradually reduce the dosage until the symptoms are under control. Once control is established, the daily dose will be doubled and given on alternate days.

Pituitary Adenomas

Several therapies are available to treat the ACTH-secreting pituitary adenomas of Cushing's disease. The most widely used treatment is removal of the tumor by surgery, known as transsphenoidal adenomectomy. Using a special microscope and very fine instruments, the surgeon approaches the pituitary gland through a nostril or an opening made in the bridge of the nose. Because this is an extremely delicate procedure, patients are often referred to centers specializing in this type of surgery. The success, or cure, rate of this procedure is over 80 percent. When surgery fails, it is usually because the CT scan or MRI is unable to identify the small adenoma. After pituitary surgery, there is a natural but temporary drop in the production of ACTH, so patients must be given a synthetic glucocorticoid hormone called hydrocortisone. Most patients can stop this replacement therapy in less than 1 year.

For patients in whom transsphenoidal surgery has failed or who are not suitable candidates for surgery, radiotherapy is another possible treatment. Radiation to the pituitary gland is given over a period of 6 weeks, with improvement occurring in 40 to 50 percent of adults and up to 80 percent of children. It may take several months before patients feel better from radiation treatment alone. However, the combination of radiation and the drug mitotane (Lysodren®) can help speed recovery. Mitotane suppresses cortisol production and lowers plasma and urine hormone levels. Treatment with mitotane alone can be successful in 30 to 40 percent of patients. Other drugs used alone or in combination to control the production of excess cortisol are aminoglutethimide, metyrapone, and ketoconazole. Like all drugs, each has its own set of side effects that doctors consider when prescribing therapy for individual patients.

Ectopic ACTH Syndrome

To cure the overproduction of cortisol caused by ectopic ACTH syndrome, it is necessary to eliminate all of the cancerous tissue that is secreting ACTH. The choice of cancer treatment—surgery, radiotherapy, chemotherapy, immunotherapy, or a combination of these treatments—depends on the type of cancer and how far it has spread. Since ACTH-secreting tumors (for example, small cell lung cancer) may be very small or widespread at the time of diagnosis, cortisol-inhibiting drugs like mitotane form an important part of treatment. In some cases, if pituitary surgery is not successful, surgical removal of the adrenal glands (bilateral adrenalectomy) may take the place of drug therapy.

Recently, researchers have found that a glucocorticoid antagonist, RU 486, is effective in fighting the excessive effects of cortisol that cause Cushing's syndrome. RU 486 is still an investigational drug, however, and its use is limited to clinical trials.

Adrenal Tumors

Surgery is the mainstay of treatment for benign as well as cancerous tumors of the adrenal glands.

Research in Cushing's Syndrome

The National Institutes of Health (NIH) is the biomedical research arm of the Federal Government. It is one of seven health agencies of the Public Health Service, which is part of the U.S. Department of Health and Human Services. Several components of NIH—the National Institute of Diabetes and Digestive and Kidney Diseases (NIDDK), the National Institute of Child Health and Human Development (NICHD), the National Institute of Neurological Disorders and Stroke, and the National Cancer Institute—conduct and support research on Cushing's syndrome and other disorders of the endocrine system.

NIH-supported scientists are conducting intensive research into the normal and abnormal function of the major endocrine glands and the many hormones of the endocrine system. One important NIDDK-supported study by Dr. Wylie W. Vale and colleagues at the Salk Institute for Biological Studies in La Jolla, California, led to the identification of corticotropin-releasing hormone (CRH), which instructs the pituitary gland to release ACTH. This finding enabled Dr. George P. Chrousos and coworkers at the NICHD to develop the CRH stimulation test, which is increasingly being used to identify the cause of Cushing's syndrome. Using the dexamethasone suppression test, doctors are able to diagnose the cause of Cushing's syndrome in 80 percent of patients. With the CRH stimulation test alone, they can accurately diagnose the cause in 85 percent of cases. By using the dexamethasone suppression test and CRH stimulation test together, they are able to diagnose Cushing's syndrome with 98 percent accuracy, according to a recent NIH study.

NIH scientists are continuing their efforts to improve the diagnosis and treatment of Cushing's syndrome. Current research is targeted not only at identifying new hormones, but also understanding their precise functions. Researchers also are focusing on the role of receptors, which are large complex molecules either on the surface of or within target cells to which hormones must attach to be effective.

One goal of future research is to find ways to cure Cushing's syndrome without surgery. For example, it may be possible to destroy pituitary tumors selectively by binding a hormone like CRH, which precisely targets pituitary tissue, with a tumor-killing toxin or monoclonal antibody.

Current NIH Studies

Scientists are treating patients with Cushing's syndrome at the NIH Warren Grant Magnuson Clinical Center in Bethesda, Maryland. Physicians who are interested in referring a patient with Cushing's syndrome may contact Dr. George P. Chrousos, Developmental Endocrinology Branch, NICHD,

Building 10, Room 10N262, Bethesda, Maryland 20892, telephone (301) 496-4686.

Suggested Reading

The following materials can be found in medical libraries, many college and university libraries, and through interlibrary loan in most public libraries.

Forsham, Peter H. and Tyrrell, J. Blake, "Cushing's Syndrome," in *Current Diagnosis,* edited by Rex B. Conn. Philadelphia, W.B. Saunders Company, 1985, pp 863-867.

Chrousos, George P., "Cushing's Syndrome," in *Conn's Current Therapy,* edited by Robert E. Rakel. Philadelphia, W.B. Saunders Company, Philadelphia, 1987, pp 495-498.

Kohler, Peter O., ed. *Clinical Endocrinology,* New York, John Wiley & Sons, 1986.

Braunwald, Eugene et al., eds. *Harrison's Principles of Internal Medicine,* 11th edition, New York, McGraw-Hill Book Company, 1987, pp 1760-1764.

NCI Research Report: Cancer of the Lung. Prepared by the Office of Cancer Communications, National Cancer Institute, NIH Publication No. 86-526.

Other Resources

National Cushing's Association
4620-1/2 Van Nuys Boulevard
Sherman Oaks, California 91403
(818) 788-9235 or (818) 788-9239
Andrea Hecht, President

This fact sheet was written by Eileen K. Corrigan of NIDDK's Office of Health Research Reports. The draft was reviewed by Dr. George P. Chrousos, National Institute of Child Health and Human Development, and by Dr. Richard Horton, University of Southern California Medical Center.

■ Document Source:
U.S. Department of Health and Human Services, Public Health Service
National Institutes of Health
National Institute of Diabetes, and Digestive and Kidney Diseases
NIH Publication No. 89-3007
April 1989

See also: Addison's Disease (page 104)

NDIC Clearinghouse Fact Sheet
DIABETES OVERVIEW

Almost everyone knows someone who has diabetes. Between 13 and 14 million people in the United States have diabetes mellitus, a serious, life-long disorder that is, as yet, incurable. Almost half of these people do not know they have diabetes and are not under medical care. Each year, 500,000 to 700,000 people are diagnosed with diabetes.

Although diabetes occurs most often in older adults, it is the second most common chronic disorder after cancer in U.S. children. Each year, 11,000 to 12,000 children and teenagers are diagnosed with diabetes.

What Is Diabetes?

Diabetes is a disorder of metabolism—the way the body uses digested food for growth and energy. Most of the food we eat is broken down by the digestive juices into chemicals including a simple sugar called glucose. After digestion, the glucose passes into the bloodstream where it is available for body cells to use for growth and energy.

For the glucose to get into the cells, insulin must be present. Insulin is a hormone produced by the pancreas.

When most people eat, the pancreas automatically produces the right amount of insulin to take care of the glucose. In people with diabetes, however, the pancreas either produces little or no insulin, or the body's cells do not respond to the insulin that is produced. As a result, glucose builds up in the blood, over-flows into the urine, and passes out of the body. Thus, the body loses its main source of fuel even though the blood contains large amounts.

There are two major types of diabetes. Type I, known as insulin-dependent diabetes (IDDM), is considered an autoimmune disease because the pancreatic cells that produce insulin, the beta cells, are destroyed by the body's own immune system. The pancreas then produces little or no insulin. To live, the person with IDDM needs daily injections of insulin. At present, scientists do not know exactly what causes the body's immune system to attack the beta cells, but they believe that both genetic factors and viruses may be involved. IDDM accounts for from 5 to 10 percent of diagnosed diabetes in the United States.

IDDM usually develops in children or young adults, although the disorder can appear at any age. Symptoms of IDDM usually develop over a short period, although beta cell destruction can begin months, or even years, earlier. Symptoms include increased thirst and urination, constant hunger, weight loss, blurred vision, and great tiredness. If not diagnosed and treated with insulin, the person can lapse into a life-threatening coma.

The most common form of diabetes is Type ll, called noninsulin-dependent diabetes (NIDDM). Ninety to 95 percent of people with diabetes have NIDDM. This form of diabetes usually develops in adults over the age of 40, and it is most common among adults over 55. About 80 percent of people with NIDDM are overweight.

In NIDDM, the pancreas usually produces insulin, but for some reason, the body cannot use the insulin effectively. The end result is the same as for IDDM—an unhealthy buildup of glucose in the blood and an inability of the body to make efficient use of its main source of fuel.

The symptoms of NIDDM appear to develop gradually, and they tend to be vague and not as noticeable as in IDDM. Symptoms include feelings of tiredness or illness, frequent urination, especially at night, unusual thirst, weight loss, blurred vision, frequent infections, and slow healing of sores.

A third form of diabetes, called gestational diabetes, develops or is discovered during pregnancy. The diabetes usually disappears when the pregnancy is over, but women who have had gestational diabetes have an increased risk of developing NIDDM later in their lives.

Diabetes is not contagious. It cannot be "caught" from another person. However, having a family history of diabetes places a person at higher risk for diabetes, especially NIDDM.

Other risk factors for NIDDM include being overweight, older, and of black, Hispanic, or Native American origin.

Scope and Impact of Diabetes

Diabetes is widely recognized as one of the leading causes of death and disability in the U.S. In 1986, diabetes caused or contributed to more than 187,000 deaths. The true toll is probably much higher because diabetes was not listed on half of the death certificates for people who had diabetes.

Diabetes is associated with long-term complications that affect almost every major part of the body. It can cause blindness, heart disease, strokes, kidney failure, amputations, nerve damage, and birth defects in babies born to women with diabetes.

In terms of medical care, treatment supplies, hospitalizations, time lost from work, disability payments, and premature death, diabetes costs this country over $40 billion annually.

Who Gets Diabetes?

Diabetes can develop in people of any age or ethnic background, although some groups appear to be at higher risk for certain types of diabetes. IDDM occurs equally among males and females, and it is more common in the white, non-Hispanic population. Although worldwide statistics are not available, it appears that IDDM is unknown or rare in some ethnic groups, including some Asian, African, and Native American populations. On the other hand, some northern European countries, including Finland and Sweden, have very high rates of IDDM. The reasons for these differences are not known.

NIDDM is more common in older people, especially older women, and it occurs more often among black, Hispanic, and Native Americans. The prevalence of NIDDM in the U.S. black population is about 60 percent higher than in non-Hispanic whites. Compared with whites, Hispanic Americans have twice the rate of diabetes. Native Americans have the highest rates of diabetes in the world. In one tribe, the Pima Indians, half of all adults have NIDDM. The rate of diabetes is likely to increase because older people, Hispanics, and other minority people make up the fastest growing parts of the U.S. population.

Treatment of Diabetes

Before the discovery of insulin in 1921, all people with IDDM died within a few years of the onset of their disease. Although insulin is not considered a cure for diabetes, its discovery was the first major breakthrough in diabetes treatment. Today, daily injections of insulin are the basic therapy for IDDM. Insulin injections must be balanced with diet and mealtimes, exercise, and daily testing of blood glucose levels. Diet, exercise, and blood or urine testing for glucose also form the basis for management of NIDDM. In addition, some people with NIDDM take oral drugs or insulin to lower their blood glucose levels.

People with diabetes are responsible for their day-to-day care. They also should be under the general care of a doctor who monitors their diabetes control and checks for diabetes complications. Doctors that specialize in diabetes are called endocrinologists or diabetologists. In addition, people with diabetes often see other specialists such as ophthalmologists for eye examinations or podiatrists for foot care. People with diabetes often consult a dietitian for dietary guidance and a diabetes educator for instruction in day-to-day care.

The goal of diabetes treatment is to keep blood glucose levels as close to the normal (nondiabetic) range as possible. Most diabetes doctors believe that trying to keep blood glucose levels near the normal range will help prevent or delay the long-term complications of diabetes.

The National Institute of Diabetes and Digestive and Kidney Diseases (NIDDK), the federal government's lead agency for diabetes research at the National Institutes of Health (NIH), is conducting a major clinical study to help answer that question. The study, called the Diabetes Control and Complications Trial (DCCT), involves more than 1,400 people with IDDM and is being carried out at 29 centers nationwide. Results from the study are expected in 1994.

Research on Diabetes

The DCCT is one of many research programs being carried out by the federal government and by nongovernment organizations to improve the health and well-being of people with diabetes and to find ways to prevent and cure the disorder.

The NIDDK supports basic and clinical research in its own laboratories, in research centers, and at hospitals throughout the U.S. NIDDK also gathers and analyzes statistics about diabetes. Other NIH Institutes carry out research on diabetes-related eye diseases, heart and vascular complications, pregnancy, and dental problems. Other government agencies that sponsor diabetes programs are the Centers for Disease Control, the Indian Health Service, the Health Resources and Services Administration, and the Department of Veterans Affairs.

Many organizations outside of the government support diabetes research and education activities. These organizations include the American Diabetes Association, the Juvenile Diabetes Foundation International, the American Association of Diabetes Educators, the Joslin Diabetes Center, the International Diabetes Center, the Barbara Davis Center for Childhood Diabetes, drug companies that develop diabetes products, and many other groups. In the past 15 years, advances in diabetes research have led to better ways to manage diabetes and treat its complications. Major advances include:

♦ New forms of purified insulin, such as human insulin produced through genetic engineering.
♦ Development of better ways for doctors to monitor blood glucose levels and for people with diabetes to test their own blood glucose levels at home.
♦ Development of external and implantable insulin pumps that deliver appropriate amounts of insulin, replacing daily injections.
♦ The use of laser treatment for diabetic eye disease, reducing the risk of blindness.
♦ Successful transplantation of kidneys in people whose own kidneys failed because of diabetes.
♦ Better ways of managing diabetic pregnancies, improving chances of a successful outcome.

♦ Development of new drugs to treat NIDDM and better ways to manage this form of diabetes through weight control.

In the future, insulin may be administered through nasal sprays or taken in the form of a pill. Devices to "read" blood glucose levels without having to prick a finger to get a blood sample also are being developed.

Research also is ongoing to find the cause or causes of diabetes and ways to prevent and cure the disorder. Scientists are searching for genes that may be involved in NIDDM and IDDM. Some genetic markers for IDDM have been identified, and it is now possible to screen relatives of people with IDDM to see if they are at risk for diabetes. Studies now are under way using drugs that stop the immune system from attacking the beta cells to try to prevent IDDM from developing in people who are at high risk for the disorder.

Transplantation of the pancreas or insulin-producing beta cells offers the best hope of cure for people with IDDM. Some successful pancreas transplants have been performed. However, people who have transplants must take powerful drugs that prevent rejection of the transplanted organ. These drugs are costly and may eventually cause serious health problems. Scientists are working to develop less harmful drugs and better methods of transplanting pancreatic tissue to prevent rejection by the body.

For NIDDM, the focus is on ways to prevent diabetes. Preventive approaches include identifying people at high risk for the disorder and encouraging them to lose weight, exercise more, and follow a healthy diet.

■ **Document Source:**
U.S. Department of Health and Human Services, Public Health Service
National Institutes of Health
National Institute of Diabetes, and Digestive and Kidney Diseases

See also: Diabetic Neuropathy: The Nerve Damage of Diabetes (page 328); Diabetic Retinopathy (page 144); Noninsulin-Dependent Diabetes (page 116); Understanding Gestational Diabetes: A Practical Guide to a Healthy Pregnancy (page 455)

INSULIN-DEPENDENT DIABETES

Insulin-dependent diabetes (IDDM) is a chronic disease that usually begins in childhood. It is not the most common form of diabetes—IDDM accounts for only 5 percent or less of diabetes in this country. Often, though, IDDM has a much greater impact on a person's life than the more common adult-onset form of diabetes, known as noninsulin-dependent diabetes (NIDDM).

The onset of IDDM is usually more swift and severe than that of NIDDM. A child with IDDM can become sick very quickly. If treatment does not begin shortly after the first symptoms, the child may need to be hospitalized. Once the diagnosis is made, a person with IDDM needs daily injections of the hormone insulin to survive.

Insulin, discovered in the 1920s, has literally made the difference between life and death for thousands of people with IDDM. Insulin is not a cure for diabetes, however. Even with careful insulin treatment, people who have had diabetes for years are at greater than average risk of developing problems that involve the heart, blood vessels, eyes, kidneys, and nerves. While most of those with IDDM can lead physically active and professionally challenging lives, they do not have the luxury of taking their health for granted.

Research is adding rapidly to our knowledge of diabetes. Besides searching for a cure, scientists are learning how to help people with diabetes enjoy a longer life with fewer health problems.

What Is Diabetes?

Diabetes mellitus impairs the way the body uses digested food for energy. The sugars and starches (carbohydrates) in the food we eat are broken down by digestive juices into a simple sugar called glucose. Glucose circulates in the blood as the major energy source for the body. For cells in muscles and other tissues to use glucose for energy, the hormone insulin must be present. Insulin is produced by the pancreas gland located behind the stomach. When the right amount of insulin is present, glucose is either used as fuel for energy or stored in the liver for future use.

In diabetes, however, the pancreas may not make enough insulin, or the body does not respond to the insulin that is present. Sometimes, a person with diabetes can have both these problems. As a result, glucose builds up in the blood and tissues, overflows into the urine, and is excreted. Thus, the body loses its main source of fuel.

In IDDM the pancreas makes little or no natural insulin, and a person with IDDM needs daily injections of the hormone to stay alive. IDDM generally occurs in children and adolescents, though it can appear at any age. An estimated 300,000 to 500,000 persons in the United States have IDDM. International statistics on IDDM are unreliable. In general, however, IDDM is unknown or rare in some ethnic groups, including the Japanese, Chinese, American Indians. Polynesians, and South African blacks. On the other hand, Sweden and Finland have very high rates: in Sweden it is estimated that 3 children in 1,000 have IDDM versus 1.6 in 1,000 in the United States. The reasons for these difference are not yet known.

NIDDM is the more common form of diabetes. Of the 11 million Americans who have diabetes, over 95 percent have NIDDM. Fully half of those with NIDDM don't know they have it. NIDDM usually occurs after age 40. In NIDDM, the pancreas can produce insulin, but the body does not use it efficiently. For this reason, most people with NIDDM can control their diabetes with careful dieting and regular exercise. When diet and exercise fail to control NIDDM, insulin or oral drugs can be used to help control the condition.

Effective treatment exists for both IDDM and NIDDM. Even with treatment, however both types of diabetes can cause long-term damage to the eyes, nerves, heart, and kidneys. These complications can lead to blindness, heart attack, stroke, kidney disease, and serious infections that may require limb amputation. In IDDM, episodes of very high or low blood sugar can cause a coma. Careful treatment of diabetes is the most effective way to minimize the chances of complications.

Symptoms

The symptoms of IDDM can be sudden and severe. They may include frequent urination, extreme thirst, constant hunger, blurred vision, and extreme fatigue. Because people with IDDM lack insulin, glucose builds up in the blood. The kidneys, trying to remove the excess sugar, excrete large amounts of water and essential body elements, causing frequent urination and thirst.

Because the body cannot use glucose, its first source of energy, it turns to stored fat and protein for fuel. As the body uses fat and protein, weight is lost. Breakdown products of fat collect in blood and raise its acid content. If levels of these products are high enough, a critical condition called ketoacidosis can develop, requiring prompt treatment.

How Is Diabetes Treated?

A person with IDDM must have insulin injections to survive. Without insulin, symptoms worsen until the patient loses consciousness and slips into a coma. With daily insulin shots and a careful diet, however, most people with IDDM can lead active lives with the same ambitions and challenges as those without diabetes.

Treatment for IDDM includes a daily routine of insulin shots or use of an insulin pump. Following a doctor's instructions, a person with IDDM buys insulin and syringes and injects himself or herself daily. (The parent of a young child with IDDM can do this for the child.) More and more people are also using home blood glucose monitoring devices to measure their blood glucose during the day. In this way, they can tailor the insulin dose more closely to changes in their hour-to-hour blood glucose. Blood glucose monitoring is a more accurate way to monitor diabetes treatment than urine testing.

Eating the right foods at the right time is an important part of treatment. A person with IDDM needs to time meals with insulin doses to keep blood glucose from getting too high or low. The foods you choose can play a role in controlling blood glucose levels, too. Increasing the proportion of fiber and complex carbohydrates in your diet and avoiding refined sugar may aid in reducing drastic changes in blood glucose and may, in some people, permit lowering of insulin dose. Foods containing fiber include beans, whole grains, and some fruits, while complex carbohydrates, or starches, include potatoes, rice, and pasta.

Reducing fats and cholesterol can help reduce the risk of heart disease, which affects people with diabetes more often than those with normal glucose metabolism.

Exercise, like diet, can help reduce the risk of heart disease. Being fit can also bring a sense of well-being and strength that has special meaning for someone with a chronic illness like diabetes.

Exercise carefully, though. Strenuous exercise increases the muscles' use of glucose, so it can lower glucose in the blood. At the same time, exercise also stimulates the body to release glucose and fats for use as energy. This stimulus can have the effect of raising blood glucose. In order to exercise safely, you should balance insulin dose, meals, and the timing of exercise to keep blood glucose levels from getting too high or too low.

What Causes Diabetes?

No one knows exactly what causes IDDM. What is clear is that the body's own immune or disease-fighting system for some reason turns against the body's own tissues. Certain substances formed by the immune system attack the beta cells of the pancreas, destroying their ability to make insulin.

Research shows that most, if not all, people with IDDM may inherit traits that put them at risk for IDDM. However, not everyone who inherits these traits develops IDDM. One or more factors in the environment are believed to trigger the immune system to destroy the insulin-producing cells. In some cases, the trigger may be a viral infection. Scientists have, in a few cases, been able to link the onset of diabetes with a virus. In most cases, however, the trigger for diabetes is unknown.

Complications of Diabetes

The discovery of insulin in 1921 lengthened the lives of people with IDDM from weeks or months to decades. In spite of insulin's life-preserving effects, diabetes remains a deadly disease. This fact is largely due to the complications of diabetes that develop over many years of insulin treatment. The complications affect the heart, eyes, kidneys, and nerves. Much of the damage done to these organs involves changes in small blood vessels throughout the body. Research is under way to determine whether very careful control of blood glucose can prevent or delay diabetic complications. Studies are also under way to determine why some people with IDDM have trouble with complications while others live long, relatively healthy lives.

Until the answers to these questions are known, it is wise for people with IDDM to follow their doctor's advice in controlling blood glucose and to be aware of the signs and risk factors for complications of diabetes.

Acute Complications

The acute complications of diabetes are the rapid effects that can occur when blood glucose levels climb too high or fall too low. If an insulin injection is missed, for example, blood glucose rises, and the person affected may start to feel weak and hungry, and may urinate frequently. Since the body can't use glucose for energy, it shifts to using fats and protein. The products of fat and protein metabolism, substances called ketones, are toxic when they reach high enough levels. This condition is called ketoacidosis, and it can cause coma and death if untreated. Ketoacidosis can develop slowly over several days. The warning symptoms may include abdominal pain, nausea and vomiting, rapid breathing and a fruity odor on the person's breath, and drowsiness.

Glucose can also fall too low in diabetes. Going too long without a meal, engaging in strenuous exercise, or taking too large a dose of insulin can cause glucose to drop, a condition called hypoglycemia, or insulin shock. Common symptoms of hypoglycemia include trembling, nervousness, sweating, hun-

ger, headache, nausea, drowsiness, or a feeling similar to drunkenness. Like ketoacidosis, hypoglycemia can cause coma and death if untreated. A quick, sugar-rich snack or drink such as orange juice or an injection of glucagon, a hormone that raises glucose levels, can restore normal glucose levels.

Long-Term Complications

In young people, acute complications pose the greatest threat to survival for people with IDDM. As people grow older, the long-term complications become more important. Diabetes can damage many organs through its effects on blood vessels. How this occurs is not well understood, but the damage can lead to kidney, heart, eye, and nerve disease.

Kidney Disease

Kidney disease is the greatest threat to life in adults with IDDM. The kidneys have a complex network of small blood vessels that filter impurities from blood for excretion in urine. Diabetes can damage these small blood vessels so that the kidneys cannot perform their waste-filtering work. The kidneys are essential to life. People can live without one kidney, but those who lose both must have their blood cleansed by a dialysis machine or have a kidney transplant.

High blood pressure can increase the chances that someone will develop kidney disease, so keeping blood pressure under control is especially important for someone with IDDM.

Heart Disease

Diabetes doubles the risk of heart disease. For reasons not yet well understood, fat and cholesterol collect more rapidly in the arteries of people with diabetes than in those without diabetes. These fatty deposits reduce the supply of blood to the heart and can lead to a heart attack.

Other risk factors for heart disease include hypertension or high blood pressure, obesity, high amounts of fats and cholesterol in blood, and cigarette smoking. The more these factors can be eliminated, the more a person reduces the risk of heart disease.

Eye Disease

The major threat to vision from diabetes is diabetic retinopathy. Retinopathy means disease of the retina, the light-sensing tissue at the back of the eye. Diabetes causes changes in the tiny vessels that supply the retina with blood. The blood vessels may swell and leak fluid. When retinopathy is more severe, new blood vessels may grow from the back of the eye and bleed into the clear gel, or vitreous, that fills the eye.

A yearly eye examination enables an eye doctor to detect changes before vision is affected and eye disease becomes harder to treat. Scientists have found that laser treatment for diabetic retinopathy can help prevent loss of vision and can, in some cases, restore vision lost as a result of this disease. A yearly eye exam by an eye doctor is the best way to make sure that changes in eyesight are diagnosed early and that effective treatment is carried out when it can be most helpful.

Diabetic Nerve Disease

Nerve damage from diabetes (diabetic neuropathy) can dull sensation in the feet, legs, and fingertips. When this happens, bruises or sores may go unnoticed until they become open or infected. Reduced blood flow caused by diabetes' effects on the blood vessels (peripheral vascular disease) can slow healing of foot sores. Because of diabetic neuropathy and peripheral vascular disease, people with diabetes are at increased risk of needing amputation when leg and foot sores become gravely infected.

Severe pain in the legs and feet sometimes comes with diabetic neuropathy. Pain-killing drugs and sometimes antidepressant drugs are used to treat painful neuropathy. In most cases, the pain subsides on its own with time.

Diabetic neuropathy can also affect body functions such as digestion. A doctor may prescribe drugs to relieve these symptoms. In addition, diabetes can, over time, affect the nerves that control erection in men. A doctor can find out whether impotence is the result of emotional or physical changes, such as diabetes, and then suggest treatment or counseling.

Pregnancy

With insulin treatment available, IDDM no longer poses the threat it once did to the health of the pregnant mother. The infant of a mother with IDDM does, however, have a higher than average risk of birth defects, stillbirth, respiratory distress, and other problems at birth. A mother's careful control of her glucose is essential to the health and life of her baby. With careful diabetes control, beginning before conception if possible, it is likely that the child will be healthy in every way.

Does Diabetes Run in Families?

A susceptibility to diabetes can be inherited. The brothers and sisters of a child with diabetes have a higher than average risk of developing IDDM. However, their risk remains small—only about 1 in 20 children with a diabetic sibling will develop IDDM. In fact, an identical twin of a child with IDDM has less than a 50 percent chance of developing the disease. Scientists are still doing research to determine how and why certain factors—both inherited and environmental—sometimes lead to diabetes.

Illness and Surgery

Illness, such as influenza, and stress, such as personal losses or conflicts, can affect the body's use of glucose. During times of illness and stress, a person needs to be even more careful about keeping glucose in control.

Surgery also places unusual stress on the body. Surgical teams take special precautions when doing surgery on a person with IDDM. The best way to ensure that doctors are aware of a patient's diabetes is to tell them.

Research in Diabetes

Diabetes research is the best hope that one day a means of curing and possibly preventing diabetes will be found. In the last 10 years, diabetes researchers have made great strides in understanding this disease. Critical to this effort has been the technology developed in genetics, microbiology, immunology, and other disciplines that have given diabetes researchers the tools they need to examine at the cell level what happens in diabetes.

The National Institute of Diabetes, and Digestive and Kidney Diseases (NIDDK) was established by Congress in 1950 as an institute of the National Institutes of Health (NIH), whose mission is to improve human health through biomedical research. The NIH is the research arm of the Public Health Service under the U.S. Department of Health and Human Services.

The NIDDK conducts and supports a variety of research in diabetes and its complications. In the past several years, scientists have identified the genetic factors that are associated with both IDDM and NIDDM. A major goal of future research will be to clarify how inherited factors affect the immune or disease-fighting system to result in IDDM. Already, scientists have identified immune factors circulating in blood that indicate increased risk of developing IDDM. This information may lead to early identification of IDDM cases and will help pave the way to understanding why the immune system goes awry in IDDM.

Scientists also have a better understanding of how insulin works in glucose metabolism. For example, groups of researchers at Memorial Sloan-Kettering Cancer Center, New York; the University of California, San Francisco; Mt. Zion Hospital and Medical Center, San Francisco; and Stanford University, Stanford, California, recently cloned and analyzed the structure of the insulin receptor, a molecule on cell surfaces to which insulin must attach in order to act. Defects in receptor function have been linked to abnormalities in glucose metabolism.

Human insulin made by recombinant DNA techniques is commercially available, as are externally worn pumps that can be programmed by the wearer to deliver insulin through a catheter in the abdomen. Research is continuing on internally implantable pumps, and clinical trials on at least one such pump have been undertaken.

New treatments are being developed for the complications of diabetes. Laser photocoagulation therapy has been shown to reduce the risk of blindness in people with diabetic retinopathy. Preventive measures and medications are available to help control high blood pressure, to avoid lower extremity amputations, and to reduce the risk of tooth loss from periodontal (gum) disease. Understanding how maternal diabetes can affect the unborn child is increasing, and with it, strategies to improve the chances that such a child will be born normal and healthy.

Research on transplantation of the insulin-producing cells of the pancreas is ongoing. The aim of this research is to provide a means of transplanting insulin-producing cells into someone with diabetes without the need to suppress the immune system to prevent rejection. If successful, the procedure would eliminate the need for daily injections of insulin.

Clinical Trials

Clinical trials are one means to test new approaches to treatment that emerge from basic research. In a clinical trial, new and existing treatments are compared with each other or with no treatment.

The NIDDK is supporting and planning clinical trials that are designed to weigh the benefits and risks of various approaches to treatment of diabetes and its complications. For information about NIDDK-supported clinical trials, contact the National Institute of Diabetes and Digestive and Kidney Diseases, National Institutes of Health, Building 31, Room 9A04, Bethesda, Maryland 20892.

Suggested Reading

The Diabetes Dictionary. Available from the National Diabetes Information Clearinghouse, Box NDIC, Bethesda, Maryland 20892, telephone (301) 468-2162.

Diabetes Mellitus: Theory and Practice, Ellenberg, M., and Rifkin, H., Editors. This book is an example of medical textbooks that provide an overview of diabetes, its symptoms, epidemiology, and treatment. This text is revised periodically and published by Medical Examination Publishing Company. It is written for readers with a medical background and is available in medical libraries and possibly university libraries or though interlibrary loan at a public library.

Diabetes and Your Eyes. Available from the National Eye Institute, of Health, Building 31, Room 6A32, Bethesda, Maryland 20892, telephone (301) 496-5248.

Other Resources

American Diabetes Association
National Service Center
1660 Duke Street
Alexandria, Virginia 22314
(703) 549-1500

Juvenile Diabetes Foundation, International
432 Park Avenue, South, 16th Floor
New York, New York 10016
(212) 889-7575

National Diabetes Information Clearinghouse
Box NDIC
Bethesda, Maryland 20892
(301) 468-2162

■ Document Source:
    U.S. Department of Health and Human Services, Public Health Service
    National Institutes of Health
    National Institute of Diabetes, and Digestive and Kidney Diseases
    NIH Publication No. 90-2098
    Revised April 1990

See also: Diabetes Overview (page 110); Diabetic Neuropathy: The Nerve Damage of Diabetes (page 328); Diabetic Retinopathy (page 144)

NONINSULIN-DEPENDENT DIABETES

Of people with diabetes, 90 to 95 percent have noninsulin-dependent or type II diabetes.

This section is about *noninsulin-dependent diabetes.* The word "diabetes" in the text refers to noninsulin-dependent diabetes unless otherwise specified.

Introduction

Of the estimated 13 to 14 million people in the United States with diabetes, between 90 and 95 percent have **noninsulin-dependent or type II diabetes**. Formerly called adult-onset, this form of diabetes usually begins in adults over age 40, and is most common after age 55. Nearly half of people with diabetes don't know it because the symptoms often develop gradually and are hard to identify at first. The person may feel tired or ill without knowing why. Diabetes can cause problems that damage the heart, blood vessels, eyes, kidneys, and nerves.

Although there is no cure for diabetes yet, daily treatment helps control blood sugar, and may reduce the risk of complications. Under a doctor's supervision, treatment usually involves a combination of weight loss, exercise and medication.

This booklet isn't a guide to treatment and it doesn't replace the advice of a doctor. It's one of many sources of extra information about diabetes. Local diabetes groups and clinics sponsor meetings and educational programs about diabetes that also can be helpful. At the end of this book is a list of groups that have information on diabetes programs.

Points to Remember

◆ Only a doctor can treat diabetes.
◆ Treatment usually involves weight loss, exercise and medication.
◆ Daily treatment helps control diabetes and may reduce the risk of complications.

What Is Diabetes?

The two types of diabetes, insulin-dependent and noninsulin-dependent, are different disorders. While the causes, short-term effects, and treatments for the two types differ, both can cause the same long-term health problems. Both types also affect the body's ability to use digested food for energy. Diabetes doesn't interfere with digestion, but it does prevent the body from using an important product of digestion, glucose (commonly known as sugar), for energy.

After a meal the digestive system breaks some food down into glucose. The blood carries the glucose or sugar throughout the body, causing blood glucose levels to rise. In response to this rise the hormone insulin is released into the bloodstream to signal the body tissues to metabolize or burn the glucose for fuel, causing blood glucose levels to return to normal. A gland called the pancreas, found just behind the stomach, makes insulin. Glucose the body doesn't use right away goes to the liver, muscle or fat for storage.

In someone with diabetes, this process doesn't work correctly. In people with insulin-dependent diabetes, the pancreas doesn't produce insulin. This condition usually begins in childhood and is also known as type I (formerly called juvenile-onset) diabetes. People with this kind of diabetes must have daily insulin injections to survive.

In people with noninsulin-dependent diabetes the pancreas usually produces some insulin, but the body's tissue don't respond very well to the insulin signal and, therefore, don't metabolize the glucose properly, a condition called insulin resistance. Insulin resistance is an important factor in noninsulin-dependent diabetes.

Points to Remember

- Diabetes interferes with the body's use of food for energy.
- While noninsulin-dependent diabetes and insulin-dependent diabetes are different disorders, they can cause the same complications.

Symptoms

The symptoms of diabetes may begin gradually and can be hard to identify at first. They may include fatigue, a sick feeling, frequent urination, especially at night, and excessive thirst. When there is extra glucose in blood, one way the body gets rid of it is through frequent urination. This loss of fluids causes extreme thirst. Other symptoms may include sudden weight loss, blurred vision, and slow healing of skin, gum and urinary tract infections. Women may notice genital itching.

A doctor also may suspect a patient has diabetes if the person has health problems related to diabetes. For instance, heart disease, changes in vision, numbness in the feet and legs or sores that are slow to heal, may prompt a doctor to check for diabetes. These symptoms do not mean a person has diabetes, but anyone who has these problems should see a doctor.

Points to Remember

- The symptoms of diabetes can develop gradually and may be hard to identify at first.
- Symptoms may include feeling tired or ill, excessive thirst, frequent urination, sudden weight loss, blurred vision, slow healing of infections, and genital itching.

What Causes Noninsulin-Dependent Diabetes?

There is no simple answer to what causes noninsulin-dependent diabetes. While eating sugar, for example, doesn't cause diabetes, eating large amounts of sugar and other rich, fatty foods, can cause weight gain. Most people who develop diabetes are overweight. Scientists do not fully understand why obesity increases someone's chances of developing diabetes, but they believe obesity is a major factor leading to noninsulin-dependent diabetes. Current research should help explain why the disorder occurs and why obesity is such an important risk factor.

A major cause of diabetes is insulin resistance. Scientists are still searching for the causes of insulin resistance, but they have identified two possibilities. The first could be a defect in insulin receptors on cells. Like an appliance that needs to be plugged into an electrical outlet, insulin has to bind to a receptor to function. Several things can go wrong with receptors. There may not be enough receptors for insulin to bind to, or a defect in the receptors may prevent insulin from binding.

A second possible cause involves the process that occurs after insulin plugs into the receptor. Insulin may bind to the receptor, but the cells don't read the signal to metabolize the glucose. Scientists are studying cells to see why this might happen.

Points to Remember

- In people with noninsulin-dependent diabetes, insulin doesn't lower blood sugar, a condition called insulin resistance.
- Obesity is a risk factor for diabetes.

Who Develops Noninsulin-Dependent Diabetes?

Age, sex, weight, physical activity, diet, lifestyle, and family health history all affect someone's chances of developing diabetes. The chances that someone will develop diabetes increase if the person's parents or siblings have the disease. Experts now know that diabetes is more common in African Americans, Hispanics, Native Americans and Native Hawaiians than whites. They believe this is the result of both heredity and environmental factors, such as diet and lifestyle. The highest rate of diabetes in the world is in an Arizona community of American Indians called the Pimas. While the chances of developing diabetes increase with age, gender isn't a risk factor, although African American women are more likely to develop diabetes than African American men.

While people can't change family history, age, or race, it is possible to control weight and physical fitness. A doctor can decide if someone is at risk for developing diabetes and offer advice on reducing that risk.

Points to Remember

- The following factors increase someone's chances of developing diabetes: obesity, family history of diabetes, and advancing age.

Diagnosing Diabetes

A doctor can diagnose diabetes by checking for symptoms such as excessive thirst and frequent urination and by testing for glucose in blood or urine. When blood glucose rises above a certain point, the kidneys pass the extra glucose in the urine. However, a urine test alone is not sufficient to diagnose diabetes.

A second method for testing glucose is a blood test usually done in the morning before breakfast (fasting glucose test) or after a meal (postprandial glucose test).

The oral glucose tolerance test is a second type of blood test used to check for diabetes. Sometimes it can detect diabetes when a simple blood test does not. In this test, blood glucose is measured before and after a person has consumed a thick, sweet drink of glucose and other sugars. Normally, the glucose in a person's blood rises quickly after the drink and then falls gradually again as insulin signals the body to metabolize the glucose. In someone with diabetes, blood glucose rises and remains high after consumption of the liquid.

A doctor can decide, based on these tests and a physical exam, whether someone has diabetes. If a blood test is borderline abnormal, the doctor may want to monitor the person's blood glucose regularly. If a person is overweight, he or she probably will be advised to lose weight. The doctor also may monitor the patient's heart, since diabetes increases the risk of heart disease.

Points to Remember

A doctor will diagnose diabetes by looking for four kinds of evidence:
- risk factors like excess weight and a family history of diabetes
- symptoms such as thirst and frequent urination
- complications like heart trouble
- signs of excess glucose or sugar in blood and urine tests.

Treating Diabetes

The goals of diabetes treatment are to keep blood glucose within normal range and to prevent long-term complications. Why control blood glucose? In the first place, diabetes can cause short-term effects: some are unpleasant and some are dangerous. These include thirst, frequent urination, weakness, lack of ability to concentrate, loss of coordination, and blurred vision. Loss of consciousness is possible with very high or low blood sugar levels, but is more of a danger in insulin-dependent than in noninsulin-dependent diabetes.

In the second place, the long-term complications of diabetes may result from many years of high blood glucose. Research is under way to find out if this is true and to learn if careful control can help prevent complications. Meanwhile, most doctors feel that if people with diabetes keep their blood glucose levels under control, they will reduce the risk of complications.

In 1986, a National Institutes of Health panel of experts recommended that the best treatment for noninsulin-dependent diabetes is a diet that helps the person maintain normal weight. In people who are overweight, losing weight is the one treatment that is clearly effective in controlling diabetes.

In some people, exercise can help keep weight and diabetes under control. However, when diet and exercise alone can't control diabetes, two other kinds of treatment are available: oral diabetes medications and insulin. The treatment a doctor suggests depends on the person's age, lifestyle, and the severity of the diabetes.

Diabetes Diet

The proper diet is critical to diabetes treatment. It can help someone with diabetes:
- Achieve and maintain desirable weight. Many people with diabetes can control their blood glucose by losing weight and keeping it off.
- Maintain normal blood glucose levels.
- Prevent heart and blood vessel diseases, conditions that tend to occur in people with diabetes.

Points to Remember

- Diabetes treatment can reduce symptoms, like thirst and weakness, and the chances of long-term problems, like heart and eye disease.
- If treatment with diet and exercise isn't effective, a doctor may prescribe oral medications or insulin.
- There is no known cure for diabetes; daily treatment must continue throughout a person's lifetime.

A doctor will usually prescribe diet as part of diabetes treatment. A dietitian or nutritionist can recommend a diet that is healthy, but also interesting and easy to follow. No one has to be limited to a preprinted, standard diet. Someone with diabetes can get assistance in the following ways:

- A doctor can recommend a local nutritionist or dietitian.
- The local American Diabetes Association, American Heart Association, and American Dietetic Association can provide names of qualified dietitians or nutritionists and information about diet planning.
- Local diabetes centers at large medical clinics, hospitals, or medical universities usually have dietitians and nutritionists on staff.

The guidelines for diabetes diet planning include the following:

- Many experts, including the American Diabetes Association, recommend that 50 to 60 percent of daily calories come from carbohydrates, 12 to 20 percent from protein, and no more than 30 percent from fat.
- Spacing meals throughout the day, instead of eating heavy meals once or twice a day, can help a person avoid extremely high or low blood glucose levels.
- With few exceptions, the best way to lose weight is gradually: one or two pounds a week. Strict diets **must never** be undertaken without the supervision of a doctor.
- People with diabetes have twice the risk of developing heart disease as those without diabetes, and high blood cholesterol levels raise the risk of heart disease. Losing weight and reducing intake of saturated fats and cholesterol, in favor of unsaturated and monounsaturated fats, can help lower blood cholesterol.

  For example, meats and diary products are major sources of saturated fats, which should be avoided; most vegetable oils are high in unsaturated fats, which are fine in limited amounts; and olive oil is a good source of monounsaturated fat, the healthiest type of fat. Liver and other organ meats and egg yolks are particularly high in cholesterol. A doctor or nutritionist can advise someone on this aspect of diet.

- Studies show that foods with fiber, such as fruits, vegetables, peas, beans, and whole-grain breads and cereals may help lower blood glucose. However, it seems that a person must eat much more fiber than the average American now consumes to get this benefit. A doctor or nutritionist can advise someone about adding fiber to a diet.
- Exchange lists are useful in planning a diabetes diet. They place foods with similar nutrients and calories into groups. With the help of a nutritionist, the person plans the number of servings from each exchange list that he

or she should eat throughout the day. Diets that use exchange lists offer more choices than preprinted diets. More information on exchange lists is available from nutritionists and from the American Diabetes Association.

Continuing research may lead to new approaches to diabetes diets. Because one goal of a diabetes diet is to maintain normal blood glucose levels, it would be helpful to have reliable information on the effects of foods on blood glucose. For example, foods that are rich in carbohydrates, like breads, cereals, fruits, and vegetables break down into glucose during digestion, causing blood glucose to rise. However, scientists don't know how each of these carbohydrates affect blood glucose levels. Research is also under way to learn whether foods with sugar raise blood glucose higher than foods with starch. Experts do know that cooked foods raise blood glucose higher than raw, unpeeled foods. A person with diabetes can ask a doctor or nutritionist about using this kind of information in diet planning.

Alcoholic Beverages

Most people with diabetes can drink alcohol safely if they drink in moderation (one or two drinks occasionally), because in higher quantities alcohol can cause health problems:

- ♦ Alcohol has calories without the vitamins, minerals, and other nutrients that are essential for maintaining good health. A doctor can discuss whether it's safe for an individual with diabetes to drink. People who are trying to lose weight need to account for the calories in alcohol in diet planning. A dietitian also can provide information about the sugar and alcohol content of various alcoholic drinks.
- ♦ Alcohol on an empty stomach can cause low blood glucose or hypoglycemia. Hypoglycemia is a particular risk in people who use oral medications or insulin for diabetes. It can cause shaking, dizziness, and collapse. People who don't know someone has diabetes may mistake these symptoms for drunkenness and neglect to seek medical help.
- ♦ Oral diabetes medications—tolbutamide and chlorpropamide—can cause dizziness, flushing, and nausea when combined with alcohol. A doctor can advise patients on the safety of drinking when taking these and other diabetes medications.
- ♦ Frequent, heavy drinking can cause liver damage over time. Because the liver stores and releases glucose, blood glucose levels may be more difficult to control in a person with liver damage from alcohol.
- ♦ Frequent heavy drinking also can raise the levels of fats in blood, increasing the risk of heart disease.

Points to Remember

- ♦ A diabetes diet should do three things: achieve ideal weight, maintain normal blood glucose levels, and limit foods that contribute to heart disease.
- ♦ A nutritionist or dietitian can help plan a diabetes diet.

Exercise

Exercise has many benefits, and for someone with diabetes regular exercise combined with a good diet can help control diabetes. Exercise not only burns calories, which can help with weight reduction, but it also can improve the body's response to the hormone insulin. As a result, following a regular exercise program can make oral diabetes medications and insulin more effective and can help control blood glucose levels.

Exercise also reduces some risk factors for heart disease. For example, exercise can lower fat and cholesterol levels in blood, which increase heart disease risk. It also can lower blood pressure and increase production of a cholesterol, called HDL, that protects against heart disease.

However, infrequent, strenuous exercise can strain muscles and the circulatory system and can increase the risk of a heart attack during exercise. A doctor can decide how much exercise is safe for an individual. The doctor will consider how well controlled a person's diabetes is, the condition of the heart and circulatory system, and whether complications require that the person avoid certain types of activity.

Walking is great exercise, especially for an inactive person, and it's easy to do. A person can start off walking for 15 or 20 minutes, three or four times a week, and gradually increase the speed or distance of the walks. The purpose of a good exercise program is to find an enjoyable activity and do it regularly. Doing strenuous exercise for six months and then stopping isn't as effective. People taking oral drugs or insulin need to remember that strenuous exercise can cause dangerously low blood glucose and they should carry a food or drink high in sugar for medical emergencies. Signs of hypoglycemia include hunger, nervousness, shakiness, weakness, sweating, headache, and blurred vision. As a precaution, a person with diabetes should wear an identification bracelet or necklace to alert a stranger that the wearer has diabetes and may need special medical help in an emergency.

A doctor may advise someone with high blood pressure or other complications to avoid exercises that raise blood pressure. For example, lifting heavy objects and exercises that strain the upper body raise blood pressure.

People with diabetes who have lost sensitivity in their feet also can enjoy exercise. They should choose shoes carefully and check their feet regularly for breaks in skin that could lead to infection. Swimming or bicycling can be easier on the feet than running.

Points to Remember

- ♦ Exercise has three major benefits: it burns calories, improves the body's response to insulin, and reduces risk factors for heart disease.
- ♦ An exercise program should be started slowly and with the advice of a doctor.

Oral Medications

Oral diabetes medicines, or oral hypoglycemics, can lower blood glucose in people who have diabetes, but are able to make some insulin. They are an option if diet and exercise don't work. Oral diabetes medications are not insulin and are not a substitute for diet and exercise. Although experts don't understand exactly how each oral medicine works, they know that they increase insulin production and affect how insulin lowers blood glucose. These medications are most effective in people who developed diabetes after age 40, have had diabetes less than 5 years, are normal weight, and have never received insulin or have taken only 40 units or less of insulin a day. Pregnant and nursing women shouldn't take oral medications because their effect on the fetus and newborn is unknown, and because insulin provides better control of diabetes during pregnancy.

There is also some question about whether oral diabetes medications increase the risk of a heart attack. Experts disagree on this point and many people with noninsulin-dependent diabetes use oral medicines safely and effectively. The Food and Drug Administration (FDA), the agency of the federal government that approves medications for use in this country, requires that oral diabetes medicines carry a warning concerning the increased risk of heart attack. Whether someone uses a medication depends on its benefits and risks, something a doctor can help the patient decide.

Six FDA-approved oral diabetes medications are now on the market. Their generic names are tolbutamide, chlorpropamide, tolazamide, acetohexamide, glyburide, and glipizide. The generic name refers to the chemical that gives each medicine its particular effect. Some of these medications are made by more than one pharmaceutical company and have more than one brand name. All six are different types of one class of medication, called sulfonylureas, but each affects metabolism differently. A doctor will choose a patient's medication based on the person's general health, the amount his or her blood glucose needs to be lowered, the person's eating habits, and the medicine's side effects.

The purpose of oral medications is to lower blood glucose. Therefore, the person taking them must eat regular meals and engage in only light to moderate exercise, to prevent blood glucose from dipping too low. Medications taken for other health problems, including illness, also can lower blood sugar and may react with the diabetes medicine. Therefore, a doctor needs to know all the medications a person is taking to prevent a harmful interaction. Lowering blood sugar too much can cause hypoglycemia with symptoms such as headache, weakness, shakiness, and if the condition is severe enough, collapse.

Oral diabetes medications usually don't cause side effects. However, a few people do experience nausea, skin rashes, headache, either water retention or diuresis (increased urination), and sensitivity to direct sunlight. These effects should gradually subside, but a person should see a doctor if they persist. For reasons that aren't always clear, sometimes oral diabetes medications don't help the person for whom they're prescribed. Investigations are under way to learn why this happens.

Points to Remember

◆ Oral diabetes medications may be used when diet and exercise alone don't control diabetes.
◆ Oral diabetes medicines aren't a substitute for diet and exercise.

Insulin

Like oral diabetes medications, insulin is an alternative for some people with noninsulin-dependent diabetes who can't control their blood glucose levels with diet and exercise. In special situations, such as surgery and pregnancy, insulin is a temporary but important means of controlling blood glucose. A section of this booklet called "special situations" discusses insulin use during pregnancy and surgery.

Sometimes it's unclear whether insulin or oral medications are more effective in controlling blood-glucose; therefore, a doctor will consider a person's weight, age, and the severity of the diabetes before prescribing a medicine. Experts do know that weight control is essential for insulin to be effective. A doctor is likely to prescribe insulin if diet, exercise, or oral medications don't work, or if someone has a bad reaction to oral medicines. A person also may have to take insulin if his or her blood glucose fluctuates a great deal and is difficult to control. A doctor will instruct a person with diabetes on how to purchase, mix, and inject insulin. Various types of insulin are available that differ in purity, concentration, and how quickly they work. They also are made differently. In the past, all commercially available insulin came from the pancreas glands of cows and pigs. Today, human insulin is available in two forms: one uses genetic engineering and the other involves chemically changing pork insulin into human insulin. The best sources of information on insulin are the company that makes it and a doctor.

Points to Remember

◆ Insulin may be used when diet, exercise, or oral medications don't control diabetes.
◆ Weight control is important when taking insulin.
◆ Insulin is taken in special situations such as surgery and pregnancy.

Checking Blood Glucose Levels

When a person's body is operating normally, it automatically checks the level of glucose in blood. If the level is too high or too low, the body will adjust the sugar level to return it to normal. This system operates in much the same way that cruise control adjusts the speed of a car. With diabetes, the body doesn't do the job of controlling blood glucose automatically. To make up for this, someone with diabetes has to check blood sugar regularly and adjust treatment accordingly.

A doctor can measure blood glucose during an office visit. However, levels change from hour to hour and someone who visits the doctor only every few weeks won't know what his or her blood glucose is daily. Do-it-yourself tests enable people with diabetes to check their blood sugar daily.

The easiest test someone can do at home is a urine test. When the level of glucose in blood rises above normal, the kidneys eliminate the excess glucose in urine. Glucose in urine, therefore, reflects an excess of glucose in blood.

Urine testing is easy. Tablets or paper strips are dipped in urine. The color change that occurs indicates whether blood glucose is too high. However, urine testing is not completely accurate because the reading reflects the level of blood glucose a few hours earlier. In addition, not everyone's kidneys are the same. Even when the amount of glucose in two people's urine is the same, their sugar levels may be different. Certain drugs and vitamin C also can affect the accuracy of urine tests.

It's more accurate to measure blood glucose directly. Kits are available that allow people with diabetes to test their blood glucose at home. The test involves pricking a finger to draw a drop of blood. A spring-operated "lancet" does this automatically. The drop of blood is placed on a strip of specially coated plastic or into a small machine that "reads" how much glucose is in the blood. A doctor may suggest that someone test his or her blood glucose several times a day. Self blood glucose monitoring can show how the body responds to meals, exercise, stress, and diabetes treatment.

Another test that measures the effectiveness of treatment is a "glycosylated hemoglobin" test. It measures the glucose that has become attached to hemoglobin, the molecule in red blood cells that gives blood its red color. Over time, hemoglobin absorbs glucose, according to its concentration in blood. Once glucose is absorbed by hemoglobin it remains there until the blood cells die and new ones replace them. With the "glycosylated hemoglobin" test, a doctor can tell whether blood glucose has been very high over the last few months.

Points to Remember

◆ Testing blood glucose levels regularly can show whether treatment is working.

Diabetes Complications

A key goal of diabetes treatment is to prevent complications because, over time, diabetes can damage the heart, blood vessels, eyes, kidneys, and nerves, although the person may not know damage is taking place. It's important to diagnose and treat diabetes early, because it can cause damage even before it makes someone feel ill.

How diabetes causes long-term problems is unclear. However, changes in the small blood vessels and nerves are common. These changes may be the first step toward many problems that diabetes causes. Scientists can't predict who among people with diabetes will develop complications, but complications are most likely to occur in someone who has had diabetes for many years. However, because a person can have diabetes without knowing it, a complication may be the first sign.

Heart Disease

Heart disease is the most common life-threatening disease linked to diabetes, and experts say diabetes doubles a person's risk of developing heart disease. In heart disease, deposits of fat and cholesterol build-up in the arteries that supply the heart with blood. If this build-up blocks blood from getting to the heart, a potentially fatal heart attack can occur.

Other risk factors include hypertension or high blood pressure, obesity, high amounts of fats and cholesterol in blood, and cigarette smoking. Eliminating these risk factors, along with treating diabetes, can reduce the risk of heart disease. The American Heart Association has literature that explains what heart disease is and how to prevent it. The association's address is in the resources section of this booklet.

Kidney Disease

People with diabetes are also more likely to develop kidney disease than other people. The kidneys filter waste products from the blood and excrete them in the form of urine, maintaining proper fluid balance in the body. While people can live without one kidney, those with out both must have special treatment, called dialysis. Most people with diabetes will never develop kidney disease, but proper diabetes treatment can further reduce the risk. High blood pressure also can add to the risk of kidney disease. Therefore, regular blood pressure checks and early treatment of the disorder can help prevent kidney disease.

Urinary tract infections are also a cause of kidney problems. Diabetes can affect the nerves that control the bladder, making it difficult for a person to empty his or her bladder completely. Bacteria can form in the unemptied bladder and the tubes leading from it, eventually causing infection. The symptoms of a urinary tract infection include frequent, painful urination, blood in the urine, and pain in the lower abdomen and back. Without prompt examination and treatment by a doctor, the infection can reach the kidneys, causing pain, fever, and possibly kidney damage. A doctor may prescribe antibiotics to treat the infection and may suggest that the person drink large amounts of water.

Kidney problems are one cause of water retention, or edema, a condition in which fluid collects in the body, causing swelling, often in the legs and hands. A doctor can decide if swelling or water retention relates to kidney function.

A nephrologist, a doctor specially trained to diagnose and treat kidney problems, can identify the cause of problems and recommend ways to reduce the risk of kidney disease.

Eye Problems

Diabetes can affect the eyes in several ways. Frequently, the effects are temporary and can be corrected with better diabetes control. However, long-term diabetes can cause changes in the eyes that threaten vision. Stable blood glucose levels and yearly eye examinations can help reduce the risk of serious eye damage.

Blurred vision is one effect diabetes can have on the eyes. The reason may be that changing levels of glucose in blood also can affect the balance of fluid in the lens of the eye, which works like a flexible camera lens to focus images. If the lens absorbs more water than normal and swells, its focusing power changes. Diabetes also may affect the function of nerves that control eyesight, causing blurred vision.

Cataract and glaucoma are eye diseases that occur more frequently in people with diabetes. Cataract is a clouding of the normally clear lens of the eye. Glaucoma is a condition in which pressure within the eye can damage the optic nerve that transmits visual images to the brain. Early diagnosis and treatment of cataract and glaucoma can reduce the severity of these disorders.

Diabetic Retinopathy

Retinopathy, a disease of the retina, the light sensing tissue at the back of the eye, is a common concern among people with diabetes. Diabetic retinopathy damages the tiny vessels that supply the retina with blood. The blood vessels may swell and leak fluid. When retinopathy is more severe, new blood vessels may grow from the back of the eye and bleed into the clear gel that fills the eye, the vitreous.

While most people with diabetes may never develop serious eye problems, people who have had diabetes for 25 years are more likely to develop retinopathy. Experts think high blood pressure may contribute to diabetic retinopathy, and that smoking can cause the condition to worsen. If someone experiences blurred vision that lasts longer than a day or so, sudden loss of vision in either eye, or black spots, lines, or flashing lights in the field of vision, a doctor should be alerted right away.

Treatment for diabetic retinopathy can help prevent loss of vision and can sometimes restore vision lost because of the disease. A yearly eye examination with dilated pupils makes it possible for an ophthalmologist, an eye doctor, to notice changes before the illness becomes harder to treat. Scientists are testing new means of treating diabetic retinopathy. For more information on eye complications of diabetes and the treatment of these conditions, see the resource list at the end of this booklet.

Legs and Feet

Leg and foot problems can arise in people with diabetes due to changes in blood vessels and nerves in these areas. Peripheral vascular disease is a condition in which blood vessels become narrowed by fatty deposits, reducing blood supply to the legs and feet. Diabetes also can dull the sensitivity of nerves. Someone with this condition, called peripheral neuropathy, might not notice a sore spot caused by tight shoes or pressure from walking. If ignored, the sore can become infected, and because blood circulation is poor, the area may take longer to heal.

Proper foot care and regular visits to a doctor can prevent foot and leg sores and ensure that any that do appear don't become infected and painful. Helpful measures include inspecting the feet daily for cuts or sore spots. Blisters and sore spots are not as likely when shoes fit well and socks or stockings aren't tight. A doctor also may suggest washing feet daily, with warm, not hot water; filing thick calluses; and using lotions that keep the feet from getting too dry. Shoe inserts or special shoes can be used to prevent pressure on the foot.

Diabetic neuropathy, or nerve disease, dulls the nerves and can be extremely painful. A person with neuropathy also may be depressed. Scientists aren't sure whether the depression is an effect of neuropathy, or if it's simply a response to pain. Treatment, aimed at relieving pain and depression, may include aspirin and other pain-killing drugs.

Any sore on the foot or leg, whether or not it's painful, requires a doctor's immediate attention. Treatment can help sores heal and prevent new ones from developing. Problems with the feet and legs can cause life-threatening problems that require amputation—surgical removal of limbs—if not treated early.

Other Effects of Diabetic Neuropathy

Nerves provide muscle tone and feeling and help control functions like digestion and blood pressure. Diabetes can cause changes in these nerves and the functions they control.

These changes are most frequent in people who have had other complications of diabetes, like problems with their feet. Someone who has had diabetes for some years and has other complications, may find that spells of indigestion or diarrhea are common. A doctor may prescribe drugs to relieve these symptoms. Diabetes also can affect the nerves that control penile erection in men, which can cause impotence that shows up gradually, without any loss of desire for sex. A doctor can find out whether impotence is the result of physical changes, such as diabetes, or emotional changes, and suggest treatment or counseling.

Skin and Oral Infections

People with diabetes are more likely to develop infections, like boils and ulcers, than the average person. Women with diabetes may develop vaginal infections more often than other women. Checking for infections, treating them early, and following a doctor's advice can help ensure that infections are mild and infrequent.

Infections also can affect the teeth and gums, making people with diabetes more susceptible to periodontal disease, an inflammation of tissue surrounding and supporting the teeth. An important cause of periodontal disease is bacterial growth on the teeth and gums. Treating diabetes and following a dentist's advice on dental care can help prevent periodontal disease.

Emergencies

Very high blood glucose levels cause symptoms that are hard to ignore: frequent urination and excessive thirst. However, in someone who is elderly or in poor health these symptoms may go unnoticed. Without treatment, a person with high blood glucose or hyperglycemia can lose fluids, become weak, confused, and even unconscious. Breathing will be shallow and the pulse rapid. The person's lips and tongue will be dry, and his or her hands and feet will be cool. A doctor should be called immediately.

The opposite of high blood glucose, very low blood glucose or hypoglycemia, is also dangerous. Hypoglycemia can occur when someone hasn't eaten enough to balance the effects of insulin or oral medicine. Prolonged, strenuous exercise in someone taking oral diabetes drugs or insulin also can cause hypoglycemia, as can alcohol.

Someone whose blood glucose has become too low may feel nervous, shaky, and weak. The person may sweat, feel hungry, and have a headache. Severe hypoglycemia can cause loss of consciousness. A person with hypoglycemia who begins to feel weak and shaky should eat or drink something with sugar in it immediately, like orange juice. If the person is unconscious, he or she should be taken to a hospital emergency room right away. An identification bracelet or necklace that states that the wearer has diabetes will let friends know that these symptoms are a warning of illness that requires urgent medical help.

Special Situations

Surgery

Surgery is stressful, both physically and mentally. It can raise blood glucose levels even in someone who is careful about control. To make sure that surgery and recovery are successful for someone with diabetes, a doctor will test blood glucose and keep it under careful control, usually with insulin. Careful control makes it possible for someone with diabetes to have surgery with little or no more risk than someone without diabetes.

Points to Remember

◆ Diabetes can cause long-term complications such as heart, kidney, eye, and nerve disease.
◆ Careful treatment of diabetes and checking for signs of complications can lower the chances that someone will be troubled by these conditions.
◆ An identification bracelet or necklace stating that the wearer has diabetes can help ensure that friends or strangers won't ignore symptoms that signal a medical emergency.

To plan a safe and successful surgery, the surgeon and attending physicians must know that the person they're treating has diabetes. While tests done before surgery can detect diabetes, the patient should inform the doctor of his or her condition. A surgical team also will evaluate the possible effect of complications of diabetes, such as heart or kidney problems.

Pregnancy

Bearing a child places extra demands on a woman's body. Diabetes makes it more difficult for her body to adjust to these demands and it can cause problems for both mother and baby. Some woman may develop a form of diabetes during pregnancy called gestational diabetes. Gestational diabetes develops most frequently in the middle and later months of pregnancy, after the time of greatest risk for birth defects. Although this kind of diabetes often disappears after the baby's birth, treatment is necessary during pregnancy to make sure the diabetes doesn't harm the mother or fetus.

A woman who knows she has diabetes should keep her condition under control before she becomes pregnant, so that her diabetes won't increase the risk of birth defects. A woman whose diabetes isn't well-controlled may have an unusually large baby. Diabetes also increases the risk of premature birth and problems in the baby, such as breathing difficulties, low blood sugar and occasionally, death.

Blood glucose monitoring and treatment with insulin can ensure that a baby born to a mother with diabetes will be healthy. Oral diabetes drugs aren't given during pregnancy because the effects of these drugs on the unborn baby aren't known. By following the advice of a doctor trained to treat gestational diabetes, the mother can make sure her blood glucose is normal and her baby is well nourished.

Approximately half of women with gestational diabetes will no longer have abnormal blood glucose tests shortly after giving birth. However, many women with gestational diabetes will develop noninsulin-dependent diabetes later in their lives.

Regular check-ups can ensure that if a woman does develop diabetes later, it will be diagnosed and treated early.

Is Diabetes Hereditary?

Scientists estimate that the child of a parent with noninsulin-dependent diabetes has approximately a 10 to 15 percent chance of developing noninsulin-dependent diabetes. If both parents have diabetes, the child's risk of having the disease increases. The child's health habits throughout his or her life will affect the risk of developing diabetes. Obesity, for example, may increase the risk of diabetes or cause it to occur earlier in life.

Noninsulin-dependent diabetes in a parent has no effect on the chances that his or her child will have insulin-dependent diabetes, the more severe form of diabetes.

Stress and Illness

One way the body responds to stress is to increase the level of blood glucose. In a person with diabetes, stress may increase the need for treatment to lower blood glucose levels. Illnesses such as colds and flu are forms of physical stress that a doctor can treat. The doctor will advise the person to drink plenty of fluids. When blood glucose is high, the body gets rid of glucose through urine, and this fluid needs to be replaced.

If nausea makes eating or taking oral diabetes drugs a problem, a doctor should be consulted. Not eating can increase the risk of low blood glucose, while stopping oral medications or insulin during illness can lead to very high blood glucose. A doctor may prescribe insulin temporarily for someone with diabetes who can't take medicine by mouth.

Great thirst, rapid weight loss, high fever, or very high urine or blood glucose are signs that blood sugar is out of control. If a person has these symptoms, a doctor should be called immediately.

Like illness, stress that results from losses or conflicts at home or on the job can affect diabetes control. Urine and blood glucose checks can be clues to the effects of stress. If someone finds that stress is making diabetes control difficult, a doctor can advise treatment and suggest sources of help.

Points to Remember

◆ Special situations such as pregnancy, surgery, and illness call for extra careful diabetes control.
◆ Special control may require the use of insulin, even in people who don't normally use insulin.

Dealing with Diabetes

Good diabetes care requires a daily effort to follow a diet, stay active, and take medicine when necessary. Talking to people who have diabetes or who treat diabetes may be helpful for someone who needs emotional support. The list of organizations at the back of this booklet can help patients find discussion groups or counselors familiar with diabetes. It's very important for people with diabetes to understand how to stay healthy, follow a proper diet, exercise, and be aware of changes in their bodies. People with diabetes can live long, healthy lives if they take care of themselves.

Points to Remember

- Good diabetes care is a daily responsibility.
- Local diabetes organizations offer programs so people with diabetes can share experiences and support.
- The good health care urged for people with diabetes is beneficial to anyone who wishes to stay healthy.

Finding Help

A person with diabetes is responsible for his or her daily care and a doctor is the best source of information on that care. A doctor in family practice or internal medicine can diagnose and treat diabetes, and may refer the patient to a doctor who specializes in treating diabetes. "Endocrinologists" and "diabetologists" are doctors with advanced training and experience in diabetes treatment. The local chapters of the American Diabetes Association or the Juvenile Diabetes Foundation have lists of doctors who specialize in diabetes. Another alternative is to contact a university-based medical center. These centers may have special diabetes clinics or may be able to suggest diabetes doctors who practice in the community.

Points to Remember

- Medical guidance is available from a variety of sources such as diabetes groups, local medical societies and hospitals, and diabetes clinics.

Printed Information

While information in books and magazines can't replace a doctor's personal advice, it can provide a clear explanation of diabetes and describe advancements in diabetes treatment. The American Diabetes Association and Juvenile Diabetes Foundation have brochures about diabetes and diabetes treatment. These publications are for people without a medical background. The addresses of these organizations are in the resources section at the back of this booklet.

Brochures and books about diabetes also are available from public libraries and bookstores. Local chapters of the American Diabetes Association, hospitals, and medical centers frequently sponsor educational programs on diabetes and diabetes treatment. Information about diabetes programs is also available from a doctor's office, a local hospital or health department, or a local diabetes organization.

Points to Remember

- Information on diabetes is available from local bookstores, libraries, and local diabetes programs and groups.

Resources on Diabetes

Agency for Health Care Policy and Research (AHCPR)
Medical Treatment Effectiveness Program
2101 East Jefferson Avenue
Rockville, MD 20852
(301) 227-8364—Division of Information and Publications

The agency supports grant and contract research on the relationship between the use of medical services and procedures and patient outcomes.

American Association of Diabetes Educators (AADE)
444 N. Michigan Avenue
Suite 1240
Chicago, IL 60611
(312) 644-2233 or 1-800-338-3633

The AADE is a multidisciplinary organization, with state and regional chapters, for health professionals involved in diabetes education. It sponsors continuing education programs on both beginning and advanced levels and a certification program for diabetes educators, and provides grants, scholarships, and awards for educational research and teaching activities. The AADE publishes a monthly journal, curriculum guides, consensus statements, self-study programs, and other resources for diabetes educators.

American Diabetes Association National Service Center
1660 Duke Street
P.O. Box 25757
Alexandria, VA 22313
(703) 549-1500 or 1-800-232-3472

A private, voluntary organization that fosters public awareness of diabetes and supports and promotes diabetes research. It publishes information on many aspects of diabetes, and local affiliates sponsor community programs. Local affiliates can be found in the telephone directory or through the national office.

American Dietetic Association
430 North Michigan Avenue
Chicago, IL 60611
(312) 822-0330

A professional organization that can help someone find a nutritionist in the community.

American Heart Association
7320 Greenville Avenue
Dallas, TX 75231
1-800-242-1793

A private, voluntary organization that has literature on heart disease and how to prevent it. Contact the local affiliate of the American Heart Association listed in telephone directories.

Centers for Disease Control (CDC) National Center for Chronic
Disease Prevention and Health Promotion
1600 Clifton Road
The Rodes Building
MS K-13
Atlanta, GA 30333
Technical Information Services Branch (404) 488-5080

The CDC is an agency of the federal government that has information on the surveillance and prevention of diabetes for health care professionals and people with diabetes.

Juvenile Diabetes Foundation International
432 Park Avenue, South
New York, NY 10016
(212) 889-7575 or 1-800-223-1138

A private, voluntary organization with an interest in type I or insulin-dependent diabetes. Local affiliates are found across the country. It also has information on noninsulin-dependent diabetes.

National Diabetes Information Clearinghouse
Box NDIC
Bethesda, MD 20892
(301) 468-2162

The National Diabetes Information Clearinghouse has a variety of publications for distribution to the public and to health professionals. The clearinghouse is a program of the National Institute of Diabetes and Digestive and Kidney Diseases, a component of the National Institutes of Health, leading the federal government's research on diabetes.

National Eye Health Education Program
National Eye Institute
National Institutes of Health
Box 20/20
Bethesda, MD 20892
(301) 496-5248

Information about how diabetes affects the eyes is available from the National Eye Institute, a component of the federal government's National Institutes of Health.

National Heart, Lung, and Blood Institute
Building 31, Room 4A21
National Institutes of Health
Bethesda, MD 20892
(301) 496-4236
    Information on heart disease is available from this component of the federal government's National Institutes of Health.

■ Document Source:
    U.S. Department of Health and Human Services, Public Health Service
    National Institutes of Health
    National Institute of Diabetes, and Digestive and Kidney Diseases
    NIH Publication No. 92-241
    September 1992

See also: Diabetes Overview (page 110); Diabetic Neuropathy: The Nerve Damage of Diabetes (page 328); Diabetic Retinopathy (page 144); Insulin-Dependent Diabetes (page 112)

CancerFax from the National Cancer Institute
THYROID CANCER

Description

What Is Cancer of the Thyroid?

Cancer of the thyroid is a disease in which cancer (malignant) cells are found in the tissues of the thyroid gland. Your thyroid gland is at the base of your throat. It has two lobes, one on the right side and one on the left. Your thyroid gland makes important hormones that help your body to function normally.

Cancer of the thyroid is more common in women than in men. Most patients are between 25 and 65 years old. People who have been exposed to large amounts of radiation, or who have had radiation treatment for medical problems in the head and neck have a higher chance of getting thyroid cancer. The cancer may not occur until 20 years or longer after radiation treatment.

Like most cancers, cancer of the thyroid is best treated when it is found (diagnosed) early. You should see your doctor if you have a lump or swelling in the front of your neck or in other parts of your neck.

If you have symptoms, your doctor will feel your thyroid and check for lumps in your neck. Your doctor may order blood tests and special scans to see whether a lump in your thyroid is making too many hormones. Your doctor may want to take a small amount of tissue from your thyroid. This is called a biopsy. To do this, a small needle is inserted into your thyroid at the base of your throat and some tissue is drawn out. The tissue is then looked at under a microscope to see whether it contains cancer.

There are four main types of cancer of the thyroid (based on how the cancer cells look under a microscope): papillary, follicular, medullary, and anaplastic. Your chance of recovery (prognosis) depends on the type of thyroid cancer you have, whether it is just in the thyroid or has spread to other parts of the body (stage), your age, and your overall health. Some types of thyroid cancer grow much faster than others.

Stage Explanation

Stages of Cancer of the Thyroid

Once cancer of the thyroid is found (diagnosed), more tests will be done to find out if cancer cells have spread to other parts of the body. This is called staging. Your doctor needs to know the stage of your disease to plan treatment.

The following stages are used for papillary cancers of the thyroid:

Stage I papillary
Cancer is only in one or both lobes of the thyroid.

Stage II papillary
Cancer has spread to lymph nodes around the thyroid (lymph nodes are small bean-shaped structures that are found throughout the body; they produce and store infection-fighting cells).

Stage III papillary
Cancer has spread outside the thyroid, but not outside of the neck.

Stage IV papillary
Cancer has spread to other parts of the body, such as the lungs and bones.

The following stages are used for follicular cancers of the thyroid:

Stage I follicular
Cancer is only in one or both lobes of the thyroid.

Stage II follicular
Cancer has spread to lymph nodes around the thyroid.

Stage III follicular
Cancer has spread outside the thyroid, but not outside of the neck.

Stage IV follicular
Cancer has spread to other parts of the body, such as the lungs and bones.

Other types or stages of thyroid cancer include the following:

Medullary
There is no staging system for medullary cancer of the thyroid.

Anaplastic
There is no staging system for anaplastic cancer of the thyroid. This type of cancer of the thyroid grows faster than the other types.

Recurrent
Recurrent disease means that the cancer has come back (recurred) after it has been treated. It may come back in the thyroid or in another part of the body.

Treatment Options Overview

How Cancer of the Thyroid Is Treated

There are treatments for all patients with cancer of the thyroid. Four types of treatment are used:

surgery (taking out the cancer)

radiation therapy (using high-dose x-rays or other high-energy rays to kill cancer cells)

hormone therapy (using hormones to stop cancer cells from growing)

chemotherapy (using drugs to kill cancer cells).

Surgery is the most common treatment for cancer of the thyroid. Your doctor may remove the cancer using one of the following operations:

♦ Lobectomy removes only the side of the thyroid where the cancer is found.

♦ Lymph nodes in the area may be taken out (biopsied) to see if they contain cancer.

♦ Near-total thyroidectomy removes all of the thyroid except for a small part.

♦ Total thyroidectomy removes the entire thyroid.

♦ Lymph node dissection removes lymph nodes in the neck that contain cancer.

Radiation therapy uses high-energy x-rays to kill cancer cells and shrink tumors. Radiation for cancer of the thyroid may come from a machine outside the body (external radiation therapy) or from drinking a liquid that contains radioactive iodine. Because the thyroid takes up iodine, the radioactive iodine collects in any thyroid tissue remaining in the body and kills the cancer cells.

Hormone therapy uses hormones to stop cancer cells from growing. In treating cancer of the thyroid, hormones can be used to stop the body from making other hormones that might make cancer cells grow. Hormones are usually given as pills.

Chemotherapy uses drugs to kill cancer cells. Chemotherapy may be taken by pill, or it may be put into the body by a needle in the vein or muscle. Chemotherapy is called a systemic treatment because the drug enters the bloodstream, travels through the body, and can kill cancer cells outside the thyroid.

Treatment by Stage

Treatment for cancer of the thyroid depends on the type and stage of your disease, your age, and your overall health.

You may receive treatment that is considered standard based on its effectiveness in a number of patients in past studies, or you may choose to go into a clinical trial. Not all patients are cured with standard therapy and some standard treatments may have more side effects than are desired. For these reasons, clinical trials are designed to find better ways to treat cancer patients and are based on the most up-to-date information. Clinical trials are going on in many parts of the country for some patients with cancer of the thyroid. If you want more information, call the Cancer Information Service at 1-800-4-CANCER (1-800-422-6237).

Treatment options: Stage I papillary thyroid cancer
Your treatment may be one of the following:
1. Surgery to remove one lobe of the thyroid (lobectomy), followed by hormone therapy. Radioactive iodine also may be given following surgery.
2. Surgery to remove almost all of the thyroid (near-total thyroidectomy).

Treatment options: Stage I follicular thyroid cancer
Your treatment may be one of the following:
1. Surgery to remove almost all of the thyroid (near-total thyroidectomy).
2. Surgery to remove one lobe of the thyroid (lobectomy), followed by hormone therapy. Radioactive iodine also may be given following surgery.

Treatment options: Stage II papillary thyroid cancer
Your treatment may be one of the following:
1. Surgery to remove one lobe of the thyroid (lobectomy) and lymph nodes that contain cancer, followed by hormone therapy. Radioactive iodine also may be given following surgery.
2. Surgery to remove almost all of the thyroid (near-total thyroidectomy) and lymph nodes that contain cancer.

Treatment options: Stage II follicular thyroid cancer
Your treatment may be one of the following:
1. Surgery to remove almost all of the thyroid (near-total thyroidectomy) and lymph nodes that contain cancer.
2. Surgery to remove one lobe of the thyroid (lobectomy) and lymph nodes that contain cancer, followed by hormone therapy. Radioactive iodine also may be given following surgery.

Treatment options: Stage III papillary thyroid cancer
Your treatment may be one of the following:
1. Surgery to remove the entire thyroid (total thyroidectomy) and tissues around the thyroid where the cancer has spread.
2. Total thyroidectomy followed by radiation therapy with radioactive iodine or external beam radiation therapy.

Treatment options: Stage III follicular thyroid cancer
Your treatment may be one of the following:
1. Surgery to remove the entire thyroid (total thyroidectomy) and tissues around the thyroid where the cancer has spread.
2. Total thyroidectomy followed by radioactive iodine or external beam radiation therapy.

Treatment options: Stage IV papillary thyroid cancer
Your treatment may be one of the following:
1. Radioactive iodine.
2. External beam radiation therapy.
3. Hormone therapy.
4. A clinical trial of chemotherapy.

Treatment options: Stage IV follicular thyroid cancer
Your treatment may be one of the following:
1. Radioactive iodine.
2. External beam radiation therapy.
3. Hormone therapy.
4. A clinical trial of chemotherapy.

Treatment options: Medullary thyroid cancer
Your treatment will probably be surgery to remove the entire thyroid (total thyoidectomy) and biopsy of the tissues around the thyroid to see if they contain cancer. If lymph nodes in the neck contain cancer, the lymph nodes in the neck will be

removed (lymph node dissection). If the cancer has spread to other parts of the body, chemotherapy may be given.

Treatment options: Anaplastic thyroid cancer
Your treatment may be one of the following:
1. Surgery to remove the thyroid and the tissues around it. Because this cancer often spreads very quickly to other tissues, your doctor may have to take out part of the tube through which you breath. Your doctor will then make an airway in the throat so you can breath. This is called a tracheostomy.
2. External beam radiation therapy or therapy with radioactive iodine.
3. Chemotherapy. Clinical trials are studying new drugs for thyroid cancer.

Treatment options: Recurrent thyroid cancer
Your choice of treatment depends on the type of thyroid cancer you have, the kind of treatment you had before, and where the cancer comes back. Your treatment may be one of the following:
1. External beam radiation therapy to relieve symptoms caused by the cancer.
2. Chemotherapy. Clinical trials are studying new drugs for thyroid cancer.

To learn more about cancer of the thyroid, call the National Cancer Institute's Cancer Information Service at 1-800-4-CANCER (1-800-422-6237). By dialing this toll-free number, you can speak with someone who can answer your questions.

■ **Document Source:**
National Cancer Institute
Building 31, Room 10A24, 9000 Rockville Pike, Bethesda, MD 20892
PDQ 208/01252
02/01/94

See also: Chemotherapy and You: A Guide to Self-Help During Treatment (page 40); Radiation Therapy: A Guide to Self-Help During Treatment (page 56); What Are Clinical Trials All About? A Booklet For Patients with Cancer, (page 68)

EAR, NOSE, AND THROAT DISORDERS

■ ■ ■

NIDCD Fact Sheet
ACOUSTIC NEURINOMA

An acoustic neurinoma is a benign tumor which may develop on the hearing and balance nerves near the inner ear. The tumor results from an overproduction of Schwann cells—small sheet-like cells that normally wrap around nerve fibers like onion skin and help support the nerves. When growth is abnormally excessive, Schwann cells bunch together, pressing against the hearing and balance nerves, often causing gradual hearing loss, tinnitus or ringing in the ears, and dizziness. If the tumor becomes large, it can interfere with the facial nerve, causing partial paralysis, and eventually press against nearby brain structures, becoming life-threatening.

Early diagnosis of an acoustic neurinoma is key to preventing its serious consequences. Unfortunately, early detection of the tumor is sometimes difficult because the symptoms may be subtle and may not appear in the beginning stages of growth. Also, hearing loss, dizziness, and tinnitus are common symptoms of many middle and inner ear problems. Therefore, once the symptoms appear, a thorough ear examination and hearing test are essential for proper diagnosis. Computerized tomography (CT) scans and magnetic resonance imaging (MRI) are helpful in determining the location and size of a tumor and also in planning its removal.

If an acoustic neurinoma is surgically removed when it is still very small, hearing may be preserved and accompanying symptoms may go away. As the tumor grows larger, surgical removal is often more complicated because the tumor may become firmly attached to the nerves that control facial movement, hearing and balance.

The removal of tumors attached to hearing, balance or facial nerves can make the patient's symptoms worse because sections of these nerves must also be removed with the tumor. As an alternative to conventional surgical techniques, radiosurgery may be used to reduce the size or limit the growth of the tumor. Radiosurgery, utilizing carefully focused radiation, is sometimes performed on the elderly, on patients with tumors on both hearing nerves, or on patients with a tumor growing on the nerve of their only hearing ear. If the tumor is not removed, MRI is used to carefully monitor its growth.

There are two types of acoustic neurinomas: unilateral and bilateral. Unilateral acoustic neurinomas affect only one ear and account for approximately 8 percent of all tumors inside the skull. Symptoms may develop at any age, but usually occur between the ages of 30 and 60 years.

Bilateral acoustic neurinomas, which affect both ears, are hereditary. Inherited from one's parents, this tumor results from a genetic disorder known as neurofibromatosis-2 (NF2). Affected individuals have a 50 percent chance of passing this disorder on to their children. Unlike those with a unilateral acoustic neurinoma, individuals with NF2 usually develop symptoms in their teens or early adulthood. Because NF2 patients usually have multiple tumors, the surgical procedure is more complicated than the removal of an unilateral acoustic neurinoma. Further research is needed to determine the best approach in these circumstances.

In addition to tumors arising from the hearing and balance nerves, NF2 patients may develop tumors on other cranial nerves associated with swallowing, speech, eye and facial movement and facial sensation. NF2 patients may also develop tumors within the spinal cord and from the brain's thin covering.

Scientists believe that both types of acoustic neurinoma form following a loss of the function of a gene on chromosome 22. A gene is a small section of DNA responsible for a particular trait like hair color or skin tone. Scientists believe that this particular gene on chromosome 22 suppresses the growth of Schwann cells. When this gene malfunctions, Schwann cells can grow out of control. Scientists also think that this gene may help suppress other types of tumor growth. In NF2 patients, the faulty gene on chromosome 22 is inherited. For individuals with unilateral acoustic neurinoma, however, some scientists hypothesize that this gene somehow loses its ability to function properly as a result of environmental factors.

Once the gene that suppresses Schwann cell growth is "mapped" or located, scientists can begin to develop gene therapy to control the overproduction of these cells in individuals with acoustic neurinoma. Also, learning more about the way genes help suppress acoustic neurinoma may help prevent brain tumors and lead to a treatment for cancer.

■ Document Source:
National Institutes of Health
National Institute on Deafness and Other Communication
  Disorders
December 1991

See also: Hereditary Deafness (page 188)

National Institute on Aging Age Page

HEARING AND OLDER PEOPLE

It is easy to take good hearing for granted. For people with hearing impairments, words in a conversation may be misunderstood, musical notes might be missed, and a ringing doorbell may go unanswered. Hearing impairment ranges from having difficulty understanding words or hearing certain sounds to total deafness.

Because of fear, misinformation, or vanity, some people will not admit to themselves or anyone else that they have a hearing problem. It has been estimated, however, that about 30 percent of adults age 65 through 74 and about 50 percent of those age 75 through 79 suffer some degree of hearing loss. In the United States alone, more than 10 million older people are hearing impaired.

If ignored and untreated, hearing problems can grow worse, hindering communication with others, limiting social activities, and reducing the choices of leisure time activities. People with hearing impairment often withdraw socially to avoid the frustration and embarrassment from not being able to understand what is being said. In addition, hearing-impaired people may become suspicious of relatives and friends who "mumble" or "don't speak up."

Hearing loss may cause an older person to be wrongly labeled as "confused," "unresponsive", or "uncooperative." At times a person's feeling of powerlessness and frustration in trying to communicate with others results in depression and withdrawal.

Older people today more often demand greater satisfaction from life, but those with hearing impairments can find the quality of their lives reduced. Fortunately, help is available in the form of treatment with medicines, special training, a hearing aid or an alternate listening device, and surgery.

Some Common Signs of Hearing Impairment

- Words are difficult to understand.
- Another person's speech sounds slurred or mumbled, worsening when there is background noise.
- Speech can be hard or impossible to understand, depending on the kind of hearing impairment.
- Certain sounds are overly loud or annoying.
- A hissing or ringing background noise may be heard constantly or the sound may be interrupted.
- TV shows, concerts, or social gatherings are less enjoyable because much goes unheard.

Diagnosis of Hearing Problems

If you have trouble hearing, see your doctor for treatment or a referral to an ear specialist. By ignoring the problem, you may be overlooking a serious medical condition. Hearing impairments may be caused by exposure to very loud noises over a long period of time, viral infections, vascular disorders (such as heart conditions or stroke), head injuries, tumors, heredity, certain medications, or age-related changes in the ear.

In some cases, the diagnosis and treatment of a hearing problem may take place in the family doctor's office. More complicated cases may require the help of specialists known as otologists, otolaryngologists, or otorhinolaryngologists—all of whom are trained to perform surgery on the head and neck. These specialists are doctors of medicine or doctors of osteopathy with extensive training in ear problems. They will take a medical history, ask about problems affecting family members, conduct a thorough exam, and order any needed tests.

An audiologist is another health professional who is trained to identify and measure hearing loss and to help with rehabilitation. However, audiologists do not prescribe drugs or perform surgery. To measure hearing they use a device that produces sounds of different pitches and loudness (an audiometer), as well as other electronic devices. These hearing measurements test a person's ability to understand speech. The tests are painless and can in a short time locate a hearing problem, allowing the doctor to recommend a course of treatment.

Types of Hearing Loss

Conductive hearing loss occurs in some older people. It involves the blocking of sounds that are carried from the ear drums (tympanic membrane) to the inner ear. This may be caused by ear wax in the ear canal, fluid in the middle ear, or abnormal bone growth or infection in the middle ear.

Sensorineural hearing loss involves damage to parts of the inner ear or auditory nerve. When sensorineural hearing loss occurs in older people, it is called presbycusis (pronounced prez-bee-KU-sis). Changes in the delicate workings of the inner ear lead to difficulties understanding speech and possibly an intolerance for loud sounds, but not total deafness. Thus, "don't shout—I'm not deaf!" is often said by older people with this type of hearing impairment.

Every year after age 50 we are likely to lose some of our hearing ability. The decline is so gradual that by age 60 or 70 as many as 25 percent of older people are noticeably hearing impaired. Just as the graying of hair occurs at different rates, presbycusis may develop differently from person to person.

Although presbycusis is usually attributed to aging, it does not affect everyone. In fact, some researchers view it as a disease. Environmental noise, certain medicines, improper diet, and genetic makeup may contribute to this disorder. The condition is permanent, but there is much a person can do to function well.

Central auditory dysfunction is a third type of hearing loss that occurs in older people, although it is quite rare even in this age group. It is caused by damage to the nerve centers within the brain. Sound levels are not affected, but understanding language usually is. The causes include extended illness with a high fever, head injuries, vascular problems, or tumors. A central auditory dysfunction cannot be treated medically or surgically; but for some, special training by an audiologist or speech pathologist can help.

Treatment

Examination and test results from the family doctor, ear specialist, and audiologist will determine the best treatment for a specific hearing problem. In some cases, medical treatment such as cleansing the ear canal to remove ear wax or surgery may restore some or all hearing ability.

At other times a hearing aid may be recommended. A hearing aid is a small device designed to make sounds louder. Before you can buy a hearing aid, you must either obtain a written statement from your doctor (saying that your hearing impairment has been medically evaluated and that you might benefit from hearing aid) or sign a waiver stating that you do not desire medical evaluation.

Many hearing aids are on the market, each offering different kinds of help for different problems. Professional advice is needed regarding the design, model, and brand of the hearing aid best for you. This advice, which is part of your hearing aid evaluation, is given by the audiologist who considers your hearing level, your understanding of speech in each ear, your ability to handle the aid and its controls and your concern about appearance and comfort.

Remember that you are buying a product and specific services, including any necessary adjustments, counseling in the use of the aid, maintenance, and repairs throughout the warranty period. Before deciding where to buy your aid, consider the quality of service as well as the quality of the product.

Buy an aid with only those features you need. The most costly hearing aid may not be the best for you while the one selling for less may offer more satisfaction. Also, be aware that the controls for many of the special features are tiny and may be difficult to adjust. Practice will make operating the aid easier. Your hearing aid dealer (usually called a "dispenser") should have the patience and skill to help you through the adjustment period. It is a good idea to take advantage of his or her help since it often takes at least a month to become comfortable with a new hearing aid.

People with certain types of hearing impairments may need special help. Speech-reading allows people to receive visual cues from lip movements as well as facial expressions, body posture and gestures, and the environment. Auditory training may include hearing aid orientation, but it is also designed to help hearing-impaired persons identify and better handle their specific communication problems. Both speech-reading and auditory training can reduce the handicapping effects of the hearing loss. If needed, counseling is also available so that people with hearing impairments can understand their communication abilities and limitations while maintaining a positive image.

If You Have Problems Hearing

If you suspect there may be a problem with your hearing, visit your doctor as soon as possible. Medicare will pay for the doctor's exam and hearing tests that are ordered by the doctor. Medicare will not pay for the hearing aid.

- Ask your doctor to explain the cause of your hearing problem and if you should see a specialist.
- Don't hesitate to ask people to repeat what they have just said.
- Try to reduce background noise (stereo, television, or radio).
- Tell people that you have a hearing problem and what they can do to make communication easier.

If You Know Someone with a Hearing Problem

- Speak at your normal rate, but not too rapidly. Do not overarticulate. This distorts the sounds of speech and makes visual clues more difficult. Shouting will not make the message any clearer and may distort it.
- Speak to the person at a distance of 3 to 6 feet. Position yourself near good light so that your lip movements, facial expressions, and gestures may be seen clearly. Wait until you are visible to the hearing-impaired person before speaking. Avoid chewing, eating, or covering your mouth while speaking.
- Never speak directly into the person's ear. This prevents the listener from making use of visual cues.
- If the listener does not understand what was said, rephrase the idea in short, simple sentences.
- Arrange living rooms or meeting rooms so that no one is more than 6 feet apart and all are completely visible. In meetings or group activities where there is a speaker presenting information, ask the speaker to use the public address system.
- Treat the hearing-impaired person with respect. Include the person in all discussions about him or her. This helps relieve the feelings of isolation common in hearing-impaired people.

For More Information

If you would like further information about hearing problems, contact the organizations listed below. Please be sure to state clearly what type of information you would like to receive.

The American Academy of Otolaryngology, Head and Neck Surgery, Inc., is a professional society of medical doctors specializing in diseases of the ear, nose, and throat. They can provide information on hearing, balance, and other disorders affecting the ear, nose, and throat. Write to One Prince Street, Alexandria, VA 22314.

The American Speech-Language-Hearing Association and the National Association of Hearing and Speech Action can both answer questions or mail information on hearing aids or hearing aids or loss and communication problems in older people. They can also provide a list of certified audiologists and speech language pathologists. Write to the American Speech-Language-Hearing Association at 10801 Rockville Pike, Dept. AP, Rockville, MD 20852; or call the National Association of Hearing & Speech Action at (800) 638-8255.

Self Help for Hard of Hearing People, Inc., is a national self-help organization for those who are hard of hearing. SHHH can help with information on coping with a hearing loss and new hearing aids and technology, and they publish the *Shhh Journal* bimonthly. Write to SHHH, 7800 Wisconsin Avenue, Bethesda, MD 20892.

The National Information Center on Deafness at Gallaudet University provides information on all areas related to deafness and hearing loss including educational programs, vocational training, sign language programs, law, technology, and barrier-free design. Write to the NICD, 800 Florida Avenue, NE., Washington, DC 20002.

The National Institute on Deafness and Other Communication Disorder at the National Institutes of Health provides information on research on hearing, balance, smell, taste, voice, speech, and language. Write to the NIDCD, Building 31, Room 1B62, Bethesda, MD 20892. Their National Information Clearinghouse also provides information to health professionals, patients, industry, and the public. Write to the NIDCD Clearinghouse, P.O. Box 37777, Washington, DC 20013-7777.

The National Institute on Aging offers information on a range of health issues that concern older people. Write to the NIA Information Center, P.O. Box 8057, Gaitherburg, MD 20898-8057.

■ **Document Source:**
U.S. Department of Health and Human Services, Public Health Service
National Institutes of Health
National Institute on Aging, National Institute on Deafness and Other Communication Disorders
1991

MENIERE'S DISEASE

What is Meniere's disease?

Meniere's disease is an abnormality of the inner ear causing a host of symptoms, including vertigo or severe dizziness, tinnitus or a roaring sound in the ears, fluctuating hearing loss, and the sensation of pressure or pain in the affected ear. The disorder usually affects only one ear and is a common cause of hearing loss. Named after French physician Prosper Meniere who first described the syndrome in 1861, Meniere's disease is now also referred to as endolymphatic hydrops.

What causes Meniere's disease?

The symptoms of Meniere's disease are associated with a change in fluid volume within a portion of the inner ear known as the labyrinth. The labyrinth has two parts: the bony labyrinth and the membranous labyrinth. The membranous labyrinth, which is encased by bone, is necessary for hearing and balance and is filled with a fluid called endolymph. When your head moves, endolymph moves, causing nerve receptors in the membranous labyrinth to send signals to the brain about the body's motion. An increase in endolymph, however, can cause the membranous labyrinth to balloon or dilate—a condition known as endolymphatic hydrops.

Many experts on Meniere's disease think that a rupture of the membranous labyrinth allows the endolymph to mix with perilymph, another inner ear fluid that occupies the space between the membranous labyrinth and the bony inner ear. This mixing, scientists believe, can cause the symptoms of Meniere's disease. Scientists are investigating several possible causes of the disease, including environmental factors, such as noise pollution and viral infections, as well as biological factors.

What are the symptoms of Meniere's disease?

The symptoms of Meniere's disease occur suddenly and can arise daily or as infrequently as once a year. Vertigo, often the most debilitating symptom of Meniere's disease, forces the sufferer to lie down. Vertigo attacks can lead to severe nausea, vomiting, and sweating and often come with little or no warning.

Some individuals with Meniere's disease have attacks that start with tinnitus, a loss of hearing, or a full feeling or pressure in the affected ear. It is important to remember that all of these symptoms are unpredictable. Typically, the attack is characterized by a combination of vertigo, tinnitus and hearing loss lasting several hours. But people experience these discomforts at varying frequencies, durations, and intensities. Some may feel slight vertigo a few times a year. Others may be occasionally disturbed by intense, uncontrollable tinnitus while sleeping. And other Meniere's disease sufferers may notice a hearing loss and feel unsteady all day long for prolonged periods. Other occasional symptoms of Meniere's disease include headaches, abdominal discomfort and diarrhea. A person's hearing tends to recover between attacks but over time becomes worse.

How is Meniere's disease treated?

There is no cure for Meniere's disease. Medical and behavioral therapy, however, are often helpful in managing its symptoms. Although many operations have been developed to reverse the disease process, their value has been difficult to establish. And, unfortunately, all operations on the ear carry risk of hearing loss.

The most commonly performed surgical treatment for Meniere's disease is the insertion of a shunt, a tiny silicone tube that is positioned in the inner ear to drain off excess fluid.

In another more reliable operation, a vestibular neurectomy, the vestibular nerve which serves balance is severed so that it no longer sends distorted messages to the brain. But the balance nerve is very close to the hearing and facial nerves. Thus, the risk of affecting a patient's hearing or facial muscle control increases with this type of surgical treatment. Also, older patients often have difficulty recovering from this type of surgery.

A labyrinthectomy, the removal of the membranous labyrinth, is an irreversible procedure that is often successful in eliminating the dizziness associated with Meniere's disease. This procedure, however, results in a total loss of hearing in the operated ear—an important consideration since the second ear may one day be affected. Also, labyrinthectomies themselves may result in other balance problems.

Some physicians recommend a change of diet to help control Meniere's symptoms. Eliminating caffeine, alcohol and salt may relieve the frequency and intensity of attacks in some people. Eliminating tobacco use and reducing stress levels may lessen the severity of the symptoms. And medications that either control allergies, reduce fluid retention or improve blood circulation in the inner ear may also help.

How is Meniere's disease diagnosed?

Scientists estimate that there are 3 to 5 million people in the United States with Meniere's disease, with nearly 100,000 new cases diagnosed each year. Proper diagnosis of Meniere's disease entails several procedures, including a medical history interview and a physical examination by a physician; hearing and balance tests; and medical imaging with magnetic resonance imaging (MRI). Accurate measurement and characterization of hearing loss are of critical importance in the diagnosis of Meniere's disease.

Through the use of several types of hearing tests, physicians can characterize hearing loss as being *sensory,* arising from the inner ear, or *neural,* arising from the hearing nerve. An auditory brain stem response, which measures electrical activity in the hearing nerve and brain stem, is useful in differentiating between these two types of hearing loss. And under certain circumstances, electrocochleography, recording the electrical activity of the inner ear in response to sound, helps confirm the diagnosis.

To test the vestibular or balance system, physicians irrigate the ears with warm and cool water. This flooding of the ears, known as caloric testing, results in nystagmus, rapid eye movements that can help a physician analyze a balance disorder. And because tumor growth can produce symptoms similar to Meniere's disease, magnetic resonance imaging is a useful test to determine whether a tumor is causing the patient's vertigo and hearing loss.

What research is being done?

Scientists are investigating environmental and biological factors that may cause Meniere's disease or induce an attack. They are also studying how fluid composition and movement in the labyrinth affect hearing and balance. And by studying hair cells in the inner ear, which are responsible for proper hearing and balance, scientists are learning how the ear converts the mechanical energy of sound waves and motion into nerve impulses. Insights into the mechanisms of Meniere's disease will enable scientists to develop preventive strategies and more effective treatment.

Where can I get more information?

The NIDCD currently supports research on Meniere's disease in medical centers and universities throughout the nation. For more information about Meniere's disease, you can contact:

American Academy of Otolaryngology-Head and Neck Surgery
One Prince Street
Alexandria, VA 22314
Telephone: (703) 836-4444

Deafness Research Foundation
9 East 38th Street
New York, NY 10016
Telephone: (212) 684-6556/(684-6559 TDD)

Ear Foundation
2000 Church Street, Box 111

Nashville, TN 37236
Telephone: (615) 329-7807/(329-7809 TDD)
(800) 545-HEAR

Vestibular Disorders Association
1015 N.W. 22nd Avenue
Portland, OR 97120
Telephone: (503) 229-7705

■ Document Source:
U.S. Department of Health and Human Services, Public Health Service
National Institutes of Health
National Institute on Deafness and Other Communication Disorders
NIH Publication No. 92-3403
January 1992

WHAT YOU NEED TO KNOW ABOUT CANCER OF THE LARYNX

Each year, more than 12,000 Americans find out they have cancer of the larynx. The National Cancer Institute (NCI) has prepared this booklet to help patients and their families and friends better understand this type of cancer. We also hope it will encourage all readers to learn more about this disease.

This booklet has information on the symptoms, diagnosis, and treatment of cancer of the larynx. Other NCI booklets about cancer, its treatment, and living with the disease are also listed. However, materials like these cannot answer every question or take the place of talks with doctors, nurses, and other members of the health care team. We hope our booklets will help with those talks.

Throughout this booklet, words that may be new to readers are printed in *italics.* Definitions of these and other terms related to cancer of the larynx are listed in the "Medical Terms" section. For some words, a "sounds-like" spelling is also given.

Knowledge about cancer of the larynx is increasing. Research is leading to better ways to treat this disease. For up-to-date information about cancer of the larynx and its treatment, call the NCI-supported Cancer Information Service (CIS) at 1-800-4-CANCER.

The Larynx

The larynx, also called the voice box, is a 2-inch-long, tube-shaped organ in the neck. We use the larynx when we breathe, talk, or swallow.

The larynx is at the top of the windpipe (*trachea*). Its walls are made of cartilage. The large cartilage that forms the front of the larynx is sometimes called the Adam's apple. The *vocal cords,* two bands of muscle, form a "V" inside the larynx.

Each time we inhale (breathe in), air goes into our nose or mouth, then through the larynx, down the trachea, and into our lungs. When we exhale (breathe out), the air goes the other way. When we breathe, the vocal cords are relaxed, and air moves through the space between them without making any sound.

When we talk, the vocal cords tighten up and move closer together. Air from the lungs is forced between them and makes them vibrate, producing the sound of our voice. The tongue, lips, and teeth form this sound into words.

The *esophagus,* a tube that carries food from the mouth to the stomach, is just behind the trachea and the larynx. The openings of the esophagus and the larynx are very close together in the throat. When we swallow, a flap called the *epiglottis* moves down over the larynx to keep food out of the windpipe.

What Is Cancer?

Cancer is a group of diseases that have one thing in common: cells become abnormal. These abnormal cells destroy body tissue and can spread to other parts of the body.

Cells make up all of the body's tissues. Healthy cells grow, divide, and replace themselves in an orderly way. This process keeps the body in good repair. If cells lose the ability to control their growth, they divide too often and without any order. They form too much tissue. The mass of extra tissue is called a *tumor.* Tumors can be *benign* or *malignant.*

- ♦ Benign tumors are not cancer. They do not spread to other parts of the body and are seldom a threat to life. Benign tumors can usually be removed, but certain types may return.
- ♦ Malignant tumors are cancer. They can invade and destroy nearby healthy tissues and organs. Cancer cells can also break away from the tumor and enter the bloodstream and the *lymphatic system.* That is how cancer spreads to other parts of the body. This spread is called *metastasis.*

Cancer of the larynx is also called *laryngeal* cancer. It can develop in any region of the larynx-the *glottis* (where the vocal cords are), the *supraglottis* (the area above the cords), or the *subglottis* (the area that connects the larynx to the trachea).

If the cancer spreads outside the larynx, it usually goes first to the *lymph nodes* (sometimes called lymph glands) in the neck. It can also spread to the back of the tongue, other parts of the throat and neck, the lungs, and sometimes other parts of the body.

Cancer that spreads is the same disease and has the same name as the original (primary) cancer. When cancer of the larynx spreads, it is called metastatic laryngeal cancer.

Symptoms

The symptoms of cancer of the larynx depend mainly on the size and location of the tumor. Most cancers of the larynx begin on the vocal cords. These tumors are seldom painful, but they almost always cause hoarseness or other changes in the voice. Tumors in the area above the vocal cords may cause a lump on the neck, a sore throat, or an earache. Tumors that begin in the area below the vocal cords are rare. They can make it hard to breathe, and breathing may be noisy.

A cough that doesn't go away or the feeling of a lump in the throat may also be warning signs of cancer of the larynx. As the tumor grows, it may cause pain, weight loss, bad breath, and frequent choking on food. In some cases, a tumor in the larynx can make it hard to swallow.

Any of these symptoms may be caused by cancer or by other, less serious problems. Only a doctor can tell for sure. People with symptoms like these usually see an ear, nose, and throat specialist (*otolaryngologist*).

Diagnosis

To find the cause of any of these symptoms, the doctor asks about the patient's personal and family medical history and does a complete physical exam. In addition to checking general signs of health, the doctor carefully feels the neck to check for lumps, swelling, tenderness, or other changes. The doctor can also look inside the larynx in two ways:

- ♦ Indirect *laryngoscopy.* The doctor looks down the throat with a small, long-handled mirror to check for abnormal areas and to see whether the vocal cords move as they should. This test is painless, but a local *anesthetic* may be sprayed in the throat to prevent gagging. This exam is done in the doctor's office.
- ♦ Direct laryngoscopy. The doctor inserts a lighted tube (*laryngoscope*) through the patient's nose or mouth. As the tube goes down the throat, the doctor can look at areas that cannot be seen with a simple mirror. A local anesthetic eases discomfort and prevents gagging. Patients may also be given a mild sedative to help them relax. Sometimes the doctor uses a general anesthetic to put the person to sleep. This exam may be done in an outpatient clinic, a hospital, or a doctor's office.

If the doctor sees abnormal areas, the patient will need to have a *biopsy.* A biopsy is the only sure way to know whether cancer is present. For a biopsy, the patient is given a local or general anesthetic, and the doctor removes tissue samples through a laryngoscope. A *pathologist* then examines the tissue under a microscope to check for cancer cells. If cancer is found, the pathologist can tell what type it is. Almost all cancers of the larynx are *squamous cell carcinomas.* This type of cancer begins in the flat, scale-like cells that line the epiglottis, vocal cords, and other parts of the larynx.

If the pathologist finds cancer, the patient's doctor needs to know the stage (extent) of the disease to plan the best treatment. To find out the size of the tumor and whether the cancer has spread, the doctor usually orders more tests, such as *x-rays,* a *CT (or CAT) scan,* and/or an *MRI scan.* During a CT scan, many x-rays are taken. A computer then puts them together to create detailed pictures of areas inside the body. An MRI scan produces pictures using a huge magnet linked to a computer.

Treatment Options

Treatment for cancer of the larynx depends on a number of factors. Among these are the exact location and size of the tumor and whether the cancer has spread. To develop a treatment plan to fit each patient's needs, the doctor also considers the person's age, general health, and feelings about the possible treatments.

The patient's doctor may want to discuss the case with other doctors who treat cancer of the larynx. Also, the patient may want to talk with the doctor about taking part in research studies of new treatment methods called *clinical trials.*

Many patients want to learn all they can about their disease and their treatment choices so they can take an active part in decisions about their medical care. The patient and the doctor should discuss the treatment choices very carefully because treatments for this disease may change the way a person looks and the way he or she breathes and talks. In many cases, the patient meets with both the doctor and a *speech pathologist* to talk about treatment options and possible changes in voice and appearance.

People with cancer of the larynx have many important questions. The doctor and other members of the health care team are the best ones to answer them. Most patients want to know the extent of their cancer, how it can be treated, how successful the treatment is expected to be, and how much it is likely to cost. These are some questions patients may want to ask the doctor:

♦ What are my treatment choices?
♦ Would a clinical trial be appropriate for me?
♦ What are the expected benefits of each kind of treatment?
♦ What are the risks and possible side effects of each treatment?
♦ How will I speak after treatment?
♦ How will I look?
♦ Will I need to change my normal activities? For how long?
♦ When will I be able to return to work?
♦ How often will I need to have checkups?

Many people find it helpful to make a list of their questions before they see the doctor. The doctor should be asked to explain anything that is not clear. Taking notes can make it easier to remember what the doctor says. Some patients also find it helps to have a family member or friend with them when they talk to the doctor, to take part in the discussion or just to listen.

Planning Treatment

Treatment decisions are complex. Before starting treatment, the patient might want a second doctor to review the diagnosis and treatment plan. A short delay will not reduce the chance that treatment will be successful. There are a number of ways to find a doctor for a second opinion:

♦ The patient's doctor may be able to suggest a doctor who has a special interest in cancer of the larynx.
♦ The Cancer Information Service, at 1-800-4-CANCER, can tell callers about cancer centers and other NCI-supported programs in their area.
♦ Patients can get the names of doctors from the local medical society, a nearby hospital, or a medical school.
♦ The *Directory of Medical Specialists* lists doctors' names and gives their background. It is in most public libraries.

Treatment Methods

Cancer of the larynx is usually treated with *radiation therapy* (also called radiotherapy) or *surgery*. These are types of local therapy; this means they affect cancer cells only in the treated area. Some patients may receive *chemotherapy,* which is called *systemic therapy,* meaning that drugs travel through the bloodstream. They can reach cancer cells all over the body. The doctor may use just one method or combine them, depending on the patient's needs.

In some cases, the patient is referred to doctors who specialize in different kinds of cancer treatment. Often several specialists work together as a team. The medical team may include a surgeon; ear, nose, and throat specialist; cancer specialist (*oncologist*); radiation oncologist; speech pathologist; nurse; and dietitian. A dentist may also be an important member of the team, especially for patients who will have radiation therapy.

Radiation therapy uses high-energy rays to damage cancer cells and stop them from growing. The rays are aimed at the tumor and the area close to it. Whenever possible, doctors suggest this type of treatment because it can destroy the tumor and the patient does not lose his or her voice. Radiation therapy may be combined with surgery; it can be used to shrink a large tumor before surgery or to destroy cancer cells that may remain in the area after surgery. Also, radiation therapy may be used for tumors that can't be removed with surgery or for patients who cannot have surgery for other reasons. If a tumor grows back after surgery, it is generally treated with radiation.

Radiation therapy is usually given 5 days a week for 5 to 6 weeks. At the end of that time, the tumor site very often gets an extra "boost" of radiation.

Surgery or surgery combined with radiation is suggested for some newly diagnosed patients. Also, surgery is the usual treatment if a tumor does not respond to radiation therapy or grows back after radiation therapy. When patients need surgery, the type of operation depends mainly on the size and exact location of the tumor.

If a tumor on the vocal cord is very small, the surgeon may use a *laser,* a powerful beam of light. The beam can remove the tumor in much the same way that a scalpel does.

Surgery to remove part or all of the larynx is a partial or total *laryngectomy.* In either operation, the surgeon performs a *tracheostomy,* creating an opening called a *stoma* in the front of the neck. (The stoma may be temporary or permanent.) Air enters and leaves the trachea and lungs through this opening. A *tracheostomy tube,* also called a trach ("trake") tube, keeps the new airway open.

A partial laryngectomy preserves the voice. The surgeon removes only part of the voice box—just one vocal cord, part of a cord, or just the epiglottis—and the stoma is temporary. After a brief recovery period, the trach tube is removed, and the stoma closes up. The patient can then breathe and talk in the usual way. In some cases, however, the voice may be hoarse or weak.

In a total laryngectomy, the whole voice box is removed, and the stoma is permanent. The patient, called a *laryngectomee,* breathes through the stoma. A laryngectomee must learn to talk in a new way.

If the doctor thinks that the cancer may have started to spread, an operation called a neck dissection may be done. The surgeon removes the lymph nodes in the neck and some of the tissue around them because these nodes are often the first place to which laryngeal cancer spreads.

Chemotherapy is the use of drugs to kill cancer cells. The doctor may suggest one drug or a combination of drugs. In some cases, anticancer drugs are given to shrink a large tumor before the patient has radiation therapy or surgery. Also, chemotherapy may be used for cancers that have spread.

Anticancer drugs for cancer of the larynx are usually given by injection into the bloodstream. Often the drugs are given in cycles—a treatment period followed by a rest period, then another treatment and rest period, and so on. Some patients have their chemotherapy in the outpatient part of the hospital, at the doctor's office, or at home. However, depending on the drugs, the treatment plan, and the patient's general health, a hospital stay may be needed. The NCI publication *Chemotherapy and You* has helpful information about this type of treatment and its possible side effects.

Treatment Studies

Researchers are looking for treatment methods that are more effective against cancer of the larynx and have fewer side effects. When laboratory research shows that a new method has promise, it is used to treat cancer patients in clinical trials. These trials are designed to answer scientific questions and to find out whether the new approach is both safe and effective. Patients who take part in clinical trials make an important contribution to medical science and may have the first chance to benefit from improved treatment methods.

Many clinical trials of new treatments for cancer of the larynx are under way. Doctors are studying new types and schedules of radiation therapy, new drugs, new drug combinations, and new ways of combining various types of treatment. Scientists are trying to increase the effectiveness of radiation therapy by giving treatments twice a day instead of once. Also, they are studying drugs called "radiosensitizers." These drugs make the cancer cells more sensitive to radiation.

People who have had cancer of the larynx have an increased risk of getting a new cancer in the larynx or in the lung, mouth, or throat. Doctors are looking for ways to prevent these new cancers. Some research has shown that a drug related to vitamin A may protect people from new cancers.

Patients interested in taking part in a trial should discuss this option with their doctor. *What Are Clinical Trials All About?* is an NCI booklet that explains some of the risks and possible benefits of treatment studies.

One way to learn about clinical trials is through PDQ, a computerized resource of cancer treatment information. Developed by NCI, PDQ contains an up-to-date list of trials in progress. Doctors can use a personal computer or the services of a medical library to get PDQ information. The Cancer Information Service, at 1-800-4-CANCER, is another source of PDQ information for doctors, patients, and the public.

Side Effects of Treatment

The methods used to treat cancer are very powerful. It is hard to limit the effects of therapy so that only cancer cells are removed or destroyed; healthy cells also may be damaged. That's why treatment often causes unpleasant side effects.

The side effects of cancer treatment vary. They depend mainly on the type and extent of the treatment. Also, each person reacts differently. Doctors try to plan the patient's therapy to keep problems to a minimum. Doctors, nurses, dietitians, and speech pathologists can explain the side effects of treatment and suggest ways to deal with them. It also may help to talk with another patient. In many cases, a social worker or another member of the medical team can arrange a visit with someone who has had the same treatment.

Radiation Therapy

During radiation therapy, healing after dental treatment may be a problem. That's why doctors want their patients to begin treatment with their teeth and gums as healthy as possible. They often recommend that patients have a complete dental exam and get any needed dental work done before the radiation therapy begins. It's also important to continue to see the dentist regularly because the mouth may be sensitive and easily irritated during cancer therapy.

In many cases, the mouth is tender during treatment, and some patients may get mouth sores. The doctor may suggest a special rinse to numb the mouth and reduce the discomfort.

Radiation to the larynx causes changes in the saliva and may reduce the amount of saliva. Because saliva normally protects the teeth, tooth decay can be a problem after treatment. Good mouth care can help keep the teeth and gums healthy and can make the patient feel more comfortable. Patients should do their best to keep their teeth clean. If it's hard to floss or brush the teeth in the usual way, patients can use gauze, a soft toothbrush, or a special toothbrush that has a spongy tip instead of bristles. A mouthwash made with diluted peroxide, salt water, and baking soda can keep the mouth fresh and help protect the teeth from decay. It also may be helpful to use a fluoride toothpaste and/or a fluoride rinse to reduce the risk of cavities. The dentist usually suggests a special fluoride program to keep the mouth healthy.

If reduced saliva makes the mouth uncomfortably dry, drinking plenty of liquids is helpful. Some patients use a special spray (artificial saliva) to relieve the dryness.

Patients who have radiation therapy instead of surgery do not have a stoma. They breathe and talk in the usual way, although the treatment can change the way their voice sounds. Also, the voice may be weak at the end of the day, and it is not unusual for the voice to be affected by changes in the weather. Voice changes and the feeling of a lump in the throat may come from swelling in the larynx caused by the radiation. The treatment can also cause a sore throat. The doctor may suggest medicine to reduce swelling or relieve pain.

During radiation therapy, patients may become very tired, especially in the later weeks. Resting as much as possible is important. It's also common for the skin in the treated area to become red or dry. The skin should be exposed to the air but protected from the sun, and patients should avoid wearing clothes that rub the area. During radiation therapy, hair usually does not grow in the treated area; if it does, men should not shave. Good skin care is important at this time. Patients will be shown how to keep the area clean, and they should not put anything on the skin before their radiation treatments. Also, they should not use any lotion or cream at other times without the doctor's advice.

Some patients complain that radiation therapy makes their tongue sensitive. They may lose their sense of taste or smell or may have a bitter taste in their mouth. Drinking plenty of liquids may lessen the bitter taste. Often, the doctor or nurse can suggest other ways to ease these problems. And it helps to keep in mind that, although the side effects of radiation therapy may not go away completely, most of them gradually become less troublesome and patients feel better when the treatment is over.

Surgery

Keeping the patient comfortable is an important part of routine hospital care. If pain occurs, it can be relieved with medicine. Patients should feel free to discuss pain control with the doctor.

For a few days after surgery, the patient isn't able to eat or drink. At first, an *intravenous (IV)* tube supplies fluids. Within a day or two, the digestive tract is getting back to normal, but the patient still cannot swallow because the throat has not healed. Fluids and nutrition are given through a feeding tube (put in place during surgery) that goes through the nose and throat to the stomach. As the swelling in the throat goes away and the area begins to heal, the feeding tube is removed. Swallowing may be difficult at first, and the patient may need the guidance of a nurse or speech pathologist. Little by little, the patient returns to a regular diet.

After the operation, the lungs and windpipe produce a great deal of mucus. To remove it, the nurse applies gentle suction with a small plastic tube placed in the stoma. Soon, the patient learns to cough and to suction mucus through the stoma without the nurse's help. For a short time, it may also be necessary to suction saliva from the mouth because swelling in the throat prevents swallowing.

Normally, air is moistened by the tissues of the nose and throat before it reaches the windpipe. After surgery, air enters the trachea directly through the stoma and cannot be moistened in the same way. In the hospital, patients are kept comfortable with a special device that adds moisture to the air.

For several days after a partial laryngectomy, the patient breathes through the stoma. Soon the trach tube is removed; within the next few weeks, the stoma closes. The patient then breathes and speaks in the usual way, although the voice may not sound exactly the same as before.

After a complete laryngectomy, the stoma is permanent. The patient breathes, coughs, and "sneezes" through the stoma and has to learn to talk in a new way. The trach tube stays in place for at least several weeks (until the skin around the stoma heals), and some people continue to use the tube all or part of the time. If the tube is removed, it is usually replaced by a smaller *tracheostomy button* (also called a stoma button). After a while, some laryngectomees get along without either a tube or a button.

After a laryngectomy, parts of the neck and throat may be numb because nerves have been cut. Also, following a neck dissection, the shoulder and neck may be weak and stiff.

Chemotherapy

The side effects of chemotherapy depend on the drugs that are given. In general, anticancer drugs affect rapidly growing cells, such as blood cells that fight infection, cells that line the digestive tract, and cells in *hair follicles*. As a result, patients may have side effects such as lower resistance to infection, loss of appetite, nausea, vomiting, or mouth sores. They may also have less energy and may lose their hair.

Effects of Treatment on Eating

Loss of appetite can be a problem for patients treated for laryngeal cancer. People may not feel hungry when they are uncomfortable or tired.

Patients who have had a laryngectomy may lose their interest in food because the operation changes the way things smell and taste. Radiation therapy also tends to affect the sense of taste. The side effects of chemotherapy can also make it hard to eat. Yet patients who eat well may be better able to withstand the side effects of their treatment, so good nutrition is important. Eating well means getting enough calories and protein to prevent weight loss, regain strength, and rebuild normal tissues.

After surgery, learning to swallow again may take some practice with the help of a nurse or speech pathologist. Some patients find liquids easier to swallow; others do better with solid foods. If eating is difficult because the mouth is dry from radiation therapy, patients may want to try soft, bland foods moistened with sauces or gravies. Others enjoy thick soups, puddings, and high-protein milkshakes. The nurse and the dietitian will help the patient choose the right kinds of food. Also, many patients find that eating several small meals and snacks during the day works better than trying to have three large meals. The NCI booklets *Radiation Therapy and You, Chemotherapy and You,* and *Eating Hints* suggest a variety of other ways to deal with eating problems.

Rehabilitation

Learning to live with the changes brought about by cancer of the larynx is a special challenge. Rehabilitation is a very important part of the treatment plan. The medical team makes every effort to help patients return to their normal activities as soon as possible.

Each laryngectomee must be able to care for the stoma. Before leaving the hospital, the patient learns to remove and clean the trach tube or stoma button, suction the trach, and care for the area around the stoma. The skin is less likely to become irritated if it is kept clean.

When shaving, men should keep in mind that the neck may be numb for several months after surgery. To avoid nicks and cuts, it may be best to use an electric shaver until normal feeling returns.

Most people continue to use a stoma cover after the area heals. Stoma covers—such as scarves, neckties, ascots, and special bibs—can be attractive as well as useful. They help keep moisture in and around the stoma. Also, laryngectomees may be sensitive to dust and smoke, and the cover filters the air that enters the stoma. The cover also catches any discharge from the windpipe when the person coughs or sneezes.

Whenever the air is too dry, as it may be in heated buildings in the winter, the tissues of the windpipe and lungs may react by producing extra mucus. Also, the skin around the stoma may get crusty and bleed. Using a humidifier at home or in the office can lessen these problems.

A person who has had a neck dissection may find that the neck is somewhat smaller. Also, the neck, shoulder, and arm may not be able to move as well as before. The doctor may advise physical therapy to help the person move more normally.

After surgery, laryngectomees work in almost every type of business and can do nearly all of the things they did before. However, they cannot hold their breath, so straining and heavy lifting may be difficult. Also, laryngectomees have to give up swimming and water skiing unless they have special instruction and equipment because it would be very dangerous for water to get into the windpipe and lungs through the stoma. Wearing a special plastic stoma shield or holding a washcloth over the stoma keeps water out when showering or shaving.

Learning to Speak Again

It's natural to be fearful and upset if the voice box must be removed. Talking is part of nearly everything we do, and losing the ability to talk—even temporarily—can be frightening. Patients and their families and friends need one another's understanding and support during this very difficult time.

Until patients learn to talk again, it's important for them to be able to communicate in other ways. In the beginning, everyone who has had a laryngectomy has to communicate by writing, gesturing, or pointing to pictures, words, or letters. Some people like to use a "magic slate" for writing notes. Others use pads of paper and pens or pencils. It's handy to have a supply of pads that fit easily in a pocket or purse. In addition, some patients use a typewriter or computer. Others carry a small dictionary or a picture book (sometimes called a picture dictionary) and point to the words they need. Patients may want to select some of these items before the operation.

Within a week or so after a partial laryngectomy, most people can talk in the usual way. After a total laryngectomy, patients must learn to speak in a new way. A speech pathologist usually meets with the patient before surgery to explain the methods that can be used. In many cases, speech lessons can begin before the person leaves the hospital.

Patients may try out various new ways of talking. One way is to use air forced into the esophagus to produce the new voice (*esophageal speech*). Or the voice can come from some type of mechanical larynx. Some people rely on a mechanical larynx only until they learn esophageal speech, some decide to use this device instead of esophageal speech, and some use both.

Even though esophageal speech may sound low-pitched and gruff, many people want to use this method instead of a mechanical larynx because it sounds more like regular speech. Also, there's nothing to carry around, and the person's hands are free. In most cases, a speech pathologist teaches the laryngectomee how to force air into the top of the esophagus and then push it out again. The puff of air is like a burp. It vibrates the walls of the throat, producing sound for the new

voice. The tongue, lips, and teeth from words as the sound passes through the mouth.

For some laryngectomees, air for esophageal speech comes through a *tracheoesophageal puncture*. The surgeon creates a small opening between the trachea and the esophagus. A plastic or silicone valve is inserted into this opening through the stoma. The valve keeps food out of the trachea.

When the stoma is covered, air from the lungs is forced into the esophagus through the valve. This air produces sound by making the walls of the throat vibrate. Words are formed in the mouth.

It takes practice and patience to learn esophageal speech, and not everyone is successful. How quickly a person learns, how natural the new voice sounds, and how understandable the speech is depend partly on the type and extent of the surgery. Other important factors are the patient's desire to learn and the help that's available. Patience and support from loved ones are important, too.

A mechanical larynx may be used until the person learns esophageal speech or if esophageal speech is too difficult. The device may be powered by batteries (*electrolarynx*) or by air (*pneumatic larynx*). The speech pathologist can help the patient choose a device and learn to use it.

One kind of electrolarynx looks like a small flashlight. It has a disk that makes a humming sound. The device is held against the neck, and the sound travels through the neck to the mouth. (This device may not be suitable for people who have had radiation therapy.) Another type of electrolarynx has a flexible plastic tube that carries sound to the person's mouth from a hand-held device.

A pneumatic larynx is held over the stoma and uses air from the lungs instead of batteries to make it vibrate. The sound it makes travels to the mouth through a plastic tube.

Followup Care

Regular followup is very important after treatment for cancer of the larynx.

The doctor will check closely to be sure that the cancer has not returned. Checkups include exams of the stoma, neck, and throat. From time to time, the doctor does a complete physical exam, blood and urine tests, and x-rays. People treated with radiation therapy or partial laryngectomy will have laryngoscopy.

People who have been treated for cancer of the larynx have a higher-than-average risk of developing a new cancer in the mouth, throat, or other areas of the head and neck. This is especially true for those who smoke. Most doctors strongly urge their patients to stop smoking to cut down the risk of a new cancer and to reduce other problems, such as coughing.

Living with Cancer

The diagnosis of cancer can change the lives of patients and the people who care about them. These changes can be hard to handle. It's natural for patients and their families and friends to have many different and sometimes confusing emotions.

At times, patients and their loved ones may feel frightened, angry, or depressed. These are normal reactions when people face a serious health problem. Most people handle their problems better if they can share their thoughts and feelings with those close to them. Sharing can help everyone feel more at ease and can open the way for people to show one another their concern and offer their support.

Worries about tests, treatments, hospital stays, learning to talk again, and medical bills are common. Doctors, nurses, speech pathologists, social workers, and other members of the health care team can help calm fears and ease confusion. They also can provide information and suggest resources.

Patients and their families are naturally concerned about what the future holds. Sometimes they use statistics to try to figure out the chance of being cured. It is important to remember, however, that statistics are averages based on large numbers of patients. They can't be used to predict what will happen to a certain patient because no two cancer patients are alike. Only the doctor who takes care of the patient knows enough about that person to discuss his or her outlook (*prognosis*).

People should feel free to ask the doctor about their prognosis, but not even the doctor knows for sure what will happen. Doctors may talk about surviving cancer, or they may use the term *remission* rather than cure. Even though many people with cancer of the larynx recover completely, doctors use these terms because the disease can recur.

Support for Cancer Patients

Living with a serious disease isn't easy. Cancer patients and those who care about them face many problems and challenges. Finding the strength to cope with these difficulties is easier when people have helpful information and support services.

People who have cancer of the larynx may have concerns about the future, family and social relationships, and finances. Sometimes they worry that changes in how they look and talk will affect the way people feel about them. They may worry about holding a job, caring for their family, or starting new friendships.

The doctor can explain the disease and give advice about treatment, going back to work, or limiting daily activities. It also may help to talk with a nurse, social worker, counselor, or member of the clergy, especially about feelings or other very personal matters.

Many patients find that it's useful to get to know other people who are facing problems like theirs. They can meet other cancer patients through self-help and support groups. Often, a social worker at the hospital or clinic can suggest local and national groups that can help with emotional support, rehabilitation, financial aid, transportation, or home care.

The American Cancer Society is one such group. This nonprofit organization has many services for patients and their families. Local offices of the American Cancer Society are listed in the white pages of the telephone book.

The International Association of Laryngectomees publishes educational materials and sponsors meetings and other activities for people who have lost their voice because of cancer. Many local laryngectomy clubs are members of this Association. For more information, patients may contact the national office, whose address and telephone number are on page 37. Information also is available from local American Cancer Society offices.

The public library is a good place to find books and articles on living with cancer. Cancer patients and their families can also find helpful suggestions in the NCI booklets *Taking Time* and *Facing Forward*.

Information about other programs and services is available through the Cancer Information Service. The toll-free number is 1-800-4-CANCER.

Cause and Prevention

Cancer of the larynx occurs most often in people over the age of 55. In the United States, it is four times more common in men than in women and is more common among black Americans than among whites. Scientists at hospitals and medical centers all across the country are studying this disease to learn more about what causes it and how to prevent it.

Doctors cannot explain why one person gets cancer of the larynx and another does not, but we are sure that no one can "catch" cancer from another person. Cancer is *not* contagious.

One known cause of cancer of the larynx is cigarette smoking. Smokers are far more likely than nonsmokers to develop this disease. The risk is even higher for smokers who drink alcohol heavily.

People who stop smoking can greatly reduce their risk of cancer of the larynx, as well as cancer of the lung, mouth, pancreas, bladder, and esophagus. Also, by quitting, those who have already had cancer of the larynx can cut down the risk of getting a second cancer of the larynx or a new cancer in another area. Special counseling or self-help groups are useful for some people who are trying to stop smoking. Some hospitals have groups for people who want to quit. Also, the Cancer Information Service and the American Cancer Society may have information about groups in local areas to help people quit smoking.

Working with asbestos can increase the risk of getting cancer of the larynx. Asbestos workers should follow work and safety rules to avoid inhaling asbestos fibers.

People who think they might be at risk for developing cancer of the larynx should discuss this concern with their doctor. The doctor may be able to suggest ways to reduce the risk and can suggest an appropriate schedule for checkups.

Medical Terms

Anesthetic (an-es-THET-ik). Drugs or gases given to cause a loss of feeling. A local anesthetic makes an area of the body numb. A general anesthetic puts the patient to sleep.

Benign (bee-NINE). Not cancer; does not spread to other parts of the body.

Biopsy (BY-op-see). The removal of a sample of tissue for examination under a microscope to check for cancer cells.

Cancer. A term for more than 100 diseases in which abnormal cells multiply without control. Cancer cells can spread through the bloodstream and lymphatic system to other parts of the body.

Carcinoma (Kar-sin-O-ma). Cancer that begins in the lining or covering of an organ.

Cartilage (KAR-ti-lij). Firm, rubbery tissue that cushions bones at joints. A more flexible kind of cartilage connects muscles with bones and makes up other parts of the body, such as the larynx and the outside parts of the ears.

Chemotherapy (Kee-mo-THER-a-pee). Treatment with anticancer drugs.

Clinical trials. Studies of new cancer treatments. Patients take part in studies designed to answer scientific questions and to find better treatments.

CT (or CAT) scan. An x-ray procedure that uses a computer to produce detailed pictures of areas inside the body.

Electrolarynx (e-LEK-tro-LAR-inks). A battery-operated instrument that makes a humming sound to help laryngectomees talk.

Epiglottis (ep-i-GLOT-is). The flap that covers the trachea during swallowing so that food does not enter the lungs.

Esophageal speech (e-SOF-a-JEE-al). Speech produced with air trapped in the esophagus and forced out again.

Esophagus (e-SOF-a-gus). The tube through which food passes from the throat to the stomach.

Glottis (GLOT-is). The middle part of the larynx; the area where the vocal cords are located.

Hair follicle (FOL-i-kul). A sac in the scalp from which a hair grows.

Humidifier (hyoo-MID-i-fy-er). A machine that puts moisture in the air.

Intravenous (IV) (in-tra-VEE-nus). Injected into a vein.

Laryngeal (la-RIN-jee-al). Having to do with the larynx.

Laryngectomee (lar-in-JEK-toe-mee). A person who has had his or her voice box removed.

Laryngectomy (lar-in-JEK-toe-mee). An operation to remove all or part of the larynx.

Laryngoscope (la-RING-go-skope). A flexible, lighted tube used to examine the larynx.

Laryngoscopy (la-ring-GOS-ko-pee). Examination of the larynx with a mirror (indirect laryngoscopy) or with a larvicides (direct laryngoscopy).

Larynx (LAR-inks). An organ in the throat used in breathing, swallowing, and talking. It is made of cartilage and muscle and is lined by a mucous membrane similar to the lining of the mouth. Also called the voice box. The larynx has three parts: the supraglottis, the glottis, and the subglottis.

Laser. A powerful beam of light used in some types of surgery.

Local therapy. Treatment that affects a tumor and the tissue near it.

Lymph (limf). The almost colorless fluid that travels through the lymphatic system and carries cells that help fight infection.

Lymph nodes. Small, bean-shaped organs located along the lymphatic system. Nodes filter bacteria or cancer cells from lymph. Also called lymph glands.

Lymphatic system (lim-FAT-ik). The tissues and organs that produce, store, and carry cells that fight infection. This system includes the bone marrow, spleen, thymus, lymph nodes, and vessels that carry lymph.

Malignant (ma-LIG-nant). Cancerous; can spread to other parts of the body.

Metastasis (me-TAS-ta-sis). The spread of cancer from one part of the body to another. Cells in the metastatic (second) tumor are like those in the primary (original) tumor.

MRI scan. A test that uses a magnet linked to a computer to create pictures of areas inside the body. Also called magnetic resonance imaging.

Oncologist (on-KOL-o-jist). A doctor who specializes in treating cancer.

Otolaryngologist (O-toe-lar-in-GOL-o-jist). A doctor who specializes in treating diseases of the ear, nose, and throat.

Pathologist (path-OL-o-jist). A doctor who identifies diseases by studying cells and tissues under a microscope.

Pneumatic larynx (noo-MAT-ik). A device that uses air to produce sound to help a laryngectomee talk.

Prognosis (prog-NO-sis). The probable outcome or course of a disease; the chance of recovery

Radiation therapy (ray-dee-AY-shun THER-a-pee). Treatment with high-energy rays from x-rays or other sources to kill cancer cells.

Remission (ree-MISH-un). Disappearance of the signs and symptoms of cancer. When this happens, the disease is said to be "in remission." A remission can be temporary or permanent.

Risk factor. Something that increases a person's chance of getting a particular type of cancer.

Speech pathologist. A specialist who evaluates and treats people with communication and swallowing problems. Also called a speech therapist.

Sputum (SPEW-tum). Mucus that comes from the throat and lungs.

Squamous cell carcinoma (SKWAY-mus). Cancer that begins in the flat, scale-like cells in the skin and in tissues that line certain organs of the body, including the larynx.

Staging. Doing exams and tests to learn the extent of the cancer, especially whether it has spread from its original site to other parts of the body.

Stoma (STOW-ma). An opening made by a surgeon. An opening into the windpipe is also called a tracheostomy. People who have had their larynx removed must breathe through this opening.

Subglottis (SUB-glot-is). The lowest part of the larynx; the area from just below the vocal cords down to the top of the trachea.

Supraglottis (SOOP-ra-GLOT-is). The upper part of the larynx, including the epiglottis; the area above the vocal cords.

Surgery. An operation.

Systemic therapy. Treatment that reaches and affects cells all over the body.

Tissue (TISH-oo). A group or layer of cells that performs a specific function.

Trachea (TRAY-kee-a). The airway that connects the larynx to the lungs. Also called the windpipe.

Tracheoesophageal puncture (TRAY-kee-o-es-OF-a-JEE-al PUNK-chur). A small opening made by a surgeon between the esophagus and the trachea. A valve keeps food out of the trachea but lets air into the esophagus for esophageal speech.

Tracheostomy (TRAY-kee-OS-toe-mee). Surgery to create an opening (stoma) into the windpipe. The opening itself may also be called a tracheostomy.

Tracheostomy button (TRAY-kee-OS-toe-mee). A 1/2- to 1-1/2-inch-long plastic tube placed in the stoma to keep it open.

Tracheostomy tube (TRAY-kee-OS-toe-mee). A 2- to 3-inch metal or plastic tube that keeps the stoma and trachea open. Also called a trach ("trake") tube.

Tumor. An abnormal mass of tissue.

Vocal cords. Two small bands of muscle within the larynx. They close to prevent food from getting into the lungs, and they vibrate to produce the voice.

X-ray. High-energy radiation. It is used in low doses to diagnose diseases and in high doses to treat cancer.

Resources

Information about cancer is available from many sources. Several are listed below. You also may wish to check your local library or contact support groups in your community.

Cancer Information Service (CIS)
1-800-4-CANCER

The Cancer Information Service, a program of the National Cancer Institute, includes a telephone service for cancer patients and their families and friends, the public, and health care professionals. The staff can answer questions and can send booklets about cancer. They also may know about local resources and services. One toll-free number, 1-800-4-CANCER, connects callers all over the country to the office that serves their area. Spanish-speaking staff members are available.

American Cancer Society (ACS)
1599 Clifton Road, N.E.
Atlanta, GA 30329
1-800-ACS-2345

The American Cancer Society is a voluntary organization with a national office (at the above address) and local units all over the country. It supports research, conducts educational programs, and offers many services to patients and their families. To obtain information about services and activities in local areas, including clubs for laryngectomees, call the society's toll-free number, 1-800-ACS-2345, or the number listed under "American Cancer Society" in the white pages of the telephone book.

International Association of Laryngectomees (IAL)
1599 Clifton Road, N.E.
Atlanta, GA 30329
1-800-ACS-2345

The International Association of Laryngectomees is sponsored by the American Cancer Society. The Association supplies printed information and sponsors meetings and other activities. It publishes a directory of speech instructors and maintains a list of sources of supplies for laryngectomees. Most Lost Chord Clubs, New Voice Clubs, and other clubs for laryngectomees are members of this organization and are listed in its directory. Information about clubs is available from the American Cancer Society.

American Speech-Language-Hearing Association (ASHA)
Consumer Division
10801 Rockville Pike
Rockville, MD 20852
1-800-638-TALK
301-897-5700 (calls from Maryland)

The American Speech-Language-Hearing Association is a professional association. Its Consumer Division provides information on all types of communication problems and can refer patients to speech therapy programs.

The National Coalition for Cancer Survivorship (NCCS)
Suite 300
1010 Wayne Avenue
Silver Spring, MD 20910
301-585-2616

The National Coalition for Cancer Survivorship is a volunteer group concerned with issues faced by people with cancer and people who have recovered from cancer. It deals with legal, financial, emotional, and social matters. This group can advise people about their rights related to jobs and insurance. It has a speakers bureau and can supply printed information, including lists of cancer support groups in many areas.

For Further Information

Cancer patients, their families and friends, and others may find the following booklets useful. They are available free of charge by calling 1-800-4-CANCER or writing:

Office of Cancer Communications
National Cancer Institute
Building 31, Room 10A24
Bethesda, MD 20892

Booklets About Cancer Treatment

- *Chemotherapy and You: A Guide to Self-Help During Treatment*
- *Radiation Therapy and You: A Guide to Self-Help During Treatment*
- *Eating Hints: Recipes and Tips for Better Nutrition During Cancer Treatment*
- *What Are Clinical Trials All About?*

Booklets About Living with Cancer

- *Taking Time: Support for People With Cancer and the People Who Care About Them*
- *Facing Forward: A Guide for Cancer Survivors*
- *When Someone in Your Family Has Cancer*
- *When Cancer Recurs: Meeting the Challenge Again*
- *Advanced Cancer: Living Each Day*

■ **Document Source:**
U.S. Department of Health and Human Services, Public Health Service
National Institutes of Health
National Cancer Institute
NIH Publication No. 92-1568
Revised July 1991. Printed March 1992

See also: Chemotherapy and You: A Guide to Self-Help During Treatment (page 40); Radiation Therapy: A Guide to Self-Help During Treatment (page 56); What Are Clinical Trials All About? A Booklet for Patients with Cancer (page 68)

EYE DISORDERS

■ ■ ■

AGE-RELATED MACULAR DEGENERATION

What is age-related macular degeneration?

Age-related macular degeneration (AMD) is an eye disease that is present to at least a mild degree in millions of older Americans. It is a leading cause of visual loss in this country.

AMD affects the macula, a small portion of the retina. The retina is the light-sensing nerve tissue that lines the inside of the eye. All parts of the retina contribute to sight, but only the macula can provide the sharp, straight-ahead vision that is needed for driving and reading small print.

As a person ages, harmful changes may occur in this small but important area of the retina, causing difficulties in reading and other tasks that require good central vision. Scientists do not know why these macular changes occur. But aging evidently plays a major role in the process. That is why it is known as age-related, or senile, macular degeneration.

Do people with age-related macular degeneration usually go blind?

No. Although AMD is a leading cause of visual loss, it is important to know that the majority of people with AMD continue to have almost normal vision throughout their lives. Even those who are severely affected do not lose all their sight, but retain enough to move about independently and make use of helpful devices called low vision aids. And for a limited number of people who develop a rapidly worsening form of AMD that seriously endangers vision, there is a sight-saving treatment developed through research.

Who gets age-related macular degeneration?

Usually, AMD does not develop until a person is 65 or older. But a few people are affected by the disease while still in their forties or fifties.

A person's chances of developing AMD are greater than average if he or she has a near relative with the disease. Scientists are now trying to learn what other factors might place a person at risk for AMD.

What are the signs and symptoms of age-related macular degeneration?

Most people with AMD have a form of the disease that develops very slowly. It is called the "dry" form. In it, tiny yellowish deposits called drusen develop beneath the macula. Also, the layer of light-sensitive cells in the macula becomes thinner as some cells break down. These changes typically cause a dimming or distortion of vision that people find most noticeable when they try to read.

Generally, if one eye has dry AMD, the other eye will also have some signs of the condition. Thus the person with dry AMD may eventually have visual problems in both eyes. However, the dry form of AMD rarely causes total loss of reading vision.

A much greater threat of visual loss arises when the dry form of AMD gives way to the "wet" or neovascular form of the disease.

This condition arises in a small percentage of AMD patients. In it, new blood vessels grow beneath the macula. These abnormal vessels leak fluid and blood, causing the light-sensitive cells near them to sicken and die. This process generally produces marked disturbance of vision in the affected eye: Straight lines look wavy, and later there may be blank spots in the field of vision.

If the leakage and bleeding from new vessels continues, much of the nerve tissue in the macula may be killed or injured within a period of a few weeks or months. Such damage cannot be repaired, because the nerve cells of the macula do not grow back once they have been destroyed.

Although only a small percentage of people with AMD develop the neovascular form, they make up the vast majority of those who experience serious visual loss from AMD.

What treatment is available for people who have new blood vessels from AMD?

A few years ago, a nationwide clinical study supported by the National Eye Institute (NEI) found that there is a treatment that can help most people whose sight is threatened by the wet or neovascular form of AMD. This treatment is called laser photocoagulation. In it, powerful light rays from a laser are directed into the eye and focused at a tiny spot on the macula. The aim of the laser treatment is to preserve vision by destroying abnormal blood vessels.

In the NEI-supported study, laser treatment reduced the risk of severe vision loss by more than half in people with neovascular AMD. However, this treatment is best applied soon after the new blood vessels develop, before they have reached and damaged the fovea—the central part of the macula.

Can everyone with AMD benefit from laser treatment?

No. Laser photocoagulation is of value only to the relatively few people who have the neovascular form of AMD, with new blood vessels actively growing in the macula and threatening to cause serious vision loss. There is no evidence that laser treatment is of any value for people with the dry form of AMD. Also, because the laser cannot restore vision already lost from AMD, an eye whose macula has been badly damaged by this disease would not benefit from laser treatment. That is why it is so important for AMD—and neovascular AMD in particular—to be detected early.

How does a person know whether AMD is present, and whether treatment is needed?

Drusen and the other macular changes typical of dry AMD cannot be seen by the person who has them, but are visible to an eye care specialist examining the eye. Anyone who is middle-aged or older should visit an eye care specialist regularly to be checked for early signs of AMD, glaucoma, and other eye diseases that are linked to aging.

Generally, when dry AMD is found, the patient is encouraged to return for further check-ups. Also, he or she may be taught to perform a simple, at-home test for visual changes. The test involves looking at a piece of paper marked with a grid of straight lines. If some of the lines begin to look curved or are not visible at all, this may be a valuable warning that new blood vessels are developing and laser treatment should be considered. Patients who use the grid are asked to look at it regularly and tell the doctor right away if they notice any changes in its appearance.

If it is suspected that neovascular AMD is developing, a procedure called fluorescein angiography is generally performed. In this procedure, a dye called fluorescein is injected into the arm. Photographs are taken to show the movement of the dye as it reaches the eye and passes through the blood vessels of the retina. If there are new vessels leaking fluid or blood in the macula, the photographs will show their exact location, and serve as a guide for treatment.

How is laser treatment performed?

Laser treatment is performed by a specially trained ophthalmologist in his office or in an eye clinic at a medical center. A local anesthetic may be used to prevent discomfort during the laser treatment session. The session generally takes only a few minutes. Soon afterwards, the patient is able to return home and continue his or her normal activities.

The patient usually will be asked to return to the doctor's office for follow-up appointments. If additional growth of new blood vessels is found, further laser treatment may be indicated. Between follow-up visits, the patient can use the home test described above to detect any visual changes that might signal renewed blood vessel growth.

Is there any way to prevent AMD?

At present, there is no proven method of preventing dry AMD or the onset of the neovascular form of the disease. Discovering effective means of prevention is a major goal of the National Eye Institute, the United States Government agency that conducts and supports research on the eye and visual disorders. NEI-supported scientists are now seeking the underlying causes of AMD, in hopes of finding some way to halt the disease in its early stages or eventually prevent it altogether. Also, a study is underway at the NEI to evaluate possible long-term protective measures that might someday be of value in reducing the risk of visual loss from AMD.

In addition, research on the treatment of neovascular AMD is continuing. A relatively new device called the krypton laser is being tested in people with neovascular AMD, especially those who have new blood vessels very close to the center of the macula.

What help is available to the person who has already lost vision from AMD?

There are many useful devices that can help a partially sighted person to make the most of his or her remaining vision. Called low vision aids, these devices have special lenses or electronic systems that produce enlarged images of nearby objects.

If you need low vision aids, your eye care specialist can generally prescribe them. Often, he or she will be able to suggest further sources you might contact to get information about counseling, training and other special services for people with low vision. Through such sources as a nearby school of medicine or optometry, or a local volunteer group devoted to helping the visually handicapped, you can learn a great deal about low vision programs in your area. It may help you to know that many organizations "for the blind" also serve people with low vision.

■ Document Source:
  U.S. Department of Health and Human Services, Public Health Service
  National Institutes of Health
  National Eye Institute
  Building 31, Room 6A32, Bethesda, MD 20892. (301) 496-5248
  NIH Publication No. 89-2294

CATARACTS

What is a cataract?

A cataract is a cloudy or opaque area in the lens of the eye. The lens is located behind the pupil and iris. It helps focus light onto the retina, the light-sensitive tissue that lines the inside of the back of the eye. Usually, the lens is transparent. But if it becomes clouded, the passage of light is obstructed and vision may be impaired.

What causes a cataract?

When a cataract forms, there is a change in the chemical composition of the lens, but scientists do not know exactly what causes these chemical changes. The most common form of cataract is related to aging, although this type can occur at age 50 or even earlier. Cataracts also may be associated with diabetes, other systemic diseases, drugs, and eye injuries. Sometimes babies are born with congenital cataracts or develop them during the early years of life.

What are the symptoms of a cataract?

Cataracts usually develop gradually, without pain, redness, or tearing in the eye. Some cataracts never progress to the point where they seriously impair vision, whereas others eventually block most or all vision in the affected eye. The effect of a cataract on vision depends on several things: 1) its size, 2) its density, 3) its location within the lens.

Among the signs that a cataract may be forming are:

- ♦ Hazy, fuzzy, or blurred vision. Double vision sometimes occurs, but this usually goes away as the cataract worsens.
- ♦ The need for frequent changes in eyeglass prescriptions. When the cataract progresses beyond a certain point, these changes no longer improve vision.
- ♦ A feeling of having a film over the eyes, or of looking through veils or a waterfall. The person with a cataract may blink a lot in an effort to see better.
- ♦ Changes in the color of the pupil, which is usually black. When the eye is examined, the pupil may look grey, yellow, or white, but color changes are not always noticeable.
- ♦ Problems with light. For example, night driving becomes harder because the cloudy part of the lens scatters the light from oncoming headlights, making these lights appear double or dazzling. Also, the person with a cataract may have trouble finding the right amount of light for reading or close work.
- ♦ "Second sight"—a temporary improvement in reading vision experienced by some people when their cataract reaches a certain stage of development. As the cataract progresses, vision again worsens.

None of these symptoms necessarily means that a person has a cataract, or if a cataract is present that it must be removed. However, people who have any of these symptoms should see an eye doctor.

When should a cataract be removed?

A cataract should be removed surgically when it has progressed to the point where resulting vision problems interfere with one's daily activities. A second reason for cataract surgery, more urgent but less common than the first, is that the cataract has become completely opaque (mature). It is possible for a mature cataract to swell and even disintegrate inside the eye. Such changes can permanently endanger vision.

With congenital cataracts, it used to be standard practice to postpone surgery until the child was at least 6 months old. Recently, however, cataracts have been removed from the eyes of newborn infants with good results. Early removal of severe congenital cataract(s) is an important advance because it reduces the risk of visual loss resulting from the disuse of one or both eyes during childhood.

How are cataracts treated?

Treating cataracts really involves two steps. The first is removal of the clouded lens by an ophthalmologist. Surgery is the only method proven effective for removing cataracts. The second is finding an appropriate substitute for the natural lens. The decision about which substitute lens to use is usually made before surgery.

There are two general methods of removing a cataract: intracapsular and extracapsular extraction of the lens. Intracapsular extraction is sometimes used to remove senile cataracts. In this method, the entire lens, including its capsule, is removed.

Extracapsular extraction involves removal of most lens tissue but the back part of the lens capsule is left in place. In infants and young children, whose lenses are relatively soft, the lens tissue may be withdrawn through a hollow needle, a procedure called aspiration. A variety of extracapsular techniques are also used to remove the lens in adults.

One technique is called phacoemulsification. High-frequency sound vibrations (ultrasound) are used to soften and liquefy the lens so it can be aspirated through the needle.

Phacoemulsification should not be confused with another form of eye surgery, photocoagulation, in which laser light—not ultrasound—is used to treat some eye disorders other than cataract. A laser cannot remove a cloudy lens or make it clear again. However, some doctors may use a laser to open the front part of the lens capsule before removing the lens or to help patients who develop "after-cataract." (See "What happens after surgery?")

How safe is cataract surgery?

Cataract surgery is one of the most successful operations done today—more than 90 percent of the people who have this surgery find that they can see better. Complications may occur, but most are treatable. Serious complications that threaten vision are rare.

Certain people may not benefit much from cataract surgery. They include people whose cataracts are not advanced enough to impair vision seriously and those whose vision is impaired by another eye disease as well.

In summary, each cataract patient should discuss the possibility of surgery with the doctor who examines his or her eyes to determine whether the potential benefits of cataract surgery outweigh the risks. It is also very important to decide in advance, with the help of the doctor, what form of substitute lens would be most suitable. Patients may want to get a second opinion on the appropriate substitute lens to use after surgery.

What are the choices for a substitute lens?

There are three options for replacing the natural lens removed in cataract surgery: eyeglasses, contact lenses, or an intraocular lens implant. Each has advantages and drawbacks.

Eyeglasses

This is a safe and time-proven solution to the problem of seeing without a natural lens. But cataract eyeglasses can have some unpleasant effects. Patients may be bothered by the fact that these glasses magnify objects 20-35 percent, affect depth perception until the person relearns how to judge distances, and limit side vision.

If only one eye requires cataract surgery, eyeglasses may well cause problems because the person is unable to fuse the different-sized images formed by the operated and unoperated eyes. Such patients are often advised before surgery that it would be best to use a contact lens, or have a lens implant.

Contact lenses

These usually provide better vision than eyeglasses and also are quite safe if handled and maintained properly. A contact lens may be especially helpful after cataract extraction in one eye. With a contact lens in the operated eye, the difference in the size of the images seen by the two eyes is much smaller. Soft contact lenses are commonly used for cataract patients.

Another option is the extended-wear contact lens. These lenses can be left in the eye for a longer period of time without being removed, even for sleep. They may be especially useful for people who have trouble inserting and removing a contact lens, because an eye care specialist can remove and clean them periodically. However, extended-wear lenses have some disadvantages: They are very fragile; some serious infections have been reported; their long-term safety is still being assessed; and they do require periodic removal, cleaning, and reinserting.

Intraocular lenses

These devices, sometimes called IOLs, are clear plastic lenses that are implanted in the eye during the cataract operation. Lens implants have certain advantages: They usually eliminate or minimize the problems with image size, side vision, and depth perception noted by people who wear cataract eyeglasses. Also, because lens implants remain in the eye and do not have to be removed, cleaned, and reinserted, they are more convenient than contact lenses. This is particularly true for people who have physical problems that would make it difficult for them to carry out the procedures involved in using contact lenses.

Because of these advantages, lens implants have been used with increasing frequency in recent years. About three-fourths of all people now undergoing cataract surgery have an IOL inserted at the same time, and the vast majority are very pleased with the results. Of course ophthalmologists will con-

tinue to study IOLs for many years in an effort to assess the long-term effects of implantation on the eye as well as the short-term complications.

What happens after surgery?

Most people who undergo cataract surgery are treated as outpatients and can go home the same day. For others, a stay in the hospital of 1-3 days may be required. In either case, during the early stages of recovery, patients need to take special care to avoid strenuous physical activity.

Sometimes people whose cataract surgery was performed by the extracapsular method develop a problem called "after-cataract." After the operation, the back part of the lens capsule left in the eye may become cloudy and interfere with passage of light to the retina.

The cloudy material must be cleared away, if possible, so that full vision can be restored. Ophthalmologists often treat after-cataract with an ophthalmic laser called the neodymium-YAG or "cold" laser. When this procedure is successful, the patient's vision is restored without additional eye surgery.

What research is being done on cataracts?

The National Eye Institute supports and conducts research on the eye and its disorders, including cataracts. The major goals of this research are to learn more about how and why cataracts develop, to find ways of preventing cataracts or slowing their progress, to evaluate the safety and effectiveness of techniques for treating cataracts, and to devise better methods of correcting vision after cataract surgery.

■ **Document Source:**
U.S. Department of Health and Human Services, Public Health Service
National Institutes of Health
National Eye Institute
Building 31, Room 6A32, Bethesda, MD 20892. (301) 496-5248
NIH Publication No. 93-201

DIABETIC RETINOPATHY

Why is it important to know how diabetes affects the eyes?

If you are among the 10 million people in the United States who have diabetes—or if someone close to you has this disease—you should know that diabetes can affect the eyes and cause visual impairment.

Fortunately, there are ways to prevent or lessen the eye damage caused by diabetes. That is why it is so important for people with this disease to have a professional eye examination as soon as their diabetes is diagnosed, and at least once a year thereafter.

Regular eye examinations are especially important for people who have had diabetes 5 years or longer, for those who have difficulty controlling the level of sugar in their blood, and for diabetic women who are pregnant. All of these people are at increased risk for diabetes-associated eye problems.

What is diabetic retinopathy?

Diabetic retinopathy is a potentially serious eye disease caused by diabetes. It affects the retina—the light-sensitive tissue at the back of the eye that transmits visual messages to the brain. Damage to this delicate tissue may result in visual impairment or blindness.

Diabetic retinopathy begins with a slight deterioration in the small blood vessels of the retina. Portions of the vessel walls balloon outward and fluid starts to leak from the vessels into the surrounding retinal tissue. Generally, these initial changes in the retina cause no visual symptoms. However, they can be detected by an eye specialist who is trained to recognize subtle signs of retinal disease.

In many people with diabetic retinopathy, the disease remains mild and never causes visual problems. But in some individuals, continued leakage from the retinal blood vessels leads to *macular edema*. This is a build-up of fluid in the macula—the part of the retina responsible for the sharp, clear vision used in reading and driving. When critical areas of the macula become swollen with excess fluid, vision may be so badly blurred that these activities become difficult or impossible.

Some people with diabetes develop an even more sight-threatening condition called *proliferative retinopathy*. It may occur in people who have macular edema, but also can develop in those who don't. In proliferative retinopathy, abnormal new blood vessels grow on the surface of the retina. These fragile new vessels can easily rupture and bleed into the middle of the eye, blocking vision. Scar tissue also may form near the retina, ultimately detaching it from the back of the eye. Severe visual loss, even permanent blindness, may result. But this happens in only a small minority of people with diabetes.

How many diabetics are affected?

Approximately 40 percent of all people with diabetes have at least mild signs of diabetic retinopathy. About 3 percent have suffered severe visual loss because of this disease.

In general, the longer one has had diabetes, the greater one's chances of developing diabetic retinopathy.

What are the symptoms of diabetic retinopathy?

As already indicated, diabetic retinopathy generally causes no symptoms in its earliest stages. For the person who develops macular edema, blurring of vision may provide a clue that something is wrong. But proliferative retinopathy can progress a long way without any warning signs. That is why a person with diabetes should make regular visits to an eye specialist, so any eye problems can be detected and treated if necessary.

How is diabetic retinopathy treated?

Recently, scientists have found that laser treatment can prevent visual loss in many people with diabetic macular edema. In this treatment, called photocoagulation, powerful beams of light from a laser are aimed at leaking retinal blood vessels in the macula. The goal of treatment is to seal the vessels and prevent further leakage. In many patients, this treatment halts the decline in vision or even reverses it.

Research also has shown that laser photocoagulation can dramatically reduce the risk of blindness in people who have proliferative retinopathy. For these patients, the laser is used in a different way: it is not directed at the macula but is aimed at hundreds of spots in other parts of the retina. The purpose of the treatment is to destroy diseased tissue and stop the retinopathy from getting worse. In fact, the treatment can reduce the risk of severe visual loss by 60 percent.

The studies which proved the value of laser treatment for people with diabetic retinopathy were supported by the National Eye Institute. It is part of the National Institutes of Health, a component of the U.S. Department of Health and Human Services.

These studies also have helped ophthalmologists determine which diabetic patients need laser treatment and when to begin it.

Who should have laser treatment?

An ophthalmologist (a medical doctor who specializes in the care of eye conditions) usually will consider laser treatment when a person with diabetes has proliferative retinopathy or retinal signs that suggest this condition may soon develop. Also, people with a significant degree of macular edema would now be considered for laser treatment.

When deciding whether to recommend laser treatment to a particular patient, the ophthalmologist weighs the potential benefits—preventing or delaying severe visual loss—against the risk of unwanted side effects. These may include some loss of central or side vision.

Unfortunately, laser treatment cannot restore sight to the person who has already suffered severe retinal damage from diabetic retinopathy. Also, the laser generally is not used when bleeding inside the eye has made it difficult or impossible for the ophthalmologist to see the areas that need treatment.

What is vitrectomy?

A few diabetic retinopathy patients—including some who have had photocoagulation—go blind from massive bleeding inside the eye. Now, ophthalmologists can remove the blood and scar tissue from the center of the eye. This procedure is known as vitrectomy.

Following vitrectomy, patients can often see well enough to move around on their own. Occasionally, vision in the operated eye recovers enough for the patient to resume reading or driving.

What research is being done on diabetic retinopathy?

The National Eye Institute is supporting a nationwide study to determine whether photocoagulation—used alone or in combination with aspirin—can benefit people who are still in the early stages of diabetic retinopathy. Almost 4,000 patients are enrolled in this 5-year clinical trial. It already has proven the value of photocoagulation for macular edema (see "How is diabetic retinopathy treated?"), and is expected to yield further valuable findings in the future.

Another clinical trial sponsored by the Institute and Pfizer, Inc., is evaluating a new drug called sorbinil to see if it can prevent eye and nerve damage in people with diabetes.

In addition to these clinical trials, the Institute is supporting an extensive program of research on the causes, detection, and treatment of diabetic retinopathy.

Who can refer you to an eye care specialist?

If you know you have diabetes, you are probably under the care of a physician who can refer you to an eye doctor for regular examinations and treatment, if needed. You may also request the name of an appropriate eye doctor from eye care centers affiliated with academic institutions, from a hospital, or from a diabetes clinic at a medical center.

You may obtain information on diabetes from the American Diabetes Association, 1660 Duke Street, Alexandria, Virginia 22314, telephone (703) 549-1500; and the Juvenile Diabetes Foundation, 432 Park Avenue South, 16th Floor, New York, New York 10016, telephone (212) 889-7575. Check your local telephone directory for their affiliates or chapters near you.

What help is available to the person who has already lost vision from diabetic retinopathy?

There are many useful devices that can help a partially sighted person to make the most of his or her remaining vision. Called low vision aids, these devices have special lenses or electronic systems that produce enlarged images of nearby objects.

If you need low vision aids, your eye care specialist can generally prescribe them. Often, he or she will be able to suggest further sources you might contact to get information about counseling, training and other special services for people with low vision. These may include a nearby school of medicine or optometry.

■ **Document Source:**
U.S. Department of Health and Human Services, Public Health Service
National Institutes of Health
National Eye Institute
Building 31, Room 6A32, Bethesda, MD 20892. (301) 496-5248.
NIH Publication No. 93-2171

See also: Diabetes Overview (page 110)

GLAUCOMA

Why you should know the facts about glaucoma

You may be among the two million adult Americans who have glaucoma. If you have this eye disease, you need treatment to prevent loss of vision. Although glaucoma cannot be cured, it can be controlled if detected and treated early.

Unfortunately, people who have glaucoma may not be aware that something is wrong with their eyes until it is too late to prevent visual impairment and even blindness. To guard against visual loss from glaucoma, people should have regular eye examinations—so their eye specialist can look for signs of this disease and determine if treatment is needed.

Regular eye check-ups are particularly important for people whose risk of glaucoma is higher than average. This includes black people, who are more likely than whites to develop glaucoma. It also includes everyone over 40, because glaucoma usually begins in middle age or later. Scientists do not yet know why aging makes a person more susceptible to glaucoma, but it is clear that the risk rises in the later decades of life. Also, there is an increased risk of glaucoma in people with diabetes or high blood pressure, and in those with a family history of glaucoma.

This brochure is mainly about the most common kind of glaucoma, which is called *open-angle glaucoma*. Other kinds of glaucoma are described briefly. In the back of the brochure, you will find out where to go for more information on glaucoma.

What is open-angle glaucoma?

In open-angle glaucoma, gradual changes within the eye lead to an internal fluid pressure that is high enough to damage delicate structures essential to vision. These changes occur in several stages:

♦ Fluid pressure inside the eye (*intraocular pressure*) begins to rise. This happens because the fluid that normally fills the inside of the eyeball flows in at the usual rate but drains too slowly. This fluid, called *aqueous humor*, is a clear liquid made continuously by cells inside the eye. Aqueous helps maintain the shape of the eyeball and bathes and nourishes the lens and cornea, transparent tissues located near the front of the eye. Aqueous leaves the eye through a spongy meshwork of tissue located at the "angle" where the cornea and iris meet.

When aqueous cannot exit fast enough, intraocular pressure rises. Why this happens is not known for certain, although scientists think the problem relates to changes in the drainage meshwork that are triggered by aging and by other factors that are still not understood. Although someone who has high intraocular pressure usually cannot feel it, an eye care specialist can detect and measure it with an instrument called a *tonometer*.

◆ Higher than normal intraocular pressure begins to destroy the tiny, delicate nerve fibers that make up the *optic nerve* at the back of the eye. Because the optic nerve relays visual messages from the eye to the brain—where seeing actually takes place—the health of this nerve is essential to sight.

Under prolonged high pressure, the optic nerve deteriorates and the patient's field of vision gradually gets narrower. Surprisingly, most people don't notice these changes until there is extensive loss of side vision.

◆ If optic nerve damage is not halted, glaucoma leads to tunnel vision and blindness. This can happen in just a few years. Glaucoma-induced vision loss is permanent and cannot be restored by treatment.

Therefore, to be fully effective, treatment must begin before there is serious damage to the optic nerve. That is why early detection is critical, for an eye specialist can detect what the glaucoma patient cannot: abnormalities of the optic nerve and subtle changes in the visual field. It is these key diagnostic signs, rather than elevated pressure, that indicate the presence of glaucoma. Although glaucoma is not contagious, if one eye is affected, the other eye will almost certainly develop the condition.

How is open-angle glaucoma controlled?

The goal of treating open-angle glaucoma is to preserve vision by lowering intraocular pressure and preventing optic nerve damage. Here are some facts about the main forms of treatment in use today:

◆ Drugs for open-angle glaucoma are the most widely used method of treating this disease. These medications are taken as eyedrops or pills. Some improve fluid drainage, while others lower pressure by inhibiting fluid formation. Most cases of glaucoma can be controlled with one or more medications, and a majority of patients tolerate these drugs well.

However, in a few patients intraocular pressure is not adequately controlled by medications. Also, some people find that the drugs' side effects—such as stinging in the eye, blurred vision, or headaches—do not go away after the first few weeks of use but continue to be a problem. The patient may have trouble adhering to the prescribed dosage schedule and may be tempted to stop taking the medication or cut back on the dosage. In this situation, the patient should contact his or her eye doctor to discuss the problem and the best means of dealing with it. Changing the treatment plan without proper medical advice may allow intraocular pressure to rise again, and the patient may suffer needless visual loss as a result.

So, in spite of the fact that glaucoma can be controlled by medications in a majority of patients, other forms of treatment also play an important role in glaucoma therapy. These are described below:

◆ Conventional surgical techniques are intended to help fluid escape from the eye, and thus reduce pressure.

Thirty years ago, before glaucoma drugs were available, surgery was the only effective treatment for glaucoma.

Now ophthalmologists generally reserve surgery for patients whose glaucoma cannot be controlled by medications for those who are unable to tolerate the side effects of these drugs. During the operation, the surgeon makes an opening to create a new drainage pathway so that aqueous can leave the eye more easily. After surgery, a few patients still need to use medication to keep their pressure under control and avoid loss of vision. And if the new drainage opening closes, a second operation may be needed.

◆ Argon laser surgery is an innovation in glaucoma treatment. The laser, a device that produces a high-energy beam of light, is used to make about 100 small burns in the drainage meshwork at the edge of the iris. Scientists think that the scars from these burns help stretch open the holes in the meshwork, making it easier for fluid to filter out. Laser surgery can be done in an ophthalmologist's office in a relatively short time. Usually, people who have this surgery must continue taking some glaucoma medication afterwards, although they may be able to lower the dosage and still keep intraocular pressure under control. However, the pressure-lowering effect of the laser treatment may wear off eventually, and for this reason patients sometimes have a second or third treatment session.

What is medical science doing about open-angle glaucoma?

In the United States, most research on glaucoma is supported by the National Eye Institute (NEI). It is part of the National Institutes of Health, a component of the U.S. Department of Health and Human Services.

The NEI is supporting a wide range of studies to learn more about the causes of glaucoma and improve its detection and treatment.

One major study now underway will further evaluate argon laser surgery for open-angle glaucoma. This nationwide study, called the Glaucoma Laser Trial, is for people whose glaucoma was recently diagnosed. Its goal is to learn whether early laser treatment offers any advantages over treatment with medications alone. Another goal is to learn what disadvantages or risks may be associated with the new laser treatment. Findings from this research will help doctors determine the best approach to preserving the vision of people with open-angle glaucoma.

Clinical research on glaucoma drugs is aimed at improving their effectiveness, safety, and ease of use, and reducing their unpleasant side effects. Some scientists are searching for new—and better—drugs, while others are experimenting with new ways of delivering drugs to the eye.

Researchers are also studying different types of lasers, as well as ultrasonic devices, for treating open-angle glaucoma that does not respond to drugs or conventional surgery. In one study they are trying to find a way to improve the effectiveness of conventional glaucoma surgery. In addition, investigators are developing new diagnostic devices to improve the early detection of glaucoma, so that doctors will be better able to determine which patients need therapy.

Eye researchers are also trying to find out why black Americans appear to be particularly susceptible to open-angle glaucoma. In fact, some studies have suggested that the risk of glaucoma-induced blindness is several times higher for blacks than for whites. Scientists are attempting to identify the factors that might account for this difference. Their research is expected to yield important information that will lead to better ways of protecting black people from glaucoma.

Information that will help to improve glaucoma treatment is also expected to emerge from basic research on the eye. Such work includes studies of the changes that occur in the eyes as it ages and the factors controlling production and drainage of aqueous humor.

What is glaucoma screening?

Many civic groups, hospitals, and community health centers in the United States offer glaucoma screening in an effort to identify people who are at high risk for glaucoma but don't know it. In screening programs, a health worker tests both eyes for increased pressure, using a tonometer. Tonometers may worry some people because part of the instrument touches the eye, but eyedrops can be used to numb the eye and the procedure is quick and painless. Some programs use non-contact tonometers which do not touch the eye, but instead measure the resistance to a puff of air blown at the eyeball.

The person who is found to have high intraocular pressure in a screening test is generally urged to make arrangements for a more thorough eye examination soon. This is because screening by tonometry can detect elevated intraocular pressure, but cannot reveal whether this condition has affected the optic nerve or side vision. To check for those key signs and thus learn whether glaucoma is present, doctors must examine the optic nerve and the field of vision. Intraocular pressure will be checked again to determine whether it is still elevated or whether it has dropped back to normal since the screening test. At the end of a complete eye examination, some people will learn that they have glaucoma and need treatment. Others will get the welcome news that they don't have the disease.

It is important to remember, however, that "passing" a screening test for glaucoma does not necessarily mean that you have no eye problems. Some cases of glaucoma are missed by screening, and other eye diseases may go undetected as well. So people who appear problem-free on the screening test should continue to have regular, thorough eye examinations to safeguard their visual health.

What is ocular hypertension?

Occasionally, eye examinations reveal that the pressure within one or both eyes is above normal, but the optic nerve and visual field are all right. This condition is called *ocular hypertension*. A person who has it is at risk of developing glaucoma; the higher the pressure, the greater the risk. If ocular hypertension is diagnosed, the eye care specialist will be able to advise whether it is better to begin treatment to lower the intraocular pressure right away, or whether it is preferable to wait, have

regular eye check-ups, and consider treatment only if definite signs of open-angle glaucoma appear.

What are the other forms of glaucoma?

- ◆ In *low-tension glaucoma*, optic nerve damage and restricted side vision occur unexpectedly in a person with normal intraocular pressure. The treatments used for this condition are the ones described in the section headed "How is open-angle glaucoma controlled?"
- ◆ In some people, an anatomical peculiarity of the eye, often inherited, makes the angle between the iris and cornea unusually narrow and easily closed off. This narrow angle can retard fluid drainage, causing numerous episodes of high pressure—a condition called *chronic narrow-angle glaucoma*. If the narrow angle closes suddenly and completely, fluid backs up fast and eye pressure goes up rapidly. This event, called *acute narrow-angle glaucoma* or *angle-closure glaucoma*, is a medical emergency. It causes severe pain and nausea as well as redness of the eye and blurred vision. Unless the patient has treatment to improve the flow of fluid, the eye can become blind in as little as one or two days. Generally, surgery is needed to restore outflow of aqueous and prevent further angle-closure attacks. Lasers have been very helpful as an alternative to conventional surgery for treating narrow-angle glaucoma.
- ◆ Some infants are born with defects in the angle of the eye that slow the normal drainage of aqueous. This relatively rare *congenital glaucoma* is easily recognized in affected infants, who have cloudy eyes, are sensitive to light, and tear excessively. Surgery is usually indicated and can prevent loss of vision if it is done soon enough.
- ◆ Glaucoma can also develop as a complication of other medical conditions. These *secondary glaucomas* are sometimes associated with eye surgery or with advanced cataracts, eye injuries, some kinds of eye tumors, or uveitis (eye inflammations). A severe form of glaucoma, called neovascular glaucoma, is linked to diabetes. Also, corticosteroid drugs—used to treat eye inflammations and a variety of other diseases—can trigger glaucoma in a few people.

How can people learn more about glaucoma?

If you are in one of the groups at special risk for glaucoma, as described in the first section of this pamphlet, you should ask your doctor about this disease. He or she can test your eyes for high intraocular pressure or refer you to an eye specialist for glaucoma tests. If you are older than age 40, you should have your eyes checked for glaucoma every two to three years.

For more information on glaucoma, check your public library, or a medical library if you live near a hospital or medical school. Also, you may wish to contact these organizations:

American Academy of Ophthalmology
655 Beach Street
P.O. Box 7424
San Francisco, California 94120-7424
(415) 561-8500

American Optometric Association
243 Lindbergh Boulevard
St. Louis, Missouri 63141
(314) 991-4100

American Foundation for the Blind
15 West 16th Street
New York, New York 10011
(212) 620-2000

National Society to Prevent Blindness
500 East Remington Road

Schaumburg, Illinois 60173
(312) 843-2020

■ **Document Source:**
U.S. Department of Health and Human Services, Public Health Service
National Institutes of Health
National Eye Institute
Building 31, Room 6A32, Bethesda, MD 20892. (301) 496-5248.
NIH Publication No. 91-651

GASTROINTESTINAL SYSTEM DISORDERS

■ ■ ■

DD Clearinghouse Fact Sheet

BLEEDING IN THE DIGESTIVE TRACT

by Paul Sherlock, M.D.

What is bleeding in the digestive tract?

Bleeding in the digestive tract is a symptom of digestive problems rather than a disease itself. Bleeding can occur as the result of a number of different conditions, many of which are not life-threatening. Most causes of bleeding are related to conditions that can be cured or controlled, for example, hemorrhoids. And in some cases, eating certain foods can give the appearance of bleeding. The cause may not be serious, but it is important to rule out other possibilities.

When doctors talk about the digestive tract, they mean the esophagus, stomach, small intestine, large intestine or colon, rectum, and anus. Bleeding can come from one or more of these areas, i.e., from a small area such as an ulcer on the lining of the small intestine or from a large surface such as an inflammation of the lining of the colon. Bleeding can sometimes occur without your being able to notice it. This type of bleeding is called "occult" or hidden. Fortunately, there are simple tests for detecting occult blood in the stool.

How common is bleeding in the digestive tract?

It is difficult to estimate the incidence of bleeding in the digestive tract. If bleeding hemorrhoids or "piles" are included, it is extremely common. Significant numbers of patients who bleed from the gastrointestinal tract have been found through the use of new methods to test the stool for occult blood. Many patients have abnormalities in the gastrointestinal tract, such as ulcer disease of polyps, that can cause bleeding. Most patients with cancer involving the gastrointestinal tract will bleed either occultly or visibly at some time during the course of their illness.

What are the causes of bleeding in the digestive tract?

There are many causes for bleeding in the digestive tract. The most common is probably hemorrhoids. Hemorrhoids are enlarged veins in the anal area that can rupture and produce bright red blood that shows up in the toilet or on toilet paper. If red blood is seen, however, it is essential to rule out other causes of bleeding. The anal area may also be the site of "cuts" (fissures) in the lining, inflammation, or tumors.

Bleeding can come from an inflammation at the *lower end of the esophagus* caused by acid or bile. This condition is called "esophagitis" or inflammation of the esophagus. Sometimes a weak muscle at the junction of the esophagus and stomach can lead to esophagitis. Enlarged veins (varices) at the lower end of the esophagus may rupture and bleed massively. Cirrhosis of the liver is the most common cause of varices.

The *stomach* is a common site of bleeding. Alcohol, aspirin, aspirin-containing compounds, and various drugs (particularly those used for arthritis) can cause individual ulcers or diffuse inflammation (gastritis). The stomach is often the site of ulcer disease. Acute or chronic ulcers may enlarge and eat through a blood vessel, causing massive bleeding. Also, patients suffering from burns, shock, head injuries, or cancer, or those who have undergone extensive surgery, may develop "stress ulcers." Bleeding can occur from benign tumors or cancer, although these disorders do not usually cause massive bleeding.

The small intestine is not a common source of bleeding, except for ulcers in the duodenum. In adults, the most common cause of bleeding from the small intestine, other than duodenal ulcers, is Crohn's disease. This disorder results in an inflammation of the bowel wall.

The large intestine (colon) and rectum are common sites of bleeding. Benign growths or polyps of the colon are very common and are thought to be forerunners of cancer. These growths can cause either bright red blood or occult bleeding. Colorectal cancer is the second most common of all cancers in the United States and usually causes bleeding at some time. Inflammation from many causes can produce extensive bleeding from the colon. Various types of intestinal infections can cause inflammation and bloody diarrhea. Ulcerative colitis can produce extensive surface bleeding from very tiny ulcerations. Crohn's disease of the large intestine can produce spotty bleeding. Diverticula—outpouches of the colon wall—can result, rarely, in massive bleeding. Finally, as one gets older, abnormalities may develop in the blood vessels of the large intestine and those may result in recurrent bleeding.

Are there genetic or lifestyle factors leading to bleeding in the digestive tract?

A variety of genetic disorders may be responsible for bleeding in the digestive tract. Certain types of cancers may tend to run in families. Some benign growths that involve the small and large intestines, such as those seen in familial polyposis, are clearly hereditary. Also, hereditary blood vessel disorders may lead to frequent bleeding in the gastrointestinal tract. Finally, there are inherited blotting disorders, such as hemophilia, that can cause bleeding anywhere in the body, with the digestive tract being a common site.

A host of lifestyle factors are thought to contribute to diseases of the digestive tract that can lead to bleeding. Alcohol, drugs, infectious agents, and stress have already been identified. Research indicates that certain dietary patterns may contribute to disorders such as diverticulosis of the colon. Tobacco and coffee may interfere with the healing responsible for bleeding. Much more research is needed, however, before the relationship between diet and disease can be established.

What are the most common causes of bleeding in the digestive tract?

Esophagus

- Inflammation (esophagitis)
- Enlarged veins (varices)

Stomach

- Ulcers
- Inflammation (gastritis)

Small Intestine

- Duodenal ulcer
- Crohn's disease

Large Intestine and Rectum

- Hemorrhoids
- Inflammation (ulcerative colitis)
- Colorectal polyps
- Colorectal cancer
- Diverticulosis

How can you recognize bleeding in the digestive tract?

The signs of bleeding in the digestive tract depend upon the site and severity of bleeding. If bleeding is coming from the rectum or the distal colon, there will be bright red blood coating the stool or mixed with the stool. The stool may be mixed with dark red blood if the bleeding is higher up in the colon or at the far end of the small intestine; however, the stool from these areas may be various shades of black. The characteristic appearance of the stool in bleeding from the esophagus, stomach, or duodenum is black or tarry. Vomited material (vomitus) may be bright red or have a coffee-grounds appearance when bleeding is from those sites. If bleeding is occult, the patient will not notice any changes in stool color.

If sudden massive bleeding occurs, there may be weakness, dizziness, faintness, shortness of breath, crampy abdominal pain, and diarrhea. Shock may occur, with a rapid pulse, drop in blood pressure, and difficulty in producing urine. The patient may become very pale. If bleeding is slower and occurs over a long period of time, there may be a gradual onset of fatigue, lethargy, shortness of breath, and pallor from the anemia that results.

How does the doctor diagnose bleeding in the digestive tract?

It is not difficult to diagnose bleeding in the digestive tract. The problem is locating the site of the bleeding. A complete history and physical examination are essential. Symptoms such as changes in bowel habits, color and consistency of the stool (whether the color is black or red), and the presence of pain or tenderness may tell the doctor which organ is affected. Because the intake of iron and foods such as beets can give the stool the same appearance as bleeding in the digestive tract, a doctor must test the stool for blood before offering a diagnosis. A blood count will indicate whether or not the patient is anemic. It will also give a rough estimate of the extent of the bleeding.

Endoscopy

Several methods are available to locate the source of bleeding. Endoscopy is a diagnostic technique that provides the advantage of direct visualization of the bleeding site. Because the endoscope can detect lesions and confirm the presence or absence of bleeding, doctors often choose this method to diagnose patients with acute bleeding.

The fiberoptic endoscope is a flexible instrument consisting of thousands of tiny glass fibers. It allows the doctor to see into the esophagus, stomach, duodenum, and colon; to perform biopsies; and to take color photographs.

Other procedures

Several other methods are available to locate the source of bleeding. The single-contrast (barium only) upper gastrointestinal series of x-rays has been found to be about one-half as accurate as endoscopy in identifying the source of bleeding. Double-contrast (barium plus air) x-rays provide a great deal of accuracy. Drawbacks of barium x-rays are that they can lead to complications in surgery, cause inaccuracies in diagnosis if there is massive bleeding, and preclude the use of other diagnostic techniques. In addition, the required number of x-rays may result in repeated exposure to radiation.

Angiography, the visualization of blood vessels after an injection of dye, is generally not as accurate or as sensitive as endoscopy or barium x-ray. The patient must be bleeding briskly for the contrast material to leak out of the blood vessel at the site of the bleeding. It is a procedure that is most useful in those situations in which injection of drugs into the veins is likely to stop the bleeding. Radioactive scanning is a promising, noninvasive, screening technique for locating sites of bleeding, especially in the lower gastrointestinal tract.

How does the doctor treat bleeding in the digestive tract?

The treatment of bleeding in the digestive tract depends on the cause of bleeding and whether the bleeding is acute or chronic. If aspirin is responsible for the bleeding, eliminate the aspirin and treat the bleeding. If cancer is the cause, removal of the tumors would usually be required. If an ulcer is the cause of the bleeding, the doctor may prescribe a drug, recommend a change in diet, or suggest a change in lifestyle. If acute, life-threatening bleeding is present, emergency measures must be used to prevent or reverse shock. Such measures include hospitalization, blood transfusions, and careful attention to the potential complications of bleeding that may affect the heart, brain, liver, or kidneys. The doctor may advise surgery to control the bleeding if medical measures are not successful.

How do you recognize blood in the stool and vomitus?

♦ Bright red blood coating the stool
♦ Dark blood mixed with the stool
♦ Black or tarry stool
♦ Bright red blood in the vomitus
♦ Coffee grounds appearance of vomitus

What are the symptoms of acute bleeding?

♦ Weakness
♦ Dizziness
♦ Faintness
♦ Shortness of breath
♦ Crampy abdominal pain
♦ Diarrhea

What are the symptoms of chronic bleeding?

♦ Fatigue
♦ Lethargy
♦ Shortness of breath
♦ Pallor

If bleeding has been slow and chronic and the bleeding has been stopped, blood transfusions may not be necessary. Iron supplements will help restore the body's supply by providing the material needed to manufacture new blood cells.

What research is being done to control bleeding in the digestive tract?

Despite increased accuracy in diagnosing the source of bleeding, bleeding in the digestive tract remains a serious problem.

A major task for researchers continues to be investigating new therapies for the different causes of bleeding.

In addition, many researchers are exploring the causes of peptic ulcer disease, gastritis, polyps, cancer, and inflammatory bowel disease. To control gastrointestinal bleeding, researchers are testing a variety of treatments including electrocoagulation and photocoagulation (lasers).

Glossary

Acute. Of short duration.

Anemia. A condition in which the number of red blood cells, the amount of hemoglobin, and the volume of packed red blood cells are less than normal.

Anus. The lower opening of the digestive tract through which fecal matter is discharged.

Barium enema. Lower gastrointestinal (GI) series. A diagnostic procedure in which x-rays are taken after barium sulfate is introduced into the patient by enema. The barium sulfate helps to outline the colon and rectum so that they show up clearly in the x-rays.

Barium meal. Upper GI series. A diagnostic procedure in which the x-rays are taken after the patient swallows barium sulfate. The barium sulfate helps to outline the upper GI tract so that it shows up clearly in the x-rays.

Benign. Noncancerous.

Biopsy. A diagnostic procedure in which a small piece of tissue is removed so that it can be examined under a microscope.

Chronic. Of long duration, often years.

Cirrhosis. A group of chronic liver diseases involving the entire liver, in which liver cells are damaged and regenerate abnormally while much of the liver substance is replaced by scar tissue.

Colitis. Inflammation of the colon.

Colon. The large intestine, the large bowel.

Colonscope. A long, flexible, narrow endoscope used to look into the colon.

Congenital. Present at the time of birth.

Crohn's disease (regional enteritis, ileitis). A chronic, recurring inflammatory disease that can affect any part of the GI tract, but most often the ileum or colon.

Diarrhea. A condition in which fecal matter is discharged from the bowel more often than usual and in a more or less liquid state.

Diffuse. Spread about and not limited to a specific area.

Distal. Farthest away from the trunk, midline, heart, or other reference point.

Diverticulitis. A condition in which diverticula become inflamed.

Diverticulosis. A condition in which there are little sacs (diverticula) on the wall of the colon. This condition is common among older people.

Diverticulum. A little sac that forms on the wall of a hollow organ, usually the colon. The plural form is diverticula.

Duodenum. The first part of the small intestine.

Endoscope. A small, flexible, tube-like instrument, consisting of thousands of tiny glass fibers, that allows a doctor to see into the esophagus, stomach, duodenum, and colon. It also allows a doctor to perform biopsies, take color photographs, and perform surgical and therapeutic procedures.

Endoscopy. A procedure in which an endoscope is used.

Enteritis. Inflammation of the small intestine.

Esophagitis. Inflammation of the small intestine.

Esophagus. The organ that connects the mouth with the stomach.

Familial polyposis. A rare, inherited disease in which many growths (polyps) occur in the colon. There is a very high risk of developing cancer of the colon among those who have this disease.

Feces (stool). Solid body wastes.

Fiber (bulk, roughage). The part of a plant that is not digested. Fiber plays a role in controlling the consistency of stool and the speed at which it is moved down the GI tract.

Fissure. A deep crack.

Gastric ulcer. An open sore on the lining of the stomach.

Gastritis. Inflammation of the stomach.

Gastroenteritis. Inflammation of the lining on both the stomach and the intestine.

Guaic test (occult blood test). A diagnostic test in which a tiny amount of the material to be tested is rubbed on a slide. A chemical reaction is performed to assess the presence or absence of blood.

Hemorrhage. Bleeding; escape of blood from blood vessels, in microscopic amounts or large volumes.

Hemorrhoids. Enlarged, swollen veins in the anal area.

Hereditary. Passed genetically from parents to children.

Heum. The lowest part or end of the small intestine.

Inflammation. A condition in which the body is trying to respond to localized injury or destruction of tissues. All or some of these signs are present: redness, swelling, pain, loss of function.

Malignant. Cancerous.

Occult bleeding (hidden bleeding). Bleeding that is not obvious.

Peptic ulcer. An open sore on the lining of the esophagus, stomach, or duodenum. An ulcer of the stomach is called a gastric ulcer; an ulcer in the duodenum, a duodenal ulcer.

Perforated ulcer. An ulcer that has extended through the full thickness of the stomach or the duodenum.

Polyp. Any mass of tissue that bulges up from the normal surface level.

Small intestine. The part of the digestive tube connecting the stomach to the colon. The small intestine is divided into the duodenum, jejunum, and ileum.

Stomach. The large, irregular sac that is found between the esophagus and the small intestine.

Stool. Feces; the waste matter discharged from the body.

Stress ulcers. Acute upper GI ulcers that occur following stressful conditions, e.g., surgery, major burns, or critical head trauma.

Varices. Abnormally dilated (stretched) veins.

Paul Sherlock, M.D. is a professor and vice chairman, Department of Medicine, Cornell University Medical College, and chairman, Department of Medicine, Memorial Sloan-Kettering Cancer Center, New York, New York.

■ Document Source:
U.S. Department of Health and Human Services, Public Health Service

National Institutes of Health
National Institute of Diabetes, and Digestive and Kidney Diseases
NIH Publication No. 89-1133
Reprinted March 1989

See also: Crohn's Disease (page 160); Diverticulosis and Diverticulitis (page 162); Ulcerative Colitis (page 176)

National Cancer Institute Research Report
CANCER OF THE PANCREAS

This publication describes current research related to the incidence, possible causes and prevention, detection and diagnosis, and treatment of cancer of the pancreas. The information presented here was gathered from the National Cancer Institute (NCI) database known as PDQ, medical textbooks, recent articles in the medical literature, and NCI scientists and other researchers. This report expands upon the information provided in the NCI pamphlet *What You Need To Know About Cancer of the Pancreas*.

Knowledge about cancer of the pancreas is increasing. Up-to-date information on this and other cancer-related subjects is available from the toll-free Cancer Information Service at 1-800-4-CANCER.

Description and Function of the Pancreas

Located in the abdomen, the pancreas is a gland surrounded by the stomach, colon, liver, gallbladder, kidneys, and that part of the small intestine called the duodenum. The pancreas is a spongy, tube-like structure about 6 inches long and 2 inches wide. Its rounded head sits next to the duodenum on the right side of the body; the narrow tail ends at the spleen on the left. The areas between the head and tail are called the neck and body of the pancreas.

The main pancreatic duct runs the length of the pancreas. At the ampulla, this duct branches like a Y turned sideways. The lower branch joins with the common bile duct from the liver and gallbladder to form the hepatopancreatic ampulla, which empties into the duodenum. The top branch, known as the accessory pancreatic duct, also empties into the duodenum above the common bile duct. Through these connections with the rest of the digestive system, the pancreas carries out its part of the digestive process.

The pancreas performs two vital functions: It supplies the intestines with enzyme-rich juices that help digest food, and it secretes insulin, glucagon, and other hormones that control the amount of sugar in the blood. The dual functions of the pancreas make it an unusual gland. Because of these two functions, the pancreas is referred to in two ways—the "exocrine pancreas" for the digestive tasks it performs and the "endocrine process" for its role in producing hormones. Exocrine glands have ducts that open on an internal or external surface of the body. Endocrine glands do not have ducts; they secrete their products (hormones and enzymes) directly into the bloodstream.

The exocrine and endocrine functions of the pancreas are handled by a network of tightly packed cells. There are far more exocrine than endocrine cells in the pancreas; in fact, exocrine cells outnumber endocrine cells by about 99 to 1. In the pancreas, some exocrine cells are arranged in clusters called acini. The acinar cells secrete pancreatic juices—water containing salts and enzymes—that flow from small ducts into the main pancreatic ducts and eventually empty into the duodenum to aid digestion.

Clusters of endocrine cells, most of which are located in the body and tail of the pancreas, are called the islets of Langerhans. These clusters secrete hormones that help regulate the way the body uses sugars and starches:

♦ Insulin causes sugar to enter the body's cells and be converted into energy; it also stimulates the conversion of sugar to glycogen, a starch stored in the liver.
♦ Glucagon triggers the reverse process. When the sugar level in the blood is below normal, glucagon converts glycogen and other nutrients in the liver into sugar, or glucose, to increase the sugar content of the blood.
♦ Somatostatin inhibits the secretion of insulin; it is also referred to as GHIF, growth hormone-inhibiting factor.

These three important hormones—glucagon, insulin, and somatostatin—are secreted by three different types of pancreatic cells: alpha cells, beta cells, and delta cells, respectively. Other kinds of endocrine cells also grow in the pancreas and produce specialized secretions, such as peptides (compounds that make up proteins) and various hormones.

The lining of the ducts—the epithelium—may be composed of several different types of cells, including squamous cells and cells referred to as giant cells.

Types of Pancreatic Cancer

Normal pancreatic cells divide and reproduce in an orderly manner, replacing wornout and injured tissue. When cell division becomes disordered, abnormal growth takes place, producing masses of tissue known as tumors. Tumors in the pancreas may be malignant (cancerous) or, in rare cases, benign (not cancerous).

Benign tumors may interfere with the normal functioning of the pancreas and may crowd nearby organs, but they do not spread to other parts of the body and generally are not life threatening. Malignant tumors, however, compress, invade, and destroy normal tissues. Also, cancer cells can break away from a tumor and spread, or metastasize, to other parts of the body, where they may form secondary tumors. When pancreatic cancer spreads, it most commonly affects the liver, lungs, and bones. The cancer cells of these secondary tumors are microscopically identical to those of the primary cancer. As such, they retain many of the characteristics of the original pancreatic cancer, despite being located in the liver, lungs, or elsewhere. These secondary tumors are referred to as "metastatic pancreatic cancer" (rather than liver, lung, or bone cancer) to indicate that they are all part of a single disease and are not new cancers originating in these parts of the body. Treatment for cancer that has spread must take into account the site and type of the primary tumor as well as the location and extent of the metastatic tumors and other factors.

Cancers of the exocrine and endocrine cells of the pancreas differ in many ways; in the symptoms they produce, the methods used to diagnose them, their tendencies to metastasize, their patterns of spread, and their responses to treatment.

Cancer of the exocrine pancreas accounts for 95 percent of all pancreatic tumors. Most exocrine cancers (about 90 percent) are duct cell carcinomas and arise in the lining of pancreatic ducts. On rare occasions, the acinar cells may become malignant; acinar cell carcinoma is characterized by changes in both the appearance and organization of these cells. In some cases, pancreatic cancer is referred to as "unclassified."

Almost three-fourths of exocrine cancers originate in the head and neck of the pancreas. Most of the rest begin in the body, and fewer than 10 percent start in the tail; in some patients, they are found throughout the pancreas.

Cancer of the endocrine pancreas, also known as islet cell carcinoma, is very rare, accounting for no more than 1,000 cases a year in the United States. Endocrine tumors are slow growing, and the outlook is usually more favorable than for exocrine pancreatic cancer.

Incidence and Mortality

Since 1950, the annual incidence of pancreatic cancer in the United States has increased from 5.3 to 9.2 cases per 100,000 population. The incidence also is rising in many other parts of the world. It is estimated that in 1991, over 28,000 new cases of pancreatic cancer were diagnosed in this country, accounting for about 3 percent of all new cancer cases.

Because the risk of developing pancreatic cancer increases steadily with age, its rising incidence may reflect the fact that the U.S. population is living longer than in 1950. Approximately four-fifths of all cases occur after the age of 60; among 80- to 84-year-olds, the annual incidence is 90.2 cases per 100,000 population, 36 times the rate for people between 40 and 44 years of age (2.5 per 100,000).

In the United States, this disease is 30 percent more common in men than in women and about 65 percent more common in blacks than in whites. It occurs more frequently in Jews than in Catholics or Protestants and least often among Mormons and Seventh-Day Adventists.

Pancreatic cancer is seen most often in developed, industrial countries. The United States and northern European countries, including Great Britain, have high rates; low rates are found in the African nations, South America, the Near East, and India; and rates for southern Europe, Asia, and the Far East are in the middle of the range. These geographic differences in incidence may be due at least in part to the substantial difficulties in diagnosing the disease, especially before the past decade, and to the ways in which medical records have been kept. However, worldwide mortality figures parallel differences in incidence.

Exocrine pancreatic cancer is the fifth leading cause of death from cancer; it accounts for about 25,000 deaths each year.

Possible Causes of Pancreatic Cancer

The most important known risk factor for pancreatic cancer is cigarette smoking. The Office of the U.S. Surgeon General reached this conclusion after a number of studies showed that the risk of pancreatic cancer for cigarette smokers is more than twice that for nonsmokers. The increase in the incidence of pancreatic cancer followed the increased use of cigarettes that began after World War II. Evidence of the relationship between smoking and pancreatic cancer is provided by the recent increase in mortality from this disease among women, whose use of cigarettes has also steadily increased. In fact, the death rate for women has gone up twice as fast as the rate for men.

Family histories of patients with pancreatic cancer have been examined to identify possible genetic factors for the disease. Some limited evidence of familial predisposition has been found—more frequently for endocrine than for exocrine tumors. Also, pancreatic cancer has been seen in patients with hereditary pancreatitis (inflammation of the pancreas), Gardner's syndrome (a hereditary condition characterized by colon polyps, various growths outside the colon, and cysts), and neurofibromatosis, sometimes called "Elephant Man" disease, which scientists believe is hereditary. In general, however, the scientific evidence suggests that most cases of pancreatic cancer are not hereditary.

Diabetes mellitus has also been investigated as a possible risk factor. Almost 15 percent of pancreatic cancer patients have a history of diabetes. However, more than half of these were diagnosed as having cancer within 3 months after being diagnosed as having diabetes. Therefore, some researchers think that the diabetes may result from the cancer. That is, they believe that when cancer affects the ability of the pancreas to function properly, diabetes may be one consequence.

Numerous studies have been conducted to determine whether food and drink can cause pancreatic cancer. Scientists have reported that a diet high in meat and fat may be related to this disease. One large study suggested that fruits and vegetables may be protective. Alcohol and coffee have been studied as possible causes, but research has not shown a clear relationship between alcohol or coffee consumption and cancer of the pancreas.

Various occupations in which workers are exposed to known carcinogens have been implicated in isolated studies, but none of these observations has been confirmed. One study reported 56 deaths from pancreatic cancer among members of the American Chemical Society, compared with 35 projected from the national rate for a group of the same size. However, in another study, no excess of pancreatic cancer deaths were found among chemists employed by a large chemical company. Still, a significant percentage of patients with cancer of the pancreas have worked in occupations where they were exposed to solvents and petroleum compounds.

Because radiation is known to cause some types of cancer, researchers have studied pancreatic cancer rates among radiologists and among Japanese atomic bomb survivors. Slightly higher rates have been reported for these groups, but the increases are considered too small to be significant.

Some epidemiologic and clinical studies have suggested that certain pancreatic tumors may depend on the female sex hormones estrogen and progesterone for growth. Researchers have found elevated amounts of estrogen in exocrine pancreatic tumors. Although the implications for prevention are not yet clear, these findings may have applications for diagnosis (through the use of hormone receptor assays) and for treatment that deprives the body of these hormones.

More research clearly is needed to identify other risk factors. At present, giving up smoking—or never starting—is the single most important step people can take to protect themselves against pancreatic cancer. The NCI also suggests that people follow the general dietary suggestions for reducing the risk of other cancers: a diet low in total fat, more poultry and fish, and more fruits, vegetables, and whole grains. Alcohol, if consumed at all, should be used in moderation.

Cancer of the Exocrine Pancreas

The pancreas is known as a "silent" organ because it is slow to signal the presence of cancer. Prompt detection is extremely difficult, because early symptoms often resemble those of other digestive disorders, like chronic pancreatitis, hepatitis, hiatal hernia, gallstones, and diabetes mellitus. By the time of diagnosis, cancer of the exocrine pancreas has often spread beyond the pancreas, usually first to nearby lymph nodes and then to the liver.

Symptoms

At first, the patient may complain of vague discomfort that comes and goes. Patients often ignore these early signs of illness, sometimes for several months. Pain is the most common symptom of either type of pancreatic cancer. The pain gradually worsens, and it is often most severe at night. Sometimes it occurs several hours after meals, once the stomach empties out. In some patients, the pain radiates to the back or is limited to that area. When the pain is far away from the real source in the digestive system, the symptom may prompt extensive and fruitless neurologic and orthopedic examinations in search of a cause for back pain.

Weight loss occurs in nearly all patients before diagnosis. The loss may be rapid, even though the person has a good appetite and eats normally. Bowel habits also may be altered. Some people have diarrhea or greasy stools; other have severe constipation.

Jaundice (a yellowish discoloration of the skin and the whites of the eyes) is present in half of pancreatic cancer patients at the time of diagnosis and in nearly all patients whose cancer is in the head of the pancreas. Jaundice usually indicates abnormal function of the common bile duct or the liver. In pancreatic cancer, it occurs when the common bile duct is blocked and does not allow passage of a substance called bilirubin, which gives bile its yellowish color. The bilirubin collects in other tissues throughout the body. Jaundice also may occur when pancreatic cancer spreads to the liver, interfering with its function.

When diabetes develops suddenly in a mature person who is not overweight and has no family history of the disease, it may be an indication that cancer is present. Diabetes appears as a symptom in 10 to 20 percent of pancreatic cancer patients.

Diagnosis

As the disease progresses, the symptoms become more pronounced. Still, physical examination, routine x-rays of the gastrointestinal tract, and blood tests may fail to reveal either exocrine or endocrine cancer.

As a rule, once pancreatic cancer is suspected, the physician prescribes a "barium swallow." In this procedure, the patient swallows barium sulfate, a contrast substance, which outlines the upper digestive tract and makes it visible on an x-ray film. Unfortunately, this test rarely reveals early tumors.

Several other tests, including ultrasonography (ultrasound) and special types of x-rays, usually are ordered. The doctor also may use a very thin needle to extract tissue from the pancreas. This procedure, known as fine-needle biopsy, allows the examination of tissue without surgery.

Ultrasonography provides pictures on a computer screen formed by the echo patterns of sound waves bounced back from the patient's organs. It has a high rate of accuracy in detecting even small tumors at the head of the pancreas but is less successful in identifying those in the body and tail. Ultrasound patterns help distinguish cancer from pancreatitis; however, the patterns sometimes fail to indicate tumors and sometimes suggest a tumor when none is present, so this test must be used with other diagnostic methods.

CT (or CAT) scans use a computer to produce cross-sectional x-ray images of an organ. They are more accurate than ultrasonography but may miss small or early tumors. This technique is good for locating cancers that have changed the shape of the pancreas and those that have spread beyond its borders.

Endoscopic retrograde cholangiopancreatography (ERCP) allows the doctor to see inside the pancreas. The doctor passes a flexible fiberoptic tube (endoscope) down the throat, through the stomach, and into the pancreas. The physician can look through the tube and guide its movement. A liquid that will show up on an x-ray is injected through the tube into the pancreas, and an x-ray picture is taken that can reveal abnormalities in the organ's shape. This procedure is highly accurate, but it can lead to such complications as infection. ERCP also is used in combination with fine-needle biopsy to obtain a sample of pancreatic cells for microscopic examination.

Percutaneous transhepatic cholangiography (PTC) is another accurate diagnostic method. A fine needle is inserted into the patient's liver, and a contrast substance is injected. This substance spreads through the gallbladder and bile ducts to reveal blockages caused by a tumor at the head of the pancreas. Complications such as hemorrhage or infection have been reported in some cases.

Because it is located behind other organs, the pancreas cannot be examined physically, except with surgery. Laparotomy, an operation that permits direct examination of the pancreas, may be needed for a conclusive diagnosis. This operation enables the doctor to confirm the site and size of the tumor. During the laparatomy, the surgeon may remove the tumor or open blockages caused by the cancer. As with any surgical procedure, there is a risk of infection and other complications.

Laparoscopy is another effective diagnostic technique. In this procedure, the doctor makes a small incision and inserts a thin, telescope-like instrument into the abdomen. Because the doctor can visually examine the pancreas without making a large incision, laparoscopy poses less risk to the patient than laparatomy. Laparoscopy can be performed under local or general anesthesia.

Tumor Markers

The need for better diagnostic tools has stimulated research to identify tumor markers for pancreatic and other types of cancer. Markers are chemical substances in the blood or other body fluids that suggest the presence of cancer. Tests to measure these substances may be used to screen people with no symptoms of the disease, to diagnose cancer in someone suspected of having it, or to monitor the course of the illness.

Scientists are investigating several substances found in the blood of patients with pancreatic cancer. One example is carcinoembryonic antigen (CEA), a substance normally present in the human embryo and found only in minute amounts in a healthy adult; high levels of CEA may signal disease. An elevated level of CEA has been reported in more than 80 percent of patients with advanced pancreatic cancer, and it is sometimes used in the diagnostic process as a check against radiologic and ultrasound tests. The CEA level is being studied as a tumor marker for several other cancers.

The level of this protein is also elevated in people with pancreatitis and other inflammatory conditions of the digestive tract. It is also much higher in disease-free smokers than in nonsmokers. For these reasons, it cannot be used as the only diagnostic tool.

Another marker under investigation is CA 19-9. In one study, the serum level of CA 19-9 was elevated in 89 percent of pancreatic cancer patients just before treatment, while 96 percent of patients had an elevated level sometime during the course of their disease. In that same study, researchers found that patients whose CA 19-9 level had returned to normal after treatment lived longer than did those whose level remained elevated. Another study showed that combining measurements of CA 19-9 with ultrasonography successfully revealed very small pancreatic cancers. In two studies that compared CA 19-9 with CEA, CA 19-9 was the more reliable indicator of pancreatic cancer. However, no study has supported the use of CA 19-9 for the diagnosis of this disease, although it is helpful in monitoring a patient's response to therapy.

Pancreatic oncofetal antigen (POA), a substance found in the pancreas of the normal fetus, may be a useful marker for pancreatic cancer. An elevated POA level has been found in 61 to 81 percent of patients known to have this disease. However, it is also present (in far lower percentages) in other malignancies, in about one-fifth of patients with pancreatitis, and even in a very few people with no disease.

Several other markers require further study:

♦ The level of AFP (alphafetoprotein, another oncofetal antigen), like that of CEA, is not elevated in normal adults. One study showed it to be elevated in 23 percent of patients with pancreatic cancer, and two other studies showed it to be higher than normal when cancer metastasized to the liver.

♦ NSE (neuron-specific enolase) is a protein that has been found in elevated amounts in patients with several types of endocrine tumors, including those arising in the pancreas. Although it has not proven useful for detecting early disease, researchers think it may be useful both as a diagnostic tool and in gauging the progress of disease or the success of treatment.

♦ CA-195 is a protein that is currently under study both for detecting and monitoring cancer of the pancreas. It is similar to CA 19-9. To date, it has been shown to be accurate in about 70 percent of cases and more accurate than CEA.

Staging

Staging, or determining the extent of disease, helps in planning appropriate treatment. A number of tests (including laparotomy) to examine the pancreas may be needed to determine how far the disease has spread.

The staging system for exocrine pancreatic cancer is still evolving. As therapies improve, determining the extent of disease will become increasingly important. Exocrine cancers are commonly identified by their location within the pancreas, and stages are based on descriptions of *tumor* (T), lymph *node* involvement (N), and degree of *metastasis* (M).

Primary tumor (T)

TX: Minimum requirements to assess the primary tumor cannot be met.

T0: No evidence of primary tumor.

T1: Tumor limited to the pancreas.

  T1a: Tumor 2 centimeters (cm) (about three-quarters of inch) or less in greatest diameter.

  T1b: Tumor more than 2 cm in greatest diameter.

T2: Tumor extends directly to the duodenum, bile duct, or tissues close to the pancreas.

T3: Tumor extends directly to the stomach, spleen, colon, or adjacent large vessels.

Nodal involvement (N)

NX: Minimum requirements to assess the regional nodes cannot be met.

N0: Regional nodes not involved.

N1: Regional nodes involved.

Distant metastasis (M)

MX: Minimum requirements to determine distant metastasis cannot be met.

M0: No known distant metastasis.

M1: Distant metastasis present.

Using the TNM system, stages of exocrine pancreatic cancer are described as follows:

Stage I: The cancer is entirely confined to the pancreas or has directly spread to involve the small intestine, bile duct, or tissues around the pancreas (T1 or T2, N0, M0)

Stage II. The cancer has spread further to involve adjacent organs such as the stomach, spleen, or colon. (T3, N0, M0)

Stage III. The cancer involves regional lymph nodes. (Any T, N1, M0)

Stage IV. The cancer has spread to distant sites, most commonly the liver or lungs. (Any T, any N, M1)

Cancer of the Endocrine Pancreas (Islet Cell Carcinoma)

Tumors that grow from endocrine cells may be classified as either functional (hormone-producing) or nonfunctional (unable to produce hormones). Researchers have found that most endocrine cell tumors are nonfunctional, and about 90 percent of nonfunctional tumors are malignant. Because there are several types of pancreatic islet cells, the term islet cell carcinoma refers to at least five separate cancers that are named for the type of secretion produced by the endocrine cells. If these islet cell cancers are functional tumors, they produce substances that cause specific disorders or symptoms. Table 1 lists the names of islet cell cancers and the disorders that they cause.

Carcinoid tumors arise from a type of interacinar cell that produces peptides and another type that produces 5-HT (5-hydroxytryptamine, or serotonin), which plays a role in regulating blood circulation and other basic functions, including sleep.

Table 1. Islet Cell Cancers

Type of Islet Cell	Secreted Active Agent	Tumor and Syndrome
Alpha	Glucagon	Glucagonoma (diabetes, dermatitis)
Beta	Insulin	Insulinoma (hypoglycemia)
Delta	Somatostatin	Somatostatinoma (mild diabetes)
D	Gastrin	Gastrinoma (peptic ulcer disease)
A -> D	Vasoactive intestinal peptide (VIP) and/or other undefined mediators	WDHA (watery diarrhea, hypokalemic acidosis)
A -> D	5-HT ACTH MSH	Carcinoid Cushing's disease Hyperpigmentation

Symptoms

Many of the symptoms are common to both exocrine and endocrine cancers; in addition, cancers of the endocrine pancreas cause other problems (as listed in Table 1). For example, when the tumor develops in beta cells, it interferes with insulin secretion and sugar regulation; patients may have attacks of hypoglycemia (low blood sugar) with restlessness, irritability, sweating, and flushing. If the hypoglycemia is not treated, the lack of glucose in the brain may result in extreme anxiety, tremor, and possibly even severe confusion. Hypoglycemia that persists may lead to convulsions, unconsciousness, and shock.

Symptoms of diabetes may result when alpha and delta cells are affected. When cancer affects gastrin-producing (D) cells (gastrinoma), patients may develop peptic ulcer disease. Diarrhea is often the most common symptom of gastrinoma, but patients may also experience pain associated with an ulcer.

When other types of endocrine cells become abnormal, patients may experience different symptoms, including those associated with Cushing's disease. This condition develops when the body improperly regulates certain hormonal processes. It results in a redistribution of fat in the body: The legs become spindly while the face becomes fat and "moon-shaped," and large fat deposits may settle on the back or abdomen. Another hormonal imbalance causes an overproduction of the skin-coloring substance melanin, and part of the body may be darkened as a result.

Diagnosis

The diagnosis of endocrine cancer includes many of the techniques used for exocrine cancer. However, identifying the precise cell type requires certain diagnostic procedures specific for each. Often it is possible for the physician to make a tentative diagnosis of cell type based on symptoms, but it is sometimes difficult to distinguish whether symptoms are caused by the size and location of the tumor or by effects of secretions of the cancer cells.

Laboratory tests are often helpful in determining the type of islet cell affected. These may include examination of blood, urine, and stool samples as well as tests to determine the chemical makeup of samples of stomach contents.

In some cases, an exploratory laparotomy and biopsy may be needed. When this procedure is done, the surgeon may also remove a sample of regional lymph nodes. Biopsy of the nodes will determine whether and how far the cancer has spread into the lymph system.

Staging

As with exocrine cancer, the staging system for endocrine pancreatic cancer is still developing. These tumors are most often divided into one of three groups:

♦ islet cell cancers occurring in one site within the pancreas;
♦ islet cell cancers occurring in several sites; and
♦ islet cell cancers that have metastasized to regional lymph nodes or distant sites.

Treatment

Although there are many similarities in approaches, treatment for pancreatic cancer depends primarily on whether the cancer affects the exocrine or endocrine (islet cell) functions. The stage of the disease is also important. In addition, doctors consider the patient's age and general health and other factors.

At present, standard treatment for all but localized pancreatic cancer is not curative. Because current therapy is frequently ineffective, patients are encouraged to consider participating in clinical trials (treatment studies) that are designed to evaluate new approaches to therapy. Researchers recommend that physicians consider these trials before attempting any treatment to relieve symptoms (palliative therapy) when it is clear that surgery will not cure the disease. Clinical trials are under way at many hospitals throughout the United States. Information about these trials is found under "Clinical Trials and PDQ," and in the NCI booklet *What Are Clinical Trials All About?*.

Surgery

The oldest operation for cancer of the pancreas is called the Whipple procedure: The head and neck of the pancreas, the duodenum, and adjacent structures are removed. This procedure, most often done for exocrine cancer, leaves enough tissue so that the pancreas can continue producing insulin, other hormones, and digestive enzymes. The Whipple procedure does not include the regional lymph nodes or major blood vessels. However, some doctors prefer complete removal of the pancreas.

Total pancreatectomy, or removal of the entire pancreas, was developed in the hope of improving the survival rate over that for the Whipple procedure and to better assure the removal of all cancer cells. In this operation, the duodenum, common bile duct, gallbladder, spleen, and most of the adjacent lymph nodes are removed along with the pancreas. To reduce the risk of peptic ulcer, the nerve that controls secretions in the stomach and pancreas is sometimes severed so activity in the stomach will be reduced. Surgeons who recommend total pancreatectomy argue that preserving the organ's function does not justify the risk of leaving stray cancer cells. When the entire pancreas has been removed, patients must be given insulin and replacement enzymes.

In a regional pancreatectomy, a more extensive operation, the pancreas, lymph nodes, and some veins and arteries that supply blood to the organ are removed. Physicians who favor this procedure believe it offers a better chance of cure, but experience is limited. Early evidence indicates that regional pancreatectomy leads to longer survival than does total pancreatectomy. It seems especially effective for small tumors at the head of the pancreas.

Surgery is a major procedure with potentially serious complications, some of which, like hemorrhaging and infection, can be life threatening. Some physicians argue that the high rate of complications with only a small chance of cure should rule out surgery altogether. Others note that surgery does provide some relief of pain and may lengthen life. For example, some patients may experience discomfort when the common bile duct is blocked by cancer. This can often be relieved by surgically inserting a catheter (a narrow tube placed into the bile duct that empties into a small bag) to drain off the bile that accumulates. Other pancreatic cancer patients may have problems with blockage of the duodenum. In this case, the surgeon may bypass it by connecting the common bile duct to another part of the small intestine called the jejunum, which is below the duodenum. Bypass procedures extend the life of many patients.

Radiation

Radiation therapy, the use of high-energy rays to destroy cancerous tissue, may help control the disease, provide relief of symptoms, and prolong survival. Radiation may be delivered by a machine outside the body (external beam therapy) or may come from radioactive material implanted in or near the tumor (interstitial therapy).

Another type of radiotherapy is high linear energy transfer of radiation (high LET), which focuses strong doses of deeply penetrating radiation on the tumor. This type of therapy, sometimes called particle beam radiation therapy, requires the use of the sophisticated cyclotron to produce and accelerate the movement of subatomic particles. So far, this type of radiotherapy, still experimental, has not significantly lengthened survival.

Intraoperative radiation therapy (IORT) is an investigational procedure that has recently shown some positive effects on survival time. This procedure involves the use of radiation during surgery, permitting a greater amount of radiation to be directed at the cancer without damage to nearby tissues.

Chemotherapy

Chemotherapy is treatment with drugs. This type of therapy has been used mainly in patients with advanced pancreatic cancer—whether exocrine or endocrine. The combination of 5-fluorouracil (5-FU) and intraoperative and standard radiation has proven effective in lengthening survival time. This approach is particularly important for patients whose tumors cannot be surgically removed. Because of evidence that drugs are effective against pancreatic cancer in animals, various agents have been tested; several have shown promise, but so far no drug regimen has provided consistently good results. Researchers are trying to learn why pancreatic cells are resistant to drugs.

Biological Therapy

Biological therapy, also known as biotherapy or immunotherapy, is the use of biological agents to fight cancer. It is a new form of cancer treatment based on the knowledge and tools of modern molecular biology, immunology, and genetics. Biological therapy works either directly against the cancer or indirectly to modify the relationship between the tumor and the patient. It may enhance a cancer patient's immune system so that the system will fight the growth of cancer cells, eliminate or suppress body responses that permit cancer growth, or make a cancer cell more sensitive to destruction by the patient's immune system.

Currently, researchers are studying a number of biological response modifiers (BRMs), including monoclonal antibodies (pure, tailored antibodies that can be mass-produced in the laboratory), in the treatment of pancreatic cancer. Monoclonal antibodies are capable of seeking out and binding to certain substances on cancer cells. They can be linked to a variety of cell-killing substances and can deliver them directly to cancer cells. The NCI is supporting studies to explore the effectiveness of monoclonal antibodies for inoperable pancreatic cancer. In addition, NCI is also supporting studies to explore the value of interferon alpha, recombinant IL-2, and combinations of these BRMs and other drug (such as 5-FU and cyclophosphamide), leucovorin, and granulo-

cyte macrophage-colony stimulating factor in patients with pancreatic cancer.

Hormone Therapy

As mentioned earlier, the fact that certain tumors show signs of being estrogen dependent has led some researchers to propose use of the estrogen-blocking drug tamoxifen in experimental adjuvant therapy (treatment given in addition to the primary treatment to kill cancer cells that might remain in the body after the primary treatment). Studies using this drug are still in their early stages.

Treatment for Exocrine Cancer

Treatment for early cancer of the exocrine pancreas involves one of several surgical procedures described earlier, depending upon the size and location of the tumor. Even when exocrine cancer is still in an early stage and the tumor can be removed surgically, additional treatment with combined radiation and chemotherapy may lengthen survival. When cancer is localized (stage 1) but the tumor cannot be surgically removed, radiation therapy helps to ease symptoms. And, although radiation alone has not greatly lengthened long-term survival, patients treated with combined surgery and IORT do show improved survival—often a year or more longer than patients not receiving radiation.

Stage II exocrine cancer may be treated with radiation therapy to relieve symptoms, and local neurosurgical procedures are often helpful is relieving pain. Some patients may get symptom relief with a combination of surgery and chemotherapy. Patients with stage III and stage IV disease may also benefit from palliative treatment (surgical or radiologic) to relieve pain and other symptoms.

All patients with advanced exocrine cancer should be considered for clinical trials. Some researchers are investigating IORT, other types of external radiation combined with chemotherapy for patients who have had a resection, and chemotherapy alone. A number of investigational drugs are under study, and researchers also are exploring the use of biological response modifiers alone or combined with chemotherapy. Therapies that combine surgery, IORT, chemotherapy, and external radiation are being studied in a few trials. Radiolabeled anti-CEA, anti-AFP, and other antibodies to tumor markers are also being explored, with the aim of delivering a large dose of radiation (iodine 131) to the tumor; these trials are appropriate only for patients whose tumors are producing these tumor markers.

Treatment for Endocrine Cancer

Islet cell carcinoma often can be cured. Surgery usually is used to remove the tumor or that part of the pancreas where the tumor is growing; in some cases, however, the entire pancreas is removed. When pancreatectomy is necessary, the patient must thereafter be given medication to replace the action of the digestive enzymes and hormones—especially insulin.

Chemotherapy is used when the cancer has spread or when surgery is either ineffective or impossible. In clinical research, streptozotocin reduced tumor size in up to 50 percent of islet cell cancer patients and lengthened survival by a few months. Streptozotocin with 5-FU is now considered the standard therapy for advanced islet cell cancer. Cimetidine (a drug used to treat ulcers) is sometimes given in addition to surgery for gastrinoma to inhibit the secretion of gastric acids. Anticancer drugs—5-FU and streptozotocin or streptozotocin alone—have been used to treat advanced gastrinoma, insulinoma, and other types of islet cell cancer. A drug called SMS 201-995, which is similar to somatostatin (the hormone that inhibits the secretion of insulin), has been used in many advanced islet cell cancer patients to inhibit the secretion of hormones by tumors. Also under study are dacarbazine, carboplatin, mitoxantrone, etoposide, doxorubicin, and human recombinant leukocyte-A interferon (alone or in combination); most of these are being evaluated in patients for whom surgery is not possible.

Clinical Trials and PDQ

To improve the outcome of treatment for patients with pancreatic cancer, NCI supports clinical studies at many hospitals throughout the United States. Patients who take part in this research make an important contribution to medical science and may have the first chance to benefit from improved treatment methods. Physicians are encouraged to inform their patients about the option of participating in such trials. To help patients and doctors learn about current trials, NCI has developed PDQ, a computerized system designed to give quick and easy access to:

♦ descriptions of current clinical trials that are accepting patients, including information about the objectives of the study, medical eligibility requirements, details of the treatment program, and the names and addresses of physicians and facilities conducting the study;

♦ up-to-date information about the standard treatment for most types of cancer; and

♦ names of organizations and physicians involved in cancer care.

To access PDQ, doctors may use an office computer with a telephone hookup and a PDQ access code, a fax machine, or the services of a medical library with online searching capability. Cancer Information Service offices (1-800-4-CANCER) provide PDQ searches to callers and can tell doctors how to obtain regular access to the database. Patients may ask their doctors to use PDQ or may call 1-800-4-CANCER to request a search themselves. Information specialists at this toll-free number use a variety of sources, including PDQ, to answer questions about cancer prevention, diagnosis, treatment, and research.

Selected References

Except as noted by an asterisk, the following materials are not available from the National Cancer Institute (NCI). They can be found in medical libraries, many college and university libraries, and some public libraries. Information about ordering NCI materials is provided at the end of this publication.

Bagne, F.R. et al. "Treatment of Cancer of the Pancreas by Intraoperative Electron Beam Therapy: Physical and Biological Aspects," *Interna-*

tional Journal of Radiation Oncology and Biological Physics, Vol. 16(1), 1989, pp. 231–242.

Chemotherapy and You: A Guide to Self-Help During Treatment. Office of Cancer Communications, National Cancer Institute. NIH Publication No. 91–1136.

Clavell, F. et al. "More on Coffee and Pancreatic Cancer," *New England Journal of Medicine*, Vol. 316(8), 1987, pp. 683–684.

DeVita V.T., Jr. et al., eds. *Cancer: Principles and Practice of Oncology*, 3rd ed. Philadelphia: Lippincott, 1989.

Dobelbower R., Jr. and Milligan, A.J., eds. "Treatment of Pancreatic Cancer by Radiation Therapy," *World Journal of Surgery*, Vol. 8(6), 1984, pp. 919–928.

Gastrointestinal Tumor Study Group. "Further Evidence of Effective Adjuvant Combined Radiation and Chemotherapy Following Curative Resection of Pancreatic Cancer," *Cancer*, Vol. 59(12), 1987, pp. 2006–2010.

Kent, R.B. et al. "Nonfunctioning Islet Cell Tumors," *Annals of Surgery*, Vol. 193(2), 1981, pp. 185–190.

Mack, T.M. et al. "Pancreas Cancer and Smoking, Beverage Consumption, and Past Medical History," *Journal of the National Cancer Institute*, Vol. 76(1), 1986, pp. 49–60.

Moossa, A.R., ed. "Pancreatic Cancer—Approach to Diagnosis, Selection for Surgery and Choice of Operation," *Cancer*, Vol. 50(11), 1982, pp. 2689–2698.

Radiation Therapy and You: A Guide to Self-Help During Treatment. Office of Cancer Communications, National Cancer Institute, NIH Publication No. 91–2227.

Tonnesen, K. and Kamp-Jensen, M. "Antiestrogen Therapy in Pancreatic Carcinoma: A Preliminary Report," *European Journal of Surgical Oncology*, Vol. 12(1), 1986, pp. 69–70.

What Are Clinical Trials All About? A Booklet for Patients with Cancer. Office of Cancer Communications, National Cancer Institute, NIH Publication No. 90–2706.

■ Document Source:
   National Institutes of Health
   National Cancer Institute
   NIH Publication No. 92-2941
   Printed August 1992

See also: Chemotherapy and You: A Guide to Self-Help During Treatment (page 40); Radiation Therapy and You: A Guide to Self-Help During Treatment (page 56); What Are Clinical Trials All About? A Booklet for Patients with Cancer (page 68)

DD Clearinghouse Fact Sheet
CROHN'S DISEASE

Inflammatory bowel disease (IBD) is a group of chronic disorders that cause inflammation or ulceration in the small and large intestines. Most often IBD is classified as ulcerative colitis or Crohn's disease but may be referred to as colitis, enteritis, ileitis, and proctitis.

Ulcerative colitis causes ulceration and inflammation of the inner lining of the colon and rectum, while Crohn's disease is an inflammation that extends into the deeper layers of the intestinal wall.

Ulcerative colitis and Crohn's disease cause similar symptoms that often resemble other conditions such as irritable bowel syndrome (spastic colitis). The correct diagnosis may take some time.

Crohn's disease usually involves the small intestine, most often the lower part (the ileum). In some cases, both the small and large intestine (colon) are affected. In other cases, only the colon is involved. Sometimes, inflammation also may affect the mouth, esophagus, stomach, duodenum, appendix, or anus. Crohn's disease is a chronic condition and may recur at various times over a lifetime. Some people have long periods of remission, sometimes for year, when they are free of symptoms. There is no way to predict when a remission may occur or when symptoms will return.

What are the symptoms?

The most common symptoms of Crohn's disease are abdominal pain, often in the lower right area, and diarrhea. There also may be rectal bleeding, weight loss, and fever. Bleeding may be serious and persistent, leading to anemia (low red blood cell count). Children may suffer delayed development and stunted growth.

What causes Crohn's disease and who gets it?

There are many theories about what causes Crohn's disease, but none has been proven. One theory is that some agent, perhaps a virus or a bacterium, affects the body's immune system to trigger an inflammatory reaction in the intestinal wall. Although there is a lot of evidence that patients with this disease have abnormalities of the immune system, doctors do not know whether the immune problems are a cause or a result of the disease. Doctors believe, however, that there is little proof that Crohn's disease is caused by emotional distress or by an unhappy childhood.

Crohn's disease affects males and females equally and appears to run in some families. About 20 percent of people with Crohn's disease have a blood relative with some form of inflammatory bowel disease, most often a brother or sister and sometimes a parent or child.

How does Crohn's disease affect children?

Women with Crohn's disease who are considering having children can be comforted to know that the vast majority of such pregnancies will result in normal children. Research has shown that the course of pregnancy and delivery is usually not impaired in women with Crohn's disease. Even so, it is a good idea for women with Crohn's disease to discuss the matter with their doctors before pregnancy. Children who do get the disease are sometimes more severely affected than adults, with slowed growth and delayed sexual development in some cases.

How is Crohn's disease diagnosed?

If you have experienced chronic abdominal pain, diarrhea, fever, weight loss, and anemia, the doctor will examine you for signs of Crohn's disease. The doctor will take a history and give you a thorough physical exam. This exam will include blood tests to find out if you are anemic as a result of blood loss, or if there is an increased number of white blood cells, suggesting an inflammatory process in your body. Examination of a stool sample can tell the doctor if there is blood loss, or if an infection by a parasite or bacteria is causing the symptoms.

The doctor may look inside your rectum and colon through a flexible tube (endoscope) that is inserted through the anus. During the exam, the doctor may take a sample of tissue (biopsy) from the lining of the colon to look at under the microscope.

Later, you also may receive x-ray examinations of the digestive tract to determine the nature and extent of disease. These exams may include an upper gastrointestinal (GI) series, a small intestinal study, and a barium enema intestinal x-ray. These procedures are done by putting the barium, a chalky solution, into the upper or lower intestines. The barium shows up white on x-ray film, revealing inflammation or ulceration and other abnormalities in the intestine.

If you have Crohn's disease, you may need medical care for a long time. Your doctor also will want to test you regularly to check on your condition.

What is the treatment?

Several drugs are helpful in controlling Crohn's disease, but at this time there is no cure. The usual goals of therapy are to correct nutritional deficiencies; to control inflammation; and to relieve abdominal pain, diarrhea, and rectal bleeding.

Abdominal cramps and diarrhea may be helped by drugs. The drug sulfasalazine often lessens the inflammation, especially in the colon. This drug can be used for as long as needed, and it can be used along with other drugs. Side effects such as nausea, vomiting, weight loss, heartburn, diarrhea, and headache occur in a small percentage of cases. Patients who do not do well on sulfasalazine often do very well on related drugs known as mesalamine or 5-ASA agents. More serious cases may require steroid drugs, antibiotics, or drugs that affect the body's immune system such as azathioprine or 6-mercaptopurine (6-MP).

Can diet control Crohn's disease?

No special diet has been proven effective for preventing or treating this disease. Some people find their symptoms are made worse by milk, alcohol, hot spices, or fiber. But there are no hard and fast rules for most people. Follow a good nutritious diet and try to avoid any foods that seem to make your symptoms worse. Large doses of vitamins are useless and may even cause harmful side effects.

Your doctor may recommend nutritional supplements, especially for children with growth retardation. Special high-calorie liquid formulas are sometimes used for this purpose. A small number of patients may need periods of feeding by vein. This can help patients who temporarily need extra nutrition, those whose bowels need to rest, or those whose bowels cannot absorb enough nourishment from food taken by mouth.

What are the complications of Crohn's disease?

The most common complication is blockage (obstruction) of the intestine. Blockage occurs because the disease tends to thicken the bowel wall with swelling and fibrous scar tissue, narrowing the passage. Crohn's disease also may cause deep ulcer tracts that burrow all the way through the bowel wall into surrounding tissues, into adjacent segments of intestine, into other nearby organs such as the urinary bladder or vagina, or into the skin. These tunnels are called fistulas. They are a common complication and often are associated with pockets of infection or abscesses (infected areas of pus). The areas around the anus and rectum often are involved. Sometimes fistulas can be treated with medicine, but in many cases they must be treated surgically.

Crohn's disease also can lead to complications that affect other parts of the body. These systemic complications include various forms of arthritis, skin problems, inflammation in the eyes or mouth, kidney stones, gallstone, or other diseases of the liver and biliary system. Some of these problems respond to the same treatment as the bowel symptoms, but others must be treated separately.

Is surgery often necessary?

Crohn's disease can be helped by surgery, but it cannot be cured by surgery. The inflammation tends to return in areas of the intestine next to the area that has been removed. Many Crohn's disease patients require surgery, either to relieve chronic symptoms of active disease that does not respond to medical therapy or to correct complications such as intestinal blockage, perforation, abscess, or bleeding. Draining of abscesses or resection (removal of a section of bowel) due to blockage are common surgical procedures.

Sometimes the diseased section of bowel is removed. In this operation, the bowel is cut above and below the diseased area and reconnected. Infrequently some people must have their colons removed (colectomy) and an ileostomy created. In an ileostomy, a small opening is made in the front of the abdominal wall, and the tip of the lower small intestine (ileum) is brought to the skin's surface. This opening, called a stoma, is about the size of a quarter or a 50-cent piece. It usually is located in the right lower corner of the abdomen in the area of the beltline. A bag is worn over the opening the collect waste, and the patient empties the bag periodically. The majority of patients go on to live normal, active lives with an ostomy.

The fact that Crohn's disease often recurs after surgery makes it very important for the patient and doctor to consider carefully the benefits and risks of surgery compared with other treatments. Remember, most people with this disease continue to lead useful and productive lives. Between periods of disease activity, patients may feel quite well and be free of symptoms. Even though there may be long-term needs for medicine and even periods of hospitalization, most patients are able to hold productive jobs, marry, raise families, and function successfully at home and in society.

Additional readings

Brandt, LJ, Steiner-Grossman, P, eds. *Treating IBD: A Patient's Guide to the Medical and Surgical Management of Inflammatory Bowel Disease*. New York: Raven Press, 1989. General guide for patients with sections on treatment and descriptions and drawings of surgical procedures. Available from the Crohn's & Colitis Foundation of America.

Clayman, CB, ed. *The American Medical Association Encyclopedia of Medicine*. New York: Random House, 1989. Reference guide for patients with sections on Crohn's disease and other intestinal disorders. Available in libraries and bookstores.

Lipshutz, WH. Exploring the causes of IBD and Crohn's disease. *Contemporary Gastroenterology* 1991; 4(4): 10-14. Review articles for physicians. Available in medical and university libraries.

Steiner-Grossman, P, Banks PA, Present, DH, eds. *The New People Not Patients: A Source Book for Living with IBD*. Dubuque, Iowa: Kendall/Hunt Publishing Company, 1992. Authoritative book for patients with sections on diagnostic tests, medications, nutrition, coping with employment and health insurance problems, and IBD in children and teenagers, older adults, and during pregnancy. Available from the Crohn's & Colitis Foundation of America.

Tapley, DF, et al., eds. *The Columbia University College of Physicians and Surgeons Complete Home Medical Guide*. New York: Crown Publishers, Inc., 1989. General medical guide with sections on Crohn's disease and other intestinal disorders. Available in libraries and bookstores.

Additional resources

Crohn's and Colitis Foundation of America, Inc., 444 Park Avenue South, 11th floor, New York, NY 10016-7374; (800) 932-2423 or (212) 685-3440.

Ileitis and Colitis Educational Foundation, Central DuPage Hospital, 24 North Winfield Road, Winfield, IL 60190; (708) 682-1600, Ext. 6493.

Wound Ostomy and Continence Nurses Society, 2755 Bristol Street, Suite 110, Costa Mesa, CA 92626; (714) 476-0268.

United Ostomy Association, 36 Executive Park, Suite 120, Irvine, CA 92714; (714) 660-8624.

■ **Document Source:**
U.S. Department of Health and Human Services, Public Health Service
National Institutes of Health
National Institute of Diabetes, and Digestive and Kidney Diseases

See also: Bleeding in the Digestive Tract (page 150); Ulcerative Colitis (page 176)

DD Clearinghouse Fact Sheet
DIVERTICULOSIS AND DIVERTICULITIS

Diverticulosis is a condition in which outpouchings form in the walls of the intestines. These pouches, known as diverticula, are about the size of large peas. They form in weakened areas of the bowels, most often in the lower part of the colon (large bowel).

What are the symptoms of diverticulosis?

Most people with diverticula do not have any symptoms from them. They may never know they have the condition. Some people feel tenderness over the affected area or muscle spasms in the abdomen. Pain may be felt on the lower left side of the abdomen or, less often, in the middle or on the right side.

Although diverticula themselves do not cause symptoms, complications such as bleeding and infection may occur. Bleeding is an uncommon symptom and is usually not severe. Sometimes the pouches become infected and inflamed, a more serious condition known as diverticulitis. When inflammation is present, there may be fever and an increased white blood cell count, as well as acute abdominal pain. Diverticulitis also may result in large abscesses (infected areas of pus), bowel blockage, or breaks and leaks through the bowel wall.

How are these disorders diagnosed?

Often diverticulosis is unsuspected and is discovered by an x-ray or intestinal examination done for an unrelated reason. The doctor may see the diverticula through a flexible tube (colonoscope) that is inserted through the anus. Through this scope, the diverticula may be seen as dark passages leading out of the normal colon wall. The doctor also may do a barium enema, an x-ray that reveals the outpouchings in the walls of the colon.

If rectal bleeding occurs, the doctor may take a special x-ray (angiography). In this procedure, dye is injected into an artery that goes to the colon, so that the site of the bleeding problem can be located. Diverticulitis may be diagnosed when a patient has pain and tenderness in the lower abdomen with disturbed bowel function and fever.

How common are these disorders?

Diverticulosis is very common, especially in older people. Studies show that about 10 percent of people over the age of 40 and nearly half of people over age 60 have diverticulosis. But among those who are found to have diverticula, only about 20 percent develop diverticulitis, and of those, only a small number have very serious or life-threatening complications.

What causes diverticula to form?

No one knows for sure why the pouches form. Scientists think they may be caused by increased pressure inside the colon due to muscle spasms or straining. The sacs might form when increased pressure acts on soft spots along the bowel wall, especially if the person has constipation problems or uses laxatives too often.

How serious are these disorders?

For most people, diverticulosis is not a problem. Diverticulitis, on the other hand, is a problem, sometimes a serious one. For instance, when one of the sacs (a diverticulum) becomes infected and inflamed, bacteria enter small tears in the surface of the bowel. This leads to small abscesses. Such an infection may remain localized and go away within a few days. In rare cases, the infection spreads and breaks through the wall of the colon causing peritonitis (infection of the abdominal cavity) or abscesses in the abdomen. Such infections are very serious and can lead to death unless treated without delay.

What are the treatments?

If you have diverticulosis with no symptoms, no treatment is needed. Some doctors advise eating a high-fiber diet and avoiding certain foods. Laxatives and enemas should not be used regularly. Patients with diverticulitis may be hospitalized and treated with bed rest, pain relievers, antibiotics, fluids given by vein, and careful monitoring.

Is surgery ever necessary?

The majority of patients will recover from diverticulitis without surgery. Sometimes patients need surgery to drain an abscess that has resulted from a ruptured diverticulum and to remove that portion of the colon. Surgery is reserved for patients with very severe or multiple attacks. In those cases, the involved segment of colon can be removed and the colon rejoined.

In some cases, the two ends of the colon cannot be rejoined right away, so more than one operation is needed. For instance, an operation may be performed to drain an abscess and remove diseased colon and a second operation done to rejoin the colon. In this case, the surgeon must connect the colon to a surgically created hole on the body's surface (colostomy) until a second operation can be done to reconnect the colon.

The delay between operations may be only a few weeks, or it might be several months if the patient needs time to overcome infection and build up strength. In rare cases, three operations are needed: the first to drain an abscess, the second to remove part of the colon, and the third to rejoin the bowel.

What about diet?

If you have diverticulosis with no symptoms, you don't need treatment, but it is a good idea to watch your diet. The diet some doctors recommend is the same kind that is healthy for most people—eat more foods high in fiber. (See *Diet, Nutrition & Cancer Prevention: The Good News* in the additional readings section.) A fiber-rich diet helps prevent constipation and promotes a healthy digestive tract. Fiber-rich foods include whole-grain cereals and breads, fruits, and vegetables. A fiber-rich diet is also thought to help prevent diverticula from forming.

Remember, diverticula usually cause no problems at all, so a diagnosis of diverticulosis should not be a serious concern.

Additional readings

Diet, Nutrition & Cancer Prevention: The Good News (NIH Publication No. 87-2878). Pamphlet available from the Cancer Information Service, Office of Cancer Communications, National Cancer Institute, 9000 Rockville Pike, Bethesda, MD 20892. 1-800-4-CANCER. Discusses high-fiber diet and fiber-rich foods.

Diverticulitis and Diverticulosis. Fact sheets available from the National Organization for Rare Disorders, Inc., P.O. Box 8923, New Fairfield, CT 06812-1783. (203) 746-6518.

Ertan A. Colonic Diverticulitis: recognizing and managing its presentations and complications. *Postgraduate Medicine* 1990; 88(3): 67-72, 77. This article for primary care physicians discusses how to recognize, evaluate, and manage diverticulitis.

Larson DE, Editor-in-chief. *Mayo Clinic Family Health Book.* New York: William Morrow and Company, Inc., 1990. General medical guide with section on diverticular disease. Available in libraries and bookstores.

Weck E. New hope for those with diverticular disease. *FDA Consumer* 1987; 21(6): 23-5. Article reprint available from the Food and Drug Administration, 5600 Fishers Lane, Rockville, MD 20857 or in libraries.

■ Document Source:
   U.S. Department of Health and Human Services, Public Health Service
   National Institutes of Health
   National Institute of Diabetes, and Digestive and Kidney Diseases
   NIH Publication 92-1163
   Reprinted October 1991

DD Clearinghouse Fact Sheet

HEMORRHOIDS

Hemorrhoids are swollen veins. Each of us has veins around the anus that tend to stretch under pressure, somewhat like varicose veins in the legs. When these veins swell, we call them "hemorrhoids." One set of veins is inside the rectum (internal), and another is under the skin around the anus (external).

Hemorrhoids also are known as "piles." As a rule, they do not cause pain or bleeding. Problems can occur, however, when these veins become swollen because pressure is raised in them. Increased pressure may result from straining to move your bowels, from sitting too long on the toilet, or from other factors such as pregnancy, obesity, or liver disease.

What are the symptoms of hemorrhoids?

The only sign you may notice from internal hemorrhoids is bright red blood on the toilet paper or in the toilet bowl. Sometimes, however, these veins stretch, and may even fall down (prolapse) through the anus to outside the body (protruding hemorrhoids). When this happens, the vein may become irritated and painful.

The set of veins around the anus causes problems when blood clots form in them, and they become large and painful. (These are called thrombosed external hemorrhoids.) You may notice bleeding and a tender lump on the edge of the anus. Bleeding starts when the swollen veins are scratched or broken by straining or rubbing. People who have external hemorrhoids may feel itching at the anus too. This might result from draining mucus and irritation caused by too much rubbing or cleaning of the anus.

How common are problems with hemorrhoids?

Hemorrhoidal problems are very common in men and in women. About half of people have hemorrhoids to some extent by the age of 50. Many people have bleeding from hemorrhoids sometimes, but most often the bleeding is not serious. Women may begin to have problems during pregnancy. The pressure of the fetus in the abdomen, as well as hormonal changes, causes hemorrhoidal veins to enlarge. These veins also are placed under severe pressure during the birth of the baby. For most women, however, such hemorrhoids are a temporary problem.

What is the treatment?

Often all that is needed to reduce symptoms is to include more fiber in your diet to soften the stool. Eat more fresh fruits, leafy vegetables, whole grain breads and cereals (especially bran). Drinking six to eight glasses of fluid (*not* alcohol) each day will also help. Softer stools make it easier to empty the bowels and lessen pressure on the veins.

Good hygiene is also important. Bathe the anus gently after each bowel movement using soft, moist toilet paper (or a commercial moist pad). Avoid a lot of wiping. If necessary, you can even use the shower as an alternative to wiping. After bathing, dry the anus gently.

When do I need to see my doctor?

It is a good idea to see your doctor any time you see bleeding from the anus. This is important to make sure you don't have cancer or some other disease of the digestive system. You will need an examination of your anus and rectum and possibly further examination of the bowel. If the doctor finds hemorrhoids, you may be advised to change your diet or to use a laxative that provides fiber and softens the stool. Your doctor might only recommend ice, warm soaks (sitz bath), or rest in bed.

If you know you are having pain from hemorrhoids, you might try putting cold packs on the anus, followed by a sitz bath, three or four times a day. To protect against irritation, cleanse the anus carefully and apply zinc oxide paste (or powder) or petroleum jelly to the area. Medicated suppositories also are available at the drug store. Any of these home treatments may relieve the symptoms, and no other treatment may be needed. If symptoms persist, see your doctor.

In some cases, internal hemorrhoids that have fallen outside of the anus (prolapsed), or that bleed too much, must be removed. Your doctor may be able to remove them during an outpatient visit to his office or to the hospital.

A number of methods besides the usual surgery with a scalpel can be used to remove or reduce the size of hemorrhoids. The surgeon may decide to use a technique in which a rubber band is put around the base of the hemorrhoid. The band cuts off circulation, and the hemorrhoid withers away within a few days. This technique is used only for internal hemorrhoids. Sometimes a chemical is injected around the vein to shrink the hemorrhoid.

Other methods include the use of freezing, electrical or laser heat, or infrared light to destroy the hemorrhoidal tissue.

How can you prevent hemorrhoids?

The best way to prevent the problem is to pass your bowel movements as soon as possible after the urge occurs. Also, don't sit on the toilet too long. This is the only time that the anus truly relaxes, allowing the veins there to fill with blood. The longer you sit, the longer pressure is put on the hemorrhoids. To avoid constipation, be active. Move around, walk, exercise to help move the stools through your body. Also, adding fiber to your diet reduces straining by helping to produce stools that are softer and easier to pass.

Remember, hemorrhoids usually do not pose a danger to your health. In most cases, hemorrhoidal symptoms will go away naturally within a few days.

Additional readings

Bleeding in the Digestive Tract. 1989. This fact sheet discusses many common causes of bleeding in the digestive tract and related diagnostic procedures and treatment. Available from the National Digestive Diseases Information Clearinghouse, Box NDDIC, 9000 Rockville Pike, Bethesda, Maryland 20892.

Finkel, Asher J., and Jeffrey R. M. Kunz, editors. *The American Medical Association Family Medical Guide.* New York: Random House. 1987. General medical guide with sections on hemorrhoids and other digestive diseases. Widely available in libraries and bookstores.

Rosenfeld, Isadore.*Second Opinion: Your Comprehensive Guide to Treatment.* New York: Bantam Books. 1988. General medical guide with sections on hemorrhoids and other digestive diseases. Available in many libraries.

Smith, Lee E. "Hemorrhoids: A Review of Current Techniques and Management. *Gastroenterology Clinics of North America* 16:1 (March 1987), 79-91. This review article for physicians is written in technical language and is available in medical libraries.

■ Document Source:
U.S. Department of Health and Human Services, Public Health Service
National Institutes of Health
National Institute of Diabetes, and Digestive and Kidney Diseases
NIH Publication No. 91-3021
February 1991

See also: Bleeding in the Digestive Tract (page 150)

DD Clearinghouse Fact Sheet
HIATAL HERNIA

A hernia is a protrusion of an organ through a wall of the cavity in which it is enclosed. In the case of a hiatal hernia, a portion of the stomach protrudes through a teardrop-

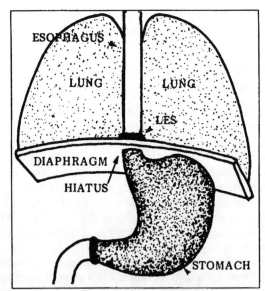

Figure 1a. Schematic drawing of normal state.

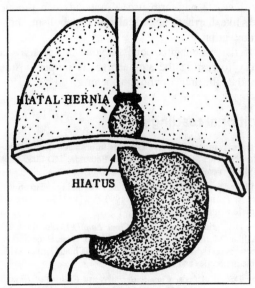

Figure 1b. Schematic drawing of hiatal hernia.

shaped hole in the diaphragm where the esophagus and the stomach join.

What causes hiatal hernia?

The most frequent known cause of hiatal hernia is an increased pressure in the abdominal cavity produced by coughing, vomiting, straining at stool, or sudden physical exertion. Pregnancy, obesity, or excess fluid in the abdomen also contribute to causing this condition.

Who gets hiatal hernia?

Hiatal hernias may develop in people of all ages and both sexes, although it is considered to be a condition of middle age. In fact, the majority of otherwise healthy people past the age of 50 have small hiatal hernias.

Are there any complications associated with hiatal hernia?

Most hiatal hernias do not need treatment. However, if the hernia is in danger of becoming strangulated (constricted in such a way as to cut off the blood supply) or is complicated by esophagitis (inflammation of the esophagus), treatment becomes necessary. To prevent strangulation, your doctor may perform surgery to reduce the size of the hernia.

Treatment of esophagitis is necessary to prevent ulcers (sores) from forming in the lining of the esophagus. When these sores heal, they can leave scars that can make it difficult or impossible to swallow. In some people, long-term esophagitis may result in Barrett's esophagus, a condition thought to be a precursor of cancer. Most cases of esophagitis respond to antacids, weight reduction, and a common sense approach to eating, drinking, and other lifestyle habits. Remember, if prolonged use of antacids becomes necessary, see your doctor. Long-term use of antacids can produce side effects like diarrhea, altered calcium metabolism, and magnesium retention.

If the esophagitis persists, your doctor may perform surgery to restore the stomach to its proper position and strengthen the area around the opening.

Additional readings

Heartburn. National Digestive Diseases Information Clearinghouse, 1986. Box NDDIC, 9000 Rockville Pike, Bethesda, MD 20892. (301) 468-6344. General information fact sheet.

Ellis FH Jr. Diaphragmatic hiatal hernias: recognizing and treating the major types. *Postgraduate Medicine,* 1990; 88(1): 113-24. General review article written for physicians.

Larson DE, Editor-in-chief. *Mayo Clinic Family Health Book.* New York: William Morrow and Company, Inc., 1990. General medical guide with sections on esophageal problems, including hiatal hernia. Widely available in libraries and bookstores.

Tapley DS, et al., eds. *Columbia University College of Physicians and Surgeons Complete Home Medical Guide,* revised edition. New York: Crown Publishers, Inc., 1990. General medical guide with sections on disorders of the esophagus, including hiatal hernia. Widely available in libraries and bookstores.

■ **Document Source:**
U.S. Department of Health and Human Services, Public Health Service
National Institutes of Health
National Institute of Diabetes, and Digestive and Kidney Diseases
NIH Publication No. 92-498
Reprinted October 1991

DD Clearinghouse Fact Sheet

IRRITABLE BOWEL SYNDROME

Irritable bowel syndrome (IBS) is a common disorder of the intestines that leads to crampy pain, gassiness, bloating, and changes in bowel habits. Some people with IBS have constipation (difficult or infrequent bowel movements); others have diarrhea (frequent loose stools, often with an urgent need to move the bowels); and some people experience both. Sometimes the person with IBS has a crampy urge to move the bowels but cannot do so.

Through the years, IBS has been called by many names—colitis, mucous colitis, spastic colon, spastic bowel, and functional bowel disease. Most of these terms are inaccurate. Colitis, for instance, means inflammation of the large intestine (colon). IBS, however, does not cause inflammation and should not be confused with ulcerative colitis, which is a more serious disorder.

The cause of IBS is not known, and as yet there is no cure. Doctors call it a functional disorder because there is no sign of disease when the colon is examined. IBS causes a great deal of discomfort and distress, but it does not cause permanent harm to the intestines and does not lead to intestinal bleeding of the bowel or to a serious disease such as cancer. Often IBS is just a mild annoyance, but for some people it can be disabling. They may be afraid to go to social events, to go out to a job, or to travel even short distances. Most people with IBS, however, are able to control their symptoms through diet, stress management, and sometimes with medications prescribed by their physicians.

What causes IBS?

The colon, which is about 6 feet long, connects the small intestine with the rectum and anus. The major function of the colon is to absorb water and salts from the digestive products that enter from the small intestine. Two quarts of liquid matter enter the colon from the small intestine each day. This material may remain there for several days until most of the fluid and salts are absorbed into the body. The stool then passes through the colon by a pattern of movements to the left side of the colon, where it is stored until a bowel movement occurs.

Colon motility (contraction of intestinal muscles and movement of its contents) is controlled by nerves and hormones and by electrical activity in the colon muscle. The electrical activity serves as a "pacemaker" similar to the mechanism that controls heart function.

Movements of the colon propel the contents slowly back and forth but mainly toward the rectum. A few times each day strong muscle contractions move down the colon pushing fecal material ahead of them. Some of these strong contractions result in a bowel movement.

Because doctors have been unable to find an organic cause, IBS often has been thought to be caused by emotional conflict or stress. While stress may worsen IBS symptoms, research suggests that other factors also are important. Researchers have found that the colon muscle of a person with IBS begins to spasm after only mild stimulation. The person with IBS seems to have a colon that is more sensitive and reactive than usual, so it responds strongly to stimuli that would not bother most people.

Ordinary events such as eating and distention from gas or other material in the colon can cause an overreaction in the person with IBS. Certain medicines and foods may trigger spasms in some people. Sometimes the spasm delays that passage of stool, leading to constipation. Chocolate, milk products, or large amounts of alcohol are frequent offenders. Caffeine causes loose stools in many people, but it is more likely to affect those with IBS. Researchers also have found that women with IBS may have more symptoms during their menstrual periods, suggesting that reproductive hormones can increase IBS symptoms.

What are the symptoms of IBS?

If you are concerned about IBS, it is important to realize that normal bowel function varies from person to person. Normal bowel movements range from as many as three stools a day to as few as three a week. A normal movement is one that is formed but not hard, contains no blood, and is passed without cramps or pain.

People with IBS, on the other hand, usually have crampy abdominal pain with painful constipation or diarrhea. In some people, constipation and diarrhea alternate. Sometimes people with IBS pass mucus with their bowel movements. Bleeding, fever, weight loss, and persistent severe pain are *not* symptoms of IBS but may indicate other problems.

How is IBS diagnosed?

IBS usually is diagnosed after doctors exclude more serious organic diseases. The doctor will take a complete medical history that includes a careful description of symptoms. A physical examination and laboratory test will be done. A stool sample will be tested for evidence of bleeding. The doctor also may do diagnostic procedures such as x-rays or endoscopy (viewing the colon through a flexible tube inserted through the anus) to find out if there is organic disease.

How do diet and stress affect IBS?

The potential for abnormal function of the colon is always present in people with IBS, but a trigger also must be present to cause symptoms. The most likely culprits seem to be diet and emotional stress. Many people report that their symptoms occur following a meal or when they are under stress. No one is sure why this happens, but scientists have some clues.

Eating causes contractions of the colon. Normally, this response may cause an urge to have a bowel movement within 30 to 60 minutes after a meal. In people with IBS, the urge may come sooner with cramps and diarrhea.

The strength of the response is often related to the number of calories in a meal, and especially the amount of fat in a meal. Fat in any form (animal or vegetable) is a strong stimulus of colonic contractions after a meal. Many foods contain fat, especially meats of all kinds, poultry skin, whole milk, cream, cheese, butter, vegetable oil, margarine, shortening, avocados, and whipped toppings.

Stress also stimulates colonic spasm in people with IBS. This process is not completely understood, but scientists point out that the colon is controlled partly by the nervous system. Mental health counseling and stress reduction (re-

laxation training) can help relieve the symptoms of IBS. However, doctors are quick to note that this does not mean IBS is the result of a personality disorder. IBS is at least partly a disorder of colon motility.

How does a good diet help IBS?

For many people, eating a proper diet lessens IBS symptoms. Before changing your diet, it is a good idea to keep a journal noting which foods seem to cause distress. Discuss your findings with your doctor. You also may want to consult a registered dietitian, who can help you make changes in your diet. For instance, if dairy products cause your symptoms to flare up, you can try eating less of those foods. Yogurt might be tolerated better because it contains organisms that supply lactase, the enzyme needed to digest lactose, the sugar found in milk products. Because diary products are an important source of calcium and other nutrients that your body needs, be sure to get adequate nutrients in the foods that you substitute.

Dietary fiber may lessen IBS symptoms in many cases. Whole grain breads and cereals, beans, fruits, and vegetables are good sources of fiber. Consult your doctor before using an over-the-counter fiber supplement. High-fiber diets keep the colon mildly distended, which may help to prevent spasms from developing. Some forms of fiber also keep water in the stools, thereby preventing hard stools that are difficult to pass. Doctors usually recommend that you eat just enough fiber so that you have soft, easily passed, painless bowel movements. High-fiber diets may cause gas and bloating, but within a few weeks, these symptoms often go away as your body adjusts to the diet.

Large meals can cause cramping and diarrhea in people with IBS. Symptoms may be eased if you eat smaller meals more often or just eat smaller portions. This should help, especially if your meals are low in fat and high in carbohydrates such as pasta, rice, whole-grain breads and cereals, fruits, and vegetables.

Can medicine relieve IBS symptoms?

There is no standard way of treating IBS. Your doctor may prescribe fiber supplements or occasional laxatives if you are constipated. Some doctors prescribe antispasmodic drugs or tranquilizers, which may relieve symptoms. Antidepressant drugs also are used sometimes in patients who are depressed.

The major concerns with drug therapy of IBS are the potential for drug dependency and the effects the disorder can have on lifestyle. In an effort to control their bowels or reduce stress, some people become dependent on laxatives or tranquilizers. If this happens, doctors try to withdraw the drugs slowly.

How is IBS linked to more serious problems?

IBS has not been shown to lead to any serious, organic diseases. No link has been established between IBS and inflammatory bowel diseases such as Crohn's disease or ulcerative colitis. IBS does not lead to cancer. Some patients have a more severe form of IBS, and the fear of pain and diarrhea may cause them to withdraw from normal activities. In such cases, doctors may recommend mental health counseling.

Additional readings

Scanlon, D, Becnel, B. *Wellness Book of IBS.* New York: St. Martin's Press, 1989. Practical patient's guide to coping with IBS written by a registered dietitian. Available in libraries and bookstores.

Shimberg, E. *Relief From IBS.* New York: M. Evans and Company, 1988. Practical book for patients offers information about IBS symptoms, diet, treatment, and self-care. Available in libraries and bookstores.

Steinhart, MJ. Irritable bowel syndrome: How to relieve symptoms enough to improve daily function. *Postgraduate Medicine* 1992; 91(6): 315-321. Article for primary care physicians includes information about relief of IBS symptoms. Available in medical and university libraries.

Thompson, WG. *Gut reactions: Understanding symptoms of the digestive tract.* New York: Plenum Publishing Corp., 1989. Clear, concise book by a digestive diseases specialist gives advice about diagnosis, diet, and treatment of IBS. Available in libraries and bookstores.

■ Document Source:
U.S. Department of Health and Human Services, Public Health Service
National Institutes of Health
National Institute of Diabetes, and Digestive and Kidney Diseases
NIH Publication No. 92-693
October 1992

DD Clearinghouse Fact Sheet

LACTOSE INTOLERANCE

Lactose intolerance is the inability to digest significant amounts of lactose, which is the predominant sugar of milk. Close to 50 million American adults are lactose intolerant. Certain ethnic and racial populations are more widely affected than others. As many as 75 percent of all African-American, Jewish, Native American, and Mexican-American adults, and 90 percent of Asian-American adults are lactose intolerant. The condition is least common among persons of northern European descent.

Lactose intolerance results from a shortage of the enzyme lactase, which is normally produced by the cells that line the small intestine. Lactase breaks down milk sugar into simpler forms that can then be absorbed into the bloodstream. When there is not enough lactase to digest the amount of lactose consumed, the results, although not usually dangerous, may be very distressing.

Common symptoms include nausea, cramps, bloating, gas, and diarrhea, which begin about 30 minutes to 2 hours after eating or drinking foods containing lactose. Many people who never have been diagnosed as lactose intolerant or "lactase deficient" may notice that milk and other diary products cause problems that don't occur when eating other foods. The severity of symptoms varies depending on the amount of lactose each individual can tolerate.

Some causes of lactose intolerance are well known. For instance, certain digestive diseases and injuries to the small intestine can reduce the amount of enzymes produced. In rare cases, children are born without the ability to produce lactase. For most people, though, lactase deficiency is a condition that develops naturally, over time. After about the age of 2 years, the body begins to produce less lactase. The reasons for this are unclear and still under study.

Diagnostic Tests

The most common tests used to measure the absorption of lactose in the digestive system are the lactose tolerance test, the hydrogen breath test, and the stool acidity test. A doctor can tell you where to go for these tests, which are performed on an outpatient basis at a hospital or clinic.

The *lactose tolerance* test can be given to older children as well as adults. Before the test, patients fast (do not eat), and blood is drawn to measure the fasting blood glucose (blood sugar) level. Patients then drink a large amount of a liquid that contains 50 grams of lactose. Blood samples are taken over a 2-hour period to determine the glucose level, which tells how well the body is able to digest lactose. When the lactose reaches the digestive system, the lactase enzyme breaks the lactose down into glucose and galactose. The liver then changes the galactose into glucose. If this process occurs normally, the glucose enters the bloodstream and raises the fasting blood glucose level. If lactose is incompletely absorbed, the blood glucose level does not rise, and a diagnosis of lactose intolerance is confirmed.

The *hydrogen breath test* measures the amount of hydrogen in the breath. Normally, no hydrogen is detectable in the breath. However, undigested lactose leads to the formation of various gases, including hydrogen, by bacteria in the colon. The hydrogen is absorbed from the intestines, carried through the bloodstream to the lungs, and exhaled. In the test, the patient drinks a lactose-loaded beverage, and the breath is analyzed at regular intervals. Hydrogen in the breath means improper digestion of lactose. Certain foods, medications, and smoking can affect the test's accuracy and may need to be avoided before.

The lactose tolerance and hydrogen breath tests are not given to infants and young children who are suspected of having lactose intolerance. Giving these patients a lactose load may be dangerous because they are more prone to the dehydration that can result from the diarrhea caused by the lactose. If a baby or young child is experiencing symptoms of lactose intolerance, many pediatricians simply recommend changing from cow's milk to soy formula and waiting for a decrease in symptoms.

If necessary, a *stood acidity test*, which measures the amount of acid in the stool and presents no risk to young children, may be given. Undigested lactose fermented by colon bacteria creates lactic acid and other short-chain fatty acids that can be detected in a stool sample. In addition, glucose may be present in the sample as a result of unabsorbable lactose in the colon.

Treatment = Control of Symptoms

Fortunately, lactose intolerance is relatively easy to treat. No known way exists to increase the amount of lactase enzyme the body can make, but symptoms can be controlled through diet.

Small children born with lactase deficiency should not be fed any foods containing lactose. Most older children and adults need not avoid lactose completely, but individuals differ in the amounts of lactose they can handle. For example, one person may suffer symptoms after drinking a small glass of milk, while another can drink one glass but not two. Others may be able to manage ice cream and aged cheeses, such as cheddar and Swiss, but not other dairy products. Dietary control of the problem depends on each person's knowing, through trial and error, *how much* milk sugar and *what forms* of it his or her body can handle.

For those who react to very small amounts of lactose or have trouble limiting their intake of foods that contain lactose, lactase additives are available from drug stores without a prescription. One form is a liquid for use with milk. A few drops are added to a quart of milk, and after 24 hours in the refrigerator, the lactose content is reduced by 70 percent. The process works faster if the milk is heated first, and adding a double amount of lactase liquid produced milk that is 90 percent lactose free. A more recent development is a lactase tablet that helps people digest solid foods that contain lactose. One to three tablets are taken just before a meal or snack.

At somewhat higher cost, shoppers can buy lactose-reduced milk at most supermarkets. The milk contains all of the other nutrients found in regular milk and remains fresh for about the same length of time.

A Nutrition Balancing Act

Milk and other dairy products are a major source of nutrients in the basic American diet. The most important of these nutrients is calcium. Calcium is needed for the growth and repair of bones throughout life, and in the middle and later years, a shortage of calcium may lead to thin, fragile bones that break easily (a condition called "osteoporosis"). A concern, then, for both children and adults with lactose intolerance is how to get enough calcium in a diet that includes little or no milk.

Although the RDA (recommended dietary allowance) for calcium, set in 1980, is 800 mg per day, many experts in bone disease believe this is too low. The results of a 1984 conference at the National Institutes of Health (NIH) suggest that women who have not yet reached menopause and older women who are taking the hormone estrogen after menopause should consume about 1,000 mg of calcium daily (roughly the amount in a quarter of milk). Pregnant women and nursing mothers need about 1,200 mg of calcium per day. Postmenopausal women not taking estrogen may need as much as 1,500 mg of calcium per day. The RDA for adult men is 1,000 mg per day and 1,500 mg per day for men in their later years.

It is important, therefore, in meal planning to make sure that each day's diet includes enough calcium, even if the diet does not contain dairy products. Quite a few foods are high in calcium and low in lactose. Many green vegetables and fish with soft, edible bones are excellent examples.

Recent research has shown that yogurt may be a very good source of calcium for many lactose intolerant people,

even though it is fairly high in lactose. There is evidence that the bacterial cultures used in making yogurt produce the lactase required for proper digestion.

Clearly, many foods can provide the calcium and other nutrients the body needs, even when intake of milk and dairy products is limited. Still, factors other than calcium and lactose content should be kept in mind when planning a diet. Some vegetables that are high in calcium (Swiss chard, spinach, and rhubarb, for instance) cannot use their calcium content. They contain substances called oxalates, which stop the calcium absorption. Remember also that calcium is absorbed and used only when there is enough vitamin D in the body. A balanced diet should provide an adequate supply of vitamin D.

Some people with lactose intolerance may think they are not getting enough calcium and vitamin D in their diet. A doctor is the best person to decide whether any dietary supplements are needed. Taking vitamins or minerals of the wrong kind or in the wrong amounts can be harmful. A dietitian can help in planning meals that will provide the most nutrients with the least chance of causing discomfort.

Calcium and Lactose in Common Foods

	Calcium Content*	Lactose Content**
Vegetables		
Broccoli (pieces cooked), 1 cup	94-177 mg	0
Chinese cabbage (bok choy, cooked), 1 cup	158 mg	0
Collard greens (cooked), 1 cup	148-357 mg	0
Kale (cooked), 1 cup	94-179 mg	0
Turnip greens (cooked), 1 cup	194-249 mg	0
Dairy Products		
Ice cream/ice milk, 8 oz.	176 mg	6-7 g
Milk (whole, low-fat, skim, buttermilk), 8 oz.	291-316 mg	12-313 g
Processed cheese, 1 oz.	159-219 mg	2-3 g
Sour cream, 4 oz.	134 mg	4-5 g
Yogurt (plain) 8 oz.	274-415 mg	12-13 g
Fish/Seafood		
Oysters (raw), 1 cup	226 mg	0
Salmon with bones (canned), 3 oz.	167 mg	0
Sardines, 3 oz.	371 mg	0
Shrimp (canned), 3 oz.	98 mg	0
Other		
Molasses, 2 tbsp.	274 mg	0
Tofu (processed with calcium salts), 3 oz.	225 mg	0

*Nutritive Value of Foods. Values vary with methods of processing and preparation.

**Derived from *Lactose Intolerance: A Resource Including Recipes,* Food Sensitivity Series, American Dietetic Association, 1985.

Watch for Hidden Lactose

Although milk and foods made from milk are the only noteworthy natural sources, lactose is often added to prepared foods. It is important for people with very low tolerance for lactose to know about the many foods that may contain lactose, even in small amounts. Grocery items that may contain lactose include:

♦ Bread and other baked goods.
♦ Processed breakfast cereals.
♦ Instant potatoes, soups, and breakfast drinks.
♦ Margarine.
♦ Lunch meats (other than kosher).
♦ Salad dressings.
♦ Candies and other snacks.
♦ Mixes for pancakes, biscuits, cookies, etc.

Some so-called nondairy products such as powdered coffee creamer and whipped topping also may include ingredients that are derived from milk and therefore contain lactose.

Smart shoppers learn to read foods labels with care, looking not only for *milk* and *lactose* among the contents but also for such words as whey, curds, milk byproducts, dry milk solids, and nonfat dry milk powder. If any of these are listed on a label, the item contains lactose.

In addition, lactose is used as the base for more than 20 percent of prescription drugs and about 6 percent of over-the-counter medicines. Many types of birth control pills, for example, contain lactose, as do some tablets for stomach acid and gas. A pharmacist can answer questions about the amounts of lactose in various medicines.

Summary

Even though lactose intolerance is a widespread problem, it need not pose a serious threat to good health. People who have trouble digesting lactose can learn, by testing themselves, which dairy products and other foods they can eat without discomfort and which ones they should avoid. Many will be able to enjoy milk, ice cream, and other such products if they take them in small amounts or eat other kinds of food at the same time. Others can use lactase liquid or tablets to help digest the lactose. Even older women and children who must avoid milk and foods made with milk can meet most of their special dietary needs by eating greens, fish, and other calcium-rich foods that are free of lactose. A carefully chosen diet (with calcium supplements if the doctor recommends them) is the key to reducing symptoms and protecting future health.

Additional Resources

American Dietetic Association. *Lactose Intolerance: A Resource Including Recipes,* Food Sensitivity Series (1985). American Dietetic Association, 216 West Jackson Blvd., Chicago, Illinois 60606. (312) 899-0040.

Martens, Richard A., and Martens, Sherlyn. *The Milk Sugar Dilemma: Living With Lactose Intolerance* (1987). Medi-Ed Press, P.O. Box 957, East Lansing, Michigan 48826-0957.

Zukin, Jane. *Dairy-free Cookbook* (1989). St. Martin's Press, 175 Fifth Avenue, New York, New York 10010. (212) 674-5151.

Zukin, Jane. *The Newsletter for People with Lactose Intolerance and Milk Allergy.* Commercial Writing Service, P.O. Box 3074, Iowa City, Iowa 52244.

■ **Document Source:**
U.S. Department of Health and Human Services, Public Health Service
National Institutes of Health
National Institute of Diabetes, and Digestive and Kidney Diseases
NIH Publication No. 91-2751
1991

DD Clearinghouse Fact Sheet

PANCREATITIS

Your pancreas is a large gland behind your stomach and close to your duodenum. The pancreas secretes powerful digestive enzymes that enter the small intestine through a duct. These enzymes help you digest fats, proteins, and carbohydrates. The pancreas also releases the hormones insulin and glucagon into the bloodstream. These hormones play an important part in metabolizing sugar.

Pancreatitis is a rare disease in which the pancreas becomes inflamed. Damage to the gland occurs when digestive enzymes are activated and begin attacking the pancreas. In severe cases, there may be bleeding into the gland, serious tissue damage, infection, and cysts. Enzymes and toxins may enter the bloodstream and seriously injure organs, such as the heart, lungs, and kidney.

There are two forms of pancreatitis. The acute form occurs suddenly and may be a severe, life-threatening illness with many complications. Usually, the patient recovers completely. If injury to the pancreas continues, such as when a patient persists in drinking alcohol, a chronic form of the disease may develop, bringing severe pain and reduced functioning of the pancreas that affects digestion and causes weight loss.

What is acute pancreatitis?

An estimated 50,000 to 80,000 cases of acute pancreatitis occur in the United States each year. This disease occurs when the pancreas suddenly becomes inflamed and then gets better. Some patients have more than one attack but recover fully after each one. Most cases of acute pancreatitis are caused either by alcohol abuse or by gallstones. Other causes may be use of prescribed drugs, trauma or surgery to the abdomen, or abnormalities of the pancreas or intestine. In rare cases, the disease may result from infections, such as mumps. In about 15 percent of cases, the cause is unknown.

What are the symptoms of acute pancreatitis?

Acute pancreatitis usually begins with pain in the upper abdomen, that may last for a few days. The pain is often severe. It may be constant pain, just in the abdomen, or it may reach to the back and other areas. The pain may be sudden and intense, or it may begin as a mild pain that is aggravated by eating and slowly grows worse. The abdomen may be swollen and very tender. Other symptoms may include nausea, vomiting, fever, and an increased pulse rate. The person often feels and looks very sick.

About 20 percent of cases are severe. The patient may become dehydrated and have low blood pressure. Sometimes the patient's heart, lungs, or kidneys fail. In the most severe cases, bleeding can occur in the pancreas, leading to shock and sometimes death.

How is acute pancreatitis diagnosed?

During acute attacks, high levels of amylase (a digestive enzymes formed in the pancreas) are found in the blood. Changes also may occur in blood levels of calcium, magnesium, sodium, potassium, and bicarbonate. Patients may have high amounts of sugar and lipids (fats) in their blood too. These changes help the doctor diagnose pancreatitis. After the pancreas recovers, blood levels of these substances usually return to normal.

What is the treatment for acute pancreatitis?

The treatment a patient receives depends on how bad the attack is. Unless complications occur, acute pancreatitis usually gets better on its own, so treatment is supportive in most cases. Usually the patient goes into the hospital. The doctor prescribes fluids by vein to restore blood volume. The kidneys and lungs may be treated to prevent failure of those organs. Other problems, such as cysts in the pancreas, may need treatment too.

Sometimes a patient cannot control vomiting and needs to have a tube through the nose to the stomach to remove fluid and air. In mild cases, the patient may not have food for 3 or 4 days but is given fluids and pain relievers by vein. An acute attack usually lasts only a few days, unless the ducts are blocked by gallstones. In severe cases, the patient may be fed through the veins for 3 to 6 weeks while the pancreas slowly heals.

Antibiotics may be given is signs of infection arise. Surgery may be needed if complications such as infection, cysts, or bleeding occur. Attacks caused by gallstones may require removal of the gallbladder or surgery of the bile duct.

Surgery is sometimes needed for the doctor to be able to exclude other abdominal problems than can simulate pancreatitis or to treat acute pancreatitis. When there is severe injury with death of tissue, an operation may be done to remove the dead tissue.

After all signs of acute pancreatitis are gone, the doctor will determine the cause and try to prevent future attacks. In some patients the cause of the attack is clear, but in others further tests need to be done.

What if the patient has gallstones?

Ultrasound is used to detect gallstones and sometimes can provide the doctor with an idea of how severe the pancreatitis is. When gallstones are found, surgery is usually needed to remove them. When they are removed depends on how severe the pancreatitis is. If it is mild, the gallstones often can be removed within a week or so. In most severe cases, the patient may wait a month or more, until he improves, before the stones are removed. The CAT (computer axial tomograph) scan also may be used to find out what is happening in and around the pancreas and how severe the problem is. This is important information that the doctor needs to determine when to remove the gallstones.

After the gallstones are removed and inflammation subsides, the pancreas usually returns to normal. Before patients leave the hospital, they are advised not to drink alcohol and not to eat large meals.

What is chronic pancreatitis?

Chronic pancreatitis usually follows many years of alcohol abuse. It may develop after only one acute attack, especially if there is damage to the ducts of the pancreas. In the early stages, the doctor cannot always tell whether the patient has acute or chronic disease. The symptoms may be the same. Damage to the pancreas from drinking alcohol may cause no symptoms for many years, and then the patient suddenly has an attack of pancreatitis. In more than 90 percent of adult patients, chronic pancreatitis appears to be caused by alcoholism. This is more common in men than women and often develops between 30 and 40 years of age. In other cases, pancreatitis may be inherited. Scientists do not know why the inherited form occurs. Patients with chronic pancreatitis tend to have three kinds of problems: pain, malabsorption of food leading to weight loss, or diabetes.

Some patients do not have any pain, but most do. Pain may be constant in the back and abdomen, and for some patients, the pain attacks are disabling. In some cases, the abdominal pain goes away as the condition advances. Doctors think this happens because pancreatic enzymes are no longer being made by the pancreas.

Patients with this disease often lose weight, even when their appetite and eating habits are normal. This occurs because the body does not secrete enough pancreatic enzymes to break down food, so nutrients are not absorbed normally. Poor digestion leads to loss of fat, protein, and sugar into the stool. Diabetes may also develop at this stage if the insulin-producing cells of the pancreas (islet cells) have been damaged.

How is chronic pancreatitis diagnosed?

Diagnosis may be difficult but is aided by a number of new techniques. Pancreatic function tests help the physician decide if the pancreas still can make enough digestive enzymes. The doctor can see abnormalities in the pancreas using several techniques (ultrasonic imaging, endoscopic retrograde cholangiopancreatography (ERCP), and the CAT scan). In more advanced stages of the disease, when diabetes and malabsorption (a problem due to lack of enzymes) occur, the doctor can use a number of blood, urine, and stool tests to help in the diagnosis of chronic pancreatitis and to monitor the progression of the disorder.

How is chronic pancreatitis treated?

The doctor treats chronic pancreatitis by relieving pain and managing the nutritional and metabolic problems. The patient can reduce the amount of fat and protein lost in stools by cutting back on dietary fat and taking pills containing pancreatic enzymes. This will result in better nutrition and weight gain. Sometimes insulin or other drugs must be given to control the patient's blood sugar.

In some cases, surgery is needed to relieve pain by draining an enlarged pancreatic duct. Sometimes, part or most of the pancreas is removed in an attempt to relieve chronic pain.

Patients must stop drinking, adhere to their prescribed diets, and take the proper medications in order to have fewer and milder attacks.

Additional reading

Banks PA, Frey CF, Greenberger NJ. The spectrum of chronic pancreatitis. *Patient Care*, 1989; 23(9): 163-96. This review article for physicians is written in technical language. Available in medical libraries.

Facts and Fallacies About Digestive Diseases. 1991. This fact sheet discusses commonly held beliefs about digestive diseases, including pancreatitis and gallbladder disease. Available from the National Digestive Diseases Information Clearinghouse, Box NDDIC, 9000 Rockville Pike, Bethesda, MD 20892. (301) 468-6344.

Clayman CB, ed. *The American Medical Association Encyclopedia of Medicine*. New York: Random House. 1989. Authoritative reference guide for patients with sections on irritable bowel syndrome and other disorders of the digestive system. Widely available in libraries and bookstores.

Frey CF, et al. Progress in acute pancreatitis. *Patient Care*, 1989; 23(5): 38-53. This review article for physicians is written in technical language. Available in medical libraries.

■ **U.S. Department of Health and Human Services, Public Health Service**
National Institutes of Health
National Institute of Diabetes, and Digestive and Kidney Diseases
NIH Publication No. 91-1596
Revised September 1991

CancerFax from the National Cancer Institute
RECTAL CANCER

Description

What Is Cancer of the Rectum?

Cancer of the rectum, a common form of cancer, is a disease in which cancer (malignant) cells are found in the tissues of the rectum. The rectum is part of the body's digestive system. The purpose of the digestive system is to remove nutrients (vitamins, minerals, and proteins) from the food you eat and to store the waste until it passes out of the body. The digestive system is made up of the esophagus, stomach, and the small and large intestines. The last 6 feet of intestine is called the large bowel or colon. The last 8 to 10 inches of the colon is the rectum.

Like all cancer, cancer of the rectum is best treated when it is found (diagnosed) early. Because of this, screening tests (such as a rectal exam, proctoscopy, and colonoscopy) may be done regularly in patients who are at higher risk to get cancer. These tests may be done in patients who are over age 50; who have a family history of cancer of the colon, rectum, or of the female organs; or who have a history of ulcerative colitis (ulcers in the lining of the large intestines). Your doctor may order these tests to look for cancer if you have a change in bowel habits or if you have any bleeding from your rectum.

Your doctor will usually begin by giving you a rectal exam. In a rectal exam your doctor, wearing thin gloves, puts a greased finger into the rectum and gently feels for lumps. Your doctor may then check the material to see if there is any blood in it.

Your doctor may also want to look inside the rectum and lower colon with a special instrument called a sigmoidoscope or proctosigmoidoscope. This exam, called a proctoscopy or procto exam, finds about half of all colon and rectal cancers. The test is usually done in a doctor's office. You may feel some pressure, but you usually do not feel pain.

Your doctor may also want to look inside the rectum and the entire colon (colonoscopy) with a special tool called a colonoscope. This test is also done in a doctor's office. You may feel some pressure but usually no pain.

If tissue that is not normal is found, the doctor will need to cut out a small piece and look at it under the microscope to see if there are any cancer cells. This is called a biopsy. Biopsies are usually done during the proctoscopy or colonoscopy in a doctor's office.

Your prognosis (chance of recovery) and choice of treatment depend on the stage of your cancer (whether it is just in the inner lining of your rectum or if it has spread to other places) and your general state of health.

Stage Explanation

Stages of Cancer of the Rectum

Once cancer of the rectum is found (diagnosed), more tests will be done to find out if cancer cells have spread to other parts of the body (staging). Your doctor needs to know the stage of your disease to plan treatment. The following stages are used for cancer of the rectum:

Stage 0 or carcinoma in situ
Stage 0 cancer of the rectum is very early cancer. Cancer is found only in the top lining of the rectum.

Stage I
Cancer has spread beyond the top lining of the rectum to the second and third layers and involves the inside wall of the rectum, but has not spread to the outer wall of the rectum or outside the rectum.

Stage I cancer of the rectum is sometimes called Dukes A rectal cancer.

Stage II

Cancer has spread outside the rectum to nearby tissue, but it has not gone into the lymph nodes. (Lymph nodes are small, bean-shaped structures that are found throughout the body. They produce and store cells that fight infection.)

Stage II cancer of the rectum is sometimes called Dukes B rectal cancer.

Stage III

Cancer has spread to nearby lymph nodes, but it has not spread to other parts of the body.

Stage III cancer of the rectum is sometimes called Dukes C rectal cancer.

Stage IV

Cancer has spread to other parts of the body.

Stage IV cancer of the rectum is sometimes called Dukes D rectal cancer.

Recurrent

Recurrent disease means that the cancer has come back (recurred) after it has been treated. It may come back in the rectum or in another part of the body. Recurrent cancer of the rectum is often found in the liver and/or lungs.

Treatment Options Overview

How Cancer of the Rectum Is Treated

There are treatments for all patients with cancer of the rectum. Three kinds of treatments are available:

surgery (taking out the cancer)
radiation therapy (using high-dose x-rays or other high-energy rays to kill cancer cells)
chemotherapy (using drugs to kill cancer cells).

Surgery is the most common treatment for all stages of cancer of the rectum.

Your doctor may take out the cancer from the rectum using one of the following:

♦ If your cancer is found at a very early stage, your doctor may take out the cancer without cutting into your abdomen. Instead, your doctor may put a tube into the rectum and cut the cancer out. This is called a local excision. Sometimes, the doctor may take out the cancer using high-energy electricity. This is called electrofulguration.

♦ If your cancer is larger, your doctor will take out the cancer and a small amount of healthy tissue around it. The healthy parts of the rectum are then sewn together (anastomosis). If only a small amount of tissue is removed, this is called a wedge resection. If a larger amount of tissue is removed, this is called a bowel resection. Your doctor will also take out lymph nodes near the rectum and look at them under the microscope to see if they contain cancer.

♦ If your doctor is not able to sew your rectum back together, he or she will make an opening (stoma) on the outside of the body for waste to pass out of the body. This is called a colostomy. Sometimes, the colostomy is only needed until the colon has healed, and then it can be reversed. However, your doctor may

have to take out the entire rectum and make the colostomy permanent. If you have a colostomy, you will need to wear a special bag to collect body wastes. This special bag, which sticks to the skin around the stoma with a special glue, can be thrown away after it is used. This bag does not show under clothing, and most people take care of these bags themselves.

Radiation therapy uses x-rays or other high-energy rays to kill cancer cells and shrink tumors. Radiation may come from a machine outside the body (external radiation therapy) or from putting materials that contain radiation through thin plastic tubes (internal radiation therapy) in the intestine area. Radiation can be used alone or in addition to surgery and/or chemotherapy.

Chemotherapy uses drugs to kill cancer cells. Chemotherapy may be taken by pill, or it may be put into the body by a needle in a vein. Chemotherapy is called a systemic treatment because the drug enters the bloodstream, travels through the body, and can kill cancer cells outside the rectum.

If your doctor removes all the cancer that can be seen at the time of the operation, you may be given chemotherapy after surgery to kill any cancer cells that are left. Chemotherapy given after an operation to a person who has no cancer cells that can be seen is called adjuvant chemotherapy.

Biological treatment tries to get your own body to fight cancer. It uses materials made by your own body or made in a laboratory to boost, direct, or restore your body's natural defenses against disease. Biological treatment is sometimes called biological response modifier (BRM) therapy.

Treatment by Stage

Treatments for cancer of the rectum depend on the stage of your disease and your overall condition.

You may receive treatments that have been proven effective in past studies, or you may choose to go into a clinical trial. Clinical trials are done to find better ways to treat cancer patients and are based on the most up-to-date information. Clinical trials are going on in most parts of the country for most stages of cancer of the rectum. If you wish to know more about clinical trials, call the Cancer Information Service at 1-800-4-CANCER (1-800-422-6237).

Treatment options: Stage 0 rectal cancer
Your treatment may be one of the following:
1. Local excision.
2. Bowel resection.
3. Radiation therapy.
4. Electrofulguration.
5. Internal radiation therapy.

Treatment options: Stage I rectal cancer
Treatment is usually surgery (bowel resection) to remove the cancer. Other treatments that may be chosen depending on the size and location of your cancer include:
1. Internal radiation therapy.
2. Electrofulguration.
3. Local resection with or without radiation therapy plus chemotherapy.

Treatment options: Stage II rectal cancer
Your treatment may be one of the following:

1. Surgery (bowel resection) to remove the cancer, followed by radiation therapy and chemotherapy.
2. Surgery (bowel resection) to remove the cancer, as well as the colon, rectum, prostate, or bladder, depending on where the cancer has spread.
3. Radiation therapy or chemotherapy followed by surgery (bowel resection) followed by chemotherapy.
4. Clinical trials evaluating all of the above treatments to find better combinations of chemotherapy drugs and better ways of combining radiation therapy with chemotherapy.
5. Radiation therapy given during surgery.

Treatment options: Stage III rectal cancer
Your treatment may be one of the following:
1. Surgery (bowel resection) to remove the cancer, followed by radiation therapy and chemotherapy.
2. Surgery (bowel resection) to remove the cancer, as well as the colon, rectum, prostate, or bladder, depending on where the cancer has spread. Surgery is followed by radiation and chemotherapy.
3. Radiation therapy or chemotherapy followed by surgery (bowel resection) followed by chemotherapy.
4. Clinical trials evaluating all of the above treatments to find better combinations of chemotherapy drugs and better ways of combining radiation therapy with chemotherapy.
5. Radiation therapy given during surgery.

Treatment options: Stage IV rectal cancer
Your treatment may be one of the following:
1. Surgery (bowel resection) to remove the cancer.
2. If the cancer has spread only to the liver, lungs, or ovaries, surgery to take out the cancer where it has spread.
3. Radiation therapy.
4. Chemotherapy.

Treatment options: Recurrent rectal cancer
If the cancer has come back (recurred) in only one part of the body, treatment may be an operation to take out the cancer. If the cancer has spread to several parts of the body, your doctor may give you either chemotherapy or radiation therapy. If your cancer is too large to be removed by surgery, your doctor may make you more comfortable by freezing the tumor to destroy as much of it as possible. You may also choose to participate in a clinical trial testing new chemotherapy drugs.

To learn more about cancer of the rectum, call the National Cancer Institute's Cancer Information Service at 1-800-4-CANCER (1-800-422-6237). By dialing this toll-free number, you can speak with someone who can answer your questions.

■ **Document Source:**
National Cancer Institute
 Building 31, Room 10A24, 9000 Rockville Pike, Bethesda, MD
  20892
 PDQ 208/00076
 02/01/94

See also: Chemotherapy and You: A Guide to Self-Help During Treatment (page 40); Radiation Therapy and You: A Guide to Self-Help During Treatment (page 56)

DD Clearinghouse Fact Sheet
STOMACH ULCERS

Stomach ulcers are sores that form in the lining of the stomach. They may vary in size from a small sore to a deep cavity 1 to 2 inches wide, surrounded by an inflamed area, and are sometimes called ulcer craters.

Stomach ulcers and ulcers that form in the esophagus and in the lining of the duodenum (the upper part of the small intestine) are called peptic ulcers because they need acid and the enzyme pepsin to form. Duodenal ulcers are the most common type, tend to be smaller than stomach ulcers, and heal more quickly. Much of what can be said about the cause, diagnosis, treatment, and future outlook for duodenal ulcers is also true for stomach ulcers. However, since stomach ulcers present both doctors and patients with unique problems, this fact sheet focuses on ulcers that develop in the stomach lining, also called gastric ulcers.

Who is at risk for stomach ulcers?

Twenty percent of the 4 million Americans with ulcers have stomach ulcers. People most at risk are those who smoke, middle-age and older men, and chronic users of alcohol, anti-inflammatory drugs including aspirin, and nonsteriodal anti-inflammatory drugs such as ibuprofen.

What is the stomach's role in digestion?

The stomach is, essentially, a bag of muscle and other tissue located near the center of the abdomen just below the rib cage. When food is swallowed, it travels into the stomach through the esophagus, the long tube that passes from the mouth to the stomach.

While in the stomach, food is crushed and mixed by the forceful contractions of the stomach muscle. The food is mixed with, and partially digested by, acid and pepsin. The presence of acid and pepsin in the stomach is normal, and in most people they do not cause problems. In some people, however, these powerful substances are responsible for forming ulcers.

What causes stomach ulcers?

Most people who develop duodenal ulcers produce more than the usual amount of stomach acid. Unlike duodenal ulcers, however, most stomach ulcers are not caused by the production of too much acid, though the presence of some acid is necessary for the ulcer to form.

Scientists suspect that the resistance of the stomach lining to acid and pepsin is lowered in those people who develop stomach ulcers and that even normal, or less than normal, amounts of these two substances can lead to the formation of an ulcer. It is thought that the lower resistance of the stomach lining allows the acid and pepsin to break down the stomach lining in much the same way that these juices digest food.

What causes the stomach lining to break down?

How or why the resistance of the stomach lining is lowered is still not known. However, it is likely that a combination of environmental and genetic factors is responsible.

Researchers believe that certain drugs (including alcohol), chemicals, smoking, and food ingredients can damage the stomach lining. This damage, in turn, lowers the resistance of the stomach lining to acid and pepsin. Substances that are normally present in the intestine and sometimes flow back into the stomach in large amounts also can damage the stomach lining, as well as harmful bacteria, which are normally killed by the acid content of the stomach.

Also, the regular use of aspirin and other related drugs used to treat arthritis such as the nonsteriodal anti-inflammatory drugs has been shown to be an important factor in stomach ulcer development. Because aspirin is an ingredient in many over-the-counter drugs, you may wish to purchase a pain reliever or other preparation that does not contain aspirin. Check with your doctor or your pharmacist for the names of suitable products.

There is mounting evidence that an S-shaped bacterium, *Helicobacter pylori*, (previously called *Campylobacter pylori*) may be a factor in the development of stomach ulcers. *H. pylori* live in the mucous lining of the stomach near the surface cells and may go undetected for years. Some researchers believe that irritation to the stomach caused by the bacteria may weaken the lining, making it more susceptible to damage by acid and resulting in the formation of ulcers.

However, the findings are still inconclusive that *H. pylori* is a cause of stomach ulcers, which seem to be caused by multiple factors under study by researchers.

Do stomach ulcers run in families?

Heredity plays a role in the development of some ulcers, although the majority of people with stomach ulcers do not have a family history of this type of ulcer. However, if a member of a family develops a stomach ulcer, it is more likely that another close family member also will develop one. The same is true of duodenal ulcers.

What are stomach ulcer symptoms?

Stomach ulcers may or may not cause any symptoms. Some stomach ulcers are found by chance during an upper gastrointestinal x-ray examination performed for some other reason. However, when symptoms do occur, the most common one is pain in the upper abdomen, which may occur after eating or during the middle of the night and may be partially or completely relieved by eating food or by taking antacids.

Other less common symptoms include nausea and vomiting and/or loss of appetite and weight. Some people have hidden or slow bleeding with weakness as the only symptom. Other people have sudden, brisk bleeding with black, tarry stools or bloody vomit.

How is a stomach ulcer diagnosed?

Because the pain of stomach ulcer is similar to that caused by other conditions, the doctor usually orders an x-ray of the esophagus, stomach, and duodenum to help make a specific diagnosis. During the x-ray examination, the patient is asked to swallow a chalky liquid (containing barium) to help make the ulcer visible on the x-ray.

If pain is present and the x-ray is negative, the doctor may order a gastroscopy, an examination of the stomach, as well. During the gastroscopy, the doctor uses an endoscope, a long, flexible tube, to see the ulcer and to obtain small pieces of tissue for examination under the microscope. Some doctors may choose to perform a gastroscopy as the first diagnostic test instead of an x-ray.

Do stomach ulcers lead to cancer?

Stomach ulcers rarely lead to cancer. However, it is sometimes hard for the doctor to tell the difference between an ulcer crater and a tumor by looking at an x-ray—another reason the doctor may order a gastroscopy. Because there is a slight chance that a cancerous growth could be missed, doctors may order another x-ray or gastroscopy 6 to 8 weeks after treatment of the ulcer begins to be sure the ulcer is healed.

How are stomach ulcers treated?

Even though the causes of ulcers are not yet known, treatments that aid in the healing of most ulcers are known. For stomach ulcers, doctors rely on drugs that work to neutralize the acid (antacids) or to reduce the amount of acid produced (cimetidine and ranitidine are two such drugs).

Each of these medications works best if the doctor's directions are followed carefully. It is important that all medications are taken in the amounts prescribed and at the times indicated on the prescription. Persons with ulcers should continue to take their medication until the doctor tells them to stop because stomach ulcer symptoms go away before the ulcer heals. Remember, the medications discussed in this section, like all medications, may have side effects. Be sure to discuss this possibility with the doctor.

Is there a diet for ulcer patients?

For a long time, having an ulcer meant that the patient had to eat a bland diet. However, it is now known that such a diet is not necessary for most patients. Also researchers have learned that while milk coats the stomach and may provide temporary relief, it also stimulates the production of acid.

Except for restricting the intake of alcohol and caffeine, there is little indication that any particular diet is helpful for most stomach ulcer patients. There is no evidence that fatty, acidic, or spicy foods are harmful to ulcer patients. Although some people with stomach ulcers may find that acidic or extremely spicy foods are bothersome, each person should find out which foods, *if any*, cause distress.

Are there complications of stomach ulcers?

Complications such as bleeding and perforation (hole) through the stomach wall are infrequent. Signs of slow or hidden bleeding from an ulcer may be present and would include dizziness, weakness, and paleness. If the bleeding is brisk, there may be vomiting of blood or passing of dark, foul-smelling stools. Perforation, which allows stomach juices to enter the abdominal cavity, causes sudden severe pain and requires emergency treatment.

Obstruction (blockage) of the stomach outlet is another possible, although uncommon, complication of stomach ulcers. Prolonged nausea and vomiting may indicate obstruction, and food eaten many hours or even days before may be vomited. The pain may spread to the back if penetration through the wall of the stomach allows juices to come in contact with another organ such as the pancreas. See your doctor right away if you have *any* of these symptoms.

When is surgery necessary?

Stomach ulcers tend to recur, though this is less likely if the right kind of drug treatment is continued. If ulcers return often, if they do not respond to medication, or if complications develop, surgery may become necessary. The failure of the ulcer to heal or to stay healed is one of the most important reasons for surgery. (In some cases, the failure to heal may indicate an ulcerating cancer.) Surgery has some risks and may have unpleasant after effects. For this reason, the doctor will help to determine whether surgery is necessary.

Points to remember

- ♦ A stomach ulcer is a sore in the lining of the stomach. Scientists do not know what causes ulcers, but they suspect that it is some combination of environmental and genetic factors.
- ♦ Whatever the cause, stomach ulcers occur when the resistance of the stomach lining to acid and pepsin is lowered.
- ♦ The regular use of aspirin and other related drugs often used to treat arthritis is an important factor leading to the formation of stomach ulcers.
- ♦ Stomach ulcers do not always cause symptoms. When they do, the most common symptom is pain in the upper abdomen. Some people have nausea, vomiting, and loss of appetite and weight.
- ♦ If a stomach ulcer is present, stools should be checked regularly for changes in color and/or odor.
- ♦ Check with a doctor before taking any over-the-counter drug; it may contain aspirin.
- ♦ There are several medications available to treat ulcers. A doctor will prescribe the one that is best suited for you. However, all drugs work best if they are taken exactly as directed by the doctor.

- ♦ Because of the slight possibility that a stomach ulcer is really a cancerous ulcer or stomach cancer, it is important to go back to the doctor 6 to 8 weeks after treatment begins to make sure that the ulcer has healed.
- ♦ Surgery may be necessary if an ulcer fails to heal, recurs, or if complications develop, like bleeding or perforation. A doctor will help to determine if surgery is necessary.
- ♦ If you have any of these symptoms, see your doctor immediately:
  - Dizziness, weakness, and paleness.
  - Vomiting of blood.
  - Passing black, foul-smelling stools.
  - Severe pain in your abdomen or back.
  - Prolonged nausea or repeated vomiting.
  - Bringing up food eaten hours or days before.

Additional readings

Johnson AG. Gastric ulcer. *Surgery* 1990; 77: 1848-51. This review article for health professionals discusses the causes, diagnosis, surgical treatment, and complications of gastric ulcers. Available in medical and university libraries.

Larson DE, Editor-in-chief. *Mayo Clinic Family Health Book*. New York: William Morrow and Company, Inc., 1990. General medical guide with sections on stomach problems and ulcers. Available in libraries and bookstores.

Modeland V. Ulcers: screaming or silent, watch them with care. *FDA Consumer* 1989; 23(5): 13-7. This article for the layperson discusses ulcer causes, symptoms, and treatment. Reprint available from the Food and Drug Administration, 5600 Fishers Lane, Rockville, MD 20857 or in libraries.

Tapley DF, et al., eds. *The Columbia University College of Physicians and Surgeons Complete Home Medical Guide*, revised edition. New York: Crown Publishers, Inc., 1990. General medical guide with section on gastrointestinal ulcers. Available in libraries and bookstores.

Ulcers under attack: the new drug arsenal. *Your Health and Fitness* 1988; 10(2): 16-7. This article for the layperson discusses drug treatments for ulcers and is available in libraries.

■ Document Source:
U.S. Department of Health and Human Services, Public Health Service
National Institutes of Health
National Institute of Diabetes, and Digestive and Kidney Diseases
NIH Publication No. 92-676
Reprinted October 1991

DD Clearinghouse Fact Sheet

ULCERATIVE COLITIS

Inflammatory bowel disease (IBD) is a group of chronic disorders that cause inflammation or ulceration in the small and large intestines. Most often IBD is classified as ulcerative colitis or Crohn's disease but may be referred to as colitis, enteritis, ileitis, and proctitis.

Ulcerative colitis causes ulceration and inflammation of the inner lining of the colon and rectum, while Crohn's disease is an inflammation that extends into the deeper layers of the intestinal wall. Crohn's disease also may affect other parts of the digestive tract, including the mouth, esophagus, stomach, and small intestine.

Ulcerative colitis and Crohn's disease cause similar symptoms that often resemble other conditions, such as irritable bowel syndrome (spastic colitis). The correct diagnosis may take some time.

In ulcerative colitis, the inner lining of the large intestine (colon) and rectum becomes inflamed. The inflammation usually begins in the rectum and lower (sigmoid) intestine and spreads upward to the entire colon. Ulcerative colitis rarely affects the small intestine except for the lower section, the ileum. The inflammation causes the colon to empty frequently, resulting in diarrhea. As cells on the surface of the lining of the colon die and slough off, ulcers (tiny open sores) form, causing pus, mucus, and bleeding.

An estimated 250,000 Americans have ulcerative colitis. It occurs most often in young people ages 15 to 40, although children and older people sometimes develop the disease, too. Ulcerative colitis affects males and females equally and appears to run in some families.

What are the symptoms of ulcerative colitis?

The most common symptoms of ulcerative colitis are abdominal pain and bloody diarrhea. Patients also may suffer fatigue, weight loss, loss of appetite, rectal bleeding, and loss of body fluids and nutrients. Severe bleeding can lead to anemia. Sometimes patients also have skin lesions, joint pain, inflammation of the eyes, or liver disorders. No one knows for sure why problems outside the bowel are linked with colitis. Scientists think these complications may occur when the immune system triggers inflammation in other parts of the body. These disorders are usually mild and go away when the colitis is treated.

What causes ulcerative colitis?

The cause of ulcerative colitis is not known, and currently there is no cure, except through surgical removal of the colon. Many theories about what causes ulcerative colitis exist, but none has been proven. The current leading theory suggests that some agent, possibly a virus or an atypical bacterium, interacts with the body's immune system to trigger an inflammatory reaction in the intestinal wall.

Although much scientific evidence shows that people with ulcerative colitis have abnormalities of the immune system, doctors do not know whether these abnormalities are a cause or result of the disease. Doctors believe, however, that there is little proof that ulcerative colitis is caused by emotional distress or sensitivity to certain foods or food products or is the result of an unhappy childhood.

How is ulcerative colitis diagnosed?

If you have symptoms that suggest ulcerative colitis, the doctor will look inside your rectum and colon through a flexible tube (endoscope) inserted through the anus. During the exam, the doctor may take a sample of tissue (biopsy) from the lining of the colon to view under the microscope.

You also may receive a barium enema x-ray of the colon to determine the nature and extent of disease. This procedure involves putting a chalky solution (barium) into the colon. The barium shows up white on x-ray film, revealing growths and other abnormalities in the colon.

The doctor will give you a thorough physical exam, including blood tests to see if you are anemic (as a result of blood loss), or if your white blood cells count is elevated (a sign of inflammation). Examination of a stool sample can tell the doctor if an infection, such as by amoebae or bacteria, is causing the symptoms.

If you have ulcerative colitis, you may need medical care for some time. Your doctor also will want to see you regularly to check on the condition.

How serious is this disease?

About half of patients have only mild symptoms. Others suffer frequent fever, bloody diarrhea, nausea, and severe abdominal cramps. Only in rare cases, when complications occur, is the disease fatal. There may be remissions—period when the symptoms go away—that last for months or even years. However, most patients' symptoms eventually return. This changing pattern of the disease can make it hard for the doctor to tell when treatment has helped.

What is the treatment?

While no special diet for ulcerative colitis is given, patients may be able to control mild symptoms simply by avoiding foods that seem to upset their intestine. In some cases, the doctor may advise avoiding highly seasoned foods or milk sugar (lactose) for a while. When treatment is necessary, it must be tailored for each case, since what may help one patient may not help another. The patient also should be given needed emotional and psychological support.

Patients with either mild or severe colitis are usually treated with the drug sulfasalazine. This drug can be used for as long as needed, and it can be used along with other drugs. Side effects such as nausea, vomiting, weight loss, heartburn, diarrhea, and headache occur in a small percentage of cases. Patients who do not do well on sulfasalazine often do very well on related drugs known as 5-ASA agents.

In some cases, patients with severe disease, or those who cannot take sulfasalazine-type drugs, are given adrenal steroids (drugs that help control inflammation and affect the immune system) such as prednisone or hydrocortisone. All of these drugs can be used in oral, enema, or suppository forms. Other drugs may be given to relax the patient or to relieve pain, diarrhea, or infection.

Patients with ulcerative colitis occasionally have symptoms severe enough to require hospitalization. In these cases, the doctor will try to correct malnutrition and to stop diarrhea and loss of blood, fluids, and mineral salts. To accomplish this, the patient may need a special diet, feeding through a vein, medications, or, sometimes, surgery.

The risk of colon cancer is greater than normal in patients with widespread ulcerative colitis. The risk may be as high as 32 times the normal rate in patients whose entire colon is involved, especially if the colitis exists for many years. However, if only the rectum and lower colon are involved, the risk of cancer is not higher than normal.

Sometimes precancerous changes occur in the cells lining the colon. These changes in the cells are called "dysplasia." If the doctor finds evidence of dysplasia through endoscopic exam and biopsy, it means the patient is more likely to develop cancer. Patients with dysplasia, or whose colitis affects the entire colon, should receive regular followup exams, which may involve colonoscopy (examination of the entire colon using a flexible endoscope) and biopsies.

About 20 to 25 percent of ulcerative colitis patients eventually require surgery for removal of the colon because of massive bleeding, chronic debilitating illness, perforation of the colon, or risk of cancer. Sometimes the doctor will recommend removing the colon when medical treatment fails or the side effects of steroids or other drugs threaten the patient's health.

Patients have several surgical options, each of which has advantages and disadvantages. The surgeon and patient must decide on the best individual option.

The most common surgery is the proctocolectomy, the removal of the entire colon and rectum, with ileostomy, creation of a small opening in the abdominal wall where the tip of the lower small intestine, the ileum, is brought to the skin's surface to allow drainage of waste. The opening (stoma) is about the size of a quarter and is usually located in the right lower corner of the abdomen in the area of the beltline. A pouch is worn over the opening to collect waste and the patient empties the pouch periodically.

The proctocolectomy with continent ileostomy is an alternative to the standard ileostomy. In this operation, the surgeon creates a pouch out of the ileum inside the wall of the lower abdomen. The patient is able to empty the pouch by inserting a tube through a small leak-proof opening in his or her side. Creation of this natural valve eliminates the need for an external appliance. However, the patient must wear an external pouch for the first few months after the operation.

Sometimes an operation that avoids the use of a pouch can be performed. In the ileoanal anastomosis ("pullthrough operation"), the diseased portion of the colon is removed and the outer muscles of the rectum are preserved. The surgeon attaches the ileum inside the rectum, forming a pouch, or reservoir, that holds the waste. This allows the patient to pass stool through the anus in a normal manner, although the bowel movements may be more frequent and watery than usual.

The decision about which surgery to have is made according to each patient's needs, expectations, and lifestyle. If you are ever faced with this decision, remembering that getting as much information as possible is important. Talk to your doctor, to nurses who work with patients who have had colon surgery (enterostomal therapists), and to other patients. In addition, read pamphlets and books, such as those available from the Crohn's & Colitis Foundation of America, before you decide.

Most people with ulcerative colitis will never need to have surgery. If surgery ever does become necessary, however, you may find comfort in knowing that after the surgery, the colitis is cured and most people go on to live normal, active lives.

Additional readings

Bleeding in the Digestive Tract. National Digestive Diseases Information Clearinghouse, 1989. Box NDDIC, 9000 Rockville Pike, Bethesda, MD 20892. (301) 468-6344. General information fact sheet.

Brandt LJ, Steiner-Grossman P, editors. *Treating IBD: A Patient's Guide to the Medical and Surgical Management of Inflammatory Bowel Disease.* New York: Raven Press. 1989. This book, produced by the Crohn's & Colitis Foundation of America, discusses many aspects of treatment and living with inflammatory bowel disease. Available in libraries and from the foundation.

Larson DE, Editor-in-chief. *Mayo Clinic Family Health Book.* New York: William Morrow and Company, Inc., 1990. General medical guide with section on ulcerative colitis. Available in libraries and bookstores.

Lipshutz WH. Exploring the causes of IBD and Crohn's Disease. *Contemporary Gastroenterology,* 1991; 4(4): 10-14. General review article written for health care professionals.

Ulcerative Colitis. National Organization for Rare Disorders, Inc., P.O. Box 8923, New Fairfield, CT 06812-1783. (203) 746-6518. General information fact sheet.

Resources

Crohn's & Colitis Foundation of American, Inc., 444 Park Avenue South, 11th floor, New York, NY 10016-7374. 1-800-343-3637.

Ileitis and Colitis Educational Foundation, Central DuPage Hospital, 25 North Winfield Road, Winfield, IL 60190. (708) 682-1600, Ext. 6493.

International Association for Enterostomal Therapy, 27241 La Paz Road, Suite 121, Laguna Niguel, CA 92656. (714) 476-0268.

United Ostomy Association (UOA), 36 Executive Park, Suite 120, Irvine, CA 92714. (714) 660-8624.

■ Document Source:
U.S. Department of Health and Human Services, Public Health Service
National Institutes of Health
National Institute of Diabetes, and Digestive and Kidney Diseases
NIH Publication No. 92-1597
Reprinted April 1992

See also: Bleeding in the Digestive Tract (page 150); Crohn's Disease (page 160)

DD Clearinghouse Fact Sheet
WHAT IS DYSPEPSIA?

Dyspepsia—often called indigestion—is a common malady that many of us have come to associate with the TV ads featuring those sorry souls who can't believe they ate the whole thing. While dyspeptic symptoms are often caused by overeating or eating the wrong foods, the disorder can be associated with a more serious problem.

Dyspepsia means painful, difficult, or disturbed digestion. The chronic recurrence and persistence of crippling dyspeptic symptoms disrupts the lives of many Americans. People suffering from the most severe symptoms can become disabled enough to miss work. Frequent doctor's visits and expensive diagnostic procedures can create a financial drain. In addition, many unnecessary operations are performed in an attempt to relieve the painful symptoms. Unfortunately, despite the surgery, many patients continue to suffer from the symptoms of dyspepsia.

The causes of dyspepsia are many and some of them are not clearly understood. Too often dyspepsia has been dismissed as a psychosomatic disorder. However, in recent years, doctors have begun to recognize that dyspepsia is often the result of a malfunctioning of either the nervous system or the muscular activity of the stomach or small intestine.

What is dyspepsia?

A person is said to have dyspepsia if she/he suffers from several of a group of symptoms which might include nausea, regurgitation (backwash of stomach contents into the esophagus or mouth), vomiting, heartburn, prolonged upper abdominal fullness or bloating after a meal, stomach discomfort or pain, and early fullness. Often people say that they have a "sick feeling in the stomach," or "indigestion," or, maybe, "nervous stomach" when they are suffering from dyspeptic symptoms. Sometimes a person will experience these symptoms after overeating or eating foods that disagree with them. Sometimes the symptoms accompany a disease such as peptic ulcer disease, gallbladder disease, or gastritis. Other people experience the symptoms for no apparent reason. The symptoms can last for 3 to 4 days, sometimes longer. In some people, dyspeptic symptoms can be severe and continuous, disrupting daily routines and causing absences from work.

Who gets dyspepsia?

Although dyspepsia can afflict men and women from all walks of life, it is most common in women ranging in age from 16 to 60. A woman is even more likely to experience dyspepsia during her childbearing years. Also, patients in whom irritable bowel syndrome (IBS) has been diagnosed comprise the majority of dyspepsia sufferers.

What causes dyspepsia?

Dyspepsia can be caused by many different things. Symptoms can accompany gastritis (inflammation of the stomach), viral gastroenteritis (stomach flu), stomach ulcer, cancer of the stomach, gallbladder disease, pancreatic diseases, and IBS. Pregnancy and advanced diabetes mellitus can also be accompanied by dyspepsia.

But dyspepsia can also occur without the presence of other digestive disorders. If no disease is apparent, doctors have, in the past, tended to diagnose patients as having a psychosomatic disorder.

In recent years, however, medical research has recognized that the stomach and small intestine are regulated by "pacemakers"—much like the heart—that coordinate the movement of the muscles of the digestive tract. During normal digestion, the muscle wall contracts and relaxes, allowing the upper part of the stomach to serve as a reservoir and the lower part to break down (digest) food. When the breakdown is complete, the stomach empties its contents into the upper part of the intestine (the duodenum).

The delicate motions of the stomach and small intestine are regulated by the brain and by a network of nerves embed-

ded in the muscle wall of the digestive tract. The coordination between these nerve endings that secrete a variety of chemical substances (called neurotransmitters), hormones, and the muscle fibers in the wall of the digestive tract regulate the movement of the tract and thereby promote the digestion, absorption, and elimination of the food we eat. Any disruption in the normal functioning of the nervous system or the muscular activity of the digestive tract can cause dyspepsia.

How is dyspepsia diagnosed?

If your symptoms are severe enough to interfere with your daily routine, you should see your doctor. To rule out diseases of the stomach, pancreas, and gallbladder, your doctor may perform an array of tests including an upper GI series, gallbladder, x-ray, endoscopy, and routine blood and urine tests.

Unfortunately, although these tests are necessary to eliminate serious gastrointestinal disorders, they offer little help in identifying dyspepsia that is caused by disruption in the normal functioning of the nervous system or the muscular activity of the digestive tract. Researchers are developing new procedures to monitor the activity of the stomach and duodenum in much the same way that EKG records the electrical activity of the heart. Also, doctors can measure gastric (stomach) emptying to determine whether there is any abnormality in the phase of the digestive process. Such an abnormality is often found in patients with severe dyspepsia. More research is needed, however, before satisfactory procedures to diagnose dyspepsia are developed.

Is dyspepsia caused by emotional tension or distress?

It is well-known that dyspepsia-like symptoms can accompany emotional upsets. However, emotional tension may not be the most common cause or even the precipitating factor. Before emotional tension or distress can be named as the culprit causing dyspepsia, your doctor will conduct a careful medical evaluation to rule out other factors.

How are symptoms controlled?

If your dyspepsia is associated with gastritis, peptic ulcer disease, gallbladder disease, or some other organic disorder, your doctor will begin by treating the specific disorder.

Most of the time, dyspepsia not associated with a specific illness can be controlled by diet. Avoiding greasy foods or solid foods containing meat often helps. And, if you are lactose intolerant, eliminating all dairy products from your diet should provide relief. (For more information about lactose intolerance, write the clearinghouse.) If your symptoms are severe, your doctor may recommend that you take only liquids or small amounts of soft foods until the symptoms subside. If these measures do not work, your doctor may prescribe medical therapies to control persistent symptoms.

In summary

Dyspepsia is a common digestive disorder among Americans which has many causes. These include intestinal diseases, inappropriate diet, or a disturbance in the delicate mechanism that govern the muscular activities of the stomach and small intestine.

If your doctor has ruled out a specific illness causing your dyspepsia, your symptoms can probably be controlled if you take the following dietary precautions:

♦ avoid greasy foods or solid foods containing meat;
♦ if you are lactose intolerant, eliminate milk and milk products; and
♦ if your symptoms are severe, follow a liquid diet or eat soft foods in small amounts until your symptoms subside.

If your symptoms persist, see your doctor. She/he may be able to prescribe a medication to control symptoms.

This fact sheet was prepared by William Y. Chey, M.D. Dr. Chey is director of the Isaac Gorden Center for Digestive Diseases and Nutrition and a clinical professor of medicine at the University of Rochester School of Medicine.

■ Document Source:
U.S. Department of Health and Human Services, Public Health Service
National Institutes of Health
National Institute of Diabetes, and Digestive and Kidney Diseases
NIH Publication No. 89-1300
Reprinted August 1989

GENETIC DISORDERS

■ ■ ■

FACTS ABOUT DOWN SYNDROME

Down syndrome, the most common genetic birth defect associated with mental retardation, occurs equally across all races and levels of society. The effects of the disorder on physical and mental development are severe and are expressed throughout the life span. The individual's family is also affected emotionally, economically and socially.

This booklet, based primarily on knowledge gained from research studies and programs developed at Mental Retardation Research Centers throughout the United States, presents current information about Down syndrome for families of children with the disorder and those who care for them. The Research Centers are supported by the National Institute of Child Health and Human Development (NICHD), National Institutes of Health (NIH), which has primary responsibility for research on mental retardation.

Genetic and Physical Aspects

Down syndrome is a combination of physical abnormalities and mental retardation characterized by a genetic defect in chromosome pair 21. All normal cells in the human body, except ova and sperm cells, have 46 chromosomes—44 autosomes and two sex chromosomes. Normal reproductive cells contain 23 chromosomes—22 autosomes and one sex chromosome.

In all other (nonreproductive) body cells, chromosomes occur in pairs. The 22 pairs of autosomes are identified by number while the remaining pair of sex chromosomes is designated XX for females or XY for males. Each autosome appears identical to its partner, but each pair is different in its genetic content, and frequently in appearance, from all other pairs.

The genetic defect associated with Down syndrome is the presence of extra material on the chromosome pair designated 21. Although other genetic disorders may be associated with an extra chromosome, only Down syndrome is characterized by extra chromosome 21 material. The forms in which this extra material can appear are classified as:

Number and Arrangement of Chromosomes in a Normal Cell

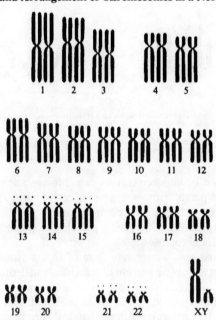

All normal cells (except ova and sperm) have 46 chromosomes—44 autosomes and 2 sex chromosomes. Scientists have given these chromosomes numbers and have paired them according to their similarities. (Note the sex chromosome: all normal males have one "X" and one "Y" chromosome; normal females have two "X" chromosomes.)

Trisomy 21—the presence of three rather than the normal pair of chromosomes designated as 21. The genetic abnormality most frequently associated with Down syndrome (95 percent of all cases), trisomy 21, results from an error in cell division during the development of the egg or sperm, or during fertilization.

Translocation—an interchange of chromosomes or parts of chromosomes which may result in a mismatched pair. Children with translocation Down syndrome, which occurs in about four percent of the cases, have an extra number 21 chromosome which has broken and become attached to another chromosome. In certain cases, a person can carry a broken chromosome 21 without showing any symptoms of Down syndrome because the correct amount of genetic material is there, even though some of it is out of place.

Trisomy 21

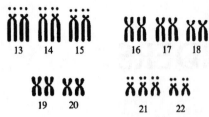

13 14 15 16 17 18

19 20 21 22

Trisomy 21 refers to a condition in which there are three rather than the usual pair of chromosomes in the "21" pair. Trisomy 21 usually results from a mistake in cell division of either the egg or the sperm and is an accidental occurrence.

Formation of a Translocation Chromosome

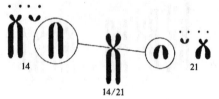

14 14/21 21

A translocation occurs when a piece of one chromosome breaks off and attaches to a different chromosome. This "translocation chromosome" has been formed by the breaking and rejoining or chromosomes 14 and 21 (with loss of the little pieces).

Normally, children receive one chromosome of pair 21 from each parent. However, a parent with a translocation can pass on his or her normal chromosome 21 *plus* the translocated chromosome 21, giving the child too much genetic material for chromosome 21.

Mosaicism—a very rare form of Down syndrome, appearing in about one percent of individuals with the disorder. Affected persons have cells with different chromosome counts (for example, 46 in some cells and 47 in others). Mosaicism is not carried in the parents' chromosomes; it is accidental, resulting from an error in cell division of the fertilized egg. Since only some of their cells have an abnormal number of chromosomes, babies with mosaic Down syndrome may have only some of the features of the disorder.

The distinct physical characteristics of Down syndrome include slanting eyes; slightly protruding lips; small ears; slightly protruding tongue; short hands, feet and trunk; and sometimes, an unusual crease on the palm of the infant's hand. Congenital heart defects are common and nystagmus (involuntary movement of the eyes), enlarged liver and spleen also occur. In 99 percent of cases, there is mild to severe mental retardation.

Surveys show the average incidence of Down syndrome to be about one in 800 live births. However, the risk of bearing a child with the disorder increases dramatically with advancing maternal age. For example, the incidence is less than one in 1,000 live births to women under 30, increasing to one in 35 to mothers aged 44.

The sharp rise in the incidence of babies with Down syndrome born to older women may occur for several reasons. Although males produce new sperm continually, women are born with all the oocytes (eggs) they will ever have. An oocyte remains in a state of incomplete development until the process

begins that results in ovulation. Thus, a 35-year-old woman has 35-year-old oocytes.

Many body functions decline with age, and oocytes in the older woman simply may be past their prime. Or they may have been exposed over the years to damaging internal and external influences, including medications, radiation or other harmful agents.

Until recently, the mother was believed to be the source of the extra genetic material. However, researchers, using new laboratory techniques, have demonstrated that in about 25 percent of cases studied, the father is the source of the extra chromosome. Because older fathers have been associated with increased incidence of other genetic disorders, researchers are looking more closely at the possible effect of the father's age on the incidence of Down syndrome. In one project, involving only a small number of cases, a paternal age effect for fathers over age 55 was reported.

Although individuals with Down syndrome are living longer than in the past, due in part to improved surgical treatment of congenital heart defects, the use of antibiotics for treating infection and avoidance of early institutionalization, their life expectancy still remains much less than for the general population.

Of special concern is the much greater risk that children with Down syndrome have of developing leukemia—20 times greater than normal children. Not only is the risk greater, but the children die earlier—the peak age of leukemia deaths in normal children is age four, but for those with Down syndrome it is one year.

Relationship of Down Syndrome to Maternal Age

Mother's Age	Incidence of Down Syndrome
under 30	less than 1 in 1,000
30	1 in 900
35	1 in 400
36	1 in 300
37	1 in 230
38	1 in 180
39	1 in 135
40	1 in 105
42	1 in 60
44	1 in 35
46	1 in 20
48	1 in 12

The Outlook

The individual with Down syndrome presents unusual and demanding problems at virtually every stage of life, beginning at birth.

In most cases, the first medical exam identifies the newborn with Down syndrome. Expecting a normal infant, most parents are intensely disappointed when the physician explains their new baby's condition to them. Parents generally experience an initial period of shock, followed by denial, grief, anger, adjustment and finally, acceptance. These events do not necessarily occur in this sequence, nor does everyone experience all of these stages.

Faced with an abrupt change in their hopes and plans for the new child, parents need early counseling and guidance to help them cope with the situation and plan for their child's future.

The presence of a retarded child in the home is not necessarily detrimental to the happiness and welfare of siblings or to the family as a whole. With professional guidance, an accepting community attitude and the help of parent support organizations, a congenial home atmosphere can evolve. All children, but especially those with Down syndrome, benefit from loving and caring homes.

In addition to help in managing medical problems, professional guidance usually includes genetic counseling for parents and a discussion of the family's plans for the future.

Since stereotypes of Down syndrome persist, early and sound information for new parents and other family members is very important. In the past, most physicians recommended placing the infant in an institution immediately upon discharge from the hospital nursery. New developments in care and treatment now permit other courses, but, unfortunately, parents are not always made aware of these approaches or to alternatives to institutionalization.

To help keep professionals and parents informed about new developments, and to provide friendly support to new Down syndrome families, parent groups have formed in many communities, sometimes as chapters of national organizations. Often, a hospital social worker will help new parents contact such groups.

In the past 20 years, through the efforts of the comprehensive, multidisciplinary University Affiliated Programs and the NICHD-supported Mental Retardation Research Centers, a new generation of professionals, skilled and knowledgeable in meeting the needs of families affected by Down syndrome, has evolved.

Work at the centers ranges from training health professionals to investigating the causes of mental retardation, particularly Down syndrome. Because the syndrome results from a chromosomal error, most studies are concerned with genetic aspects. However, because of the complexity of the studies and the need for additional research, preventing Down syndrome through genetics research remains a distant goal.

Research has provided strategies for recognizing Down syndrome and other genetic defects through advances in prenatal diagnosis. For example, NICHD-supported studies have demonstrated the safety and efficiency of amniocentesis and related technologies.

Health and Development

Since significant health and developmental problems occur in the child with Down syndrome during the first few years of life, close monitoring is necessary throughout this period.

Medical management and surgical correction, when indicated, of the life-threatening congenital defects frequently associated with Down syndrome are essential to assure the child's optimal health and well-being. Today, most experts agree that surgical procedures to correct defects should not be withheld, as occasionally happens, simply because the child has Down syndrome. In a few cases, cosmetic surgery has been used to alter the distinct physical characteristics of

the syndrome; however, the use of cosmetic surgery does not appeal to everyone.

Children with Down syndrome are more susceptible to infections than normal children and, as a result, often suffer chronic respiratory infection, recurrent pneumonia and repeated bouts of tonsillitis. Researchers believe that children with the disorder have a deficient immune response. According to several studies, they not only have fewer of the cells needed for normal immunologic response to infection, but the cells they have do not function well.

Hearing loss occurs more frequently among individuals with Down syndrome than in the normal population. Because affected persons are particularly vulnerable to deficiencies in speech and language development, careful screening and testing for hearing loss should be done and corrective procedures started as early as possible.

Development delays are evident from the early months of life. Infants are slow to turn over, sit, stand, speak and respond, and parents or others caring for them may not interact with them—smiling and talking while feeding them or changing their diapers, for example—as readily as with normally developing babies.

Such early interaction is even more important for Down syndrome children, however, because their weak motor development reduces their own self-initiated activities, like rolling over or reaching for objects. Proponents of home care point out that children reared in a home atmosphere function better than those reared in institutions, because opportunities for early interaction in institutions are generally inadequate.

Compared with early delay in postural motor development (sitting, standing, walking), the delay in speech and language development encountered by the child with Down syndrome is more noticeable. In addition, beginning in the second year of life, there is an apparent decline in intelligence because language and speech become increasingly more important in intelligence tests.

The reasons for the special difficulty that Down syndrome children have in speech and language are not fully understood. Part of the difficulty stems from the characteristic overlarge and protruding tongue, and in some instances surgical correction of this condition has been helpful. The acquisition of speech and language also depends upon the patterns of vocal and verbal interactions between child and parents and upon cognitive processes.

At this time, there is no known medical regimen that can reverse the pattern of early developmental delay observed in children with the syndrome. Various forms of medication, including chemicals and vitamins, have been tested, without success. Most often, the gains observed are attributed to changes in the quality and quantity of parental care associated with the treatment being tested. This has led to increased interest by researchers and parents in early intervention programs.

Preliminary results from one early intervention program, operating at the Mental Retardation Research Center, University of Washington, Seattle, is encouraging. Children with Down syndrome who entered the project as infants are now in elementary school, or about to begin. Researchers are finding that in a variety of developmental tasks, children in the program exceed the development of other children with

Down syndrome not in the program. In addition, the program appears to reduce the severity of retardation.

On the other hand, a 6-month, less intensive intervention program at McGill University in Montreal did not produce beneficial gains—contrasting results that only point to the need for more information about early intervention efforts.

Not all families have easy access to specialized resources for their handicapped child. In these situations, efforts have focused on enhancing the ability of parents to teach their children speech and language and self-help and social skills through home-based programs.

If effective early intervention programs can be designed and used in the preschool years, the subsequent educational progress of a child with Down syndrome may be altered significantly. A child may then be classified as educable, rather than trainable, and therefore qualified for different educational opportunities and strategies.

An "educable" person is defined as one who is capable of learning such basic skills as reading and arithmetic and is quite capable of self care and independent living (those with mild retardation are generally considered educable). Although trainable (moderately retarded) persons are very limited in educational attainments, they can profit from simple training for self care and vocational tasks.

The Elementary School Years

Under Public Law 94-12, each state is required to have a goal that "all handicapped children have available to them . . . a free public education and related services designed to meet their unique needs."

School entry for children with Down syndrome brings with it the need to determine what is an *appropriate* education designed to meet their special situation. Because the physical characteristics associated with the syndrome easily identify and label the child, the old stereotype of a trainable but uneducable person is readily aroused and can affect early school placement.

As increasing numbers of children with Down syndrome are cared for in their home communities and receive school instruction, the demand for research on their unique learning problems is expected to increase. And as expectations rise for their academic achievement, increased research concern for special educational strategies can also be expected.

Adolescence

At adolescence, children with Down syndrome tend to be overweight. This may be due to general body type (short stature and decreased muscle tone), lack of physical activity associated with social isolation and reduced outlets for activity, and excessive eating of high-calorie foods. In addition to detracting from the adolescent's appearance, the weight gain has negative implications for later health and longevity. A supervised regimen of diet and exercise through the elementary school years, or even earlier, may have a beneficial effect.

Parental concern for the social and sexual life of their child with Down syndrome usually intensifies at adolescence. Unless earlier efforts have been highly successful, the child's social isolation increases outside of structured school and other group situations. Although persons with Down syndrome seldom reproduce, it is necessary to provide them with a healthy understanding and orientation toward sexuality. Pregnancy has been rare, probably as a result of sexual isolation in institutions, but sometimes does occur. About half the infants born of such pregnancies have Down syndrome. Males with trisomy 21 not associated with mosaicism or translocation have not been known to reproduce.

Generally, few services and programs exist for adolescents with the disorder and their families. In the past, both research and service efforts have concentrated on younger persons. The national trend toward "mainstreaming" is a fairly recent development, and the present generation of adolescents with Down syndrome is the first raised under conditions of greater educational and community opportunity. The long-range effects of these new opportunities on adolescents and upon community attitudes remain to be determined.

The Adult Years

For more than a century, researchers have observed that individuals born with Down syndrome tend to age prematurely. This phenomenon has become more apparent with the increased longevity of affected persons. Because intellectual deterioration—a striking symptom in the senile dementias—is more difficult to assess in retarded individuals, the judgment of premature aging in a person with Down syndrome is generally based on emotional deterioration as shown by changes in personality and behavior.

Neurological signs such as tremors, incoordination and changes in reflexes are often noted among older persons with Down syndrome. Brain tissue research has revealed the same type of degenerative changes in Down syndrome as in Alzheimer's disease, the most common form of the senile dementias, but the relationship between Alzheimer's disease and Down syndrome is not yet well understood. Studies underway at NIH and elsewhere are expected to yield more knowledge about both disorders.

Parents who elect to raise a child with Down syndrome at home face many problems and demands throughout the child's life. As the child grows older, and as the parents age, parents become more concerned about who will care for their child in case they become ill or die.

In some cases, families arrange for the older child or adult to move into a group home for mentally retarded persons in the community. In this way, family ties are maintained, yet the child is no longer totally dependent on the parents.

Still to be determined are the effects of deinstitutionalization on adults with Down syndrome and their families.

NICHD continues to support research into the causes of mental retardation. Through its Mental Retardation Research Centers, the Institute also funds research on better management, treatment and programs for individuals and families affected by Down syndrome.

Voluntary agencies, like those listed below, comprised of interested persons and parents and families of individuals with Down syndrome are excellent sources of information:

March of Dimes Birth Defects Foundation, 1275 Mamaroneck Avenue, White Plains, New York 10605

Down's Syndrome Congress, 1640 West Roosevelt Road, Room 156-E, Chicago, Illinois 60608

National Association for Retarded Citizens, 2709 Avenue E East, Arlington, Texas 76011

National Down Syndrome Society, 146 East 57th Street, New York, New York 10022

Mental Retardation Research Centers Supported by the NICHD

Child Development Research and Evaluation Center, Boston Children's Hospital Medical Center; 300 Longwood Avenue; Boston, Massachusetts 02115

Eunice Kennedy Shriver Center for Mental Retardation; 200 Trapelo Road; Waltham, Massachusetts 02154

Rose F. Kennedy Center for Research in Mental Retardation and Human Development, Albert Einstein College of Medicine, 1410 Pelham Parkway South, Bronx, New York 10461

Child Development Research Institute, Frank Porter Graham Child Development Center, University of North Carolina, Chapel Hill, North Carolina 27514

Mental Retardation Research Center, Neuropsychiatric Institute, Center for the Health Sciences, University of California at Los Angeles; 760 Westwood Plaza; Los Angeles, California 90024

The John F. Kennedy Child Development Center, University of Colorado Health Sciences Center, B.F. Stolinsky Research Laboratories, 4200 East Ninth Avenue, Denver, Colorado 80220

The Joseph P. Kennedy, Jr., Mental Retardation Research Center, School of Medicine, University of Chicago, Wyler's Children's Hospital, Chicago, Illinois 60637

Center for Research in Human Development, University of Kansas, New Haworth Hall, University of Kansas, Lawrence, Kansas 66045

The John F. Kennedy Center for Research on Education and Human Development, George Peabody College of Vanderbilt University, Nashville, Tennessee 37203

Child Development and Mental Retardation Research Center, University of Washington, WJ-10, Seattle, Washington 98195

Harry A. Waisman Center on Mental Retardation and Human Development, University of Wisconsin, 1500 Highland Avenue, University of Wisconsin, Madison, Wisconsin 53706

Cincinnati Mental Retardation Research Center, Children Hospital Research Foundation, Elland and Bethesda Avenues, Cincinnati, Ohio 45229

"Facts About Down Syndrome" was prepared by Drs. Theodore Tjossem and Felix De La Cruz of the Mental Retardation and Disabilities Branch, and Ms. Joan Z. Muller of the Office of Research Reporting, National Institute of Child Health and Human Development (NICHD), and is reprinted from the November/December 1983 issue of *Children Today* magazine.

The Institute, part of the federal government's National Institutes of Health, conducts and supports research on the various processes that determine the health of children, adults, families and populations. For more copies of this fact sheet or others in this series, write to the Office of Research Reporting, NICHD, NIH, Building 31, Room 2A32, 9000 Rockville Pike, Bethesda, Maryland 20205.

Other Publications in This Series:

- ♦ *Facts About Anorexia Nervosa*
- ♦ *Facts About Cesarean Childbirth*
- ♦ *Facts About Dysmenorrhea and Premenstrual Syndrome*
- ♦ *Facts About Oral Contraceptives*
- ♦ *Facts About Precocious Puberty*
- ♦ *Facts About Pregnancy and Smoking*
- ♦ *Facts About Premature Birth*

■ Document Source:
U.S. Department of Health and Human Services, Public Health Service
National Institutes of Health
National Institute of Child Health and Human Development

FACTS ABOUT DYSLEXIA

Developmental dyslexia is a specific learning disability characterized by difficulty in learning to read. Some dyslexics also may have difficulty learning to write, to spell, and, sometimes, to speak or to work with numbers. We do not know for sure what causes dyslexia, but we do know that it affects children who are physically and emotionally healthy, academically capable, and who come from good home environments. In fact, many dyslexics have the advantages of excellent schools, high mental ability, and parents who are well-educated and value learning.

School children are subject to a broad range of reading problems and researchers have discovered the causes of many problems. Today, most teachers accept these research findings and use them in planning their instruction, but there remains a small group of children who have difficulty in learning to read for no apparent reason. These children are called dyslexic. Although estimates of the prevalence of dyslexia are hard to find, some researchers estimate that as many as 15 percent of American students may be classified as dyslexic.

Defining Dyslexia

Over the years, the term dyslexia has been given a variety of definitions, and for this reason, many teachers have resisted using the term at all. Instead, they have used such terms as "reading disability" or "learning disability" to describe conditions more correctly designated as dyslexia. Although there is no universally recognized definition of dyslexia, the one presented by the World Federation of Neurology has won broad respect: "A disorder manifested by difficulty in learning to read despite conventional instruction, adequate intelligence and sociocultural opportunity."

Symptoms

Children with dyslexia are not all alike. The only trait they share is that they read at levels significantly lower than is typical for children of their age and intelligence. This reading lag usually is described in terms of grade level. For example, a fourth grader who is reading at a second grade level is said to be two years behind in reading. (Such a child may or may not be dyslexic; there are many nondyslexic children who experience problems in reading.)

Referring to grade level as a measure of reading is convenient but it can be misleading. A student who has a two-year lag when he is in fourth grade has a much more serious problem than a tenth grader with a two-year lag. The fourth grader has learned few of the reading skills which have been taught in the early grades, while the tenth grader, by this measure, has mastered eight years or 80 percent of the skills needed to be a successful reader.

Samuel T. Orton, a neurologist who became interested in the problems of learning to read in the 1920s, was one of the first scientific investigators of dyslexia. In his work with students in Iowa and New York, he found that dyslexics commonly have one or more of the following problems:

- ♦ difficulty in learning and remembering printed words;
- ♦ letter reversal (b for d, p for q) and number reversals (6 for 9) and changed order of letters in words (tar for rat, quite for quiet) or numbers (12 for 21);
- ♦ leaving out or inserting words while reading;
- ♦ confusing vowel sounds or substituting one consonant for another;
- ♦ persistent spelling errors;
- ♦ difficulty in writing.

Orton noted that many dyslexics are lefthanded or ambidextrous and that they often have trouble telling left from right. Other symptoms he observed include: (a) delayed or inadequate speech; (b) trouble with picking the right word to fit the meaning desired when speaking; (c) problems with direction (up and down) and time (before and after, yesterday and tomorrow); and (d) clumsiness, awkwardness in using hands, and illegible handwriting. Orton also found that more boys than girls show these symptoms and that dyslexia often runs in families. Fortunately, most dyslexics have only a few of these problems, but the presence of even one is sufficient to create unique educational needs.

Possible Causes

When researchers first began searching for the cause of dyslexia, they looked for one factor as the exclusive source of the problem. Now most experts agree that a number of factors probably work in combination to produce the disorder. Possible causes of dyslexia may be grouped under three broad categories: educational, psychological, and biological.

Educational Causes

Teaching Methods: Some experts believe that dyslexia is caused by the methods used to teach reading. In particular, they blame the whole-word (look-say) method that teaches children to recognize words as units rather than by sounding out letters. These experts think that the phonetic method, which teaches children the names of letters and their sounds first, provides a better foundation for reading. They claim that the child who learns to read by the phonetic method will be able to learn new words easily and to recognize words in print that are unfamiliar as well as to spell words in written form after hearing them pronounced. Other reading authorities believe that combining the whole-word and the phonetic approaches is the most effective way to teach reading. Using this method children memorize many words as units, but they also learn to apply phonetic rules to new words.

Whatever method they support, experts who think that instructional practices may cause dyslexia agree that strengthening the beginning reading programs in all schools would significantly decrease the number and the severity of reading problems among school children.

Nature of the English Language: Many common English words do not follow phonetic principles, and learning to read and to spell these words can be difficult, especially for the dyslexic. Words such as cough, was, where, and laugh are typical of those words that must be memorized since they cannot be sounded out. While such words undoubtedly contribute to reading problems, they constitute only a small percent of words in English and so cannot be considered a primary cause of dyslexia.

Intelligence Tests: The commonly accepted definition of dyslexia as a reading disability affecting children of normal intelligence is based on the assumption that we can measure intelligence with a fair degree of accuracy. Intelligence test results, usually referred to as IQ scores, must be interpreted carefully. IQ scores may be affected by factors other than intelligence. Those IQ tests which require the child to read or write extensively pose special problems for the dyslexic. Scores from such tests may reflect poor language skills rather than actual intelligence. Even those IQ tests that are individually administered and demand little or no reading and writing may fail to give a fair measure of intelligence; dyslexics often develop negative attitudes toward all testing situations. In addition, conditions such as noise, fatigue, or events immediately preceding the testing session may adversely affect test results. With such a range of possible influences on IQ scores, we must regard these scores as, at best, an estimate of the range of the child's scholastic aptitude, and at worst, a meaningless number that can unjustly label the student.

Psychological Causes

Some researchers attribute dyslexia to psychological or emotional disturbances resulting from inconsistent discipline, absence of a parent, frequent change of schools, poor relationships with teachers or other causes. Obviously a child who is unhappy, angry, or disappointed with his or her relations with parents or other children may have trouble learning. Sometimes such a child is labelled lazy or stupid by parents and friends—even by teachers and doctors. Emotional problems may result from rather than cause reading problems. Although emotional stress may not produce dyslexia, stress can aggravate any learning problem. Any effective method of treatment must deal with the emotional scars of dyslexia.

Biological Causes

A number of investigators believe that dyslexia results from alterations in the function of specific parts of the brain.

They claim that certain brain areas in dyslexic children develop more slowly than is the case for normal children, and that dyslexia results from a simple lag in brain maturation. Others consider the high rate of lefthandedness in dyslexics as an indication of differences in brain function. This theory has been widely debated, but recent evidence indicates that it may have some validity. Another theory is that dyslexia is caused by disorders in the structure of the brain. Few researchers accepted this theory until very recently when brains of dyslexics began to be subjected to postmortem examination. These examinations have revealed characteristic disorders of brain development. It now seems likely that structure disorders may account for a significant number of cases of severe dyslexia.

Genetics probably play a role as well. Some studies have found that 50 percent or more of affected children come from families with histories of dyslexia or related disorders. The fact that more boys than girls are affected means that nongenetic biological factors as well as environmental/sociological factors could contribute to the problem.

Treatment

Educators and psychologists generally agree that the remedial focus should be on the specific learning problems of dyslexic children. Therefore, the usual treatment approach is to modify teaching methods and the educational environment. Just as no two children with dyslexia are exactly alike, the teaching methods used are likewise varied.

Children suspected of being dyslexic should be tested by trained educational specialists or psychologists. By using a variety of tests, the examiners are able to identify the types of mistakes the child commonly makes. The examiner is then able to diagnose the problem and if the child is dyslexic, make specific recommendations for treatment such as tutoring, summer school, speech therapy, or placement in special classes. The examiner may also recommend specific remedial approaches. Since no method is equally effective for all children, remediation should be individually designed for each child. The child's educational strengths and weaknesses, estimated scholastic aptitude (IQ), behavior patterns, and learning style, along with the suspected causes of the dyslexia, should all be considered when developing a treatment plan. The plan should spell out those skills the child is expected to master in a specific time period, and it should describe the methods and materials that will be used to help the child achieve those goals.

Treatment programs for dyslexic children fall into three general categories: developmental, corrective, and remedial. Some programs combine elements from more than one category.

The *developmental* approach is sometimes described as a "more of the same" approach: Teachers use the methods that have been previously used believing that these methods are sound, but that the child needs extra time and attention. Small-group or tutorial sessions in which the teacher can work on reading with each child allow for individual attention. Some researchers and educators believe, however, that this method is not effective for many children.

The *corrective* reading approach also uses small groups in tutorial sessions, but it emphasizes the child's assets and interests. Those who use this method hope to encourage children to rely on their own special abilities to overcome their difficulties.

The third approach, called *remedial,* was developed primarily to deal with shortcomings of the first two methods. Proponents of this method try to resolve the specific educational and psychological problems that interfere with learning. The instructor recognizes a child's assets but directs teaching mainly at the child's deficiencies. Remedial teachers consider it essential to determine the skills that are the most difficult and then to apply individualized techniques in a structured, sequential way to remedy deficits in those skills. Material is organized logically and reflects the nature of the English language. Many educators advocate a multisensory approach, involving all of the child's senses to reinforce learning: Listening to the way a letter or word sounds; seeing the way a letter or word looks; and feeling the movement of hand or mouth muscles in producing a spoken or written letter, word or sound.

Prognosis

For dyslexic children, the prognosis is mixed. The disability affects such a range of children and presents such a diversity of symptoms and such degrees of severity that predictions are hard to make.

Parents of dyslexic children may be told such things as "the child will read when he is ready" or "she'll soon outgrow it." Comments like these fail to recognize the seriousness of the problem. Recent research shows that dyslexia does not go away, that it is not outgrown and that extra doses of traditional teaching have little impact.

Fortunately, educators are becoming more aware of the complexities of dyslexia, placing greater emphasis on choosing the most appropriate teaching method for each child. Teachers are more willing to provide remedial teaching over longer periods of time, whereas prior practice often has been to cut off services if observable changes fail to occur in a limited time. Some dyslexics improve quickly, others make steady but very slow progress, and still others are highly resistant to instruction. Many have persistent spelling problems. Some acquire a basic reading skill but cannot read fluently.

A child's ability to conquer dyslexia depends on many things. An appropriate remedial program is critical. However, environmental and social conditions can undermine any treatment program. The child's relationships with family, peers, and teachers have a major effect on the outcome of instruction. In a supportive atmosphere, a child's chance of success is enhanced. Attitudes such as "expectancy," the degree to which a teacher expects a child to learn, are important. Children who sense that they are not expected to succeed seldom do. Since slight progress in reading ability can make an enormous difference in academic success and vocational pursuits, children need to know that they are expected to progress.

The earlier dyslexia is diagnosed and treatment started, the greater the chance that the child will acquire adequate language skills. Untreated problems are compounded by the time a child reaches the upper grades, making successful treatment more difficult. Older students may be less motivated because of repeated failure, adding another obstacle to the course of treatment. The time at which remediation is given also affects a dyslexic's chances. Often, remedial programs are offered only in the early grades even though they may be needed through high school and college. Remedial programs should be available as long as the student makes gains and is motivated to learn. Adults can make significant progress, too, although there are fewer programs for older students.

A dyslexic child's personality and motivation may influence the severity of the condition. Because success in reading is so vital to a child, dyslexia can affect his or her emotional adjustment. Repeated failure takes its toll. The child with dyslexia may react to repeated failure with anger, guilt, depression, resignation, and even total loss of hope and ambition; he or she may require counseling to overcome these emotional consequences of dyslexia. With help a dyslexic child can make gains but the assistance must be timely and thorough, dealing with everything that affects progress. For the child whose dyslexia is identified early, with supportive family and friends, with a strong self-image, and with a proper remedial program of sufficient length, the prognosis is good.

NICHD Research Support

The National Institute of Child Health and Human Development (NICHD) supports many studies designed to determine how most children learn to read and what may interfere with or prevent some children from acquiring this important skill. Some investigators are attempting to develop language tests that can predict which 5- or 6-year-old children have the necessary skills to learn to read and those who are at risk for reading failure. If these investigators are successful it is likely that many cases of dyslexia can be prevented. Other scientists are attempting to identify children at risk for dyslexia through the use of modern neurological examination procedures, including electroencephalography and PET scans (Positron Emission Tomography, an imaging technique that measures brain activity.)

Some scientists supported by the NICHD are studying the children from families that have a higher than normal incidence of dyslexia and related language disorders to determine a possible genetic cause of the reading disorder. Other investigators are concentrating their research efforts on the development of specific descriptions of various subtypes of dyslexia with the hope that more appropriate therapies can then be planned.

Although a number of important advances have been made through research, many unanswered questions remain about this developmental disorder of childhood. Our ultimate goal is the complete prevention of dyslexia as well as other specific learning disabilities. Intermediate to that goal is the early identification of all children who are at risk for dyslexia so that prompt and appropriate procedures can be administered which will preclude the manifestation of dyslexic symptoms, or minimize their effects on the child's intellectual, academic, psychological or social development.

Although impressive evidence exists concerning the specific behaviors and neurological characteristics of dyslexia, continued research is essential. Such medical and educational research along with sound diagnostic techniques and individually designed educational programs can open the doors through which the dyslexic may enter into full participation in our literate society.

Other Sources of Information

The Orton Dyslexia Society, 8600 LaSalle Road, Suite 382, Chester Building, Baltimore, MD 21286-2044. Phone: (410) 296-0232

LDA (Learning Disabilities Association of America), 4156 Library Road, Pittsburgh, PA 15234. Phone: (412) 341-1515

CEC (The Council for Exceptional Children), 1920 Association Drive, Reston, VA 22091. Phone: (703) 620-3660

American Academy of Pediatrics, P.O. Box 927, 141 Northwest Point Boulevard, Elk Grove Village, IL 60009-0927. Phone (800) 433-9016 or (708) 228-5005

ASHA (American Speech-Language-Hearing Association), 10801 Rockville Pike, Rockville, MD 20852. Phone: (301) 897-5700

Other Publications in This Series

- ♦ *Facts About Anorexia Nervosa*
- ♦ *Facts About Cesarean Childbirth*
- ♦ *Facts About Down Syndrome*
- ♦ *Facts About Down Syndrome for Women over 35*
- ♦ *Facts About Endometriosis*
- ♦ *Facts About McCune-Albright Syndrome*
- ♦ *Facts About Oral Contraceptives*
- ♦ *Facts About Precocious Puberty*
- ♦ *Facts About Vasectomy Safety*

■ Document Source:
 U.S. Department of Health and Human Services Public Health Service
 National Institutes of Health
 National Institute of Child Health and Human Development
 NIH Publication No. 93-3534
 April 1993

HEREDITARY DEAFNESS

What Is Hereditary Deafness?

Hereditary deafness is hearing loss that is inherited or passed down from parents to their children. This type of hearing loss may be inherited from one or both parents who may or may not have a loss of hearing themselves.

Hereditary material or genes are located on chromosomes which are found in each cell of the body. Genes provide instructions for specific traits or characteristics such as hair color or blood type. Defective genes can also pass along traits such as hearing loss or speech and language disorders.

The hereditary hearing loss that results from defective genes may be syndromic or nonsyndromic, dominant or recessive. Syndromic hearing loss is associated with specific traits additional to hearing impairment. For example, hearing, balance and visual problems occur in Usher syndrome. Nonsyndromic hearing impairment has hearing loss as its only characteristic. Dominant transmission of deafness requires only one faulty gene, from either the mother or father to cause the hearing loss, whereas recessive transmission of deafness requires a faulty gene from both the mother and father.

Of the more than 4,000 infants born deaf each year, more than half have a hereditary disorder. However, not all hereditary hearing loss is present at birth. Some infants may inherit the tendency to acquire hearing loss later in life.

Scientists supported by the National Institute on Deafness and Other Communication Disorders (NIDCD) are on the forefront of research on the molecular bases of hearing and deafness, continuing to explore the genetics of hearing loss in a variety of disorders, including Waardenburg syndrome, Usher syndrome, nonsyndromic hereditary deafness, otosclerosis, adult-onset hearing loss and presbycusis and the hereditary predisposition to noise-induced hearing loss and otitis media. This research should lead to a better understanding of how hearing impairment or deafness is transmitted from parent to child, making it possible to identify and characterize the genes in which changes or mutations cause hearing impairment. Through these efforts it may be possible to discover how genes work, what proteins they manufacture and the role they play in the development and maintenance of normal hearing. These discoveries should lead to early diagnosis, prevention and treatment, such as gene transfer therapy.

Research on Hereditary Deafness

Syndromic Hearing Impairment

There are more than 200 forms of syndromic hereditary hearing impairment. NIDCD-supported scientists have been able to map or locate the abnormal genes on their chromosomes for three of these hereditary syndromic forms of hearing loss: Waardenburg syndrome (WS) type 1 and Usher syndrome types 1 and 2. WS type 1, which accounts for two to three percent of all cases of congenital deafness, has been mapped to a narrow band on the long arm of chromosome 2. Usher syndrome type 2 has been mapped to chromosome 1 and type 1 has been mapped to chromosome 11. These two types account for approximately ten percent of all cases of congenital deafness.

Both Usher syndrome types 1 and 2 are recessive disorders which cause congenital hearing loss and late-onset blindness due to retinitis pigmentosa. Usher syndrome type 1 is characterized by severe hearing loss, complete loss of balance and blindness. Usher syndrome type 2 is characterized by moderate hearing loss, normal balance function and blindness. More than half of the approximately 16,000 deaf and blind people in the United States are believed to have Usher syndrome.

WS types 1 and 2 are dominant disorders which are often characterized by hearing impairment and changes in skin and hair pigmentation. Hearing impairment is present in approximately 20 percent of those with WS type 1. In addition, individuals with WS type 1 have an unusually wide space between the inner corners of their eyes. In contrast, approximately 50 percent of individuals with WS type 2 have hearing impairment but they do not have the wide spacing between the inner corners of their eyes.

To accelerate research on WS, an international consortium was formed by the NIDCD in September 1990. The consortium consists of the following six research teams: Boston University Medical School Center for Human Genetics, Boston, Massachusetts; Michigan State University Department of Zoology, East Lansing, Michigan; Laboratory of Molecular Biology, NIH-NIDCD, Bethesda, Maryland; De-

partment of Medical Genetics, University of Manchester, United Kingdom; Molecular Genetics Laboratory, Virginia Commonwealth University, Richmond, Virginia; and Department of Human Genetics, University of Cape Town Medical School, Cape Town, South Africa.

One team from the consortium recently studied 60 members from six generations of a Brazilian family, 26 of whom were diagnosed with WS type 1. This team discovered that each affected family member had a defect in the gene called PAX 3 on chromosome 2. This defect was due to one amino acid substitution in the gene that was not found in 17 other WS type 1 families unrelated to the Brazilian family, indicating that other mutations may cause the syndrome in other families. Seventy-eight percent of the members of this Brazilian family had noticeable hearing loss which is well above the 20 percent found in most WS type 1 cases placing additional importance on the significance of this gene in the development of hearing loss in WS.

A group of scientists has discovered a defective gene in disordered mice referred to as Pax-3 (lowercase to distinguish it from the human symbol PAX 3). These mice have hearing loss, pigmentary disturbances and facial changes. The Pax-3 gene, which regulates early development of the mice in the womb, is comparable to the PAX 3 gene found on chromosome 2 in humans. Another team from the consortium has found another mutation in the PAX 3 gene in several families with WS type 1.

Nonsyndromic Recessive Hearing Impairment

Approximately 80 percent of the nonsyndromic hereditary hearing disorders are recessive. Another international collaboration will provide NIDCD scientists with a rare opportunity to study nonsyndromic recessive hearing impairment in a large segment of the population in southern India where scientists report that 40 to 50 percent of the children in schools for the deaf have this type of hearing impairment. This type of hearing loss has been difficult to study in the United States because of the difficulty in making a definitive diagnosis.

Nonsyndromic Dominant Hearing Impairment

A team of NIDCD-supported scientists has located the gene responsible for a nonsyndromic dominant form of hearing impairment in a large family from Costa Rica who develop hearing impairment in late childhood. Hearing loss for the affected members of this family becomes severe between 30 and 40 years of age. These scientists were able to analyze the genetic material of 86 descendents of Felix Monge, an 18th-century ancestor who had a hearing loss similar to his 20th-century descendents. The gene is located on a specific portion of chromosome 5. Since hearing loss in this family begins later in childhood, rather than at birth, it is possible that this gene is responsible for the maintenance of auditory hair cells during early life.

About the NIDCD

The NIDCD is one of the institutes of the National Institutes of Health (NIH). The NIDCD conducts and supports biomedical and behavioral research and research training on normal and disordered mechanisms of hearing, balance, smell, taste, voice, speech and language.

About the Recent Research Series

This series is intended to inform health professionals, patients, and the public about progress in understanding the normal and disordered processes of human communication through recent advances made by NIDCD-supported scientists in each of the Institute's seven program areas of hearing, balance, smell, taste, voice, speech and language.

For additional information on hereditary deafness, write to: National Institute on Deafness and Other Communication Disorders, NIDCD Clearinghouse, PO Box 37777, Washington, DC 20013-7777

■ Document Source:
   U.S. Department of Health and Human Services, Public Health Service
   National Institute on Deafness and Other Communication Disorders
   August 1992

HEART DISEASES AND BLOOD VESSEL DISORDERS

■ ■ ■

FACTS ABOUT ANGINA

What is angina?

Angina pectoris ("Angina") is a recurring pain or discomfort in the chest that happens when some part of the heart does not receive enough blood. It is a common symptom of coronary heart disease (CHD), which occurs when vessels that carry blood to the heart become narrowed and blocked due to atherosclerosis.

Angina feels like a pressing or squeezing pain, usually in the chest under the breast bone, but sometimes in the shoulders, arms, neck, jaws, or back. Angina is usually precipitated by exertion. It is usually relieved within a few minutes by resting or by taking prescribed angina medicine.

What brings on angina?

Episodes of angina occur when the heart's need for oxygen increases beyond the oxygen available from the blood nourishing the heart. Physical exertion in the most common trigger for angina. Other triggers can be emotional stress, extreme cold or heat, heavy meals, alcohol, and cigarette smoking.

Does angina mean a heart attack is about to happen?

An episode of angina is not a heart attack. Angina pain means that some of the heart muscle is not getting enough blood temporarily—for example, during exercise, when the heart has to work harder. The pain does **NOT** mean that the heart muscle is suffering irreversible, permanent damage. Episodes of angina seldom cause permanent damage to heart muscle.

In contrast, a heart attack occurs when the blood flow to a part of the heart is suddenly and permanently cut off. This causes permanent damage to the heart muscle. Typically, the chest pain is more severe, lasts longer, and does not go away with rest or with medicine that was previously effective. It may be accompanied by indigestion, nausea, weakness, and sweating. However, the symptoms of a heart attack are varied and may be considerably milder.

When someone has a repeating but stable pattern of angina, an episode of angina does not mean that a heart attack is about to happen. Angina means that there is underlying coronary heart disease. Patients with angina are at an increased risk of heart attack compared with those who have no symptoms of cardiovascular disease, but the episode of angina is not a signal that a heart attack is about to happen. In contrast, when the pattern of angina changes—if episodes become more frequent, last longer, or occur without exercise—the risk of heart attack in subsequent days or weeks is much higher.

A person who has angina should learn the pattern of his or her angina—what causes an angina attack, what it feels like, how long episodes usually last, and whether medication relieves the attack. If the pattern changes sharply or if the symptoms are those of a heart attack, one should get medical help immediately, perhaps best done by seeking an evaluation at a nearby hospital emergency room.

Is all chest pain "angina"?

No, not all. Not all chest pain is from the heart, and not all pain from the heart is angina. For example, if the pain lasts for less than 30 seconds or if it goes away during a deep breath, after drinking a glass of water, or by changing position, it almost certainly is **NOT** angina and should not cause concern. But prolonged pain, unrelieved by rest and accompanied by other symptoms may signal a heart attack.

How is angina diagnosed?

Usually the doctor can diagnose angina by noting the symptoms and how they arise. However, one or more diagnostic tests may be needed to exclude angina or to establish the severity of the underlying coronary disease. These include the electrocardiogram (ECG) at rest, the stress test, and x-rays of the coronary arteries (coronary "arteriogram" or "angiogram").

The ECG records electrical impulses of the heart. These may indicate that the heart muscle is not getting as much oxygen as it needs ("ischemia"); they may also indicate abnormalities in heart rhythm or some of the other possible abnormal features of the heart. To record the ECG, a technician positions a number of small contacts on the patient's arms, legs, and across the chest to connect them to an ECG machine.

For many patients with angina, the ECG at rest is normal. This is not surprising because the symptoms of angina occur during stress. Therefore, the functioning of the heart may be tested under stress, typically exercise. In the simplest stress test, the ECG is taken before, during, and after exercise to look for stress-related abnormalities. Blood pressure is also measured during the stress test and symptoms are noted.

A more complex stress test involves picturing the blood flow pattern in the heart muscle during peak exercise and after rest. A tiny amount of a radioisotope, usually thallium, is injected into a vein at peak exercise and is taken up by normal heart muscle. A radioactivity detector and computer record the pattern of radioactivity distribution to various parts of the heart muscle. Regional differences in radioisotope concentration and in the rates at which the radioisotopes disappear are measures of unequal blood flow due to coronary artery narrowing, or due to failure of uptake in scarred heart muscle.

The most accurate way to assess the presence and severity of coronary disease is a coronary angiogram, an x-ray of the coronary artery. A long thin flexible tube (a "catheter") is threaded into an artery in the groin or forearm and advanced through the arterial system into one of the two major coronary arteries. A fluid that blocks x-rays (a "contrast medium" or "dye") is injected. X-rays of its distribution show the coronary arteries and their narrowing.

How is angina treated?

The underlying coronary artery disease that causes angina should be attacked by controlling existing "risk factors." These include high blood pressure, cigarette smoking, high blood cholesterol levels, and excess weight. If the doctor has prescribed a drug to lower blood pressure, it should be taken as directed. Advice is available on how to eat to control weight, blood cholesterol levels, and blood pressure. A physician can also help patients to stop smoking. Taking these steps reduces the likelihood that coronary artery disease will lead to a heart attack.

Most people with angina learn to adjust their lives to minimize episodes of angina, by taking sensible precautions and using medications if necessary.

Usually, the first line of defense involves changing one's living habits to avoid bringing on attacks of angina. Controlling physical activity, adopting good eating habits, moderating alcohol consumption, and not smoking are some of the precautions that can help patients live more comfortably and with less angina. For example, if angina comes on with strenuous exercise, exercise a little less strenuously, but do exercise. If angina occurs after heavy meals, avoid large meals and rich foods that leave one feeling stuffed. Controlling weight, reducing the amount of fat in the diet, and avoiding emotional upsets may also help.

Angina is often controlled by drugs. The most commonly prescribed drug for angina is nitroglycerin, which relieves pain by widening blood vessels. This allows more blood to flow to the heart muscle and also decreases the work load of the heart. Nitroglycerin is taken when discomfort occurs or is expected. Doctors frequently prescribe other drugs, to be taken regularly, that reduce the heart's workload. Beta blockers slow the heart rate and lessen the force of the heart muscle contraction. Calcium channel blockers are also effective in reducing the frequency and severity of angina attacks.

What if medications fail to control angina?

Doctors may recommend surgery or angioplasty if drugs fail to ease angina or if the risk of heart attack is high. Coronary artery bypass surgery is an operation in which a blood vessel is grafted onto the blocked artery to bypass the blocked or diseased section so that blood can get to the heart muscle. An artery from inside the chest (an "internal mammary" graft) or a long vein from the leg (a "saphenous vein" graft) may be used.

Balloon angioplasty involves inserting a catheter with a tiny balloon at the end into a forearm or groin artery and threading its tip into the narrowed coronary artery. The balloon is inflated briefly to open the vessel in places where the artery is narrowed. Other catheter techniques are also being developed for opening narrowed coronary arteries, including laser and mechanical devices applied by means of catheters.

Can a person with angina exercise?

Yes. It is important to work with the doctor to develop an exercise plan. Exercise may increase the level of pain-free activity, relieve stress, improve the heart's blood supply, and help control weight. A person with angina should start an exercise program only with the doctor's advice. Many doctors tell angina patients to gradually build up their fitness level—for example, start with a 5-minute walk and increase over weeks or months to 30 minutes or 1 hour. The idea is to gradually increase stamina by working at a steady pace, but avoiding sudden bursts of effort.

What is the difference between "stable" and "unstable" angina?

It is important to distinguish between the typical, stable pattern of angina and "unstable" angina. Angina pectoris often recurs in a regular or characteristic pattern. Commonly a person recognizes that he or she is having angina only after several episodes have occurred, and a pattern has evolved. The level of activity or stress that provokes the angina is somewhat predictable, and the pattern changes only slowly. This is "stable" angina, the most common variety.

Instead of appearing gradually, angina may first appear as a very severe episode or as frequently recurring bouts of angina. Or, an established stable pattern of angina may change sharply; it may be provoked by far less exercise than in the past, or it may appear at rest. Angina in these forms is referred to as "unstable angina" and needs prompt medical attention.

The term "unstable angina" is also used when symptoms suggest a heart attack but hospital tests do not support that diagnosis. For example, a patient may have typical but prolonged chest pain and poor response to rest and medication, but there is no evidence of heart muscle damage either on the electrocardiogram or in blood enzyme tests.

Are there other types of angina?

There are two other forms of angina pectoris. One, long recognized but quite rare, is called Prinzmetal's or variant angina. This type is caused by vasospasm, a spasm that narrows the coronary artery and lessens the flow of blood to the heart. The other is a recently discovered type of angina called microvascular angina. Patients with this condition experience chest pain but have no apparent coronary artery blockages. Doctors have found that the pain results from poor function of tiny blood vessels nourishing the heart as well as the arms and legs. Microvascular angina can be treated with some of the same medications used for angina pectoris.

For further information:

- ♦ *Eating to Lower Your High Blood Cholesterol* (reprinted 1992), NIH Publication No. 92-2920
- ♦ *Facts About Blood Cholesterol* (revised 1990), NIH Publication No. 90-2696
- ♦ *Facts About Coronary Artery Bypass Surgery*, NIH Publication No. 87-2891
- ♦ *Facts About Coronary Heart Disease* (revised 1992), NIH Publication No. 92-2265
- ♦ *High Blood Pressure and What You Can Do About It*, NN222
- ♦ *Questions About Weight, Salt, and High Blood Pressure* (reprinted 1988), NIH Publication No. 88-1459

■ Document Source:
U.S. Department of Health and Human Services, Public Health Service
National Institutes of Health
National Heart, Lung, and Blood Institute
NIH Publication No. 92-2890
Reprinted May 1992

See also: Facts About Coronary Heart Disease (page 195); Managing Unstable Angina (page 202)

FACTS ABOUT ARRHYTHMIAS/RHYTHM DISORDERS

What is an arrhythmia?

An arrhythmia is a change in the regular beat of the heart. The heart may seem to skip a beat or beat irregularly or very fast or very slowly.

Does having an arrhythmia mean that a person has heart disease?

No, not necessarily. Many arrhythmias occur in people who do not have underlying heart disease.

What causes arrhythmia?

Many times, there is no recognizable cause of an arrhythmia. Heart disease may cause arrhythmia. Other causes include: stress, caffeine, tobacco, alcohol, diet pills, and cough and cold medicines.

In some people, arrhythmias are associated with heart disease. In these cases, heart disease, not the arrhythmia, poses the greatest risk to the patient.

In a very small number of people with serious symptoms, arrhythmias themselves are dangerous. These arrhythmias require medical treatment to keep the heartbeat regular. For example, a few people have a very slow heartbeat (bradycardia), causing them to feel lightheaded or faint. If left untreated, the heart may stop beating and these people could die.

How common are arrhythmias?

Arrhythmias occur commonly in middle-age adults. As people get older, they are more likely to experience an arrhythmia.

What are the symptoms of an arrhythmia?

Most people have felt their heart beat very fast, experienced a fluttering in their chest, or noticed that their heart skipped a beat. Almost everyone has also felt dizzy, faint, or out of breath or had chest pains at one time or another. One of the most common arrhythmias is sinus arrhythmia, the change in heart rate that can occur normally when we take a breath. These experiences may cause anxiety, but for the majority of people, they are completely harmless.

You should not panic if you experience a few flutters or your heart races occasionally. But if you have questions about your heart rhythm or symptoms, check with your doctor.

What happens in the heart during an arrhythmia?

Describing how the heart beats normally helps to explain what happens during an arrhythmia.

The heart is a muscular pump divided into four chambers, two atria located on the top and two ventricles located on the bottom.

Normally each heartbeat starts in the right atrium. Here, a specialized group of cells called the sinus node, or natural pacemaker, sends an electrical signal. The signal spreads throughout the atria to the area between the atria called the atrioventricular (AV) node.

The AV node connects to a group of special pathways that conduct the signal to the ventricles below. As the signal travels through the heart, the heart contracts. First the atria contract, pumping blood into the ventricles. A fraction of a second later, the ventricles contract, sending blood throughout the body.

Usually the whole heart contracts between 60 and 100 times per minute. Each contraction equals one heartbeat.

An arrhythmia may occur for one of several reasons:

- ♦ Instead of beginning in the sinus node, the heartbeat begins in another part of the heart.

♦ The sinus node develops an abnormal rate or rhythm.
♦ A patient has a heart block.

Arrhythmia Types

Originating in the Atria

Sinus arrhythmia. Cyclic changes in the heart rate during breathing. Common in children and often found in adults.

Sinus tachycardia. The sinus node sends out electrical signals faster than usual, speeding up the heart rate.

Sick sinus syndrome. The sinus node does not fire its signals properly, so that the heart rate slows down. Sometimes the rate changes back and forth between a slow (bradycardia) and fast (tachycardia) rate.

Premature supraventricular contractions or premature atrial contractions (PAC). A beat occurs early in the atria, causing the heart to beat before the next regular heartbeat.

Supraventricular tachycardia (SVT), paroxysmal atrial tachycardia (PAT). A series of early beats in the atria speed up the heart rate (the number of times a heart beats per minute). In paroxysmal tachycardia, repeated periods of very fast heartbeats begin and end suddenly.

Atrial flutter. Rapidly fired signals cause the muscles in the atria to contract quickly, leading to a very fast, steady heartbeat.

Atrial fibrillation. Electrical signals in the atria are fired in a very fast and uncontrolled manner. Electrical signals arrive in the ventricles in a completely irregular fashion so the heart beat is completely irregular.

Wolff-Parkinson-White syndrome. Abnormal pathways between the atria and ventricles cause the electrical signal to arrive at the ventricles too soon and to be transmitted back into the atria. Very fast heart rates may develop as the electrical signal ricochets between the atria and ventricles.

Originating in the Ventricles

Premature ventricular complexes (PVC). An electrical signal from the ventricles causes an early heart beat that generally goes unnoticed. The heart then seems to pause until the next beat of the ventricle occurs in a regular fashion.

Ventricular tachycardia. The heart beats fast due to electrical signals arising from the ventricles (rather than from the atria).

What is a heart block?

Heart block is a condition in which the electrical signal cannot travel normally down the special pathways to the ventricles. For example, the signal from the atria to the ventricles may be (1) delayed, but each one conducted; (2) delayed with only some getting through; or (3) completely interrupted. If there is no conduction, the beat generally originates from the ventricles and is very slow.

What are the different types of arrhythmias?

There are many types of arrhythmias. Arrhythmias are identified by where they occur in the heart (atria or ventricles) and by what happens to the heart's rhythm when they occur.

Arrhythmias arising in the atria are called atrial or supraventricular (above the ventricles) arrhythmias. Ventricular arrhythmias begin in the ventricles. In general, ventricular arrhythmias caused by heart disease are the most serious.

Tests for Detecting Arrhythmias

♦ **Electrocardiogram (ECG or EKG).** A record of the electrical activity of the heart. Disks are placed on the chest and connected by wires to a recording machine. The heart's electrical signals cause a pen to draw lines across a strip of graph paper in the ECG machine. The doctor studies the shapes of these lines to check for any changes in the normal rhythm. The types of ECGs are:

  • **Resting ECG.** The patient lies down for a few minutes while a record is made. In this type of ECG, disks are attached to the patient's arms and legs as well as to the chest.

  • **Exercise ECG (stress test).** The patient exercises either on a treadmill machine or bicycle while connected to the ECG machine. This test tells whether exercise causes arrhythmias or makes them worse or whether there is evidence of inadequate blood flow to the heart muscle ("ischemia").

  • **24-hour ECG (Holter) monitoring.** The patient goes about his or her usual daily activities while wearing a small, portable tape recorder that connects to the disks on the patient's chest. Over time, this test shows changes in rhythm (or "ischemia") that may not be detected during a resting or exercise ECG.

  • **Transtelephonic monitoring.** The patient wears the tape recorder and disks over a period of a few days to several weeks. When the patient feels an arrhythmia, he or she telephones a monitoring station where the record is made. If access to a telephone is not possible, the patient has the option of activating the monitor's memory function. Later, when a telephone is accessible, the patient can transmit the recorded information from the memory to the monitoring station. Transtelephonic monitoring can reveal arrhythmias that occur only once every few days or weeks.

♦ **Electrophysiologic study (EPS).** A test for arrhythmias that involves cardiac catheterization. Very thin, flexible tubes (catheters) are placed in a vein of an arm or leg and advanced to the right atrium and ventricle. This procedure allows doctors to find the site and type of arrhythmia and how it responds to treatment.

How does the doctor know that I have an arrhythmia?

Sometimes an arrhythmia can be detected by listening to the heart with a stethoscope. However, the electrocardiogram is the most precise method for diagnosing the arrhythmia.

An arrhythmia may not occur at the time of the exam even though symptoms are present at other times. In such cases, tests will be done if necessary to find out whether an arrhythmia is causing the symptoms.

What test can be done?

First the doctor will take a medical history and do a thorough physical exam. Then one or more tests may be used to check for an arrhythmia and to decide whether it is caused by heart disease. The box on the previous page gives details about these tests.

How are arrhythmias treated?

Many arrhythmias require no treatment whatsoever.

Serious arrhythmias are treated in several ways depending on what is causing the arrhythmia. Sometimes the heart disease is treated to control the arrhythmia. Or, the arrhythmia itself may be treated using one or more of the following treatments.

- ♦ **Drugs.** There are several kinds of drugs used to treat arrhythmias. One or more drugs may be used.

    Drugs are carefully chosen because they can cause side effects. In some cases, they can cause arrhythmias or make arrhythmias worse. For this reason, the benefits of the drug are carefully weighed against any risks associated with taking it. It is important not to change the dose or type of your medication unless you check with your doctor first.

    If you are taking drugs for an arrhythmia, one of the following tests will probably be used to see whether treatment is working: a 24-hour electrocardiogram (ECG) while you are on drug therapy, an exercise ECG, or a special technique to see how easily the arrhythmia can be caused. Blood levels of antiarrhythmic drugs may also be checked.
- ♦ **Cardioversion.** To quickly restore a heart to its normal rhythm, the doctor may apply an electrical shock to the chest wall. Called cardioversion, this treatment is most often used in emergency situations. After cardioversion, drugs are usually prescribed to prevent the arrhythmia from recurring.
- ♦ **Automatic implantable defibrillators.** These devices are used to correct serious ventricular arrhythmias that can lead to sudden death. The defibrillator is surgically placed inside the patient's chest. There, it monitors the heart's rhythm and quickly identifies serious arrhythmias. With an electrical shock, it immediately disrupts a deadly arrhythmia.
- ♦ **Artificial pacemaker.** An artificial pacemaker can take charge of sending electrical signals to make the heart beat if the heart's natural pacemaker is not working properly or its electrical pathway is blocked. During a simple operation, this electrical device is placed under the skin. A lead extends from the device to the right side of the heart, where it is permanently anchored.
- ♦ **Surgery.** When an arrhythmia cannot be controlled by other treatments, doctors may perform surgery. After locating the heart tissue that is causing the arrhythmia, the tissue is altered or removed so that it will not produce the arrhythmia.

How can arrhythmias be prevented?

If heart disease is not causing the arrhythmia, the doctor may suggest that you avoid what is causing it. For example, if caffeine or alcohol is the cause, the doctor may ask you not to drink coffee, tea, colas, or alcoholic beverages.

Is research on arrhythmias being done?

The National Heart, Lung, and Blood Institute (NHLBI) supports basic research on normal and abnormal electrical activity in the heart to understand how arrhythmias develop. Clinical studies with patients aim to improve the diagnosis and management of different arrhythmias. These studies will someday lead to better diagnostic and treatment strategies.

Where can I find publications about heart disease?

To obtain publications about heart disease, you may want to contact your:

- ♦ local American Heart Association chapter.
- ♦ local or state health department.

The National Heart, Lung, and Blood Institute also has publications about heart disease. For more information, contact:

- ♦ NHLBI Communications and Public Information Branch, Building 31, Room 4A21, Bethesda, Maryland 20892.

■ **Document Source:**
U.S. Department of Health and Human Services, Public Health Service
National Institutes of Health
National Heart, Lung, and Blood Institute
NIH Publication No. 91-2264
April 1991

FACTS ABOUT CORONARY HEART DISEASE

Some 7 million Americans suffer from coronary heart disease, the most common form of heart disease. This type of heart disease is caused by a narrowing of the coronary arteries that feed the heart.

Coronary heart disease (CHD) is the number one killer of both men and women in the U.S. Each year, more than 500,000 Americans die of heart attacks caused by CHD.

Many of these deaths could be prevented because CHD is related to certain aspects of lifestyle. Risk factors for CHD include high blood pressure, high blood cholesterol, smoking, obesity, and physical inactivity—all of which can be controlled. Although medical treatments for heart disease have come a long way, controlling risk factors remains the key to preventing illness and death from CHD.

Who is at risk for CHD?

Risk factors are conditions that increase your risk of developing heart disease. Some can be changed (left column), and some cannot (right column). Although these factors each increase the risk of CHD, they do not describe all the causes of coronary heart disease; even with none of these risk factors, you might still develop CHD.

Controllable	Uncontrollable
High blood pressure	Gender
High blood cholesterol	Heredity (family history of CHD)
Smoking	Obesity
Physical inactivity	Age
Diabetes	
Stress*	

*Although stress may be a risk factor for CHD, scientists still do not know exactly how stress might be involved in heart disease.

What is coronary heart disease?

Like any muscle, the heart needs a constant supply of oxygen and nutrients that are carried to it by the blood in the coronary arteries. When the coronary arteries become narrowed or clogged and cannot supply enough blood to the heart, the result is CHD. If not enough oxygen-carrying blood reaches the heart, the heart may respond with a pain called angina. The pain is usually felt in the chest or sometimes in the left arm and shoulder. (However, the same inadequate blood supply may cause no symptoms, a condition called silent angina.)

When the blood supply is cut off completely, the result is a heart attack. The part of the heart that does not receive oxygen begins to die, and some of the heart muscle may be permanently damaged.

What causes CHD?

CHD is caused by a thickening of the inside walls of the coronary arteries. This thickening, called atherosclerosis, narrows the space through which blood can flow, decreasing and sometimes completely cutting off the supply of oxygen and nutrients to the heart.

Atherosclerosis usually occurs when a person has high levels of cholesterol, a fat-like substance, in the blood. Cholesterol and fat, circulating in the blood, build up on the walls of the arteries. This buildup narrows the arteries and can slow or block the flow of blood. When the level of cholesterol in the blood is high, there is a greater chance that it will be deposited onto the artery walls. This process begins in most people during childhood and the teenage years and worsens as they get older.

In addition to high blood cholesterol, high blood pressure and smoking also contribute to CHD. On the average, each of these doubles your chance of developing heart disease. Therefore, a person who has all three risk factors is eight times more likely to develop heart disease than someone who has none. Obesity and physical inactivity are other factors that can lead to CHD. Overweight increases the likelihood of developing

high blood cholesterol and high blood pressure, and physical inactivity increases the risk of heart attack. Regular exercise, good nutrition, and smoking cessation are key to controlling the risk factors for CHD.

What are the symptoms of CHD?

Chest pain (angina) or shortness of breath may be the earliest signs of CHD. A person may feel heaviness, tightness, pain, burning, pressure or squeezing, usually behind the breastbone but sometimes also in the arms, neck, or jaw. These signs usually bring the patient to a doctor for the first time. Nevertheless, some people have heart attacks without ever having any of these symptoms.

It is important to know that there is a wide range of severity for CHD. Some people have no symptoms at all, some have mild intermittent chest pain, and some have more pronounced and steady pain. Still others have CHD that is severe enough to make normal everyday activities difficult.

Because CHD varies so much from one person to another, the way a doctor diagnoses and treats CHD will also vary a lot. The following descriptions are general guidelines to some tests and treatments that may or may not be used, depending on the individual case.

Are there tests for CHD?

There is no one simple test—some or all of the following procedures may be needed. These diagnostic procedures are used to establish CHD, to determine its extent and severity, and to rule out other possible causes of the symptoms.

After taking a careful medical history and doing a physical examination, the doctor may use some tests to see how advanced the CHD is. The only certain way to diagnose and assess the extent of CHD is coronary angiography (see below); other tests can indicate a problem but do not show exactly where it is.

An examination for CHD may include the following tests:

- An **electrocardiogram** (ECG or EKG) is a graphic record of the electrical activity of the heart as it contracts and rests. Abnormal heartbeats and some areas of damage, inadequate blood flow, and heart enlargement can be detected on the records.
- A **stress test** (also called a treadmill test or exercise ECG) is used to record the heartbeat during exercise. This is done because some heart problems only show up when the heart is working hard. In the test, an ECG is done before, during, and after exercising on a treadmill; breathing rate and blood pressure may be measured as well. Exercise tests are useful but are not completely reliable; false positives (showing a problem where none exists) and false negatives (showing no problem when something is wrong) are fairly common.
- **Nuclear scanning** is sometimes used to show damage areas of the heart and expose problems with the heart's pumping action. A small amount of radioactive material is injected into a vein, usually in the arm. A scanning camera records the nuclear material that is taken up by

heart muscle (healthy areas) or not taken up (damaged areas).

♦ **Coronary angiography** (or arteriography) is a test used to explore the coronary arteries. A fine tube (catheter) is put into an artery of an arm or leg and passed through this blood vessel to the heart. A fluid that shows up on x-rays is injected through the tube into the arteries of the heart. The heart and blood vessels are then filmed while the heart pumps. The picture that is seen, called an **angiogram** or **arteriogram**, will show problems such as a blockage caused by atherosclerosis.

How is CHD treated?

Coronary heart disease is treated in a number of ways, depending on the seriousness of the disease. For many people, CHD is managed with lifestyle changes and medications. Others with severe CHD may need surgery. In any case, once CHD develops, it requires lifelong management.

What kind of lifestyle changes can help a person with CHD?

Although great advances have been made in treating coronary heart disease, changing one's habits remains the single most effective way to stop CHD from progressing.

If you know that you have CHD, changing your diet to one low in fat, especially saturated fat, and cholesterol will help reduce high blood cholesterol, a primary cause of atherosclerosis. In fact, it is even more important to keep your cholesterol low after a heart attack to help lower your risk of having another one. Eating less fat should also help you lose weight. If you are overweight, losing weight can help lower blood cholesterol and is the most effective lifestyle way to reduce high blood pressure, another risk factor for atherosclerosis and heart disease.

People with CHD can also benefit from exercise. Recent research has shown that even moderate amounts of physical activity are associated with lower death rates from CHD. However, people with severe CHD may have to restrict their exercise somewhat. If you have CHD, check with your doctor to find out what kinds of exercise are best for you.

Smoking is one of the three major risk factors for CHD. Quitting smoking dramatically lowers the risk of a heart attack and also reduces the risk of a second heart attack in people who have already had one.

What medications are used to treat coronary heart disease?

Medications are prescribed according to the nature of the patient's CHD and other problems. The symptoms of angina can generally be controlled by "beta-blocker" drugs that decrease the workload on the heart, by nitroglycerin and other "nitrates" and by "calcium-channel blockers" that relax the arteries, and by other classes of drugs. The tendency to form clots is reduced by aspirin or by other platelet inhibitory and anticoagulant drugs. Beta-blockers are given to decrease the recurrence of heart attack. For those with elevated blood cholesterol that is unresponsive to dietary and weight loss measures, cholesterol-lowering drugs may be prescribed, such as lovastatin, colestipol, cholestyramine, gemfibrozil, and niacin. Impaired pumping function of the heart may be treated with digitalis drugs or ACE inhibitors. If there is high blood pressure or fluid retention, these conditions are also treated.

Ask your doctor which medication you are taking, what it does, and whether there are any side effects. Knowing more about this will help you stick to the schedule that has been prescribed for you.

What types of surgery are used to treat CHD?

Many patients can control CHD with lifestyle changes and medication. Surgery may be recommended for patients who continue to have frequent or disabling angina despite the use of medications, or people who are found to have severe blockages in their coronary arteries.

Coronary angioplasty or **balloon angioplasty** begins with a procedure similar to that described under angiography. However, the catheter positioned in the narrowed coronary artery has a tiny balloon at its tip. The balloon is inflated and deflated to stretch or break open the narrowing and improve the passage for blood flow. The balloon-tipped catheter is then removed.

Strictly speaking, angioplasty is not surgery. It is done while the patient is awake and may last 1 to 2 hours. If angioplasty does not widen the artery or if complications occur, bypass surgery may be needed.

In a **coronary artery bypass operation**, a blood vessel, usually taken from the leg or chest, is grafted onto the blocked artery, bypassing the blocked area. If more than one artery is blocked, a bypass can be done on each. The blood can then go around the obstruction to supply the heart with enough blood to relieve chest pain.

Bypass surgery relieves symptoms of heart disease but does not cure it. Usually you will need to make a number of changes in your lifestyle after the operation. If your normal lifestyle includes smoking, a high-fat diet, or no exercise, changes are advised.

Several experimental catheter-surgical procedures for unblocking coronary arteries are under study; their safety and effectiveness have not yet been established. They include:

♦ **Arthrectomy**, a procedure in which surgeons shave off thin strips of the plaque blocking the artery and remove these strips.

♦ **Laser angioplasty;** instead of using a balloon to open up the blocked artery, doctors insert a catheter with a laser tip that burns or breaks down the plaque.

♦ Insertion of a **stent**, a metal coil that can be permanently implanted in a narrowed part of an artery to keep it propped open.

For more information

The following brochures and fact sheets are available by writing to the National Heart, Lung, and Blood Institute

(NHLBI) Information Center, P.O. Box 30105, Bethesda, MD 20824-0105:

- *Check Your Healthy Heart I.Q.* (revised 1992), NIH Publication No. 92-2724
- *Check Your Smoking I.Q.: An Important Quiz for Older Smokers,* NIH Publication No. 91-3031
- *Check Your Weight and Heart Disease I.Q.,* NIH Publication No. 90-3034
- *Eat Right to Lower Your Blood Cholesterol* (reprinted 1992), NIH Publication No. 92-2972
- *Eat Right to Lower Your High Blood Pressure,* NIH Publication No. 92-3289
- *Facts About Angina* (reprinted 1992), NIH Publication No. 92-2890
- *Facts About Arrhythmias/Rhythm Disorders* (reprinted 1992), NIH Publication No. 92-2264
- *Facts About Coronary Artery Bypass Surgery* (revised 1992), NIH Publication No. 92-2891

■ **Document Source:**
U.S. Department of Health and Human Services, Public Health Service
National Institutes of Health
National Heart, Lung, and Blood Institute
NIH Publication No. 92-2265
Revised July 1992

See also: Facts About Angina (page 191); Facts About Mitral Valve Prolapse (page 200); High Blood Pressure: A Common but Controllable Disorder (page 201); Managing Unstable Angina (page 202)

FACTS ABOUT HEART AND HEART/LUNG TRANSPLANTS

In the two decades since the performance of the first human heart transplant in December 1967, the procedure has changed from an experimental operation to an established treatment for advanced heart disease. Approximately 1,600 heart transplants are performed each year in the United States.

Since 1981, combined heart and lung transplants have been used to treat patients with conditions that severely damage both these organs. As of 1990, about 800 people worldwide have received heart/lung transplants.

In 1983, a major barrier to the success of transplantation—rejection of the donor organ by the patient—was overcome. The drug cyclosporine was introduced to suppress rejection of a donor heart or heart/lung by the patient's body. Cyclosporine and other medications to control rejection have significantly improved the survival of transplant patients. About 80 percent of heart transplant patients survive 1 year or more. About 60 percent of heart/lung transplants live at least 1 year after surgery. Research is under way to develop even better ways to control transplant rejection and improve survival.

Organ availability is the second barrier to increasing the number of successful transplantations. Efforts by hospitals and organizations nationwide aim to increase public awareness of this problem and improve organ distribution.

What happens during a heart or heart/lung transplant?

A transplant is the replacement of a patient's diseased heart or heart and lungs with a normal organ(s) from someone who has died, called a donor. The donor's organ(s) is completely removed and quickly transported to the patient, who may be located across the country. Organs are cooled and kept in a special solution while being taken to the patient.

During the operation, the patient is placed on a heart/lung machine. This machine allows surgeons to bypass the blood flow to the heart and lungs. The machine pumps the blood throughout the rest of the body, removing carbon dioxide (a waste product) and replacing it with oxygen needed by body tissues. Doctors remove the patient's heart except for the back walls of the atria, the heart's upper chambers. The backs of the atria on the new heart are opened and the heart is sewn into place. A similar process is followed in heart/lung transplants, except doctors remove the heart and lungs as a unit from the donor; the new lungs are attached first, followed by the heart.

Surgeons then connect the blood vessels and allow blood to flow through the heart and lungs. As the heart warms up, it begins beating. Sometimes, surgeons must start the heart with an electrical shock. Surgeons check all the connected blood vessels and heart chambers for leaks before removing the patient from the heart/lung machine.

Patients are usually up and around a few days after surgery, and if there are no signs of the body immediately rejecting the organ(s), patients are allowed to go home within 2 weeks.

Why are transplants done?

A transplant is considered when the heart is failing and does not respond to all other therapies, but health is otherwise good. The leading reasons why people receive heart transplants are:

- Cardiomyopathy, a weakening of the heart muscle.
- Severe coronary artery disease, in which the heart's blood vessels become blocked and the heart muscle is damaged.
- Birth defects of the heart.

Heart/lung transplants are performed on patients who will die from end-stage lung disease that also involves the heart. Alternative therapies for these patients have been tried or considered. Leading reasons people receive heart/lung transplants are:

- Severe pulmonary hypertension—a large increase in blood pressure in the vessels of the lungs that limits blood flow and delivery of oxygen to the rest of the body.
- A birth defect of the heart that results in Eisenmenger's complex, which is acquired pulmonary hypertension.

Who can have a transplant?

Patients under age 60 are the most likely heart transplant candidates. Patients under age 45 are generally accepted for heart/lung transplants. In both cases, patients must be suffering from end-stage disease and be in good health otherwise. The doctor, patient, and family must address the following four basic questions to determine whether a transplant should be considered:

- ♦ Have all other therapies been tried or excluded?
- ♦ Is the patient likely to die without the transplant?
- ♦ Is the person in generally good health other than the heart or heart and lung disease?
- ♦ Can the patient adhere to the lifestyle changes—including complex drug treatments and frequent examinations—required after a transplant?

Patients who do not meet the above considerations or who have additional problems—other severe diseases, active infections, or severe obesity—are not good candidates for a transplant.

How are donors found?

Donors are individuals who are brain-dead, meaning that the brain shows no signs of life while the person's body is being kept alive by a machine. Donors have often died as a result of an automobile accident, a stroke, a gunshot wound, suicide, or a severe head injury. Most hearts come from those who died under the age of 45. Donor organs are located through the United Network for Organ Sharing (UNOS).

Not enough organs are available for transplant. At any given time, almost 2,000 patients are waiting for a heart or heart/lung transplant. Patients may wait months for a transplant. More than 25 percent do not live long enough. Yet, only a fraction of those who could donate organs actually do.

Does a person lead a normal life after a transplant?

After a heart or heart/lung transplant, patients must take several medications. The most important are those to keep the body from rejecting the transplant. These medications, which must be taken for life, can cause significant side effects, including hypertension, fluid retention, tremors, excessive hair growth, and possible kidney damage. To combat these problems, additional drugs are often prescribed.

A transplanted heart functions differently from the old one. Because the nerves leading to the heart are cut during the operation, the transplanted heart beats faster (about 100 to 110 beats per minute) than the normal heart (70 beats a minute). The new heart also responds more slowly to exercise and doesn't increase its rate as quickly as before.

A patient's outlook depends on many factors, including age, general health, and response to the transplant. Recent figures show that 73 percent of heart transplant patients live at least 4 years after surgery. Nearly 85 percent of patients return to work or other activities they like. Many patients enjoy swimming, cycling, running, or other sports.

About 60 percent of patients who receive combined heart/lung transplants survive at least 1 year, and 50 percent live at least 5 years.

What are the risks from transplants?

The most common causes of death following a transplant are infection or rejection of the heart. Patients on drugs to prevent transplant rejection are at risk for developing kidney damage, high blood pressure, osteoporosis (weakness of the major bones such as the hips and spine), and lymphoma (a type of cancer that affects cells of the immune system).

Coronary artery disease is a problem that develops in almost half the patients who receive transplants. Normally, patients with this disease experience chest pain and/or other symptoms when their hearts are under stress. This is called angina and is an early warning sign of a blocked heart artery. However, transplant patients may have no early pain symptoms of a blockage building up because they have no sensations in their new hearts.

Thirty to fifty percent of patients who receive a heart/lung transplant develop destructive changes in the lung tissue, bronchiolitis obliterans.

What does rejection mean?

The body's immune system protects the body from infection. Cells of the immune system move throughout the body, checking for anything that looks foreign or different from the body's own cells. Immune cells recognize the transplanted organ(s) as different from the rest of the body and attempt to destroy it; this is called rejection. If left alone, the immune system would damage the cells of a new heart and eventually destroy it. In a heart/lung transplant, immune cells may also destroy healthy lung tissue.

To prevent rejection, patients receive immunosuppressants, drugs that suppress the immune system so that the new organ(s) is not damaged. Because rejection can occur anytime after a transplant, immunosuppressive drugs are given to patients the day before their transplants and thereafter for the rest of their lives. To avoid complications, patients must strictly adhere to their drug regimen. The three main drugs now being use are cyclosporine, azathioprine, and prednisone. Researchers are working on safer, more effective immunosuppressants for future testing.

Doctors must balance the dose of immunosuppressive drugs so that a patient's transplanted organ(s) is protected, but his or her immune system is not completely shut down. Without an active enough immune system, a patient can easily develop severe infections. For this reason, medications are also prescribed to fight any infections.

To carefully monitor transplant patients for signs of heart rejection, small pieces of the transplanted organ are removed for inspection under a microscope. Called a biopsy, this procedure involves advancing a thin tube called a catheter through a vein to the heart. At the end of the catheter is a bioptome, a tiny instrument used to snip off a piece of tissue. If the biopsy shows damaged cells, the dose and kind of immunosuppressive drug may be changed. Biopsies of the heart muscle are usually performed weekly for the first 3 to 6 weeks, every 3 months for the first year, and yearly thereafter.

How much do transplants cost?

According to the Health Resources and Services Administration, the average cost of a heart transplant ranges from $57,000 to $110,000. In most cases these costs are paid by private insurance companies. More than 80 percent of commercial insurers and 97 percent of Blue Cross/Blue Shield plans offer coverage for heart transplants. Medicaid programs in 33 states and the District of Columbia also reimburse for transplants. Heart transplants are covered by Medicare for Medicare-eligible patients if the operation is performed at approved centers.

Approximately 70 percent of commercial insurance companies and 93 percent of Blue Cross/Blue Shield plans cover heart/lung transplants. Medicaid coverage for heart/lung transplants is available in 20 states.

What will transplants be like in 5 to 10 years?

Hospitals nationwide are trying to set up a better system for distributing organs to patients in need. Researchers are looking for easier methods to monitor rejection to replace the regular biopsies that are needed now. Work is progressing to make immunosuppressive drugs with fewer long-term side effects so that coronary artery disease development and lung destruction may be prevented.

Where can I get more information on transplants?

Information is available 24 hours a day, 7 days a week from the United Network for Organ Sharing at 1-800-24-DONOR. This hotline provides general information on transplants, current statistics, and listings of transplant centers.

Information on organ donation can be obtained from the American Council on Transplantation at 1-800-ACT-GIVE. The address is P.O. Box 1709, Alexandria, VA 22313.

Additional information is available from the Division of Organ Transplantation, Health Resources and Services Administration, Room 11A-22, 5600 Fishers Lane, Rockville, MD 20857.

■ Document Source:
   U.S. Department of Health and Human Services, Public Health Service
   National Institutes of Health
   National Heart, Lung, and Blood Institute
   NIH Publication No. 90-2990
   September 1990

FACTS ABOUT MITRAL VALVE PROLAPSE

Mitral valve prolapse is frequently diagnosed in healthy people and is, for the most part, harmless. Most people suffer no symptoms whatsoever from mitral valve prolapse. Estimates are that 1 in 10 to 1 in 20 individuals has mitral valve prolapse. It is also called floppy valve syndrome, Barlow's or Reid-Barlow's syndrome, ballooning mitral valve, mid-systolic-click-late systolic murmur syndrome, or click murmur syndrome.

Mitral valve prolapse can be present from birth or develop at any age. It occurs in both men and women, but is more common in women. Mitral valve prolapse is one of the most frequently made cardiac diagnoses in the United States.

What Is Mitral Valve Prolapse?

Although in general healthy hearts are structurally similar, like other parts of the body, there are individual variations. The heart's valves work to maintain the flow of blood in one direction, ensuring proper circulation. The mitral valve controls the flow of blood into the left ventricle. Normally when the left ventricle contracts the mitral valve closes and blood flows out through the aortic valve. In mitral valve prolapse the shape or dimensions of the leaflets of the valve are not ideal; they may be too large and fail to close properly or balloon out, hence the term "prolapse." When the valve leaflets flap, a clicking sound may be heard. Sometimes the prolapsing of the mitral valve allows a slight flow of blood back into the left atrium, which is called "mitral regurgitation," and this may cause a sound called a murmur. Some people with mitral valve prolapse have both a click and a murmur and some have only a click. Many have no unusual heart sounds at all; those who do may have clicks and murmurs which come and go.

Diagnosis

Mitral valve prolapse is commonly diagnosed by listening to the sounds that the heart makes or occasionally is discovered through echocardiographic tests. Sometimes once a physician has heard the characteristic sounds of mitral valve prolapse through a stethoscope, other tests may be ordered. Echocardiography is a common and painless test which uses sound waves of a very high frequency which travel through the layers of the skin and muscle to produce an image of the heart which can be seen on a screen. In this sense it is a technique similar to radar or sonar imaging.

Symptoms

The vast majority of people with mitral valve prolapse have no discomfort whatsoever. Most are surprised to learn that their heart is functioning in any way abnormally. Some individuals report mild and common symptoms such as shortness of breath, dizziness, and either "skipping" or "racing" of the heart. More rarely chest pain is reported. However, these are symptoms which may or may not be related to the mitral valve prolapse.

Treatment

In most cases no treatment is needed. For a small proportion of individuals with mitral valve prolapse, beta blockers or other drugs are used to control specific symptoms. Serious problems are rare, can easily be diagnosed and if necessary, treated surgically.

Preventing Complications

The overwhelming majority of people with mitral valve prolapse are free of symptoms and never develop any noteworthy problems. However, it is important to understand that in some cases mitral regurgitation, that is, the flow of blood back into the left atrium, can occur. Where mitral regurgitation has been diagnosed, there is an increased risk of acquiring bacterial endocarditis, an infection in the lining of the heart. To prevent bacterial endocarditis many physicians and dentists prescribe antibiotics before certain surgical or dental procedures.

Historical Background

It may seem that mitral valve prolapse is becoming more common but actually it has probably always been around and was simply less well recognized. For instance, some historians cite the observation of "soldier's heart" made by Dr. J.M. Dacosta during the Civil War as the first description of mitral valve prolapse. Contemporary understanding of this condition advanced, however, with the work in 1966 of Dr. J.B. Barlow in South Africa when he related the characteristic sounds to the specific anatomical characteristics of the leaflets in mitral valve prolapse. More precise identification became possible as increasingly sophisticated diagnostic tools were available.

The increased visibility of this disorder has also come from one-time or cross-sectional studies of healthy people as well as longitudinal studies which follow individuals over years such as the Framingham Study where routine tests have shown that it is commonly present. No one knew quite how common, and unnoticed, mitral valve prolapse was until 1976 when researchers examined 100 presumably healthy young students at a woman's school. Their finding, that it occurred frequently and that as many as 1 in 10 have mitral valve prolapse, was then underscored by findings from the Framingham study in 1983, as well as by reports from other research.

Clinical Significance

The overwhelming majority of people with mitral valve prolapse are free of symptoms and never develop any noteworthy problems. Whether or not there is any discomfort, health care providers should be notified of the existence of mitral

valve prolapse so that recommendations can be made about the advisability of using antibiotics to protect against bacterial endocarditis.

■ Document Source:
  U.S. Department of Health and Human Services, Public Health Service
  National Institutes of Health
  National Heart, Lung, and Blood Institute

See also: Facts About Coronary Heart Disease (page 195)

National Institute on Aging Age Page

HIGH BLOOD PRESSURE: A COMMON BUT CONTROLLABLE DISORDER

You may be surprised if your doctor says you have high blood pressure (HBP) because it does not cause symptoms and can occur in an otherwise healthy person. Fortunately, there are simple ways to control the condition by bringing blood pressure (BP) readings down to safe levels.

What is HBP? As blood flows from the heart out to the blood vessels, it creates pressure against the blood vessel walls. Your BP reading is a measure of this pressure, and it tells you if the pressure is normal (normotensive), high (hypertensive), or low (hypotensive). Thus, another name for HBP is hypertension.

BP readings are given in two numbers, such as 120/80. Although the average BP reading for adults is 120/80, a slightly higher or lower reading (for either number) is not necessarily abnormal or unsafe. Lower BP readings (for example 110/70) are usually considered safe for most people. For older people, many experts feel that readings up to 140/90 are acceptable. Once the BP goes above this level, however, some form of treatment may be needed.

The BP test is painless and takes only a few minutes. When your doctor takes your BP reading, he or she may want you to stand, sit, or both. The doctor should take several readings on different days before deciding if your BP is too high. All of these steps are necessary because BP changes so quickly and is affected by many factors, including the normal feelings of anxiety during a visit to the doctor.

As many as 58 million Americans may have HBP. About 40 percent of whites and more than 50 percent of blacks age 65 and older suffer from some form of HBP. Because this disease is so common, everyone should have a BP test once a year.

Although some cases of HBP are caused by other illnesses, these cases account for very few of the total number of patients with HBP. This kind of HBP is referred to as "secondary hypertension," and it is often cured by treating the original medical problem. Most HBP, however, cannot be cured, but can be controlled by continuous treatment. These cases of HBP fall into the category known as "essential" or "primary" hypertension.

Most experts agree that there are some things that increase a person's risk of developing HBP. For example, it appears that HBP runs in families. Also, HBP is more common in blacks than whites, and it tends to be more severe in blacks. Other possible risk factors include obesity, excessive alcohol consumption, and diets high in salt. Many doctors now feel that a combination of many factors may be responsible for HBP.

Hypertension occurs not only in tense people or during periods of tension; BP will go up in all people during periods of stress or increased physical activity. Still, you can have HBP even though you are usually a calm, relaxed person.

The good news about HBP is that it can be controlled by drugs and often by changes in daily habits. The type and severity of a patient's HBP, as well as his or her other medical problems, will determine which treatment is best for that person.

Some people incorrectly believe that once BP is brought down to normal levels treatment is no longer needed. If your doctor has prescribed an antihypertensive drug, you may have to take the medicine for the rest of your life, although the amount you take may be reduced.

If you have mild HBP, your doctor might recommend that you lose weight and keep it off, eat less salt, reduce alcohol intake, and get more exercise. It may be possible to lower you BP simply by making some of these changes in your daily habits. Your doctor may suggest that you follow this advice even if drugs are needed to control your BP. These changes may help your medication work better.

If you have HBP, help yourself by remembering these facts:

- ♦ You may not feel sick, but HBP is serious and should be treated by a doctor.
- ♦ BP can be lowered with medicines, but it will rise again if the medicine is not used. If one day's dose is missed, do not "double-up" the next day. Instead, call your doctor for his or her advice.
- ♦ Try to take your medicine at the same time each day— for example, in the morning or evening after brushing your teeth. This will help you set a regular, easy-to-remember routine.
- ♦ Weight loss, reduced salt and alcohol intake, and exercise may be helpful, but only as recommended by your doctor. Do not assume that these actions are substitutes for drugs unless your doctor specifically says they are.

HBP can lead to many serious conditions including stroke, heart disease, and kidney failure. You can reduce your risk of developing these problems by getting proper treatment. Have your BP checked by a doctor or nurse or at a health clinic. If HBP is diagnosed, follow your doctor's advice closely.

Resources

For more information on HBP, write to the National High Blood Pressure Education Program, 4733 Bethesda Avenue, Suite 530, Bethesda, MD 20814-4820.

For more information about health and aging, contact the National Institute on Aging (NIA) Information Center, P.O. Box 8057, Gaithersburg, MD 20898-8057. The NIA distrib-

utes free Age Pages on a number of topics, including information about nutrition, exercise, and how to stop smoking.

■ Document Source:
   U.S. Department of Health and Human Services, Public Health Service
   National Institute on Aging
   P.O. Box 8057, Gaithersburg, MD 20898-8057
   1991

See also: Facts About Coronary Heart Disease (page 195); Stroke: Prevention and Treatment (page 207)

MANAGING UNSTABLE ANGINA

Purpose of this booklet

The purpose of this booklet is to describe unstable angina and how it relates to other heart conditions, answer some common questions about this condition, and describe the main types of treatments available.

This booklet is written for people who have been told they have unstable angina, have been treated before for coronary artery disease, or think they might have coronary artery disease. It is also for people with a family member or friend who has unstable angina or stable angina.

This booklet also suggests some questions to ask your doctor, as well as the best time to ask them.

What is unstable angina?

Unstable angina is a type of coronary artery disease. The coronary arteries bring oxygen-rich blood to your heart. Because your heart is a muscle, it needs oxygen to work well. In coronary artery disease, one or more of these arteries may be partially or even completely blocked.

The type of coronary artery disease you have usually depends on the amount of blockage in your arteries. A heart attack, called a myocardial infarction, means the heart muscle has been damaged by not getting enough blood. Stable angina usually does not damage the heart. Unstable angina is worse than stable angina and may progress to a heart attack if not treated.

Angina is caused by a lack of oxygen in the heart muscle. The symptoms of angina include pain or discomfort in the chest, arms, back, neck, or jaw. Sometimes, anginal pain may feel like a tightness or crushing sensation, or it may be a stabbing pain or seem like numbness. Some people mistake anginal pain for indigestion or gas pain.

Having either stable or unstable angina does not always mean you will have a heart attack. But, unstable angina can be serious and should be treated by a doctor.

How are stable and unstable angina different?

Anginal discomfort may be different for different people. Some people have anginal discomfort when they overexert themselves (for example, when they shovel snow). Other people feel anginal pain when they get very upset or excited. Over time, they can usually tell which activities will give them discomfort. Usually, the discomfort will go away in a few minutes. This type of chest discomfort is called stable angina.

Stable angina attacks usually have a regular pattern. But in some people the pattern of angina is different—it becomes unstable.

Unstable angina is more serious than stable angina because the risk of having a heart attack is greater.

People with unstable angina include those who:

- Have anginal discomfort when they are resting or that awakens them from sleep.
- Suddenly develop moderate or severe discomfort on exertion when they have never had angina before.
- Have a marked increase in the frequency or severity of their discomfort.

What causes unstable angina?

In coronary artery disease, blockages—made up of fats, such as cholesterol, and other debris—form on the inside walls of the coronary arteries. In patients who have stable angina, the blockages may not seriously block the flow of blood.

In unstable angina, the blockages may be large. Sometimes, the blockage cracks open. When this happens, your body tries to heal the crack in the blockage by making a blood clot around the damage. If the clot is big enough to block the artery, the clot will keep blood flow from getting through. This can cause a heart attack.

Do I need to see a doctor?

This may depend on whether or not your doctor has ever told you that you have coronary artery disease.

People without known coronary artery disease

Many people do not know if they have heart disease. Any new or severe chest discomfort that is not related to an injury, such as a pulled muscle, could be unstable angina or a heart attack.

Unstable angina is not dangerous to most people who get medical care right away, but it can be very serious if it is not treated. Even anginal pain that goes away with rest can be serious. Only your doctor will be able to tell how serious it is and what should be done.

People with known coronary artery disease

If you have coronary artery disease, your past symptoms are the best guide to whether you should call your doctor about new symptoms. Call your doctor if the discomfort you are having is more severe or lasts longer than the discomfort you have had before, has begun to happen more frequently or with less effort, or happens when you are resting or asleep.

Chest pain can be an emergency

Here are some signs that your angina is very serious and you should go to the hospital right away:

- Pain or discomfort that is very bad, gets worse, and lasts longer than 20 minutes.
- Pain or discomfort along with weakness, feeling sick to your stomach, or fainting.
- Pain or discomfort that does not go away when you take three nitroglycerin tablets.
- Pain or discomfort that is worse than you have ever had before.

If you live in an area where ambulance service is not quickly available, have someone drive you to the nearest hospital. You should not drive yourself to the hospital.

It is a good idea to talk with your family, friends, or neighbors about your heart condition and have them read this booklet. They should be familiar with warning signs that signal when you should go to the hospital. You also may want to tell them which medicines you are taking and where you keep them.

What will happen in the emergency room?

At your hospital emergency room, the doctors and nurses will decide if you have unstable angina. If you do have unstable angina, they will give you medicines through a vein in your arm to stop your pain and prevent injury to your heart. These medicines will help prevent blood clots and help your heart work more easily. You probably will be given oxygen to help you breathe and get more oxygen in your blood.

The doctors and nurses will ask how you are feeling and if the medicines have stopped your discomfort. It is important to tell them how you really feel. If the medicines do not stop your discomfort, there are other things they can do to help you.

These things need to be done quickly. The doctors and nurses may not be able to explain everything as it is happening. There will be time for you to ask questions after your doctor finds out how serious your condition is.

What is an electrocardiogram?

When you are in the emergency room you may have an electrocardiogram, called an ECG or EKG. An ECG records on paper the electrical activity of your heart beat. The ECG may show your doctor if your heart muscle is getting enough oxygen-rich blood.

Will I have to stay in the hospital?

Your ECG, past medical history, and the nature of your pain tell your doctor how serious your problem is.

If your doctor does not consider your condition to be serious enough to admit you to the hospital, he or she may make an appointment to see you in a day or two for more tests. If your chest discomfort comes back before this appointment and is like that described in "Chest Pain Can Be an Emergency," you should return immediately to the hospital.

It is not easy to accurately diagnose unstable angina, and your doctor may need to see you more than once to be sure.

If your doctor suggests admission to a hospital, you may be put in a regular bed or in an intensive care unit. In either case, treatment will continue while your doctor does more tests.

The tests you have will depend on how serious your condition is and how well the medicines control your discomfort.

What tests will I have?

There is more than one kind of test your doctor can do to decide how badly your coronary arteries are blocked. Some of these tests are usually done while you are in the hospital. Other tests can be done in the hospital, but you do not have to stay overnight. Some tests can be done in your doctor's office.

Stress tests

You may have an exercise tolerance test. In this test you will be asked to ride a stationary bicycle or walk on a treadmill while a doctor takes an ECG. Your doctor may give you an injection of a radioactive drug that shows up on special cameras. This allows your doctor to make pictures of how your heart moves and the way your blood flows.

This test will let the doctor see the changes that take place in your heart when you exercise. Trained personnel or the doctor will watch your condition by asking how you are feeling during the test. Be sure to follow their instructions carefully and tell them exactly how you feel.

If you have other health problems, you may be given another kind of stress test that does not use exercise. If you have this test, you will be given a special type of drug that makes your heart beat faster and opens your coronary arteries. An ECG will be taken at the same time. This test gives the doctor the same type of information as the exercise tolerance test.

The exercise tolerance test or other stress test will help your doctor tell how well your heart is functioning. Although stress tests are useful, they cannot tell your doctor exactly where your arteries are blocked or how bad the blockages may be. Also, these tests are accurate no more than 90 percent of the time. In some cases, doctors will want to do a cardiac catheterization.

Cardiac catheterization

An angiogram or cardiac catheterization (sometimes called a cath) lets the doctor see the coronary arteries. A thin tube, called a catheter, is placed in an artery in either your arm or leg. The catheter is threaded up to your heart while your doctor watches on a screen.

The catheter will measure the blood pressure in your heart to see how well it is pumping blood. Then, a liquid is injected through the catheter into the artery, and x-rays are taken. The x-rays allow the doctor to see how much blockage there is and where it is located.

Cardiac catheterization is a test and not a treatment for unstable angina. A treatment called angioplasty looks and

feels a lot like cardiac catheterization. Angioplasty is described later in this booklet.

What can these tests show?

Stress testing may help your doctor decide how much of the heart could be in danger from blockages in your arteries. An angiogram shows how severe the blockages are and where they are. If you are told that you have single, two-, or three-vessel disease, it means that one, two, or three of the major coronary arteries have a blockage. Your doctor may also talk about the percentage of blockage in the vessel.

The number of blocked arteries and the percentage of blockage are used to measure the severity of your coronary artery disease. Generally, the greater the number of vessels that are blocked, the higher the percentage of blockage, and the more poorly your heart pumps blood, the more severe the disease.

These tests will give your doctor a lot of information about your condition. At this point, he or she can start to give you more information about how serious your condition is and the types of treatment available.

Treatment of unstable angina

After your tests, you and your doctor can decide on which treatment you should have. The treatment that is best for you will depend on the results of your tests, whether or not you are still having discomfort, and your own preferences. In general you will have three choices: medical therapy, angioplasty, or bypass surgery.

Medical therapy

You may have been given medicine in the hospital or emergency room. Some of these medicines, such as heparin which is used to decrease blood clotting, are given to you only in the hospital.

Many other medicines used to treat unstable angina can be taken at home. They come in the form of pills or creams that you can use by yourself.

Many people do very well on medicine alone. If you decide to use medicine to treat your unstable angina, and it does not control all your discomfort, you can still have bypass surgery or angioplasty later.

Almost everyone who has unstable angina will be given some type of medicine. The nurses or doctors caring for you will explain how and when to take all your medicines.

Several types of medicine can help to relieve the discomfort of unstable angina. Many of these drugs also make it easier for the heart to work. Medical therapy may be used alone or in combination with the other treatments described later in this booklet.

Medical therapy alone also may be the right treatment for people with other illnesses and people who do not want to have surgery or other procedures.

Here are some questions to ask your doctor about medical treatment.

♦ What side effects will I have from the medicine?

◆ Will I have to take medicine for the rest of my life?

> ## Medical therapy alone may benefit patients who:
>
> ◆ Have a blockage or blockages in only one vessel
> ◆ Have a less severe blockage
> ◆ Do not have severe anginal discomfort
> ◆ Have stabilized in the hospital

Some people have uncomfortable side effects from the medicine, but most people feel better because they have less anginal discomfort. If you do have a reaction to a medicine, be sure to tell your doctor about it. Often the reaction goes away or becomes less severe with time. If not, your doctor may be able to change your medicine to make you more comfortable.

Remember, none of these drugs removes any of the blockages from your arteries. They do relieve anginal discomfort by bringing more blood to your heart or by making it easier for your heart to work.

Some of the most common medicines given to patients with unstable angina include aspirin, nitrates, and beta blockers.

Aspirin

How it works: Most people think of aspirin as something to relieve a headache or a fever. But aspirin also can prevent blood clots from forming. These are the same kind of blood clots that can block the coronary arteries and cause a heart attack.

Research in patients with unstable angina has proven that taking an aspirin every day reduces the risk of heart attack or death. Acetaminophen (for example, Tylenol®) and ibuprofen (for example, Advil®) are not the same as aspirin and should not be used in place of aspirin.

Side effects: Most patients with unstable angina will be told to take aspirin every day. Your doctor will tell you how much to take. When coated or buffered aspirin is used there are few major side effects. Aspirin should not be used if you are allergic to it or if you have had an ulcer or any other bleeding problem.

Nitrates

How they work: Nitrates (usually nitroglycerin and isosorbide) are used to open blood vessels. Nitrates increase blood flow to the heart muscle and the blood vessels and make it easier for the heart to work. Nitrates can relieve most anginal discomfort very quickly.

Nitrates come in tablets that you put under your tongue or a different type of tablet that you swallow, as a patch that you wear on your skin, or as a cream that you apply on your skin.

Nitrate tablets, cream, and patches all have a limited shelf life after which they will no longer work. Ask your pharmacist how long they will last and when you should replace them.

Nitrate cream and patches are for maintenance therapy only. If you are using a nitrate patch or cream, you should still use nitrate tablets if you have anginal discomfort.

Take one nitroglycerin tablet as soon as you feel discomfort. If the discomfort does not go away in 5 minutes, take a second tablet. If the discomfort does not go away after 5 more minutes, take a third tablet.

If the discomfort has not gone away after taking three tablets in 15 minutes, go to the hospital immediately. Do not wait!

Persistent discomfort that does not go away could be a sign that you are having a heart attack. You should see a doctor immediately.

Side effects: You may feel dizzy or lightheaded right after taking nitrates. Patients are usually told to take nitrate tablets while sitting down. Some people may also get a headache when they take nitrates.

Beta blockers

How they work: This drug decreases the amount of work your heart has to do and the amount of oxygen your heart needs.

Side effects: Beta blockers are very powerful drugs that can have many side effects. About 10 percent of patients taking beta blockers will feel tired or dizzy. Depression, diarrhea, or skin rash may also happen in about 5 percent of patients. Mental confusion, headaches, heartburn, and shortness of breath are much less common.

Angioplasty

This procedure is done like an angiogram. A thin tube called a catheter is inserted into an artery in the groin and threaded up to the blocked artery. This catheter has a very small balloon attached on the end. When the catheter gets to the blockage, the doctor inflates the balloon. When the balloon is deflated, the blockage should be open enough for the blood to get through, stopping the anginal discomfort.

> ## Benefits and risks of angioplasty
>
> ### Possible benefits
>
> ◆ Relieve anginal pain
> ◆ Increase activity/exercise
> ◆ Allow return to former activities
> ◆ Reduce amount of medicine
> ◆ Decrease anxiety/fear
>
> ### Possible risks
>
> ◆ Worsened angina
> ◆ Emergency bypass surgery
> ◆ Heart attack
> ◆ Damage to the artery
> ◆ Re-blockage of the artery
> ◆ Death

Questions to ask your doctor about angioplasty include:

◆ Will I need additional angioplasty or bypass surgery in the future?
◆ What will it feel like to have angioplasty?
◆ What is the chance that I might die during the angioplasty procedure or have other problems?

Bypass surgery

Surgery is usually recommended for patients who have severe blockages in the left main coronary artery or disease in several vessels. Surgery is also an option when medicines do not control anginal symptoms.

Coronary artery bypass surgery can be a very effective way to increase the amount of blood getting to your heart and stop your discomfort.

In this operation, a piece of a vein, usually from your leg or an artery from your chest, is removed and used to "bypass" the section of your artery that has the most blockage. One end of the blood vessel is placed into your aorta. The aorta is the artery that supplies all the blood going out of your heart into your body. The other end is sewn into the artery below the blocked section to bypass the blockage.

Here are some questions to ask your doctor about bypass surgery:

♦ What will it feel like to have bypass surgery?
♦ Is it normal to be afraid of having surgery?
♦ What is the chance that I might die during surgery or have other problems?
♦ Will I need more surgery in the future?

Benefits and risks of coronary artery bypass surgery

Possible benefits

♦ Prolong life
♦ Relieve anginal pain
♦ Increase activity/exercise
♦ Allow return to former activities
♦ Reduce need for medicine
♦ Decrease anxiety/fear

Possible risks

♦ Bleeding, requiring more surgery
♦ Wound infection
♦ Stroke
♦ Blood clots
♦ Organ failure (liver, kidney, lung)
♦ Heart attack
♦ Death

Angioplasty or bypass surgery?

Both angioplasty and bypass surgery are designed to do the same thing. They both can increase the supply of blood to your heart muscle. Depending on the severity of your disease, you may have a choice between the two.

How will you know which one is right for you? Your doctor will help you make this decision. But in general, angioplasty:

♦ Is not as major a procedure as bypass surgery.
♦ Results in a shorter hospital stay.
♦ Will allow you to return to normal activities sooner.

You should also know that:

♦ In about 2 to 5 percent of cases, angioplasty does not work, and emergency bypass surgery will be necessary.
♦ About 40 percent of the time, the arteries become blocked again within 6 months of the angioplasty. If this happens, you may have to have angioplasty again or have bypass surgery.

Talking with your health care team

Some people think that their doctors are too busy to answer questions. Other people do not know how to ask their questions. But talking with the doctors, nurses, and other health care providers is an important part of your care.

Your questions are important, and the people taking care of you should make the time to answer your questions and listen to what you have to say. Your preferences for the type of treatment you receive are very important.

You may feel more comfortable if a family member or friend is there when you talk to your doctors, nurses, and other health care providers. This person can help to make sure that you understand what is happening, ask questions, and tell the doctor your concerns and preferences for care.

Here are some questions to ask your doctor before you decide what the best treatment might be for you.

♦ Am I a candidate for medical treatment, angioplasty, or bypass surgery?
♦ What are the chances that my arteries will become blocked again if I have angioplasty or bypass surgery? How soon might this happen?
♦ Will I have to change my job or retire?
♦ How soon can I resume my normal activities? What about resuming sexual activity?
♦ How much will my treatment cost?
♦ Do I have to go on a low-sodium or low-fat diet? If so, for how long?
♦ Will I have a heart attack? Will I always have chest pain?

Can blockages come back?

Neither angioplasty nor bypass surgery is a cure for coronary artery disease. Blockages continue to build up on artery walls even after angioplasty or bypass surgery.

Both angioplasty and bypass surgery can be repeated if the arteries become blocked again. The only way to stop coronary artery disease is to prevent the blockages from building up.

Although doctors do not know for sure why blockages form, they do know, from studies of large numbers of patients, that some people are more likely to have blocked arteries than others.

Your doctor may recommend that you attend a cardiac rehabilitation program. These programs usually are offered by local hospitals and very often they are covered by insurance. In a rehabilitation program, nurses, exercise specialists, and doctors will help you to change behaviors that put you at higher risk. They will also teach you how to exercise safely and help you gain confidence in your ability to live with heart disease.

Preventing blockages

The best way to prevent blockages from forming is to:

- Take aspirin every day
- Stop smoking
- Eat foods that are lower in fat
- Keep weight down
- Increase physical activity
- Control blood pressure if it is high
- Lower stress

Living with coronary artery disease

It is normal for you to worry about your health and your future. But, you should know that most people with unstable angina do not have heart attacks. Usually, angina becomes more stable within 8 weeks. In fact, people who are treated for their unstable angina can live productive lives for many years.

Coronary artery disease does not go away. Your behavior and lifestyle will affect your condition. This is why it is so important to follow the advice of your doctor and the other health care professionals who treat you.

Every year, thousands of people are told they have coronary artery disease. This may come as a shock, especially if they have never felt ill before. Often, they become anxious about their future and wonder if they will still be able to take care of their families or other responsibilities. It is normal to feel a loss of control, as if something has taken over your life.

Doctors, nurses, members of the clergy, and counselors all have experience in helping people with coronary artery disease. They can help you and your family. It is important to talk about how you feel, not just physically, but emotionally.

The best way to feel like you are in control is to learn more about coronary artery disease—what it is and the choices you have. When you see your doctor or other health care provider, be prepared to ask questions.

How can I learn more about unstable angina?

Organizations that can provide additional information include:

American Heart Association
7272 Greenville Avenue
Dallas, TX 75231-4596
Phone: (800) AHA-USA1

National Heart, Lung, and Blood Institute Information Center
P.O. Box 30105
Bethesda, MD 20824
Phone: (301) 251-1222

The Mended Hearts, Inc.
7272 Greenville Avenue
Dallas, TX 75231-4596
Phone: (214) 373-6300

For further information

The information in this booklet was based on the *Clinical Practice Guideline on Unstable Angina.* The guideline was developed by a private-sector panel of experts, including physicians, surgeons, nurses, and people with unstable angina.

Support for this guideline was provided by the Agency for Health Care Policy and Research and the National Heart, Lung,. and Blood Institute. Other guidelines on common health problems are available, and more are being developed.

For more information on guidelines or to receive another copy of this booklet, call toll free (800) 358-9295 or write to:

Agency for Health Care Policy and Research
Publications Clearinghouse
P.O. Box 8547
Silver Spring, MD 20907

■ **Document Source:**
U.S. Department of Health and Human Services, Public Health Service
Agency for Health Care Policy and Research
Executive Office Center, Suite 501, 2101 East Jefferson Street, Rockville, MD 20852
AHCPR Publication No. 94-0604
March 1994

See also: Facts About Angina (page 191)

National Institute on Aging Age Page

STROKE: PREVENTION AND TREATMENT

Stroke can often be prevented today. In fact, the death rate from stroke has fallen as much as 50 percent since 1970. This decline in deaths has come about, in part, because of new diagnostic tests and treatments. In addition, many Americans are adopting sensible health habits such as controlling their high blood pressure. These new habits may lower the risk of stroke.

Yet stroke remains a leading cause of death among older people and is the cause of a large number of nursing home admissions.

What Is a Stroke?

A stroke is a sudden disruption in the flow of blood to an area of the brain. Deprived of blood, the affected brain cells either become damaged or die. While cell damage can often be repaired and the lost function regained, the death of brain cells is permanent and results in disability. There are three major types of stroke:

The **thrombotic** stroke is most common. Fatty deposits (plaques) build up in the arteries (blood vessels) that supply blood to the brain. This severely reduces the blood flow until, eventually, a clot or clump (called a thrombus) in an artery entirely blocks the path of blood.

An **embolic** stroke results when a blood clot forms somewhere else in the body (usually in arteries of the heart or neck), and the clot travels through the circulatory system to the brain. The traveling clot is an embolus.

A **hemorrhagic** stroke is the most severe type of stroke. It occurs when a blood vessel in the brain bursts, allowing blood to pour into the brain outside of normal channels.

Diagnosis and Treatment

A stroke is a medical condition that requires immediate care in a hospital. Patients may be treated by a family doctor, internist, or geriatrician and may then be referred to a neurologist—a doctor specializing in the diagnosis and treatment of disorders of the brain and nervous system. The neurologist first evaluates the patient to determine if a stroke in progress has been completed. The entire episode can last from minutes to hours and sometimes (although rarely) days.

An early diagnosis is made by evaluating symptoms, reviewing the patient's medical history, and performing routine tests. Tests that may be given include an electrocardiogram (a test that measures the electrical activity of the heart), an electroencephalogram (a test that measures nerve cell activity in the brain), a computerized tomography scan (a 3-dimensional x-ray technique making pictures that look like slices), and a magnetic resonance imager (a test that can show, for example, blockage of the main artery in the neck).

Treatment begins as soon as the stroke is diagnosed to ensure that no further damage to brain cells occurs. Anticoagulant drugs may be prescribed to prevent blood clots from becoming larger; or, in the case of a hemorrhagic stroke, drugs may be prescribed to lower the blood pressure, which is usually high.

What You Can Do to Prevent Stroke

Stroke was once viewed as a single devastating attack, but we now know it develops over a period of many years. The risk factors or conditions that lead to stroke include high blood pressure, atherosclerosis, heart disease, diabetes, smoking, and being overweight.

You can help prevent stroke by taking these steps:

♦ Control your blood pressure. Have your blood pressure checked regularly, and if it is high follow your doctor's advice on how to lower it.
♦ Stop smoking.
♦ Eat a healthy diet: choose, prepare, and eat foods that contain lower amounts of total fat, saturated fatty acids, and cholesterol.
♦ Exercise regularly. There is evidence that exercise strengthens the heart and improves circulation. It will also help in weight control; being overweight increases the chance of developing high blood pressure, heart disease, and atherosclerosis.
♦ Control diabetes. If untreated, diabetes can cause destructive changes in the blood vessels throughout the body.
♦ Promptly report warning signs to your doctor. Sometimes people experience "little strokes" (transient ischemic strokes—TIAs) which are the clearest warning that a stroke may occur. TIAs produce symptoms of a stroke that disappear completely within hours.

Rehabilitation for Stroke

Rehabilitation should begin as soon as possible after the patient's condition is stable and for most, continues at home. It consists of various types of therapy: physical therapy to strengthen muscles and improve balance and coordination; speech and language therapy; and occupational therapy to improve eye-hand coordination and skills needed for tasks such as bathing and cooking. A team of health care experts (physicians, physical and occupational therapists, nurses, social workers, and speech and language specialists) coordinates activities for the patient and family.

Progress in rehabilitation varies from person to person. For some, recovery is completed within weeks following a stroke; for others, it may take many months or years.

Where to Get Help

For more information on high blood pressure or other stroke risk factors, contact the National High Blood Pressure Education Program, 4733 Bethesda Avenue, Suite 530, Bethesda, MD 20814-4820.

For information on treatment or rehabilitation services, call a university teaching hospital in your area or write to the American Heart Association, 7320 Greenville Avenue, Dallas, TX 75231.

The National Institute of Neurological Disorders and Stroke can answer your questions on stroke research. Write to the NINDS Information Office, Building 31, Room 8A06, Bethesda, MD 20892.

The National Stroke Association can also answer questions about stroke. Their address is 300 East Hampden Avenue, Suite 240, Englewood, CO 80110; or call (800) 367-1990.

■ **Document Source:**
U.S. Department of Health and Human Services, Public Health Service
National Institutes of Health
National Institute on Aging
National Heart, Lung, and Blood Institute
1991

See also: High Blood Pressure: A Common but Controllable Disorder (page 201); Women: Heart Disease and Stroke (page 211)

VARICOSE VEIN TREATMENTS

Fast facts

♦ Varicose veins are bulging veins that become enlarged when they fail to circulate the blood properly.
♦ Spider veins are the smaller threadlike or "starburst" vessels appearing on the surface of the skin.
♦ Doctors use a variety of methods to treat venous disease. Problem veins may be surgically removed or injected with a solution.

- Varicose veins and spider veins may recur following treatment by any known method. New varicose and spider veins also may appear.
- Question doctors carefully about the cosmetic side effects and health risks for each type of treatment.
- Be wary of claims promising "major breakthroughs," "permanent results," "unique treatments," "painless," or "absolutely safe" treatments.

Thousands of people every year consider getting treatment for varicose veins and spider veins. Advertisements for treating venous disease often tout "unique," "permanent," "painless," or "absolutely safe" methods—making it difficult to decide on the best treatment. If you are considering this procedure, the following information may help.

Remember, though, this cannot substitute for a consultation with a properly trained physician.

What are varicose veins?

Veins can become enlarged with pools of blood when they fail to circulate the blood properly. These visible and bulging veins, called varicose veins, are often associated with symptoms such as tired, heavy, or aching limbs. In severe cases, varicose veins can rupture, or open sores (called "ulcers") can form on the skin. Varicose veins are most common in the legs and thighs.

What are spider veins?

Small "spider veins" also can appear on the skin's surface. These may look like short, fine lines, "starburst" clusters, or a web-like maze. Spider veins are most common in the thighs, ankles, and feet. They may also appear on the face.

Who gets varicose and spider veins?

Varicose and spider veins can occur in men or women of any age but most frequently affect women of childbearing years and older. Family history of the problem and aging increase one's tendency to develop varicose and spider veins.

What causes varicose and spider veins?

The causes of varicose and spider veins are not entirely understood. In some instances, the absence or weakness of valves in the veins, which prevent the backward flow of blood away from the heart, may cause the poor circulation. In other cases, weaknesses in the vein walls may cause the pooling of the blood. Less commonly, varicose veins are caused by such diseases as phlebitis or congenital abnormalities of the veins. Venous disease is generally progressive and cannot be prevented entirely. However, in some cases, wearing support hosiery and maintaining normal weight and regular exercise may be beneficial.

Is treatment always necessary?

No. Varicose and spider veins may be primarily a cosmetic problem. Severe cases of varicose veins, especially those involving ulcers, typically require treatment. Check with a doctor if you are uncertain.

What procedures are available to treat varicose and spider veins?

Varicose veins are frequently treated by eliminating the "bad" veins. This forces the blood to flow through the remaining healthy veins. Various methods can be used to eliminate the problem veins, including, most commonly, surgery or sclerotherapy. Less commonly, laser or electro-cautery treatments have been used to treat the smallest spider veins, especially on the face.

Surgery to treat varicose veins, commonly referred to as "stripping," is usually done under local or partial anesthesia, such as an "epidural." Here, the problematic veins are "stripped" out by passing a flexible device through the vein and removing it through an incision near the groin. Smaller tributaries of these veins also are stripped with this device or removed through a series of small incisions. Those veins that connect to the deeper veins are then tied off. This stripping method has been used since the 1950s.

Spider veins cannot be removed through surgery. Sometimes, they disappear when the larger varicose veins feeding the spider veins are removed. Remaining spider veins also can be treated with "sclerotherapy."

"Sclerotherapy" uses a fine needle to inject a solution directly into the vein. This solution irritates the lining of the vein, causing it to swell and the blood to clot. The vein turns into scar tissue that fades from view. Some doctors treat both varicose and spider veins with sclerotherapy. Today, the substances most commonly used in the United States are hypertonic saline or Sotradecol (sodium tetradactyl sulfate). Polidocanol (aethoxyskerol) is undergoing FDA testing but has not yet been approved in the U.S. for sclerotherapy.

During sclerotherapy, after the solution is injected, the vein's surrounding tissue is generally wrapped in compression bandages for several days, causing the vein walls to stick together. Patients whose legs have been treated are put on walking regimens, which forces the blood to flow into other veins and prevents blood clots. This method and variations of it have been used since the 1920s. In most cases, more than one treatment session will be required.

Do these procedures hurt?

For all of these procedures, the amount of pain an individual feels will vary, depending on the person's general tolerance for pain, how extensive the treatments are, which parts of the body are treated, whether complications arise, and other factors. Because surgery is performed under anesthesia, you will not feel pain during the procedure. After the anesthesia wears off, you will likely experience pain near the incisions.

For sclerotherapy, the degree of pain will also depend on the size of the needle used and which solution is injected. Most people find hypertonic saline to be the most painful solution and experience a burning and cramping sensation for several minutes when it is injected. Some doctors mix a mild local anesthetic in with the saline solution to minimize the pain.

What types of doctors provide treatments for varicose and spider veins?

Doctors providing surgical treatment include general and vascular surgeons. Sclerotherapy is often performed by dermatologists. Some general, vascular, and plastic surgeons also perform sclerotherapy treatments. You may want to consult more than one doctor before deciding on a method of treatment. Be sure to ask doctors about their experience in performing the procedure you want.

What are the side effects of these treatments?

Carefully question doctors about the safety and side effects for each type of treatment. Thoroughly review any "informed consent" forms your doctor gives you explaining the risks of a procedure.

For surgical removal of veins, the side effects are those for any surgery performed under anesthesia, including nausea, vomiting, and the risk of wound infection. Surgery also results in scarring where small incisions are made and may occasionally cause blood clots.

For sclerotherapy, the side effects can depend on the substance used for the injection. People with allergies may want to be cautious. For example, Sotradecol may cause allergic reactions, occasionally severe. Hypertonic saline solution is unlikely to cause allergic reactions. Either substance may burn the skin (if the needle is not properly inserted) or permanently mark or "stain" the skin. (These brownish marks are caused by the scattering of blood cells throughout the tissue after the vein has been injected and may fade over time.) Occasionally, sclerotherapy can lead to blood clots.

Laser and electro-cautery treatments can cause scarring and changes in the color of the skin.

How long do results last?

Many factors will affect the rate at which treated veins recur. These include the diagnosis, the method used and its suitability for treating a particular condition, and the skill of the physician. Sometimes the body forms a new vein in place of the one removed by a surgeon. An injected vein that was not completely destroyed by sclerotherapy may reopen, or a new vein may appear in the same location as a previous one. Many studies have found that varicose veins are more likely to recur following sclerotherapy than following surgery. However, no treatment method has been scientifically established as free from recurrences. For all types of procedures, recurrence rates increase with time. Also, because venous disease is typically progressive, no treatment can prevent the appearance of new varicose or spider veins in the future.

Is one treatment better than another?

The method you select for treating venous disease should be based on your physician's diagnosis, the size of the veins to be treated, your treatment history, your age, your history of allergies, and your ability to tolerate surgery and anesthesia, among other factors. As noted above, small spider veins cannot be surgically removed and can only be treated with sclerotherapy. On the other hand, larger varicose veins may, according to many studies, be more likely to recur if treated with sclerotherapy.

Be wary of claims touting "major breakthroughs," "permanent results," "unique treatments," "brand-new," "painless," or "absolutely safe" methods. Always ask for specific documentation for claims made about particular recurrence rates or fewer health risks or cosmetic side effects.

How expensive is the procedure?

Sclerotherapy can cost anywhere from a few hundred dollars to several thousand dollars, depending on the number of injections and treatment sessions required and the area of the country where the procedure is performed.

Surgery can cost approximately $600-$2,000 per leg for the surgeon's fee, plus charges for anesthesia and hospitalization. Most vein surgery can be performed on an outpatient basis. Costs can vary depending on how many veins must be removed and the area of the country where the procedure is performed.

You may want to check to see if the procedure is covered under your medical insurance. Many policies do not cover costs for elective cosmetic surgery.

For more information

If you need to resolve a problem with a doctor regarding treatment for varicose veins, you may want to contact your county medical society, state medical board, or local consumer protection agency.

You also may want to report any concerns about advertising claims to the Federal Trade Commission (FTC). Write: Correspondence Branch, Federal Trade Commission, Washington, DC 20580. Although the FTC does not generally intervene in individual disputes, the information you provide may indicate a pattern of possible law violations requiring action by the Commission or referral to state authorities.

For a free brochure on Cosmetic Surgery, write: Public Reference, Federal Trade Commission, Washington, DC 20580; 202-326-2222. You also may request Best Sellers, which lists all of the FTC's consumer publications.

FTC Headquarters
6th & Pennsylvania Avenue, N.W.
Washington, DC 20580
(202) 326-2222
TDD (202) 326-2502

FTC Regional Offices
1718 Peachtree Street, NW, Suite 1000
Atlanta, GA 30367
(404) 347-4836

10 Causeway Street, Suite 1184
Boston, MA 02222-1073

(617) 565-7240

55 East Monroe Street, Suite 1437
Chicago, IL 60603
(312) 353-4423

668 Euclid Avenue, Suite 520-A
Cleveland, OH 44114
(216) 522-4207

100 N Central Expressway, Suite 500
Dallas, TX 75201
(214) 767-5501

1405 Curtis Street, Suite 2900
Denver, CO 80202-2393
(303) 844-2271

11000 Wilshire Blvd, Suite 13209
Los Angeles, CA 90024
(310) 575-7575

150 William Street, Suite 570
San Francisco, CA 94103
(415) 744-7920

2806 Federal Bldg., 915 Second Ave
Seattle, WA 98174
(206) 220-6363

■ Document Source:
**Federal Trade Commission
Bureau of Consumer Protection
Office of Consumer and Business Education
(202) 326-3650
#F030421
January 1994**

WOMEN: HEART DISEASE AND STROKE

Heart disease (specifically, coronary heart disease) usually is considered a disease of middle-aged men, so it may be surprising to learn that it is also the number one cause of death among women. More than 550,000 Americans die each year of heart-related causes; more than 250,000 of them are women. That is a larger number by far than die of all forms of cancer combined. In addition, more than 100,000 women die of stroke each year.

Risk Factors

A risk factor is a characteristic that increases the probability of developing a disease. Some risk factors, such as age, sex, and family history for a disease cannot be changed, but others can.

The three major risk factors for the development of coronary heart disease are elevated blood cholesterol, high blood pressure, and cigarette smoking. Furthermore, high blood pressure is the single most important risk factor for stroke, the third leading cause of death among women. More than 100,000 women die of stroke each year.

Research has shown that black women are at increased risk for heart disease and stroke. Black women have nearly double the stroke risk of white women and from two to three times the risk of death from heart disease than do white women.

Awareness of these risk factors and of their prevention and control is the first step toward reducing the chances of developing these diseases. In fact, death rates from heart attacks and stroke have been declining over the past few decades. In 1980, the death rate for women from heart disease was 25 percent lower than in 1970. During the same period, the death rate for stroke went down 39 percent, and this favorable trend is continuing. Now, what are these risk factors and what can you do about them?

Elevated Blood Cholesterol

What is cholesterol?

Cholesterol is a waxy substance that is made in our body cells. Despite a bad reputation, cholesterol is important to us as an essential ingredient in cell manufacture and growth. It is found in all foods of animal origin.

What is the relationship between diet and blood cholesterol?

Cholesterol is obtained directly from foods of animal origin. However, an even more important factor in elevating blood cholesterol is the saturated fat in the diet, some of which is converted into cholesterol in the body. Most saturated fat also is obtained from foods of animal origin. Reducing the amount of dietary saturated fat is an important means of lowering blood cholesterol.

Why should I be concerned about my blood cholesterol level?

Too much blood cholesterol increases your risk of heart disease. Although cholesterol is manufactured normally in your body, eating foods containing high levels of cholesterol or saturated fat raises the level of blood cholesterol. Over time this excess cholesterol may build up in the blood vessels of your heart, reduce the blood supply to the heart muscle and possibly lead to a heart attack. Evidence shows that the higher your blood cholesterol level, the higher your risk of heart disease. For example, women between 45 and 74 years of age who have a cholesterol level over 265 mg/dl have more than twice the risk of developing heart disease as do women with a blood cholesterol level below 205 mg/dl. The measure "mg/dl" means milligrams per deciliter, the weight of cholesterol in a deciliter of blood. A deciliter is approximately one-tenth of a quart.

What is the relationship between my age and my cholesterol level?

Blood cholesterol levels generally increase with age. The blood cholesterol level in women younger than age 45 generally is lower than in men of the same age. From about the ages of 45 to 55 (roughly the age of menopause) the average cholesterol level of women increases to a level higher than that of men. An estimated 15 million American women have cholesterol levels of 260 mg/dl or above, which place them at substantially increased risk of developing heart disease.

What are the different kinds of cholesterol and why are they important?

Cholesterol is carried in the blood with several other substances which can be separated based on their density or relative weight. When blood cholesterol is measured, several parts of the total cholesterol can be determined. The total cholesterol level is the measure of all forms of cholesterol floating in the blood—200 mg/dl, for example. The two parts thought to be the most important are the low density lipoprotein (LDL) cholesterol, often thought of as the cholesterol fraction that is most dangerous to arteries, and the high density lipoprotein (HDL) cholesterol, which is believed to have a protective function by ridding the body of LDL. Recent research indicates that the proportion of HDL cholesterol to total cholesterol is a stronger predictor of heart disease than is the total blood cholesterol level itself. The higher the proportion of HDL, the lower the risk of heart disease.

High Blood Pressure

What is blood pressure? What is high blood pressure? What is hypertension?

Blood pressure, the force exerted by the blood against the walls of the arteries, generally is expressed as two numbers such as 120/70 and is measured in millimeters of mercury (mm Hg). The first or top number, called the systolic blood pressure, is the force exerted when the heart beats. The second number, or diastolic blood pressure, is the pressure that remains in the arteries between heartbeats.

Blood pressure varies up and down during the day depending upon a person's activities. However, high blood pressure, which is the same thing as hypertension, occurs when the blood pressure *stays too high—140/90 mm Hg or above.*

Who gets high blood pressure?

Anyone can have high blood pressure. An estimated 25 million American women have hypertension, which is defined as having elevated blood pressure (i.e., 140/90 mm Hg or higher) or currently taking antihypertensive medication. Of these hypertensive women, almost 17 percent are successfully controlling their blood pressure to below 140/90 mm Hg.

The likelihood of high blood pressure increases steadily with age, with more than half of all women over the age of 55 having this condition. Black women, on average, are almost one and a half times more likely to have high blood pressure as are white women. In addition, several recent studies have shown that oral contraceptives (birth control pills) or estrogen replacement therapy may raise some women's blood pressure.

Blood pressure can be determined quickly, easily and painlessly by means of the familiar inflatable cuff and stethoscope. It takes but a few minutes and can be done by many health professionals. A single reading in which the blood pressure measurement is high is not a diagnosis of hypertension. But a high reading means you should consult your physician to determine whether you have high blood pressure and what you should do about it.

Does having high blood pressure increase my chances of having heart disease or stroke?

High blood pressure is one of the major risk factors for developing heart disease or stroke. For example, women between the ages of 45 and 74 whose diastolic blood pressure (the lower of the two numbers) is between 100 and 104 mm Hg have about twice the risk of developing heart disease and almost triple the risk of having a stroke as do women whose diastolic blood pressure is between 75 and 79 mm Hg.

What are the symptoms of high blood pressure?

High blood pressure usually has no symptoms. You can feel fine, but still have this very serious disease.

Does controlling my blood pressure reduce my risk?

Yes, controlling your high blood pressure reduces your chances of suffering from the complications of high blood pressure—stroke, heart disease and kidney disease. Several studies have shown that those who controlled their hypertension had fewer strokes and less heart disease than did those who had uncontrolled high blood pressure. Although more remains to be done, it is encouraging to note that, compared to 20 years ago, a substantially greater proportion of hypertensive women now have their blood pressure under control.

Cigarette Smoking

How many women in the United States smoke cigarettes? Has cigarette smoking behavior changed in women over the past 15 years?

Almost 30 percent (more than 25 million) of all adult women in the United States smoke cigarettes. The percentage of women smoking still is less than that of men, but trends show that women are smoking more heavily now than they did in the past. For example, the percentage of both black and white women who smoke more than 25 cigarettes a day increased steadily from 1965 to 1980. The number of teenaged girls who smoke also has increased, especially among 17- to 18-year-olds, and now surpasses the number of teenaged boys who smoke.

One theory has suggested that the increasingly heavy smoking is related to the greater number of women in the workforce. However, recent studies show that it is homemakers—not working women—who are more likely to be heavy smokers.

Does smoking cigarettes increase a woman's risk of heart disease?

Yes. Studies indicate that cigarette smoking increases the risk of heart disease among women and that risk increases with the number of cigarettes smoked per day. Women who smoke are from 2 to 6 times more likely to suffer a heart attack as are nonsmokers.

However, heart disease is not the only problem. Lung diseases such as emphysema and chronic bronchitis and lung and many other cancers are much more common among smokers. Also, pregnant women who smoke are more likely to have stillborn babies, spontaneous abortions or premature deliveries than are women who do not smoke. Babies born to women who smoke usually are smaller than those born to nonsmoking mothers.

What happens if I smoke and use oral contraceptives (birth control pills)?

The combination of cigarette smoking and the use of birth control pills greatly increases the risk of heart disease among women. Recent studies have shown women smokers who used oral contraceptives were up to 39 times more likely to have a heart attack and up to 22 times more likely to have a stroke than were women who neither smoked nor used birth control pills.

Risk Factors in Combination

If I have more than one risk factor present is my risk even greater?

Yes, a combination of two or more of the major risk factors—elevated blood cholesterol and high blood pressure, for example—can seriously increase your chances of having a heart attack. If you have all three major risk factors—high blood pressure, elevated blood cholesterol and you smoke cigarettes—your risk is increased even more.

Resources to Help You Alter These Risks

Consult your physician to determine the extent of your risk factors and the ways to control them. As you consider ways to reduce your cholesterol, stop smoking and control your blood pressure, the following list may help guide you to useful resources.

National Organization Resources

Action on Smoking and Health (ASH)
2013 H Street, NW
Washington, DC 20006

American Cancer Society
777 Third Avenue
New York, NY 10017

American Dietetic Association
430 North Michigan Avenue
Chicago, IL 60611

American Heart Association
7320 Greenville Avenue
Dallas, TX 75321

American Lung Association
1749 Broadway
New York, NY 10019

National Nutrition Education Clearinghouse
1736 Franklin Street
Oakland, CA 94612

Federal Government Resources

Cancer Information Clearinghouse
National Cancer Institute
Office of Cancer Communications
Building 31, Room 10A18
9000 Rockville Pike
Bethesda, MD 20205

Center for Health Promotion and Education
Centers for Disease Control
Atlanta, GA 30333

Consumer Information Center
Pueblo, CO 81009

Food and Nutrition Information Center
3101 Park Center Drive
Alexandria, VA 22302

National Heart, Lung, and Blood Institute
Public Inquiries and Reports Branch
Building 31, Room 4A21
9000 Rockville Pike
Bethesda, MD 20205

Office on Smoking and Health Technical Information Center
Park Building
5600 Fishers Lane, Room 110
Rockville, MD 20857

■ Document Source:
  U.S. Department of Health and Human Services, Public Health Service
  National Institutes of Health
  National Heart, Lung, and Blood Institute

See also: Facts About Coronary Heart Disease (page 195); High Blood Pressure: A Common but Controllable Disorder (page 201); Stroke: Prevention and Treatment (page 207)

INFECTIOUS DISEASES

■ ■ ■

CHICKEN POX (VARICELLA) DISEASE INFORMATION

Chickenpox is a common, highly contagious disease of childhood. Most Americans will have been infected by the virus by age 15, and it is estimated that approximately 4 million cases occur each year. Children between 5 and 9 years of age account for the majority of all cases, with more cases occurring during the winter and spring than during other times of the year.

Chickenpox is easily transmitted between household members or classmates at schools or day-care centers through the drainage from the open sores, respiratory droplets, or airborne particles. The virus can also be transmitted indirectly through contact with articles containing fresh drainage from the sores. Persons are most contagious from 1 to 2 days before the rash appears through the first 5 to 6 days after the rash. Generally, patients are no longer contagious after the sores have crusted over.

Persons exposed to chickenpox are most likely to develop symptoms 14 to 16 days after exposure, However, for normal individuals, symptoms may appear any time after 10 days and up to 21 days.

Chickenpox is characterized by 1 to 2 days of fever up to 102 degrees, general body weakness, and a rash, which in many children is the first sign of the disease. Only rarely will a person have chickenpox without a rash. Often, the rash begins on the scalp, moves to the trunk, and then to the arms and legs.

The chickenpox rash usually is generalized, itchy, and progresses to blisters, which become open sores before crusting. The blisters contain a clear fluid that can transmit the virus to others. Successive crops of blisters appear over several days.

In normal children, chickenpox is generally a mild disease although the following complications do occur. Sometimes bacterial skin infections will develop from the open sores associated with chickenpox. Other complications that are more rare but serious include pneumonia, infection of the brain (encephalitis), infections of the covering of the brain (meningitis), Reye syndrome, and death.

Serious chickenpox disease and complications are more likely to occur in the following types of patients:

1. Those whose immune systems are not functioning normally, such as persons with certain leukemias or cancers, persons with AIDS, or persons taking drugs, including steroids, which suppress their immune systems;
2. Newborn infants whose mother developed the chickenpox rash close to the time of delivery; and
3. To a lesser degree, normal adults.

After a chickenpox infection, persons generally have lifelong immunity to chickenpox and do not have a second episode of chickenpox. However, the virus can reactivate later in life as a different problem—zoster or shingles. This is particularly likely to happen if a person has a problem with their immune system such as can occur with older age, disease, or drugs.

■ Document Source:
Centers for Disease Control and Prevention
Document #248001
July 8, 1992

See also: Shingles/Zoster (page 240)

CHRONIC FATIGUE SYNDROME

The Centers for Disease Control and Prevention is actively engaged in chronic fatigue syndrome research. This document reflects current and reliable information. At this time CDC is not equipped to handle counseling, but suggests that you call your nearest support group.

General Description

Chronic fatigue syndrome, or CFS, is characterized by persistent and debilitating fatigue and additional nonspecific symptoms such as sore throat, headache, tender muscles, joint pains, difficulty thinking and loss of short-term memory. On physical examination, patients may have nonspecific findings such as low grade fever and redness in the throat, but frequently no abnormalities are found. No laboratory test or panel of tests is available to diagnose CFS, so the diagnosis is made solely on clinical grounds. The cause of CFS is unknown.

In some individuals, CFS appears to develop after an acute illness like influenza or infectious mononucleosis, both of which usually resolve within a few months, or after periods of unusual stress. In other persons, however, CFS appears to develop gradually with no precipitating event. Symptoms are usually most severe early in the course of illness. Later in the illness, periods of partial improvement may be followed by relapses or recovery. While some patients have recovered after several months of illness, others have remained ill for many years. The average duration and full clinical picture of CFS over time is unknown. The degree to which CFS patients are disabled varies widely. Some patients continue to function at home and at work, although at a reduced level of activity, while others become severely disabled and cannot perform many of the routine activities of daily living.

CFS affects females and males, and adolescents as well as adults. Most reported cases, however, have occurred in young to middle-aged adults with females diagnosed more frequently than males. It is unclear to what extent these demographic characteristics reflect biases among reported cases. CFS does not appear to be directly transmissible from person to person, and there is no justification for CFS patients to be isolated. No deaths from CFS have been reported. Epidemiologic studies of CFS have not documented clear and consistent risk factors.

The total number of persons with CFS in the United States is unknown. CDC has conducted surveillance for CFS in four cities across the United States since 1989. Preliminary analysis of the first three years of data indicates that in these sites, two to seven adults out of 100,000 have CFS. These figures, or prevalence rates, are based upon persons who meet all of the criteria in the CFS research case definition, which was published in the Annals of Internal Medicine in 1988. Because this case definition was deliberately designed to be restrictive for purposes of research, these prevalence rates probably represent low estimates. They should not be used to estimate the overall number of CFS patients in the rest of the United States because the cities chosen for CFS surveillance were not selected randomly.

Case Definition of CFS

In 1987, a panel of experts met at CDC in order to define chronic fatigue syndrome for research purposes. The criteria chosen to define CFS cases were deliberately selected to be restrictive in order to facilitate research. The goal of the case definition was to identify CFS patients who were relatively similar in terms of their illness. The case definition was not designed to diagnose all persons with CFS or to process CFS-associated disability claims. This research case definition, which was published in March 1988 in the Annals of Internal Medicine, essentially requires:

1) the presence of new and debilitating persistent or relapsing fatigue for at least 6 months, and
2) the exclusion, by medical examination and laboratory testing, of other clinical conditions (including psychiatric disorders) that may also cause prolonged fatigue, and

3) the presence of a combination of 8 or more symptom and physical sign criteria during 6 or more months of illness. The symptom criteria are mild fever, sore throat, painful lymph nodes, generalized muscle weakness, muscle aches, prolonged fatigue following exercise, generalized headaches, joint pains, various nervous system complaints, sleep alterations, and development of the symptom complex over a few hours to a few days. The physical examination criteria are low grade fever, an inflamed pharynx without pus, and enlarged lymph nodes.

Diagnostic Evaluation

Severe persistent fatigue and other CFS symptoms can be associated with many other illnesses. These illnesses include underlying major depression and anxiety disorders, autoimmune diseases such as systemic lupus erythematosus, malignancies such as ovarian cancer, lymphoma or leukemia, infectious diseases such as endocarditis, hepatitis, syphilis, or AIDS, and a variety of other diseases such as anemia, diabetes, and diseases of the thyroid, heart, lungs, liver, kidneys, gastrointestinal tract, and endocrine system.

The exclusion of other possible diseases as a cause of CFS symptoms is the most important part of the diagnostic evaluation. Since many of these diseases can be treated or managed appropriately following diagnosis, and since some of these conditions can be progressive or even fatal if untreated, it is absolutely imperative that a thorough medical evaluation be done before a diagnosis of CFS is made.

The role of laboratory and radiologic testing in the diagnostic workup of CFS is to exclude other possible diseases. There are no laboratory tests currently available, including tests for infections, tests for activation of the body's natural defenses against infection, or tests for immune function, that can identify CFS. In particular, tests for Epstein-Barr virus or EBV, human T-cell lymphotropic virus type-II or HTLV-II, human spumavirus, and immunologic abnormalities should not be used to diagnose CFS. Such tests do not distinguish people with CFS from healthy people and are expensive. Some physicians have reported finding brain abnormalities in CFS patients using radiologic tests such as magnetic resonance imaging, known as MRI scans, or nuclear medicine brain scans such as PET or SPECT scans. The meaning of these findings is unknown. They are not unique to CFS and are not found in all CFS patients. Therefore MRI and nuclear medicine scans, which are very expensive, should not be routinely used to diagnose CFS. These radiologic scans should only be used, when clinically warranted, to exclude the possibility of another brain disease.

CDC cannot recommend specific physicians for referral. Our general recommendation is to contact the county medical society, closest university, or a local CFS patient support group for a referral to an internist, infectious disease specialist, or other physician who is knowledgeable about CFS.

Possible Causes of CFS

The cause of CFS is unknown. It is also unknown whether or not CFS is a single illness or a group of different illnesses that share common symptoms. A number of theories about the underlying cause or causes of CFS have been proposed. Some theories have focused on possible underlying viral infections, while others have focused on possible underlying immunologic, hormonal, neurologic, and psychological dysfunction. Some of the more prominent theories are discussed in more detail.

Possible Viral Causes

Epstein-Barr virus or EBV, which is the virus that causes mononucleosis, was widely thought to be responsible for CFS in the 1980s. Later studies, however, indicated that EBV was not the cause of CFS. Most adults have antibody to EBV, and a positive test for EBV, even at a high level of antibody, does not diagnose CFS. In addition to EBV, several other viruses have been proposed as possible causes of CFS, including cytomegalovirus, coxsackie B virus, adenovirus type 1, and human herpesvirus 6 or HHV-6. Although it is possible that viral infections play a role in causing CFS in some patients, none of these viruses has been consistently associated with CFS. More recently, there have been reports suggesting associations between CFS and human retroviruses. These reports, which suggested that CFS may be associated with human spumavirus and viruses like human T-cell lymphotropic virus type-II, received a great deal of attention and generated a great deal of excitement. Since then, however, three published studies have failed to verify an association between CFS and any known human retroviruses. At present there does not appear to be an association between human retroviruses and CFS. The only role for retroviral testing in the diagnosis of CFS should be to exclude the possibility of infection with human immunodeficiency virus or HIV.

Possible Immunologic Causes

Several subtle immunologic abnormalities have been described in some patients with CFS. Results of immunologic studies as a whole have been confusing, and the results of some published findings are in conflict. Recently a panel of distinguished immunologists and virologists from the National Chronic Fatigue Syndrome Advisory Council issued an official statement regarding immunologic and virologic aspects of chronic fatigue syndrome. In their statement, the following points were made:

1) No test is diagnostic for CFS.
2) There is evidence of immune abnormalities in CFS studies, which suggests a pattern of chronic immune activation. However, similar findings can be found in other chronic disorders such as chronic infections, autoimmune disorders, and allergies.
3) Among the most frequently identified abnormalities are the following: chronic activation of T-cells, decreased function of natural killer cells, reduction of subsets of CD8 positive suppressor cells, and increased levels of antibody to Epstein-Barr virus early antigen.
4) Other immune abnormalities have been inconsistently reported. These include: failure to respond to skin tests, deficiencies of immunoglobulin subclasses, and abnormal CD4 and CD8 numbers and ratios.

Recently researchers at the National Institutes of Health reported finding slightly lower percentages of native CD4 T-cells circulating in the blood of CFS patients than in controls.

The significance of these reported immunologic abnormalities is uncertain, but to keep these reports in perspective, the following points should be kept in mind. While it is possible that immunologic abnormalities may be part of the process that causes CFS, these abnormalities may also represent nonspecific immune changes that occur as part of many chronic diseases. It is clear, however, that severe suppression of the immune system such as that seen in AIDS, does not occur in CFS. The opportunistic infections common to AIDS are not seen in CFS.

Possible Psychological Causes

The role of psychological factors and psychiatric diseases in causing CFS is highly controversial and particularly difficult to study. It is clear that psychiatric disease, and especially depression, is frequently found in individuals with persistent fatigue and among patients referred for evaluation for CFS.

Approximately half of the individuals referred to the CDC's CFS surveillance system have evidence of psychiatric illness, which was present before the start of their CFS symptoms. It is also clear that CFS patients commonly experience depression or anxiety sometime during the course of their illness.

These kinds of findings have led some researchers to conclude that CFS is one specific manifestation of underlying psychiatric illness. Other researchers, however, point out that many patients who develop CFS do not have evidence of prior psychiatric disease, and that the depression or anxiety that develops after the start of CFS symptoms may be a part of the CFS disease process or simply a natural reaction to any chronic illness.

Treatment

Treatment for CFS should be initiated only after the possibility of another disease has been excluded as thoroughly as possible. No medication has been shown to be effective for curing CFS in well-conducted clinical trials. The current standard of treatment is to treat the symptoms of CFS.

Most experts begin by recommending a regimen of adequate rest, balanced diet, and physical conditioning. Moderate exercise is generally helpful to minimize loss of physical conditioning, but patients should take care to avoid overexertion since this can lead to relapses of severe fatigue and other symptoms. Nonsteroidal anti-inflammatory medications can be useful for treating headaches, and muscle and joint pains. Since all medications can have side effects, a physician should be consulted for specific recommendations regarding drugs.

Among the numerous medications claimed to be effective for treating CFS are a variety of antiviral and immune system modulating drugs, vitamins, and holistic remedies. While some of these treatments may be of benefit to some patients, other treatments are expensive, are of no proven use, and are potentially harmful to the patient. If you are in doubt about a specific therapy, one or more reputable physicians in your area should be consulted.

Acyclovir and gamma globulin are two medications that have undergone rigorous clinical testing in CFS patients. Acyclovir, which is usually used to treat herpes infections, was shown to be no more effective than a placebo in treating CFS patients. Gamma globulin, which is composed of antibodies pooled from many individuals, was tested in two trials. One trial conducted in the U.S. showed no benefit. The other trial conducted in Australia showed minimal benefit, but this benefit was lost after the trial ended. Currently, two other medications, cortisol and ampligen are undergoing controlled trials.

For Further Information

There are several national and local nonprofit support groups for persons with chronic fatigue syndrome. These groups publish periodic newsletters, provide lists of interested physicians, and facilitate contact between affected persons. The CDC does not endorse these organizations or their published information but provides the names and addresses of the two largest national organizations for further information. These are:

1) The National CFS Association, 919 Scott Avenue, Kansas City, KS 66105, (913) 321-2278.

2) The CFIDS Association, Community Health Services, P.O. Box 220398, Charlotte, NC 28222-0398, (704) 362-2343

■ Document Source:
   Centers for Disease Control and Prevention
   Document # 362100
   May 8, 1993

See also: Epstein-Barr Virus (page 220)

DIPHTHERIA, TETANUS, AND PERTUSSIS: WHAT YOU NEED TO KNOW

What are these diseases?

PERTUSSIS, sometimes called whooping cough, may be a mild or serious disease. It is very easily passed from one person to another. Pertussis can cause spells of coughing and choking that make it hard to eat, drink, or breathe. The coughing can last for several weeks.

The information on pertussis that follows is based on cases that were reported from doctors and health care providers. In recent years, as many as 4,200 cases of pertussis have been reported yearly in the United States and outbreaks still occur. Many cases, including those with less serious illness, do not get reported.

Pertussis is most dangerous to babies (children less than 1 year old). Even with modern medical care, complications occur. About half of the babies reported to have pertussis are so sick that they must go into the hospital. As many as 16 out of 100 babies with pertussis get pneumonia, and as many as 2 out of 100 may have convulsions (seizures, fits, spasms, twitching, jerking, or staring spells). About 1 baby out of 200 has brain problems that may last all his or her life. About 1 out of every 200 babies with pertussis dies of it. Serious illness is less likely in older children and adults.

DIPHTHERIA is a very serious disease. It can make a person unable to breathe, cause paralysis, or heart failure. About 1 out of every 10 people who get diphtheria dies of it.

Only a few cases of diphtheria were reported in the United States during the past few years. This is mostly because people have had shots to protect them.

TETANUS, sometimes called lockjaw, is a very serious disease that can occur after a cut or wound lets the germ into the body. Tetanus makes a person unable to open his or her mouth or swallow, and causes serious muscle spasms. People with tetanus usually have to stay in the hospital for a long time. In the United States, tetanus kills 3 out of every 10 people who get the disease. Since 1975, only 50 to 90 cases of tetanus have been reported each year.

Almost no cases occur in children or young adults because children and young adults have taken the shots and are usually protected.

What about the vaccines and their benefits?

The vaccines to protect children younger than 7 years old against all 3 diseases are usually given together as one shot. This is called the **DTP** vaccine (**D**iphtheria, **T**etanus, and **P**ertussis). Most children should get 5 DTP shots before they go to school. Most babies should get 3 DTP shots by 6 months of age.

Three or more DTP shots keep:

♦ 70 to 90 children out of 100 from getting **pertussis** if exposed to it, and usually protect the child through the elementary school years. The others who have had the DTP vaccine but get pertussis usually have a milder illness than if they had not had the vaccine.

♦ At least 85 children out of 100 from getting **diphtheria** for at least 10 years.

♦ At least 95 children out of 100 from getting **tetanus** for at least 10 years.

Pertussis vaccine should not be given to a few children. Other vaccines are available for these children and for adults:

♦ **DT** vaccine (Diphtheria and Tetanus) is given to children under age 7 years who should not receive pertussis vaccine.

♦ **Td** vaccine (Tetanus and diphtheria) is specially made for children age 7 years and older and for adults.

What are the risks of these vaccines?

DTP

Most children have little or no problem from the DTP shot. Many children will have fever or soreness, swelling, and redness where the shot was given. Usually these problems are mild and last 1 to 2 days. Some children will be cranky, drowsy, or not want to eat during this time.

Less often—that is, following 1 DTP shot in 100 to 1 shot in 1,000—a more serious problem can happen:

- Crying without stopping for 3 hours or longer
- A temperature of 105°F or higher
- An unusual, high-pitched cry

Even less often—following 1 DTP shot in 1,750—a child may have:

- A convulsion (seizures, fits, spasms, twitching, jerking, or staring spells), usually from high fever that may happen after the shot
- Shock-collapse (become blue or pale, limp, and not responsive)

Rarely, brain damage that lasts for the child's life has been reported after getting DTP. However, most experts now agree that DTP has not been shown to be a cause of brain damage. If DTP ever causes brain damage, then such an event would be very rare. There is no test that can tell in advance if your child will have any of these problems following DTP vaccination.

DT, Td, and T

DT, Td, and T vaccines cause few problems. They may cause mild fever or soreness, swelling, and redness where the shot was given. These problems usually last for 1 to 2 days, but this does not happen nearly as often as with DTP vaccine. Sometimes, adults who get these vaccines too often can have a lot of soreness and swelling where the shot was given.

There is a rare chance that other serious problems or even death could occur after getting DTP, Pertussis, DT, T, or Td. Such problems could happen after taking any medicine or after receiving any vaccine.

Are the benefits of the vaccines greater than the risks?

Yes, for almost all people.

Children, especially infants, who catch pertussis are often seriously ill. People with diphtheria or tetanus usually are seriously ill. Most people who have had 3 or more shots of DTP are protected from these diseases for many years. If children have the DTP shots but get pertussis, the illness is usually milder than if they had not had the shots. The number of children who have had a serious problem after receiving DTP is unknown, but is probably very small.

Experts believe that most children should receive DTP shots. If a child should not receive DTP, the child should usually receive DT. After reading this pamphlet and talking with your doctor or nurse, you can decide together what is best for your child.

When should your child get the DTP vaccines and other vaccines?

Below are **all** of the vaccines that most infants and children should get and the age when most experts suggest they should get each dose of vaccine.

Recommended Schedule of Vaccinations for All Children						
Vaccine		2 Months	4 Months	6 Months	12 Months	15 Months	4-6 Years (Before School Entry)
DTP		DTP	DTP			DTP*	DTP
Polio		Polio	Polio			Polio*	Polio
MMR						MMR†	MMR¶
Option 1§		HIB	HIB	HIB		HIB	
Option 2§		HIB	HIB		HIB		
Vaccine	Birth	1-2 Months	4 Months	6-18 Months			
HB Option 1	HB	HB‡		HB‡			
Option 2		HB‡	HB‡	HB‡			

DTP: Diptheria, Tetanus, and Pertussis Vaccine
Polio: Live Oral Polio Vaccine drops (OPV) or Killed (Inactivated) Polio Vaccine shots (IPV)
MMR: Measles, Mumps, and Rubella Vaccine
HIB: *Haemophilus* b Conjugate Vaccine
HB: Hepatitis B Vaccine
* Many experts recommend these vaccines at 18 months.
† In some areas this dose of MMR vaccine may be given at 12 months.
¶ Many experts recommend this dose of MMR vaccine be given at entry to middle school or junior high school.
§ HIB vaccine is given in either a 4-dose schedule (1) or a 3-dose schedule (2), depending on the type of vaccine used.
‡ Hepatitis B vaccine can be given simultaneously with DTP, Polio, MMR, and *Haemophilus* b Conjugate Vaccine at the same visit.

When should a shot be delayed?

There are several reasons for a child to delay getting the DTP shot. If the child:

- Is sick with something more serious than a minor illness such as a common cold, delay the vaccination until your child is better.
- Has **ever** had a convulsion or other brain problem or seems not to be developing normally (until it is clear that your child is not getting worse or having more convulsions).

Such children should be carefully examined by a doctor before a decision is made.

If your child is sick or if you are not sure if a shot should be delayed, talk to your doctor or nurse. Then you can decide together what is best for your child.

When should the DTP vaccine not be given?

Your child should not get another DTP shot if any of the problems listed below happened after an earlier DTP and had no other obvious cause. Talk with your doctor or nurse about any of these problems.

- Serious problems of the brain within 7 days after getting DTP.
- Serious allergic problem (swelling in the mouth, throat, or face, or difficulty breathing) within a few hours after getting DTP.
- The presence of a brain problem that is getting worse, such as uncontrolled convulsions.

Many experts believe that a child should not get another DTP shot if any of the problems listed below happened after an earlier DTP shot and had no other obvious cause. However, for some children, the benefits outweigh the risks. Talk with your doctor or nurse about any of these problems.

- Temperature of 105°F or higher within 2 days after getting DTP.
- Shock-collapse (becoming blue or pale, limp and not responsive) within 2 days after getting DTP.
- Convulsion within 3 days after getting DTP.
- Crying that cannot be stopped and which lasts for more than 3 hours at a time within the 2 days after getting DTP.

If you know or think that any of these problems happened after getting DTP, tell a doctor or nurse before that child receives another DTP or any other vaccine. If a child should not be given DTP, usually the child should get DT vaccine instead.

Should pregnant women receive Td?

Babies born under unclean conditions to women who have no protection against tetanus have an increased risk of getting tetanus as newborns. This can be prevented by giving Td vaccine to women. Women who have not received Td or T earlier should be given the vaccine when they are pregnant.

Td and T vaccines are not known to cause special problems for pregnant women or their unborn babies. While doctors usually do not recommend giving any drugs or vaccines to pregnant women, a pregnant woman who needs Td vaccine should get it.

Which children may be more likely to have a convulsion after receiving DTP?

The chance of a child having a convulsion with fever after receiving DTP vaccine is up to 9 times greater if the child has had a convulsion before. It is about 3 times greater if the child's brother, sister, or parent has ever had a convulsion.

Most experts agree that unless the convulsion occurred within 3 days after getting DTP vaccine, children who have had a convulsion should still get the DTP vaccine. Also children who have a family member who has had a convulsion should get the DTP vaccine.

It is usually the fever that causes the convulsion. Most experts believe that convulsions with fever do not cause any permanent damage to the child.

Be sure to tell the doctor or nurse who is giving the shot about any history of convulsions. Talk with them about the medicines or other measures to reduce fever and soreness from the vaccines.

What to look for and to do after the shot

Talk with the doctor or nurse who gives the shot about taking medicines or other measures to reduce fever and soreness from the vaccine.

This pamphlet lists the problems that may occur after receiving DTP or other shots for diphtheria, tetanus, or pertussis.

As with any serious medical problem, if the person has a serious or unusual problem after getting the vaccine, **CALL A DOCTOR OR GET THE PERSON TO A DOCTOR PROMPTLY.**

If you or your child does have a reaction to the vaccine, you can help your doctor by writing down exactly what happened. Write on a piece of paper exactly what happened, what day it happened, and the time it happened.

Have the problem reported

The Public Health Service is interested in finding out if any serious problems may be related to DTP, Pertussis, DT, T, or Td vaccines, especially those that occur within 4 weeks after the shot.

If you believe that the person receiving the vaccine had a serious problem or died because of the shot, call your doctor or health department to report the problem.

If you think the problem was not reported, you should report the problem yourself. You can do so by calling this toll-free number: **1-800-822-7967.**

Get information about possible help

A U.S. government program provides compensation for some persons injured by vaccines. For more information, call this toll-free number:

    1-800-338-2382

    OR contact:

The U.S. Claims Court
717 Madison Place, NW
Washington, DC 20005
(202) 633-7257

What vaccines does your state require?

To protect as many children as possible from these diseases, all states require certain vaccines before the child goes to child-care or school. Ask you doctor or nurse what vaccines your state requires.

Addendum to "Diphtheria, Tetanus, and Pertussis: What You Need to Know"

What you need to know about the new pertussis vaccine

After the 1991 pamphlet "Diphtheria, Tetanus, and Pertussis: What You Need to Know" was prepared, a new pertussis vaccine became available for the fourth and fifth shots against diphtheria, tetanus, and pertussis. The information below provides up-to-date information about the new vaccine.

What is the new vaccine?

DTP vaccine is usually given 5 times before a child reaches age 7 years. Until now, pertussis vaccine has been made from killed whole pertussis cells and mixed with diphtheria and tetanus vaccines to make the whole-cell DTP shot. The new acellular pertussis vaccine, DTaP, is made of only a few parts of the pertussis cell and is also combined with diphtheria and tetanus vaccines.

When should it be used?

The fourth and fifth shots of the DTP vaccine series are usually given to children 15-18 months old and 4-6 years old. The DTaP vaccine can be used only for the fourth and fifth shots. Testing is now in progress to show that DTaP is safe and effective for the first three doses. Until these studies are completed, this vaccine cannot be considered for use for the first three doses of the vaccine series. Whole-cell DTP vaccine should still always be used for the first three shots, and can still be used for the fourth and fifth DTP shots, although most experts will prefer to use DTaP vaccine.

■ Document Source:
U.S. Department of Health and Human Services, Public Health Service
Centers for Disease Control and Prevention
Atlanta, Georgia 30333
April 1992

See also: Pertussis (page 231); Tetanus (page 241)

EPSTEIN-BARR VIRUS

Disease Information

The Epstein-Barr virus frequently referred to as EBV, is one of the most common human viruses, and it occurs worldwide. The Epstein-Barr virus is in the herpes family of viruses, and most people will become infected with EBV sometime during their lives. In the United States, as many as 95% of adults between 35 and 40 years of age have been infected. Infants become susceptible to EBV as soon as the maternal protection present at birth disappears. Many children are infected, with EBV and these infections usually cause no symptoms or are indistinguishable from the other mild, brief illnesses of childhood.

In the United States and in other developed countries, many persons are not infected with EBV in their childhood years. In these people infection with Epstein-Barr virus during adolescence or young adulthood commonly causes infectious mononucleosis.

Symptoms of infectious mononucleosis are fever, sore throat, and swollen lymph glands. Sometimes there is also a swollen spleen or liver infection. Heart problems or involvement of the central nervous system occur only rarely, and infectious mononucleosis is almost never fatal. There are no known associations between active Epstein-Barr virus infection and problems during pregnancy, such as miscarriages or birth defects. Although the symptoms of infectious mononucleosis usually resolve in one or two months, the Epstein-Barr virus remains dormant in cells in the throat and blood for the rest of the person's life. Periodically, the virus can reactivate and can be found in the saliva of infected persons. This reactivation usually occurs without symptoms of illness.

EBV also establishes a lifelong dormant infection in some cells of the body's immune system. A late event in a very few viral carriers is the emergence of Burkitt's lymphoma and nasopharyngeal carcinoma, two rare cancers that are not normally found in the United States. EBV appears to play an important role in these malignancies, but is probably not the sole cause of disease.

Most individuals exposed to people with infectious mononucleosis have previously been infected with EBV and are not at risk of developing infectious mononucleosis. In addition, transmission of EBV requires contact with the saliva (found in the mouth) of an infected person. Transmission of this virus through the air or blood does not normally occur. The incubation period, or the time from infection to appearance of symptoms, ranges from 4 to 6 weeks. Thus persons with infectious mononucleosis may be able to spread the infection to others for a period of time. However, no special precautions or isolation procedures are recommended since the virus is also found frequently in the saliva of healthy people. In fact, many healthy people can carry and spread the virus intermittently for life. These people are usually the primary reservoir for person-to-person transmission. For this reason, transmission of the virus is almost impossible to prevent.

The diagnosis of infectious mononucleosis is suggested on the basis of the clinical symptoms of fever, sore throat, swollen lymph glands, and the age of the patient. Usually, laboratory tests are needed for confirmation.

Blood findings with infectious mononucleosis include an elevated white blood cell count, an increased percentage of certain white blood cells, and a positive reaction to a "mono spot test."

There is no specific treatment for infectious mononucleosis, other than treating the symptoms. No antiviral drugs or vaccines are available. Some physicians have prescribed a five-day course of steroids to control the swelling of the tonsils. The use of steroids has also been reported to decrease the overall length and severity of ♦ illness, but these reports have not been published.

Please note: Symptoms related to infectious mononucleosis due to EBV, as confirmed in the laboratory seldom last for more than 3 or 4 months. When such an illness lasts more than 6 months, it is frequently called chronic EBV infection. However, valid evidence for continued active EBV infection is found very seldom in these patients, and their illness is usually more appropriately described as chronic fatigue syndrome, or CFS.

■ Document Source:
   Centers for Disease Control and Prevention
   Document #362501
   November 19, 1992

FOOD AND WATER BORNE BACTERIAL DISEASES

Foodborne Bacterial Diseases—General Information

More than 250 different diseases have been described that can be caused by contaminated food or drink. The most common foodborne diseases are infections caused by bacteria, such as salmonella and campylobacter, or by the Norwalk family of viruses. A foodborne disease outbreak is defined as a group of people developing the same illnesses after ingesting the same food. Most cases of foodborne disease are single cases not associated with a recognized outbreak.

The great majority of food items which cause foodborne diseases are raw or undercooked foods of animal origin such as meat, milk, eggs, cheese, fish, or shellfish.

In 1983, it was estimated that there were approximately 6 million cases of infectious foodborne diseases which caused 9,000 deaths. Some foodborne diseases such as botulism and trichinosis are becoming less common, while others such as salmonellosis are becoming more common. Thus, the spectrum of foodborne disease is changing. New infections not previously known to be foodborne diseases are emerging.

Approximately 400-500 foodborne disease outbreaks are reported each year. Not all outbreaks or diseases are equally likely to be reported, and many cases of foodborne diseases are sporadic.

To prevent contracting foodborne diseases, the consumer can do the following:

1) Make sure that food from animal sources (meat, dairy, eggs) is thoroughly cooked or pasteurized. Avoid eating such foods raw or undercooked.

2) Be careful to keep juices or drippings from raw meat, poultry, shellfish or eggs, from contaminating other foods.

3) Do not leave potentially contaminated foods for extended periods of time at temperatures that permit bacteria to grow. Promptly refrigerate leftovers and food prepared in advance.

Thorough cooking kills almost all foodborne bacteria, viruses and parasites, and is the single most important step in preventing foodborne disease. Preventing spread of contamination from raw foods in the kitchen is also important. Washing one's hands, cutting board, and knife with soap and water immediately after handling raw meat, raw poultry, raw seafood or raw eggs will help keep the food handler from contaminating any other foods in the kitchen. Persons who are ill with diarrhea or vomiting should not prepare food for others. Special care is needed in the preparation of food for infants, the elderly, and persons whose immune systems are compromised by underlying illness or medical treatment of illness.

While foodborne diseases, their causes and effects are better understood today, emerging risks need to be monitored for several reasons.

First, the food supply of the United States is changing dramatically. The conditions under which food animals are raised have changed greatly. We now import 30 billion tons of food a year, including fruit, vegetables, seafoods, and canned goods; these imported foods are an increasing proportion of the diet, and often come from developing countries where food hygiene and basic sanitation is less advanced. Food processing technologies are constantly evolving. The centralization of the food industry means that a single contaminated product may appear in many different foods and many different forms, and infect a considerable number of people before it is identified.

Second, consumers are changing; there are increasing numbers of elderly or immunosuppressed persons who are at higher risk of severe illness; consumers spend less time cooking than before, and may have received less instruction in food handling in home or school than before.

Finally, new and emerging foodborne pathogens have been identified, which can cause diseases unrecognized 50 years ago. These include bacteria, parasites, and viruses, along with toxic causes of foodborne illnesses. Constant vigilance is necessary to identify new problems requiring new solutions as they emerge.

However, despite these new risks, the food supply of the United States is probably safer now than ever.

Botulism

Botulism is a rare but serious foodborne disease. It is caused by contamination of certain foods by the botulism bacterium commonly found in the soil. There are two different illnesses: adult botulism and infant botulism. An adult may become ill by eating spoiled food containing the botulism toxin. This toxin is produced when the bacteria grow in improperly canned foods and occasionally in contaminated fish. Infant botulism is caused by eating the spores of the botulinum bacterium. For infants one source of these spores is honey.

When contaminated food is eaten by adults, toxin is absorbed from the intestines and attaches to the nerves causing the signs and symptoms of botulism. Early symptoms include blurred vision, dry mouth, difficulty in swallowing or speaking, general weakness, and shortness of breath. The illness may progress to complete paralysis, respiratory failure, and death. When infants eat contaminated food, the spores grow in the intestines and release toxin.

Diagnosis is made by the presence of appropriate neurologic symptoms and by laboratory tests that detect toxin or by culture of *Clostridium botulinum* bacterium from the patient's stool.

Although there are very few cases of botulism poisoning each year, prevention is extremely important. Home canning should follow strict hygienic recommendations to reduce contamination of foods. In addition, because the botulism toxin is destroyed by boiling for 10 minutes, people who eat home-canned foods should consider boiling the food before eating it to ensure safety. A county extension home economist can provide specific instructions on safe home canning techniques. To help prevent infant botulism, infants less than 12 months old should not be fed honey.

Treatment for adults requires care in an intensive care unit; botulism antitoxin can be helpful if given soon after symptoms begin. Treatment for infants requires hospitalization and possibly care in an intensive care unit. Antitoxin is not recommended for infants.

In 1989, 23 adult and 75 infant botulism cases were reported to CDC from 23 states.

Additional Sources of Information

More detailed information on foodborne disease can be found in encyclopedias, in medical and public health textbooks, and in textbooks on food microbiology. CDC surveillance summaries on foodborne diseases and their outbreaks are published as supplements to the Morbidity and Mortality Weekly Report, the MMWR, and are available at many public libraries, and all medical libraries. These surveillance summaries include information on salmonellosis, campylobacteriosis, trichinosis, and viral hepatitis, as well as on foodborne disease outbreaks. They can also be obtained by writing this office: Public Inquiries, Office of Public Affairs, Centers for Disease Control, 1600 Clifton Road, Atlanta, Georgia, 30333.

Questions about the safe handling of food can be addressed to your county health department or county extension home economist.

Questions about the safety of a specific food can be answered by the FDA Consumer Hotline: 1-301-443-1240.

Questions specifically about meat and poultry can be answered by the USDA Meat and Poultry Hotline: 1-800-535-4555.

■ Document Source:
  Centers for Disease Control and Prevention
  Document #310100; #310107
  November 19, 1992

HAEMOPHILUS INFLUENZAE TYPE b (HIB)

Disease Information

Haemophilus Influenzae type b disease, also called Haemophilus b or "Hib" disease can be a serious disease, especially among children under 5 years of age. Before vaccines recently became available to prevent Hib disease the numbers of cases and deaths due to Hib disease in the United States were similar to those of paralytic polio during the peak epidemic years from 1951 to 1955.

The Hib bacteria are found universally throughout the population, and can cause a serious bacterial infection that should not be confused with the viral infection called influenza or flu. In many cases the Hib organism lives, along with other bacteria, in the upper respiratory tract of an individual without causing illness.

The most commonly recognized and severe manifestation of Hib disease is meningitis (an inflammation and swelling in the covering of the brain), but it can cause other distinct diseases such as pneumonia, and infections of the blood, joints, bones, throat, soft tissues and the covering of the heart.

In the prevaccine era in the United States Hib caused about 12,000 cases of meningitis, and about 20,000 episodes of all types of diseases combined. In the absence of effective vaccination about 1 in 200 children is affected with Hib before their fifth birthday. Of those 12,000 children who are affected by meningitis, about 1 in 4 suffers permanent brain damage, and around 1 in 20 dies.

Hib disease occurs most frequently in children between 6 months and 1 year of age. As children grow older they are less likely to develop Hib disease. Very few cases of Hib are found in persons older than 5 years of age. Hib cases are more frequent in the fall and spring of the year.

Recently, two vaccines have been licensed and are now recommended for infants 2 months or older. This is very important because it allows those young children who are most susceptible to the bacteria to be protected from this serious disease.

Vaccine Information

Children as young as 2 months can now safely be immunized against Hib disease. The recent approval of two vaccines for children under 15 months of age means that those most likely to get Hib disease can now be protected from it. Depending on the vaccine chosen by a doctor, infants just 2 months old can and should begin the primary vaccine series. Normally doses are spaced about 2 months apart, and a booster dose is given either at 12 or 15 months. Your doctor or clinic can give you the details on the vaccine and schedule which is right for your child.

Whichever vaccine is chosen, it is best to use the same vaccine for all doses. Good record keeping can insure this.

All children under 5 years old should be vaccinated for Hib disease. If your child is not immunized against Hib, then consult with your doctor for details on immunization dosage and schedule. The Hib vaccine is usually not recommended for children after their 5th birthday.

The Hib vaccines are some of the safest of all vaccine products. The vaccine cannot cause meningitis, and has not been associated with any other serious reaction. Two or three children per 100 children receiving the vaccine will develop either a slight redness, or swelling with warmth, or fever higher than 101. These reactions begin within 24 hours after the shot, and usually go away in 2 to 3 days. The Hib vaccine and other childhood vaccines like measles-mumps-rubella vaccine (MMR), diphtheria-tetanus-pertussis (DTP), and oral poliovirus vaccine (OPV), can safely be given during the same visit to a doctor or clinic.

■ Document Source:
   Centers for Disease Control
   Document #247001; #247003
   July 8, 1992

See also: What to do About Flu (page 242)

LYME DISEASE: THE FACTS, THE CHALLENGE

Introduction

In the early 1970s, a mysterious clustering of arthritis occurred among children in Lyme, Connecticut, and surrounding towns. Medical researchers soon recognized the illness as a distinct disease, which they called Lyme disease. They subsequently described the clinical features of Lyme disease, established the usefulness of antibiotic therapy in its treatment, identified the deer tick as the key to its spread, and isolated the bacterium that caused it.

Lyme disease is still mistaken for other ailments, and it continues to pose many other challenges: it can be difficult to diagnose because of the inadequacies of today's laboratory tests; it can be troublesome to treat in its later phases; and its prevention through the development of an effective vaccine is hampered by the elusive nature of the bacterium.

The National Institutes of Health (NIH), a part of the U.S. Public Health Service, conducts and supports biomedical research aimed at meeting the challenges of Lyme disease. This brochure presents the most recently available information on the diagnosis, treatment, and prevention of Lyme disease.

How Lyme Disease Became Known

Lyme disease was first recognized in 1975 after researchers investigated why unusually large numbers of children were being diagnosed with juvenile rheumatoid arthritis in Lyme and two neighboring towns. The investigators discovered that most of the affected children lived near wooded areas likely to harbor ticks. They also found that the children's first symptoms typically started in the summer months coinciding with the height of the tick season. Several of the patients interviewed reported having a skin rash just before developing their arthritis and many also recalled being bitten by a tick at the rash site.

Further investigations resulted in the discovery that tiny deer ticks infected with a spiral-shaped bacterium or spirochete (which was later named *Borrelia burgdorferi*) were responsible for the outbreak of arthritis in Lyme.

In Europe, a skin rash similar to that of Lyme disease had been described in medical literature dating back to the turn of the century. Lyme disease may have spread from Europe to the United States in the early 1900s but only recently became common enough to be detected.

Ticks That Most Commonly Transmit B. burgdorferi in the U.S.

(These ticks are all quite similar in appearance.)
Ixodes dammini—most common in the northeast and mid-west
Ixodes scapularis—found in south and southeast
Ixodes pacificus—found on west coast

The ticks most commonly infected with *B burgdorferi* usually feed and mate on deer during part of their life cycle. The recent resurgence of the deer population in the northeast and the influx of suburban developments into rural areas where deer ticks are commonly found have probably contributed to the disease's rising prevalence.

The number of reported cases of Lyme disease as well as the number of geographic areas in which it is found has been increasing. Lyme disease has been reported in nearly all states in this country, although most cases are concentrated in the coastal northeast, mid-Atlantic states, Wisconsin and Minnesota, and northern California. Lyme disease is endemic in large areas of Asia and Europe. Recent reports suggest that it is present in South America too.

Symptoms of Lyme Disease

Erythema Migrans. In most people the first symptom of Lyme disease is a red rash known as erythema migrans (EM). The telltale rash starts as a small red spot that expands over a period of days or weeks, forming a circular, triangular, or oval-shaped rash. Sometimes the rash resembles a bull's eye because it appears as a redning surrounding a central clear area. The rash which can range in size from that of a dime to the entire width of a person's back appears within a few weeks of a tick bite and usually occurs at the site of a bite. As infection spreads, several rashes can appear at different sites on the body.

Erythema migrans is often accompanied by symptoms such as fever, headache, stiff neck, body aches, and fatigue. Although these flulike symptoms may resemble those of common viral infections, Lyme disease symptoms tend to persist or may occur intermittently.

Arthritis. After several months of being infected by B. burgdorferi, slightly more than half of those people not treated with antibiotics develop recurrent attacks of painful and swollen joints that last a few days to a few months. The arthritis can shift from one joint to another; the knee is most commonly affected. About 10 to 20 percent of untreated patients will go on to develop chronic arthritis.

Neurological Symptoms. Lyme disease can also affect the nervous system, causing symptoms such as stiff neck and severe headache (meningitis), temporary paralysis of facial muscles (Bell's palsy), numbness, pain or weakness in the limbs, or poor motor coordination. More subtle changes such as memory loss, difficulty with concentration, and a change in mood or sleeping habits have also been associated with Lyme disease.

Nervous system abnormalities usually develop several weeks, months, or even years following an untreated infection. These symptoms often last for weeks or months and may recur.

Heart Problems. Fewer than one out of ten Lyme disease patients develops heart problems, such as an irregular heartbeat, which can be signalled by dizziness or shortness of breath. These symptoms rarely last more than a few days or weeks. Such heart abnormalities generally surface several weeks after infection.

Other Symptoms. Less commonly, Lyme disease can result in eye inflammation, hepatitis, and severe fatigue, although none of these problems is likely to appear without other Lyme disease symptoms being present.

How Lyme Disease Is Diagnosed

Lyme disease may be difficult to diagnose because many of its symptoms mimic those of other disorders. In addition, the only distinctive hallmark unique to Lyme disease—the erythema migrans rash—is absent in at least one-fourth of the people who become infected. Although a tick bite is an important clue for diagnosis, many patients cannot recall having been bitten recently by a tick. This is not surprising because the tick is tiny, and a tick bite is usually painless.

When a patient with possible Lyme disease symptoms does not develop the distinctive rash, a physician will rely on a detailed medical history and a careful physical examination for essential clues to diagnosis, with laboratory tests playing a supportive role.

Blood Tests. Unfortunately, the Lyme disease microbe itself is difficult to isolate or culture from body tissues or fluids. Most physicians look for evidence of antibodies against *B. burgdorferi* in the blood to confirm the bacterium's role as the cause of a patient's symptoms. Antibodies are molecules or small substances tailor-made by the immune system to lock onto and destroy specific microbial invaders.

Some patients experiencing nervous system symptoms may also undergo a spinal tap. Through this procedure doctors can detect brain and spinal cord inflammation and can look for antibodies in the spinal fluid.

The inadequacies of the currently available antibody tests may prevent them from firmly establishing whether the Lyme disease bacterium is causing a patient's symptoms. In the first few weeks following infection, antibody tests are not reliable because a patient's immune system has not produced enough antibodies to be detected. Antibiotics given to a patient early during infection may also prevent antibodies from reaching detectable levels, even though the Lyme disease bacterium is the cause of the patient's symptoms.

Because some tests cannot distinguish Lyme disease antibodies from antibodies to similar organisms, patients may test positive for Lyme disease when their symptoms actually stem from other bacterial infections. A lack of standardization of antibody tests and poor quality control also contribute to inaccuracies in test results.

Due to these pitfalls, physicians must rely on their clinical judgment in diagnosing someone with Lyme disease even though the patient does not have the distinctive erythema migrans rash. Such a diagnosis would be based on the history of a tick bite, the patient's symptoms, a thorough ruling out of other diseases that might cause those symptoms, and other implicating evidence. This evidence could include such factors as an initial appearance of symptoms during the summer months when tick bites are most likely to occur, outdoor exposure in an area where Lyme disease is common, and a clustering of Lyme disease symptoms among family members.

Most Common Symptoms of Lyme Disease (One or more may be present at different times during infection)

Early Infection

- Rash (erythema migrans)
- Muscle and joint aches
- Headache
- Stiff neck
- Significant fatigue
- Fever
- Facial paralysis (Bell's palsy)
- Meningitis
- Brief episodes of joint pain and swelling

Less common:

- Eye problems such as conjunctivitis
- Heart abnormalities such as heart block and myocarditis

Late Infection

- Arthritis, intermittent or chronic

Less common:

- Neurologic conditions such as encephalitis or confusion
- Skin disorders

New Tests under Development. To improve the accuracy of Lyme disease diagnosis, NIH-supported researchers are developing a number of new tests that promise to be more reliable than currently available procedures. Some of these detect distinctive protein fragments of the Lyme disease bacterium in fluid samples.

NIH scientists are developing tests that use the highly sensitive genetic engineering technique, known as polymerase chain reaction (PCR), to detect extremely small quantities of the genetic material of the Lyme disease bacterium in body tissues and fluids.

Several new methods to detect infection are under development in NIH laboratories. Scientists have isolated a protein of *B. burgdorferi*, called p39, that reacts strongly on blood tests. The presence of antibodies to this protein was found to be a strong indicator of the presence of *B. burgdorferi*. Although further research will be needed to determine how soon after infection it can detect the bacterium, p39 may prove to be an ideal test for Lyme disease.

A somewhat different approach is the use of an assay based on two closely related spirochetal proteins that are not found in other species of bacterial spirochetes. This assay differs from blood tests now in use because it detects products of the spirochete itself rather than detecting human antibodies to the bacterium.

How Lyme Disease Is Treated

Nearly all Lyme disease patients can be effectively treated with an appropriate course of antibiotic therapy. In general, the sooner such therapy is begun following infection, the quicker and more complete the recovery.

Antibiotics, such as doxycycline or amoxicillin taken orally for a few weeks, can speed the healing of the erythema migrans rash and usually prevent subsequent symptoms such as arthritis or neurological problems.

Patients younger than 9 years or pregnant or lactating women with Lyme disease are treated with amoxicillin or penicillin because doxycycline can stain the permanent teeth developing in young children or unborn babies. Patients allergic to penicillin are given erythromycin.

Lyme disease patients with neurological symptoms are usually treated with the antibiotic ceftriaxone given intravenously once a day for a month or less. Most patients experience full recovery.

Lyme arthritis may be treated with oral antibiotics. Patients with severe arthritis may be treated with ceftriaxone or penicillin given intravenously. To ease these patients' discomfort and further their healing, the physician might also give anti-inflammatory drugs, draw fluid from affected joints, or surgically remove the inflamed lining of the joints.

Lyme arthritis resolves in most patients within a few weeks or months following antibiotic therapy, although it can take years to disappear completely in some people. Some Lyme disease patients who are untreated for several years may be cured of their arthritis with the proper antibiotic regimen. If the disease has persisted long enough, however, it may irreversibly damage the structure of the joints.

Physicians prefer to treat Lyme disease patients experiencing heart symptoms with antibiotics such as ceftriaxone or penicillin given intravenously for about 2 weeks. If these symptoms persist or are severe enough, patients may also be treated with corticosteroids or given a temporary internal cardiac pacemaker. People with Lyme disease rarely experience long-term heart damage.

Following treatment for Lyme disease, some people still have persistent fatigue and achiness. This general malaise can take months to subside, although it generally does so spontaneously without requiring additional antibiotic therapy.

Researchers are currently conducting studies to assess the optimal duration of antibiotic therapy for the various manifestations of Lyme disease. Investigators are also testing newly developed antibiotics for their effectiveness in countering the Lyme disease bacterium.

Unfortunately, a bout with Lyme disease is no guarantee that the illness will be prevented in the future. The disease can strike more than once in the same individual if he or she is reinfected with the Lyme disease bacterium.

Lyme Disease Prevention

Avoidance of Ticks. At present, the best way to avoid Lyme disease is to avoid deer ticks. Although generally only about one percent of all deer ticks are infected with the Lyme disease bacterium, in some areas more than half of them harbor the microbe.

Most people with Lyme disease become infected during the summer, when immature ticks are most prevalent. Except in warm climates, few people are bitten by deer ticks during winter months.

Deer ticks are most often found in wooded areas and nearby grasslands, and are especially common where the two areas merge. Because the adult ticks feed on deer, areas where deer are frequently seen are likely to harbor sizable numbers of deer ticks.

To help prevent tick bites, people entering tick-infested areas should walk in the center of trails to avoid picking up ticks from overhanging grass and brush.

To minimize skin exposure to both ticks and insect repellents, people outdoors in tick-infested areas should wear long pants and long-sleeved shirts that fit tightly at the ankles and wrists. As a further safeguard, people should wear a hat, tuck pant legs into socks, and wear shoes that leave no part of the feet exposed. To make it easy to detect ticks, people should wear light-colored clothing.

To repel ticks, people can spray their clothing with the insecticide permethrin, which is commonly found in lawn and garden stores. Insect repellents that contain a chemical called DEET (N, N-diethyl-M-toluamide) can also be applied to clothing or directly onto skin. Although highly effective, these repellents can cause some serious side effects, particularly when high concentrations are used repeatedly on the skin. Infants and children may be especially at risk for adverse reactions to DEET.

Pregnant women should be especially careful to avoid ticks in Lyme disease areas because the infection can be transferred to the unborn child. Such a prenatal infection can make the woman more likely to miscarry or deliver a stillborn baby.

Checking for Ticks. Once indoors, people should check themselves and their children for ticks, particularly in the hairy regions of the body. The immature deer ticks that are most likely to cause Lyme disease are only about the size of a poppy seed, so they are easily mistaken for a freckle or a speck of dirt. All clothing should be washed. Pets should be checked for ticks before entering the house, because they, too, can develop symptoms of Lyme disease. In addition, a pet can carry ticks into the house. These ticks could fall off without biting the animal and subsequently attach to and bite people inside the house.

If a tick is discovered attached to the skin, it should be pulled out gently with tweezers, taking care not to squeeze the tick's body. An antiseptic should then be applied to the bite. Studies by NIH-supported researchers suggest that a tick must be attached for many hours to transmit the Lyme disease bacterium, so prompt tick removal could prevent the disease.

The risk of developing Lyme disease from a tick bite is small, even in heavily infested areas, and most physicians prefer not to treat patients bitten by ticks with antibiotics unless they develop symptoms of Lyme disease.

Vaccine Development. Because Lyme disease is difficult to diagnose and sometimes does not respond to treatment, researchers are trying to create a vaccine that will protect people from the disorder. Vaccines work in part by prompting the body to generate antibodies. These custom-shaped molecules lock onto specific proteins made by a virus or bacterium—often those proteins lodged in the microbe's outer coat. Once antibodies attach to an invading microbe, other immune defenses are evoked to destroy it.

Development of an effective vaccine for Lyme disease has been difficult to create for a number of reasons. Scientists need to find out how the immune system protects against the bacterium because people who have been infected once can acquire the infection again. In addition, there are several different strains of the bacterium, each with its own distinct set of proteins, and bacteria within an individual strain may change the shape of their proteins over time so that antibodies can no longer identify and lock onto them.

Tick Eradication. In the meantime, researchers are trying to develop an effective strategy for ridding areas of deer ticks. Studies show that a single fall spraying of pesticide in wooded areas can substantially reduce the number of adult deer ticks residing there for as long as a year. Spraying on a large scale, however, may not be economically feasible and may prompt environmental or health concerns.

Scientists are also pursuing biological control of deer ticks by introducing tiny stingerless wasps, which feed on immature ticks, into tick-infested areas. Researchers are currently assessing the effectiveness of this technique.

Successful control of deer ticks will probably depend on a combination of tactics. More studies are needed before wide-scale tick control strategies can be implemented.

Tips for Personal Protection

♦ Avoid tick-infested areas, especially in May, June, and July.*

♦ Wear light-colored clothing so that ticks can be easily spotted.

♦ Wear long-sleeved shirts and closed shoes and socks.

♦ Tuck pant legs into socks or boots and tuck shirt into pants.

♦ Apply insect repellent containing permethrin to pants, socks, and shoes, and compounds containing DEET on exposed skin. Do not overuse these products.

♦ Walk in the center of trails to avoid overgrown grass and brush.

♦ After being outdoors in a tick-infested area, remove, wash, and dry clothing.

♦ Inspect the body thoroughly and remove carefully any attached ticks.

♦ Check pets for ticks.

*Local health departments and park or agricultural extension services may have information on the seasonal and geographic distribution of ticks in your area.

How to Remove a Tick

♦ Tug gently but firmly with blunt tweezers near the "head" of the tick until it releases its hold on the skin.

♦ To lessen the chance of contact with the bacterium, try not to crush the tick's body or handle the tick with bare fingers.

♦ Swab the bite area thoroughly with an antiseptic to prevent bacterial infection.

Research—The Key to Progress

Although Lyme disease poses many challenges, they are challenges the medical research community is well equipped to meet. New information on Lyme disease is accumulating at a rapid pace, thanks to the scientific research being conducted around the world.

■ **Document Source:**
U.S. Department of Health and Human Services, Public Health Service
National Institutes of Health
National Institute of Allergy and Infectious Diseases, National Institute of Arthritis and Musculoskeletal and Skin Diseases
NIH Publication No. 92-3193
April 1992

MALARIA

General Information

Malaria is caused by a parasite that is transmitted from person to person by the bite of an infected mosquito. Only certain mosquitoes can transmit malaria. These mosquitoes are present in almost all countries in the tropics and subtropics. They are active only during the evening and night, from dusk to dawn. Therefore, it is very unlikely that you will be infected with malaria during daylight hours. The symptoms of malaria include fever, chills, headache, muscle ache, and malaise. Early stages of malaria may resemble the flu.

Malaria can often be prevented by the use of drugs, and by using individual protection measures against mosquitoes. The need for malaria prevention and the kind of measures depend on the itinerary of the traveler, the duration of travel, and the place where the traveler will spend the evenings and nights.

Travelers to malarious areas should use drugs to prevent malaria and take measures to avoid being bitten by mosquitoes. However, they can still get malaria, despite use of prevention measures. Malaria symptoms can develop as early as 6 days after the first exposure to infected mosquitoes in a malaria endemic area, or as late as several months after departure from a malarious area, even after preventive drugs are discontinued. Malaria can be treated effectively in its early stages, but delaying treatment can have serious consequences. Persons who become ill with a fever during or after travel in a malarious area should seek prompt medical attention and should inform their physician of their recent travel. Neither the traveler nor the physician should assume that the traveler has the flu or some other disease without doing a laboratory test to determine if the symptoms are caused by malaria.

Prescription Drugs for Malaria

All travelers to areas of the world where malaria is present are advised to use the appropriate drug regimen and personal protection measures to prevent malaria. The regional information provided by this travel service specifies both the appropriate drug regimen and personal protection measures for geographical regions and countries. (See the CDC FAX Travel Directory.)

Prevention

Drugs Used in Chloroquine-Resistant Areas:

Mefloquine. This drug is marketed in the United States under the name Lariam™. The adult dosage is 250 mg (one tablet) once a week, mefloquine should be taken one week before leaving, weekly while in the malarious area, and weekly for 4 weeks after leaving the malarious area.

Minor side effects one may experience while taking mefloquine include gastrointestinal disturbances and dizziness, which tend to be mild and temporary. More serious side effects at the recommended dosage have rarely occurred. Mefloquine is **not recommended** for use by:

♦ pregnant women
♦ children under 30 pounds
♦ travelers with a history of epilepsy or psychiatric disorder
♦ travelers with a known hypersensitivity to mefloquine

Doxycycline. Travelers who cannot take Mefloquine should take doxycycline to prevent malaria if they are traveling in a malarious area. This drug is taken every day at an adult dose of 100 mg, to begin on the day before entering the malarious area, while there, and continued for 4 weeks after leaving. If doxycycline is used, there is no need to take other preventive drugs, such as chloroquine.

Possible side effects include skin photosensitivity that may result in an exaggerated sunburn reaction. This risk can be minimized by wearing a hat and using sunblock. Women who take doxycycline may develop vaginal yeast infections and should discuss this with their doctor before using doxycycline. Doxycycline **should not be used** by:

♦ pregnant women
♦ children under 8 years of age
♦ travelers with a known hypersensitivity to doxycycline

Chloroquine & Proguanil. Chloroquine is used to prevent malaria for travelers who cannot take mefloquine or doxycycline. Chloroquine is often marketed in the United States under the brand name Aralen™. The adult dosage is 500 mg (salt) once a week. This drug should be taken one week before entering a malarious area, weekly while there, and weekly for 4 weeks after leaving the malarious area. Travelers who use Chloroquine should, if possible, also consider taking *simultaneously,* proguanil. The adult dose of proguanil is 200 mg/day. Proguanil is not available in the United States, but can be purchased abroad.

Rare side effects to chloroquine include upset stomach, headache, dizziness, blurred vision, and itching. Generally these effects do not require the drug to be discontinued.

Drugs Used in Chloroquine-Sensitive Areas:

Chloroquine. Chloroquine alone is used to prevent malaria for travelers going to specific geographical regions such as North Africa, the Caribbean, temperate South America, most of Central America, and part of the Middle East. In these regions Chloroquine is still effective in preventing malaria. Chloroquine is often marketed in the United States under the brand name Aralen™. The adult dosage is 500 mg (salt) once a week. This drug should be taken one week before entering a malarious area, weekly while there, and weekly for 4 weeks after leaving the malarious area. Rare side effects to chloroquine include upset stomach, headache, dizziness, blurred vision, and itching. Generally these effects do not require the drug to be discontinued.

Drugs Used for Temporary Self-Treatment

Fansidar. Chloroquine may not prevent malaria (in areas where there is chloroquine-resistant malaria) and travelers who use chloroquine must take additional measures. In addition to stringent personal protection measures, they should also take with them one or more treatment doses of Fansidar. **NO ONE WITH A HISTORY OF SULFA ALLERGY SHOULD TAKE FANSIDAR**. Each treatment dose for an adult consists of 3 tablets. These 3 tablets should be taken as a single dose to treat any fever during the travel if **professional** medical care is not available within 24 hours. **Such presumptive self-treatment of a possible malaria infection is only a temporary measure; the traveler should seek medical care as soon as possible**. Travelers should continue taking the weekly dose of chloroquine after treatment with Fansidar.

Preventing Mosquito Bites

In addition to using drugs to prevent malaria, travelers should use measures to reduce exposure to malaria-carrying mosquitoes, which bite during the evening and night. To reduce mosquito bites travelers should remain in well-screened areas, use mosquito nets, and wear clothes that cover most of the body. Travelers should also take insect repellent with them to use on any exposed areas of the skin. The most effective repellent is DEET (N,N-diethyl meta-toluamide) an ingredient in most insect repellents. However, DEET containing insect repellents should always be used according to label directions and sparingly on children. Avoid applying high-concentration (greater than 35%) products to the skin, particularly on children. Rarely toxic reactions or other problems have developed after contact with DEET. Travelers should also purchase a flying insect-killing spray to use in living and sleeping areas during the evening and night. For greater protection, clothing and bednets can be soaked in or sprayed with permethrin, which is an insect repellent licensed for use on clothing. If applied according to the directions, permethrin will repel insects from clothing for several weeks. Portable mosquito bednets, DEET containing repellents, and permethrin can be purchased in hardware, backpacking, or military surplus stores.

■ Document Source:
   Centers for Disease Control and Prevention
   Document #221011; #221010
   March 8, 1993; April 8, 1993

See also: Preventing 'Turista' and Other Travelers' Ailments (page 235)

MEASLES

Disease Information

Measles is caused by a virus, and may be serious or even fatal. It usually causes a rash, high fever, cough, runny nose and watery eyes lasting 1 to 2 weeks. Its more serious effects are diarrhea, middle ear infections, pneumonia, and, less frequently, encephalitis leading to convulsions, deafness, mental retardation, or death.

Before 1963, when measles vaccine was first used, an average of about 500,000 cases were reported in the United States each year. Due to an aggressive vaccination program, measles cases reached their lowest point, less than 1500 cases in 1983. Since then the number of measles cases has risen to over 27,000 in 1990, with outbreaks occurring in schools, colleges, universities, and in children less than 5 years of age living in inner-city areas.

Measles is one of the most highly contagious infectious diseases. The virus is transmitted by airborne droplets, and is easily spread from person to person. The virus enters the body through the upper respiratory tract. Ten to 12 days after becoming infected, a person develops fever, cough, runny nose, red, watery eyes, and becomes contagious. The characteristic measles rash begins 2-4 days after the onset of fever. The rash usually begins on the face and over 2-3 days spreads to the trunk and abdomen, and finally to the arms and legs. A person becomes contagious at the time the fever begins, and remains contagious for 7 to 9 days after fever begins, or 4-5 days after the rash appears.

The diagnosis of measles is often made based on the signs and symptoms. Measles symptoms are usually distinctive and include fever, runny nose, cough, and red, watery eyes, often with sensitivity to light. The most definitive method of diagnosing measles is by either isolating the virus from the throat, or by a blood test for antibodies.

Once a person develops measles, treatment includes bedrest, maintenance of intake of fluids, and medication for fever and headache. The preventive use of antibiotics is of no value, and may increase the risk of severe secondary bacterial infection. Presently, there are no antiviral drugs available for treatment of measles.

Measles Immunity

In general you can consider yourself immune to measles if you meet one of the following four criteria:

(1) You have received, after your first birthday, at least one dose of live measles vaccine,

(2) You have documentation of prior physician-diagnosed measles disease,

(3) You have had laboratory testing which indicates immunity, or

(4) You were born before 1957.

Many states now require that children must have received a second dose of measles vaccine before they enter either kindergarten, first grade, or some other grade as determined by individual state policy.

Some adults, who are at higher risk of measles infection, including college students, health-care workers, and international travelers may need two doses of measles vaccine. Some people who have been vaccinated against measles may not be immune. These include children who were vaccinated before their first birthday and have not received another dose, or some adults who received the killed measles virus vaccine, which was used from 1963 through 1967. If you are in doubt as to your immune status, consult with your doctor. In many cases the easiest way to ensure you are immune is to be vaccinated, for there is no risk in taking an additional dose if you are already immune to measles.

If you have been exposed to measles and you are uncertain about your immune status, call your doctor. He may ask you to do one of the following:

(1) have your immune status verified by laboratory testing,

(2) receive the measles vaccine if less than 72 hours have passed since exposure,

(3) receive immune globulin (or IG) if it has been more than 72 hours but less than 6 days since exposure,

(4) monitor your health from the 5th day after exposure till the 21st day, if laboratory tests indicate no immunity.

Vaccine Information

There is only one measles vaccine currently used in the United States. However, in the past other measles vaccines have been used. The measles virus vaccine used in the United States is prepared in chick-embryo-cell culture. It is a live weakened virus vaccine available in three forms: (1) by itself, (2) in a measles-rubella combination vaccine, and (3) most commonly in a measles-mumps-rubella combination vaccine. The vaccine is equally effective and safe in any of the combinations. Measles vaccine produces an inapparent or mild infection, which cannot be transmitted to another person. Ninety-five percent or more of persons vaccinated at age 15 months or older will be protected from measles.

Who Should Be Vaccinated & Dosing Schedule

Generally, two doses of live measles vaccine are recommended, one shot at 15 months of age and the second shot before entering either kindergarten or first grade (or at some other age as required by laws in your state).

Measles Re-Vaccination Information

Certain situations warrant special attention.

1. Persons vaccinated with live measles vaccine before their first birthday should be considered unvaccinated, and should receive at least one dose of measles vaccine.

2. Persons given one or more doses of inactivated or killed measles vaccine, used from 1963 to 1967,

should receive the live measles vaccine in use today. This is because, if these vaccinated persons are infected with the wild virus, some may develop severe illness.

3. Finally, persons who received measles vaccine between 1963 and 1967, but are not sure what type of vaccine it was, can either ask their doctor about their immune status, or receive at least one additional dose of vaccine.

If you are in doubt about your immune status, consult your doctor.

Children

For children, a routine two-dose measles vaccination schedule is recommended. The first dose is given at age 15 months, and the second dose given at school entry (age 4-6 years). Three situations can alter this normal schedule.

First, for persons living in areas at high risk of measles, the first dose may be administered at 12 months. These high-risk areas have been defined by public health officials and can either be areas of recent measles activity or areas with large inner-city urban populations. Check with your local health department or doctor to see if you live in a high-risk area.

Secondly, some states require the second dose of measles vaccine at entry into middle school, not at entry into kindergarten or first grade. Check with your local health department or school health officials to see which requirement applies to your area.

Thirdly, during a measles outbreak infants may be vaccinated at a younger age. Measles vaccine without mumps or rubella vaccine is recommended for infants as young as 6 months of age when exposure to natural measles is considered likely. Measles-mumps-rubella (MMR) vaccine, may be used if the measles-only vaccine is not available.

Measles vaccine given to children less than 12 months of age may not produce immunity to measles. As a result, children vaccinated with measles vaccine before their first birthday should be considered unvaccinated, and should receive 2 doses of measles vaccine according to the standard schedule.

Preschool children visiting health-care professionals for any reason should have their measles vaccination status checked and vaccine should be given, if needed. Unless a medical reason exists for postponing vaccinations, all appropriately aged, unvaccinated children should not be rescheduled for vaccination; rather, they should be vaccinated immediately. Measles-mumps-rubella (MMR), diphtheria-tetanus-pertussis (DTP), oral polio vaccine (OPV), and Haemophilus influenzae b conjugate vaccine (Hib) can be given at the same time.

Adults

All adults born during or after 1957 should have had at least one dose of the live measles vaccine. Those born before 1957 are likely to have had measles disease as children and generally do not require vaccination.

Person vaccinated between 1963 and 1967 may have received the inactivated or killed virus vaccine, or may not be sure what type of vaccine they received. Such individuals

should consult their doctor, and possibly receive one dose of the live measles vaccine.

For anyone in doubt about their immune status, we recommend at least one dose of vaccine—preferably as combined measles-mumps-rubella MMR vaccine. There is no risk in receiving the additional vaccine dose, even if you are already immune to measles.

Special Situations—College Students, Travelers, Health-Care Workers

Some groups of adults are at higher risk of measles than others. These high-risk groups include (1) health-care workers who have direct contact with patients, (2) students attending colleges, junior colleges, technical schools, and other institutions of post-high school education, and (3) international travelers. Because of the increased risk of measles, it is very important that persons in these groups be certain that they are immune to measles.

You can be certain that you are immune to measles if one or more of the following criteria apply to you: (1) you have received 2 doses of live measles vaccine after your first birthday, with the doses spaced at least one month apart; or (2) you have documented evidence of prior physician-diagnosed measles disease; or (3) you have laboratory test results that indicate immunity.

For anyone in doubt as to their immune status, we recommend at least one dose of vaccine, either as combined Measles-mumps-rubella vaccine or the measles vaccine by itself. There is no risk in taking the additional dose, if you are already immune to measles.

Pregnancy

Measles infection during pregnancy has been associated with an increased risk of miscarriages or premature delivery. Although birth defects have rarely been reported among children of women who had measles while they were pregnant, measles has not been proven to be the cause of the defects. On the other hand, rubella (sometimes called German measles) does cause birth defects, particularly if contracted during the first three months of pregnancy.

Measles vaccine should not be given to a woman known to be pregnant or who is considering becoming pregnant within the next few months. This precaution is based on the theoretical risk of fetal infection, although there is no evidence that this occurs.

A pregnant woman who is not immune and who is exposed to measles should receive immune globulin, or IG, as soon as possible after known exposure. Immune globulin can either prevent development of measles or result in a milder infection.

If a woman is pregnant and inadvertently receives a dose of measles vaccine, then consult with a doctor. Remember, the precaution not to vaccinate a pregnant women is based on the theoretical risk of fetal infection, although there is no actual evidence that measles vaccine can harm the fetus. Measles vaccination during pregnancy should not be a reason to consider interruption of the pregnancy.

The children of pregnant women can receive the vaccine. This will pose no risk to the pregnant mother.

■ Document Source:
   Centers for Disease Control and Prevention
   Document #241001; #241002
   July 7, 1992

See also: Rubella (page 239)

MUMPS

General Information

Mumps infection is caused by a virus similar in nature to the influenza virus.

Mumps usually causes fever, headache, and swollen, painful glands under the jaw. The initial symptoms of mumps include neck or ear pain, loss of appetite, tiredness, headache, and low-grade fever. Up to one-third of infected persons have minimal or no manifestations of disease. Swelling of salivary glands in the lower jaw is the most common symptom with the involved gland soon becoming visibly enlarged. Salivary glands on either side of the face may be affected and any combination of single or multiple salivary gland involvement may occur. Severe pain can accompany the swelling, which tends to occur within the first 2 days, and may first be noted as an earache with tenderness to touch. These symptoms tend to decrease after 1 week and are usually gone within 2 weeks. Additional symptoms include a headache, and mild meningitis, which is an inflammation in the covering of the brain or spinal cord, and about 1 out of every 4 teenage or adult males with mumps will have a painful swelling of the testicles for several days. This usually does not make a person sterile and unable to father children.

Mumps can also cause several more severe complications such as swelling or inflammation of the brain (encephalitis), or hearing loss. Before there was a mumps vaccine, many children had hearing loss caused by mumps. Mumps has been one of the leading causes of acquired deafness in childhood; onset may be sudden or gradual and deafness may be complete or permanent. Other complications involve organs such as the heart, pancreas, and ovaries. Transient arthritis has been reported in some males. Complete recovery is the rule. While deaths due to mumps have been reported, fatalities from mumps are rare.

No conclusive evidence exists to link birth defects with mumps infection during pregnancy.

Prior to the licensing of the mumps vaccine in the 1960s, more than 200,000 cases of mumps occurred each year. In recent years, 4,500 to 13,000 cases of mumps have been reported each year in the United States and outbreaks still occur. Vaccination has resulted in a decline in mumps by more than 90%. The number of mumps cases peaks during the winter-spring, but cases occur year-round. Outbreaks have been common wherever there are large groups of children or young adults in close contact with each other, such as in schools, prisons, orphanages, etc.

In recent years older children and teenagers have developed mumps. Mumps is uncommon in infants less than 1 year of age. Mumps is equally common in males and females.

Teenagers and adults, especially males, who catch mumps are often much sicker for a longer period of time than younger children with a mumps infection.

Mumps is not as contagious as measles or chickenpox. A person is considered to be contagious from 3 days before to the 4th day of active disease, and even those who have few or no symptoms can transmit the disease. During mumps infection, the virus can been found in many parts of the body including fluids such as, saliva, urine, blood, breast milk, as well as in infected body tissues. Transmission of the virus is through direct contact with infected fluids, or contaminated objects such as toys, dishes, etc. Symptoms can appear 14 to 25 days after exposure to an infected person, with an average waiting time of between 16 and 18 days.

Immunity

In general a person can be considered immune to mumps only if they meet one of the following four criteria:

(1) They have documentation of receipt of 1 dose of live mumps vaccine on or after 12 months of age;
(2) They have documentation of physician-diagnosed mumps disease;
(3) They have documentation of laboratory testing which indicates immunity; or
(4) They were born before 1957.

If you are in doubt as to your immune status, consult with your doctor. In many cases, the appropriate action is to receive a dose of vaccine; there is no increased risk for getting local or other reactions from mumps vaccination if you are already immune to mumps.

Vaccine Information

Live mumps virus vaccine was licensed in December 1967. The current vaccine results in protective immunity in over 90% of vaccinated persons. The slight infection induced by the vaccine can not be transmitted to other persons.

Most adverse events following mumps vaccination consist of fever or swollen glands. Rare cases of neurologic problems have been reported. No long-term effects have been reported.

Recently a higher rate of serious adverse side effects have been reported for a mumps vaccine used in Japan and other countries. However, this is not the vaccine used in the United States. The mumps vaccine used in the United States is one of the safest live viral vaccines.

Who Should Be Vaccinated & Dosing Schedule

All infants 12 months of age or older should receive the mumps vaccine, preferably in combination with measles and rubella vaccines (MMR vaccine). If MMR vaccine is used, normal vaccination usually occurs around 15 months of age. All older children not previously immunized should receive the vaccine. Only a single dose of vaccine is currently recommended.

Since most persons born before 1957 are likely to have been infected naturally by mumps virus, persons born before 1957 can generally be considered immune.

All adolescents and adults, who are not considered immune to mumps and are therefore susceptible to mumps infection, should receive the vaccine. Testing for immunity is not necessary (or recommended) since revaccination of those who are immune (either by prior infection or vaccination) is safe.

Vaccination after exposure, while not effective in preventing mumps if significant exposure to mumps has already occurred, is not harmful and may possibly avert later disease. Neither mumps immune globulin nor immune globulin is effective in preventing mumps after a person has been exposed.

Who Should Not Be Vaccinated with Mumps Vaccine

Women who are pregnant, or who are considering pregnancy within the next 3 months, should not receive the mumps vaccine given either by itself or in combination with measles and rubella vaccines (MMR). This precaution is based on the theoretical risk of adverse effects on the unborn child after vaccination during pregnancy, although there is no evidence that this occurs.

Persons with defective immune systems should not be given mumps vaccine. This would include persons with leukemia, lymphoma, certain cancers, or therapy with certain cancer treatment drugs, radiation, or large doses of steroids. A physician should be consulted before a patient with a defective immune system is given mumps vaccine. However, a person who has contact with or lives in a household with an immunosuppressed person may be given mumps vaccine.

Patients with leukemia in remission who have not received chemotherapy for at least three months may receive live-virus vaccines, including mumps vaccine. Short-term, (less than 2 weeks,) low to moderate-dose steroid therapy, topical steroid therapy, long-term alternate-day treatment with moderate doses of short-acting steroids, and joint or tendon injections of steroids are not reasons to withhold the vaccine.

Persons with HIV infection, whether symptoms of AIDS are present or not, may be given the combined measles-mumps-rubella vaccine (MMR). Available information or vaccination of HIV-infected children indicate that MMR has not been associated with severe or unusual adverse events, although the response to the vaccine may be less than in a normal child.

Persons with severe allergy to eggs should not receive the vaccine. Severe allergy means an intense life-threatening reaction requiring medical attention. Persons who have egg allergies that are not life threatening in nature can be vaccinated. If a person can eat eggs, then the allergy is not considered to be severe.

All mumps vaccines contain trace amounts of the antibiotic neomycin. Persons who have experienced a severe allergic reaction to neomycin requiring medical attention should not be given the vaccine. Persons who have only a history of skin inflammation after contact with neomycin can be vaccinated. Live mumps vaccine does not contain penicillin, so persons allergic to penicillin can safely take the vaccine.

Persons with a moderate or severe illness can be vaccinated as soon as they have recovered. Children with minor illness, such as a mild upper-respiratory infection with or without low-grade fever, can be vaccinated.

Mumps vaccine should not be given for at least 6 weeks, and preferably for 3 months, after a person has been given immune globulin, sometimes known as IG or gamma globulin, whole blood, or other antibody containing blood products. IG should not be given within 14 days of administration of mumps vaccine. In either situation, IG may interfere with response to the vaccine.

A family history of diabetes is not a reason to withhold vaccination.

■ **Document Source:**
Centers for Disease Control and Prevention
Document #242001; #242003
July 8, 1992

PERTUSSIS

Disease Information

The introduction and widespread use of pertussis vaccine in the United States has been associated with a 99% reduction in the reported number of pertussis cases. Currently, the number of reported pertussis cases in the United States ranges from 1,000 to 4,000 annually. In unimmunized populations in the world, however, pertussis remains a major childhood health problem, with millions of cases and an estimated 600,000 deaths per year due to the disease.

The bacteria that causes pertussis attaches to the cells in the lungs and produces a poison that cripples the lungs. Thus, the lungs are not able to clear themselves of mucus, and are in danger of developing pneumonia.

For pertussis the time between exposure to the disease and the first symptoms of illness is usually 5 to 10 days, but can be as long as 21 days. The first symptoms are similar to those of a common cold—a runny nose, sneezing, low-grade fever, and a mild, occasional cough. Thus, at first there is no particular reason to think of pertussis unless the patient was known to be exposed to someone with active pertussis. The cough gradually becomes more severe, and after 1-2 weeks the patient has spasmodic bursts of numerous, rapid coughs, apparently due to difficulty expelling thick mucous from the lungs. The characteristic high-pitched whoop comes from breathing in after a coughing episode. During such an attack, the patient may turn blue, vomit, or become exhausted. Children and young infants may appear very ill and distressed. Between coughing attacks the patient usually appears normal.

Coughing attacks occur more frequently at night, with an average of 15 attacks per 24 hours. The coughing attacks increase in frequency for a couple of weeks, then remain at the same level for 2 to 3 weeks, and then gradually decrease. Coughing may last as long as 10 weeks. Recovery is gradual, but coughing episodes can recur with subsequent respiratory infections for many months after the onset of pertussis. Older people and those partially protected by vaccine may lack the whoop and have fewer episodes of coughing, making their symptoms difficult to distinguish from those of other upper respiratory infections.

Young infants are at highest risk for acquiring pertussis and for pertussis-associated complications. The most common complication and the cause of most pertussis-related deaths is bacterial pneumonia. Less serious complications include ear infections, loss of appetite, and dehydration. Although infrequent, complications affecting the brain such as convulsions and inflammation may occur, especially in infants. These problems with the brain can lead to long-term problems or death.

Pertussis is easily transmitted from person to person; 70-90% of susceptible household contacts of a person with pertussis will develop the disease. It is most easily transmitted from 7 days following exposure to 3 weeks after onset of the spasmodic coughing. Antibiotics can shorten the length of this period. Transmission from person to person most commonly occurs through coughing or sneezing.

The treatment of pertussis cases is primarily supportive. The use of antibiotics, especially early in the illness, may decrease the patient's chance of transmitting pertussis to others and may make the patient's illness less severe. Household contacts of pertussis patients should receive antibiotics to minimize transmission of the disease.

Vaccine Information

Late in 1991 a new pertussis vaccine became available for the fourth and fifth doses of pertussis vaccine, which is customarily combined with diphtheria and tetanus toxoids in the diphtheria, tetanus, pertussis vaccine, known as DTP. This new pertussis vaccine can only be given for the fourth and fifth doses in the DTP vaccine series.

Pertussis—New Vaccine

Diphtheria, tetanus, and pertussis vaccine, known as DTP vaccine, is usually given 5 times before a child reaches the 7th birthday. The new vaccine only can be used for the fourth and fifth doses—the old vaccine must be used for the first three doses.

Whereas the old vaccine is made from killed whole pertussis germ cells, the new vaccine is made from only a few parts of the pertussis germ, and is termed the acellular pertussis vaccine. When combined with diphtheria and tetanus it is know as DTaP, capital D, capital T, small a, capital P.

The new acellular vaccine has proven to result in fewer local reactions, such as swelling, soreness, or fever, and yet is as effective in preventing pertussis infection.

Normally, the fourth and fifth doses of the DTP vaccine are given to children 15-18 months old and 4 to 6 years old, respectively. The new acellular DTaP vaccine can only be used for these vaccinations. The old whole-cell DTP vaccine should always be used for the first 3 doses and can be used for the fourth and fifth dose as well. However, most experts prefer to use the new acellular DTaP for those fourth and fifth vaccinations.

The following children should not receive the new acellular DTaP vaccine: Children under 15 months of age or children after their seventh birthday. If a child should not

receive the old whole-cell DTP vaccine, the new acellular DTaP also should not be received. Children who should not receive either pertussis vaccine instead may receive the combined diphtheria-tetanus vaccine (DT vaccine).

Old Whole-Cell Pertussis Vaccine Information

The following information applies to the old whole-cell pertussis vaccine.

Pertussis vaccines have been used since the mid-1940s. The whole-cell killed bacterial vaccine is provided in combination with diphtheria and tetanus toxoid as DTP.

The pertussis vaccine has proven to be effective in 70-90 percent of those who receive it. In those cases where the vaccine does not prevent the disease it often makes it milder.

Routine vaccination against pertussis is recommended until the seventh birthday. It is not normally recommended for individuals after that time because pertussis-associated disease and death decrease with increasing age, and because vaccine reactions are thought to be more frequent in older age groups.

During outbreaks of pertussis disease, pertussis vaccine may be given to infants as young as 4 weeks of age.

Who Should Receive the Vaccine & Dosing Schedule—Laymen

The following information applies to the old whole-cell pertussis vaccine. In the United States, pertussis vaccination, usually given as DTP, is recommended for children 6 weeks through 6 years of age. For most infants and children up to age seven, the primary immunizing series consists of four doses of DTP. The recommended schedule for DTP doses is the first shot at 2 months of age, the second shot at 4 months of age, and the third shot at 6 months of age. These first three doses are usually spaced at 4 to 8 week intervals. The fourth dose is given 6-12 months after the third to maintain adequate immunity during the ensuing preschool years. Children who received all four primary immunizing doses before the fourth birthday should receive a fifth dose of DTP just before entering school. This fifth dose is not necessary if the fourth dose in the primary series was given on or after the fourth birthday. This last dose increases protective antibody levels and may decrease the risk of school-age children transmitting the disease to younger siblings who may not be fully vaccinated.

If the recommended immunizing schedule is interrupted or delayed, then complete the required number of doses. There is no need to restart the series, and normally there is no reduction in immunity once the primary series is completed.

Routine vaccination against pertussis is recommended until the seventh birthday. Pertussis-associated disease and death decrease with increasing age, and because vaccine reactions are thought to be more frequent in older age groups, pertussis vaccination is not normally recommended for individuals after their seventh birthday.

If a child has a medical reason not to receive pertussis vaccine, then tetanus and diphtheria toxoids should be given. Children not receiving the pertussis vaccine should receive the combined diphtheria-tetanus toxoid using the normal DTP schedule. Medical reasons for not receiving the vaccine are given in the section titled "Who should not receive the vaccine."

Children who have recovered from physician documented pertussis do not need pertussis vaccine. When such confirmation is lacking, DTP vaccination should be completed.

Reduced Dose—Laymen

Recently some physicians have advocated using more frequent but smaller doses of DTP in the belief that this will reduce adverse reactions. This procedure may be called split doses or half doses. However, the Immunization Practices Advisory Committee recommends giving only full doses of DTP vaccine. The attempt to reduce adverse side effects through the use of a reduced dosage of DTP has not proven effective, and may produce less protective immunity. Increasing the number of doses to equal the total volume of the five standard doses is also not recommended.

Remember, the number of doses and amount of vaccine in each dose has been carefully formulated on the basis of scientific information obtained during clinical trials of the vaccines. Altering these recommendations without scientific basis is both unwise and unwarranted.

Normal Side Effects and Adverse Reactions—Laymen

Acetaminophen is frequently given by physicians to lessen fever and irritability associated with DTP immunization. It may also be useful in preventing seizures in children who have a tendency to have seizures associated with a fever. However, fever which starts 24 hours or more after a DTP immunization, or persists more than 24 hours, should not be assumed to be due to the immunization.

Local reactions such as redness, pain and swelling are common. Occasionally, a lump can be felt at the injection site for several weeks. Reactions such as fever, drowsiness, fretfulness, and loss of hunger occur frequently. Most of these problems resolve by themselves.

Less frequently, high fever, persistent inconsolable crying lasting more than 3 hours, fainting or an unresponsive collapsed-like state, and convulsions can occur. Most of these events have no long-term consequences. Very rarely severe nervous system problems have been reported.

Local reactions and fever tend to increase with the number of DTP immunizations given, while other reactions such as fretfulness and vomiting become less frequent.

More severe reactions following pertussis vaccination have been reported and include encephalitis, which is inflammation of the brain, with or without permanent neurologic damage. However, based on thorough review of scientific studies, the Immunization Practices Advisory Committee, known as ACIP, concludes:

A relationship of cause and effect between DTP vaccine and brain damage has not been demonstrated. If the vaccine ever causes brain damage, then the occurrence of such an event must be exceedingly rare.

A similar conclusion has been reached by the American Academy of Pediatrics, the Child Neurology Society, the Canadian National Advisory Committee on Immunization, the British Joint Committee on Vaccination and Immunization, and the British Pediatric Association.

There has also been a suggested link between DTP vaccination and sudden infant death syndrome (SIDS). However, several recent large studies have found no association between receiving DTP vaccine and SIDS.

Finally, claims that DTP may be responsible for transverse myelitis, hyperactivity, learning disorders, infantile autism, and progressive degenerative central nervous system conditions have no scientific basis.

Who Should Not Receive the Vaccine

Children with minor illness, such as a mild upper-respiratory infection with or without low-grade fever, can be vaccinated. Children with a moderate or severe illness with or without fever should not receive DTP vaccine until they have recovered from their illness. A short wait allows underlying illness to resolve.

Immunosuppressive drugs, such as those used for cancer treatment, and long-term steroid use may reduce a persons' immune response to vaccines. If these drugs will be discontinued shortly, it is reasonable to wait to vaccinate until the patient has been off the drug for 1 month. Otherwise, the patient should be vaccinated while still taking the immunosuppressive drug.

Short-term (less than 2 weeks) steroid treatment should not suppress the immune response and DTP vaccine may be given during treatment time.

Certain events following a DTP immunization are reasons not to receive additional doses of pertussis vaccine. These include:

1. An immediate severe allergic reaction, such as difficulty in breathing.
2. Severe problems with the brain without another identifiable cause occurring within 7 days of vaccination. For example, loss of consciousness and responsiveness, or generalized or focal seizures.

Certain other events may be reason not to receive additional doses of DTP depending on specific individual medical counsel. If any of the following events occur soon after a DTP vaccination, the decision to give subsequent doses of vaccine containing pertussis should be carefully considered.

1. A fever equal to or greater than 105°F within 48 hours of vaccination.
2. An episode of limpness, collapse or shock-like state within 48 hours of vaccination.
3. Persistent crying lasting 3 or more hours occurring within 48 hours of vaccination.
4. Convulsions with or without fever occurring within 3 days after vaccination.

Whether and when to administer DTP to children with proven or suspected underlying neurologic disorders must be decided on an individual basis. In the presence of an evolving neurologic disorder (e.g., uncontrolled epilepsy, infantile spasms, and progressive encephalopathy) it is prudent to delay DTP vaccination until the child's status has been fully assessed. Infants and children with a history of seizures are more likely to have a seizure following DTP than those without a history of seizures. Static neurologic conditions (such as cerebral palsy or developmental delay) or a family history of seizures or other neurologic diseases are not reasons to deny a child DTP vaccination. If DTP is to be administered to a child with a neurologic or suspected neurologic disorder, then acetaminophen, found in products such as Tylenol should be given at the time of DTP vaccination and every four hours for 24 hours.

■ Document Source:
Centers for Disease Control and Prevention
Document #246001; #246002
March 31, 1993; July 8, 1992

See also: Diptheria, Tetanus, and Pertussis: What You Need to Know (page 217)

POLIO: WHAT YOU NEED TO KNOW

What is polio?

Polio is a very dangerous disease caused by a virus. Some children and adults who get a serious case of polio become paralyzed. This means that they are unable to move parts of their bodies. They may even die from the disease.

The serious cases of polio cause severe muscle pain and sometimes make the person unable to move one or both legs or arms and may make it difficult to breathe without the help of a machine. Mild cases of polio may last only a few days and may cause the person to have a fever, sore throat, stomachache, and headache.

There are no drugs or other special treatments that will cure people who get polio. How sick people get with the disease and how much they recover are different for each person. Most people who are paralyzed by polio will have some weakness in an arm or leg for the rest of their lives. Many of these people will be seriously disabled.

Although there are few cases of polio in the United States now, there are still many thousands of cases of polio each year in other countries. Therefore, it is important to protect our children with vaccines so that they cannot get the disease when someone brings the virus into the United States from another country.

What about the vaccines and their benefits?

There are 2 types of polio vaccines. Most experts recommend the live **o**ral **p**olio **v**accine, which is called **OPV**. "Live" means that the polio virus used in the vaccine is still alive but has been made very weak. This type of vaccine is given as drops in the mouth. The other vaccine is called **IPV** (Inactivated **p**olio **v**accine). "Inactivated" means that the polio virus used in the vaccine has been killed. This type of vaccine is given as a shot.

At least 90 out of every 100 people who get 3 or more doses of either OPV or IPV will be protected against polio. For healthy children and teenagers up to their 18th birthday, most experts recommend OPV drops rather than IPV shots. This is because OPV is easier to take and is more effective in preventing the spread of polio.

The best way to be protected against polio is to get 4 doses of polio vaccine. Most babies should get 2 doses by 4 months of age and a third dose at 15 to 18 months of age. The fourth dose is given at 4 to 6 years of age.

These doses may be the drops given in the mouth (OPV) or the shots (IPV).

If there is a case of polio in your neighborhood or where your child goes to school or child-care, your child may need another dose of vaccine. Your doctor may also suggest that your child get another dose before taking a trip to any country where polio is common.

Adults who are going to countries where polio is common should also get at least one dose of either OPV (if they have had this type of vaccine before) or IPV. If an adult has never had OPV, he or she should get IPV. It would be best to get 3 doses before going. If there is only enough time to get one dose, either OPV or IPV should be given before leaving the country.

What are the risks of these vaccines?

Both OPV and IPV vaccines cause problems in very few people.

OPV drops:

- ♦ Very rarely, OPV causes polio *in the person who gets the drops.*
- ♦ *For the person who gets the vaccine,* the chance of becoming paralyzed is higher after getting the first dose of vaccine than after the second, third, or fourth doses. Paralysis after the first dose happens about once for every 1-1/2 million doses of drops given. But paralysis after later doses happens only about once for every 40 million doses given.
- ♦ OPV drops very rarely can cause polio *in people who are in close contact with the person who gets the vaccine.* This happens only to people not already protected by polio vaccine.
- ♦ The chance of *a person in close contact with the one who gets the vaccine* becoming paralyzed is higher after the first dose of vaccine than after the second, third, or fourth doses. Paralysis after the first dose happens about once for every 2 million doses of drops given. But paralysis after later doses happens only about once for every 14 million doses given. If the parent or other adult household contact of a child receiving OPV has never received polio vaccine, this person should consider, if possible, being vaccinated with IPV before or at the same time as the child. Vaccination of the child should not be delayed. Talk with your doctor or nurse if you have any questions.

IPV shots:

- IPV can cause a little soreness and redness where the shot was given.

There is a very rare chance that other serious problems or even death could occur after getting either vaccine. Such problems could happen after taking any medicine or after receiving any vaccine.

When should your child get the polio vaccine and other vaccines?

For a list of **all** of the vaccines that most infants and children should get and the age when most experts suggest they should get each dose of vaccine, see page 218.

Are the benefits of the vaccines greater than the risks?

Yes, for almost all people.

Polio can be a very serious disease. Almost all people who get the vaccines are protected from this disease. Only a small number of people have problems after getting the vaccines. The problems that may happen after receiving vaccine occur much less often than when the person has the disease.

Experts believe that most people should receive polio vaccine. After reading this pamphlet and talking with your doctor or nurse, you can decide whether there is any reason for you or your child to delay or not get the polio vaccine.

There are several reasons why some people may need to delay getting polio vaccine or should not get it at all.

When should the vaccines be delayed?

Polio drops (OPV) **or** shots (IPV) should be delayed for any person who:

- Is sick with something more serious than a minor illness such as a common cold. Delay the vaccination until the person is better.

When should the vaccines not be given?

IPV should be given instead of OPV to a person who:

- Is born with or develops any disease that makes it hard for the body to fight infection, such as cancer, leukemia, or lymphoma (cancer of the lymph glands).
- Has AIDS or infection with the virus that causes AIDS.
- Is taking special cancer treatments such as x-rays or drugs or is taking other drugs, such as prednisone or steroids, that make it hard for the body to fight infection.

The close contact that occurs in the home makes it possible for the virus that is present in OPV drops to be passed on to another member of the household. Doctors usually advise that if any person in the home has any of the medical conditions listed above, IPV should be used instead of OPV.

IPV should not be given to a person who:

- Has had an allergy problem with the antibiotics neomycin or streptomycin so serious that it required treatment by a doctor.

Be sure to talk to the doctor or nurse about which polio vaccine you or your child should get.

Should pregnant women receive the vaccines?

The polio vaccines are not known to cause any problems to the unborn babies of pregnant women. Doctors usually do not recommend giving any drugs or vaccines to pregnant women unless there is a special need. However, if a pregnant woman needs immediate protection, OPV is recommended.

What to look for and to do after getting the polio vaccine:

This pamphlet lists the problems that may occur after receiving either OPV or IPV.

As with any other serious medical problem, if the person has a serious or unusual problem after getting the vaccine, **CALL A DOCTOR OR GET THE PERSON TO A DOCTOR PROMPTLY.**

■ Document Source:
U.S. Department of Health and Human Services, Public Health Service
Centers for Disease Control and Prevention
Atlanta, Georgia 30333
10/15/91

PREVENTING 'TURISTA' AND OTHER TRAVELERS' AILMENTS

by Jeffrey P. Cohn

I was in my hotel room in Guatemala when it hit. That sudden urge to go to the bathroom, right now. If it had been the first time that morning I would not have thought twice about it. But it was the fourth time in less than an hour. I knew I had it, that dreaded affliction of American tourists overseas—travelers' diarrhea.

Travelers' diarrhea is the affliction most likely to strike the 8 million Americans who travel abroad each year, but it is not the only disease or medical condition they should be wary of.

There are also a number of other diseases or medical conditions that are rare or nonexistent in the United States but common abroad, especially in developing countries. These include the ancient scourges of malaria, typhoid, cholera, and yellow fever. Other exotic ailments like schistosomiasis can also strike the unsuspecting.

But should Americans or any other of the estimated 250 million-a-year worldwide travelers change their itineraries to include only safe areas or limit their travel to within their own country's borders because of a fear of such diseases?

"Oh, no," responds Hans Lobel, M.D., of the Centers for Disease Control in Atlanta. "What's the purpose of living if you can't enjoy it?" he asks.

Fortunately, travelers can take many precautionary measures to reduce the risk of getting most diseases Americans are likely to be exposed to in other countries. Vaccines and drugs are also available to prevent or treat those diseases. Some are prescription medications, but others are sold over the counter.

Simple precautions include, experts say, knowing what health conditions might be encountered, making sure immunizations are up to date, taking along a supply of medicines, and being careful about what you eat, drink or do abroad. Travelers, especially older ones or those with diseases such as diabetes, are also advised to discuss their travel plans and any special medical needs with their physicians before leaving.

"People should travel with care," says Pamela Prindle, administrative director of immunizations at Foxhall Internists, a Washington, D.C., medical practice specializing in travelers' health. "Travel as wisely and as healthy as you can," Prindle advises Foxhall's patients.

The specific diseases or medical conditions any traveler might be exposed to depend on where that individual is going, how long he or she will be staying, and how that person will be living once there, says Theodore Nash, M.D., a senior scientist at the National Institutes of Health's Laboratory of Parasitic Diseases.

Traveling in Europe is safer, for example, than in tropical Africa or Asia. But staying in a London or Paris hotel for a few days differs from spending weeks in rural Yugoslavia or Greece. Similarly, there is a big difference between going to an African city such as Nairobi and undertaking a wildlife safari in the bush. And traveling for business or sightseeing is not the same as living in a rural area for weeks, months or years.

In general, the diseases that concern most travelers are found largely in tropical Central and South America, Africa and Asia, says R. Bradley Sack, M.D., director of the international travel clinic at the Johns Hopkins University School of Medicine in Baltimore. The bacteria, viruses and parasites that cause such diseases thrive in hot climates and in countries or areas where sanitation and medical care usually fall below U.S. standards.

Even so, the chances of getting a serious tropical disease are remote for most tourists and business travelers, especially if precautions are taken. For example, each year, only a thousand or so Americans traveling abroad get malaria, says Lobel, chief of CDC's malaria surveillance program. In East Africa, where most American tourists to that continent go, the risk is 1 in about 200. In India and southern Asia, it is 1 in 50,000.

Travelers' Diarrhea

Some 20 to 50 percent of Americans visiting the tropics get what is called "Montezuma's revenge," the "skitters" or, in Spanish-speaking countries, "turista," says Martin Wolfe, M.D., director of the Travelers' Medical Service in Washington, D.C.

Its symptoms include loose and watery stools, nausea, bloating, abdominal cramps, and sometimes fever and malaise. Fortunately, it is a self-limiting disease. Even if untreated, its symptoms usually go away in three or four days. If diarrhea lasts more than four days or is accompanied by severe cramps, bloody stools, or foul-smelling gas, the individual should see a physician.

Most travelers' diarrhea is caused by a special strain of the common intestinal bacteria *Escherichia coli*. This strain of *E. coli*, as it is usually known, accounts for at least 40 percent of all travelers' diarrhea. Other bacteria, such as the ones responsible for salmonellosis and shigellosis, can also cause diarrhea, as can such parasitic conditions as giardiasis and amebiasis.

Whatever the cause, the best way to treat travelers' diarrhea, the experts say, is to prevent it. Most diarrhea-causing organisms are waterborne, passed on in untreated water or by food handlers who have not washed their hands adequately.

Savvy tourists will avoid using untreated or suspect water in areas where travelers' diarrhea is common. This includes not drinking tap water or using it to brush your teeth (even in good hotels), not using ice in sodas or alcoholic drinks, and not mixing alcohol with water. It's also smart to skip milk and other dairy products unless you are sure they have been pasteurized.

For brushing your teeth or drinking in your hotel room, boil the water you intend to use for at least five minutes or add water purification tablets. Avoid bottled water unless it is carbonated—the carbonation process inhibits bacterial growth. Drink carbonated beverages, beer, wine, and coffee or tea. And wipe off bottle or can tops before drinking from them.

Also, be cautious about food, especially in developing countries. Don't eat raw vegetables, fruits, meats, or seafood. Avoid cold buffets left in the sun for several hours, garden or potato salads, and food from street vendors. Eat only hot cooked meals, fruits you have peeled yourself, and packaged foods.

If, despite all your best efforts, travelers' diarrhea strikes, medical experts and experienced travelers alike recommend drinking plenty of fluids to replace water and adding oral rehydration packets to fluids to replace lost minerals. Additionally, several prescription and over-the-counter drugs will relieve diarrhea symptoms or kill bacteria that cause the disease.

The first line of defense now for early treatment of travelers' diarrhea is the antibiotic trimethoprim/sulfamethoxazole (Bactrim). Long used for other illnesses, it is the only antibiotic approved by the Food and Drug Administration for travelers' diarrhea. Bactrim is 90 percent effective against the organisms that cause the disease, says John Hopkins' Sack. It usually shortens the illness and makes it less severe. Travelers can ask their physicians for a prescription to take along so it will be available at the first signs of travelers' diarrhea.

Physicians may also prescribe other drugs for travelers' diarrhea. These include doxycycline (Vibramycin), diphenoxylate (Lomotil), and the newer quinolone drugs, ciprofloxacin and norfloxacin. However, none of these drugs has been approved by FDA specifically for travelers' diarrhea due to *E. coli*. Moreover, doxycycline is not approved for children younger than 8, and the two newer quinolone drugs may be dangerous when taken by those under 18.

Perhaps the most widely used antidiarrheal medications are the over-the-counter drugs bismuth subsalicylate (Pepto Bismol) and loperamide (Imodium). Several scientific studies have been published on the effectiveness of these products in treating travelers' diarrhea. These products are approved for treating diarrhea, and FDA is reviewing their effectiveness for treating travelers' diarrhea as well. Both products treat diarrhea symptoms rather than killing the bacteria. "This is an infection and you need to get rid of it," Sack says.

Bismuth subsalicylate may take a few hours to work and cannot stop severe diarrhea. Nor should it be used by people taking a lot of aspirin or other blood thinners, pregnant women, or people subject to seizures, says Celia Maxwell, M.D., a medical officer in FDA's anti-infective drug division.

Products containing bismuth subsalicylate also should be avoided by children and teenagers recovering from flu, chicken pox, or other viral infections, because of the risk of Reye syndrome.

Malaria

If travelers' diarrhea is the disease most likely to strike Americans abroad, malaria is the most serious ailment they are likely to encounter. Once thought to be under control and perhaps even close to eradication, malaria has made a remarkable comeback in the past decade or two, says CDC's Lobel.

Malaria is caused by a single-cell blood parasite called plasmodium. The parasite is usually transmitted to people by the bite of an infected *Anopheles* mosquito. Symptoms start with a listless feeling, loss of appetite, muscle aches, and a low fever. After a few days, the classic symptoms appear: a fever that can reach 105 degrees Fahrenheit and teeth-rattling chills that can last 20 to 60 minutes. The fever may break and then return again in a 48-to-72-hour cycle, and it may be accompanied by nausea, diarrhea and vomiting.

Worldwide, some 200 million people are estimated to have malaria, Lobel says. Those numbers are guesses, he admits, since reliable figures are hard to come by. In Africa, he says, "most everybody has been infected." In this country, about 1,000 malaria cases a year are reported to CDC, a figure Lobel thinks represents only a third of the true numbers. According to Bruce Burlington, M.D., deputy director of FDA's Office of Drug Evaluation II, people living in Africa come "more or less into equilibrium" with malaria and don't get as sick as travelers who are newly infected.

Malaria is prevalent throughout the tropics, but the traveler's risk of contracting the disease is greatest in Africa and the island of Papua New Guinea in the Pacific near Australia. It is common but less of a risk in India and southeastern Asia, central and northeastern South America, and in Haiti. It is less prevalent in China and the Middle East. Even in high-risk regions, Lobel adds, the chances of getting malaria are much greater in rural areas than in cities.

The reasons for malaria's comeback are a familiar refrain nowadays. The mosquitoes that transmit the disease now resist what had been the most effective pesticides, and many of the parasites themselves now resist what had been the most effective drug used to prevent and treat the disease.

Actually, malaria is four diseases caused by four different species of the plasmodium organism. In particular, the form known as falciparum now widely resists chloroquine (Aralen), the drug developed in the 1940s to prevent and treat malaria. Often called "malignant malaria" or "black-water fever," falciparum is the most serious form of the disease and the one most likely to kill its victims. Resistance began to appear in the 1960s and is widespread in most places falciparum malaria is found today.

Fortunately, malaria can still be prevented and cured in most cases if diagnosed properly, Lobel says. While chloroquine remains an effective antimalarial drug in nonresistant areas and for the nonfalciparum forms, mefloquine (Lariam), approved by FDA in 1989, is now also recommended.

Travelers going to chloroquine-resistant areas who cannot take mefloquine—people taking beta blocker drugs for heart conditions or who are subject to seizures, FDA's Maxwell says—can use pyrimethamine/sulfadoxine (Fansidar) or doxycycline. Doxycycline is as effective as mefloquine, Lobel says, but cannot be used for as long a time because of its potential side effects. Doxycycline must also be taken daily rather than weekly as with chloroquine and mefloquine. Fansidar can cause an uncommon but potentially fatal rash as a side effect, so it is generally used only when other drugs aren't appropriate.

Several other drugs are sometimes prescribed for malaria by physicians in other countries. One, proguanil (Paludrine), is widely used in Great Britain and Kenya. Others include pyrimethamine (Daraprim) and pyrimethamine-dapsone (Maloprim). None are as broadly effective as mefloquine or chloroquine, some need to be used with other antimalarial drugs, and a few have serious side effects. Nor have any been approved by FDA for malaria.

As with travelers' diarrhea, the best treatment for malaria is prevention. Americans are advised to avoid the mosquitoes that transmit the disease. Stay inside at dusk and dawn, wear long pants or long-sleeved shirts when in mosquito-infested areas, sleep in well-screened rooms or under mosquito nets, and use an insect repellant such as DEET (N,N-diethyl-m-tolumide) on exposed skin.

Other Diseases

Most other diseases or medical conditions to which American travelers are likely to be exposed are rare and easily avoided. Schistosomiasis, for example, occurs in much of Africa, the Middle East, northeastern South America, and some Caribbean islands. Also called bilharzia or snail fever, it is caused by a freshwater snailborne parasite. Schistosomiasis can be prevented by staying out of freshwater lakes and streams in infested areas. Salt water and adequately chlorinated swimming pools are okay, though.

Sleeping sickness is a serious illness that is transmitted by the bite of tsetse flies. It is confined to areas of Africa usually not on most American tourists' itineraries. For travelers visiting such areas, the best advice for prevention is to wear long pants and long-sleeved shirts when outside.

Giardiasis, a parasitic disease, most common in the Soviet Union, Mexico, western South American, South and Southeast Asia, and the Middle East, is also increasing in

North America, particularly among mountain hikers who drink untreated water from streams contaminated with feces from infected animals such as beavers.

Giardiasis can range from a mild intestinal discomfort that disappears in a few days to a severe debilitating disease. Its symptoms include the sudden onset of explosive diarrhea and foul-smelling gas. Giardiasis can be treated with metronidazole (Flagyl), quinacrine (Atabrine), or furazolidone (Furoxone). Quinacrine can cure 90 percent of the disease's victims, Wolfe says, but can cause nausea, headaches and diarrhea in children and, rarely, toxic psychosis in adults, FDA's Maxwell says.

In several cases, vaccination can prevent diseases travelers may be exposed to. FDA approved an oral vaccine for typhoid in 1989 that has significantly fewer side effects than the injectable vaccines previously used. Typhoid is caused by the bacterial organism *Salmonella typhi,* usually transmitted through contaminated food or water. Rare in the United States, most of the 400 to 500 typhoid cases a year reported in this country have been contracted abroad, usually in less developed areas where sanitation is poor. Immunization is therefore recommended, but only for travelers going to areas where the disease is common.

Yellow fever, still endemic through much of tropical Africa and South America, is easily preventable by vaccination, as is meningitis. The cholera vaccine, on the other hand, is only about 50 percent effective. As a result, the World Health Organization advises against its use. Three countries—Pakistan, Sudan and Pitcairn Island (best remembered as where mutineers from the British ship *Bounty* hid out 200 years ago)—still require it for entrance, however. Fortunately, few tourists are likely to get cholera.

There is also a vaccine for hepatitis B, which can be transmitted sexually, by blood transfusions, and by intravenous drug use. For hepatitis A, experts recommend immunization with immune globulin for travelers going to rural areas with poor sanitation. Hepatitis E, which is transmitted similarly to hepatitis A, has caused epidemics in Africa, Asia and, most recently, Mexico. It is not known whether gamma globulin can prevent it. Polio immunizations should also be brought up-to-date since the disease has recently resurged in Israel and parts of Africa and Mexico.

Finally, a word about acquired immune deficiency syndrome. AIDS, which is transmitted the same ways as hepatitis B, is now widespread throughout much of the world, but especially in sub-Saharan Africa and Brazil. In Africa, it is commonly spread through heterosexual contact, often with prostitutes. The only sure way to avoid the sexual transmission of AIDS is to abstain from sexual contact. Otherwise, safe sex practices, including the use of a latex condom, are advised. (See "Latex Condoms Lessen Risks of STDs" in the September 1990 *FDA Consumer.*)

For tourists wanting to learn more about travelers' illnesses, the Centers for Disease Control publishes an annual "Health Information for International Travel." Copies are available for $5 from the U.S. Government Printing Office by writing the Superintendent of Documents, Washington, D.C. 20402.

CDC also maintains a recorded telephone message system with general and geographic-specific information on travelers' diseases. The number is (404) 332-4559. Information on malaria and other specific diseases can be obtained by calling (404) 332-4555.

Jeffrey P. Cohn is a freelance writer in Takoma Park, Md. His most recent trip abroad was in 1988, when he traveled to Guatemala.

■ **Document Source:**
U.S. Department of Health and Human Services, Public Health Service
Food and Drug Administration
FDA Consumer
March 1991

See also: Malaria (page 226)

RABIES

General Information

Rabies is a disease that can affect all mammals, and each year over 4,000 animals—most of them wild—are diagnosed as having the disease in the United States. The disease is found in all states except Hawaii, and also is found in Canada and Mexico and many other countries around the world.

Rabies can be given to people and other animals if they are bitten or scratched by a rabid animal. Although rabies in humans is very rare in this country, about 18,000 people still receive treatment to prevent it each year. There are several ways for you and your family to avoid the need for the treatments to prevent rabies.

Since contact with wild animals is the main way people and their pets get exposed to rabies, avoid any direct contact with wild animals—especially skunks, raccoons, and bats.

Also, make sure your pets are vaccinated against rabies. This includes your cats as well as dogs, since more cats than dogs were reported rabid for 8 of the last 10 years.

Signs in an animal which should lead you to suspect that it may be rabid are:

♦ nervousness,
♦ aggressiveness,
♦ excessive drooling and foaming at the mouth,
♦ abnormal behavior such as wild animals loosing their fear of human beings, or animals normally active at night being seen in the daytime.

If you suspect that an animal has rabies, notify your animal warden or health department so the animal can be captured. *Do not attempt to catch the animal yourself.*

If you are bitten or seriously scratched by any animal, you should wash the wound thoroughly with soap and water as soon as possible and contact your doctor immediately. Also, notify your state or local health department.

Rabies Vaccine Information

To report a vaccine reaction call one of the following two numbers:

For persons receiving HDCV (Imovax), call Connaught Laboratories, Inc., at 1 (800) VACCINE or (717) 839-7187.

For persons receiving Rabies Vaccine, Absorbed (RVA), call the Michigan Department of Public Health in Lansing at (517) 335-8085.

For serologic testing call either:

The Department of Veterinary Diagnosis, Kansas State University at (913) 532-5650, or

The Maryland Department of Health and Mental Hygiene at (301) 225-6167.

■ Document Source:
Centers for Disease Control and Prevention
Document #361501
November 19, 1992

ROCKY MOUNTAIN SPOTTED FEVER

Rocky Mountain spotted fever affects about 800 people in the United States each year. The disease usually occurs in the eastern U.S. from New York to Florida, and from Alabama to Texas in the south. It is most commonly seen from April through September but can occur anytime during the year when there is warm weather.

Rocky Mountain spotted fever is spread to people by the bites of some ticks. Signs of the disease usually begin 3 to 12 days after a tick bite. The most common symptoms are fever, headache, rash, and nausea or vomiting. If the disease is not treated, it can cause death.

Although there is no vaccine for Rocky Mountain spotted fever, it can be prevented. The best way to avoid getting the disease is to avoid areas such as the woods or fields where ticks are found. If this is not possible, the following precautions are suggestions:

1) Whenever going into the woods, or if you live or work near woods, you should use tick repellents and wear proper clothing such as long-sleeved shirts and pants that fit tightly around your wrists, waist, and ankles;

2) When you are in the woods, check yourself and your companions at least twice a day for ticks which may have gotten onto you. If you do find a tick on yourself, remove it immediately with tweezers. Gently grasp the tick as close as possible to your skin and slowly pull it away. If tweezers are not available, fingers covered with tissue paper can be used. Do not attempt to remove the tick with vaseline, hot objects such as matches or cigarettes, or by other methods. After handling ticks, be sure to wash your hands thoroughly with soap and water.

If you get a fever, headaches, rash, or nausea within two weeks of a possible tick bite or exposure you should see your doctor immediately.

■ Document Source:
Centers for Disease Control and Prevention
Document #361701
November 19, 1992

RUBELLA

Disease Information

Rubella, also called German measles, is a viral infection of children and adults, and most often occurs in late winter and early spring. Before rubella vaccine was used in the United States, children 5 to 9 years old accounted for most of the cases. The most serious consequence of rubella infection is the birth defects (called congenital rubella syndrome, or CRS) which commonly occur if a woman is infected in the first trimester (the first three months) of her pregnancy. Since the licensure of rubella vaccine, rubella and CRS have declined dramatically. However, recently, there has been a moderate increase in rubella and a dramatic increase in CRS. The increase in rubella has occurred in unvaccinated adolescents and adults as well as in children and adults in religious communities with low levels of vaccination.

Rubella is only a moderately contagious illness compared to more infectious diseases such as measles. It is passed directly from person to person via coughing, sneezing, and talking. The disease is most contagious as the rash is appearing, but can be spread from 1 week before to 5-7 days after rash onset. Infants with congenital rubella syndrome, who were infected with rubella before birth, may be able to infect others for usually about a year, and can therefore transmit rubella to those susceptible persons caring for them. Rubella may be transmitted by infected persons who exhibit no signs or symptoms, and 30%-50% of all rubella infections are not recognized as rubella disease.

The period from exposure to rubella to actual onset of rubella symptoms, called the incubation period, varies from 12-23 days, with an average of 16-18 days.

Children are apt to have a milder case of rubella than adults. For rubella illness developed after birth, symptoms are often mild with 30-50% of cases having no sign of symptoms. In children, rash is often the first manifestation. In older children and adults, there is often 1-5 days of low-grade fever, tiredness, and upper-respiratory infection preceding the rash.

There are a number of common symptoms.

1. A fever of 99-101°F, which lasts about 2 days, is common.

2. The rash usually begins on the face, progresses from head to foot, and lasts about 3 days. The rash, which is usually fainter than a measles rash and is often itchy, may not be easy to identify as a rubella rash. Rubella can be confused with many other rash illnesses.

3. The lymph nodes may begin swelling 1 week before the rash and remain swollen for several weeks.

4. Joint pain and temporary arthritis, which are uncommon in children, occur frequently in adults, especially in women.

Complications of rubella infection occurring after birth are uncommon but tend to occur more often in adults than in children. Arthritis and joint pain may occur in up to 60% or more of adult women who contract rubella. Fingers, wrists, and knees tend to be affected. These effects may take up to months to resolve, but rarely lead to long-term problems.

Swelling of the brain occurs rarely, and is more frequently found in adults (especially in females) than in children. Problems with blood clotting can occur more often in children than in adults. Effects may last weeks to months.

The developing unborn child is at high risk to develop severe rubella with lasting consequences, if the illness is passed from the mother to the unborn baby early in the pregnancy. Developing unborn infants infected with rubella in utero have a number of problems and symptoms which are called congenital rubella syndrome or CRS. Some common manifestations of congenital rubella syndrome include: deafness; eye problems, including cataracts and glaucoma; congenital heart disease; mental retardation; and many others.

After an attack of rubella, lifelong protection against the disease develops in most persons. However, reinfection with rubella virus can occur. The overwhelming majority of these reinfections occur without symptoms, but occasionally rash or joint pain have been observed. Rubella reinfection has also occurred in persons who received the rubella vaccine. Rubella reinfection during pregnancy can rarely result in transmission of the virus to the unborn child. Rare cases have been reported in which infants with congenital rubella syndrome were born to mothers who were reinfected during pregnancy.

Proof of Immunity

Persons can be considered immune only if they have documentation of:

1. Laboratory evidence of rubella immunity, or
2. Documented evidence of adequate immunization with at least one dose of rubella vaccine on or after their first birthday.

Unlike measles, neither birth before 1957 nor physician diagnosis of rubella constitute proof of immunity.

Persons who may be immune to rubella, but who lack adequate documentation of immunity, should be vaccinated.

Rubella vaccine may be given alone, but is preferably given in combination with measles and mumps vaccines. The combined measles-mumps-rubella vaccine is called MMR, and it is routinely given to children 15 months of age or older.

■ **Document Source:**
   Centers for Disease Control and Prevention
   Document #243001
   July 8, 1992

SHINGLES/ZOSTER

Disease Information

Shingles is caused by a reactivation of the same virus that causes chickenpox. After chickenpox, which normally occurs in childhood, the chickenpox virus can remain in the body for the life of the individual. It is usually dormant and causes no signs or symptoms. However, due to circumstances not fully understood, the virus may reactivate and produce a localized skin condition. In many instances, shingles begins with a localized rash which progresses rapidly to blister-like lesions. These lesions may appear in crops in irregular fashion along a nerve pathway on one side of the body. The lesions continue to form for a period of 3 to 5 days, with a total duration of the disease being 10 to 15 days. Generally the lesions are more deeply seated and more closely grouped than chickenpox. Severe pain and/or itching often occurs.

Shingles has been reported to be associated with aging, a suppression or malfunction of the immune system, trauma, sun exposure, or chickenpox in children exposed either before birth or before 18 months of age. For those with malfunctioning immune systems, the disease can be severe and spread throughout the body, causing problems in many organs of the body.

Shingles, although sometimes painful or very itchy, usually resolves without complications. Sometimes more serious effects occur, especially if the lesion involves the eye or nerves in the head.

Persons with shingles should seek professional medical care if the lesions occur on the head. A high fever, difficulty in eating or drinking, problems with hearing or balance, or persistence of symptoms are reasons to visit a doctor.

It is estimated that approximately 300,000 cases of shingles occur annually, with approximately 5% of the cases being repeat episodes. States do not require reporting of shingles; therefore little data on the occurrence of shingles exist.

Treatment

There is no treatment that prevents shingles. Once shingles develop, treatment of shingles provides varying degrees of benefit. The best source of treatment information is a local physician who is familiar with the treatment of shingles. Treatments include topical agents, antiviral drugs, and steroids. Varicella-Zoster Immune Globulin, known as VZIG, has no value in treating or preventing shingles.

Transmission

Transmission of the shingles virus results in a chickenpox infection in a susceptible person who has never had chickenpox. The main risk of transmission is through contact with drainage of the lesions (the fluid in the blisters of shingles contains infectious virus) or from articles containing fresh drainage from the lesions. Thus, a local covering of the lesions can prevent transmission of the virus to others. Isolation of a person with localized shingles is not recommended.

■ **Document Source:**
  Centers for Disease Control and Prevention
  Document #248007
  July 8, 1992

See also: Chicken Pox (Varicella) Disease Information (page 214); Measles (page 228)

TETANUS

Disease Information

Tetanus, sometimes known as lockjaw, is a disease manifested by uncontrolled muscle spasms. The disease is frequently fatal especially to the very old or very young, and is preventable by immunization. It occurs predominantly in developing countries among newborn infants, children, and young adults, but it is still encountered in the United States, especially in unimmunized or inadequately immunized adults over 50 years of age.

The tetanus bacterium depends upon the introduction of its spores into damaged tissue along with foreign bodies and/or other bacteria to provide the necessary conditions favorable for its growth.

Tetanus is not directly transmitted from person to person. Instead tetanus spores may be introduced into the body through a puncture wound contaminated with soil, street dust, animal feces, injected contaminated street drugs, lacerations, burns and even trivial or unnoticed wounds.

Tetanus disease is due to a potent poison produced by the bacteria. The poison has a stimulating effect on certain muscle groups. Most of the time the muscles of the jaw, face, and neck are affected first and then progressively more distant muscles such as the arms and legs. In this type of generalized tetanus which is the most frequent form of the disease, the release of larger quantities of poison from a wound into the bloodstream will tend to produce both a quicker onset and a more rapid progression of symptoms, as well as more severe disease.

The tetanus bacteria spores are found everywhere. Any wound can serve as an entry point for the disease. The number of cases of tetanus in any given population decreases as more of the population receives effective immunization. Thus, tetanus is a major problem in developing countries where compulsory immunization of children is not required or enforced. It is often among the 10 most frequent causes of death in such countries, and the number of cases per year worldwide has been estimated at 1 million.

In the United States, tetanus cases average between 50 and 100 per year, mostly in under-immunized older adults, and the source is usually a wound. About 30% of the people who get tetanus die from it.

The time between an injury and the occurrence of first symptoms is typically less than 2 weeks but may range from 2 days to months. Usually the shorter the period the more severe the disease.

Initial symptoms of tetanus may include such complaints as localized or generalized weakness, stiffness or cramping, or difficulty chewing and swallowing food. An early sign is often the complaint of "lockjaw." Increasing muscle rigidity follows in the generalized disease and progressively involves more muscle groups.

For patients who survive tetanus, recovery can be long (1-2 months) and arduous. Muscle spasms may begin to decrease after 10-14 days and disappear after another week or two. Residual weakness, stiffness, and other complaints may persist for a prolonged period, but complete recovery can occur from uncomplicated tetanus.

Patients with tetanus are hospitalized in an intensive care unit until it is clear that progression of disease has stabilized at a level that does not interfere with vital functions and therapy can be managed outside the unit.

Human tetanus immune globulin (TIG) is administered intramuscularly as soon as possible to neutralize the toxin that has not gained entry to the nervous system.

Illness with tetanus usually does not result in immunity, therefore immunization for all recovered patients is recommended.

Vaccine Information

Tetanus toxoid has proved to be safe and effective since its introduction during the 1920s. Tetanus toxoid consists of inactivated tetanus toxin. For practical purposes tetanus should be considered a disease against which there is no naturally acquired immunity and one that is entirely preventable with appropriate immunization and wound care.

Tetanus toxoid is very effective in preventing illness. There are two types of tetanus toxoid available, and both produce immunity to the tetanus toxin poison. Tetanus toxoid is available by itself, or frequently is administered as one of two or three components in a vaccine. It can be combined as follows:

1. with diphtheria toxoid and pertussis vaccine (DTP) for primary immunization of children younger than 7 years old,
2. with full-dose diphtheria toxoid (DT) for children who are younger than 7 years old and have a medical reason not to receive pertussis vaccination, and
3. with reduced-dose diphtheria toxoid (Td) for immunization of older children and adults.

Completion of the primary series will produce immunity to tetanus for at least 10 years in 95 percent or more of the vaccinees. Booster doses are recommended every 10 years to ensure the maintenance of protective antitoxin levels.

However, anyone who sustains a wound other than a minor cut—and especially a wound that is deep or becomes contaminated with dirt—should receive a tetanus booster if more than 5 years have elapsed since the last dose. If you aren't sure whether your wound is serious enough to require a dose of tetanus toxoid, check with your doctor.

Who Should Receive the Vaccine & Dosing Schedule

Primary tetanus immunization, usually the combined diphtheria, tetanus, pertussis (DTP) shot, is recommended for all persons at least 6 weeks old, but less that 7 years of age who do not have a medical reason to be exempted from immunization. The recommended five-dose routine schedule calls for DTP vaccinations at 2 months, 4 months, 6 months, 15 months, and 4 to 6 years. After the initial dose of the primary series, the second and third doses are spaced 4-8 weeks apart. The fourth dose of the primary series should be given approximately one year after the third dose. Normally, a fifth dose should be given after the fourth birthday but before the seventh birthday. The fifth dose is not required for children who receive their fourth dose after their fourth birthday.

For persons over 7 years old, a different, adult formulated vaccine, containing tetanus and diphtheria, but no pertussis, is recommended. For primary immunization a series of three doses of adult formulated tetanus and diphtheria toxoid is recommended. The second dose is given 4 to 8 weeks after the first, and the third dose is given 6 to 12 months after the second.

If a dose is given as part of wound management, the next booster dose is not needed for an additional 10 years. More frequent boosters are not needed and have been reported to increase the number and severity of adverse reactions.

Booster Doses

A booster dose of the adult formulated combined tetanus and diphtheria toxoids is recommended for all persons over 7 years of age. Normally the first booster dose is given 10 years after the last dose in the primary series (usually between 14 and 16 years of age), and then every 10 years thereafter.

If a dose is given as part of wound management, the next booster dose is not needed for an additional 10 years. More frequent boosters are not needed and have been reported to increase the number and severity of adverse reactions.

Normal Side Effects and Adverse Reactions

Reactions to tetanus vaccine are generally minor and local, such as redness, swelling or tenderness at the site of injection, but the administration of more frequent booster vaccinations increases the risk of these and also generalized reactions such as fever.

Local reactions are similar to DTP, but are generally milder. They are usually self-limited and require no therapy.

Severe local reactions, for example painful swelling from shoulder to elbow, generally beginning 2-8 hours after injections, have been reported in some adults, particularly those who have received frequent, which means annual, doses of tetanus toxoid. Persons experiencing these severe reactions should not get routine or emergency booster doses of adult formula tetanus-diphtheria toxoid more frequently than every 10 years. Less severe local, allergic reactions may occur in persons who have had multiple prior boosters. Rarely, severe reactions such as generalized rashes, difficulty in breathing, or nervous system problems have been reported after receipt of tetanus toxoid.

Who Should Not Receive the Vaccine

Children with moderate or severe fever can be vaccinated as soon as they have recovered. Children with minor illness, such as a mild upper-respiratory infection with or without low-grade fever, can be vaccinated.

Persons on immunosuppressive therapies given for cancer or other treatments may not develop the same immune response as a normal person. Therefore, if immunosuppressive therapy is to be discontinued shortly, it is reasonable to defer immunization until the patient has been off the therapy for one month, otherwise, give it now.

Any person who experienced difficulty in breathing following a previous dose of tetanus toxoid should not receive further doses of tetanus toxoid. If there is reason to suspect a sensitive reaction to tetanus toxoid, skin testing may be useful before deciding whether to discontinue tetanus toxoid immunization altogether.

Persons who develop encephalitis, which is a swelling of the covering of the brain, within 7 days of DTP immunization should not receive additional immunizations containing the pertussis vaccine. It may be desirable to postpone further doses of diphtheria-tetanus toxoid until the child's neurologic status becomes clear.

Immunizing children with known or suspected problems with the brain must be decided on an individual basis. A family history of convulsions or other central nervous system disorders does not justify withholding DTP immunization.

■ **Document Source:**
   Centers for Disease Control and Prevention
   Document #245001; #245004
   March 31, 1993

National Institute on Aging Age Page
WHAT TO DO ABOUT FLU

Each winter, millions of people suffer from the unpleasant effects of the "flu." For most people, a few days in bed, a few more days of rest, aspirin, and plenty to drink will be the best treatment.

Flu—the short name for influenza—is usually a mild disease in healthy children, young adults, and middle-age people. However, flu can be life-threatening in older people and in those of any age who have chronic illnesses (such as heart disease, emphysema, asthma, bronchitis, kidney disease, and diabetes). By lowering a person's resistance, flu may allow more serious infections to occur, especially pneumonia.

It is easy to confuse a common cold with influenza. An important difference is that flu causes fever, which is usually absent during a cold. Also, a stuffy nose occurs more often with a cold than with the flu. Cold symptoms generally are milder and don't last as long as symptoms of the flu.

Flu is a viral infection of the nose, throat, and lungs. It spreads quickly from one person to another, particularly in crowded places such as buses, theaters, hospitals, and schools.

Because of its ability to spread rapidly, flu was once believed to be caused by the influence of the stars and planets.

In the 1500s, the Italians gave the disease the name "influenza," their word for "influence."

What Causes Flu?

Not until the 1930s and 1940s did scientists discover that flu is caused by ever changing types of viruses. These tiny parasites enter animals and humans and begin to grow rapidly. Disease appears when their number is too large for the body's immune system to fight off immediately.

The flu can be passed easily from one person to another. When someone infected with the flu coughs or sneezes, droplets with the virus may reach another person, entering their body through the respiratory system. There, the viruses can multiply and cause flu.

Symptoms

Flu symptoms can differ from person to person. Sometimes flu will cause no obvious symptoms. Often, however, the patient will feel weak and will develop a cough, a headache, and a sudden rise in temperature. Fever can last anywhere from 1 to 6 days. Other symptoms include aching muscles, chills, and red, watery eyes.

Complications of Flu

Flu is rarely a fatal illness. But while the immune system is busy fighting off the flu, a person is less able to resist a second infection. If this second infection is in the lungs, it can be life-threatening. Older people and people with chronic diseases have the greatest risk of developing secondary infections. The most serious of these is pneumonia, one of the five leading causes of death among people 65 and older.

Pneumonia—an inflammation of the lungs—may be caused by a flu virus. More often, however, it results from bacteria that grew in the system during the flu infection.

The symptoms of pneumonia are somewhat similar to those of the flu but are much more severe. Shaking chills are very common, and coughing becomes more frequent and may produce a colored discharge. The fever that accompanied the flu will continue during pneumonia and will stay high. Pain in the chest may occur as the lungs become more inflamed.

Bacterial pneumonia is usually treated with antibiotics, such as penicillin. Antibiotic drugs, which kill bacteria, are very effective when given early enough in the course of the disease. During the most serious phase of pneumonia, the body loses fluids. Patients often receive extra fluids to prevent shock, a dangerous condition marked by inadequate blood flow.

Prevention

Because older people are prone to develop pneumonia along with the flu, they should get a flu shot (or vaccination) in the early fall according to many doctors. Side effects will sometimes occur, such as a low fever or redness at the injection site. But in most people the dangers from getting flu and possibly pneumonia are greater than the dangers from the side effects of the flu shot. One exception is people who are allergic to eggs; flu vaccines are made in egg products and may cause serious reactions in those who have such allergies.

Preventing flu is hard because flu viruses change all the time and in unpredictable ways. This year's virus usually is slightly different from last year's. Therefore, flu shots are effective for only 1 year.

Treatment

Vaccination remains the most commonly used method of preventing influenza. An antiviral drug, amantadine, also is recommended to prevent and treat many types of influenza, particularly in high-risk people. In addition, the usual treatment for the aches and pains is to take aspirin, drink plenty of fluids, and stay in bed until the fever has been gone for 1 or 2 days. It is very important to rest, since the fever may return if you become too active too soon. Call your doctor if the fever lasts; this may mean a more serious infection is present.

Scientists continue to look for ways to prevent and treat influenza. In the meantime, the Public Health Service's Advisory Committee on Immunization Practices encourages people 65 and older and others with chronic illnesses to get a yearly vaccination.

For More Information

The National Institute of Allergy and Infectious Diseases has prepared the brochure *Flu*. For single copies, write to the NIAID, Building 31, Room 7A32, Bethesda, MD 20892.

For more information about health and aging, contact the National Institute on Aging Information Center, P.O. Box 8057, Gaithersburg, MD 20898-8057. The NIA distributes free *Age Pages* on a number of topics, including the *Age Page* "Shots for Safety."

■ **Document Source:**
U.S. Department of Health and Human Services, Public Health Service
National Institutes of Health
National Institute on Aging
1992

See also: Haemophilus Influenzae Type b (HIB) (page 222)

LIVER AND GALLBLADDER DISORDERS

■ ■ ■

CancerFax from the National Cancer Institute
ADULT PRIMARY LIVER CANCER

Description

What Is Adult Primary Liver Cancer?

Adult primary liver cancer is a disease in which cancer (malignant) cells start to grow in the tissues of the liver. The liver is one of the largest organs in the body, filling the upper right side of the abdomen and protected by the rib cage. The liver has many functions. It plays an important role in making your food into energy. The liver also filters and stores blood.

Primary liver cancer is different from cancer that has spread from another place in the body to the liver (liver metastases). (A separate PDQ statement is available for childhood liver cancer.)

Adult primary liver cancer is very rare in the United States. People who have hepatitis B or C (viral infections of the liver) or a disease of the liver called cirrhosis are more likely than other people to get adult primary liver cancer.

Like most cancers, liver cancer is best treated when it is found (diagnosed) early. You should see your doctor if you have a hard lump just below the rib cage on the right side where the liver has swollen, you feel discomfort in your upper abdomen on the right side, you have pain around your right shoulder blade, or your skin turns yellow (jaundice).

If you have symptoms, your doctor may order special x-rays, such as a CT scan or a liver scan. If a lump is seen on an x-ray, your doctor may remove a small amount of tissue from your liver using a needle inserted into your abdomen. This is called a needle biopsy and is usually done using an x-ray to guide your doctor. Your doctor will have the tissue looked at under the microscope to see if there are any cancer cells. Before the test, you will be given a local anesthetic (a drug that causes loss of feeling for a short period of time) in the area so that you do not feel pain.

Your doctor may also want to look at the liver with an instrument called a laparoscope, which is a small tube-shaped instrument with a light on the end. For this test, a small cut is made in the abdomen so that the laparoscope can be inserted. Your doctor may also take a small piece of tissue (biopsy) during the laparoscopy and look at it under the microscope to see if there are any cancer cells. You will be given an anesthetic so you do not feel pain.

Your doctor may also order an exam called an angiography. During this exam, a tube (catheter) is inserted into the main blood vessel that takes blood to the liver. Dye is then injected through the tube so that the blood vessels in the liver can be seen on an x-ray. Angiography can help your doctor tell whether the cancer is primary liver cancer or cancer that has spread from another part of the body. This test is usually done in the hospital.

Certain blood tests (such as alpha fetoprotein, or AFP) may also help your doctor diagnose primary liver cancer.

Your chance of recovery (prognosis) and choice of treatment depend on the stage of your cancer (whether it is just in the liver or has spread to other places) and your general state of health.

Stage Explanation

Stages of Adult Primary Liver Cancer

Once adult primary liver cancer is found, more tests will be done to find out if the cancer cells have spread to other parts of the body (staging). The following stages are used for adult primary liver cancer:

Localized resectable
Cancer is found in one place in the liver and can be totally removed in an operation.

Localized unresectable
Cancer is found only in one part of the liver, but the cancer cannot be totally removed.

Advanced
Cancer has spread through much of the liver or to other parts of the body.

Recurrent
Recurrent disease means that the cancer has come back (recurred) after it has been treated. It may come back in the liver or in another part of the body.

Treatment Options Overview

How Adult Primary Liver Cancer Is Treated

There are treatments for all patients with adult primary liver cancer. Three kinds of treatment are used:

surgery (taking out the cancer in an operation)
radiation therapy (using high-dose x-rays to kill cancer cells)
chemotherapy (using drugs to kill cancer cells).

Hyperthermia (warming the body to kill cancer cells) and biological therapy (using the body's immune system to fight cancer) are being tested in clinical trials.

Surgery may be used to take out the cancer or to replace the liver.

- ♦ Resection of the liver takes out the part of the liver where the cancer is found.
- ♦ A liver transplant removes the entire liver and replaces it with a healthy liver donated from someone else. Only a very few patients with liver cancer are eligible for this procedure.

Chemotherapy uses drugs to kill cancer cells. Chemotherapy for liver cancer is usually put into the body by a needle in a vein or artery. This type of chemotherapy is called a systemic treatment because the drug enters the bloodstream, travels through the body, and can kill cancer cells outside the liver. In another type of chemotherapy called regional chemotherapy, a small pump containing drugs is placed in the body. The pump puts drugs directly into the blood vessels that go to the tumor.

If your doctor removes all the cancer that can be seen at the time of the operation, you may be given chemotherapy after surgery to kill any remaining cells. Chemotherapy given after surgery when your doctor has removed the cancer is called adjuvant chemotherapy.

Radiation therapy uses x-rays or other high-energy rays to kill cancer cells and shrink tumors. Radiation may come from a machine outside the body (external radiation therapy) or from putting materials that contain radiation through thin plastic tubes (internal radiation therapy) in the area where the cancer cells are found. Drugs may be given with the radiation therapy to make the cancer cells more sensitive to radiation (radiosensitization).

Radiation may also be given by attaching radioactive substances to antibodies (radiolabeled antibodies) that search out certain cells in the liver. Antibodies are made by your body to fight germs and other harmful things; each antibody fights specific cells.

Hyperthermia uses a special machine to heat your body for a certain period of time to kill cancer cells. Because cancer cells are often more sensitive to heat than normal cells, the cancer cells die and the tumor shrinks.

Biological therapy tries to get your own body to fight cancer. It uses materials made by your own body or made in a laboratory to boost, direct, or restore your body's natural defenses against disease. Biological therapy is sometimes called biological response modifier (BRM) therapy or immunotherapy.

Treatment by Stage

Treatments for adult primary liver cancer depend on the stage of your disease the condition of your liver, your age, and your general health. You may receive treatment that is considered standard based on its effectiveness in a number of patients in past studies, or you may choose to go into a clinical trial. Many patients are not cured with standard therapy and some standard treatments may have more side effects than are desired. For these reasons, clinical trials are designed to find better ways to treat cancer patients and are based on the most up-to-date information. Clinical trials are going on in most parts of the country for most stages of adult liver cancer. If you want more information, call the Cancer Information Service at 1-800-4-CANCER (1-800-422-6237).

Treatment options: Localized resectable adult primary liver cancer
Treatment is usually surgery (resection). Clinical trials are testing adjuvant systemic or regional chemotherapy following surgery.

Treatment options: Localized unresectable adult primary liver cancer
Your treatment may be one of the following:
1. A clinical trial of external radiation therapy plus chemotherapy followed by radiolabeled antibodies.
2. A clinical trial of regional chemotherapy.
3. A clinical trial of systemic chemotherapy.
4. A clinical trial of surgery followed by chemotherapy. Hyperthermia or radiation therapy with or without drugs to make the cancer cells more sensitive to radiation may be given in addition to chemotherapy.
5. A clinical trial of radiation therapy.
6. A clinical trial of liver transplantation (in certain patients).

Treatment options: Advanced adult primary liver cancer
Your treatment may be one of the following:
1. A clinical trial of biological therapy.
2. A clinical trial of chemotherapy.
3. A clinical trial of chemotherapy, radiation therapy, and drugs to make the cancer cells more sensitive to radiation (radiosensitizers).
4. A clinical trial of external radiation therapy plus chemotherapy followed by radiolabeled antibodies.

Treatment options: Recurrent adult primary liver cancer
Treatment for recurrent adult primary liver cancer depends on what treatment you received before, the part of the body where the cancer has come back, whether the liver has cirrhosis, and other factors. You may wish to consider taking part in a clinical trial.

■ Document Source:
National Cancer Institute
  Building 31, Room 10A24, 9000 Rockville Pike, Bethesda, MD 20892
  PDQ 208/01195
  02/01/94

See also: Chemotherapy and You: A Guide to Self-Help During Treatment (page 40); Radiation Therapy and You: A Guide to Self-Help During Treatment (page 56)

DD Clearinghouse Fact Sheet

CIRRHOSIS OF THE LIVER

The liver weighs about 3 pounds and is the largest organ in the body. It is located in the upper right side of the abdomen, below the ribs. When chronic diseases cause the liver to become permanently injured and scarred, the condition is called cirrhosis.

The scar tissue that forms in cirrhosis harms the structure of the liver, blocking the flow of blood through the organ. The loss of normal liver tissue slows the processing of nutrients, hormones, drugs, and toxins by the liver. Also slowed is production of proteins and other substances made by the liver.

What is the impact of cirrhosis?

Cirrhosis is the seventh leading cause of death by disease. About 25,000 people die from cirrhosis each year. There also is a great toll in terms of human suffering, hospital costs, and the loss of work by people with cirrhosis.

What are the major causes of cirrhosis?

Cirrhosis has many causes. In the United States, chronic alcoholism is the most common cause. Cirrhosis also may result from chronic viral hepatitis (types B, C, and D). Liver injury that results in cirrhosis also may be caused by a number of inherited diseases such as cystic fibrosis, alpha-1 antitrypsin deficiency, hemochromatosis, Wilson's disease, galactosemia, and glycogen storage diseases.

Two inherited disorders result in the abnormal storage of metals in the liver leading to tissue damage and cirrhosis. People with Wilson's disease store too much copper in their livers, brains, kidneys, and in the corneas of their eyes.

In another disorder, known as hemochromatosis, too much iron is absorbed, and the excess iron is deposited in the liver and in other organs, such as the pancreas, skin, intestinal lining, heart, and endocrine glands.

If a person's bile duct becomes blocked, this also may cause cirrhosis. The bile ducts carry bile formed in the liver to the intestines, where the bile helps in the digestion of fat. In babies, the most common cause of cirrhosis due to blocked bile ducts is a disease called biliary atresia. In this case, the bile ducts are absent or injured, causing the bile to back up in the liver. These babies are jaundiced (their skin is yellowed) after their first month in life. Sometimes they can be helped by surgery in which a new duct is formed to allow bile to drain again from the liver.

In adults, the bile ducts may become inflamed, blocked, and scarred due to another liver disease, primary biliary cirrhosis. Another type of biliary cirrhosis also may occur after a patient has gallbladder surgery in which the bile ducts are injured or tied off.

Other, less common, causes of cirrhosis are severe reactions to prescribed drugs, prolonged exposure to environmental toxins, and repeated bouts of heart failure with liver congestion.

What are the symptoms of cirrhosis?

People with cirrhosis often have few symptoms at first. The two major problems that eventually cause symptoms are loss of functioning liver cells and distortion of the liver caused by scarring. The person may experience fatigue, weakness, and exhaustion. Loss of appetite is usual, often with nausea and weight loss.

As liver function declines, less protein is made by the organ. For example, less of the protein albumin is made, which results in water accumulating in the legs (edema) or abdomen (ascites). A decrease in proteins needed for blood clotting makes it easy for the person to bruise or to bleed.

In the later stages of cirrhosis, jaundice (yellow skin) may occur, caused by the buildup of bile pigment that is passed by the liver into the intestines. Some people with cirrhosis experience intense itching due to bile products that are deposited in the skin. Gallstones often form in persons with cirrhosis because not enough bile reaches the gallbladder.

The liver of a person with cirrhosis also has trouble removing toxins, which may build up in the blood. These toxins can dull mental function and lead to personality changes and even coma (encephalopathy). Early signs of toxin accumulation in the brain may include neglect of personal appearance, unresponsiveness, forgetfulness, trouble concentrating, or changes in sleeping habits.

Drugs taken usually are filtered out by the liver, and this cleansing process also is slowed down by cirrhosis. The liver does not remove the drugs from the blood at the usual rate, so the drugs act longer than expected, building up in the body. People with cirrhosis often are very sensitive to medications and their side effects.

A serious problem for people with cirrhosis is pressure on blood vessels that flow through the liver. Normally, blood from the intestines and spleen is pumped to the liver through the portal vein. But in cirrhosis, this normal flow of blood is slowed, building pressure in the portal vein (portal hypertension). This blocks the normal flow of blood, causing the spleen to enlarge. So blood from the intestines tries to find a way around the liver through new vessels.

Some of these new blood vessels become quite large and are called "varices." These vessels may form in the stomach and esophagus (the tube that connects the mouth with the stomach). They have thin walls and carry high pressure. There is great danger that they may break, causing a serious bleeding problem in the upper stomach or esophagus. If this happens, the patient's life is in danger, and the doctor must act quickly to stop the bleeding.

How is cirrhosis diagnosed?

The doctor often can diagnose cirrhosis from the patient's symptoms and from laboratory tests. During a physical exam, for instance, the doctor could notice a change in how your liver feels or how large it is. If the doctor suspects cirrhosis, you will be given blood tests. The purpose of these tests is to find out if liver disease is present. In some cases, other tests that take pictures of the liver are performed such as the computerized axial tomography (CAT) scan, ultrasound, and the radioisotope liver/spleen scan.

The doctor may decide to confirm the diagnosis by putting a needle through the skin (biopsy) to take a sample of tissue from the liver. In some cases, cirrhosis is diagnosed during surgery when the doctor is able to see the entire liver. The liver also can be inspected through a laparoscope, a viewing device that is inserted through a tiny incision in the abdomen.

What are the treatments for cirrhosis?

Treatment of cirrhosis is aimed at stopping or delaying its progress, minimizing the damage to liver cells, and reducing complications. In alcoholic cirrhosis, for instance, the person must stop drinking alcohol to halt progression of the disease. If a person has hepatitis, the doctor may administer steroids or antiviral drugs to reduce liver cell injury.

Medications may be given to control the symptoms of cirrhosis, such as itching. Edema and ascites (fluid retention) are treated by reducing salt in the diet. Drugs called "diuretics" are used to remove excess fluid and to prevent edema from recurring. Diet and drug therapies can help to improve the altered mental function that cirrhosis can cause. For instance, decreasing dietary protein results in less toxin formation in the digestive tract. Laxatives such as lactulose may be given to help absorb toxins and speed their removal from the intestines.

The two main problems in cirrhosis are liver failure, when liver cells just stop working, and the bleeding caused by portal hypertension. The doctor may prescribe blood pressure medication, such as a beta blocker, to treat the portal hypertension. If the patient bleeds from the varices of the stomach or esophagus, the doctor can inject these veins with a sclerosing agent administered through a flexible tube (endoscope) that is inserted through the mouth and esophagus. In critical cases, the patient may be given a liver transplant or another surgery (such as a portacaval shunt) that is sometimes used to relieve the pressure in the portal vein and varices.

Patients with cirrhosis often live healthy lives for many years. Even when complications develop, they usually can be treated. Many patients with cirrhosis have undergone successful liver transplantation.

Additional readings

Biliary Atresia. This fact sheet presents information on biliary atresia and cirrhosis, including discussions of diagnosis, treatment, and complications. Available from the American Liver Foundation. 1428 Pompton Avenue, Cedar Grove, NJ 07009. (201) 256-2550 or 1-800-223-0179.

Cirrhosis: Many Causes. This fact sheet presents general information on cirrhosis of the liver, research, and the work of the American Liver Foundation. Available from the foundation.

Clayman CB, ed. *The American Medical Association Encyclopedia of Medicine.* New York: Random House. 1989. Authoritative reference guide for patients, with sections on cirrhosis, hepatitis, and other disorders affecting the liver. Widely available in libraries and bookstores.

Primary Biliary Cirrhosis. This fact sheet presents information on PBC and cirrhosis, including discussions of diagnosis, treatment, and liver transplantation. Available from the American Liver Foundation.

Rosenfeld I. *Second Opinion: Your Comprehensive Guide to Treatment.* New York: Bantam Books, 1988. General medical guide with sections on cirrhosis and other disorders affecting the liver. Widely available in libraries and bookstores.

Resources

The Children's Liver Foundation, Inc. 14245 Ventura Boulevard, Suite 201, Sherman Oaks, CA 91423. (818) 906-3021 or (800) 526-1593.

United Network for Organ Sharing. 1100 Boulders Parkway, Suite 500, P.O. Box 13770, Richmond, VA 23225-8770. (804) 330-8500.

■ **Document Source:**
  U.S. Department of Health and Human Services, Public Health Service
  National Institutes of Health
  National Institute of Diabetes, and Digestive and Kidney Diseases
  NIH Publication 92-1134
  Reprinted November 1991

CancerFax from the National Cancer Institute
GALLBLADDER CANCER

Description

What Is Cancer of the Gallbladder?

Cancer of the gallbladder, an uncommon cancer, is a disease in which cancer (malignant) cells are found in the tissues of the gallbladder. The gallbladder is a pear-shaped organ that lies just under the liver in the upper abdomen. Bile, a fluid made by the liver, is stored in the gallbladder. When food is being broken down (digested) in the stomach and the intestines, bile is released from the gallbladder through a tube called the bile duct that connects the gallbladder and liver to the first part of the small intestine. The bile helps to digest fat.

Cancer of the gallbladder is more common in women than in men. It is also more common in people who have hard clusters of material in their gallbladder (gallstones).

Cancer of the gallbladder is hard to find (diagnose) because the gallbladder is hidden behind other organs in the abdomen. Cancer of the gallbladder is sometimes found after the gallbladder is removed for other reasons. The symptoms of cancer of the gallbladder may be like other diseases of the gallbladder, such as gallstones or infection, and there may be no symptoms in the early stages. You should see your doctor if you have pain above the stomach, you lose weight without trying to, you have a fever that won't go away, or your skin turns yellow (jaundice).

If you have such symptoms, your doctor may order x-rays and other tests to see what is wrong. However, usually the cancer cannot be found unless you have surgery. During surgery, a cut is made in your abdomen so that the gallbladder and other nearby organs and tissues can be examined.

Your chance of recovery (prognosis) and choice of treatment depend on the stage of cancer (whether it is just in the gallbladder or has spread to other places) and your general state of health.

Stage Explanation

Stages of Cancer of the Gallbladder

Once cancer of the gallbladder is found, more tests will be done to find out if cancer cells have spread to other parts of the body. Your doctor needs to know the stage to plan treatment. The following stages are used for cancer of the gallbladder:

Localized
Cancer is found only in the tissues that make up the wall of the gallbladder, and it can be removed completely in an operation.

Unresectable
All of the cancer cannot be removed in an operation. Cancer has spread to the tissues around the gallbladder, such as the liver, stomach, pancreas, or intestine and/or to lymph nodes in the area. (Lymph nodes are small, bean-shaped structures that are found throughout the body. They produce and store infection-fighting cells.)

Recurrent
Recurrent disease means that the cancer has come back (recurred) after it has been treated. It may come back in the gallbladder or in another part of the body.

Treatment Options Overview

How Cancer of the Gallbladder Is Treated

There are treatments for all patients with cancer of the gallbladder. Three treatments are used:

surgery (taking out the cancer or relieving symptoms of the cancer in an operation)
radiation therapy (using high-dose x-rays to kill cancer cells)
chemotherapy (using drugs to kill cancer).

Surgery is a common treatment for cancer of the gallbladder if it has not spread to surrounding tissues. Your doctor may take out the gallbladder in an operation called a cholecystectomy. Part of the liver around the gallbladder and lymph nodes in the abdomen may also be removed.

If your cancer has spread and it cannot be removed, your doctor may do surgery to relieve symptoms. If the cancer is blocking the bile ducts and bile builds up in the gallbladder, your doctor may do surgery to go around (bypass) the cancer. During this operation, your doctor will cut the gallbladder or bile duct and sew it to the small intestine. This is called biliary bypass. Surgery or other procedures may also be done to put in a tube (catheter) to drain bile that has built up in the area. During these procedures, your doctor may make the catheter

drain through a tube to the outside of your body or the catheter may go around the blocked area and drain the bile to the small intestine.

Radiation therapy uses high-energy x-rays to kill cancer cells and shrink tumors. Radiation for gallbladder cancer usually comes from a machine outside the body (external beam radiation therapy). Radiation may be used alone or in addition to surgery.

Chemotherapy uses drugs to kill cancer cells. Chemotherapy for cancer of the stomach is usually put into the body by a needle in the vein. Chemotherapy is called a systemic treatment because the drug enters the bloodstream, travels through the body, and can kill cancer cells outside the gallbladder. Chemotherapy or other drugs may be given with radiation therapy to make cancer cells more sensitive to radiation (radiosensitizers).

Treatment by Stage

Treatments for cancer of the gallbladder depend on the stage of the disease and your general health.

You may receive treatment that is considered standard based on its effectiveness in a number of patients in past studies, or you may choose to go into a clinical trial. Most patients with gallbladder cancer are not cured with standard therapy and some standard treatments may have more side effects than are desired. For these reasons, clinical trials are designed to find better ways to treat cancer patients and are based on the most up-to-date information. Clinical trials are going on in many parts of the country for patients with cancer of the gallbladder. If you want more information, call the Cancer Information Service at 1-800-4-CANCER (1-800-422-6237).

Treatment options: Localized gallbladder cancer
Your treatment may be one of the following:
1. Surgery to remove the gallbladder and some of the tissues around it (cholecystectomy).
2. External beam radiation therapy.
3. Surgery followed by external beam radiation therapy.
4. Clinical trials of radiation therapy plus chemotherapy or drugs to make the cancer cells more sensitive to radiation (radiosensitizers).

Treatment options: Unresectable gallbladder cancer
Your treatment may be one of the following:
1. Surgery or other procedures to relieve symptoms.
2. External beam radiation therapy with or without surgery or other procedures to relieve symptoms.
3. Chemotherapy to relieve symptoms. Clinical trials are testing new chemotherapy drugs.
4. Clinical trials of radiation therapy plus chemotherapy or drugs to make the cancer cells more sensitive to radiation (radiosensitizers).

Treatment options: Recurrent gallbladder cancer
Treatment for recurrent cancer of the gallbladder depends on the type of treatment you received before, the place where the cancer has recurred, and other facts about your cancer

and your general health. You may wish to consider taking part in a clinical trial.

To learn more about cancer of the gallbladder, call the National Cancer Institute's Cancer Information Service at 1-800-4-CANCER (1-800-422-6237). By dialing this toll-free number, you can speak with someone who can answer your questions.

■ **Document Source:**
   National Cancer Institute
      Building 31, Room 10A24, 9000 Rockville Pike, Bethesda, MD
         20892
      PDQ 208/01186
      02/01/94

See also: Chemotherapy and You: A Guide to Self-Help During Treatment (page 40); Radiation Therapy and You: A Guide to Self-Help During Treatment (page 56)

DD Clearinghouse Fact Sheet
GALLSTONES

The gallbladder is a small pear-shaped organ located beneath the liver on the right side of the abdomen. The gallbladder's primary functions are to store and concentrate bile, and secrete bile into the small intestine at the proper time to help digest food.

The gallbladder is connected to the liver and the small intestine by a series of ducts, or tube-shaped structures, that carry bile. Collectively, the gallbladder and these ducts are called the biliary system.

Bile is a yellow-brown fluid produced by the liver. In addition to water, bile contains cholesterol, lipids (fats), bile salts (natural detergents that break up fat), and bilirubin (the bile pigment that gives bile and stools their color). The liver can produce as much as three cups of bile in one day, and at any one time, the gallbladder can store up to a cup of concentrated bile.

As food passes from the stomach into the small intestine, the gallbladder contracts and sends its stored bile into the small intestine through the common bile duct. Once in the small intestine, bile helps digest fats in foods. Under normal circumstances, most bile is recirculated in the digestive tract by being absorbed in the intestine and returning to the liver in the bloodstream.

What are gallstones?

Gallstones are pieces of solid material that form in the gallbladder. Gallstones form when substances in the bile, primarily cholesterol and bile pigments, form hard, crystal-like particles.

Cholesterol stones are usually white or yellow in color and account for about 80 percent of gallstones. They are made primarily of cholesterol.

Pigment stones are small, dark stones made of bilirubin and calcium salts that are found in bile. They account for the other 20 percent of gallstones. Risk factors for pigment stones include cirrhosis, biliary tract infections, and hereditary blood cell disorders, such as sickle cell anemia.

Gallstones vary in size and may be as small as a grain of sand or as large as a golf ball. The gallbladder may develop a single, often large, stone or many smaller ones, even several thousand.

What causes gallstones?

Progress has been made in understanding the process of gallstone formation. Researchers believe that gallstones may be caused by a combination of factors, including inherited body chemistry, body weight, gallbladder motility (movement), and perhaps diet.

Cholesterol gallstones develop when bile contains too much cholesterol and not enough bile salts. Besides a high concentration of cholesterol, two other factors seem to be important in causing gallstones. The first is how often and how well the gallbladder contracts; incomplete and infrequent emptying of the gallbladder may cause the bile to become overconcentrated and contribute to gallstone formation. The second factor is the presence of proteins in the liver and bile that either promote or inhibit cholesterol crystallization into gallstones.

Other factors also seem to play a role in causing gallstones but how is not clear. Obesity has been shown to be a major risk factor for gallstones. A large clinical study showed that being even moderately overweight increases one's risk for developing gallstones. This is probably true because obesity tends to cause excess cholesterol in bile, low bile salts, and decreased gallbladder emptying. Very low-calorie, rapid weight-loss diets, and prolonged fasting, seem to also cause gallstone formation.

In addition, increased levels of the hormone estrogen as a result of pregnancy, hormone therapy, or the use of birth control pills, may increase cholesterol levels in bile and also decrease gallbladder movement, resulting in gallstone formation.

No clear relationship has been proven between diet and gallstone formation. However, low-fiber, high-cholesterol diets, and diets high in starchy foods have been suggested as contributing to gallstone formation.

Who is at risk for gallstones?

This year, more than 1 million people in the United States will learn they have gallstones. They will join the estimated 20 million Americans—roughly 10 percent of the population—who already have gallstones.

Those who are most likely to develop gallstones are:

♦ Women between 20 and 60 years of age. They are twice as likely to develop gallstones than men.
♦ Men and women over age 60.
♦ Pregnant women or women who have used birth control pills or estrogen replacement therapy.
♦ Native Americans. They have the highest prevalence of gallstones in the United States. A majority of Native American men have gallstones by age 60. Among the

Pima Indians of Arizona, 70 percent of women have gallstones by age 30.
- Mexican-American men and women of all ages.
- Men and women who are overweight.
- People who go on "crash" diets or who lose a lot of weight quickly.

What are the symptoms of gallstones?

Most people with gallstones do not have symptoms. They have what are called silent stones. Studies show that most people with silent stones remain symptom free for years and require no treatment. Silent stones usually are detected during a routine medical checkup or examination for another illness.

What problems can occur?

A gallstone attack usually is marked by a steady, severe pain in the upper abdomen. Attacks may last only 20 or 30 minutes but more often they last for one to several hours. A gallstone attack also may cause pain in the back between the shoulder blades or in the right shoulder and may cause nausea or vomiting. Attacks may be separated by weeks, months, or even years. Once a true attack occurs, subsequent attacks are much more likely.

Sometimes gallstones may make their way out of the gallbladder and into the cystic duct, the channel through which bile travels from the gallbladder to the small intestine. If stones become lodged in the cystic duct and block the flow of bile, they can cause cholecystitis, an inflammation of the gallbladder. Blockage of the cystic duct is a common complication caused by gallstones.

A less common but more serious problem occurs if the gallstones become lodged in the bile ducts between the liver and the intestine. This condition can block bile flow from the gallbladder and liver, causing pain and jaundice. Gallstones may also interfere with the flow of digestive fluids secreted from the pancreas into the small intestine, leading to pancreatitis, an inflammation of the pancreas.

Prolonged blockage of any of these ducts can cause severe damage to the gallbladder, liver, or pancreas, which can be fatal. Warning signs include fever, jaundice, and persistent pain.

How are gallstones diagnosed?

Many times gallstones are detected during an abdominal x-ray, computerized axial tomography (CT) scan, or abdominal ultrasound that has been taken for an unrelated problem or complaint.

When actually looking for gallstones, the most common diagnostic tool is ultrasound. An ultrasound examination, also known as ultrasonography, uses sound waves. Pulses of sound waves are sent into the abdomen to create an image of the gallbladder. If stones are present, the sound waves will bounce off the stones, revealing their location.

Ultrasound has several advantages. It is a noninvasive technique, which means nothing is injected into or penetrates the body. Ultrasound is painless, has no known side effects, and does not involve radiation.

How are gallstones treated?

Surgery

Despite the development of nonsurgical techniques, gallbladder surgery, or cholecystectomy, is the most common method for treating gallstones. Each year more than 500,000 Americans have gallbladder surgery. Surgery options include the standard procedure, called open cholecystectomy, and a less invasive procedure, called laparoscopic cholecystectomy.

The standard cholecystectomy is a major abdominal surgery in which the surgeon removes the gallbladder through a 5- to 8-inch incision. Patients may remain in the hospital about a week and may require several additional weeks to recover at home.

Laparoscopic cholecystectomy is a new alternative procedure for gallbladder removal. Some 15,000 surgeons have received training in the technique since its introduction in the United States in 1988. Currently about 80 percent of cholecystectomies are performed using laparoscopes.

Laparoscopic cholecystectomy requires several small incisions in the abdomen to allow the insertion of surgical instruments and a small video camera. The camera sends a magnified image from inside the body to a video monitor, giving the surgeon a close-up view of the organs and tissues. The surgeon watches the monitor and performs the operation by manipulating the surgical instruments through separate small incisions. The gallbladder is identified and carefully separated from the liver and other structures. Finally the cystic duct is cut and the gallbladder removed through one of the small incisions. This type of surgery requires meticulous surgical skill.

Laparoscopic cholecystectomy does not require the abdominal muscles to be cut, resulting in less pain, quicker healing, improved cosmetic results, and fewer complications such as infection. Recovery is usually only a night in the hospital and several days recuperation at home.

The most common complication with the new procedure is injury to the common bile duct, which connects the gallbladder and liver. An injured bile duct can leak bile and cause a painful and potentially dangerous infection. Many cases of minor injury to the common bile duct can be managed nonsurgically. Major injury to the bile duct, however, is a very serious problem and may require corrective surgery. At this time it is unclear whether these complications are more common following laparoscopic cholecystectomy than following standard cholecystectomy.

Complications such as abdominal adhesions and other problems that obscure vision are discovered during about 5 percent of laparoscopic surgeries, forcing surgeons to switch to the standard cholecystectomy for safe removal of the gallbladder.

Many surgeons believe that laparoscopic cholecystectomy soon will totally replace open cholecystectomy for routine gallbladder removals. Open cholecystectomy will probably remain the recommended approach for complicated cases.

A Consensus Development Conference panel, convened by the National Institutes of Health in September 1992, endorsed laparoscopic cholecystectomy as a safe and effective surgical treatment for gallbladder removal, equal in efficacy to the traditional open surgery. The panel noted, however, that laparoscopic cholecystectomy should only be performed by experienced surgeons and only on patients who have symptoms of gallstones.

In addition, the panel noted that the outcome of laparoscopic cholecystectomy is greatly influenced by the training, experience, skill, and judgment of the surgeon performing the procedure. Therefore, the panel recommended that strict guidelines be developed for training and granting credentials in laparoscopic surgery, determining competence, and monitoring quality. According to the panel, efforts should continue toward developing a noninvasive approach to gallstone treatment that will not only eliminate existing stones, but also prevent their formation or recurrence.

What are the alternatives to gallbladder surgery?

In addition to surgery, nonsurgical approaches have been pursued but are only used in special situations and only for gallstones that are predominantly cholesterol.

Oral dissolution therapy with ursodiol (Actigall) and chenodiol (Chenix) works best for small, cholesterol gallstones. These medicines are made from the acid naturally found in bile. They most often are used in individuals who cannot tolerate surgery. Treatment may be required for months to years before gallstones are dissolved.

Mild diarrhea is a side effect of both drugs; chenodiol may also temporarily elevate the liver enzyme transaminase and mildly elevate blood cholesterol levels.

Two therapies, contact dissolution with methyltert butyl ether instillation through a catheter placed into the gallbladder and extracorporeal shock-wave lithotripsy (ESWL), are still experimental.

Each of these alternatives to gallbladder surgery leaves the gallbladder intact; so stone recurrence, which happens in about one-half the cases, is a major drawback.

■ Document Source:
   U.S. Department of Health and Human Services, Public Health Service
   National Institutes of Health
   National Institute of Diabetes, and Digestive and Kidney Diseases

VIRAL HEPATITIS

General Information

If you've been exposed to hepatitis, it is important to know exactly which type of hepatitis you have. The best thing you can do is talk to your doctor or someone from your local health department about the specific circumstances of exposure.

Hepatitis A

Hepatitis A is transmitted by the fecal-oral route. This means that you must get something in your mouth which is contaminated with stool from an infected person. Most infections result from contact with a household member or sexual partner who has hepatitis A. Sometimes, infection results from eating food or drink which is contaminated with the hepatitis A virus. Gamma globulin, if given within 2 weeks of exposure, can prevent infection. It is given to people who live in the same house as a person with hepatitis A, to sexual contacts of a person with hepatitis A, or to other children in the same day care center with a child with hepatitis A. Gamma globulin is NOT given to casual contacts of a person with hepatitis A, such as friends or coworkers, because the risk of infection in these situations is extremely small.

Hepatitis B

Hepatitis B is a bloodborne infection. It is transmitted by exposure to the blood of an infected person or by sexual contact with an infected person. Infants become infected by exposure to an infected mother's blood during birth. Hepatitis B can be prevented by the hepatitis B vaccine. Hepatitis B is NOT transmitted by stool contamination of food or beverages or by casual contact with friends or coworkers. If you have been exposed, a special type of gamma globulin, called hepatitis B immune globulin, can help prevent infection, and is usually given along with hepatitis B vaccine.

Hepatitis B Vaccine

Two companies have a hepatitis B vaccine licensed for use in the United States and both are synthetically produced and do not contain blood products. Three doses of vaccine are required and will provide protection in 80 to 95 per cent of persons who get all three doses. The vaccination schedule most often used is 3 intramuscular injections, with the second and third doses administered at 1 and 6 months after the first.

Adults and older children should receive the injections in the upper arm. Infants should receive the injections in the thigh. Hepatitis B vaccine should never be given in the buttock. Hepatitis B vaccine should only be give intramuscularly.

Hepatitis B vaccine may be given with other vaccines at the same time, in a different location.

Universal Infant Hepatitis B Immunization

As part of a national effort to eliminate hepatitis B virus transmission in the United States, the Advisory Committee on Immunization Practices, with the concurrence of the American Academy of Pediatrics and the American Academy of Family Physicians, has recommended that all infants receive hepatitis B vaccine as part of their childhood immunization schedule.

The previous strategy for preventing hepatitis B emphasized immunization of selected adults with identified risk factors. Efforts to vaccinate these individuals has had limited success.

There are two hepatitis B vaccines available in the United States and both provide good protection against the disease.

There are two schedules for hepatitis B vaccine administration in children born to mothers not infected with the hepatitis B virus. Under one schedule, the first dose of the hepatitis B vaccine is given soon after birth before the infant is discharged from the hospital. The second dose is given between 1 and 2 months of age and the last dose between 6 and 18 months of age. Under the other schedule, the first dose of hepatitis B vaccine is given between 1 and 2 months of age, the second dose at 4 months of age and the last dose between 6 and 18 months of age.

Infants born to mothers infected with hepatitis B virus should be treated with hepatitis B immune globulin and hepatitis B vaccine within 12 hours of birth, with the second and third doses of vaccine given at 1 and 6 months of age.

Information for Pregnant Women

All pregnant women should be screened for hepatitis B using the hepatitis B surface antigen test.

Infants born to mothers infected with hepatitis B virus should receive hepatitis B immune globulin intramuscularly within 12 hours of birth for maximum effectiveness. Hepatitis B vaccine should be given at the same time but at a different site. The vaccine series should be completed by receiving a second dose at one month of age and the final dose at six months of age. Hepatitis B vaccine may be administered at the same time with other childhood vaccines.

Infants born to infected mothers should have blood tests three to nine months after the last dose of vaccine to determine if the treatment was effective.

If the mother is first identified as infected with the hepatitis B virus more than one month after delivery, the infant should be tested. If testing is negative for hepatitis B virus, hepatitis B immune globulin should be given with the first dose of the hepatitis B vaccine.

The Safety of Immune Globulin

Gamma globulin, hepatitis B immune globulin, and hepatitis B vaccine are safe when administered to infants, children, and adults. All of these products can be administered during pregnancy and breast-feeding. No instance of transmission of human immunodeficiency virus, the virus that causes AIDS, or other viruses has been observed with any of these products. Only limited data are available on the safety of hepatitis B vaccine for the developing fetus. However, because the vaccine contains only noninfectious material, there should be no risk to the fetus. In contrast, hepatitis B virus infection in a pregnant woman may result in severe disease for the mother and long-lasting infection in the newborn.

Hepatitis C

Hepatitis C is a viral infection which causes inflammation in the liver. Hepatitis C, also called non-A, non-B hepatitis, is another bloodborne infection, and may result from exposure to blood or body fluids that contain the hepatitis C virus. Persons at increased risk of acquiring hepatitis C include injecting drug users, health-care workers with occupational exposure to blood, hemodialysis patients, and blood transfusion recipients. Hepatitis C is transmitted by exposure to the blood of a person with hepatitis C. It may also be transmitted by sexual contact. Hepatitis C is NOT transmitted by casual contact with coworkers or friends. There is no known treatment to prevent infection.

Hepatitis C Tests

A blood test was recently developed that detects antibodies to the hepatitis C virus. Currently, this test is mainly being used to screen blood donors for hepatitis C virus infection. The test cannot distinguish between recent infection, or infection that has been present for a long time. Also, the test can not tell the difference between those who are infectious and can pass the disease, and those who have recovered and are no longer infectious.

It is recommended that persons who have a positive test for hepatitis C should see their physician for further evaluation and counseling. Because some tests may be wrong, your physician may need to repeat the test in order to decide what the positive test means.

Counselling for Persons Whose Hepatitis C Tests Are Positive

Persons who have a positive test for hepatitis C should see their physicians for further evaluation and counselling. If you have a positive hepatitis C test you should be considered potentially infectious and:

1. should not donate blood, plasma, body organs, other tissue, or sperm
2. should not share toothbrushes, razors, or other items that could become contaminated with blood
3. should cover open sores or other breaks in the skin.

The risk of infecting someone else by sexual intercourse is unknown, however, in order to prevent sexually transmitted diseases, including hepatitis and AIDS, it is recommended that:

1. the number of sexual partners be reduced
2. infected persons inform prospective sexual partners so they can prevent exchange of body fluids.

The effectiveness of latex condoms in preventing infection with hepatitis C virus is unknown, but their proper use may reduce transmission. In order to decide whether you should change your sexual practices you should consult your physician.

The risk of transmission of the hepatitis C virus from an infected mother to her infant appears to be very low. At the present time, there is no evidence to support advising against pregnancy based on a positive hepatitis C test, or to advise any special treatments or precautions for pregnant women or their offspring.

Viral Hepatitis Treatment

If you think you were exposed to any type of hepatitis and need additional information, we recommend that you talk to your doctor or someone in your local health department.

The Centers for Disease Control is not a patient treatment center. For information on currently available treatment methods for chronic hepatitis B and chronic hepatitis C, we recommend that you contact your family physician or a physician specializing in gastroenterology, or hepatology, or a specialist in infectious disease.

■ Document Source:
Centers for Disease Control and Prevention
Document #361300
November 19, 1992

WHY DOES MY BABY NEED HEPATITIS B VACCINE?

Hepatitis B vaccination is recommended as a routine childhood vaccination by the Advisory Committee on Immunization Practices (ACIP) of the U.S. Public Health Service and the Committee on Infectious Diseases of the American Academy of Pediatrics. All people—no matter how old they are or where they live—may be at risk for hepatitis B virus (HBV) infection. Babies who are vaccinated against HBV infection will be protected from the disease.

What is hepatitis B?

Hepatitis B, a serious disease of the liver, is caused by HBV. HBV infects and damages the liver. The disease can lead to severe illness, lifelong HBV infection, cirrhosis of the liver, liver failure, liver cancer, and even death. Hepatitis B is the most common cause of liver cancer worldwide.

Here are the facts about HBV infection. Each year in the United States

♦ more than 240,000 people become infected with HBV
♦ more than one million people carry HBV in their blood
♦ approximately 5,000 people die of HBV-related cirrhosis of the liver
♦ approximately 1,500 people die of HBV-related liver cancer

How can I get hepatitis B?

HBV is found in the blood and body fluids of people who have hepatitis B. You can get hepatitis B by direct contact with the blood or body fluids of an infected person. Contact with even small amounts of infected blood can cause infection.

A baby can get HBV from an infected mother during birth. You are at risk for HBV if you

♦ share needles for injecting drugs
♦ have sex with an infected person
♦ live in the same household with someone who has lifelong HBV infection
♦ have a job that exposes you to human blood

What is a hepatitis B carrier?

Some people who are infected with HBV never fully recover and carry the virus in their blood for the rest of their lives. These people are known as carriers. Many HBV carriers look and feel well. They do not know they are infected, yet they pass the infection to others throughout their lives. Approximately 5% to 10% of adults who get infected with HBV become carriers and have a lifelong infection. The risk for lifelong infection is much higher for infants and children who become infected. HBV carriers are at risk for chronic liver disease, cirrhosis, and liver cancer.

What happens to babies and children who become hepatitis B carriers?

Of babies who get HBV from their infected mothers at birth, as many as 90% may become carriers and have lifelong HBV infection. Of children who become infected with HBV before the age of 5 years, 30% to 60% may become carriers.

At first, babies may not look or feel sick, they grow up, they may have serious damage. Approximately one of four who become HBV carriers dies of disease, cirrhosis, or liver cancer.

Why does my baby need a shot now?

Hepatitis B vaccination is an investment in your baby's future. All babies should receive hepatitis B vaccine to be protected from HBV—a virus that they can come in contact with at any time in life. Hepatitis vaccination is recommended for all infants because of the high risk that children younger than 5 years of age, if infected, will become HBV carriers. This vaccination also protects your children from HBV if they are exposed to infection as teenagers or adults. Although HBV infection has no cure, it can be prevented with hepatitis B vaccine.

How is hepatitis B vaccine given?

Hepatitis B vaccine is given in a series of three shots. If a mother does not have HBV in her blood, her baby may get the first shot of hepatitis B vaccine before leaving the hospital. Or the baby may get the first shot at the doctor's office or clinic. The next two shots will be given with the other baby shots.

If a mother has HBV in her blood when her baby is born, her baby will need the first shot of hepatitis B vaccine within 12 hours after birth. Hepatitis B immune globulin, called HBIG, is also given. The baby will get the next two shots of hepatitis B vaccine as recommended by the doctor or clinic.

Why should all babies receive hepatitis B vaccine?

Health experts believe that HBV infection cannot be prevented by vaccinating only adults who are at high risk for infection. Babies who are vaccinated against HBV are no longer at risk of becoming infected. They are protected from the serious problems caused by HBV—liver cancer, liver damage, and the danger of infecting other people. As more and more people become immune to HBV infection through hepatitis B vaccination, the number of new infections will decrease. This is part of the plan to eliminate HBV infection as a health problem in the United States.

For more information call the CDC hotline (404) 332-4555

■ **Document Source:**
U.S. Department of Health and Human Services, Public Health Service
Centers for Disease Control and Prevention
September 1993

See also: Viral Hepatitis (page 251)

LUNG AND RESPIRATORY DISEASES

■ ■ ■

CYSTIC FIBROSIS: TESTS, TREATMENTS IMPROVE SURVIVAL

by Ricki Lewis, Ph.D.

Alex Deford had been ill almost from the moment of her birth on Oct. 30, 1971. Her frequent colds and ear infections coupled with her small size, despite a healthy appetite, prompted doctors to vaguely diagnose "failure to thrive." When Alex developed double pneumonia at 4 months, it was clear that something was very wrong.

That something turned out to be cystic fibrosis, the most common inherited illness among white people of Northern and Western European ancestry, although it is seen in all ethnic groups. Symptoms include thick, sticky mucus clogging the lungs, impairing breathing and attracting infection; a blocked pancreas that cannot release digestive enzymes, causing pain after eating; stubbed fingers from poor circulation; infertility; salty sweat; and other problems. Patients may have any or all of these symptoms—Alex had quite a list.

When she was diagnosed at Boston Children's Hospital early in 1972, Alex was so ill that she was expected to live only days. She survived eight years, but not easily.

Alex began each day by inhaling a decongestant. Then her parents took turns providing "postural drainage," a 30- to 60-minute pounding and pressing on each of 11 segments of the lungs, to loosen the mucus, which she coughed up. Alex would then take drugs—antibiotics to prevent lung infection and powdered digestive enzymes mixed into applesauce.

Despite this daily regimen, Alex died in January 1980. Her father, sportswriter and commentator Frank Deford, tells her story in his book, *Alex, the Life of a Child.*

Cystic fibrosis (CF) is inherited and affects 30,000 Americans. In 1989, scientists discovered the gene that causes cystic fibrosis. This discovery is enabling researchers to develop new diagnostic tests that will help identify those who can benefit from traditional as well as several new treatment approaches being evaluated by FDA.

How CF Is Inherited

CF is typically passed from parents who each carry the gene, to children of either sex. Carriers have one faulty copy of the gene, which is responsible for the illness, plus one normal copy, which prevents symptoms. Each child of carrier parents has a 1 in 4 chance of inheriting CF; a 1 in 4 chance of being completely free of the mutant gene; and a chance of 1 in 2 of being a carrier, like the parents.

Couples usually learn that they carry CF when they have an affected child. By 1985, individuals who had a sibling with CF could find out if they carried the gene by taking a "genetic marker" (linkage analysis) test that spots a particular family's CF-carrying chromosome, but not the gene itself. Finding the CF gene makes it possible to detect most carriers, even if there are no affected relatives.

The Office of Technology Assessment estimates that 100 million to 200 million people in the United States might want to take a CF carrier test. About 8 million people in the United States, or 1 in 25 whites, may be carriers.

Diagnosing CF

The same gene discovery that has led to developing carrier tests is expected to help more quickly diagnose CF, whose symptoms resemble those of other illnesses.

The most widely used and best-known CF test is the electrolyte sweat test. It detects the excess sodium, potassium and chloride (charged chemicals called electrolytes) found on the skin of many people with CF. A physician would perform a sweat test in a child with unexplained failure to gain weight, or with very frequent respiratory infections.

The sweat test evolved from the observations made by a physician, Dr. Paul di Sant' Agnese, during a 1953 heat wave in New York City. He was curious why so many children with CF were being brought to Babies and Children's Hospital, where he worked, with heat prostration. The youngsters were unable to cope with the heat because too much salt exited their bodies in sweat. The fact that the sweat of a person with CF contains two to six times as much salt as normal sweat gave him the idea for the sweat test.

The sweat test became widely used by the mid-1950s, and is the only CF test cleared by FDA for marketing. (A forerunner of the sweat test was the observation that a child's brow was salty when kissed. At the turn of the century, this is how midwives identified babies with cystic fibrosis.)

Although the sweat test is a critical part of a CF diagnostic work-up, salty sweat can indicate any of several disorders. Other tests help focus the diagnosis. Some of these tests are based on methodologies developed by reference laboratories, which perform medical tests and send the results to physicians. According to Freda Yoder of FDA's Center for Devices and Radiological Health, methodologies developed in-house have not traditionally been regulated by the agency.

Explains Tom Tsakeris, director of the division of clinical laboratory devices at FDA, "FDA regulates products, not laboratories. As long as they are not marketing the test itself, we do not regulate the lab." However, he adds, the Clinical Laboratory Improvement Act, signed into law in 1988 but not yet fully implemented, will regulate reference laboratories.

One test developed by reference labs measures the amount of the protein trypsinogen in a newborn's blood. Trypsinogen is manufactured by the pancreas and sent to the intestine, where it is snipped to a shorter form, trypsin, which helps digest proteins. If the pancreas is clogged by the sticky mucus of CF, trypsinogen levels are elevated, because the longer protein cannot be cut down to size.

In one study conducted by researchers at the University of Colorado School of Medicine and Children's Hospital in Denver, the trypsinogen test identified 95.2 percent of infants with CF who did not have the earliest sign, a greenish discharge called meconium ileus indicating intestinal blockage. But in the study there were many false positives—of 96 infants who tested high for trypsinogen on two tests, only 31 had CF. So, although the trypsinogen test alone is not perfect, combined with a sweat test and observing symptoms, it can begin to paint a portrait of CF.

Another test detects the level of certain fetal intestinal enzymes in the amniotic fluid (the liquid surrounding the fetus). Amniotic fluid is collected for testing by a procedure called amniocentesis (see "Genetic Screening: Fetal Signposts on a Journey of Discovery" in the December 1990 *FDA Consumer*). In a fetus with CF, these enzymes are decreased. Again, however, other disorders besides CF can produce this finding, and therefore it is not a specific disease marker. Researchers have turned to the genetic material to develop a definitive CF test.

Enter Genetic Testing

Developing a test to detect the gene that causes CF would provide a definitive diagnosis, because this mutant gene is the only cause of the disorder. The first step was to find out where the gene behind CF lies among the 23 pairs of chromosomes.

By 1985, several research teams had narrowed the search to a part of chromosome 7 (the seventh largest chromosome). Until the CF gene itself was isolated and characterized in 1989, relatives of patients could take an indirect test that uses linkage analysis. Because of the complexity of test interpretation, these tests are primarily performed at academic centers.

A genetic linkage test tracks a known DNA sequence (a genetic marker) that, within a family, always occurs in people with CF, and never in those who do not have the illness. A genetic marker and the gene responsible for the disorder behave like two inseparable friends. If you see one at a party, you know the other is nearby. Genetic linkage testing is based on the observation that genes carried close together on the same chromosome tend to be inherited together.

Ray White at the Howard Hughes Medical Institute at the University of Utah in Salt Lake City and Robert Williamson of St. Mary's Hospital Medical School in London each found a marker, one on either side of the CF gene. Using these two markers, a couple who already had a child with CF could have fetal chromosomes tested in a subsequent pregnancy. If the two markers on the two chromosome 7's in the fetus matched those of the affected child, then it, too, has likely inherited the disease.

A major limitation of linkage tests is that they only work on families known to have CF. Because people can carry CF without having symptoms, a disease-causing gene can be in a family without anyone in recent memory being ill. Finding the CF gene itself, however, may make possible a test useful on anyone, so that carriers could be detected in families where no one has CF.

Like other genetic tests, CF tests can be performed on any type of tissue, because all human cells (except red blood cells) contain two copies of all of the genes, and sperm and egg have one copy of each. The first CF tests used white blood cells. Then Williamson's group in London came up with a pleasanter alternative—a mouthwash! After swishing a saltwater solution in the mouth, the person spits into a bottle. The CF gene can be spotted in cells dislodged from the inside of the cheek.

Taking a cue from London, Genzyme Corp. (Cambridge, Mass.) developed a cheekbrush test for CF, which is investigational. A patient swabs cheek cells onto a brush, and the physician sends the sample to Genzyme. The presence of both normal and mutant CF genes indicates carrier status. If only mutant genes are there, CF is indicated.

To Test or Not to Test?

A carrier test provides information to couples who are not ill but whose children are at high risk of inheriting the condition.

Many experts predict that the day of universal CF screening is approaching, with several companies developing CF tests that simultaneously screen for several CF mutations.

Two factors contribute to the sensitivity of a CF carrier test. The first is the number of mutations that can be detected. The more mutations tested for, the more carriers will be spotted.

Ethnic background is the other important factor, says Marisa Ladoulis, a genetic counselor at Collaborative Diagnostic Services in Waltham, Mass. For example, a 12-mutation test that spots 84 percent of whites with a Northern or Western European background will detect 92 to 95 percent of Ashkenazi Jews, and the 16-mutation test finds 96 to 98 percent of them.

All CF Mutations Are Not Equal

Checking for an errant CF gene may be easy, but interpreting the results may not be. Researchers are finding that different CF mutations cause different degrees of sickness. Alex Deford probably had two copies of delta F508, the most common and one of the more serious mutations that can cause

CF. But a researcher in the laboratory of Francis Collins, the co-discoverer of the CF gene, has a milder case of CF because he inherited the delta F508 mutation as well as a different one.

This young man must perform postural drainage on himself and take antibiotics and digestive enzymes, but he also plays the trumpet, bikes, and sings. Still, a respiratory infection can send him to the hospital for a week or longer. Clinicians are finding that some people who have frequent bouts of pneumonia and other respiratory infections actually have CF.

Some people with CF may not even have lung or digestive symptoms. Aubrey Milunsky, D.Sc., Director of the Center for Human Genetics at the Boston University School of Medicine, found that some men who were referred to him because they were having difficulty fathering a child actually had CF. In examining x-rays that had been taken as part of a standard fertility work-up, Milunsky noticed the men lacked the vas deferens, the paired tubes that deliver sperm from the body. Knowing this is a symptom in 90 percent of men with CF, Milunsky tested their genes and found they had inherited CF.

"Cystic fibrosis is not a simple single mutation to look for," says Margaret Wallace, Ph.D., assistant professor in the division of genetics in the department of pediatrics at the University of Florida in Gainesville. "There will be a lot of problems in doing the diagnosis and giving an idea of what it means," she adds.

Treating CF

CF symptoms are controlled with a number of drugs. Antibiotic drugs combat infections to which CF patients are prone, including *Pseudomonas aeruginosa* bacteria, a type of microbe that is attracted to the sticky mucus in the lungs. The combination of animal enzymes, called Viokase, that Alex Deford took regularly is still used today by CF patients. It is approved as a prescription digestive aid for CF patients and others with pancreatic insufficiencies. Combined with a high-calorie diet, this enzyme preparation aids digestion, helping the patient to maintain weight.

Many patients also take anti-inflammatory prescription drugs, such as ibuprofen (Motrin and others), prednisone (Deltasone, Winpred, Orason, and others), and naproxen (Anaprox, Naprosyn and others).

The drug amiloride (Midamor, Moduretic), introduced in 1967 and approved as an adjunct to treatment with some diuretic drugs, is now being tested as a treatment for CF. Scientists believe amiloride thins lung secretions by blocking sodium uptake by lung cells. Clinical studies are under way to assess amiloride as a CF treatment alone, and in combination with the biological products adenosine triphosphate (ATP) and uridine triphosphate (UTP). (ATP and UTP are components of the nucleic acids DNA and RNA.)

Other investigational products are aimed at tempering the body's immune response to lung infection, which can be excessive. One such product is deoxyribo-nuclease. The March 19, 1992, *New England Journal of Medicine* reported that in a pilot study, this protein biologic given in an aerosol helped clear the lungs of 16 adult CF patients. It is being tested in 900 CF patients at 50 medical centers in the United States.

For more information, contact:

The Cystic Fibrosis Foundation
6000 Executive Blvd., Suite 510
Rockville, MD 20852
Telephone (1-800) FIGHTCS.

Gene Therapy

FDA has designated recombinant cystic fibrosis transmembrane conductance regulator (the gene's protein product, abbreviated CFTR) as well as gene therapy as orphan products. This gives their sponsors special incentives because they are developing products for a condition affecting relatively few people.

The first human gene therapy study of CF got under way last April 17 at the National Heart, Lung, and Blood Institute after FDA gave the go-ahead the previous day. An engineered cold virus (adenovirus) was introduced into the cells lining the nose and airways of a 23-year-old man with CF. The virus was altered to carry the normal CFTR gene and lacks the genes to cause a cold and to replicate.

The research was the first use of gene therapy for a common genetic disorder and the first use of a cold virus to transport genes. The study includes 10 patients 21 or older who have mild to moderate CF symptoms.

Previous experiments in rats indicated that replacing the CF genes in just 10 percent of the lung lining cells improves lung function. However, because the genes go to the patients' lungs but not their sex cells, CF can still be passed to the patients' children.

New knowledge of CF is coming so fast that the goals of carrier screening may change even before the tests are cleared for marketing.

Soon, detecting the gene for CF may be a way of finding who needs treatment, as early as possible, just as is presently done for high blood pressure and elevated blood cholesterol. Says Wallace, "CF research is moving so quickly, with a lot of hope for treatment in the near future. It will be treatable, and possibly easily."

Advances and Stumbling Blocks

The symptoms of CF were first described in medical journals in 1938. The malady was attributed to a defect in the channels leading from certain glands—a remarkably accurate description, it would turn out. But the disorder was recognized before it was given a name, as illustrated by the 17th-century English saying, "A child that is salty to taste will die shortly after birth."

In 1960, a CF patient rarely lived past the age of 12. By 1970, only half lived to see their 18th birthdays. In the 1970s, when postural drainage began to be implemented and FDA approved enzyme replacement and antibiotic therapy, the average lifespan began to creep upwards. Today, it is 29 years, according to the Cystic Fibrosis Foundation. New, more targeted therapies may raise survival age higher.

Cystic fibrosis researchers marked a medical milestone on Oct. 8, 1989, when *Science* magazine published a report by Francis Collins and his coworkers at the University of Michigan at Ann Arbor and Lap-chee Tsui at the Hospital for

Sick Children in Toronto on precisely how a specific gene disrupts a certain protein to cause CF.

The researchers named the protein the "cystic fibrosis transmembrane conductance regulator," or CFTR for short. CFTR is normally manufactured inside cells lining glands in the respiratory passages, small intestine, pancreas, and sweat glands. The protein travels to the cell's surface, where it controls the flow of salt in and out of the cell like a gateway in the cell membrane.

In the disorder, CFTR protein is abnormal in a way that prevents it from reaching the cell's surface. Without the gateway in the membrane, salt is trapped inside cells. Following a natural chemical tendency to try to dilute the salty interiors of cells, moisture is drawn inside them through other gateways. This dries out the surrounding secretions, causing symptoms. In most people with CF, the protein is missing just one amino acid building block out of 1,480—a tiny, but devastating, glitch.

Almost as soon as Collins and Tsui described the mutation that causes CF, dubbed delta F508, a difficulty arose. Delta F508 was not the only way that the gene could be altered. (A gene consists of sequences of four types of building blocks. Just as a sentence can have an error in any of its letters, a gene can be altered in many ways. A person with CF inherits two abnormal forms.)

But within days of the publication of the *Science* report, several biotechnology firms were already devising carrier tests for delta F508. A test for the disease-causing gene variant became available on an investigational basis by November 1989. But on Feb. 1, 1990, Collins, Tsui, and several others reported in *The New England Journal of Medicine* that only 75.9 percent of white CF patients of Northern and Western European backgrounds had the delta F508 variant. How useful would a test for delta F508 be, researchers worried, if this wasn't the only variant responsible for CF? At current count, more than 200 variants of the gene are known.

The multiple guises of the CF gene meant that a test to spot delta F508 would miss about 24 percent of Northern or Western European descended whites in the United States who do carry a CF gene. This, in turn, meant that the test would find only about half the couples in the United States who risk passing CF to a child (this figure is derived by multiplying the chances of each parent having delta F508). But it would be too costly to develop a test for more than 200 different mutations, when only a few of them are common.

Adding to the complexity is that different populations have different proportions of the CF gene variants. For example, delta F508 occurs in only 35 percent of African-Americans and Jews of Central and Eastern European ancestry (called Ashkenazi) who carry CF, making the test for this mutation even less valuable than it is for non-Jewish whites. For Hispanics and Italians, the frequency of delta F508 is 50 percent.

The potential powder keg of a carrier test for a common genetic disease that would, at best, only work three-quarters of the time set off a flurry of statements by professional medical organizations. On Nov. 13, 1989, the American Society of Human Genetics urged caution in carrier testing until a greater percentage of the CF-carrying population could be identified, calling for pilot programs to test the tests. Mean-

while, they suggested the test only for those with a close affected relative.

In early March 1990, a panel of physicians, geneticists, genetic counselors, and attorneys met at the National Institutes of Health in Bethesda, Md., to develop guidelines for CF carrier testing. This group echoed the earlier call for pilot programs, adding that widespread testing should wait until tests could detect 90 to 95 percent of carriers.

In December 1992, the American Society of Human Genetics reevaluated their 1989 statement, in light of the ability to detect many CF mutations. Their advice remains unchanged—for now, CF testing should be offered only to those with a relative who has the disorder. The organization also calls for informed consent and genetic counseling, confidentiality of results, and quality control of the laboratory performing the test.

Ricki Lewis is a genetic counselor and is the author of textbooks on biology and human genetics.

■ Document Source:
   FDA Consumer
   June 1993

FACTS ABOUT ASTHMA

What is asthma?

Asthma is a chronic, inflammatory lung disease charactized by recurrent breathing problems. People with asthma have acute episodes (some people say "attack" or "flare") when the air passages in their lungs get narrower, and breathing becomes more difficult. These problems are caused by an oversensitivity of the lungs' airways, which overreact to certain "triggers" and become inflamed and clogged.

Asthma varies a great deal from one person to another. Symptoms can range from mild to moderate to severe and can be life threatening. The episodes can come only occasionally or often. The symptoms of asthma are a major cause of time lost from school and work and sleep disturbances. However, with proper treatment these symptoms can almost always be controlled.

Asthma cannot be cured, but it can be controlled with proper treatment. People with asthma can use medicine prescribed by their doctor to prevent or relieve their symptoms, and they can learn ways to manage episodes. They also can learn to identify and avoid the things that trigger an episode. By educating themselves about medications and other asthma management strategies, most people with asthma can gain control of the disease and live an active life.

What causes it?

The basic cause of the lung abnormality in asthma is not yet known. Through research, scientists have established that this lung abnormality is a special type of inflammation of the airway that leads to contraction of airway muscle, mucus production, and swelling in the airways. The airways become "twitchy," overly responsive to environmental changes. This results in wheezing and coughing. Some researchers think that the wheezing and coughing may be set off by an abnormal reaction of sensory nerves—part of the overall inflammatory reaction.

A variety of known triggers can set off an asthma episode. They include:

- allergens (substances to which some people are allergic) such as pollens, foods, dust, mold, feathers, or animal dander (small scales from animal hair or feathers);
- irritants in the air such as dirt, cigarette smoke, gases, and odors;
- respiratory infections such as colds, flu, sore throats, and bronchitis;
- too much exertion such as running upstairs too fast or carrying heavy loads;*
- emotional stress such as excessive fear or excitement;
- weather such as very cold air, windy weather, or sudden changes in weather;
- medication such as aspirin or related drugs and some drugs used to treat glaucoma and high blood pressure.

Each person with asthma reacts to a different set of triggers. Identifying one's own triggers is a major step towards learning to control asthma attacks.

Although episodes can sometimes be brought on by strong emotions, it is important to know that asthma is not *caused* by emotional factors such as a troubled parent-child relationship. Some people believe that asthma is "all in one's head" and therefore not a "real" illness. This is wrong. Asthma is a disease, not a psychosomatic illness or a sign of emotional disturbance.

Who gets asthma?

Asthma has been diagnosed in nearly 10 million Americans; of these, 3 million are children under age 18. About the same number of men and women have asthma. Slightly, a higher percent of blacks have asthma than whites—4.4 percent of American blacks have asthma, while 4.0 percent of American whites have the disease.

The reported number of cases of asthma is increasing. Between 1979 and 1987, the percent of Americans with asthma increased by about one-third, from 3 percent to 4 percent of the population. This increase is occurring in all age, race, and sex groups.

The number of reported deaths from asthma has increased from about 2,600 in 1979 to about 4,600 in 1988. The racial disparity in asthma deaths is significant and continues to increase: in 1979, blacks were about twice as likely as whites to die from asthma, but by 1987 the asthma death rate was almost three times as great among blacks as among whites. However, the death rate for asthma in the U.S. is still one of the lowest in the world, and is very small compared with the number of deaths from major killers such as heart disease, cancer, and stroke.

How is asthma diagnosed?

Asthma is sometimes hard to diagnose because it can resemble other respiratory problems such as emphysema, bronchitis, and lower respiratory infections. For that reason, it is underdiagnosed—many people with the disease do not know they have it—and therefore undertreated. Sometimes the only symptom is a chronic cough, especially at night. Or, coughing or wheezing may occur only with exercise. Some people think they have recurrent bronchitis, since respiratory infections usually settle in the chest in a person predisposed to asthma.

To diagnose asthma and distinguish it from other lung disorders, physicians rely on a combination of a medical history, a thorough physical examination, and certain laboratory tests. These tests include spirometry (using an instrument that measures the air taken into and out of the lungs), peak flow monitoring (another measure of lung function), chest x-rays, and sometimes blood and allergy tests.

Is there any warning of an asthma episode?

Usually, certain signs occur hours or days before audible wheezing or before an episode is fully in progress. These early signs vary a great deal among individuals. Some people have an itchy chin or throat or a dry mouth. Others may feel very tired or grouchy. Common warning signs include light wheezing or coughing pain or a tight feeling in the chest, shortness of breath, or restlessness.

Becoming aware of these signals helps patients use self-management techniques as soon as possible. This early action may ward off a severe episode.

What happens during an episode?

An asthma episode feels somewhat like taking deep breaths of very cold air on a winter day. Breathing becomes harder and may hurt, and there may be coughing. The air may make a wheezing or whistling sound.

These problems occur because the airways of the lungs are getting narrower. The muscles that surround the airways tighten, the inner lining of the airways swells and pushes inward, and the membranes that line the airways secrete extra mucus, which can form plugs that block the air passages. The rush of air through the narrowed airways produces the wheezing sounds that are typical of asthma.

Asthma episodes range in severity from slight wheezing, coughing, or problems with breathing, to moderate episodes that can be handled at home, to severe episodes that require emergency treatment from a physician. Some episodes are life threatening and require immediate medical attention.

---

* However, a moderate amount of exercise has been shown to benefit many asthma patients; exercise should not be avoided just because one has asthma.

What can people with asthma do to avoid or lessen episodes?

The key to asthma management is monitoring one's condition, preventing episodes, and controlling an episode once it starts.

To prevent episodes, people with asthma should avoid asthma triggers and should take preventive medication appropriately. If they are to be exposed to a known trigger, such as animals or exercise, they can take medicine beforehand to avoid an attack.

To monitor lung function, asthma patients can use a peak flow meter. This is a small, inexpensive device for measuring breathing that can be used at home, at work, or at school. Because lung function decreases even before symptoms of an attack begin, the meter works as an early warning sign of an attack. Like a thermometer or a blood pressure cuff, when used properly it can be an objective measure of illness. Using a peak flow meter gives the patient information to share with the physician, so both can make decisions about the treatment plan.

At the first sign of an oncoming episode, a person with asthma should stop and rest, and take asthma medicines as prescribed. It is important to do these things as soon as one is aware of the early warning signs. This way, a serious episode often can be prevented. Different types of medicines are used for asthma episodes, so it is important to understand how to use whatever medicines are prescribed and how long they take to work.

If symptoms still do not get better, a doctor should be called. People with asthma should know how to get medical help quickly in case of a severe episode, and should have a partner or friend who can help them get to an emergency room or clinic. Patients and their physicians should develop a written action plan to guide the overall asthma treatment and to specify treatment when acute symptoms develop. This plan should spell out which medicines to take, when to call a doctor, and when to go to the emergency room.

To sum up, here are a few general guidelines that may help prevent or lessen episodes:

- ♦ identify and avoid personal asthma triggers. However, if exercise is a trigger, consider medication before exercise.
- ♦ take prescribed medicines on time, in the correct way, and in the correct dose.
- ♦ recognize early warning signs of asthma.
- ♦ take peak flow meter readings to monitor lung function.
- ♦ take action when warning signs occur.
- ♦ have a personal plan for managing attacks, worked out with a physician.
- ♦ try to stay calm if an episode may be coming on—know what to do, and do it.
- ♦ do not wait too long to get a doctor's help if needed.
- ♦ stay healthy—get enough rest, eat properly, drink plenty of liquids, and exercise regularly.

How is asthma treated?

Environmental control

Eliminating trigger factors is the first step towards achieving long-term control of asthma. For example, upper respiratory infections, cigarette smoke, and allergens are triggers for many people with asthma. Both cigarette smoking and exposure to other people's tobacco smoke should be avoided. Simple measures to reduce exposure to colds may help, such as avoiding close contact with people who have colds and frequent hand washing during the "cold season."

The most common triggers are often allergic ones. At least 90 percent of children with asthma and half of all adults with asthma have allergies that aggravate their asthma. Almost all allergens (allergy-causing substances) that affect asthma are inhaled. These include microscopic pollen and mold particles outdoors; and dust mites, animal dander, and mold indoors. Allergens in the workplace may also be important—for example, dust and vapors from plastics, grains, metal, and wood.

Taking steps to avoid or eliminate some of these allergens may dramatically improve asthma symptoms, even for people with severe asthma. In general, people whose asthma symptoms are not well controlled, who are exposed to allergens at home or work, or who suspect specific allergic factors should have a physician evaluate the possible role of allergies in their asthma. Appropriate environmental changes can then be recommended which will improve control of one's asthma.

Medication

Medication is the mainstay of asthma treatment. Since patterns of asthma are different for different people, the specific type of drug treatment varies a lot depending on the frequency, severity, and particular triggers of each patient's episodes. For example, people with mild, intermittent asthma may take medicine only before exposure to an asthma trigger or when they feel symptoms coming on. Those with more regular symptoms may take regular daily medicine to prevent episodes as well as using medicine for specific symptoms. Those whose asthma is severe and persistent may need two or more daily medications.

Although drug companies sell asthma medicines under many brand names, there are only a few major types. These are:

Anti-inflammatory agents

- ♦ *Corticosteroids.* These are increasingly important anti-asthma drugs that act directly to reduce the inflammatory response of the airways. They come as pills and in an aerosolized (inhaled) form. Because of potentially serious side effects, prolonged use of oral steroids is usually reserved for severe asthma. Inhaled steroids, however, have far fewer side effects, are very effective in reducing symptoms and airway reactivity, and seem to be safe for most patients.
- ♦ *Anti-allergy drugs.* Cromolyn sodium is the best known, with others such as nedocromil and ketotifen now under clinical testing. Anti-allergy drugs are used to prevent episodes, but do not work after an episode

starts. These drugs are best used daily as a preventive measure, but do not work for everyone. They are most effective in people with mild or moderate asthma.

♦ *Bronchodilators.*

Adrenergic bronchodilators (beta agonists). These are medicines that relax the muscles of the airways and open them up. Aerosolized (inhaled) bronchodilators are breathed into the lungs using an inhaler or a compressor nebulizer. Adrenergic bronchodilators also are made in tablet form; however, these work more slowly than aerosols and have more side effects, so the inhaled version is usually preferred. Bronchodilators are best used as needed— either alone, if symptoms are infrequent, or as a supplement to regular anti-inflammatory agents.

A note of caution: it is dangerous to rely too much on using inhaled bronchodilators only when an episode is starting. Bronchodilators do provide temporary relief of symptoms—but they do not work on the underlying inflammation that actually causes the episode, and so are not long-term solutions.

Theophylline is another type of bronchodilator. It comes in liquid, capsule, or tablet form. Although theophylline is not as strong a bronchodilator as the adrenergic medications, it can be effective for some people—for example, patients with nighttime asthma—because its effects tend to last longer than the effects of adrenergic bronchodilators. Side affects are more common than with other bronchodilators, and may include nausea, vomiting, and heart rhythm abnormalities.

Anticholinergic agents, such as atropine, are the oldest forms of bronchodilator therapy for asthma. However, other medications are now preferred because they have fewer side effects and act more quickly to relieve asthma symptoms than anticholinergics.

A word about over-the-counter medicines: although they may relieve symptoms temporarily, in the long run they are inadequate, and may make things worse by masking a real need for medical care. Many asthma patients mistakenly try to treat themselves with these medicines, only to find that when they really need help, these medicines are not enough. The only effective drug treatments for asthma are those that are prescribed, monitored, and adjusted by a physician.

Immunotherapy

For some allergic people who cannot control their asthma symptoms with enviromental changes and medication, immunotherapy (allergy desensitization shots) may be beneficial. Allergies to dust mites, pollen, and cats seem to be the allergies most successfully treated with immunotherapy.

What can asthma patients reasonably expect from treatment?

With proper treatment, most people with asthma can expect to achieve:

♦ a full night's sleep with no awakenings due to coughing,

♦ a clear chest in the morning,
♦ the ability to go to work or school regularly,
♦ full physical activity with a normal lifestyle,
♦ no emergency room visits or hospitalizations, and
♦ no significant side effects from medication.

In treating asthma, physicians aim for long-term suppression of the airway inflammation that triggers asthma attacks. Because asthma is now understood to be an inflammatory disease, and not simply abnormal airway constriction, treatment is aimed at reducing the inflammation in the long run as well as opening up the airways when they do constrict.

Can people with asthma exercise?

Generally, people with asthma can and should exercise when they are feeling well. Special care may be needed when the air is cold or during a pollen season. It is always best to start slowly and build up, and it is essential to consult one's physician before starting any type of regular exercise. Often, using an inhaled adrenergic bronchodilator before exercise can prevent exercise-induced symptoms and allow people to be fully active. People with asthma should not assume that they must limit physical activity simply because they have the disease—after all, some Olympic athletes have severe asthma. People should not be restricted from physical activity simply because they have asthma.

Are scientists doing research that could help people with asthma?

Researchers are working on several fronts to solve some of the many unanswered questions about asthma. At the National Institutes of Health, research on asthma is conducted and supported by two units, the National Heart, Lung, and Blood Institute (NHLBI) and the National Institute of Allergy and Infectious Diseases. Projects supported by these agencies focus on identifying the basic abnormality that causes asthma, on developing better drug treatments and emergency measures, and on educating people with asthma to help themselves.

Research supported by NHLBI has established that education programs can greatly reduce asthma hospitalizations and disability. In these programs, patients are trained in asthma self-management techniques while under medical supervision. Building on this and other research-derived knowledge, the NHLBI started the National Asthma Education Program in March 1989. This national effort aims to increase public awareness of asthma as a serious chronic disease, to ensure proper diagnosis of asthma, and to allow effective control of the disease by promoting a partnership between patients, physicians, and other health care professionals through modern treatment and education programs.

For more information on asthma:

National Asthma Education Program Information Center
4733 Bethesda Avenue, Suite 530
Bethesda, MD 20814
(301) 951-3260

Ask for the asthma reading and resource list, which gives many sources for more specific information on various aspects of the disease.

■ Document Source:
U.S. Department of Health and Human Services, Public Health Service
National Institutes of Health
National Heart, Lung and Blood Institute
NIH Publication No. 90-2339
October 1990

See also: Allergic Diseases (page 15); Something in the Air: Airborne Allergens (page 20)

CancerFax from the National Cancer Institute

NONSMALL CELL LUNG CANCER

Description

What Is Nonsmall Cell Lung Cancer?

Lung cancers can be divided into two types: small cell lung cancer and nonsmall cell lung cancer. The cancer cells of each type grow and spread in different ways, and they are treated differently. Nonsmall cell lung cancer is usually associated with prior smoking, passive smoking, or radon exposure. (See the PDQ "Information for Patients: Small Cell Lung Cancer" for information on treatment of this disease).

There are three main kinds of nonsmall cell lung cancer. They are named for the type of cells found in the cancer: squamous cell carcinoma (also called epidermoid carcinoma), adenocarcinoma, and large cell carcinoma.

Nonsmall cell lung cancer is a common disease. It is usually treated by surgery (taking out the cancer in an operation) or radiation therapy (using high-dose x-rays to kill cancer cells).

Your prognosis (chance of recovery) and choice of treatment depend on the stage of your cancer (whether it is just in the lung or has spread to other places), tumor size, the type of lung cancer, and your general health.

Stage Explanation

Stages of Nonsmall Cell Lung Cancer

Once lung cancer has been found (diagnosis), more tests will be done to find out if the cancer has spread from the lung to other parts of the body (staging). The doctor needs to know the stage to plan treatment. The following stages are used for nonsmall cell lung cancer:

Occult stage
Cancer cells are found in sputum, but no tumor can be found in the lung.

Stage 0
Cancer is only found in a local area and only in a few layers of cells. It has not grown through the top lining of the lung. Another term for this type of lung cancer is carcinoma in situ.

Stage I
The cancer is only in the lung, and normal tissue is around it.

Stage II
Cancer has spread to nearby lymph nodes.

Stage III
Cancer has spread to the chest wall or diaphragm near the lung; or the cancer has spread to the lymph nodes in the area that separates the two lungs (mediastinum); or to the lymph nodes on the other side of the chest or in the neck. Stage III is further divided into stage IIIA (can be operated on) and stage IIIB (cannot be operated on).

Stage IV
Cancer has spread to other parts of the body.

Recurrent
Cancer has come back (recurred) after previous treatment.

Treatment Options Overview

How Nonsmall Cell Lung Cancer Is Treated

Surgery and radiation therapy are used to treat nonsmall cell lung cancer. However, these treatments often do not cure the disease.

If you have lung cancer, you may want to think about taking part in one of the many clinical trials being done to improve treatment. Clinical trials are going on in most parts of the country for all stages of nonsmall cell lung cancer. Talk with your doctor about your treatment choices.

Patients with nonsmall cell lung cancer can be divided into three groups, depending on the stage of the cancer and the treatment that is planned. The first group (stages 0, I, and II) includes patients whose cancers can be taken out by surgery. The operation that takes out only a small part of the lung is called a wedge resection. When a whole section (lobe) of the lung is taken out, the operation is called a lobectomy. When one whole lung is taken out, it is called a pneumonectomy.

Radiation therapy may be used to treat patients in this group who cannot have surgery because they have other medical problems. Like surgery, radiation therapy is called local treatment because it works only on the cells in the area being treated.

The second group of patients has lung cancer that has spread to nearby tissue or to lymph nodes. These patients can be treated with radiation therapy alone or with surgery and radiation.

The third group of patients has lung cancer that has spread to other parts of the body. Radiation therapy may be used to shrink the cancer and to relieve pain.

Chemotherapy (using drugs to kill cancer cells) for nonsmall cell lung cancer is being studied in many clinical trials.

Chemoprevention uses drugs to prevent a second cancer from occurring.

Cryosurgery freezes the tumor and kills it.

Photodynamic therapy uses a certain type of light and a special chemical to kill cancer cells.

Treatment options: Occult nonsmall cell lung cancer
Tests are done to find the main tumor (cancer). Lung cancer that is found at this early stage can be cured by surgery.

Treatment options: Stage 0 nonsmall cell lung cancer

Your treatment may be one of the following:

1. Surgery to cure these very early cancers. However, these patients may get a second lung cancer that may not be able to be taken out by surgery.
2. Photodynamic therapy used internally.

Treatment options: Stage I nonsmall cell lung cancer

Your treatment may be one of the following:

1. Surgery.
2. Radiation therapy (for patients who cannot be operated on).
3. Clinical trials of chemotherapy following surgery.
4. Clinical trials of chemoprevention following other therapy.
5. Clinical trials of photodynamic therapy used internally.

Treatment options: Stage II nonsmall cell lung cancer

Your treatment may be one of the following:

1. Surgery to take out the tumor and lymph nodes.
2. Radiation therapy (for patients who cannot be operated on).
3. Surgery and/or radiation therapy with or without chemotherapy.

Treatment options: Stage III nonsmall cell lung cancer

Stage IIIA nonsmall cell lung cancer

Your treatment may be one of the following:

1. Surgery alone.
2. Surgery and radiation therapy.
3. Radiation therapy alone.
4. Surgery and/or radiation therapy plus chemotherapy.

Stage IIIB nonsmall cell lung cancer

Your treatment may be one of the following:

1. Radiation therapy alone.
2. Chemotherapy plus radiation therapy.
3. Chemotherapy plus radiation therapy followed by surgery.
4. Chemotherapy alone.
5. Cryotherapy plus radiation therapy.

Treatment options: Stage IV nonsmall cell lung cancer

Your treatment may be one of the following:

1. Radiation therapy.
2. Chemotherapy.
3. Chemotherapy and radiation therapy.
4. Other kinds of care to control pain and other problems.

Treatment options: Recurrent nonsmall cell lung cancer

When lung cancer comes back again (recurs), radiation therapy and/or chemotherapy can help to control pain.

To learn more about lung cancer, call the National Cancer Institute's Cancer Information Service at 1-800-4-CANCER (1-800-422-6237). By dialing this toll-free number, you can speak with someone who can answer your questions.

■ Document Source:
National Cancer Institute
Building 31, Room 10A24, 9000 Rockville Pike, Bethesda, MD 20892

PDQ 208/00039
02/01/94

See also: Chemotherapy and You: A Guide to Self-Help During Treatment (page 40); Radiation Therapy and You: A Guide to Self-Help During Treatment (page 56); What Are Clinical Trials All About? A Booklet for Patients with Cancer (page 68); What You Need to Know About Lung Cancer (page 266)

CancerFax from the National Cancer Institute
SMALL CELL LUNG CANCER

DESCRIPTION

What Is Small Cell Lung Cancer?

Small cell lung cancer is a disease in which cancer (malignant) cells are found in the tissues of the lungs. Small cell lung cancer is sometimes called oat cell lung cancer. The lungs are a pair of cone-shaped organs that take up much of the room inside the chest. The lungs bring oxygen into the body and take out carbon dioxide, which is a waste product of the body's cells. Tubes called bronchi make up the inside of the lungs.

There are two kinds of lung cancer based on how the cells look under a microscope: small cell and nonsmall cell. If you have nonsmall cell lung cancer, see the PDQ patient information statement on nonsmall cell lung cancer.

Small cell lung cancer is usually found in people who smoke or who used to smoke cigarettes. Like most cancer, small cell lung cancer is best treated when it is found (diagnosed) early. You should see your doctor if you have any of the following problems: a cough or chest pain that doesn't go away, a wheezing sound in your breathing, shortness of breath, coughing up blood, hoarseness, or swelling in your face and neck.

If you have symptoms, your doctor may want to look into the bronchi through a special instrument, called a bronchoscope, that slides down the throat and into the bronchi. This test, called bronchoscopy, is usually done in the hospital. Before the test, you will be given a local anesthetic (a drug that makes you lose feeling for a short period of time) in the back of your throat. You may feel some pressure, but you usually do not feel pain. Your doctor can take cells from the walls of the bronchi tubes or cut small pieces of tissue to look at under the microscope to see if there are any cancer cells. This is called a biopsy.

Your doctor may also use a needle to remove tissue from a place in the lung that may be hard to reach with the bronchoscope. A cut will be made in your skin and the needle will be put in between your ribs. This is called a needle aspiration biopsy. Your doctor will look at the tissue under the microscope to see if there are any cancer cells. Before the test, you will be given a local anesthetic to keep you from feeling pain.

Your chance of recovery (prognosis) and choice of treatment depend on the stage of your cancer (whether it is just in the lung or has spread to other places) and your general state of health.

Stage Explanation

Stages of Small Cell Lung Cancer

Once small cell lung cancer has been found, more tests will be done to find out if cancer cells have spread from one or both lungs to other parts of the body (staging). Your doctor needs to know the stage of your disease to plan treatment. The following stages are used for small cell lung cancer:

Limited stage
Cancer is found only in one lung and in nearby lymph nodes. (Lymph nodes are small, bean-shaped structures that are found throughout the body. They produce and store infection-fighting cells.)

Extensive stage
Cancer has spread outside of the lung where it began to other tissues in the chest or to other parts of the body.

Recurrent stage
Recurrent disease means that the cancer has come back (recurred) after it has been treated. It may come back in the lungs or in another part of the body.

Treatment Options Overview

How Small Cell Lung Cancer Is Treated

There are treatments for all patients with small cell lung cancer. Three kinds of treatment are used:

surgery (taking out the cancer)
radiation therapy (using high-dose x-rays or other high-energy rays to kill cancer cells)
chemotherapy (using drugs to kill cancer cells).

Chemotherapy is the most common treatment for all stages of small cell lung cancer. Chemotherapy may be taken by pill, or it may be put into the body by a needle in the vein or muscle. Chemotherapy is called a systemic treatment because the drug enters the bloodstream, travels through the body, and can kill cancer cells outside the lungs.

Radiation therapy uses x-rays or other high-energy rays to kill cancer cells and shrink tumors. Radiation therapy for small cell lung cancer usually comes from a machine outside the body (external beam radiation therapy). It may be used to kill cancer cells in the lungs. Radiation therapy may also be used to prevent the cancer from growing in the brain. This is called prophylactic cranial irradiation (PCI). Radiation therapy can be used alone or in addition to surgery and/or chemotherapy.

Surgery may be used if the cancer is found only in one lung and in nearby lymph nodes. Your doctor may take out the cancer in one of the following operations:

- ◆ Wedge resection removes only a small part of the lung.
- ◆ Lobectomy removes an entire section (lobe) of the lung.
- ◆ Pneumonectomy removes the entire lung.

During surgery, your doctor will also take out lymph nodes to see if they contain cancer.

Treatment by Stage

Treatment for small cell lung cancer depends on the stage of the disease, your age, and your overall condition.

You may receive treatment that is considered standard based on its effectiveness in a number of patients in past studies, or you may choose to go into a clinical trial. Most patients are not cured with standard therapy and some standard treatments may have more side effects than are desired. For these reasons, clinical trials are designed to find better ways to treat cancer patients and are based on the most up-to-date information. Clinical trials are going on in most parts of the country for most stages of small cell lung cancer. If you wish to know more about clinical trials, call the Cancer Information Service at 1-800-4-CANCER (1-800-422-6237).

Treatment options: Limited stage small cell lung cancer
Your treatment may be one of the following:
1. Chemotherapy and radiation therapy to the chest with or without radiation therapy to the brain to prevent spread of the cancer (prophylactic cranial irradiation).
2. Chemotherapy with or without prophylactic cranial irradiation.
3. Surgery followed by chemotherapy with or without prophylactic cranial irradiation.

Clinical trials are testing new drugs and new ways of giving all of the above treatments.

Treatment options: Extensive stage small cell lung cancer
Your treatment may be one of the following:
1. Chemotherapy with or without radiation therapy to the brain to prevent spread of the cancer (prophylactic cranial irradiation).
2. Chemotherapy and radiation therapy to the chest with or without prophylactic cranial irradiation.
3. Radiation therapy to places in the body where the cancer has spread, such as the bone or spine, to relieve symptoms.

Clinical trials are testing new drugs and new ways of giving all of the above treatments.

Treatment options: Recurrent small cell lung cancer
Your treatment may be one of the following:
1. Radiation therapy to reduce discomfort.
2. A clinical trial testing new drugs.

To learn more about small cell lung cancer, call the National Cancer Institute's Cancer Information Service at 1-800-4-CANCER (1-800-422-6237). By dialing this toll-free number, you can speak with someone who can answer your questions.

■ **Document Source:**
National Cancer Institute
   Building 31, Room 10A24, 9000 Rockville Pike, Bethesda, MD
     20892
   PDQ 208/00040
   02/01/04

See also: Chemotherapy and You: A Guide to Self-Help During Treatment (page 40); Nonsmall Cell Lung Cancer (page 262); Radiation Therapy and You: A Guide to Self-Help During Treatment (page 56); What Are Clinical Trials All About? A Booklet for Patients with Cancer (page 68); What You Need to Know About Lung Cancer (page 266)

National Institute on Aging Age Page

SMOKING: IT'S NEVER TOO LATE TO STOP

"I've smoked two packs of cigarettes a day for 40 years—what's the use of quitting now?"

At any age there are many reasons to stop smoking. Some of the benefits for older people include:

♦ Reduced risk of cancer and lung disease
♦ Healthier heart and lungs
♦ Improved blood circulation
♦ Better health for nonsmoking family members, particularly children.

Smoking doesn't just cut a few years off the end of each smoker's life—it prematurely kills 390,000 people each year and seriously disables millions of others.

What Smoking Does

Cigarette smoke affects a smoker's lungs and air passages, causing irritation, inflammation, and excess production of mucus. These smoking effects can result in a chronic cough and, in more severe cases, the lung disease known as chronic bronchitis. Long-term lung damage can lead to emphysema, which prevents normal breathing.

Smoking, high blood pressure (HBP), and high blood cholesterol (a fatty substance in the blood) are major factors that contribute to coronary heart disease. A person with HBP or high cholesterol who also smokes has a much greater risk of heart attack than a person who has only one of these risk factors.

When a person stops smoking, the benefits to the heart and circulatory system begin right away. The risk of heart attack, stroke, and other circulatory diseases drops. Circulation of blood to the hands and feet improves. Although quitting smoking won't reverse chronic lung damage, it may slow the disease and help retain existing lung function.

Smoking causes several types of cancer, including those of the lungs, month, larynx, and esophagus. It also plays a role in cancers of the pancreas, kidney, and bladder. A smoker's risk of cancer depends in part on the number of cigarettes smoked, the number of years of smoking, and how deeply the smoke is inhaled. After a smoker quits, the risk of smoking-related cancer begins to decline and within a decade the risk is reduced to that of a nonsmoker.

Smokers have a higher risk than non-smokers of getting influenza, pneumonia, and other respiratory conditions such as colds. Influenza and pneumonia can be life-threatening in older people.

One woman in four over age 60 develops osteoporosis, a bone-thinning disorder that leads to fractures. There is evidence that cigarette smoking may increase the risk of developing this disabling condition.

Passive Smoking

There is growing evidence about the harmful effects of secondhand tobacco smoke on the health of nonsmokers. This should be an especially important concern if the husband or wife of a smoker has asthma, another lung condition, or heart disease. In addition, smoke in the home poses a health hazard for babies and young children. Passive smoking (exposure to another's smoke) by nonsmokers has been linked to a higher incidence of bronchitis, pneumonia, asthma, and inner ear infections in children. This is a good reason for a parent or grandparent to consider quitting or to avoid smoking while in the presence of young children and infants. New studies report that passive smoking increases the nonsmoker's risk for cancer.

How to Stop Smoking

Over 30 million Americans have been able to quit smoking, and recent surveys suggest that this decline in smoking is continuing. By giving up cigarettes, you can be healthier and feel healthier, regardless of how many years or how many cigarettes you have smoked.

There are many ways to stop smoking. No single method works for everyone, so each person must try to find what works best. Many people can stop on their own, but others need help from doctors, clinics, or organized groups. Some studies have found that older people who take part in programs to stop smoking have higher success rates than younger ones do.

Withdrawal symptoms reported by some people who quit smoking include anxiety, restlessness, drowsiness, difficulty concentrating, and digestive problems. Some people have no withdrawal symptoms at all.

Nicotine chewing gum can be prescribed by a physician to help people who are dependent on nicotine (a substance present in tobacco) overcome withdrawal symptoms. When prescribing the gum, many doctors also recommend joining an organized support group or using self-help materials to assist in quitting smoking. Nicotine chewing gum is not recommended for people who have certain forms of heart disease. Denture wearers may find it difficult to chew.

Where to Get Help

Organizations, doctors, and clinics offering stop-smoking programs are listed in telephone books under "Smokers' Treatment and Information Centers." Further information can be obtained from organizations such as the American Cancer Society, 1599 Clifton Road, Atlanta, GA 30329; the American Heart Association, 7320 Greenville Avenue, Dallas, TX 75231; and the American Lung Association, 1740 Broadway, P.O. Box 596, New York, NY 10019-4374. For all three organizations, consult your local telephone directory for listings of local chapters.

The Office on Smoking and Health collects and distributes information on health risks associated with smoking and methods for quitting. Write to the OSH at 5600 Fishers Lane, Park Building, Room 1-10, Rockville, MD 20857.

You may also contact the Office of Cancer Communications, National Cancer Institute, Bethesda, MD 20892. Or call the Cancer Information Service at (800) 4-CANCER.

The National Institute on Aging offers a variety of information on health and aging. Write to the NIA Information Center, P.O. Box 8057, Gaithersburg, MD 20898-8057.

■ Document Source:
U.S. Department of Health and Human Services, Public Health Service
National Institutes of Health
National Institute on Aging
1991

WHAT YOU NEED TO KNOW ABOUT LUNG CANCER

The National Cancer Institute (NCI) has prepared this booklet to help patients and their families better understand and cope with cancer of the lung. We also hope that it will encourage all readers to learn more about this disease. The information presented here—on the symptoms, diagnosis, and treatment of lung cancer and the outlook for lung cancer patients—is intended to add to information supplied by doctors, nurses, and other members of the medical team.

Our knowledge about lung cancer and other types of cancer is increasing rapidly. Research sponsored by the NCI and by other groups has led to better methods of diagnosing and treating cancer, and it offers hope that in the future more patients with lung cancer will be treated successfully.

Throughout this booklet, words that may be new to readers are printed in *italics*. Definitions of these and other terms related to lung cancer are found in the "Medical Terms" section. For some words, a simple, "sounds-like" spelling is also given.

Other NCI publications about cancer, its treatment, and living with the disease are listed at the back of this booklet along with the toll-free telephone numbers for the NCI-supported Cancer Information Service (CIS). The CIS can provide information about cancer and cancer-related resources to patients, their families, and the general public.

The Lungs

The lungs, a major part of the respiratory system, are a pair of cone-shaped organs made up of pinkish-gray, spongy tissue. They occupy most of the chest cavity and are separated from each other by the *mediastinum,* which is an area in the chest containing the heart, trachea (windpipe), esophagus, and *lymph nodes.* The right lung has three sections, called *lobes,* and is a little larger than the left lung, which has only two lobes. The lungs exchange gases between the body and the air. They remove carbon dioxide, a waste product of the body's cells, and take in oxygen, which is necessary for cells to live and carry out normal activities.

Air enters the body through the nose and mouth and travels down the throat, through the larynx (voice box), and into the lungs through tubes called *bronchi.* One bronchus goes to the right lung and one to the left lung. The bronchi divide into smaller and smaller tubes called *bronchioles,* which end in tiny air sacs called *alveoli.*

What Is Cancer?

Cancer is a group of diseases. There are more than 100 different types of cancer, but they all have one thing in common—the abnormal growth of cells that destroy body tissue rather than build and repair it.

Healthy cells that make up the body's tissues grow, divide, and replace themselves in an orderly manner. This process keeps the body in good repair. Sometimes, however, normal cells lose the ability to limit and direct their growth. They divide and grow without any order and form tumors. Tumors can be one of two types:

- ♦ Tumors that are not cancers are called *benign.* They do not spread to other parts of the body and are seldom a threat to life. Often, benign tumors can be removed by surgery, and they are not likely to return.
- ♦ Cancerous tumors are called *malignant.* They invade and destroy nearby healthy tissues and organs. Cancers can also *metastasize,* or spread, to other parts of the body causing new tumors.

Because cancer can grow and spread, it is important for the doctor to find out as early as possible if a tumor is present and whether it is benign or malignant. As soon as a diagnosis of cancer is made, the doctor can begin treatment to control the disease.

Types of Lung Cancer

Lung cancers are generally divided into two types: *small cell lung cancer* and *nonsmall cell lung cancer*. The tumor cells of each type grow and spread differently, and they are treated differently.

Small cell lung cancer is sometimes called *oat cell cancer* because the cancer cells look like oats when they are viewed under a microscope. This type of lung cancer makes up about 20 to 25 percent of all cases. It is a rapidly growing cancer that spreads very early to other organs. It is generally found in people who are heavy smokers.

There are three main kinds of nonsmall cell lung cancer, and they are named for the type of cells found in the cancer.

- ♦ Epidermoid carcinoma, which is also called *squamous cell carcinoma,* makes up about 33 percent of all lung cancer cases. (*Carcinoma* is a cancer that begins in the lining or covering tissues of an organ.) This type of lung cancer often begins in the bronchi and may remain in the chest without spreading for longer periods than the other types. It is the most common type of lung cancer.

♦ *Adebicarcinoma* accounts for about 25 percent of all lung cancers. It often grows along the outer edges of the lungs and under the tissue lining the bronchi.

♦ *Large cell carcinomas* make up about 16 percent of all lung cancer cases. These cancers are found most often in the smaller bronchi.

More information about the types of lung cancers can be found in the NCI publication *Research Report: Lung Cancer.*

Symptoms

Lung cancer may cause a number of symptoms. A cough is one of the more common symptoms and is likely to occur when a tumor grows and blocks an air passage. Another symptom is chest pain, which feels like a constant ache that may or may not be related to coughing. Other symptoms may include shortness of breath, repeated pneumonia or bronchitis, coughing up blood, hoarseness, or swelling of the neck and face.

In addition, there may be symptoms that do not seem to be at all related to the lungs. These may be caused by the spread of lung cancer to other parts of the body. Depending on which organs are affected, symptoms can include headache, weakness, pain, bone fractures, bleeding, or blood clots.

Sometimes symptoms may be caused by hormones that are produced by lung cancer cells. For example, certain lung cancer cells produce a hormone that causes a sharp drop in the level of salt (sodium) in the body. A decrease in sodium level can produce many symptoms, including confusion and sometimes even coma. Like all cancers, lung cancer can also cause fatigue, loss of appetite, and loss of weight.

These symptoms may be caused by a number of problems. They are not a sure sign of cancer. However, it is important to see a doctor if any of these symptoms lasts as long as 2 weeks. Any illness should be diagnosed and treated as early as possible, and this is especially true for cancers.

Diagnosing Lung Cancer

If lung cancer is suspected, a patient undergoes a series of tests to confirm whether cancer is present. Once cancer is diagnosed, doctors do more tests to learn if the disease has spread. This process is called staging.

When symptoms suggest that there might be cancer growing in the lungs, the first step for all patients is a complete physical examination. This includes telling about any health problems, work history, and anything else that might be important in learning the cause of the symptoms. The physical examination is usually followed by chest x-rays. Next, the doctor may want to collect cells from the lungs so that they can be examined under a microscope. This is important because it is the only sure way to know if cancer is present and, if it is, to identify the type of lung cancer. Doctors may collect cells by *biopsy* using a needle, surgery, or other methods.

In addition to chest x-rays, the patient may have other x-ray tests. For example, a lung tomogram is a series of x-rays of sections of the lung. In computed tomography (*CT* or *CAT scans),* a computer helps produce the pictures. The CT scan is useful in finding out if the tumor has spread from the lung to other parts of the chest or to more distant organs such as the brain or liver.

A test called *bronchoscopy* permits the doctor to see the breathing passages through a thin, hollow, lighted tube. The tube is inserted through the patient's nose or mouth into the lung. The doctor can collect cells from the bronchial walls or snip small pieces of tissue for study under the microscope. This test generally is done in a hospital. The patient, who is given a local anesthetic and is awake during the test, usually can go home a few hours later.

A new procedure, used to collect cells that are hard to reach with the bronchoscope, is called needle aspiration biopsy guided by *fluoroscopy.* Fluoroscopy is an x-ray test that uses a television screen so that internal organs, such as the heart, can be viewed while they are in motion. Using the picture on the screen as a guide, the doctor inserts a needle into the tumor to withdraw cells for examination.

The doctor may use a test called *mediastinoscopy* to learn if cancer cells have spread to lymph nodes in the mediastinum. This test requires an incision in the chest, so the patient is given a general anesthetic. *Mediastinotomy* is similar to mediastinoscopy, except the incision is made in another part of the chest.

Doctors also may perform *scans* to locate lung cancer cells that may have spread to the brain, bone, or liver. In these tests, a substance that is mildly radioactive is injected into the blood, and a machine then scans the body to measure radiation and detect abnormal areas.

Treating Lung Cancer

Treatment for lung cancer depends on the type of cancer cells, the location of the tumor, and the stage of the cancer (whether it is just in the lungs or it has spread to other organs). After diagnosis and staging, the doctor develops a treatment plan to fit the type and location of the cancer as well as the patient's medical history and general health.

Treatment Planning

Before starting treatment, the patient might want a second doctor to review the diagnosis and treatment plan. If so, there are a number of ways to get a second opinion:

♦ The doctor can discuss a patient's case with other physicians who treat lung cancer. Names of these doctors are available from PDQ (Physician Data Query). This NCI computerized system also contains up-to-date treatment information for more than 80 different types of cancer. (Information about PDQ is found at the end of this booklet.)

♦ Patients can get the names of doctors to consult about their treatment plan from the local medical society, nearby medical schools, or the *Directory of Medical Specialists,* a book available in many libraries.

♦ The Cancer Information Service, whose telephone number is listed at the back of this booklet, also may be able to help patients locate doctors to consult for a second opinion.

Treating Lung Cancer

There are three basic ways to treat lung cancer: surgery, *radiation therapy,* and *chemotherapy.* The type of surgery that the doctor recommends depends on the size and location of the tumor. Radiation therapy (also called x-ray therapy, radio-therapy, or irradiation) uses high-energy rays to kill cancer cells. The use of anticancer drugs to treat cancer is called chemotherapy. Sometimes, a combination of these methods is used.

Treating Small Cell Lung Cancer

Small cell lung cancer spreads quickly to distant parts of the body. Often these second tumors cannot be found by routine tests. Thus, treatment with surgery or radiation therapy to the chest usually is not effective in controlling small cell lung cancer.

Patients with small cell lung cancer are commonly treated with a combination of several anticancer drugs or with anticancer drugs plus radiation to the chest. The radiation is directed to the original (primary) tumor in the lungs, while chemotherapy is used to reach tumors in other parts of the body.

Treating Nonsmall Cell Lung Cancer

Patients with nonsmall cell lung cancer generally can be divided into three groups. The first group includes patients whose cancer is only in the lung and whose tumor can be removed by surgery. An operation that removes only a small part of the lung is called a wedge resection. When an entire lobe of the lung is removed, the procedure is called a *lobectomy. Pneumonectomy* is the removal of the entire lung. Radiation therapy may be used to treat patients in this group who cannot have surgery because of other medical problems.

The second group is nonsmall cell lung cancer patients whose cancer has spread to nearby tissue or lymph nodes. The usual treatment for these patients is radiation therapy to the chest. This treatment is sometimes combined with other forms of treatment, especially surgery.

The third group includes patients whose cancer has spread to distant parts of the body. Radiation therapy and chemotherapy are used to shrink the cancer and to relieve symptoms.

Side Effects of Treatment

Because cancer can spread rapidly and threaten life, the treatments used against this disease must be very powerful. It is rarely possible to limit the effects of cancer treatment so that only cancer cells are destroyed; normal, healthy cells may be damaged at the same time. For this reason, many patients experience unpleasant side effects while they are having cancer treatments. Doctors try to plan treatments to keep such side effects to a minimum. Most side effects end soon after treatment.

Certain problems can occur following surgery to remove cancer in the lungs. For example, blood loss during an operation on the chest may be greater than blood loss during other types of surgery. Other complications are caused by damage

to or removal of lung tissue. In such cases, patients may have difficulty breathing and sometimes can become drowsy.

Radiation at high levels destroys the ability of cells to grow and divide. Both normal cells and cancer cells are affected, but most normal cells are able to recover quickly. Radiation therapy is usually given 5 days a week for several weeks. This schedule helps to protect healthy tissues by spreading out the total dose of radiation and by giving rest breaks so that normal cells can recover. During radiation therapy, the side effects that patients notice most often are unusual tiredness, painful swallowing, and skin reactions in the area being treated.

Drugs used to treat cancer are given to patients in different ways: some are given by mouth; others are injected into a muscle, a vein, or an artery. The anticancer drugs travel through the bloodstream to almost every part of the body, helping to stop the growth of cancer cells. Chemotherapy is most often given in cycles—a treatment period, followed by an "off" or "rest" period, then another treatment period, and so on.

Depending on which drugs the doctor orders, the patient may need to stay in the hospital for a few days so that the drugs' effects on the body can be watched. Sometimes, the patient may receive treatments as an outpatient at the hospital, at the doctor's office, or at home.

Chemotherapy affects not only cancer cells but also other rapidly growing cells, such as blood cells, hair cells, and cells that line the digestive tract. As a result, the patient may have side effects such as anemia, an increased risk of infection or bleeding, hair loss, nausea, and vomiting. Fatigue also may occur during treatment with anticancer drugs.

Loss of appetite can be a serious problem for cancer patients. Researchers are learning that patients who eat well are better able to stand the side effects of treatment. Therefore, nutrition is an important part of the treatment plan. Eating well means getting enough calories to prevent weight loss and having enough protein in the diet to build and repair skin, hair, muscles, and organs. Many patients find that eating several small meals during the day is easier than eating three large meals.

Doctors, nurses, dietitians, and other members of the medical team can provide advice about the side effects that might occur during cancer treatment and how best to deal with them. Further information on cancer treatment and side effects is given in the NCI publications *Radiation Therapy and You, Chemotherapy and You,* and *Eating Hints.*

Adjusting to the Disease

In addition to providing information about lung cancer and its treatment, this booklet was written to help people better understand and be more sensitive to the feelings of lung cancer patients and those who care about them. It is very stressful for a person to learn that he or she has cancer, and it is common for many different and sometimes confusing emotions to appear when cancer is found.

Sometimes, cancer patients and family members may be depressed or angry. At other times, their feelings may vary from hope to despair or from courage to fear. These feelings are normal reactions for people dealing with a disturbing change in their lives. Patients usually are better able to cope with emotional stresses if they can talk openly about their illness and their feelings with family members and friends.

Concerns about treatments, tests, or a hospital stay are common. Talking to doctors, nurses, or others of the health care team can help to ease fear and confusion. Patients can take an active part in decisions about their medical care by asking questions about lung cancer and its treatment. Patients and family members often find it helpful to write down questions as they think of them to ask the doctor. Taking notes during visits to the doctor can help them remember what was talked about. Patients should ask the doctor to repeat or explain more fully anything that is not clear.

Most patients want to know what kind of lung cancer they have, how it can be treated, and how successful the treatment is likely to be. The patient's doctor is the best person to answer these questions. Other questions for the doctor might include:

- ♦ What are the benefits of treatment?
- ♦ What are the risks and side effects of treatment?
- ♦ How often are checkups needed?
- ♦ Is it possible to keep working?
- ♦ What changes in normal activities will be required?
- ♦ How much will the treatment cost?

People being treated for lung cancer may need to change their lifestyle. The ability to work or carry on other activities may be altered—perhaps for a short time, perhaps permanently. The patient's doctor is the best person to give advice about limits on specific activities, but it may be hard for some patients and family members to talk to the doctor about their feelings and other very personal matters. However, sharing these concerns with the doctor often makes it possible for him or her to respond with understanding and useful guidance. In the same way, sharing feelings with family members and friends can open the way for others to show their concern and offer support. In addition, many patients feel better when they can talk with people who are facing problems similar to their own. This kind of help is available through self-help and support groups such as those described in the next section.

For patients and their families who find it hard to talk with others, it may be helpful to seek professional counseling. Also, if emotional problems of the patient or family become severe, it's best to get help from a mental health professional.

Coping with any serious disease can be difficult. Cancer patients and their families can find suggestions about adjusting to their new situation in the NCI booklets *Taking Time, When Cancer Recurs,* and *Advanced Cancer: Living Each Day.* Also, the public library is a good source for books and articles on living with cancer.

Support for Cancer Patients

Adapting to the changes brought about by having lung cancer is easier for both patients and their families when they get good information and support services. Often, the hospital or clinic social service office can suggest agencies that will help with emotional support, financial aid, home care, or transportation. Also, the American Cancer Society (ACS) provides patient services and education. Local offices of the ACS are listed in the telephone book under American Cancer Society, Inc.

Information about other resources and services is available through the Cancer Information Service toll-free telephone numbers, which are listed at the end of this booklet.

What the Future Holds

The outlook for a person with lung cancer depends on the type of cancer, the stage of the disease, and the patient's age, general health, and response to treatment. Researchers are working to find better ways to diagnose and treat lung cancer, and the chances of controlling the disease are improving every day.

Doctors usually talk about "surviving" cancer, or they may use the words "remission" and "disease-free interval" rather than "cure." These terms are used because cancer may show up again at a later time. Patients often try to figure out their own chances of survival from statistics they have heard or read about. It is important to remember that statistics describe an average of many, many people, and no two cancer patients are alike. Only the doctor who cares for a patient knows enough about that person to discuss the course of the disease.

The Promise of Cancer Research

With financial support from the National Cancer Institute, scientists at hundreds of hospitals and medical centers around the country are studying cancer. Other public agencies and private groups are also conducting cancer research. Among the areas that are under study are the cause, prevention, diagnosis, and treatment of lung cancer.

Cause and Prevention of Lung Cancer

Cigarette smoking causes about 85 percent of lung cancer deaths. If the number of smokers could be substantially reduced, thousands of lives could be saved before the end of this century. The NCI's goal is to reduce the percentage of adults and youths who smoke to 15 percent by the year 2000.

About 10 to 20 percent of all cases of lung cancer occur in people who do not smoke. Work-related hazards, air pollution, and other environmental factors may be involved. Workers who are exposed to cancer-causing substances, such as asbestos, face an even greater chance of developing lung cancer if they smoke cigarettes.

In addition to many studies on the health hazards caused by the use of tobacco, the NCI is supporting research in the area of chemoprevention of lung cancer. Chemoprevention is the use of natural and manmade substances to prevent cancer. One goal of this research is to find ways to stop or reverse the development of cancer in people already exposed to known cancer-causing substances, such as those found in cigarette smoke.

Diagnosis

A new technique known as magnetic resonance imaging (MRI) produces images of the organs inside the body without exposing the person to radiation. Scientists are studying MRI to learn if it may prove useful in diagnosing and staging lung cancer.

Treatment

The NCI is supporting studies of new treatments for lung cancer, including drug combinations and *immunotherapy,* which uses the body's natural defense system to fight disease. Scientists will study these methods closely to learn whether they can be of value in future treatment.

When research on animals shows that a new treatment method has promise for use against cancer in people, the method is then studied in a clinical trial. A clinical trial is conducted with cancer patients and is designed to answer scientific questions and to find out if a promising new treatment is safe and effective. More information about clinical trials is found in the NCI booklet *What Are Clinical Trials All About?*

The NCI has developed the PDQ database to help doctors across the country learn about these trials. A doctor may obtain information from PDQ by using an office computer or the services of a medical library. Most Cancer Information Service offices provide a physician with one free PDQ search and can tell doctors how to obtain regular access to the database. More information about current research is available through the Cancer Information Service.

Medical Terms

Adenocarcinoma (AD-eh-no-kar-si-NO-mah). A cancer that develops in the lining or inner surface of an organ.

Alveoli (al-VEE-o-li). Tiny air sacs at the end of the bronchioles.

Benign tumor (bee-NINE). A growth that is not a cancer and does not spread to other parts of the body.

Biopsy (BY-op-see). Removal of a sample of tissue to see if cancer cells are present.

Bronchi (BRON-ki). The large air tubes leading to the lungs.

Bronchioles (BRON-kee-ols). The tiny branches of air tubes in the lungs.

Bronchoscopy (bron-KOS-ko-pee). A test that permits the doctor to see the breathing passages through a hollow, lighted tube.

Cancer. A general term for more than 100 diseases that are characterized by uncontrolled, abnormal growth of cells. Cancer cells can spread through the blood and lymph (the clear fluid that bathes body cells) to start new cancers in other parts of the body.

Carcinoma (kar-sin-O-mah). Cancer that begins in the lining or covering tissues of an organ.

CAT or CT scan. An x-ray procedure that uses a computer to produce a detailed picture of a section of the body.

Chemotherapy (kee-mo-THER-a-pee). Treatment with anticancer drugs.

Epidermoid carcinoma (ep-i-DER-moid). The most common type of lung cancer; also called squamous cell carcinoma.

Fiberoptic bronchoscope. A thin, flexible instrument used to view the air passages of the lung.

Fluoroscopy (floor-OS-ko-pee). An x-ray test that makes it possible to see internal organs in motion.

Immunotherapy (IM-myoo-no-THER-uh-pee). Treatment that uses the body's immune defense system to fight cancer.

Large cell carcinoma. A type of lung cancer in which the cells are large and do not resemble the cells of other types of lung cancer.

Lobe. A portion of the lung.

Lobectomy (lo-BEK-to-mee). An operation that removes an entire lobe of the lung.

Lymph nodes (limf). Bean-shaped structures located throughout the body. Nodes act as filters, collecting bacteria or cancer cells that may travel through the lymphatic system.

Lymphatic system (lim-FAT-ik). The lymphoid organs (such as the lymph nodes, spleen, and thymus) that produce and store infection-fighting cells and the network of channels carrying lymph (the almost colorless fluid that bathes body cells).

Malignant (me-LIG-nant). Cancerous (see Cancer).

Mediastinoscopy (mee-dee-ah-steh-NOS-ko-pee) and *Mediastinotomy* (mee-dee-ah-steh-NOT-o-mee). Procedures that permit the doctor to view the organs in the mediastinum.

Mediastinum (mee-dee-ah-STY-num). The area that separates the lungs from each other. It contains the heart and its large veins and arteries, the trachea (wind-pipe), the esophagus, the thymus gland, and lymph nodes.

Metastasis (meh-TAS-ta-sis). The spread of cancer from one part of the body to another. Cells in the new cancer are like those in the original tumor.

Mucous membrane. The tissue lining the inside of the lungs and several other organs.

Mucus. A thick fluid produced by the inner lining of some organs of the body.

Nonsmall cell carcinoma. Epidermoid carcinoma, adenocarcinoma, and large cell carcinoma are grouped under this general classification.

Oat cell cancer. Lung cancer whose cells look like oats when they are viewed under the microscope; also called small cell lung cancer.

Oncologist (on-KOL-o-jist). A doctor who is a specialist in treating cancers.

Paraneoplastic syndrome (pa-ra-nee-o-PLAS-tic). A group of symptoms caused by hormones produced by some lung cancer cells.

Pneumonectomy (nu-mo-NEK-to-mee). An operation that removes the right or left lung.

Radiation therapy. Treatment with high-energy radiation from x-rays or other sources of radiation.

Scan. A test using a radioactive substance to locate tumors.

Small cell carcinoma. A type of lung cancer in which the cells are small and round; also called oat cell carcinoma.

Sputum. Mucus from the bronchial tubes.

Squamous cell carcinoma (SKWA-mus). The most common type of lung cancer; also called epidermoid carcinoma.

Thoracotomy (thor-ah-KOT-o-mee). An operation in which an incision is made into the chest and the lung to look for cancer or other diseases.

Trachea (TRA-kee-ah). Windpipe.

Resources

General information about cancer is widely available. Some of the resources and publications listed below may be helpful to patients and their families.

Cancer Information Service

The Cancer Information Service of the National Cancer Institute is a telephone service that responds to inquiries from cancer patients and their families, health care professionals, and the public. Information specialists in CIS offices are available to provide answers to questions about cancer. The toll-free telephone number of the CIS is 1-800-4-CANCER. Spanish-speaking CIS staff members are also available.

American Cancer Society

1599 Clifton Road, NE
Atlanta, GA 30329
(404) 320-3333

The American Cancer Society (ACS) is a voluntary organization offering a variety of patient services. The ACS also is involved in cancer education and research. Local units are listed in the telephone directory.

American Lung Association

1740 Broadway
New York, NY 10019
(212) 315-8700

The American Lung Association is a voluntary organization interested in the prevention and control of lung disease.

American Red Cross

421 18th Street, NW
Washington, DC 20006
(202) 737-8300

The American Red Cross is a network of local chapters that provides various community services including nursing health programs.

For Further Information

The following printed materials may be helpful to cancer patients, their families, and others. They are available free of charge from:

Office of Cancer Communications
National Cancer Institute
Building 31, Room 10A24
Bethesda, MD 20892

- ◆ *Advanced Cancer: Living Each Day*
- ◆ *Answers to Your Questions About Metastatic Cancer*
- ◆ *Chemotherapy and You: A Guide to Self-Help During Treatment*
- ◆ *Eating Hints: Recipes and Tips for Better Nutrition During Cancer Treatment*
- ◆ *Radiation Therapy and You: A Guide to Self-Help During Treatment*
- ◆ *Research Report: Lung Cancer*
- ◆ *Taking Time: Support for People with Cancer and the People Who Care About Them*
- ◆ *What Are Clinical Trials All About?*
- ◆ *When Cancer Recurs: Meeting the Challenge Again*

■ **Document Source:**
U.S. Department of Health and Human Services, Public Health Service
National Institutes of Health
National Cancer Institute
NIH Publication No. 91-1553
Revised August 1987. Reprinted October 1990

See also: Chemotherapy and You: A Guide to Self-Help During Treatment (page 40); Nonsmall Cell Lung Cancer (page 262); Radiation Therapy and You: A Guide to Self-Help During Treatment (page 56); Small Cell Lung Cancer (page 263); What Are Clinical Trials All About? A Booklet for Patients with Cancer (page 68); When Cancer Recurs: Meeting the Challenge Again (page 74)

MENTAL AND EMOTIONAL HEALTH

■ ■ ■

BIPOLAR DISORDER: MANIC-DEPRESSIVE ILLNESS

Bipolar disorder (also called manic-depressive illness) is a mental illness involving episodes of serious mania and depression. The person's mood usually swings from overly "high" and irritable to sad and hopeless and then back again, with periods of normal mood in between.

Bipolar disorder typically begins in adolescence or early adulthood and continues throughout life. It is often not recognized as an illness, and people who have it may suffer needlessly for years or even decades.

Effective treatments are available that greatly alleviate the suffering caused by bipolar disorder and can usually prevent its devastating complications [which] include marital break-ups, job loss, alcohol and drug abuse, and suicide.

Here are some facts about bipolar disorder.

Awareness

Bipolar disorder has a devastating impact on many people.

- Almost 2 million Americans suffer from bipolar disorder.
- For those afflicted with the illness, it is extremely distressing and disruptive.
- Like other serious illnesses, bipolar disorder is also hard on spouses, family members, friends, and employers.
- Family members of people with bipolar disorder often have to cope with serious behavioral problems (such as wild spending sprees) and the lasting consequences of these behaviors.
- Bipolar disorder tends to run in families, and is believed to be inherited in many cases. Progress has been made in identifying a specific genetic defect associated with the disease.

D/ART: A National Educational Program

The National Institute of Mental Health (NIMH) has launched the Depression/Awareness, Recognition and Treatment (D/ART) campaign to help people:

- recognize the symptoms of depressive disorders, including bipolar disorder.
- obtain an accurate diagnosis.
- obtain effective treatments.

D/ART also:

- encourages and trains health care professionals to recognize the signs of bipolar disorder and utilize the most up-to-date treatment approaches.
- organizes citizens' advocacy groups to extend the D/ART program.
- works with business and industry to improve recognition, treatment, and insurance coverage for depressive disorders.

Recognition

Bipolar disorder involves cycles of mania and depression.

Signs and symptoms of mania include:

- excessive "high" or euphoric feelings.
- a sustained period of behavior that is different from usual.
- increased energy, activity, restlessness, racing thoughts, and rapid talking.
- decreased need for sleep.
- unrealistic beliefs in one's abilities and powers.
- extreme irritability and distractibility.
- uncharacteristically poor judgment.
- increased sexual drive.
- abuse of drugs, particularly cocaine, alcohol, and sleeping medications.
- obnoxious, provocative, or intrusive behavior.
- denial that anything is wrong.

Signs and symptoms of depression include:

- persistent sad, anxious, or empty mood.
- feelings of hopelessness or pessimism.
- feelings of guilt, worthlessness, or helplessness.
- loss of interest or pleasure in ordinary activities, including sex.
- decreased energy, a feeling of fatigue or of being "slowed down."
- difficulty concentrating, remembering, making decisions.

- restlessness or irritability.
- sleep disturbances.
- loss of appetite and weight, or weight gain.
- chronic pain or other persistent bodily symptoms that are not caused by physical disease.
- thoughts of death or suicide; suicide attempts.

Some people with untreated bipolar disorder have repeated depressions and only an occasional episode of mania. In others, mania or hypomania (a mild form of mania) may be the main symptom and depression may occur only infrequently.

Symptoms of mania and depression may be mixed together in a single episode of bipolar disorder.

Recognition of the disorder is essential so that the person who has it can obtain effective treatment and avoid the harmful consequences of the disease, which include destruction of personal relationships, loss of employment, and suicide.

- An early sign of bipolar disorder may be hypomania—a state in which the person shows a high level of energy, excessive moodiness or irritability, and impulsive or reckless behavior.
- Hypomania may feel good to the person who experiences it. Thus, even when family and friends learn to recognize the mood swings, the individual often will deny that anything is wrong.
- Also in its early stages, bipolar disorder may masquerade as some problem other than mental illness. For example, it may first appear as alcohol or drug abuse, or poor school or work performance.
- If left untreated, bipolar disorder tends to worsen, and the person experiences episodes of full-fledged mania and clinical depression.

Treatment

Most people with bipolar disorder can be helped with treatment.

- Almost all people with bipolar disorder—even those with the most severe forms—can obtain substantial relief from their symptoms.
- One medication, lithium, is usually very effective in controlling mania and preventing the recurrence of both manic and depressive episodes. Other medications are also available and may be of significant value.
- For the treatment of depression, several effective medications are available.
- Electroconvulsive therapy (electroshock) is often helpful in the treatment of severe depression that does not respond to medications.
- Psychotherapy may be very helpful in providing support, education, and guidance to the patient and his or her family.

Getting Help

Anyone with bipolar disorder should be under the care of a knowledgeable physician, typically a psychiatrist. The physician should be skilled in the diagnosis and treatment of this disease.

Other mental health professionals, such as psychologists and psychiatric social workers, can assist in providing the patient and his or her family with additional approaches to treatment.

Help can be found at:

- university- or medical school-affiliated programs.
- hospital departments of psychiatry.
- private psychiatric offices and clinics.
- health maintenance organizations.
- offices of family physicians, internists, and pediatricians.

People with bipolar disorder often need help to get help.

- Often people with bipolar disorder do not recognize how impaired they are or blame their problems on some cause other than mental illness.
- People with bipolar disorder need encouragement from family and friends to seek treatment.
- Family and friends and the family physician can "propel" the person toward treatment by insisting that something is wrong and that the attention of a mental health professional must be sought.
- Some people need even more help, and must be taken for treatment. If the person is in the midst of a severe episode, he or she may have to be committed to a hospital for his or her own protection and for much-needed treatment.
- Ongoing encouragement and support are needed after the person obtains treatment, because it may take a while to discover what therapeutic regimen is best for that particular patient.
- It is important for patients to understand that bipolar disorder will not go away, and continued compliance with treatment is needed to keep the disease under control.
- Many people receiving treatment also benefit from joining mutual support groups such as those sponsored by the National Alliance for the Mentally Ill (NAMI), the National Depressive and Manic Depressive Association (NDMDA), and the National Mental Health Association.
- Families and friends of people with bipolar disorder can also benefit from mutual support groups such as those sponsored by NAMI and NDMDA.

For Further Information

National Institute of Mental Health
5600 Fishers Ln.
Rockville, MD 20857
(301) 443-4513

National Alliance for the Mentally Ill
1901 N. Fort Myer Dr., Ste. 500
Arlington, VA 22209
(703) 524-7600

National Depressive and Manic Depressive Association
Merchandise Mart, Box 3395
Chicago, IL 60654
(312) 939-2442

National Foundation for Depressive Illness
245 Seventh Ave., 5th Floor
New York, NY 10001
(212) 620-7637 or (800) 248-4344

National Mental Health Association
1201 Prince St.
Alexandria, VA 22314-2971
(703) 684-7722

■ Document Source:
   U.S. Department of Health and Human Services, Public Health Service
   Alcohol, Drug Abuse, and Mental Health Administration
   National Institute of Mental Health

See also: Lithium (page 288)

DEPRESSION IS A TREATABLE ILLNESS: A PATIENT'S GUIDE

Purpose of This Booklet

This booklet talks about major depressive disorder, which is only one form of depressive illness. If you are not sure that you have major depressive disorder, this booklet may help to answer your questions and give you information.

This booklet has two sections:

Section 1 answers some of the common questions about depression and gives some basic information.

Section 2 gives more detailed information about depression and its treatment.

This is your booklet; use it any way that will help you. You may want to:

◆ Take this booklet with you when you visit your health care provider. Your notes and records can help you get the best possible treatment for your depression.
◆ Share this booklet with a family member or close friend. It can help them to better understand your depression and its treatment.

The information in the booklet is based on evaluation of research studies. Other treatments for depression that are available, while effective for some people, have not been carefully studied.*

Finding Help

Depression is a serious illness, but it can be successfully treated with the help of a health professional. If you think you are depressed, there are many places to get the help you need. You can:

◆ Call your family physician or other health care provider.

◆ Call your local health department, community mental health center, hospital, or clinic. They can help you or tell you where else you can go for help.
◆ Contact a local university medical center (many have special programs for the treatment of depression).
◆ Contact one of the national health groups listed below. They can refer you to a health professional where you live. They can also give you more information about depression, provide you with books and pamphlets, and tell you about support groups.

National Alliance for the Mentally Ill (NAMI)
2101 Wilson Blvd., Ste. 302
Arlington, VA 22201
Toll free: (800) 950-6264

National Depressive and Manic Depressive Association (NDMDA)
730 N. Franklin St., Ste. 501
Chicago, IL 60610
Toll free: (800) 82-NDMDA

National Foundation for Depressive Illness, Inc. (NFDI)
P.O. Box 2257
New York, NY 10116-2257
Toll free: (800) 248-4344

National Mental Health Association (NMHA)
National Mental Health Information Center
1021 Prince St.
Alexandria, VA 23314-2971
Toll free: (800) 969-6642

What You Need to Know

Who Gets Depressed?

Major depressive disorder—often referred to as depression—is a common illness that can affect anyone. About 1 in 20 Americans (over 11 million people) get depressed every year. Depression affects twice as many women as men.

What Is Depression?

Depression is not just "feeling blue" or "down in the dumps." It is more than being sad or feeling grief after a loss. Depression is a medical disorder (just like diabetes, high blood pressure, or heart disease are medical disorders) that day after day affects your thoughts, feelings, physical health, and behaviors.

Depression may be caused by many things, including:

◆ Family history and genetics.
◆ Other general medical illnesses.
◆ Certain medicines.
◆ Drugs or alcohol.
◆ Other psychiatric conditions.

Certain life conditions (such as extreme stress or grief) may bring on a depression or prevent a full recovery. In some people, depression occurs even when life is going well.

Depression is not your fault. It is not a weakness. It is a medical illness. Depression is treatable.

* In this booklet, the word "depression" is used to describe major depressive disorder.

How Will I Know If I Am Depressed?

People who have major depressive disorder have a number of symptoms nearly every day, all day, for at least 2 weeks. These always include at least one of the following:

♦ Loss of interest in things you used to enjoy.
♦ Feeling sad, blue, or down in the dumps.

You may also have at least three of the following symptoms:

♦ Feeling slowed down or restless and unable to sit still.
♦ Feeling worthless or guilty.
♦ Increase or decrease in appetite or weight.
♦ Thoughts of death or suicide.
♦ Problems concentrating, thinking, remembering, or making decisions.
♦ Trouble sleeping or sleeping too much.
♦ Loss of energy or feeling tired all the time.

With depression, there are often other physical or psychological symptoms, including:

♦ Headaches.
♦ Other aches and pains.
♦ Digestive problems.
♦ Sexual problems.
♦ Feeling pessimistic or hopeless.
♦ Feeling anxious or worried.

What Should I Do If I Have These Symptoms?

Too often people do not get help for their depression because they don't recognize the symptoms, have trouble asking for help, blame themselves, or don't know that treatments are available.

Family practitioners, clinics, or health maintenance organizations are often the first places that people go for help. These health care providers will:

♦ Find out if there is a physical cause for your depression.
♦ Treat the depression.
♦ Refer you to a mental health specialist for further evaluation and treatment.

If you do not have a regular health care provider, contact your local health department, community mental health clinic, or hospital. University medical centers also provide treatment for depression.

How Will Treatment Help Me?

Treatment reduces the pain and suffering of depression. Successful treatment removes all of the symptoms of depression and returns you to your normal life. The earlier you get treatment for your depression, the sooner you will begin to feel better. As with other medical illnesses, the longer you have the depression before you seek treatment, the more difficult it can be to treat.

Most people who are treated for depression feel better and return to daily activities in several weeks. Because it takes several weeks for treatment to work fully, it is important to get treatment early before your depression gets worse.

As with any medical condition, you may have to try one or two treatments before finding the best one. It is important not to get discouraged if the first treatment does not work. In almost every case, there is a treatment for the depression that will work for you.

What Types of Treatment Will I Get?

The major treatments for depression are:

♦ Antidepressant medicine.
♦ Psychotherapy.
♦ Antidepressant medicine combined with psychotherapy.

In some cases of depression, other treatments, such as electroconvulsive therapy (ECT) and light therapy, are also useful.

> Thoughts of suicide or death are often a part of depression. If you have these thoughts, tell someone you trust now. Ask them to help you find professional help right away. Once your depression is properly treated, these thoughts will go away.

Who Should See a Mental Health Specialist?

Many people with depression can be successfully treated by their general health care provider. However, some people need specialized treatment because the first treatment does not work, because they need a combination of treatments, or because the depression is severe or it lasts a long time. Many times, a second opinion or consultation is all that is needed. If the mental health specialist provides treatment, it is most often on an outpatient basis (not in the hospital). If you think you need to see a mental health specialist, tell your health care provider, or contact one of the mental health organizations listed in this booklet.

Section 2 of this booklet will tell you more about depression, its diagnosis, and its treatment.

People Who Treat Depression

The following health care providers can treat depression:

♦ General Health Care Provider

Physician—A medical health care provider who has some training in treating mental or psychiatric disorders.

Physician Assistant—An individual with medical training and some training in treating mental or psychiatric disorders.

Nurse Practitioner—A registered nurse (R.N.) with additional nursing training and some training in treating mental or psychiatric disorders.

These health care providers listed above can refer you to one of the health care providers specializing in mental health listed below:

♦ Mental Health Specialists

Psychiatrist—A physician who specializes in the diagnosis and treatment of mental or psychiatric disorders.

Psychologist—A person with a doctoral degree (PhD or PsyD) in psychology and training in counseling, psychotherapy, and psychological testing.

Social Worker—A person with a degree in social work. A social worker with a master's degree often has specialized training in counseling.

Psychiatric Nurse Specialist—A registered nurse (R.N.) usually with a master's degree in psychiatric nursing who specializes in treating mental or psychiatric disorders. *

Symptoms of Depression

When someone is depressed, that person may have several of the symptoms listed below nearly every day, all day, that last at least 2 weeks.

- Loss of interest in things you used to enjoy, including sex.**
- Feeling sad, blue, or down in the dumps.**
- Feeling slowed down or restless and unable to sit still.
- Feeling worthless or guilty.
- Changes in appetite or weight loss or gain.
- Thoughts of death or suicide; suicide attempts.
- Problems concentrating, thinking, remembering, or making decisions.
- Trouble sleeping or sleeping too much.
- Loss of energy or feeling tired all of the time.

Other symptoms include:

- Headaches.
- Other aches and pains.
- Digestive problems.
- Sexual problems.
- Feeling pessimistic or hopeless.
- Being anxious or worried.

If you have had five or more of these symptoms **including at least one of the first two symptoms marked with a asterisk (**)** for at least 2 weeks, you may have major depressive disorder. See your health care provider for diagnosis.

If you have some depressive symptoms, you should also tell your health care provider.

Sometimes a few symptoms can go on to become major depressive disorder. Some forms of depression are mild, but persistent or chronic. Chronic symptoms of depression also need treatment.

Another Form of Depression

Some people with depression have mood cycles. They have terrible "lows" (depression) and inappropriate "highs" (mania) that can last from several days to months. In between the highs and lows, they feel completely normal. This condition is called bipolar disorder or manic-depressive disorder.

Bipolar disorder affects about 1 in 100 people. Just as eye or hair color are inherited, bipolar disorder in most cases is inherited. It can also be caused by other general medical problems, such as head injury or neurologic or other general medical conditions.

You can use this list to learn the systems of mania.

- Feeling unusually "high," euphoric, or irritable.**
- Needing less sleep.
- Talking a lot or feeling that you can't stop talking.
- Being easily distracted.
- Having lots of your ideas go through your head very quickly at one time.
- Doing things that feel good but have bad effects (spending too much money, inappropriate sexual activity, foolish business investments).
- Having feelings of greatness.
- Making lots of plans for activities (at work, school, or socially) or feeling that you have to keep moving.

If you have had four of these symptoms at one time for at least 1 week, **including the first symptom marked with an asterisk (**),** then you may have had a manic episode. Tell your health care provider about the episode. There are effective treatments for this form of depression.

Causes of Depression

Major depressive disorder is not caused by any one factor. It is probably caused by a combination of biological, genetic, psychological, and other factors. Certain life conditions (such as extreme stress or grief) may bring out a natural psychological or biological tendency toward depression. In some people, depression occurs even when life is going well.

Drinking too much alcohol or using drugs can sometimes cause depression. When the drug and alcohol use is stopped, the depression usually goes away. Talk to your health care provider if you have a problem with drugs or alcohol. It can be treated.

> Remember, major depressive disorder is not caused by personal weakness, laziness, or lack of will power. It is a medical illness that can be treated.

Diagnosing Depression

Before depression can be treated, it must be accurately diagnosed. Your health care provider will:

- Ask about your symptoms.
- Ask about your general health.
- Ask about your family history of general medical and mental disorders.
- Give you a physical examination.
- Conduct some basic laboratory tests.

---

* **Note:** In this booklet, the term "health care provider" is used to describe any general health care provider or mental health specialist listed above.

Information About My Health

If you have been working along in this booklet, you already have a record of your symptoms to talk to your health care provider about. Here are some examples of the kinds of things your health care provider will ask you about your health.

1. General medical illnesses that I have now or have had (for example, cancer; arthritis; heart, thyroid, neurologic disease; or other illness).
2. Other depressions or mental illnesses that I have had.
3. Drugs and/or alcohol that I use on a regular basis.
4. Prescription or over-the-counter medicines that I am now taking or take regularly.
5. Allergies that I have to foods, medicines, or other things.
6. General medical illnesses that run in my family (such as diabetes, heart disease, and others).
7. Family history of mental illnesses (such as suicide, manic-depressive illness, hospitalization for mental illness, and neurologic conditions) or a relative who had an "unexplained illness" or stayed in seclusion.
8. Recent changes or stresses that I have had in my life.

Preparing for Your First Visit

You can help your health care provider diagnose and treat you by giving as much information as possible about your health. Information that you share with a health care provider is confidential.

> If your depression is causing you to have a hard time talking and remembering, take a family member or friend along on your first visit to help.

A general medical history, physical examination, and basic laboratory tests can help find out if a general medical disorder is the cause of your depression. About 10 to 15 percent of all depressions are caused by general medical illness (such as thyroid disease, cancers, or neurologic diseases) or medicines. Once the condition is treated or the medicines are changed or adjusted, the depression will usually go away.

If you have a general medical illness and feel depressed, it is important to tell your health care provider. Sometimes depression is a reaction to a life-threatening condition. Getting help during a difficult time in your life may help you to cope with your general medical illness.

If your first episode of major depressive disorder occurred after age 40, a very thorough medical evaluation is important.

Severe? Moderate? Mild?

In the treatment section of this booklet, the terms severe, moderate, and mild depression are used. In general . . .

♦ **Severe depression** is present when a person has nearly all the symptoms of depression, and the depression almost always keeps them from doing their regular day-to-day activities.
♦ **Moderate depression** is present when a person has many symptoms of depression that often keep them from doing things that they need to do.
♦ **Mild depression** is present when a person has some of the symptoms of depression and it takes extra effort to do the things they need to do.

For each type of depression there is a treatment that works best. You should talk with your health care provider about your depression and the best treatment for you.

Treating Depression

Depression is usually treated in two steps.

♦ **First:** Acute treatment.
♦ **Second:** Continuation treatment.

The aim of acute treatment is to remove the symptoms of depression until you feel well. Continuation treatment (continuing the treatment for some time even after you are well) is important because it keeps the episode of depression from coming back. Depending on the type of treatment you have, your chances of staying well for 6 months on continuation treatment are extremely good.

In cases of recurrent depression (three or more episodes), a third step, called maintenance treatment, is used to treat the depression. In maintenance treatment, you stay on the treatment for a longer period of time. The purpose of maintenance treatment is to prevent a recurrence of the depression. With maintenance treatment, the chances of staying well are also extremely good.

Types of Treatment

The major types of treatment for depression are:

♦ Antidepressant medicine.
♦ Psychotherapy.
♦ Antidepressant medicine combined with psychotherapy.
♦ Other treatments, including electroconvulsive therapy (ECT) and light therapy.

For severe depression, research studies show that medicine is very effective. Psychotherapy has not been well studied for the more severe forms of depression.

How Treatment Works

Treatment for depression works gradually over several weeks. With medicine, most people see some benefits by 3 or 4 weeks; with psychotherapy alone, it can sometimes take longer. There is a very good chance that your first treatment will work well for you. If treatment is not effective after a certain amount of time, it can be changed or adjusted. There are other treatments to try, and your chances for effective treatment are still very good.

Choosing a Treatment

You and your health care provider can work together to find the best treatment for you. In choosing which acute treatment is best for you, you should weigh the chances of getting better (benefits) against the chances of possible harms, as well as the expense of the treatment offered and the costs of the depression (time from work, effect on personal relationships, etc.). Here are some questions you may want to ask when discussing treatment.

1. What are the chances of getting better with this treatment?
2. What are the possible risks and side effects of treatment?
3. What are the costs of treatment?

About Hospitalization

Most people with depression get their treatment through regular outpatient visits to a health care provider. However, sometimes treatment in the hospital is needed. This is because other medical conditions could affect your treatment. Another reason is that people with severe depression may need hospital care (for example, to adjust medicine). Also, people who are at great risk for suicide are hospitalized until those feelings pass and treatment begins to work.

If you go to the hospital for treatment, it is often only for a few days or a week or two. Early treatment, before the depression becomes severe or chronic, can lower the chances of hospitalization.

Why Depression Must Be Treated

Without treatment, a major depressive episode can last 6 to 12 months. In between the episodes, most people feel better or are completely well (without symptoms).

Even though some people are able to struggle through an episode of depression without treatment, most find that it is much easier to get some help for their pain and suffering. It is important to get treatment for your depression because:

♦ Early treatment may help to keep the depression from becoming more severe or chronic.
♦ Thoughts of suicide are common in depression, and the risk of suicide is increased when patients are not treated and the depression recurs. When depression is successfully treated, the thoughts of suicide will go away.
♦ Between episodes, about 1 out of 4 people with depression will still have some symptoms and trouble doing their daily activities. These people, if not treated, have a greater chance of having another episode of depression.
♦ Treatment (especially medicines) can prevent recurrences of depression. The more episodes of depression you have had, the greater the chance that you will have another. About half of the people who have had one episode of depression will have a second. Without treatment, after two episodes, the chances of having a third episode (recurrent depression) are even greater. After three episodes, the chances of having a fourth are 90 percent.

If You Have Concerns About Your Treatment . . .

If at any time you are worried about your treatment or you don't think that things are going well, tell someone about your concerns. You can:

♦ Talk to your health care provider.
♦ Ask for a second opinion.
♦ Talk to someone you trust.

Health care providers are interested in your concerns and will help you. This may mean getting a second opinion or even finding another health care provider.

Antidepressant Medicines

There are many different types of antidepressant medicines that can be used to treat depression. Each of these types of medicine work a little differently. Your symptoms, medical history, and family history often give clues about the best medicine for you. Still, it may take some time to find the one that works best for you and has the least side effects. Together, you and your health care provider will find the exact type and amount of medicine that you need.

> Antidepressant medicines are not addictive or habit forming. They work in severe depression and may be useful in mild to moderate depression.

Many people begin to feel the effects of medicine even in the first few weeks of treatment. After about 6 weeks, more than half of the people who begin antidepressant medicine will feel more like their usual self.

At the beginning of treatment, your health care provider will want to see you more often (possibly every week). The purpose of these visits is to check the dosage (how much and how often you take the medicine), to watch for side effects (problems caused by the medicine), and to see how the treatment is working on your depression.

Once you begin to feel better, you probably will visit the health care provider less often. In continuation treatment, you will probably visit your health care provider every month or two. In maintenance treatment, visits are usually every 2 to 3 months.

You will get the most help from your treatment if you do five things:

1. Keep all of your appointments.
2. Ask questions.
3. Take your medicine as your health care provider tells you.
4. Tell your health care provider right away about any side effects you have.
5. Tell your health care provider how the medicine is working.

Keep all of your appointments whether you are feeling better or worse. If you are taking antidepressant medicines, you must keep all of your appointments to check the dosage and watch for side effects. You can copy this record and keep it on your refrigerator door.

Ask questions. Talk to your health care provider if you have concerns about the medicine. The answer to some of your questions may help you and your health care provider to choose the treatment that is best for you personally. Remember: There is no such thing as a "dumb" question when it comes to your health.

My Questions About Medicine

Here are some questions that patients often ask when they are taking medicine.

1. When and how often do I take the medicine?
2. What are the side effects of the medicine? Will I be tired, hungry, thirsty?
3. Are there any foods I should not eat while taking the medicine?
4. Can I have beer, wine, or other alcoholic drinks?
5. Can I take the medicine with other medicines I am taking?
6. What do I do if I forget to take my medicine?

Other questions:

7. How long will I have to take the medicine?
8. What are the chances of getting better with this treatment?
9. How will I know if the medicine is working or not working?
10. What is the cost of the medicine?

Take your medicine as directed, even when you begin to feel better. It is important to continue to take the medicine in order to keep feeling well. You may want to write down the name of the medicine you are taking and keep a weekly record of how and when you should take your medicine.

Tell your health care provider right away about any side effects you have. Even though all medicines have some side effects, not all people get them. Some patients have different side effects than others. With antidepressant medicines, up to half of the people have some side effects early in treatment (in the first 4 to 6 weeks). Side effects are usually not a problem after that. For a small number of people, side effects are bad enough to stop the medicine.

The side effects you might get depend on many things. These are:

♦ The type and amount of medicine you take.
♦ Your body chemistry.
♦ Your age.
♦ Other medicines you take.
♦ Other medical conditions you may have.

If side effects are a problem for you, there are a number of things your health care provider can do. Changes can be made in:

♦ The amount of medicine you take. Sometimes side effects can be lessened by reducing the amount of medicine you take.

♦ The type of medicine you take. Your health care provider may try a different medicine to see if there are fewer or less bothersome side effects.
♦ The time of day you take your medicine. Sometimes side effects can be lessened by taking medicine at night instead of in the morning.
♦ How the medicine is taken. Your health care provider may suggest dividing a single daily dose into smaller amounts to take more than once a day.

> Changing medicine is a complicated medical decision. It is dangerous to make changes in your medicine on your own!

Here are some common side effects of antidepressant medicines:

♦ Dry mouth.
♦ Dizziness.
♦ Constipation.
♦ Skin rash.
♦ Sleepiness.
♦ Trouble sleeping.
♦ Weight gain/loss.
♦ Restlessness.

More serious side effects are rare. As with minor side effects, they usually happen in the first few weeks of treatment. They include difficulty passing urine, heart trouble, sexual problems, seizures, fainting, or other effects. Both the common and rare side effects are nearly always treatable.

If you are having side effects, call your health care provider. Do not wait for the next appointment.

About 1 in 10 people who have a close relative with bipolar disorder can develop manic symptoms in the first few weeks of taking the medicine. Only a very small number (1 or 2 out of 100) of people without a relative with bipolar disorder experience manic symptoms when taking antidepressant medicine. An early sign that manic symptoms may be coming is that you feel that you have a lot of energy or feel very "high" or euphoric. Tell your health care provider about these changes right away.

Tell your health care provider how the medicine is working. One way to know how the medicine is working is to keep a record of your symptoms. If the medicine is not working for you (your symptoms are getting worse or not getting better), your health care provider may recommend a blood test to see whether you are getting the right amount of medicine in your body.

There are many things that can be done if the medicine is not working. These are:

♦ Adjust the dose.
♦ Change the medication.
♦ Add psychotherapy.
♦ Add a medicine.

Feeling Better

Continuation treatment. Once you are feeling better for a while, you and your health care provider will decide if this episode of depression has ended. In most cases, you should continue to take the antidepressant medicine for several months. Research clearly shows that continuation treatment with medicine helps prevent a relapse (return) of the depression episode.

After 4 to 9 months of continuation treatment, if you continue to feel good, you have recovered from this episode of depression. If you have had only a single episode of depression, continuation treatment can be stopped with a good chance that you will remain well. Nearly all patients who are on continuation treatment will stay well during that time.

Maintenance treatment. Some people with depression need maintenance (long-term) treatment. If you have had at least three episodes of depression or if you have bipolar disorder, you will need maintenance treatment to stay well. Research clearly shows that maintenance treatment with medicine prevents a new episode of depression. Some antidepressant medicines have been used by patients for 30 or more years with no bad effects.

Before starting maintenance treatment, you and your health care provider should discuss its costs and benefits.

Psychotherapy

The aim of acute treatment with psychotherapy is to remove all symptoms of depression and return you to your normal life. In psychotherapy, you work with a qualified health care provider (therapist) who listens, talks, and helps you solve your problems. Psychotherapy is usually brief and often has a time limit (for example, 8 to 20 visits).

Types of Psychotherapy

Psychotherapy can be individual (only you and a therapist); it can be group therapy (with a therapist, you, and other people with similar problems); or it can be family or marriage therapy (with a therapist, you, and family members, loved ones, or spouse).

Your health care provider will help you decide if psychotherapy is the right treatment for your depression.

Three psychotherapies have been most well studied for their effectiveness in reducing symptoms of major depressive disorders. They are:

♦ **Behavior therapy**—focuses on current behaviors.
♦ **Cognitive therapy**—focuses on thoughts and beliefs.
♦ **Interpersonal therapy**—focuses on current relationships.

> Psychotherapy alone is not recommended as the only treatment for severe depression or for bipolar (manic-depressive) disorder. Medicine is needed for these types of depression.

Choosing Psychotherapy

If you choose psychotherapy you need to:

♦ Keep your appointments.
♦ Be honest and open.
♦ Try to do the tasks if assigned to you as part of your therapy.
♦ Tell your health care provider how the treatment is working.

The cognitive, behavioral, and interpersonal therapies usually work gradually. Although psychotherapy may begin to work right away, for some people it may take 8 to 10 weeks to show a full effect. More than half of the patients with mild to moderate forms of major depression respond well to psychotherapy.

As with medicine, it is important to remember that people can react differently to similar treatments. While many people find psychotherapy effective, others do not. This usually means that another treatment is needed.

If you do not feel any better at all after 6 weeks, or if you are not completely well by 12 weeks, talk to your health care provider about other treatments.

Continuation psychotherapy. If your depression gets better with psychotherapy, you and your health care provider can decide if your therapy should continue and for how long.

Maintenance psychotherapy. In general, maintenance (long-term) psychotherapy by itself is not recommended unless there are reasons, such as pregnancy or severe side effects, that keep you from taking medicine. While maintenance psychotherapy does not prevent another episode of depression, some research suggests that it can delay a recurrence.

Combining Medicine and Psychotherapy

In combined treatment, medicine is used to treat the symptoms of depression, and psychotherapy is used to help with ways in which depression causes problems in your life. Some people find that combining treatment is very helpful. With combined treatment, more than half of the patients feel better after 6 to 8 weeks. Combined treatment may be most helpful for longer lasting depression, for those with symptoms between episodes, or for those who do not respond fully to medication or psychotherapy alone.

Other Treatments

Electroconvulsive Therapy

Most depressions, even severe depressions, can be treated completely with medicine, psychotherapy, or the combination of both. Electroconvulsive therapy (ECT) works to remove the symptoms of depression. It is mostly used for severely depressed patients who have not responded to antidepressant medicines. It can also be used for patients who are severely depressed and have other severe general medical illnesses. ECT is much safer than in years past. General anesthesia and special muscle relaxing medicines are used to prevent physical harm and pain during the ECT. The choice of ECT as a treatment and the possible side effects should be discussed with a psychiatrist. As with other treatments, the psychiatrist will monitor the ECT treatment and check for side effects.

Light Therapy

In light therapy, a special kind of light called broad-spectrum light is used to give people the effect of having a few extra hours of daylight each day. Specially made light boxes or light visors are used to provide this light. Light therapy may help people who have mild or moderate seasonal depression. This treatment should only be given by a specialist until it has been studied more thoroughly.

Taking Care of Yourself

When you are depressed, it is important to:

♦ Pace yourself. Do not expect to do all of the things you were able to do in the past. Set a schedule that is realistic for you.

♦ Remember that negative thinking (blaming yourself, feeling hopeless, expecting failure, and other such thoughts) is a part of a depression. As the depression lifts, the negative thinking will go away, too.

♦ Avoid making major life decisions during a depression. If you must make a major decision about your life, ask your health care provider or someone you trust to help you.

♦ Avoid drugs and alcohol. Research shows that drinking too much alcohol and use of drugs can cause or worsen a depression. It can also lower the effectiveness of antidepressant medicines or cause dangerous side effects.

♦ Understand that it took time for the depression to develop and it will take time for it to go away.

There is also evidence in milder cases of depression that exercise can be a helpful addition to treatment.

You can get information about other ways to help yourself during treatment from the organizations listed in this booklet. Your public library also has books about depression.

Benefits and Harms of Treatment

The treatments for major depressive disorder discussed in detail in this booklet are:

♦ Antidepressant medicine.
♦ Psychotherapy.
♦ Antidepressant medicine combined with psychotherapy.

How well each of these treatments works depends on the type of depression, how severe the depression is, how long you have been depressed, how you as an individual may react to treatment, and other factors. The risks and benefits described below are based on current medical knowledge using studies of large numbers of depressed patients and expert opinion.

Talking to Others About Depression

When people have major depressive disorder, they often have difficulty at work, school, and with family members. With treatment, almost everyone returns to their normal life.

Some jobs (where the safety of others is involved) require that you report treatment for medical illnesses (including depression). You and your health care provider should talk about how and what to tell your supervisor, teacher, or friends.

Treatment	Antidepressant medicine*	Psychotherapy	Antidepressant medicine* combined with psychotherapy
Chances that treatment will work (benefit)	50 to 65 percent	45 to 60 percent	50 to 65 percent
Chances for immediate side effects or complications (risks)	Minor side effects: 50 percent. Side effects bad enough to stop treatment: 3 to 10 percent.	None.	Minor side effects: 50 percent. Side effects bad enough to stop treatment: 3 to 10 percent.
Chances for medically dangerous harms (risks)	Less than 1 percent (less than 1 in 100).	None.	Less than 1 percent (less than 1 in 100).

*The chances given are for the *first* medicine tried. The chances that a second medicine will work are also very good.

Your Family and Friends

Ask your friends for their support, understanding, and patience during your depression. It may be helpful to talk to your friends about your feelings and treatment and to spend time with friends in social activities. Keep the name and phone number of people that you can talk to and ask to help you. Some people with depression find it difficult to be with others during this time. If you feel this way, do whatever lifts your mood and makes you feel better. If you find yourself alone and unable to be with others, tell your health care provider. Many people find that family members are very supportive and helpful, especially those who have received education about depression.

Your Children

Parents often worry about whether depression is inherited. Most children of people with depression will not get this illness. Overall, research shows that only about 1 in 7 children with one parent who has had several episodes of major depressive disorder or bipolar disorder will develop major depressive disorder. Another 1 in 7 children with one parent who has bipolar disorder will develop bipolar disorder. If you have questions about your child's mental health talk to a health care provider.

Additional Resources

In addition to the organizations listed in this booklet, the National Institute of Mental Health has free publications about depression for persons of all ages, including teenagers and the elderly. Write:

DEPRESSION Awareness, Recognition, and Treatment (D/ART) Program
Department GL, Rm. 10-85
5600 Fishers Lane
Rockville, MD 20857
Toll free: 800-421-4211

For More Information

The information in this booklet was taken from the *Clinical Practice Guideline on Depression in Primary Care, Volumes*

1 and 2. The guideline was developed by a private, non-federal expert panel of physicians, psychologists, psychiatrists, social workers, nurses, counselors, and persons who have depression. The development of the guideline was sponsored by the Agency for Health Care Policy and Research (AHCPR), an agency of the U.S. Public Health Service. Other guidelines on common health problems are being developed and will be released in the near future.

To receive additional copies of this booklet or the depression guidelines call: Toll free: 800-358-9295

or write:

AHCPR Publications Clearinghouse
PO Box 8547
Silver Spring, MD 20907

■ **Document Source:**
  U.S. Department of Health and Human Services, Public Health Service
  Agency for Health Care Policy and Research
  Executive Office Center, 2101 E. Jefferson St., Ste. 501, Rockville, MD 20852
  Publication No. AHCPR 93-0553
  April 1993

See also: Bipolar Disorder: Manic-Depressive Illness (page 272); Lithium (page 288)

DRUG TREATMENT TAMES OBSESSIVE-COMPULSIVE DISORDER

By Evelyn Zamula

In the late 1980s, a number of people appeared on TV shows to talk about a condition that had nearly wrecked their lives: obsessive-compulsive disorder (OCD). They wanted to tell fellow sufferers how they were being helped, even cured, of this distressing disorder by an experimental drug.

At that time, OCD was thought to be comparatively rare. But, surprisingly, in response to the TV programs, thousands of people called or wrote in from all over the country, expressing relief that there were others with the same problem. When Ann Landers ran a column about OCD, she was deluged with 8,000 letters in one week.

If people with OCD didn't know they had a lot of company—maybe as many as 5 million people in the United States—it's because most feel ashamed and try as much as possible to keep their behavior hidden from other people.

And they succeed remarkably well. Sigmund Freud noted that people who have this disorder are adept at concealment because they function well during a part of the day, once they have devoted a number of hours to their "secret doings."

What are the secret doings that Freud speaks of? They are repetitive acts called compulsions, performed to relieve anxiety caused by obsessive thoughts or urges or images. Individuals with OCD realize that these thoughts are senseless and struggle unsuccessfully to resist them. They know that the compulsive actions, or rituals, they perform are also senseless, but feel that if they don't do them, something bad will happen to them or others.

Common Obsessions

The most common obsessions include:

♦ fear of contagion or contamination: "Everything I touch is full of germs."
♦ fear of violent or aggressive actions toward oneself or others: "I'm going to stab my mother."
♦ doubt: "Did I hit that child with my car at that last intersection?"

Other frequent obsessions are concerned with:

♦ orderliness: "I can't go to school until everything in my room is in perfect order."
♦ continual sexual fantasies that dominate thought processes.
♦ thoughts the person considers blasphemous.
♦ repetition of numbers, tunes, words, or sounds.

In response to fears of contagion, the person with OCD goes overboard about cleanliness and is compelled to wash hands or shower for several hours a day. Michael A. Jenike, M.D., of Boston's Massachusetts General Hospital, writes in the Aug. 24, 1989, *New England Journal of Medicine*, that a recent study revealed that 37 percent of the patients who visited a dermatology clinic with nonspecific dermatitis had OCD, though none had sought treatment for it. "Cleaners," as these compulsive washers are called, constitute about 85 percent of those afflicted.

Less familiar are "checkers," who, because they doubt the evidence of their senses, are compelled, for example, to continually check with their mothers to make sure they haven't stabbed them, or repeatedly visit the scene of an imagined accident to be certain they have not run over a child.

"Hoarders" may save every piece of mail they've ever received—every scrap of paper they've picked up on the street, even Christmas trees from years past—for fear that they'll throw out something valuable.

Other compulsions take the form of routines: Some OCD sufferers are compelled to jump over every crack in the sidewalk (shades of childhood), touch ever light pole they pass, or go from the car to the door in a certain way—four steps forward, two steps back, sing one refrain of "Yankee Doodle Dandy," four steps forward, and so forth, to the despair of their families and possible amusement of the neighbors. Such a routine may stretch a 20-second walk to 20 minutes.

Everybody feels obsessive or compulsive at times. These can be positive traits. At their grandest, they may be magnificent obsessions that result in cures for disease or scientific discoveries that benefit all. On a less significant level, they can be an occasional illogical thought, or certain habitual and rigid ways of doing things. Some people must straighten every crooked picture on the walls or they are not comfortable. Others can't rest until every used dish or glass is washed and put away for the night. This is not OCD. The American Psychiatric Association says that the essential feature of OCD is recurrent obsessions or compulsions, or both, sufficiently severe to cause marked distress, be time-consuming (over one hour a day), or significantly interfere with a person's normal routine.

Degrees of Disorder

There are degrees of the disorder. Most people with OCD carry on with their lives, giving in to their compulsions temporarily, usually in the privacy of the home. Others go through phases of OCD behavior with complete remission between episodes. Family members often become involved in the rituals to keep peace in the household, for example, rising from their beds at night to aid the "checker"—for the twentieth time—in seeing that all the doors are locked and all the appliances are off.

For about 10 percent of those affected, the disorder is chronic and disabling. Days, even nights, are consumed by rituals that prevent them from functioning normally, if at all. Many cannot hold down a job, others are afraid to marry, because their rituals would be revealed. OCD people find no pleasure in their rituals, only temporary relief from anxiety. Without treatment, OCD may last a lifetime.

In childhood, boys with OCD outnumber girls by about 3 to 1. OCD may appear as early as 2 years of age as compulsions, though it usually begins in adolescence. Compulsions may take different forms at different ages. Judith L. Rapoport, M.D., author of *The Boy Who Couldn't Stop Washing*, tells of a boy who walked in circles around manhole covers at the age of 2. At 12 he was unable to attend school because of a bizarre compulsion to draw O's.

While diagnosis in children is easy when symptoms are obvious, parents should be alert to more subtle signs, such as too much time spent on homework with no results, frequent erasures on homework or tests, a puzzling increase in laundry and utility bills, stopped-up toilets because of overuse of toilet paper, overlong bedtime rituals, hoarding of useless things, or frequent requests for reassurance.

In adulthood, the disorder is divided almost evenly between men and women, and the average age of onset is about 22. OCD affects people in all ethnic groups and cultures worldwide.

Biochemical Origin?

No one knows exactly what causes OCD, but researchers believe it is biochemical in origin, at least in the most severe cases. About 20 percent of people with OCD have family members who also have the disorder, although different rituals may be practiced by each affected family member.

Researchers have found considerable evidence suggesting abnormalities in functioning of one or more neurotransmitters, chemicals that act as messengers between brain cells. The neurotransmitter thought to be most prominently involved in OCD is serotonin, which plays an important role in the brain in regulating activities such as sleep, mood, aggression, and repetitive behaviors. Investigators using imaging techniques—such as positron emission tomography (PET), x-ray computer tomography (CT), or magnetic resonance imaging (MRI)—have reported abnormalities in the brains of people with OCD, especially in the frontal lobe. Researchers think that overactivity in this part of the brain leads to excessive concern with fastidiousness, order and meticulousness.

Some who suffer from OCD display other neurological symptoms. About 20 percent have tics, such as eye-blinking or facial grimacing. People with Sydenham's chorea (characterized by movements of the face and extremities), epilepsy, and postencephalitic Parkinson's disease may exhibit symptoms of OCD because these conditions involve the same part of the brain. Ten percent of schizophrenics display OCD symptoms.

"OCD is as much an illness as diabetes," says John S. March, M.D., M.Ph., director of the program in child and adolescent anxiety disorders at Duke University. "On the other hand, the concordance rates for OCD between identical twins aren't 100 percent, so there are obviously some environmental factors that play a role as well. People have families and stories and life histories that contribute to whether or not the child with OCD has an easy time of it or a more difficult time. There is a kind of interplay between environmental factors and the biological vulnerability that is required for the disturbance, but it's not treating strep throat with penicillin. Each kid is different."

Several Treatments

Some experts believe that a technique called behavior therapy works better than traditional psychotherapy in treating OCD. The therapist exposes the individual to what is feared, but prevents the usual response, or rituals. Simply explained, someone who cannot bear shaking hands without washing 20 times a day agrees to shake hands with one person, but not to wash afterward. As the treatment progresses, the therapist encourages the patient to do more and more handshaking, also without washing. As the patient realizes nothing bad has happened from being unwashed, anxiety levels diminish and rituals disappear. When successful, treatment goes quickly, with improvement seen in a matter of weeks for 60 to 70 percent of patients.

Help is also available in the form of medication. Anafranil (clomipramine), the drug taken by the OCD sufferer appearing on TV talk shows several years back, was approved by FDA late in 1989 specifically for OCD. Another drug, Prozac (fluoxetine), approved for depression but not for OCD, has been reported to be effective. Both Anafranil and Prozac were developed as antidepressants and appear to increase the availability of serotonin in the brain.

While some patients on Anafranil show improvement in a matter of weeks, it may take as long as three months for the drug to take effect. Side effects include constipation, dry mouth, blurred vision, sexual dysfunction, dizziness, and weight gain. Other drugs being investigated include fluvoxamine, sertraline and paroxetine.

It is not know at this time whether OCD patients will have to remain on drugs indefinitely. Some are so improved that they stop medication after a year or two, gradually reducing the doses. Other patients seem to need medication on a more prolonged basis. A small percentage of patients cannot take either drug because of side effects.

While either behavior therapy or drug therapy can be used alone, some experts report that a combination of the two produces the best outcome. Patricia Perkins, the president of the OCD Foundation, says: "You've got two things going on here. You've got a biochemical imbalance, plus all of these behaviors that are coping mechanisms put in place since childhood to cope with the anxiety that is the real disease. You need behavior therapy to get rid of the habit side. The brain is not O.K., but if for 15 years you haven't touched a doorknob because it's full of germs, someone has to help you touch it the first time to realize that no longer are you going to feel the terrible anxiety you used to feel."

Evelyn Zamula is a freelance writer in Potomac, MD.

More information about the disorder is available from the OCD Foundation, Inc., P.O. Box 9573, New Haven, CT 06535. The telephone number is (203) 772-0565.

■ **Document Source:**
  FDA Consumer
  May 1992

EATING DISORDERS

Each year millions of people in the United States develop serious and sometimes life-threatening eating disorders. The vast majority—more than 90 percent—of those afflicted with eating disorders are adolescent and young adult women. One reason that women in this age group are particularly vulnerable to eating disorders is their tendency to go on strict diets to achieve an "ideal" figure. Researchers have found that such stringent dieting can play a key role in triggering eating disorders.

Approximately 1 percent of adolescent girls develop *anorexia nervosa*, a dangerous condition in which they can literally starve themselves to death. Another 2 to 3 percent of young women develop *bulimia nervosa*, a destructive pattern of excessive overeating followed by vomiting or other "purging" behaviors to control their weight. These eating disorders also occur in men and older women, but much less frequently.

The consequences of eating disorders can be severe, with 1 in 10 leading to death from starvation, cardiac arrest, or suicide. Fortunately, increasing awareness of the dangers of eating disorders—sparked by medical studies and extensive media coverage of the illness—has led many people to seek help. Nevertheless, some people with eating disorders refuse to admit that they have a problem and do not get treatment. Family members and friends can help recognize the problem and encourage the person to seek treatment.

This brochure provides valuable information to individuals suffering from eating disorders, as well as to family members and friends trying to help someone cope with the illness. The publication describes the symptoms of eating disorders, possible causes, treatment options, and how to take the first steps toward recovery.

Scientists funded by the National Institute of Mental Health (NIMH) are actively studying ways to treat and understand eating disorders. In NIMH-supported research, scientists have found that people with eating disorders who get early treatment have a better chance of full recovery than those who wait years before getting help.

Anorexia Nervosa

People who intentionally starve themselves suffer from an eating disorder called *anorexia nervosa*. The disorder, which usually begins in young people around the time of puberty, involves extreme weight loss—at least 15 percent below the individual's normal body weight. Many people with the disorder look emaciated but are convinced they are overweight. Sometimes they must be hospitalized to prevent starvation.

Deborah developed anorexia nervosa when she was 16. A rather shy, studious teenager, she tried to please everyone. She had an attractive appearance, but was slightly overweight. Like many teenage girls, she was interested in boys but concerned that she wasn't pretty enough to get their attention. When her father jokingly remarked that she would never get a date if she didn't take off some weight, she took him seriously and began to diet relentlessly—never believing she was thin enough even when she became extremely underweight.

Soon after the pounds started dropping off, Deborah's menstrual periods stopped. As anorexia tightened its grip, she became obsessed with dieting and food, and developed strange eating rituals. Every day she weighed all the food she would eat on a kitchen scale, cutting solids into minuscule pieces and precisely measuring liquids. She would then put her daily ration in small containers, lining them up in neat rows. She also exercised compulsively, even after she weakened and became faint. She never took an elevator if she could walk up steps.

No one was able to convince Deborah that she was in danger. Finally, her doctor insisted that she be hospitalized and carefully monitored for treatment of her illness. While in the hospital, she secretly continued her exercise regimen in the bathroom, doing strenuous routines of sit-ups and knee-bends. It took several hospitalizations and a good deal of individual and family outpatient therapy for Deborah to face and solve her problems.

Deborah's case is not unusual. People with anorexia typically starve themselves, even though they suffer terribly from hunger pains. *One of the most frightening aspects of the disorder is that people with anorexia continue to think they are overweight even when they are bone-thin.* For reasons not yet understood, they become terrified of gaining any weight.

Food and weight become obsessions. For some, the compulsiveness shows up in strange eating rituals or the refusal to eat in front of others. It is not uncommon for people with anorexia to collect recipes and prepare gourmet feasts for family and friends, but not partake in the meals themselves. Like Deborah, they may adhere to strict exercise routines to keep off weight. Loss of monthly menstrual periods is typical in women with the disorder. Men with anorexia often become impotent.

Bulimia Nervosa

People with *bulimia nervosa* consume large amounts of food and then rid their bodies of the excess calories by vomiting, abusing laxatives or diuretics, taking enemas, or exercising obsessively. Some use a combination of all these forms of purging. Because many individuals with bulimia "binge and purge" in secret and maintain normal or above average normal body weight, they can often successfully hide their problem from others for years.

> Lisa developed bulimia nervosa at 18. Like Deborah, her strange eating behavior began when she started to diet. She too dieted and exercised to lose weight, but unlike Deborah, she regularly ate huge amounts of food and maintained her normal weight by forcing herself to vomit. Lisa often felt like an emotional powder keg—angry, frightened, and depressed.
>
> Unable to understand her own behavior, she thought no one else would either. She felt isolated and lonely. Typically, when things were not going well, she would be overcome with an uncontrollable desire for sweets. She would eat pounds of candy and cake at a time, and often not stop until she was exhausted or in severe pain. Then, overwhelmed with guilt and disgust, she would make herself vomit.
>
> Her eating habits so embarrassed her that she kept them secret until, depressed by her mounting problems, she attempted suicide. Fortunately, she didn't succeed. While recuperating in the hospital, she was referred to an eating disorders clinic where she became involved in group therapy. There she received medications to treat the illness and the understanding and help she so desperately needed from others who had the same problem.

Family, friends, and physicians may have difficulty detecting bulimia in someone they know. Many individuals with the disorder remain at normal body weight or above because of their frequent binges and purges, which can range from once or twice a week to several times a day. Dieting heavily between episodes of binging and purging is also common. Eventually, half of those with anorexia will develop bulimia.

As with anorexia, bulimia typically begins during adolescence. The condition occurs most often in women but is also found in men. Many individuals with bulimia, ashamed of their strange habits, do not seek help until they reach their thirties or forties. By this time, their eating behavior is deeply ingrained and more difficult to change.

Binge Eating Disorder

An illness that resembles bulimia nervosa is *binge eating disorder*. Like bulimia, the disorder is characterized by episodes of uncontrolled eating or bingeing. However, binge eating disorder differs from bulimia because its sufferers do not purge their bodies of excess food.

Individuals with binge eating disorder feel that they lose control of themselves when eating. They eat large quantities of food and do not stop until they are uncomfortably full. Usually, they have more difficulty losing weight and keeping it off than do people with other serious weight problems.

Most people with the disorder are obese and have a history of weight fluctuations. Binge eating disorder is found in 2 percent of the general population—more often in women than men. Recent research shows that binge eating disorder occurs in about 30 percent of people participating in medically supervised weight control programs.

Medical Complications

Eating disorders have among the highest mortality rates of all mental disorders, killing up to 10 percent of their victims. *Individuals with eating disorders who use drugs to stimulate vomiting, bowel movements, or urination are in the most danger, as this practice increases the risk of heart failure.*

In patients with anorexia, starvation can damage vital organs such as the heart and brain. To protect itself, the body shifts into "slow gear": monthly menstrual periods stop, breathing, pulse, and blood pressure rates drop, and thyroid function slows. Nails and hair become brittle; the skin dries, yellows, and becomes covered with soft hair called lanugo. Excessive thirst contributes to constipation, and reduced body fat leads to lowered body temperature and the inability to withstand cold.

Mild anemia, swollen joints, reduced muscle mass, and light-headedness also commonly occur in anorexia. If the disorder becomes severe, patients may lose calcium from their bones, making them brittle and prone to breakage. They may also experience irregular heart rhythms and heart failure. In some patients, the brain shrinks, causing personality changes. Fortunately, this condition can be reversed when normal weight is reestablished.

In NIMH-supported research, scientists have found that many patients with anorexia also suffer from other psychiatric illnesses. While the majority have co-occurring clinical depression, others suffer from anxiety, personality or substance abuse disorders, and many are at risk for suicide. Obsessive-compulsive disorder (OCD), an illness characterized by repetitive thoughts and behaviors, can also accompany anorexia. Individuals with anorexia are typically compliant in personality but may have sudden outbursts of hostility and anger or become socially withdrawn.

Bulimia nervosa patients—even those of normal weight—can severely damage their bodies by frequent binge eating and purging. In rare instances, binge eating causes the stomach to rupture; purging may result in heart failure due to the loss of vital minerals, such as potassium. Vomiting causes other less deadly, but serious problems—the acid in vomit wears down the outer layer of the teeth and can cause scarring on the backs of hands when fingers are pushed down the throat to induce vomiting. Further, the esophagus becomes inflamed and the glands near the cheeks become swollen. As in anorexia, bulimia may lead to irregular menstrual periods. Interest in sex may also diminish.

Some individuals with bulimia struggle with addictions, including abuse of drugs and alcohol, and compulsive stealing. Like individuals with anorexia, many people with bulimia suffer from clinical depression, anxiety, OCD, and other psychiatric illnesses. These problems, combined with their impulsive tendencies, place them at increased risk for suicidal behavior.

People with binge eating disorder are usually overweight, so they are prone to the serious medical problems associated with obesity, such as high cholesterol, high blood pressure, and diabetes. Obese individuals also have a higher risk for gallbladder disease, heart disease, and some types of cancer. Research at NIMH and elsewhere has shown that individuals with binge eating disorder have high rates of co-occurring psychiatric illnesses—especially depression.

Causes of Eating Disorders

In trying to understand the causes of eating disorders, scientists have studied the personalities, genetics, environments, and biochemistry of people with these illnesses. As is often the case, the more that is learned, the more complex the roots of eating disorders appear.

Personalities

Most people with eating disorders share certain personality traits: low self-esteem, feelings of helplessness, and a fear of becoming fat. In anorexia, bulimia, and binge eating disorder, eating behaviors seem to develop as a way of handling stress and anxieties.

Symptoms	Anorexia Nervosa*	Bulimia Nervosa*	Binge Eating Disorder
Excessive weight loss in relatively short period of time	■		
Continuation of dieting although bone-thin	■		
Dissatisfaction with appearance; belief that body is fat, even though severely underweight	■		
Loss of monthly menstrual periods	■		
Unusual interest in food and development of strange eating rituals	■		
Eating in secret	■	■	
Obsession with exercise	■	■	
Serious depression	■	■	■
Binging—consumption of large amounts of food		■	■
Vomiting or use of drugs to stimulate vomiting, bowel movements, and urination		■	
Binging but no noticeable weight gain		■	
Disappearance into bathroom for long periods of time to induce vomiting		■	
Abuse of drugs or alcohol		■	■

*Some individuals suffer from anorexia and bulimia and have symptoms of both disorders.

People with anorexia tend to be "too good to be true." They rarely disobey, keep their feelings to themselves, and tend to be perfectionists, good students, and excellent athletes. Some researchers believe that people with anorexia restrict food—particularly carbohydrates—to gain a sense of control in some area of their lives. Having followed the wishes of others for the most part, they have not learned how to cope with the problems typical of adolescence, growing up, and becoming independent. Controlling their weight appears to offer two advantages, at least initially: they can take control of their bodies and gain approval from others. However, it eventually becomes clear to others that they are out-of-control and dangerously thin.

People who develop bulimia and binge eating disorder typically consume huge amounts of food—often junk food—to reduce stress and relieve anxiety. With binge eating, however, comes guilt and depression. Purging can bring relief, but it is only temporary. Individuals with bulimia are also impulsive and more likely to engage in risky behavior such as abuse of alcohol and drugs.

Genetic and Environmental Factors

Eating disorders appear to run in families—with female relatives most often affected. This finding suggests that genetic factors may predispose some people to eating disorders; however, other influences—both behavioral and environmental—may also play a role. One recent study found that mothers who are overly concerned about their daughters' weight and physical attractiveness may put the girls at increased risk of developing an eating disorder. In addition, girls with eating disorders often have fathers and brothers who are overly critical of their weight.

Although most victims of anorexia and bulimia are adolescent and young adult women, these illnesses can also strike men and older women. Anorexia and bulimia are found most often in Caucasians, but these illnesses also affect African Americans and other racial ethnic groups. People pursuing professions or activities that emphasize thinness—like modeling, dancing, gymnastics, wrestling, and long-distance running—are more susceptible to the problem. In contrast to other eating disorders, one-third to one-fourth of all patients with binge eating disorder are men. Preliminary studies also show that the condition occurs equally among African Americans and Caucasians.

Biochemistry

In an attempt to understand eating disorders, scientists have studied the biochemical functions of people with the illnesses. They have focused recently on the neuroendocrine system—a combination of the central nervous and hormonal systems. Through complex but carefully balanced feedback mechanisms, the neuroendocrine system regulates sexual function, physical growth and development, appetite and digestion, sleep, heart and kidney function, emotions, thinking, and memory—in other words, multiple functions of the mind and body. Many of these regulatory mechanisms are seriously disturbed in people with eating disorders.

In the central nervous system—particularly the brain—key chemical messengers known as neurotransmitters control hormone production. Scientists have found that the neurotransmitters *serotonin* and *norepinephrine* function abnormally in people affected by depression. Recently, researchers funded by NIMH have learned that these neurotransmitters are also decreased in acutely ill anorexia and bulimia patients and long-term recovered anorexia patients. Because many people with eating disorders also appear to suffer from depression, some scientists believe that there may be a link between these two disorders. This link is supported by studies showing that antidepressants can be used successfully to treat some people with eating disorders. In fact, new research has suggested that some patients with anorexia may respond well to the antidepressant medication fluoxetine, which affects serotonin function in the body.

People with either anorexia or certain forms of depression also tend to have higher than normal levels of *cortisol*, a brain hormone released in response to stress. Scientists have been able to show that the excess levels of cortisol in both anorexia and depression are caused by a problem that occurs in or near a region of the brain called the hypothalamus.

In addition to connections between depression and eating disorders, scientists have found biochemical similarities between people with eating disorders and obsessive-compulsive disorder (OCD). Just as serotonin levels are known to be abnormal in people with depression and eating disorders, they are also abnormal in patients with OCD. Recently, NIMH researchers have found that many patients with bulimia have obsessive-compulsive behavior as severe as that seen in patients actually diagnosed with OCD. Conversely, patients with OCD frequently have abnormal eating behaviors.

The hormone *vasopressin* is another brain chemical found to be abnormal in people with eating disorders and OCD. NIMH researchers have shown that levels of this hormone are elevated in patients with OCD, anorexia, and bulimia. Normally released in response to physical and possibly emotional stress, vasopressin may contribute to the obsessive behavior seen in some patients with eating disorders.

NIMH-supported investigators are also exploring the role of other brain chemicals in eating behavior. Many are conducting studies in animals to shed some light on human disorders. For example, scientists have found that levels of *neuropeptide Y* and *peptide YY*, recently shown to be elevated in patients with anorexia and bulimia, stimulate eating behavior in laboratory animals. Other investigators have found that *cholecystokinin* (CCK), a hormone known to be low in some women with bulimia, causes laboratory animals to feel full and stop eating. This finding may possibly explain why women with bulimia do not feel satisfied after eating and continue to binge.

Treatment

Eating disorders are most successfully treated when diagnosed early. Unfortunately, even when family members confront the ill person about his or her behavior, or physicians make a diagnosis, individuals with eating disorders may deny that they have a problem. Thus, people with anorexia may not receive medical or psychological attention until they have already become dangerously thin and malnourished. People with bulimia are often normal weight and are able to hide their illness from others for years. Eating disorders in males may be overlooked because anorexia and bulimia are relatively rare in boys and men. Consequently, getting—and keeping—people with these disorders into treatment can be extremely difficult.

In any case, it cannot be overemphasized how important treatment is—the sooner, the better. The longer abnormal eating behaviors persist, the more difficult it is to overcome the disorder and its effects on the body. In some cases, long-term treatment may be required. Families and friends offering support and encouragement can play an important role in the success of the treatment program.

If an eating disorder is suspected, particularly if it involves weight loss, the first step is a complete physical examination to rule out any other illnesses. Once an eating disorder is diagnosed, the clinician must determine whether the patient is in immediate medical danger and requires hospitalization. While most patients can be treated as outpatients, some need hospital care. Conditions warranting hospitalization include excessive and rapid weight loss, serious metabolic disturbances, clinical depression or risk of suicide, severe binge eating and purging, or psychosis.

The complex interaction of emotional and physiological problems in eating disorders calls for a comprehensive treatment plan, involving a variety of experts and approaches. Ideally, the treatment team includes an internist, a nutritionist, an individual psychotherapist, a group and family psychotherapist, and a psychopharmacologist—someone who is knowledgeable about psychoactive medications useful in treating these disorders.

To help those with eating disorders deal with their illness and underlying emotional issues, some form of psychotherapy is usually needed. A psychiatrist, psychologist, or other mental health professional meets with the patient individually and provides ongoing emotional support, while the patient begins to understand and cope with the illness. Group therapy, in which people share their experiences with others who have similar problems, has been especially effective for individuals with bulimia.

Use of individual psychotherapy, family therapy, and cognitive-behavioral therapy—a form of psychotherapy that teaches patients how to change abnormal thoughts and behavior—is often the most productive. Cognitive-behavior therapists focus on changing eating behaviors, usually by rewarding or modeling wanted behavior. These therapists also help patients work to change the distorted and rigid thinking patterns associated with eating disorders.

NIMH-supported scientists have examined the effectiveness of combining psychotherapy and medications. In a recent study of bulimia, researchers found that both intensive group therapy and antidepressant medications, combined or alone, benefited patients. In another study of bulimia, the combined use of cognitive-behavioral therapy and antidepressant medications was most beneficial. The combination treatment was particularly effective in preventing relapse once medications were discontinued. For patients with binge eating disorder, cognitive-behavioral therapy and antidepressive medications may also prove to be useful.

Antidepressant medications commonly used to treat bulimia include desipramine, imipramine, and fluoxetine. For anorexia, preliminary evidence shows that some antidepressant medications may be effective when combined with other forms of treatment. Fluoxetine has also been useful in treating some patients with binge eating disorder. These antidepressants may also treat any co-occurring depression.

The efforts of mental health professionals need to be combined with those of other health professionals to obtain the best treatment. Physicians treat any medical complications, and nutritionists advise on diet and eating regimens. The challenge of treating eating disorders is made more difficult by the metabolic changes associated with them. Just to maintain a stable weight, individuals with anorexia may actually have to consume more calories than some of similar weight and age without an eating disorder.

This information is important for patients and the clinicians who treat them. Consuming calories is exactly what the person with anorexia wishes to avoid, yet must do to regain the weight necessary for recovery. In contrast, some normal weight people with bulimia may gain excess weight if they consume the number of calories required to maintain normal weight in others of similar size and age.

Helping the Person with an Eating Disorder

Treatment can save the life of someone with an eating disorder. Friends, relatives, teachers, and physicians all play an important role in helping the ill person start and stay with a treatment program. Encouragement, caring, and persistence, as well as information about eating disorders and their dangers, may be needed to convince the ill person to get help, stick with treatment, or try again.

Family members and friends can call local hospitals or university medical centers to find out about eating disorder clinics and clinicians experienced in treating these illnesses. For college students, treatment programs may be available in school counseling centers.

Family members and friends should read as much as possible about eating disorders, so they can help the person with the illness understand his or her problem. Many local mental health organizations and the self-help groups listed below provide free literature on eating disorders. Some of these groups also provide treatment program referrals and information on local self-help groups. Once the person gets help, he or she will continue to need lots of understanding and encouragement to stay in treatment.

NIMH continues its search for new and better treatments for eating disorders. Congress has designated the 1990s as the Decade of the Brain, making the prevention, diagnosis, and treatment of all brain and mental disorders a national research priority. This research promises to yield even more hope for patients and their families by providing a greater understanding of the causes and complexities of eating disorders.

For Further Information

For additional information on eating disorders, check local hospitals or university medical centers for an eating disorders clinic, or contact:

National Association of Anorexia Nervosa and Associated Disorders (ANAD)
P.O. Box 7
Highland Park, IL 60035
(708) 831-3438

Anorexia Nervosa and Related Eating Disorders, Inc. (ANRED)
P.O. Box 5102
Eugene, OR 97405
(503) 344-1144

American Anorexia/Bulimia Association, Inc. (AABA)
418 E. 76th St.
New York, NY 10021
(212) 734-1114

Center for the Study of Anorexia and Bulimia
1 W. 91st St.
New York, NY 10024
(212) 595-3449

National Anorexic Aid Society (NAAS)
Harding Hospital
1925 E. Dublin Granville Rd.
Columbus, OH 43229
(614) 436-1112

Foundation for Education about Eating Disorders
P.O. Box 16375
Baltimore, MD 21210
(410) 467-0603

Bulimia Anorexia Self Help, Inc. (BASH)
6125 Clayton Ave., Ste. 215
St. Louis, MO 63139
(314) 567-4080

Overeaters Anonymous
P.O. Box 92870
Los Angeles, CA 90009
(310) 618-8835

For information on other mental disorders, contact:

Information Resources and Inquiries Branch
National Institute of Mental Health
5600 Fishers Ln., Rm. 15C-05
Rockville, MD 20857

This pamphlet was rewritten by Lee Hoffman, Office of Scientific Information (OSI), National Institute of Mental Health (NIMH). An earlier version was prepared by OSI staff member Marilyn Sargent. Scientific review was provided by NIMH staff Susan J. Blumenthal, M.D.; Harry E. Gwirtsman, M.D.; and Susan Z. Yanovski, M.D.

■ Document Source:
   U.S. Department of Health and Human Services, Public Health Service
   National Institutes of Health
   National Institute of Mental Health
   NIH Publication No. 93-3477
   January 1993

LITHIUM

If a doctor has prescribed lithium for you or someone close to you, you may wish to know more about the medication: Is it safe? Will it cause discomfort? Most importantly, will it work? Chances are you've been told that lithium may prevent future bouts of your illness. You can benefit from this remarkable effect only if you continue to take the drug exactly as the doctor prescribes. You may have to take it for long periods of time, perhaps indefinitely. That means lithium is as important to you as insulin is to a diabetic or other kinds of daily medications are to people with high blood pressure. Like a diabetic or hypertensive person, you may question whether you need to continue taking the medication day after day, especially if you feel well. But lithium can save your life as surely as those other drugs save theirs. This pamphlet will help you learn more about lithium.

Lithium: Mineral and Drug

Pure lithium, like sodium, calcium, or potassium, is a naturally occurring mineral. Lithium is found abundantly in certain rocks and the sea and in minute amounts in plant and animal tissues. Lithium also shows up in water, notably in the springs and spas where in earlier times people "took the waters," bathing in and drinking the lithium-rich water for its soothing effects. Whether lithium actually calmed 19th-century ladies and gentlemen has never been documented. What we do know is that, from time to time since antiquity, doctors have noticed that lithium can control overexcitement in some of their patients.

Today, lithium is administered to patients as a lithium salt, usually as lithium carbonate or lithium citrate, which is taken by mouth in capsule, tablet, or syrup form. Pharmaceutical companies often assign a "trade name" to their products. Examples of trade names for lithium are Cibalith, Eskalith, Lithane, and Lithobid.

Some companies use only the chemical name, that is, lithium carbonate or lithium citrate.

Modern physicians rely on these various forms of lithium to treat serious mental illness. Properly administered, it is one of the most powerful medications available for mood disorders.

What Are Mood Disorders?

Patients with mood disorders, also called *affective disorders,* suffer from depression. In contrast to "the blues" that we all go through, a depressive episode is a true illness, often referred to as *clinical depression.* Some patients also experience episodes of *mania*—intense excitement and mental disorganization that usually require immediate hospitalization. Although mania is popularly thought of as a state of excess euphoria, patients report that a depressive mood is as frequent as euphoria during a manic episode, and irritability is the most common symptom.

According to the National Institute of Mental Health (NIMH)—the federal agency that supports research nationwide on the causes, treatment, and prevention of mental illness—depression is one of the most common mental disorders. The latest NIMH surveys indicate that during the course of a year, 5 in every 100 Americans has an episode of clinical depression and another 1.2 percent has an episode of *manic-depressive illness* that might consist of mania, depression, or the combination of both.

Unlike the ups and downs of everyday life, clinical depression envelops a person in a dark cloud of gloom and lethargy. Often, no cause can be found for the extreme sadness—no death or financial setback or ruined romance. Although such losses can trigger a depressive episode, the

sadness and apathy of clinical depression are deeper and go on far longer than is usual when a person grieves a loss. Without treatment, depression can continue for years, but typically it will last from 4 to 12 months.

During a depressive episode, thinking slows down, concentration and memory are impaired, decisions are difficult to make, eating and sleeping habits may become disrupted, and anxiety—sometimes in the form of panic attacks—can add to the individual's overall misery. People with depression usually feel that they have lost their value, that they are no good to anyone. When they also lose all hope of regaining their sense of self-worth, some may come to feel that suicide is the only option left to them. In fact, about one in five individuals with depression will attempt suicide.

In some people, the "lows" of depression more or less alternate with the "highs" of mania. In its early stages, mania may feel much like waking on a sunny day full of energy, good will, and high spirits, with a head full of ideas. These periods of *hypomania*—that is, something less than full-blown mania—pleasurable as they are, can quickly progress to true mania. By the time a person has reached that stage, thoughts are racing so fast that it is impossible to carry through any one idea. Good judgment vanishes. Manic individuals may spend the family into bankruptcy, engage in multiple sexual liaisons, pick fights with the boss, start grandiose projects that have no chance of success, grow angry too quickly, drink far too much, and generally convey the impression that they are not bound by earthly limitations on time, the need for sleep, or consideration of others.

As this strange mix of symptoms implies, depression and mania are part of the same illness, *bipolar disorder,* which is also called *manic-depressive illness.* The mix of depression and mania varies tremendously from one patient to the next, as does the timing of episodes and their duration. Some people may experience both depression and mania at the same time; these are the mixed states that doctors sometimes refer to. Some patients cycle rapidly from one state to the other, sometimes within the course of a day. Some people have episodes of clinical depression alternating with hypomania that never progresses to mania; this form is usually called *bipolar-II* illness. Severe depression that occurs without mania is usually referred to as *unipolar depression, clinical depression, major depression* or, sometimes, the classic term, *melancholia.*

Left untreated, manic-depressive illness nearly always recurs. A first episode in the late teens or early twenties, the typical age of onset, tends to be followed by episodes that get closer and closer and then settle into a somewhat regular pattern of recurrences. Unipolar depression may also recur. In either case, these illnesses rob the patient of years of life. Much of that suffering can be avoided with lithium and other treatments.

Mania and clinical depressions, especially the forms that tend to recur, clearly reflect some malfunction in the brain. Scientists have been able to use new brain imaging technologies to picture such differences. In addition, research on the biochemical aspects of these illnesses suggests that faulty regulation of neurotransmitters, the chemical messengers that help nerve cells to communicate, is involved in depression and mania. Also important are various hormones, especially those that regulate the body's response to stress.

Scientists have learned enough about these processes to realize that, so far, they know only part of the story. They have also developed a profound respect for the complexity of the human brain.

One surprisingly complex aspect of the brain is its capacity to change, to be influenced by the person's experience—losing a parent at a critical age in childhood, for example, or feeling under great pressure at home or work from time to time. Such experiences can produce physical changes in the central nervous system and affect the brain's capacity to regulate mood. In some people, these adverse experiences may trigger the changes that end in clinical illness.

The Development of Lithium Treatment

John Cade, an Australian physician, introduced lithium into psychiatry in 1949 when he reported that lithium carbonate was an effective treatment for manic excitement. Unfortunately, Dr. Cade's discovery coincided with reports of several deaths from the unrestricted use of lithium chloride as a salt substitute for cardiac patients. Four patients died, and several developed toxic reactions. It was not known at that time that lithium can accumulate to dangerous levels in the body or that lithium has to be used with special caution in patients with cardiac disorders.

As a result of these experiences, lithium was virtually neglected in this country until the early 1960s. Research by European psychiatrists, especially Dr. Mogens Schou in Denmark, hastened acceptance of lithium in the United States. Renewed interest in the compound led to numerous clinical trials, including pivotal studies conducted by NIMH. These studies showed how lithium could be used safely and effectively to treat psychiatric disorders.

In addition, research—both in animals and humans—showed that lithium influences several functions in the body, including the distribution of sodium and potassium, which regulate impulses along the nerve cells. Lithium can affect the activity of neurotransmitters and biological systems because it alters the way in which a variety of messages are transmitted after they reach their target. Although scientists have many promising leads, they have yet to explain the biochemical actions of depression.

In 1970, the U.S. Food and Drug Administration (FDA) approved lithium as a treatment for mania. Four years later, the FDA also approved the use of lithium as a preventive, or prophylactic, treatment for manic-depressive illness.

Lithium's Uses

Psychiatrists use lithium in two ways: to treat episodes of mania and depression and to prevent their recurrence. Lithium can often subdue symptoms when a patient is in the midst of a manic episode, and it may also ameliorate the symptoms of a depressive episode. The single most important use for lithium, though, is in preventing new episodes of mania and depression. Lithium is also being used experimentally to treat other disorders.

A Checklist for Patients Taking Lithium

1. Take the medication on a regular basis as prescribed by the doctor. Ask the doctor for instructions on what to do if one or more doses are missed. Unless the doctor advises otherwise, do not catch up on a missed dose by doubling the next dose. This may produce a dangerously high blood level of lithium.
2. Obtain regular blood tests for lithium levels.
3. Have the doctor take blood tests for lithium levels 12 hours after the last dose. Inform the doctor if it has been less than 11 hours or more than 13 hours since the last dose.
4. Inform the doctor if other medications are being taken, since they can change lithium levels.
5. Notify the doctor whenever there is a significant change in weight or diet. It is especially important to tell the doctor if you plan to begin a rapid weight-loss diet, since lithium levels in the body may be drastically affected.
6. Advise the doctor about any changes in frequency of urination, loss of fluids through diarrhea, vomiting, excessive sweating, or physical illness, particularly if there is a fever, because adjustment of dosage or further testing may be required.
7. If planning to become pregnant, advise the doctor.
8. If another doctor is being seen or an operation is planned, be sure to inform that doctor that you are taking lithium.
9. Because it may take time for mood swings to be completely controlled by lithium, try not to get discouraged. Continue taking the medicine as prescribed until advised otherwise by the doctor. However, be sure to notify the doctor of recurrences in mania or depression because it may be necessary to increase the dose or to receive additional medication for a time. Psychotherapy can help you to recognize manic or depressive episodes early in their course, as well as help you to express and understand your feelings about having manic-depressive illness.
10. Ask the doctor any questions about the treatment program or any procedures that you do not understand. A well-informed patient and family are important factors contributing to a successful treatment outcome. Also, if your psychotherapist is someone other than the doctor prescribing the medication, it is important for the two professionals to exchange information about your progress and problems as needed.

Manic and Depressive Episodes

Lithium is highly effective in treating acute episodes of mania, especially when symptoms are mild. Patients going through severe manic episodes need to be calmed as quickly as possible, however, and lithium may take 1 to 3 weeks to achieve its full effect. Therefore, physicians most often treat very disturbed patients by first combining lithium with a different type of drug, a tranquilizer, such as haloperidol or chlorpromazine. When lithium has had a chance to act, the tranquilizer may be gradually withdrawn. Lithium can normalize the manic disorder without causing the drugged feeling that often occurs with tranquilizers. Also, tranquilizers may produce troublesome side effects that limit their usefulness as a long-term treatment.

Lithium is also effective in treating depressive episodes in some patients with manic-depressive illness. For these patients, some doctors prefer to treat mild to moderate depressive episodes with lithium alone because of the possibility that conventional antidepressant drugs such as imipramine may trigger a hypomanic or manic attack. If the depression is severe, treatment is usually begun with a conventional antidepressant in combination with lithium. That same combination is sometimes used in unipolar depressions that do not respond to antidepressant medications alone.

Lithium's Role in Preventing Manic and Depressive Episodes

As noted, lithium's greatest value is in preventing or reducing the occurrence of future episodes of bipolar disorder. The effectiveness of this *lithium prophylaxis* or *lithium prophylactic treatment* has been demonstrated in more than two decades of careful research. In related research, several major studies indicate that lithium can decrease the frequency or severity of new depressive episodes in recurrent unipolar disorder. This suggests that lithium may also have prophylactic value in treating this mood disorder. Conventional antidepressants also have been shown to be effective prophylactic treatments for recurrent unipolar depression.

There are patients who are not helped at all by lithium. About one in ten patients with bipolar disorder who takes lithium does not respond to the medication, but continues to have manic-depressive episodes at the same frequency and severity as before. Doctors cannot predict with certainty how lithium will work in any individual case. This can be determined only by actual use of the medication.

In prophylactic treatment, lithium is administered after a manic or depressive episode to prevent or dampen future attacks. Some patients respond quickly and have no further episodes. Others respond more slowly and continue to have moderate mood swings even months after therapy is started. These highs or lows usually become progressively less severe with continued lithium treatment; often they disappear. With other patients, lithium may not prevent all future manic and depressive episodes, but may reduce or lessen their severity so that the individual can continue to lead a productive life.

When deciding whether a patient should start lithium prophylactic therapy, a psychiatrist or other physician considers the likelihood of a new episode in the near future; the impact that the episode might have on the patient, family, and job; the patient's willingness to commit himself or herself to a long-term treatment program; and the presence of medical conditions that may rule out lithium treatment. Usually, a doctor prescribes lithium prophylactic therapy only after a patient has had two or three well-defined episodes requiring treatment. Patients who have had only a single attack, mild attack, or a long interval between episodes—for example, over 5 years—usually do not receive prophylactic treatment unless the second episode would be life threatening or highly disruptive to the patient's career or family relations.

Such rules, though, serve as only broad guidelines. Patients must act as the doctor's partner in weighing the circumstances and making the decision. Each patient should understand the reasons for lithium prophylaxis as well as the benefits and risks and be an informed participant in the treatment program.

When lithium fails or when a patient has another medical condition that precludes its use, the doctor may consider an alternative prophylactic drug treatment. First, however, he or she will reevaluate why lithium failed: Was dosage adequate? Did the patient take the medication as prescribed? Does the patient have a problem with thyroid function? Many patients with mood disorders have malfunctioning thyroid glands, a problem that can be successfully treated with a thyroid hormone or related preparations without withdrawing lithium.

For manic-depressive patients, the anticonvulsant drugs carbamazepine (trade name Tegretol) and valproate (trade name Depakote) seem to be the best alternatives to lithium. Sometimes the anticonvulsant drugs are given alone, sometimes in combination with lithium, to prevent or dampen future episodes.

Patients with unipolar disorder who fail on lithium often are given an antidepressant drug alone or in combination with lithium. A severe episode may be treated with electroconvulsive therapy. Information on alternatives to lithium treatment can be found in the literature listed at the end of the pamphlet.

Other Disorders

Lithium may also be useful for treating other mental illnesses. Research psychiatrists have evaluated lithium as a treatment for a variety of psychiatric disorders, including schizophrenia, schizoaffective disorder, alcoholism, premenstrual depression, and periodic aggressive and explosive behavior. Lithium appears to produce the best responses in patients who have mood swings, a tendency to have intermittent bouts of illness, or a family history of mood disorder.

Lithium's Side Effects

Most patients do not experience serious side effects when they begin lithium therapy. Initially, the patient may have slight nausea, stomach cramps, diarrhea, thirstiness, muscle weakness, and feelings of being somewhat tired, dazed, or sleepy. A mild hand tremor may emerge as the dose is increased. These effects are normally minimal and usually subside after several days of treatment. But some of the initial side effects may carry over into long-term therapy and others may emerge. Some patients continue to have a slight hand tremor. Many drink more fluids than usual—without always being aware of it—and urinate more frequently, while still others may gain weight. Weight gain often can be controlled with proper diet. Crash diets should be avoided, however, since they may adversely affect lithium levels. Also, to avoid excessive weight gain, excessive amounts of drinks with high sugar content should be avoided.

In patients who have low amounts of thyroid hormone, enlargement of the thyroid gland may develop, but this condition is generally not serious if monitored closely by a physician. It can be successfully treated with supplementary thyroid medication without withdrawing lithium.

Because of physiological changes in kidneys observed in some lithium-treated patients, any past or current kidney disorder or changes in frequency of urination should be reported to the physician. Long-term lithium therapy can also worsen certain skin conditions, especially acne and psoriasis, and may produce edema, or swelling, which is due to accumulation of water in tissues.

Lithium must be taken with care, with attention to taking the proper dose, having regular blood tests, and reporting changes in diet, exercise, and the occurrence of illness. Toxic levels of lithium in the blood can cause vomiting, severe diarrhea, extreme thirst, weight loss, muscle twitching, abnormal muscle movement, slurred speech, blurred vision, dizziness, confusion, stupor, or pulse irregularities. Sudden physical or mental changes should be reported to the doctor immediately. These problems can almost always be avoided when the doctor's instructions are followed carefully.

Periodic Blood Tests

The amount of lithium needed to treat or prevent manic and depressive symptoms effectively differs greatly from one patient to another. The doctor determines how much lithium a patient needs by taking a sample of blood from time to time. The blood is analyzed to determine how much lithium is present. Testing for the lithium blood level is a vital part of treatment with lithium. It aids the doctor in selecting and maintaining the most effective dose. Just as important, lithium blood levels assure the doctor that a patient is not taking a toxic dose—that is, a poisonous dose.

Lithium is an unusual drug because the amount needed to be effective is only slightly less than the amount that is toxic. For that reason, patients must be very careful not to take more lithium than prescribed.

Lithium levels in the blood can change even when the patient takes the same dose every day. The concentration of lithium can increase when a person becomes ill with another medical condition, especially influenza or other illnesses that result in fever or changes in diet and loss of body fluids. Surgery, strenuous exercise, and crash diets are other circumstances that can lead to dangerously increased lithium levels in the blood. The doctor should be informed of illness or changes in eating habits, and a regular blood testing schedule should be set up and followed rigorously.

If a patient stops taking lithium for only one day, the blood level of the drug falls to half that needed for effective therapy. A forgotten dose should not, however, be taken with the regular dose the next day, because it could raise the lithium level too much. Furthermore, the lower lithium level that results from missing one dose is unlikely to jeopardize therapeutic response.

Because the blood level of lithium rises rapidly for a few hours after swallowing a lithium pill and then slowly levels off, having a blood test right after taking the drug can mislead the doctor into thinking that the dose is too high. To gauge the average blood level accurately, it is important to have blood drawn about 12 hours after the last dose of lithium. Otherwise, the results will be misleading and possibly dangerous. Most patients take their nighttime dose of lithium and then come to the doctor's office the next morning to have a blood test before taking their first dose for the day. Some patients are able to take their full daily dose at bedtime and don't have to worry about the morning dose when getting a blood test.

Precautions in Taking Lithium

Lithium is excreted from the body almost entirely by the kidneys. If, for some reason, the kidneys are unable to get rid of the proper amount of lithium, the drug may accumulate to dangerous levels in the body. The excretion of lithium in the kidneys is closely linked to that of sodium. The less sodium, or salt, in the body, the less lithium is excreted, and the greater chance of lithium buildup to toxic levels. Diuretics cause the kidneys to excrete sodium; as a result, lithium levels rise. The reason that many illnesses can increase lithium levels is that increased sweating, fever, a low-salt diet, vomiting, and diarrhea all result in less sodium present in the body, thus producing higher levels.

Lithium should not be taken by patients with severely impaired kidney function. Patients with heart disease and others who have a significant change in sodium in their diet or periodic episodes of heavy sweating should be especially careful to have their lithium blood levels monitored regularly.

For women in the fertile age range, the possibility of harmful effects on the unborn child may pose problems for continued use of lithium. Children of mothers who received lithium during the first 3 months of pregnancy have been reported in some, but not all, studies to have a slightly increased frequency of malformations of the heart and blood vessels. Even though this risk is low and uncertain, it is strongly recommended that women discontinue lithium during the first 3 months of pregnancy. The decision to stop the medication, however, must be weighed against the possible consequences of an untreated manic or depressive attack, which may result in injury, physiological stress, dehydration and malnutrition, sleep deprivation, or possibly even suicide. Because of the risk of postpartum depression or mania, lithium is sometimes restarted during the final weeks before birth is expected. Women should not breast feed when they are taking lithium, except in rare circumstances when the potential benefits to the mother outweigh possible hazards to the child.

Taking Lithium: How Long?

When fully effective, lithium can control manic-depressive illness for the rest of a person's life. But it is not a cure. Like antihypertensive medications for controlling high blood pressure, lithium should not be discontinued without consulting the physician.

Unfortunately, some patients stop taking their lithium when they find that it diminishes the wonderful sense of well-being they felt when hypomanic; most resume taking their medication when disabling manic episodes return.

Other patients discontinue lithium because they feel they no longer need it. Such reasoning is perfectly understandable. When a person remains well week after week, there is a tendency to forget to take lithium or to deliberately stop taking the medication, believing that the illness has been cured. Lithium's effects, however, last only when patients regularly take the medication. If patients stop taking lithium—no matter if they've been taking it for 5 weeks or 5 years—the chances of having another manic or depressive attack increase. In fact, patients who stop taking the medication are just as likely as patients who have never been treated to fall back into a manic or depressive episode.

This does not mean, though, that all patients must take lithium for a lifetime. After a long period of treatment without a recurrence of mania or depression, the doctor and patient may consider withdrawal of medication under close supervision. That decision will depend upon several factors, including the impact that a subsequent episode may have on the patient's marriage or other significant relationships, career, and general functioning; the likelihood that an emerging recurrence will be detected early enough to prevent a full-blown attack; and the patient's tolerance of lithium.

Information Resources

Suggested Reading

Bohn, J., and Jefferson, J. *Lithium and Manic Depression: A Guide.* Rev. ed. Madison, WI: Lithium Information Center, University of Wisconsin, 1990.

Fieve, R. *Moodswing: The Third Revolution in Psychiatry.* Rev. ed. New York: William Morrow and Company, 1989.

Gold, M. *The Good News About Depression.* New York: Villard Books, 1987.

Goodwin, F.K., and Jamison, K.R. *Manic-Depressive Illness.* New York and Oxford: Oxford University Press, 1990.

Jefferson, J., and Greist, J. *Valproate and Manic Depression: A Guide.* Madison, WI: Lithium Information Center, University of Wisconsin, 1991.

Jefferson, J.; Greist, J.; Ackerman, D.; and Carroll, J. *Lithium Encyclopedia for Clinical Practice.* Rev. ed. Washington, DC: American Psychiatric Press, Inc., 1987.

Johnson, F.N., ed. *Handbook of Lithium Therapy.* Lancaster, England: MTP Press Ltd., and Baltimore, MD: University Park Press, 1980.

Johnson, F.N. *Depression and Mania: Modern Lithium Therapy.* Oxford: IRL Press, 1987.

Medenwald, J.; Greist, J.; and Jefferson, J. *Carbamazepine and Manic Depression: A Guide.* Rev. ed. Madison, WI: Lithium Information Center, University of Wisconsin, 1990.

Post, R., and Uhde, T. Refractory manias and alternatives to lithium treatment. In: Georgotis, A., and Cancro, R., eds. *Depression and Mania.* New York: Elsevier, 1988.

Prien, R.F., and Potter, W.Z. National Institute of Mental Health workshop report on treatment of bipolar disorder. *Psychopharmacology Bulletin* 26(4): 409-427, 1990.

Schou, M. Lithium treatment of manic-depressive illness: Past, present, and perspectives. *Journal of the American Medical Association* 259:1834-1836, 1988.

Schou, M. *Lithium Treatment of Manic-Depressive Illness: A Practical Guide.* Rev. ed. New York and Basel: Karger, 1989.

For More Information on Mood Disorders and Lithium

There are a number of consumer advocacy and support organizations for people with mood disorders. The underlying philosophy of these organizations is that the best helpers are often those who have experienced similar problems. These groups typically provide a variety of forms of practical help for dealing with problems that their members share in common. Organizations that have chapters in many communities are:

The National Alliance for the Mentally Ill
2101 Wilson Boulevard, Suite 302
Arlington, VA 22201
(703) 524-7600
1-800-950-NAMI

National Depressive and Manic Depressive Association
730 N. Franklin, Suite 501
Chicago, IL 60610
(312) 642-0049
1-800-826-2632

National Mental Health Association
1021 Prince Street
Alexandria, VA 22314-2971
(703) 684-7722
1-800-969-NMHA

For further information on lithium contact:

Lithium Information Center
Dean Foundation
8000 Excelsior Drive, Suite 203
Madison, WI 53717-1914
(608) 836-8070

This booklet was written by Robert F. Prien, Ph.D., and William Z. Potter, M.D., Ph.D., psychopharmacology and manic-depressive illness experts, National Institute of Mental Health. Editors were Bette Runck and Lynn J. Cave, NIMH.

■ **Document Source:**
   U.S. Department of Health and Human Services, Public Health Service
   National Institutes of Health
   National Institute of Mental Health
   NIH Publication No. 93-3476
   January 1993

See also: Bipolar Disorder: Manic-Depressive Illness (page 272); Depression is a Treatable Illness: A Patient's Guide (page 274)

MEDICATIONS FOR THE TREATMENT OF SCHIZOPHRENIA: QUESTIONS AND ANSWERS

Introduction

Schizophrenia, a severe mental disorder characterized by psychotic symptoms (thought disorder, hallucinations, delusions, paranoia) and impairment in job and social functioning, affects more than two million Americans. Current treatment programs for schizophrenia include combinations of medication, psychotherapy, education, and social-vocational rehabilitation.

This booklet was prepared in response to inquiries reflecting a growing public need for information on the medications used to treat schizophrenia and related illnesses. In this booklet, meant to serve as a companion to *Schizophrenia: Questions and Answers*, we have addressed concerns and questions from the public that are frequently directed to us.

General information about antipsychotic medications

The primary medications used to treat schizophrenic disorders are the antipsychotic medications, also called neuroleptics. Although these medications are not a cure for schizophrenia, they are effective in alleviating or reducing symptoms. Chlorpromazine (Thorazine), the first medication of this kind, became available for use in the United States during the early 1950s. Since its discovery, several other classes of antipsychotic medications have been developed.

All of the widely used traditional antipsychotic medications are equally effective in treating schizophrenia; however, some individuals may prefer one medication to another because they experience different side effects. Some patients may respond better or experience fewer side effects with those traditional antipsychotic medications that are available in a long-acting, injectable form. Long-acting, injectable medication may also be helpful to patients who do not take their medication reliably.

On the other hand, clozapine (Clozaril), an atypical antipsychotic medication, was first marketed in February 1990 and has been found to be superior to traditional antipsychotic medications for some patients with treatment-resistant schizophrenia. Clozapine appears to cause less muscle stiffness and restlessness (extrapyramidal side effects) than traditional antipsychotic medications and is less likely to produce tardive dyskinesia (TD). However, close monitoring via weekly blood testing is necessary for patients who are treated with clozapine.

The traditional antipsychotic medications are believed to help relieve psychotic symptoms by blocking the binding sites (receptors) for certain chemicals (neurotransmitters) found in the brain. The neurotransmitter dopamine has been the focus of much interest in learning how many of the antipsychotic medications work. Receptors for dopamine and other chemical transmitters in the brain are targets of the antipsychotic medications, different classes of which may affect one receptor type more than another. Specific side effects may result because a particular binding site is affected by a certain medication.

One way to classify antipsychotic agents is by the dosage of medication, or the potency (strength) in milligrams, that is typically recommended. Antipsychotic agents are often classified on this basis as high, middle, or low potency. Individual doses of medication taken by patients may vary because of differences among individuals in both the severity of their illness and the rate at which they metabolize (break down) medication. This latter factor is influenced by age, race, sex, body build, diet, use of cigarettes or alcohol, and other medications being taken.

The lowest possible dosage of medication effective in relieving symptoms is usually prescribed. Sometimes symptoms of schizophrenia will flare up, requiring a temporary (weeks to months) increase in medication dosage. After an initial or acute episode of illness has been treated with medication, the doctor usually will taper the dosage very slowly to the lowest possible level necessary to keep the symptoms from returning. In a few circumstances, especially when symptoms are mild, some individuals may not require medication. Others may be able to use very low doses except when symptoms are severe. Because of all these factors, it is important that patients consult with their doctor before making changes in medication dose.

Can a patient become addicted to antipsychotic medications?

Addiction to antipsychotic medications does not occur. However, some individuals who have taken such medications for more than a few weeks experience mild, unpleasant symptoms such as nausea, vomiting, abdominal cramps, diarrhea, or sweating when the medication is abruptly stopped. If it becomes necessary to stop medication, the dosage should be slowly tapered to avoid an increase in psychotic symptoms or the effects mentioned above.

How long will a patient have to take antipsychotic medication?

Duration of therapy with antipsychotic medication is highly individual. Most patients with chronic schizophrenia require some type of medication, usually antipsychotic, for most of their lives. However, some individuals, especially those who have insight into the nature of their illness and understand that increased symptoms may be a warning sign for relapse, are able to take a reduced dose or discontinue medication periodically.

What are the major side effects of antipsychotic medications?

As noted previously, the side effects of antipsychotic medications are a result of their action on chemical receptors. The different classes of antipsychotic medications may affect one receptor more than another, causing different side effects. For example, the lower potency antipsychotic medications are more likely to produce sedation, dry mouth, episodic low blood pressure, and dizziness, whereas the higher potency agents are more likely to produce drooling and muscle stiffness.

Other side effects of antipsychotic medications include constipation, skin rash, sun sensitivity, cholestatic jaundice (slowing of bile flow in the liver), and lowered white blood cell count (agranulocytosis). For all of the currently available antipsychotic medications except clozapine, the risk for lowered white blood cell count is extremely low. With clozapine, however, the risk is high enough (1% to 2% during the first year) to require weekly blood cell monitoring to ensure early detection of this disorder.

Antipsychotic medications are also capable of lowering the seizure threshold. This is an especially critical side effect of clozapine, as patients taking higher doses are at greater risk for seizures than patients taking lower doses. Additional important side effects (e.g., movement disorders, including muscle stiffness and TD; neuroleptic malignant syndrome;

and side effects involving the reproductive system) are discussed separately.

Although most patients develop some mild side effects to antipsychotic medications, the risk for developing severe side effects is relatively low overall, and most such side effects can be controlled or tolerated with another medication.

What types of movement disorders are produced by antipsychotic medications?

Antipsychotic medications may produce several types of abnormal movements and muscle stiffness. Dystonia is the powerful, involuntary contraction or spasm of a muscle or group of muscles. It may occur in any muscle group and may be dramatic in appearance. Dystonia typically occurs within the first week of treatment with, or during an increase in dose of, the antipsychotic medication. Akathisia is a feeling of internal restlessness, which may result in continuous leg movements and leaves some patients feeling compelled to pace. Both dystonia and akathisia are reversible when antipsychotic medication is lowered or stopped, and both can be treated with anticholinergic medications such as benztropine mesylate (Cogentin) and trihexyphenidyl (Artane). Akathisia is also sometimes treated with propranolol (Inderal), amantadine (Symmetrel), or lorazepam (Ativan).

Antipsychotic medications can also produce slowed or stiff movements resulting in a condition resembling Parkinson's disease called pseudoparkinsonism. This condition can occur during the first few weeks of treatment and is characterized by stiffness or rigidity of arms and legs, shuffling when walking, a tremor occurring at rest, and slowed movements of facial muscles causing a lack of facial expression. Pseudoparkinsonism caused by antipsychotic medication may improve with time, is reversible when medication is lowered or stopped, and may be treated with anticholinergic medication.

TD is another movement disorder that can result from the use of antipsychotic medications. This syndrome is discussed in the next section.

What is TD?

TD is a syndrome of abnormal involuntary muscle movements that occurs in some patients who take antipsychotic medications. Research studies show the risk of developing TD is about 5 percent per year, with 25 to 40 percent of patients developing TD after several years of taking these medications. Certain factors such as being older, being female, and having a diagnosis of affective or organic mental disorder may increase the risk of developing TD. In addition, a high total cumulative dose (the total of all the doses and length of time that medications were taken by a patient) may increase the risk of developing TD.

The muscles of the face, especially those of the mouth and tongue, are most frequently involved in TD, although muscles of the neck, trunk, and extremities may also be affected. TD may appear in various forms and degrees of severity, from mild to severe and disabling. The abnormal muscle movements may appear as muscle spasms, twitching, chorea, or athetosis. The movements characteristic of chorea are sudden and brisk, appearing as a flicking or jerking in the trunk, pelvis, arms, and legs, or as a grimace, frown, tic, or smirk in the muscles of the face. Athetosis is a slow twisting or writhing movement of the muscles. Chorea and athetosis may occur alone or together in TD and other neuropsychiatric conditions.

Because other neuropsychiatric disorders may be mistaken for TD, a doctor must take a history of the patient to include information about past and present use of antipsychotic medications, neurological and psychiatric symptoms, medical illnesses, and psychiatric and medical illnesses in the family. The doctor should also do a complete physical examination with emphasis on the nervous system. It may be necessary to perform blood tests and a magnetic resonance imaging examination of the brain to rule out other causes of the abnormal movements.

Patients who take antipsychotic medications should be examined periodically for TD. Whenever possible, an evaluation for the presence of abnormal movements should be performed before such medication is started. Examinations should then be performed after 3 months, 6 months, and at least every 6 months thereafter. Patients who develop TD should be examined every 3 months.

In some patients, symptoms of TD may be reversed or reduced when antipsychotic medication is reduced to the lowest dosage possible that will still control psychotic symptoms. Similarly, TD symptoms may lessen or disappear (i.e., be "masked") when antipsychotic medication dosages are increased. Some patients experience brief symptoms of TD, known as withdrawal dyskinesia, when antipsychotic medication is stopped or lowered.

However, anticholinergic medications, such as trihexyphenidyl (Artane) and benztropine mesylate (Cogentin), which are useful for treating muscle stiffness, may worsen the symptoms of TD. Anxiety and emotional distress may aggravate the symptoms of TD; therefore, antianxiety medications may be helpful to reduce TD symptoms in anxious patients. Recent research studies on medications effective in treating TD suggest that some medications may reduce symptoms in some patients, so any patients identified as having TD should consult their doctor regarding possible treatments.

What is neuroleptic malignant syndrome (NMS)?

NMS is a relatively rare but potentially serious side effect of antipsychotic (neuroleptic) medications. It is characterized by muscle rigidity, fever, and dysfunction of the autonomic nervous system (a part of the nervous system that helps regulate blood pressure and body temperature) leading to changes in blood pressure and heart rate, and to increased sweating. Breakdown of muscle tissue can occur in severe cases of NMS, causing high levels of an enzyme creatinine phosphokinase, also called CPK, to accumulate in the bloodstream. Patients who develop severe NMS usually need to be immediately admitted to a medical facility for treatment with intravenous fluids to prevent dehydration, and they may be given muscle-relaxing medications to treat muscle rigidity. Antipsychotic medications should be used very cautiously in patients with a history of NMS.

Questions frequently asked about the effect of antipsychotic medications on the reproductive system

Will taking antipsychotic medications affect sexual performance?
Some men and women who take antipsychotic medications experience a lowering of their sexual drive. Antipsychotic agents may slightly lower blood levels of testosterone, the hormone responsible for maintaining the libido (sex drive) in both men and women. The lower potency antipsychotic medications, such as thioridazine (Mellaril) and chlorpromazine (Thorazine), occasionally cause delayed or retrograde ejaculation in men. During retrograde ejaculation, orgasm is reached without the simultaneous emission of semen; semen is instead propelled backwards into the bladder and eliminated with the next urination (which may appear cloudy as a result).

Will antipsychotic medications affect the menstrual cycle or the ability to have children?
Antipsychotic medications lead to an increased level of the hormone prolactin. High prolactin levels may cause irregularity or lengthening of the menstrual cycle, breast swelling, and lactation (breast milk production) in women. Breast enlargement may also occur in men taking antipsychotic medications; this is called gynomastia. These changes are reversible when the dose of antipsychotic medication is reduced or stopped, causing prolactin levels to be lowered or return to normal.

Women with schizophrenia, regardless of their medication status, may have a lower level of fertility compared with nonschizophrenic women. Conceiving a child may be even more difficult for a woman taking antipsychotic medications because of lowered fertility or menstrual irregularities associated with such medications. Therefore, it is important for women taking these medications to discuss family planning with their doctor and other clinicians.

Do antipsychotic medications cause birth defects?
There are no birth malformations known to be caused by antipsychotic medications. As previously discussed in this booklet, antipsychotic medications are thought to reduce symptoms of schizophrenia by helping to correct chemical imbalances in the brain; it is unknown if the changes in neurochemical levels or their receptors that occur in the brain of a developing fetus exposed to antipsychotic medications will affect the developing nervous system connections of the fetus. Further research is needed in this important area.

As all circumstances are not the same and each patient may have different medical and emotional needs, any woman who takes antipsychotic medications (or other medications) and considers becoming pregnant should seek advice from her physician to discuss the risks and benefits for her.

What additional medications are available for patients who do not achieve full relief of their symptoms with antipsychotic medications?

Some patients receive only partial relief of their symptoms from antipsychotic medications. Research studies suggest that three other medications—lithium, carbamazepine (Tegretol), and some of the benzodiazepine antianxiety medications—may be useful in the treatment of schizophrenic patients when taken in conjunction with traditional antipsychotic medications. Lithium may help to reduce psychotic symptoms further; may increase the length of time between episodes of illness; may reduce excitement; and may lead to improved social functioning, cooperation with treatment, and personal hygiene. Patients do not need to have mood swings to benefit from lithium treatment. Research studies of carbamazepine, an antiseizure medication also used to treat bipolar affective disorder (manic-depressive illness), have found this medication useful in reducing hostile and aggressive behavior in some schizophrenic patients. Benzodiazepines such as lorazepam (Ativan) and alprazolam (Xanax), which are primarily used to treat anxiety, have been found to help reduce agitation during acute episodes of schizophrenic illness and may, if given early in the course of an acute episode of schizophrenia, prevent relapse. Results from research studies of the use of benzodiazepines in patients with chronic schizophrenia show mixed results as to the benefit of these medications for long-term use. Benzodiazepines may help to reduce symptoms of psychosis in very anxious patients, but further research needs to be done into the types and dosages of these medications and the symptoms that may best respond to treatment with benzodiazepines.

Antidepressant medications are often helpful in treating depression when it occurs in schizophrenic patients. More recently, clozapine has been used to treat patients with chronic schizophrenia who do not respond well to traditional treatment regimens. Clozapine is more thoroughly discussed in the next section.

Many other medications have been studied for their effectiveness in treating schizophrenia, with inconsistent results. Medications not generally considered useful for treatment of schizophrenia include propranolol (Inderal), levodopa, vitamins in high dosages, and valproate (Depakote, Depakene).

Electroconvulsive therapy (ECT) was one of the earliest treatments of schizophrenia. Although ECT is not useful for most schizophrenic patients, it may be useful in treating acute symptoms in certain patients who are in severe states of withdrawal (catatonia) or who present with significant affective symptoms such as uncontrolled mania.

Clozapine and other atypical antipsychotic medications

As a group, the atypical antipsychotic medications differ from the traditional antipsychotic medications in two ways. First, atypical antipsychotic medications are believed to produce less muscle stiffness and may be less likely to cause TD than the traditional antipsychotic agents. Accordingly, because they are less likely to produce neurological side effects, they do not compound or worsen negative symptoms such as flat affect, lack of motivation, and poverty of thought and speech. Second, they do not cause an increase in the hormone prolactin. Thus, specific endocrine side effects, such as enlarged breast tissue and menstrual irregularities, occur to a much lesser extent. (See section on "Questions Frequently Asked About the Effect of Antipsychotic Medications on the Reproductive System.")

Clozapine (Clorzaril), the only atypical antipsychotic agent currently marketed in the United States, has been found to be beneficial to some patients who have not responded to treatment with traditional antipsychotic medications or could not tolerate traditional antipsychotic medication because of severe side effects. In a large research study conducted at several medical centers across the United States, it was found that 30 percent of chronic schizophrenic patients who had not responded to treatment with traditional antipsychotic agents improved at least somewhat on clozapine. While there have been a few reports of seriously ill schizophrenic patients making a dramatic recovery from treatment with clozapine, this is a relatively rare event. As previously noted, clozapine can also cause agranulocytosis (low white blood cell count), a serious side effect that can lead to death if not diagnosed and treated immediately. The risk of developing some degree of agranulocytosis on clozapine is between 1 and 2 percent during the first year. If detected and promptly treated, however, this condition is completely reversible. Therefore, patients who take clozapine must have blood tests done every week. Because the high cost of this medication and the weekly blood test requirements have limited its availability, government agencies, consumer groups, and the manufacturer of clozapine have been seeking ways to make this medication more available to patients who may benefit from it.

Will any new antipsychotic medications be available soon?

Research is ongoing to develop newer, safer antipsychotic medications. Two promising medications, remoxipride (available in Europe under the trade name Roxiam) and risperidone, appear to be as effective as the traditional antipsychotic medications and they may cause less muscle stiffness and other movement disorders. These medications are still being tested in the United States and are not expected to be available here for some time.

Questions frequently asked about drugs of abuse and their effects on schizophrenia

Do street drugs cause schizophrenia?
Abusing drugs does not cause schizophrenia, but certain street drugs can produce symptoms similar to acute schizophrenia, such as hallucinations (both visual and auditory), paranoia, delusions, disorganized thinking, and excited behavior. Psychostimulant medications (amphetamines and cocaine) and hallucinogenic drugs such as lysergic acid diethylamide (LSD), phencyclidine (PCP), mescaline, and marijuana (especially marijuana high in tetrahydrocannabi-

nol or laced with other drugs) are more likely to produce psychosis than other street drugs. Individuals with a biological vulnerability toward schizophrenia or other psychotic illness may be at greater risk for developing drug-induced psychosis.

What effects do drugs of abuse or alcohol have on patients with schizophrenia?
Drugs of abuse or alcohol may worsen schizophrenic symptoms or lead to a relapse. Therefor, schizophrenic patients who abuse drugs or alcohol may require a higher dose of antipsychotic medication to control their schizophrenic symptoms.

Comments

Although the antipsychotic medications are not a cure for schizophrenia, they help to relieve the symptoms of illness and prevent the recurrence of those symptoms for many patients. Since the introduction of these medications in the 1950s, many individuals have been able to lead improved lives outside mental institutions. Some of the newer medications under development are as effective as the traditional agents and are likely to produce fewer extrapyramidal side effects. This may result in better medication compliance in patients who experience troubling side effects. Researchers are working to find new medications that are more effective than the traditional antipsychotic agents, especially for the treatment of negative symptoms of schizophrenia, and to find ways to produce the best possible treatment outcome using the currently available medications.

Antipsychotic medications available in the United States		
Generic name	*Trade name*	*PDR dose range (mg/day)[1]*
Chlorpromazine	Thorazine	100-1000
Chlorprothixene	Taractan	75-600
Clozapine	Clozaril	300-900
Fluphenazine	Prolixin, Permitil	1-20
Haloperidol	Haldol	1-15
Loxapine	Loxatane	60-100
Molindone	Moban	15-225
Mesoridazine	Serentil	100-400
Perphenazine	Trilafon	8-64
Thiothixene	Navane	20-60
Thioridazine	Mellaril	200-800
Trifluoperazine	Stelazine	10-40

Note—PDR = *Physician's Desk Reference*
[1]As discussed in this booklet, the daily dosage of medication varies among individuals. The lowest dosage possible to relieve symptoms should be prescribed.

■ **U.S. Department of Health and Human Services, Public Health Service**
National Institute of Mental Health
5600 Fishers Ln., Rockville, MD 20857
DHHS Publication No. (ADM) 92-1950
1992

SLEEP DISORDERS

Introduction

One-third of all adult Americans—about 50 million people—complain about their sleep. Some sleep too little, some fitfully, and some too much. Although one-third of our lives is spent asleep, most of us don't know much about sleep, not even our own. We don't even know exactly why we sleep, other than—like an overnight battery recharge—sleep promotes daytime alertness. Sleep problems profoundly disturb both sleeping and waking life. What is the significance of these problems and what can be done about them? Recent scientific research is beginning to provide some of the answers.

The Balm of the Bard

Sleep was, for Shakespeare, the "balm of hurt minds, great nature's second course, chief nourisher in life's feast." For centuries, science knew little more: sleep was a magical phenomenon. Not until the 1930s was it shown to possess a secret life. Only then did investigators, using the electroencephalogram (EEG), measure the brain's electrical activity in sleeping subjects. On rivers of graph paper, they could watch the rhythm of activity in the brain during sleep. They discovered that these biological rhythms naturally fall into different states, stages, and cycles. Instead of being a quiet and peaceful period of rest and recuperation, as most of us think of it, sleep is a very complex, dynamic activity. Your body may be the picture of tranquillity while you sleep. But, in fact, numerous biochemical, physiological, and psychological events are constantly taking place.

How Long to Sleep

Most adults sleep between 7 and 8 hours. But no one really knows how much sleep we need. A natural "short sleeper" may sleep for only 3 or 4 hours, and actually function worse with more sleep. A "long sleeper," on the other hand, may need more than 10 hours. "Variable sleepers" seem to need more sleep at times of stress and less during peaceful times. Changes with age also contribute to changes in the ability to sleep continuously and soundly. A newborn infant may sleep 16 hours a day, an adolescent may sleep very deeply for 9 or 10 hours straight, while an elderly person may take daytime naps and then sleep only 5 hours a night. With advancing age, some people switch to shorter days and some to longer ones. Such a switch may be simply a normal condition of aging. Or, it may result from shifts in daily patterns, retirement, or changes in the person's physical or mental health.

In general, sleep is helped by two factors—being tired at bedtime and being in tune with your own internal clock. Sleep may be difficult or less satisfying if it occurs at a time when the biological clock says, "It's time to be awake."

To find out how much sleep you need, try to determine your own sleep pattern. You should feel sleepy about the same time every evening. If you frequently have trouble staying awake in the daytime, you may not be sleeping long enough. Or perhaps you are not sleeping well enough. Both the quantity and quality of sleep and wakefulness are important. You are sleeping as much as you need if, during your waking hours, you are alert and have a sense of well-being.

Insomnia: A Symptom, Not an Illness

Insomnia, the most common sleep complaint, is the feeling that you have not slept well or long enough. It occurs in many different forms. Most often it is characterized by difficulty falling asleep (taking more than 30 or 45 minutes), awakening frequently during the night, or waking up early and being unable to get back to sleep.

With rare exception, insomnia is a *symptom* of a problem, and not the problem itself. Good sleep is a sign of health. Poor sleep is often a sign of some malfunctioning and may signal either minor or serious medical or psychiatric disorders. Insomnia can begin at any age. And, it can last for a few days (transient insomnia), a few weeks (short-term insomnia), or indefinitely (long-term insomnia).

Causes of Insomnia

Transient insomnia may be triggered by stress—say, a hospitalization for surgery, a final exam, a cold, headache, toothache, bruised muscles, backache, indigestion, or itchy rash. It can also be caused by jet travel that involves rapid time-zone change.

Short-term insomnia, lasting up to 3 weeks, may result from anxiety, nervousness, and physical and mental tension. Typical are worries about money, the death of a loved one, marital problems, divorce, looking for or losing a job, weight loss, excessive concern about health, or plain boredom, social isolation, or physical confinement.

Long-lasting distress over lack of sleep is sometimes caused by the environment, such as living near an airport or on a noisy street. Working a night shift can also cause problems: sleeping during the day may be difficult on weekdays, especially when the person sleeps at night on weekends. But more often, long-term insomnia stems from such medical conditions as heart disease, arthritis, diabetes, asthma, chronic sinusitis, epilepsy, or ulcers. Long-term impaired sleep can also be brought on by chronic drug or alcohol use, as well as by excessive use of beverages containing caffeine and abuse of sleeping pills.

Sometimes (as we shall see), long-term sleep difficulty can result from a number of other directly sleep-related medical ailments that are more directly related to sleep. Some examples are sleep apnea, nocturnal myoclonus, or "restless legs" syndrome.

Many patients with long-term insomnia may be suffering from an underlying psychiatric condition, such as depression or schizophrenia. Depression, in particular, is often accompanied by sleep problems (which usually disappear when the depression is treated). People with phobias, anxiety, obsessions, or compulsions are often awakened by their fears and worries, sometimes by nightmares and feelings of sadness, conflict, and guilt.

Sleep Hygiene: A First Move Against Insomnia

Insomnia is a complex problem, not given to simple solutions. Most experts agree that treatment should start with assessing and correcting sleep hygiene and habits.

Exercise

Regular exercise tends to benefit sleep, but not right at bedtime. Vigorous exercise, especially just before sleep, can cause arousal and delay sleep. You cannot force sleep on a given night by exercising excessively during the day. Exercise in the morning also has little beneficial effect on sleep. The best time to exercise is in the afternoon or early evening. But, even then, it probably won't help you sleep unless you exercise on a regular schedule.

Trying Too Hard

Trouble falling asleep, the most common form of sleep disturbance, may be brought on simply by going to bed too early. Sleep cannot be forced. You should not go to sleep until you are sleepy. If you turn in too early—even if you *do* fall asleep you could experience a disturbed night's rest or could wake early without feeling refreshed. If you go to bed when you feel sleepy but find that you can't fall asleep, don't stay in bed brooding about being awake. It is best to get out of bed. Leave the bedroom. Read, sew, watch TV, take a warm bath, or find some other way to relax before slipping between the sheets once more.

Naps

Laboratory tests have shown that daytime naps disrupt normal nighttime sleep. Although many people feel like napping between 2 and 4 p.m. (siesta time), most sleep better if they don't nap during the day. Naps should not be used as a substitute for poor sleep at night. However, there are exceptions to this general rule. Many older people, in particular, do sleep better at night when they take daytime naps. But if you are a napper who sleeps poorly at night, your nighttime sleep might improve if you skip the nap.

Bedtime Snacks

If hunger keeps you awake, a light snack might help you sleep, unless it causes problems with digestion. Avoid heavy meals, alcohol, and caffeine-containing coffee, tea, and cola. For those who can tolerate milk, that old, time-tested remedy may work best.

Smoking at Bedtime

Nicotine stimulates the nervous system and can interfere with sleep. In one sleep laboratory study, smokers experienced greater difficulty than nonsmokers. Sleep patterns also improved significantly among chronic smokers when they abstained from smoking.

Alcohol

The effect of alcohol is deceiving. It may induce sleep, but chances are it will be a fragmented sleep. The sleeper will probably wake up in the middle of the night when the alcohol's relaxing effect wears off.

Regular Bedtime

The best way to sleep better is to keep a regular schedule for sleeping. Go to bed at about the same time every night, but only when you are tired. Set your alarm clock to awaken you about the same time every morning—including weekends and regardless of the amount of sleep you have had. If you have a poor night's sleep, don't linger in bed or oversleep the next day. If you awaken before it is time to rise, get out of bed and start your day. Most insomniacs stay in bed too long and get up too late in the morning. By establishing a regular wakeup time, you help solidify the biological rhythms that establish your periods of peak efficiency during the 24-hour day.

Sleeping Pills: A Temporary Solution

According to the latest evidence, the medical profession is becoming increasingly conservative in prescribing sleep-promoting medications. Over the past decade, prescriptions filled in drugstores have dropped from 42 to 21 million. Only about 10 percent of people with insomnia receive prescribed sleeping pills. Another 5 percent buy over-the-counter sleep compounds that don't require a prescription. Still others use drugs intended for other purposes—for example, daytime sedatives, antihistamines, anticholinergic drugs, and tranquilizers.

None of these drugs should be used without consulting a physician first. Their misuse or outright abuse poses a danger. All sleeping medications should be used sparingly, for the shortest possible time, and in the smallest effective dose.

Prescribed Sleeping Pills

All brands of prescribed sleeping pills are hypnotics—that is, drugs that depress the central nervous system and put users to sleep. A variety of hypnotics are now on the market, including barbiturates, benzodiazepines, and several classes of drugs generally referred to as the nonbarbiturates/nonbenzodiazepines.

The barbiturates usually lose their effectiveness within 2 or 3 weeks of daily use. Doctors today tend not to prescribe the barbiturates. Most prefer to treat their patients with one of the benzodiazepines or a variant class of drug, which are considered less addictive and safer in overdose than barbiturates. The benzodiazepines are still *very* toxic, however, when taken in combination with alcohol, or when overdoses are taken by persons with respiratory disorders. Benzodiazepine drugs sometimes can aid sleep for up to 30 days. The benzodiazepines are not all alike, though. Some work faster than others, some produce effects that last longer, and some are eliminated from the body sooner.

Which type of sleeping pill is prescribed depends on a person's particular problem and needs. One pill might be right for problems in falling asleep and another for problems in maintaining sleep or insomnia associated with anxiety.

Do Sleeping Pills Help?

When taken for a brief period and under a doctor's guidance, prescription sleeping pills may help you sleep better. But insomnia cannot be corrected with pills. At best, sleeping pills have only a limited usefulness. They provide a temporary solution to insomnia. Thus, only when a person's health, safety, and well-being are threatened should sleep-promoting drugs be considered—and then only after the doctor takes a medical history and does a physical examination. He or she might identify conditions that should not be treated with sleeping pills and weigh other risks of drug treatment.

Hazards

Although temporarily helpful, sleep-promoting medications can eventually cause disturbed sleep, side effects, a sleep "hangover" during the day, and dependence on the drug. Furthermore, once the drugs are stopped, sleep problems return, at least temporarily, and may be even more severe than they were before the medication was first taken. Clearly, the regular, long-term use of sleeping pills should usually be avoided.

Sleeping pills can be fatal when taken in combination with alcohol or other drugs. Even when not fatal, combining drugs and alcohol can be perilous to driving and the use of other machinery. Long-acting sleeping pills, by themselves, may also impair driving performance the day after they are taken. People who are taking sleeping pills should *never* drink for a couple of days afterward.

Sleeping Pills for the Elderly

Many people over 60 are dissatisfied with their sleep. While they make up about 14 percent of the population, they consume about 20 to 45 percent of all sleep medications.

Toxic (poisonous) drug reactions occur more frequently in the elderly than in the young. In addition to their frequent use of sleeping pills, many older people also take other medications prescribed by their doctors. Combining sleeping pills and other drugs poses an increased hazard for the elderly because of changes in bodily functioning that accompany aging. The elderly tend to absorb and excrete all medications more slowly than younger people and usually require smaller doses. Their nervous systems may also be more sensitive, which, in turn, may increase the effects of combining drugs.

Sleeping pills may cause older people to stumble or fall, feel groggy or hung-over, or appear forgetful and senile. Before turning to sleep medications, older people (like people of any age) should consult their doctor and first seek help for the underlying *cause* of the sleep problem.

Sleeping Pills and Pregnant Women

Pregnant women should be aware that sleeping pills may be harmful to their infants. If a woman is pregnant or intends to become pregnant, she should ask her physician whether it is safe or advisable to use any drug. She also should learn about the effects of every drug, including cigarettes and alcohol, on her and her unborn baby.

Sleep Disorders: A National Health Problem

Sleep disturbances place an uncalculated, but enormous, burden on the American public. Many industrial and automobile accidents are related to undiagnosed and untreated disorders of sleep. School and job performance, and even everyday social relationships, are also affected. Most sleep disorders, whether caused by physical or mental factors, can be treated or managed effectively once they are properly diagnosed.

Anxiety, Depression, and Sleep

In a recent national survey, 47 percent of those reporting severe insomnia reported a high level of emotional distress. Psychological factors, such as fears, phobias, and compulsions, can so occupy the mind that sleep is delayed, disturbed, or shortened. Chronically tense people are frequently so restless, hyperactive, and apprehensive that they expect not to sleep when they go to bed.

In depressed people, an overwhelming feeling of sadness, hopelessness, worthlessness, or guilt can be associated with abnormal sleep patterns. Often, the depressed person awakens early and cannot return to sleep. Yet, sometimes, just the opposite is true. Some depressed people find relief in sleeping, denying or escaping from the problems of living by sleeping. The loss of a sense of purpose in life may be associated with an overwhelming urge to sleep, a constant feeling of tiredness, or nighttime sleep marked by an irregular sleep/wake pattern.

Many depressed people complain of insomnia without recognizing they are depressed. If you have lost interest in activities you used to enjoy, or if you have feelings of hopelessness or suicidal thoughts, you may be one of them. You should discuss the problem with your physician, who may recommend psychiatric consultation. While the complaint may be insomnia, the underlying depression, not the insomnia, must be treated. Antidepressant medications and/or psychotherapy can produce remarkable improvement, both in mood and sleep patterns.

Snoring

Snoring is a sign of impaired breathing during sleep. The older you get, the more apt you are to snore. Almost 60 percent of males in their 60s and 45 percent of females are habitual snorers—in all, one in eight Americans. Light snoring may be no more than a nuisance. But, snoring that is loud, disruptive, and accompanied by extreme daytime sleepiness or sleep attacks should be taken very seriously. Such snoring may be a sign that a person is suffering from the life-threatening condition called sleep apnea—a blockage of breathing during sleep.

Sleep Apnea

Discovered only recently, sleep apnea is believed to affect at least 1 out of every 200 Americans—70 to 90 percent of them men, mostly middle-aged, and usually overweight. But the condition can afflict both men or women at any age.

People with this disorder actually may stop breathing while asleep—even hundreds of times—without being aware of the problem. During an apnea attack, the snorer may seem to gasp for breath, and the oxygen level in the blood may become abnormally low. In severe cases, a sleep apnea victim may actually spend more time *not* breathing than breathing and may be at risk for death.

In the most common form of the condition, obstructive apnea (also called upper airway apnea), air stops flowing through the nose and mouth, but throat and abdominal breathing efforts are uninterrupted. The snoring that results is produced when the upper rear of the mouth (the soft palate and the cone-shaped tissue—the uvula—that descends from it) relaxes and vibrates as air passes in and out. This sets up an air current between the palate and the base of the tongue, resulting in snoring. Typically, the individual will wake up, emit a vigorous snort or grunt while gasping for air, then immediately fall back to sleep, only to repeat the cycle.

In another form of the disorder, central apnea, both oral breathing and throat and abdominal breathing efforts are simultaneously interrupted. In a third type of apnea, mixed apnea, a brief period of central apnea is followed by a longer period of obstructive apnea.

Sleep apnea can be recognized by a number of symptoms. As mentioned, loud and intermittent snoring is one warning signal. The person who has sleep apnea may experience a choking sensation, early-morning headaches, or extreme daytime sleepiness, as well. His bed partner or roommate might comment on his excessive body movements or his snoring or gasping for breath during sleep.

If the condition is suspected, it should be reported to a physician, who may recommend evaluation by a specialist in sleep disorders. Since sleeping pills may be harmful for people with sleep apnea, they should not be taken if the condition is suspected.

Many people with such conditions as obesity, deviated nasal septum, polyps, enlarged tonsils, large adenoids, or a host of other problems may be particularly likely to develop sleep apnea. Doctors can reliably diagnose the disorder only by monitoring oxygen intake, breathing, and other physical functions while the patient is sleeping.

In mild cases, sleep apnea often responds to medication. Or, in the case of overweight middle-aged males, losing weight may lessen the problem. Another procedure, known as continuous positive air pressure, involves the use of a machine that blows air into the nose during the night, opening the air passages in the throat. Patients with severe sleep apnea may require surgery. One procedure widens the throat. In another, a tracheostomy, which is used in very severe cases, a small hole is made at the base of the neck, below and in front of the Adam's apple. At night, a valve on a hollow tube in the hole is opened so that the air can flow directly to the lungs, bypassing the sleep-induced upper airway blockage. During the day, the valve is closed, allowing the patient to breathe and speak normally.

Narcolepsy—Sleep Attacks

A sleepy feeling during the day could be caused by insufficient, inadequate, or fragmented sleep, by insomnia, or by boredom, social isolation, physical confinement, or depression. But, if you continually experience excessive daily daytime sleepiness—sometimes expressed as tiredness, lack of energy, and/or irresistible sleepiness—you could be suffering from another little-known, chronic sleep disorder called narcolepsy.

According to the American Narcolepsy Association, 1 out of every 100 Americans is afflicted by this disorder. Yet, between 50 and 80 percent of them remain undiagnosed. People with narcolepsy suffer from sleep apnea more often than the general population, although apnea is not a core feature of the disorder.

During a narcoleptic attack, the person may find it physically impossible to stay awake and sleeps for periods ranging from a few seconds to a half hour. An attack can occur while watching TV, reading, or listening to a lecture. More surprising, these sudden attacks of sleep can also strike while walking, eating, riding a bike, or carrying on a conversation.

Despite modern medical knowledge about narcolepsy, people who have such attacks typically do not seek medical attention for years—an average of 5 to 7 years. Usually, narcolepsy starts in the early teen years, but it can strike anyone at any age. At first, the symptoms are rather mild. Gradually, over a period of years, they increase in severity.

Narcolepsy with Cataplexy

Besides the presence of excessive sleepiness, which usually is the first symptom noted, the person suffering from narcolepsy may experience a sudden weakness of the muscles called cataplexy. A cataplectic attack is usually triggered by such emotions as laughter, anger, elation, or surprise. It may be experienced as partial muscle weakness lasting a few seconds or as almost complete loss of muscle control lasting for 1 or 2 minutes. During this period, the victim may be in a state of nearly total physical collapse, unable to move or speak, but still conscious and at least partially aware of activity in the immediate environment.

Sometimes, narcolepsy is misdiagnosed as epilepsy. But while epilepsy is often accompanied by loss of bladder and bowel control and tongue biting, narcolepsy is not. More often, the symptoms of narcolepsy are attributed to laziness, malingering, or psychiatric disorder. Job and home life usually suffer when narcolepsy goes untreated.

Narcolepsy, believed to be caused by a defect in the central nervous system, has no known cure. However, after proper diagnosis, the disorder can be effectively managed with drugs.

Hazards of Narcolepsy

People who have narcolepsy but don't know it represent a serious safety hazard to themselves and others when they drive. They may doze off while waiting for a traffic signal to change, or they may drive to some destination and be completely unable to recall how they got there. At least one in every 500 drivers is estimated to be suffering from narcolepsy.

Tragically, many of the drivers may not survive to be diagnosed or counted among the sufferers. Yet, narcolepsy is a major traffic safety problem with a low-cost and easy solution: proper diagnosis and medical care. Diagnosed patients who understand their symptoms appear to be very safe drivers, and their driving can be coordinated with the use of medication.

Nocturnal Myoclonus—Unusual Movement During Sleep

Just before some people fall asleep, they experience an uncomfortable, but not always painful, sensation deep in the thigh, calf, or feet. They usually find that vigorous movement eases the discomfort enough to fall asleep, but they complain of sleepiness and fatigue during the day. These people are generally not aware that such episodes of repetitive leg muscle jerks or muscle twitches—nocturnal myoclonus—are followed throughout the night by hundreds of related awakenings. People with nocturnal myoclonus may have involuntary movement in their legs, in addition to twitches, while trying to relax. This condition, known as "restless leg syndrome," usually occurs in people who have nocturnal myoclonus.

Like many other sleep disorders, nocturnal myoclonus often goes unrecognized by the person who has it. It is most common in middle-aged and older people. And, it may be inherited. Often a bed partner or roommate must call attention to the characteristic twitches—repeated muscle jerks in which the big toes extends, while the ankle, knee, and occasionally, the hip flex. Upon awakening, some people with nocturnal myoclonus complain of an itching-crawling sensation in their legs, like "current going through them."

In some cases, these disorders have been associated with too little vitamin E, iron, or calcium, and vitamin and mineral supplements have been used as treatment. In other cases, drugs have been found effective, and, in still other, less severe cases, relief has come from leg exercises.

Sleep Problems of Children

Most childhood sleep disturbances occur only at certain ages, are temporary, and disappear as the child grows older. While annoying or frightening, they usually are not serious. In some cases, however, abnormal sleeping habits can be a sign of more serious problems requiring medical consultation.

Sleepwalking

Sleepwalking (somnambulism) is fairly common, especially among children. An estimated 15 percent of all children between the ages of 5 and 12 have walked in their sleep at least once, and most outgrow the disorder. Typically, the child (or adult) sleepwalker sits up, gets out of bed, and moves about in an uncoordinated manner. Less frequently, the sleepwalker may dress, open doors, eat, or go to the bathroom without incident and usually will avoid obstacles. But sleepwalkers don't always make their rounds in safety. They sometimes hurt themselves, stumbling against furniture and losing their balance, going through windows, or falling down stairs.

In children, sleepwalking is not believed to be influenced by psychological factors. In adults, it could indicate a personality disturbance.

Usually, it is enough for parents of sleepwalkers to provide their children with emotional support. They should also lock windows and doors and make sure the child does not sleep near stairways and potentially dangerous objects. For severe cases, a doctor may prescribe drugs.

Night Terrors versus Nightmares

Night terrors (known as *pavor nocturnus* in children) are relatively short nocturnal episodes during which the child sits up in bed, emits a piercing scream or cry, looks frightened, and sweats and breathes profusely. Episodes usually occur between the ages of 4 and 12, are more common in boys than girls, and can be expected to disappear as the child grows older. Typically, they occur during the first third of the night. The disorder may progress to sleepwalking, but generally that only happens when the child is made to stand up. Later the child will forget the entire episode. Parents should comfort and provide warmth and support to children who experience night terrors. The condition does not indicate any personality disorder.

Nightmares, unlike night terrors, can be recalled afterward and are accompanied by much less anxiety and movement. These frightening dream experiences, which tend to occur at times of insecurity, emotional turmoil, depression, or guilt, can occur in all age groups. They are rarely accompanied by the anguished, terrified scream of the night-terror arousal. A person experiencing a nightmare will usually recount in detail a threat which ultimately led to the awakening. Some people rarely have nightmares, while others seem predisposed to them.

Bedwetting

Bedwetting (enuresis) is a common childhood sleep disorder which, contrary to popular belief, is almost never emotionally or psychologically caused; less than 1 percent of bedwetting has an emotional source. About 5 to 17 percent of children aged 3 to 5 wet their beds; usually the condition will stop by the age of 4 or 5. However, a bedwetting child may feel guilty or ashamed. Waking the child up in the middle of the night or handing out punishments and rewards may only serve to increase the problem.

In most cases, the cause is unknown, but a congenitally small bladder, a bladder infection, or some other physical problem may be responsible. Bedwetting that continues into adolescence or adulthood may be attributed to emotional problems, but neurological disease or diabetes also can be the cause. If the disorder persists, a physician should be consulted. For some children, drugs or time away from home may be prescribed for short periods, such as a week at camp or a weekend with friends or relatives.

Help for Sleep Disorders

If your sleep is continually disrupted and you lack initiative and energy during the day, you should seek professional help. In most cases of sleep disorder, it's best to see your own physician first, in order to sort out the general nature and severity of a sleep problem. The physician may conduct a thorough physical examination, ask you questions about your sleep habits and emotional state, and can often determine whether the sleep difficulty is related to treatable causes. However, if necessary, a referral to a mental health specialist or facility, a sleep clinic, or a sleep disorders center may be made.

The same basic service is provided by both sleep clinics and sleep disorders centers. Generally, sleep clinics are set up as a part of hospitals. Sleep disorders centers may be associated with hospitals, medical centers, universities, or psychiatric or neurological institutes. Most clinics or centers primarily treat patients on referral from general practitioners and internists. However, it is possible to obtain information on specific sleep problems directly from a clinic or to make an appointment for a consultation.

Specialized sleep facilities usually have on their staffs experts called somnologists with training in a variety of medical and scientific fields. A sleep disorders team will often include a physician, a psychologist, a psychiatrist, and a surgeon.

Patients are typically seen as outpatients. They are interviewed thoroughly, given a battery of psychological tests and, if indicated, have their sleep patterns recorded in the laboratory for one night (sometimes two or three consecutive nights) to determine the cause of the sleep disturbance.

Fees vary, depending on the clinic or center. An entire analysis can range from a few hundred to about a thousand dollars. Insurance companies or Medicare may cover some of the cost. (This can be determined by consulting the center or your insurance company.)

Special sleep facilities are scattered throughout the country. Your physician or nearest hospital should be able to help you locate the nearest sleep clinic or center. Or, for a complete roster of accredited and provisional sleep disorders centers and clinics, write to:

Association of Professional Sleep Societies
604 2nd St., SW
Rochester, MN 55902

American Narcolepsy Association
P.O. Box 1187
San Carlos, CA 94070

Narcolepsy Network
155 Van Brackle Rd.
Aberdeen, NJ 07747

For Further Information

American Medical Association. *Drugs Used for Anxiety and Sleep Disorders.* Chapter 5. Chicago: AMA, 1986.

Better Sleep Council, Inc. *A Guide to Better Sleep.* Burtonsville, MD: the Council, 1984.

Berger, G. *Addiction: Its Causes, Problems, and Treatment.* New York: Watts, 1982.

Dement, W.C. *Some Must Watch While Some Must Sleep.* Gailfort, CT: Norton, 1978.

Ferber, R. *Solve Your Child's Sleep Problems.* New York: Simon & Schuster, 1985.

Fort, J. *The Addicted Society.* New York: Grove Press, 1981.

Hartmann, E. *The Sleep Book: Understanding and Preventing Sleep Problems in People Over 50.* Glenview, IL: Scott, Foresman, & Co., 1987.

Kales, A.; Kales, J.; and Soldatos, C. Insomnia and other sleep disorders. *Medical Clinics of North America,* 66(5): 971-991, 1982.

Lamberg, L. *The AMA Guide to Better Sleep.* New York: Random House, 1984.

Medelson, W.B. *The Use and Misuse of Sleeping Pills: A Clinical Guide.* New York: Plenum, 1980.

Nicholi, A.M., Jr., ed. *The Harvard Guide to Modern Psychiatry.* Cambridge: Harvard U. Press, 1978.

This pamphlet was written by science writer Gerald S. Snyder, on contract with the Science Communication Branch, Office of Scientific Information, National Institute of Mental Health (NIMH). The Science Communication Branch wishes to thank the following sleep experts who made valuable comments on drafts of the pamphlet: Richard P. Allen, Ph.D., A.C.P., Baltimore Regional Sleep Disorders Center; Mitchell Balter, Ph.D., formerly of NIMH; J. Christian Gillin, M.D., San Diego VA Medical Center; Peter Hauri, Ph.D., Sleep Disorders Center, Dartmouth-Hitchcock Medical Center; J. Allan Hobson, M.D., Harvard Medical School; J. Stephen Kennedy, Ph.D., NIMH; David Kupfer, M.D., University of Pittsburgh Department of Psychiatry; Wallace Mendelson, M.D., NIMH; and Thomas Roth, Ph.D., University of Michigan Sleep Disorders and Research Center.

■ **Document Source:**
U.S. Department of Health and Human Services, Public Health Service
Alcohol, Drug Abuse, and Mental Health Administration
National Institute of Mental Health
DHHS Publication No. (ADM) 87-1541
Printed 1987

See also: Facts About Narcolepsy (page 332)

UNDERSTANDING PANIC DISORDER

Fear . . . heart palpitations . . . terror, a sense of impending doom . . . dizziness . . . fear of fear. The words used to describe panic disorder are often frightening. But there is great hope: Treatment can benefit virtually everyone who has this condition. It is extremely important for the person who has panic disorder to learn about the problem and the availability of effective treatments and to seek help.

The encouraging progress in the treatment of panic disorder reflects recent, rapid advances in scientific understanding of the brain. In fact, the President and the U.S. Congress have declared the 1990s the Decade of the Brain. In addition to supporting intensified research on brain disorders, the federal government is working to bring information about these conditions to the people who need it.

The National Institute of Mental Health (NIMH), the federal agency responsible for conducting and supporting research related to mental disorders, mental health, and the brain, is conducting a nationwide education program on panic disorder. The program's purpose is to educate the public and health care professionals about the disorder and encourage people with it to obtain effective treatments.

What Is Panic Disorder?

In panic disorder, brief episodes of intense fear are accompanied by multiple physical symptoms (such as heart palpitations and dizziness) that occur repeatedly and unexpectedly in the absence of any external threat. These "panic attacks," which are the hallmark of panic disorder, are believed to occur when the brain's normal mechanism for reacting to a threat—the so-called "fight or flight" response—becomes inappropriately aroused. Most people with panic disorder also feel anxious about the possibility of having another attack and avoid situations in which they believe these attacks are likely to occur. Anxiety about another attack, and the avoidance it causes, can lead to disability in panic disorder.

Who Has Panic Disorder?

In the United States, 1.6 percent of the adult population, or more than 3 million people, will have panic disorder at some time in their lives. This disorder typically begins in young adulthood, but older people and children can be affected. Women are affected twice as frequently as men. While people of all races and social classes can have panic disorder, there appear to be cultural differences in how individual symptoms are expressed.

Panic Attack Symptoms

During a panic attack, some or all of the following symptoms occur:

♦ Terror—a sense that something unimaginably horrible is about to happen and one is powerless to prevent it
♦ Racing or pounding heartbeat
♦ Chest pains
♦ Dizziness, lightheadedness, nausea
♦ Difficulty breathing
♦ Tingling or numbness in the hands
♦ Flushes or chills
♦ Sense of unreality
♦ Fear of losing control, going "crazy," or doing something embarrassing
♦ Fear of dying

Symptoms and Course of Panic Disorder

Initial panic attack. Typically, a first panic attack seems to come "out of the blue," occurring while a person is engaged in some ordinary activity like driving a car or walking to work. Suddenly, the person is struck by a barrage of frightening and uncomfortable symptoms. These symptoms often include terror, a sense of unreality, or a fear of losing control.

This barrage of symptoms usually lasts several seconds, but may continue for several minutes. The symptoms gradually fade over the course of about an hour. People who have experienced a panic attack can attest to the extreme discomfort they felt and to their fear that they had been stricken with some terrible, life-threatening disease or were "going crazy." Often people who are having a panic attack seek help at a hospital emergency room.

Initial panic attacks may occur when people are under considerable stress, from an overload of work, for example,

or from the loss of a family member or close friend. The attacks may also follow surgery, a serious accident, illness, or childbirth. Excessive consumption of caffeine or use of cocaine or other stimulant drugs or medicines, such as the stimulants used in treating asthma, can also trigger panic attacks.

Nevertheless panic attacks usually take a person completely by surprise. This unpredictability is one reason they are so devastating. Sometimes people who have never had a panic attack assume that panic is just a matter of feeling nervous or anxious—the sort of feelings that everyone is familiar with. In fact, even though people who have panic attacks may not show any outward signs of discomfort, the feelings they experience are so overwhelming and terrifying that they really believe they are going to die, lose their minds, or be totally humiliated. These disastrous consequences don't occur, but they seem quite likely to the person who is suffering a panic attack.

Some people who have one panic attack, or an occasional attack, never develop a problem serious enough to affect their lives. For others, however, the attacks continue and cause much suffering.

Panic disorder. In panic disorder, panic attacks recur and the person develops an intense apprehension of having another attack. As noted earlier, this fear—called *anticipatory anxiety* or *fear of fear*—can be present most of the time and seriously interfere with the person's life even when a panic attack is not in progress. In addition, the person may develop irrational fears called *phobias* about situations where a panic attack has occurred. For example, someone who has had a panic attack while driving may be afraid to get behind the wheel again, even to drive to the grocery store.

People who develop these panic-induced phobias will tend to avoid situations that they fear will trigger a panic attack, and their lives may be increasingly limited as a result. Their work may suffer because they can't travel or get to work on time. Relationships may be strained or marred by conflict as panic attacks, or the fear of them, rule the affected person and those close to them.

Also, sleep may be disturbed because of panic attacks that occur at night, causing the person to awaken in a state of terror. The experience is so harrowing that some people who have nocturnal panic attacks become afraid to go to sleep and suffer from exhaustion. Also, even if there are no nocturnal panic attacks, sleep may be disturbed because of chronic, panic-related anxiety.

Many people with panic disorder remain intensely concerned about their symptoms even after an initial visit to a physician yields no indication of a life-threatening condition. They may visit a succession of doctors seeking medical treatment for what they believe is heart disease or a respiratory problem. Or their symptoms may make them think they have a neurological disorder or some serious gastrointestinal condition. Some patients see as many as 10 doctors and undergo a succession of expensive and unnecessary tests in the effort to find out what is causing their symptoms.

This search for medical help may continue a long time, because physicians who see these patients frequently fail to diagnose panic disorder. When doctors do recognize the condition, they sometime explain it in terms that suggest it is of no importance or not treatable. For example, the doctor may say, "There's nothing to worry about, you're just having a panic attack" or "It's just nerves." Although meant to be reassuring, such words can be dispiriting to the worried patient whose symptoms keep recurring. The patient needs to know that the doctor acknowledges the disabling nature of panic disorder and that it can be treated effectively.

Agoraphobia. Panic disorder may progress to a more advanced stage in which the person becomes afraid of being in any place or situation where escape might be difficult or help unavailable in the event of a panic attack. This condition is called *agoraphobia*. It affects about a third of all people with panic disorder.

Typically, people with agoraphobia fear being in crowds, standing in line, entering shopping malls, and riding in cars or public transportation. Often, these people restrict themselves to a "zone of safety" that may include only the home or the immediate neighborhood. Any movement beyond the edges of this zone creates mounting anxiety. Sometimes a person with agoraphobia is unable to leave home alone, but can travel if accompanied by a particular family member or friend. Even when they restrict themselves to "safe" situations, most people with agoraphobia continue to have panic attacks at least a few times a month.

People with agoraphobia can be seriously disabled by their condition. Some are unable to work, and they may need to rely heavily on other family members, who must do the shopping and run all the household errands, as well as accompany the affected person on rare excursions outside the "safety zone." Thus the person with agoraphobia typically leads a life of extreme dependency as well as great discomfort.

Treatment for Panic Disorder

Treatment can bring significant relief to 70 to 90 percent of people with panic disorder, and early treatment can help keep the disease from progressing to the later stages where agoraphobia develops.

Before undergoing any treatment for panic disorder, a person should undergo a thorough medical examination to rule out other possible causes of the distressing symptoms. This is necessary because a number of other conditions, such as excessive levels of thyroid hormone, certain types of epilepsy, or cardiac arrhythmias, which are disturbances in the rhythm of the heartbeat, can cause symptoms resembling those of panic disorder.

Several effective treatments have been developed for panic disorder and agoraphobia. In 1991, a conference held at the National Institutes of Health (NIH) under the sponsorship of the National Institute of Mental Health and the Office of Medical Applications of Research, surveyed the available information on panic disorder and its treatment. The conferees concluded that a form of psychotherapy called cognitive-behavioral therapy and medications are both effective for panic disorder. A treatment should be selected according to the individual needs and preferences of the patient, the panel said, and any treatment that fails to produce an effect within 6 to 8 weeks should be reassessed.

Cognitive-behavioral therapy. This is a combination of *cognitive therapy*, which can modify or eliminate thought

patterns contributing to the patient's symptoms, and *behavioral therapy*, which aims to help the patient to change his or her behavior.

Typically the patient undergoing cognitive-behavioral therapy meets with a therapist for 1 to 3 hours a week. In the cognitive portion of the therapy, the therapist usually conducts a careful search for the thoughts and feelings that accompany the panic attacks. These mental events are discussed in terms of the "cognitive model" of panic attacks.

The cognitive model states that individuals with panic disorder often have distortions in their thinking, of which they may be unaware, and these may give rise to a cycle of fear. The cycle is believed to operate this way: First the individual feels a potentially worrisome sensation such as an increasing heart rate, tightened chest muscles, or a queasy stomach. This sensation may be triggered by some worry, an unpleasant mental image, a minor illness, or even exercise. The person with panic disorder responds to the sensation by becoming anxious. The initial anxiety triggers still more unpleasant sensations, which in turn heighten anxiety, giving rise to catastrophic thoughts. The person thinks "I am having a heart attack" or "I am going insane," or some similar thought. As the vicious cycle continues, a panic attack results. The whole cycle might take only a few seconds, and the individual may not be aware of the initial sensations or thoughts.

Proponents of this theory point out that, with the help of a skilled therapist, people with panic disorder often can learn to recognize the earliest thoughts and feelings in this sequence and modify their responses to them. Patients are taught that typical thoughts such as "This terrible feeling is getting worse!" or "I'm going to have a panic attack" or "I'm going to have a heart attack" can be replaced with substitutes such as "It's only uneasiness—it will pass" that help to reduce anxiety and ward off a panic attack. Specific procedures for accomplishing this are taught. By modifying thought patterns in this way, the patient gains more control over the problem.

Often the therapist will provide the patient with simple guidelines to follow when he or she can feel that a panic attack is approaching. One therapist has offered a set of strategies that have helped some of her patients to cope with panic attacks.

In cognitive therapy, discussions between the patient and the therapist are not usually focused on the patient's past, as is the case with some forms of psychotherapy. Instead, conversations focus on the difficulties and successes the patient is having at the present time, and on skills the patient needs to learn.

The behavioral portion of cognitive-behavioral therapy may involve systematic training in relaxation techniques. By learning to relax, the patient may acquire the ability to reduce generalized anxiety and stress that often sets the stage for panic attacks.

Breathing exercises are often included in the behavioral therapy. The patient learns to control his or her breathing and avoid *hyperventilation*—a pattern of rapid, shallow breathing that can trigger or exacerbate some people's panic attacks.

Another important aspect of behavioral therapy is exposure to internal sensations called *interoceptive exposure*.

During interoceptive exposure the therapist will do an individual assessment of internal sensations associated with panic. Depending on the assessment, the therapist may then encourage the patient to bring on some of the sensations of a panic attack by, for example, exercising to increase heart rate, breathing rapidly to trigger lightheadedness and respiratory symptoms, or spinning around to trigger dizziness. Exercises to produce feelings of unreality may also be used. Then the therapist teaches the patient to cope effectively with these sensations and to replace alarmist thoughts such as "I am going to die," with more appropriate ones, such as "It's just a little dizziness—I can handle it."

Another important aspect of behavioral therapy is *in vivo* or *real-life exposure*. The therapist and the patient determine whether the patient has been avoiding particular places and situations, and which patterns of avoidance are causing the patient problems. They agree to work on the avoidance behaviors that are most seriously interfering with the patient's life. For example, fear of driving may be of paramount importance for one patient, while inability to go to the grocery store may be most handicapping for another.

Some therapists will go to an agoraphobic patient's home to conduct the initial sessions. Often therapists take their patients on excursions to shopping malls and other places the patients have been avoiding. Or they may accompany their patients who are trying to overcome fear of driving a car.

The patient approaches a feared situation gradually, attempting to stay in spite of rising levels of anxiety. In this way the patient sees that as frightening as the feelings are, they are not dangerous, and they do pass. On each attempt, the patient faces as much fear as he or she can stand. Patients find that with this step-by-step approach, aided by encouragement and skilled advice from the therapist, they can gradually master their fears and enter situations that had seemed unapproachable.

Many therapists assign the patient "homework" to do between sessions. Sometimes patients spend only a few sessions in one-on-one contact with a therapist and continue to work on their own with the aid of a printed manual.

Often the patient will join a therapy group with others striving to overcome panic disorder or phobias, meeting with them weekly to discuss progress, exchange encouragement, and receive guidance from the therapist.

Cognitive-behavioral therapy generally requires at least 8 to 12 weeks. Some people may need a longer time in treatment to learn and implement the skills. This kind of therapy, which is reported to have a low relapse rate, is effective in eliminating panic attacks or reducing their frequency. It also reduces anticipatory anxiety and the avoidance of feared situations.

Treatment with medications. In this treatment approach, which is also called *pharmacotherapy,* a prescription medication is used both to prevent panic attacks or reduce their frequency and severity, and to decrease the associated anticipatory anxiety. When patients find that their panic attacks are less frequent and severe, they are increasingly able to venture into situations that had been off-limits to them. In this way, they benefit from exposure to previously feared situations as well as from the medication.

Strategies for Coping with Panic

1. Remember that although your feelings and symptoms are very frightening, they are not dangerous or harmful.
2. Understand that what you are experiencing is just an exaggeration of your normal bodily reactions to stress.
3. Do not fight your feelings or try to wish them away. The more you are willing to face them, the less intense they will become.
4. Do not add to your panic by thinking about what "might" happen. If you find yourself asking "What if?" tell yourself "So what!"
5. Stay in the present. Notice what is really happening to you as opposed to what you think might happen.
6. Label your fear level from zero to ten and watch it go up and down. Notice that it does not stay at a very high level for more than a few seconds.
7. When you find yourself thinking about the fear, change your "what if" thinking. Focus on and carry out a simple and manageable task such as counting backwards from 100 by 3's or snapping a rubber band on your wrist.
8. Notice that when you stop adding frightening thoughts to your fear, it begins to fade.
9. When the fear comes, expect and accept it. Wait and give it time to pass without running away from it.
10. Be proud of yourself for your progress thus far, and think about how good you will feel when you succeed this time.

Courtesy Jerilyn Ross, M.A., L.I.C.S.W., The Ross Center for Anxiety and Related Disorders, Inc., Washington, DC. Adapted from the Mathews et al., 1981.

The three groups of medications most commonly used are the *tricyclic antidepressants,* the *high-potency benzodiazepines,* and the *monoamine oxidase inhibitors* (MAOIs). Determination of which drug to use is based on considerations of safety, efficacy, and the personal needs and preferences of the patient. Some information about each of the classes of drugs follows.

The tricyclic antidepressants were the first medications shown to have a beneficial effect against panic disorder. Imipramine is the tricyclic most commonly used for this condition. When imipramine is prescribed, the patient usually starts with small daily doses that are increased every few days until an effective dosage is reached. The slow introduction of imipramine helps minimize side effects such as dry mouth, constipation, and blurred vision. People with panic disorder, who are inclined to be hypervigilant about physical sensations, often find these side effects disturbing at the outset. Side effects usually fade after the patient has been on the medication a few weeks.

It usually takes several weeks for imipramine to have a beneficial effect on panic disorder. Most patients treated with imipramine will be panic-free within a few weeks or months. Treatment generally lasts from 6 to 12 months. Treatment for a shorter period of time is possible, but there is substantial risk that when imipramine is stopped, panic attacks will recur. Extending the period of treatment to 6 months to a year may reduce this risk of a relapse. When the treatment period is complete, the dosage of imipramine is tapered over a period of several weeks.

The high-potency benzodiazepines are a class of medications that effectively reduce anxiety. Alprazolam, clonazepam, and lorazepam are medications that belong to this class. They take effect rapidly, have few bothersome side effects, and are well-tolerated by the majority of patients. However, some patients, especially those who have had problems with alcohol or drug dependency, may become dependent on benzodiazepines.

Generally, the physician prescribing one of these drugs starts the patient on a low dose and gradually raises it until panic attacks cease. This procedure minimizes side effects.

Treatment with high-potency benzodiazepines is usually continued for 6 months to a year. One drawback of these medications is that patients may experience withdrawal symptoms—malaise, weakness, and other unpleasant effects—when the treatment is discontinued. Reducing the dose gradually generally minimizes these problems. There may also be a recurrence of panic attacks after the medication is withdrawn.

Of the MAOIs, a class of antidepressants which have been shown to be effective against panic disorder, phenelzine is the most commonly used. Treatment with phenelzine usually starts with a relatively low daily dosage that is increased gradually until panic attacks cease or the patient reaches a maximum dosage of about 100 milligrams a day.

Use of phenelzine or any other MAOI requires the patient to observe exacting dietary restrictions, because there are foods and prescription drugs and certain substances of abuse that can interact with the MAOI to cause a sudden, dangerous rise in blood pressure. All patients who are taking MAOIs should obtain their physician's guidance concerning dietary restrictions and should consult with their physician before using any over-the-counter or prescription medications.

As in the case of the high-potency benzodiazepines and imipramine, treatment with phenelzine or another MAOI generally lasts 6 months to a year. At the conclusion of the treatment period, the medication is gradually tapered.

Newly available antidepressants such as fluoxetine (one of a class of new agents called serotonin reuptake inhibitors), appear to be effective in selected cases of panic disorder. As with other antipanic medications, it is important to start with very small doses and gradually raise the dosage.

Scientists supported by NIMH are seeking ways to improve drug treatment for panic disorder. Studies are underway to determine the optimal duration treatment with medications, who they are most likely to help, and how to moderate problems associated with withdrawal.

Combination treatments. Many believe that a combination of medication and cognitive-behavioral therapy represents the best alternative for the treatment of panic disorder. The combined approach is said to offer rapid relief, high effectiveness, and a low relapse rate. However, there is a need for more research studies to determine whether this is in fact the case.

Comparing medications and psychological treatments, and determining how well they work in combination, is the goal of several NIMH-supported studies. The largest of these is a 4-year-old clinical trial that will include 480 patients and involve four centers at the State University of New York at Albany, Cornell University, Hillside Hospital/Columbia University, and Yale University. This study is designed to determine how treatment with imipramine compares with a cognitive-behavioral approach, and whether combining the two yields benefits over either method alone.

What to Do If a Family Member Has an Anxiety Disorder

1. Don't make assumptions about what the affected person needs; ask them.
2. Be predictable; don't surprise them.
3. Let the person with the disorder set the pace for recovery.
4. Find something positive in every experience. If the affected person is only able to go part way to a particular goal, such as a movie theater or party, consider that an achievement rather than a failure.
5. Don't enable avoidance; negotiate with the person with panic disorder to take one step forward when he or she wants to avoid something.
6. Don't sacrifice your own life and build resentments.
7. Don't panic when the person with the disorder panics.
8. Remember that it's all right to be anxious yourself; it's natural for you to be concerned and even worried about the person with the panic disorder.
9. Be patient and accepting, but don't settle for the affected person being permanently disabled.
10. Say: "You can do it no matter how you feel. I am proud of you. Tell me what you need now. Breathe slow and low. Stay in the present. It's not the place that's bothering you, it's the thought. I know that what you are feeling is painful, but it's not dangerous. You are courageous."

    Don't say: "Relax. Calm down. Don't be anxious. Let's see if you can do this (i.e., setting up a test for the affected person). You can fight this. What should we do next? Don't be ridiculous. You *have* to stay. Don't be a coward."

Adapted from Sally Winston, Psy.D., The Anxiety and Stress Disorders Institute of Maryland, Towson, MD, 1992.

Psychodynamic treatment. This is a form of "talk therapy" in which the therapist and the patient, working together, seek to uncover emotional conflicts that may underlie the patient's problems. By talking about these conflicts and gaining a better understanding of them, the patient is helped to overcome the problems. Often, psychodynamic treatment focuses on events of the past and making the patient aware of the ramifications of long-buried problems.

Although psychodynamic approaches may help to relieve the stress that contributes to panic attacks, they do not seem to stop the attacks directly. In fact, there is no scientific evidence that this form of therapy by itself is effective in helping people to overcome panic disorder or agoraphobia. However, if a patient's panic disorder occurs along with some broader and pre-existing emotional disturbance, psychodynamic treatment may be a helpful addition to the overall treatment program.

When Panic Recurs

Panic disorder is often a chronic, relapsing illness. For many people, it gets better at some times and worse at others. If a person gets treatment, and appears to have largely overcome the problem, it can still worsen later for no apparent reason. These recurrences should not cause a person to despair or consider himself or herself a "treatment failure." Recurrence can be treated effectively, just like an initial episode.

In fact, the skills that a person learns in dealing with the initial episode can be helpful in coping with any setbacks. Many people who have overcome panic disorder once or a few times find that, although they still have an occasional panic attack, they are now much better able to deal with the problem. Even though it is not fully cured, it no longer dominates their lives, or the lives of those around them.

Coexisting Conditions

At the NIH conference on panic disorder, the panel recommended that patients be carefully evaluated for other conditions that may be present along with panic disorder. These may influence the choice of treatment, the panel noted. Among the conditions that are frequently found to coexist with panic disorder are:

Simple phobias. People with panic disorder often develop irrational fears of specific events or situations that they associate with the possibility of having a panic attack. Fear of heights and fear of crossing bridges are examples of simple phobias. Generally, these fears can be resolved through repeated exposure to the dreaded situations, while practicing specific cognitive-behavioral techniques to become less sensitive to them.

Social phobia. This is a persistent dread of situations in which the person is exposed to possible scrutiny by others and fears acting in a way that will be embarrassing or humiliating. Social phobia can be treated effectively with cognitive-behavioral therapy or medications, or both.

Depression. About half of panic disorder patients will have an episode of clinical depression sometime during their lives. Major depression is marked by persistent sadness or feelings of emptiness, a sense of hopelessness, and other symptoms (see box).

Symptoms of Depression

- ◆ Persistent sadness or feelings of emptiness
- ◆ A sense of hopelessness
- ◆ Problems sleeping
- ◆ Loss of interest or pleasure in ordinary activities
- ◆ Fatigue or decreased energy
- ◆ Difficulty concentrating, remembering, and making decisions

---

Obsessive-compulsive disorder (OCD). In OCD, a person becomes trapped in a pattern of repetitive thoughts and behaviors that are senseless and distressing but extremely difficult to overcome. Such rituals as counting, prolonged handwashing, and repeatedly checking for danger may occupy much of the person's time and interfere with other activities. Today, OCD can be treated effectively with medications or cognitive-behavioral therapies.

Alcohol abuse. About 30 percent of people with panic disorder abuse alcohol. A person who has alcoholism in addition to panic disorder needs specialized care for the alcoholism along with treatment for the panic disorder. Often the alcoholism will be treated first.

Drug abuse. As in the case of alcoholism, drug abuse is more common in people with panic disorder than in the population at large. In fact, about 17 percent of people with panic disorder abuse drugs. The drug problems often need to be addressed prior to treatment for panic disorder.

Suicidal tendencies. Recent studies in the general population have suggested that suicide attempts are more common in people who have panic attacks than among those who do not have a mental disorder. Also, it appears that people who have both panic disorder and depression are at elevated risk for suicide. (However, anxiety disorder experts who have treated many patients emphasize that it is extremely unlikely that anyone would attempt to harm himself or herself during a panic attack.)

Anyone who is considering suicide needs immediate attention from a mental health professional or from a school counselor, physician, or member of the clergy. With appropriate help and treatment, it is possible to overcome suicidal tendencies.

There are also certain physical conditions that are often associated with panic disorder.

Irritable bowel syndrome. The person with this syndrome experiences intermittent bouts of gastrointestinal cramps and diarrhea or constipation, often occurring during a period of stress. Because the symptoms are so pronounced, panic disorder is often not diagnosed when it occurs in a person with irritable bowel syndrome.

Mitral valve prolapse. This condition involves a defect in the mitral valve, which separates the two chambers on the left side of the heart. Each time the heart muscle contracts in people with this condition, tissue in the mitral valve is pushed for an instant into the wrong chamber. The person with the disorder may experience chest pain, rapid heartbeat, breathing difficulties, and headache. People with mitral valve prolapse may be at higher than usual risk of having panic disorder, but many experts are not convinced this apparent association is real.

Causes of Panic Disorder

The National Institute of Mental Health supports a sizable and multifaceted research program on panic disorder—its causes, diagnosis, treatment, and prevention. This research involves studies of panic disorder in human subjects and investigations of the biological basis for anxiety and related phenomena in animals. It is part of a massive effort to overcome the major mental disorders, an effort that is taking place during the 1990s—the Decade of the Brain. Here is a description of some of the most important new research on panic disorder and its causes.

Genetics. Panic disorder runs in families. One study has shown that if one twin in a genetically identical pair has panic disorder, it is likely that the other twin will also. Fraternal, or nonidentical, twin pairs do not show this high degree of "concordance" with respect to panic disorder. Thus, it appears that some genetic factor, in combination with environment, may be responsible for vulnerability to this condition.

NIMH-supported scientists are studying families in which several individuals have panic disorder. The aim of these studies is to identify the specific gene or genes involved in the condition. Identification of these genes may lead to new approaches for diagnosing and treating panic disorder.

Brain and biochemical abnormalities. One line of evidence suggests that panic disorder may be associated with increased activity in the hippocampus and locus ceruleus, portions of the brain that monitor external and internal stimuli and control the brain's responses to them. Also, it has been shown that panic disorder patients have increased activity in a portion of the nervous system called the adrenergic system, which regulates such physiological functions as heart rate and body temperature. However, it is not clear whether these increases reflect the anxiety symptoms or whether they cause them.

Another group of studies suggests that people with panic disorder may have abnormalities in the benzodiazepine receptors, brain components that react with anxiety-reducing substances within the brain.

In conducting their research, scientists can use several different techniques to provoke panic attacks in people who have panic disorder. The best-known method is intravenous administrations of sodium lactate, the same chemical that normally builds up in the muscles during heavy exercise. Other substances that can trigger panic attacks in susceptible people include caffeine (generally 5 or more cups of coffee are required). Hyperventilation and breathing air with a higher-than-usual level of carbon dioxide can also trigger panic attacks in people with panic disorder.

Because these provocations generally do *not* trigger panic attacks in people who do *not* have panic disorder, scientists have inferred that individuals who have panic disorder are biologically different in some way from people who do not. However, it is also true that when the people prone to panic attacks are told in advance about the sensations these provocations will cause, they are much less likely to panic. This suggests that there is a strong psychological component, as well as a biological one, to panic disorder.

NIMH-supported investigators are examining specific parts of the brain and central nervous system to learn which ones play a role in panic disorder, and how they may interact to give rise to this condition. Other studies funded by the Institute are under way to determine what happens during "provoked" panic attacks, and to investigate the role of breathing irregularities in anxiety and panic attacks.

Animal studies. Studies of anxiety in animals are providing NIMH-sponsored researchers with clues to the underlying causes of this phenomenon. One series of studies involves and inbred line of pointer dogs that exhibit extreme, abnormal fearfulness when approached by humans or startled by loud noises. In contrast with normal pointers, these nervous dogs have been found to react more strongly to caffeine and to have brain tissue that is richer in receptors for adenosine, a naturally occurring sedative that normally exerts a calming effect within the brain. Further study of these

animals is expected to reveal how a genetic predisposition toward anxiety is expressed in the brain.

Other animal studies involve macaque monkeys. Some of these animals exhibit anxiety when challenged with an infusion of lactate, much like people with panic disorder. Other macaques do not exhibit this response. NIMH-supported scientists are attempting to determine how the brains of the responsive and nonresponsive monkeys differ. This research should provide additional information on the causes of panic disorder.

In addition, research with rats is exploring the effect of various medications on the parts of the brain involved in anxiety. The aim is to develop a clearer picture of which components of the brain are responsible for anxiety, and to learn how their actions can be brought under better control.

Cognitive factors. Scientists funded by NIMH are investigating the basic thought processes and emotions that come into play during a panic attack and those that contribute to the development and persistence of agoraphobia. The institute also supports research evaluating the impact of various versions of cognitive-behavioral therapy to determine which variants of the procedure are effective for which people. The NIMH panic disorder research program will also explore the effects of interpersonal stress such as marital conflict on panic disorder with agoraphobia and determine if including spouses in the cognitive-behavioral treatment of the condition improves outcome.

Finding Help for Panic Disorder

Often the person with panic disorder must undertake a strenuous search to find a therapist who is familiar with the most effective treatments for the condition. A list of places to start follows. The Anxiety Disorders Association of America can provide a list of professionals in your area who specialize in the treatment of panic disorder and other anxiety disorders.

Self-help and *support groups* are the least expensive approach to managing panic disorder, and are helpful for some people. A group of about 5 to 10 people meet weekly and share their experiences, encouraging each other to venture into feared situations and cope effectively with panic attacks. Group members are in charge of the sessions. Often family members are invited to attend these groups, and at times a therapist or other panic disorder expert may be brought in to share insights with group members. Information on self-help groups in specific areas of the country can be obtained from the Anxiety Disorders Association of America.

Help for the Family

When one member of a family has panic disorder, the entire family is affected by the condition. Family members may be frustrated in their attempts to help the affected member cope with the disorder, overburdened by taking on additional responsibilities, and socially isolated. Family members must encourage the person with panic disorder to seek the help of a qualified mental health professional. Also, it is often helpful for family members to attend an occasional treatment or self-help session or seek the guidance of the therapist in dealing with their feelings about the disorder.

Sources of Referral to Professional Help for Panic Disorder

Here are the types of people and places that will make a referral to, or provide, diagnostic and treatment services for a person with symptoms resembling those described in this brochure. Also check the *Yellow Pages* under "mental health," "health," "anxiety," "suicide prevention," "hospitals," "physicians," "psychiatrists," "psychologists," or "social workers" for phone numbers and addresses.

- Family doctors
- Mental health specialists, such as psychiatrists, psychologists, social workers, or mental health counselors
- Health maintenance organizations
- Community mental health centers
- Hospital psychiatry departments and outpatient clinics
- University- or medical school-affiliated programs and clinics
- State hospital outpatient clinics
- Family service/social agencies
- Private clinics and facilities
- Employee assistance programs
- Local medical, psychiatric, or psychological societies

Certain strategies, such as encouraging the person with panic disorder to go at least partway toward a place or situation that is feared, can be helpful. The director of one anxiety disorder clinic has developed a list of suggestions for family members who want to help loved ones cope with an anxiety disorder. By their skilled and caring efforts to help, family members can aid the person with panic disorder in making a recovery.

Also it may be valuable for family members to join or form a support group to share information and offer mutual encouragement.

For More Information on Panic Disorder and Related Conditions

American Psychiatric Association
1400 K St., N.W.
Washington, DC 20005

American Psychological Association
750 First St., N.E.
Washington, DC 20002
Anxiety Disorders Association of America
6000 Executive Blvd., Ste. 513
Rockville, MD 20852

Association for the Advancement of Behavior Therapy
305 7th Ave.
New York, NY 10001

National Alliance for the Mentally Ill
2101 Wilson Blvd, Ste. 302
Arlington, VA 22201

National Anxiety Foundation
3135 Custer Dr.
Lexington, KY 40517-4001

National Depressive and Manic Depressive Association
740 N. Franklin St., Ste. 501
Chicago, IL 60601

National Institute of Mental Health Publications List
Room 7C-02, 5600 Fishers Ln.
Rockville, MD 20857

National Mental Health Association
1201 Prince St.
Alexandria, VA 22314-2971

References

Barlow, D.H., and Craske, M.G. *Mastery of Your Anxiety and Panic*. Albany, NY: Graywind Publications, 1988.

Beck, A.T.; Emery, G.; and Greenberg, R. *Anxiety Disorders and Phobias: A Cognitive Perspective*. New York: Basic Books, 1985.

Gold, M.S. *The Good News About Panic, Anxiety, and Phobias*. New York: Bantam, 1989.

Greist, J.H., and Jefferson, J.W. *Panic Disorder and Agoraphobia: A Guide*. Madison, WI: Anxiety Disorders Center and Information Centers, University of Wisconsin, 1992.

Hecker, J.E., and Thorpe, G.L. *Agoraphobia and Panic: A Guide to Psychological Treatment*. Needham Heights, MA: Allyn and Bacon, 1992.

Katon, W. *Panic Disorder in the Medical Setting*. DHHS Pub. No. (ADM) 92-1629. Washington, DC: Supt. of Docs., U.S. Govt. Print. Off., 1992.

Kernodle, W.D. *Panic Disorder*. Richmond, VA: William Byrd Press, 1991.

Klerman, G.L., et al., eds. *Panic Anxiety and Its Treatments*. Washington, DC: American Psychiatric Press, 1993.

Mathews, A.M.; Gelder, M.G.; and Johnston, D.W. *Agoraphobia: Nature and Treatment*. New York and London: Guilford Press, 1981.

National Institutes of Health. NIH Consensus Development Conference Statement, Vol. 9, No. 2. *Treatment of Panic Disorder*. Bethesda, MD: NIH, September 1991.

Rachman, S., and Maser, J.D. *Panic: Psychological Perspectives*. Hillsdale, NJ: Lawrence Erlbaum Associates, 1988.

Sheehan, D.V. *The Anxiety Disease*. New York: Bantam, 1986.

Wilson, R.R. *Don't Panic: Taking Control of Anxiety Attacks*. New York: Harper and Row, 1986.

This booklet was written by Mary Lynn Hendrix, science writer in the Office of Scientific Information, National Institute of Mental Health. Scientific review was provided by Frederick K. Goodwin, M.D., Hagop Akiskal, M.D., David Barlow, Ph.D., Bernard Beitman, M.D., Susan Blumenthal, M.D., Alan Leshner, Ph.D., Jack Maser, Ph.D., Larry Michelson, Ph.D., Jerilyn Ross, M.A., L.I.C.S.W., Michael Telch, Ph.D., Gary Tucker, M.D., Thomas Uhde, M.D., Myrna Weissman, Ph.D., and Sally Winston, Psy.D.

■ Document Source:
U.S. Department of Health and Human Services, Public Health Service
National Institutes of Health
National Institute of Mental Health
NIH Publication No. 93-3509
September 1993

See also: Useful Information on Phobias and Panic (page 311)

USEFUL INFORMATION ON PHOBIAS AND PANIC

The Varieties of Fear

Phobias take many forms. Some people are terrified of dogs, even tiny dogs with wagging tails. Some people stiffen with fright at the mere thought of talking in front of a group. Some can't fly. Some tremble and hide at the crack of thunder. Some can't ride an escalator. Some are struck by panic attacks for no apparent reason. And some never leave their homes.

Fears such as these are very common. Millions of Americans are afflicted with phobias or panic disorder. They suffer intensely. To escape their fear, they go to great lengths to avoid the object, place, or situation that provokes it. They change jobs merely to avoid an elevator ride, for example, or cut back their social life. Some wear down their families with their clinging dependency. Nearly all lose out on much of life.

Many people go from doctor to doctor seeking cures for the physical symptoms that accompany their phobias. Often, even the doctor fails to recognize that stomach pains, high blood pressure, rapid heart beat, and other symptoms may be related to intense fear. Unless questioned, patients may not think to mention their fears. Doctors may not ask. While the bills keep mounting, the medical condition fails to improve.

The many phobic people who think their fears are silly, childish, or trivial often try to conceal them. While hiding from their fears, they hide their phobias from others, further limiting their experience of life.

It is better to tell someone. Much of the pain and disruption—perhaps most of it—can be remedied. New treatments for phobias are remarkably effective. But few people, including doctors, know about them.

If you or someone you know is excessively fearful—afraid out of all proportion to the cause—then you may gain some understanding of the problem from this pamphlet. It describes what experts know about phobias and panic. It may help you.

Phobias and Panic—Anxiety Disorders

Anxiety is the emotion you feel when a person, object, situation, or impulse seems dangerous to you. If you're crossing a street and suddenly notice a car speeding toward you, you feel afraid that you will be hit, and you dash out of the way. This fear and the behavior it provokes probably saved your life. If you're fed up with your boss and want to hit him, the sick feeling in the pit of your stomach—the anxiety you feel when you anticipate the consequences of slugging your boss—keep you from carrying through on your impulse. The anxiety and your control of your behavior probably saved your job.

While "normal" anxiety is adaptive—that is, it helps you to survive and be productive—too much anxiety can be crippling. People who suffer from certain patterns of signs and symptoms related to anxiety are considered by mental health specialists to have anxiety disorders. Phobias and panic attacks are the most common of these disorders.*

Both phobias and panic disorders are marked not only by great anxiety in situations that are relatively safe, but also by an exaggerated avoidance of the source of distress. Depending on the type of phobia or panic, the person may shy away from floor-to-ceiling windows in a highrise, refuse an invitation to speak in front of a church group, or stay out of crowded shopping malls. People with these disorders don't actually have to encounter what they fear.

They become intensely anxious just by anticipating that they might soon be in the feared situation, brooding over it in their imagination.

The fears can start in childhood or adulthood. Some people have suddenly become terrified of things they've been doing for years. For example, a flight attendant began having panic attacks on her 500th flight.

Some people can sidestep the thing they fear without much difficulty. Some, especially adults, can hide their distress and conceal their phobias. Even those who usually adjust their lives to fit their phobias are sometimes able to confront what they fear, "toughing it out," suffering all the while. While children may outgrow their phobias, adults usually do not get rid of them unless they receive treatment.

Recognized even in ancient times, phobias and panic are known around the world, probably in every human culture. The most recent and thorough studies show that, in the United States, phobias are the most common of all mental disorders. Seven out of every hundred Americans have phobias. Eight out of every thousand have panic disorder. Compared to men, women more often suffer from most types of phobia and panic disorder.

The reason that phobias and panic are more common in women is not known. Investigators speculate that men may be more likely to drown their fears, since alcohol abuse is more common in men than women. This is just one of the many possible explanations, however. Differences in biological makeup or social and psychological experiences may also be responsible. For example, in our society some girls are encouraged to be more fearful and less independent than males.

Types of Phobias and Panic

Mental health professionals now recognize three types of phobia—simple phobia, social phobia, and agoraphobia (with and without panic attacks)—and a separate diagnosis for people who repeatedly experience severe attacks of panic.

---

* Other anxiety disorders—generalized anxiety disorder, obsessive-compulsive disorder, posttraumatic stress disorder, and atypical anxiety disorder—are each characterized by somewhat different symptoms. They will not be discussed here.

Simple Phobias

The most common of the various phobias is simple phobia, the unreasonable fear of some object or situation. Bees, germs, heights, odors, illness, and storms are examples of the things commonly feared in simple phobias.

If you have a simple phobia, it might have begun when you actually did face a risk that realistically provoked anxiety. Perhaps, for example, you found yourself in deep water before you learned to swim. Extreme fear was appropriate in such a situation. But if you continue to avoid even the shallow end of a pool, your anxiety is excessive and may be of phobic proportions.

Simple phobias, especially animal phobias, are common in children, but they occur at all ages. The best evidence to date suggests that between 5 to 12 percent of the population have phobic disorders in any 6-month period.

The recognition by most phobics that their fears are unreasonable doesn't make them feel any less anxious. Simple phobias do not often interfere with daily life or cause as much subjective distress as most other anxiety disorders.

Social Phobias

The person with social phobia is intensely afraid of being judged by others. Even at a gathering of many people, the social phobic expects to be singled out, scrutinized, and found wanting. Thus, the person with a social phobia feels compelled to avoid social situations associated with such apprehensions.

If you have a social phobia, you might be afraid to go to a party because you fear that other people will laugh at your clothing or think you are hopeless stupid because you won't be able to think of anything to say. Like people with simple phobias, you work hard to avoid these anxiety-provoking situations.

People with social phobias are usually most anxious over feeling humiliated or embarrassed by showing fear in front of others. Ironically, they are often so crippled by the inhibitions resulting from such fears that they, in fact, may have difficulty thinking clearly, remembering facts, or expressing themselves in words. Even success in social situations fails to make them feel more confident. They are likely to think something like, "Next time I'll fall on my face."

Although studies of the incidence of social phobias are so far only preliminary, most experts believe social phobias are not as common as simple phobias. But because they result in considerable distress, people who suffer from them are more likely to seek treatment than are people with simple phobias. Social phobias tend to begin between the ages of 15 to 20 and, if left untreated, continue through much of the person's life. Often, social phobics suffer from symptoms of depression, and many also become dependent on alcohol.

Panic Disorder

Another group of anxious people are subject to devastating episodes of panic that are unexpected and seemingly without cause. Such unpredictable panic attacks are marked by an overwhelming sense of impending doom and a host of bodily symptoms. The person's heart races and breathing quickens, as he gasps for air. Sweating, weakness, dizziness, and feelings of unreality are also common. The person having the panic attack fears he is going to die, go crazy, or at least lose control. *

Panic disorder is diagnosed when patients experience repeated episodes of such panic. Although people with simple or social phobias may sometimes experience panic, they are clearly responding to an encounter—or an anticipated encounter—with the object or situation they fear. Such is not the case with panic disorder, when the fear strikes from nowhere, seemingly "out of the blue."

People with simple and social phobias can also predict that they will feel fear every time they come close to a cat, climb to the roof of a tall building, or encounter whatever else they fear. People with panic disorder, by contrast, never can predict when they will suddenly be struck by panic. Some situations may seem more "dangerous," especially those that make escape difficult, but an attack does not invariably occur in those situations.

Panic disorder, which runs in families, afflicts some 1.2 million Americans. For most, panic attacks begin sometime between the ages of 15 and 19.

Agoraphobia

Many people who suffer from panic attacks go on to develop agoraphobia, a severely handicapping disorder that often prevents its victims from leaving their homes unless accompanied by a friend or relative—a "safe" person. The first panic attack may follow some stressful event, such as a serious illness or the death of a loved one. (The agoraphobic often doesn't make this connection, though.) Fearing more attacks, the person develops a more-or-less continual state of anxiety, anticipating the next attack, avoiding situations where he would be helpless if a panic attack occurred. It is this avoidance behavior that distinguishes agoraphobia from panic disorder. Two different types of anxiety appear to afflict the person with agoraphobia—panic and the "anticipatory anxiety" engendered by expectations of future panic attacks.

If you have agoraphobia, chances are it developed something like this: One ordinary day, while tending to some chore, taking a walk, driving to work—in other words, just going about your usual business—you were suddenly struck by a wave of awful terror. Your heart started pounding, you trembled, you perspired profusely, and you had difficulty catching your breath. You became convinced that something terrible was happening to you, maybe you were going crazy, maybe you were having a heart attack, maybe you were about to die. You desperately sought safety, reassurance from your family, treatment at a clinic or emergency room. Your doctor could

---

* In the interest of brevity and grace of style, the pronoun "he" will be used throughout this pamphlet when either sex could be the topic of discussion.

find nothing wrong with you, so you went about your business, until a panic attack struck you again. As the attacks became more frequent, you spent more and more time thinking about them. You worried, watched for danger, and waited for the next one to hit.

You began to avoid situations where you had experienced an attack, then others where you would find it particularly difficult to cope with one—to escape and get help. You started by making minor adjustments in your habits—going to a supermarket at midnight, for example, rather than on the way home from work when the store tends to be crowded.

Gradually, you got to the point where you couldn't venture outside your immediate neighborhood, couldn't leave the house without your spouse, or maybe couldn't leave at all. What started out as an inconvenience turned into a nightmare. Like a creature in a horror movie, fear expanded until it covered the entire screen of your life.

To the outside observer, a person with agoraphobia may look no different from one with a social phobia. Both may stay home from a party. But their reasons for doing so are different. While the social phobic is afraid of the scrutiny of other people, many investigators believe that the agoraphobic is afraid of his or her own internal cues. The agoraphobic is afraid of feeling the dreadful anxiety of a panic attack, afraid of losing control in a crowd. Minor physical sensations may be interpreted as the prelude to some catastrophic threat to life.

Agoraphobics may abuse alcohol in an effort to keep the anticipatory anxiety in check. Their pattern of abuse appears to be different from the binging characteristic of alcoholism, however. The agoraphobic usually takes small amounts of alcohol, avoiding loss of control. Other drugs may also be abused.

Agoraphobia typically begins during the late teens or twenties. The best surveys done to date show that between 2.7 percent and 5.8 percent of the U.S. adult population suffer from agoraphobia. Women are affected two to four times more often than men. The condition tends to run in families.

Recent surveys have found that many people are afraid to leave their homes. Most likely, they are not all suffering from agoraphobia. Some people may stay confined because of depression, fear of street crime, or other reasons. These surveys also show, however, that many agoraphobics have never suffered a panic attack. This finding suggests that their agoraphobia may have developed in ways different from that outlined above.

Panic and agoraphobia have received a great deal of attention from clinical investigators in recent years. Some believe that panic attacks are a severe expression of general anxiety, while others think that they constitute a biologically distinct disorder, possibly related to depression, possibly indistinguishable from agoraphobia. This controversy will probably be resolved through more research in the coming years.

The Masquerade: Phobias and Other Conditions

Given the dramatic symptoms of phobic and panic disorder, it is surprising that they are sometimes difficult to recognize, even for medical professionals. Some patients, especially those with simple phobias, are able to conceal the severity of their handicap. Agoraphobia is often not detected because its physical symptoms become the center of concern for both patient and doctor. Health problems, such as peptic ulcer, high blood pressure, skin rashes, tics, tooth grinding, hemorrhoids, headaches, muscle aches, and heart disease, often occur together with anxiety disorders.

Phobias may cover up other problems. School phobia, a complex condition in which a youngster refuses to attend school, is one example; often the underlying problem is the child's anxiety over separating from his parents. (A mental health professional can easily distinguish between school phobia and other causes of missing school.)

Just as panic and phobias can masquerade as other illnesses, some physical diseases may be mistaken for anxiety disorders. For example, people can become anxious as a result of such medical conditions as head injury, withdrawal from alcohol or drugs, and even pneumonia. In these cases, the panicky feelings usually disappear when the condition clears up. Phobic behavior also occurs in conditions that are not diagnosed as phobias, such as the phobic-like avoidance of sexual contact in a person whose principal problem is sexual.

Reactive hypoglycemia—a rapid decline in blood sugar followed by compensatory changes in adrenaline and other hormones—can produce many symptoms of panic, such as sweating, heart palpitations, and tremor. Most likely, this medical condition mimics panic disorder.

More puzzling is the relationship between panic attacks and agoraphobia, on the one hand, and depression, on the other. About half of people subject to phobias and panic are demoralized or depressed more often than the average person. Many agoraphobic patients develop their symptoms shortly after suffering a loss (which can trigger depression), and some either have histories of depressive episodes themselves or have relatives who do.

Whether phobias cause depression or depression causes phobias is unknown. Panic and anxiety can wear down a person until he or she feels demoralized. Alternatively, phobia and panic might result from depression and its symptoms—difficulties with sleep, appetite, and concentration, fatigue, lack of pleasure, and feelings of worthlessness.

Yet another possibility is the simple coexistence of anxiety and depression, neither causing the other. Some underlying biological process—an inherited vulnerability, perhaps—may be common to both anxiety and depression.

Causes of Phobia and Panic

Phobias and panic, like all anxiety disorders, disturb many areas of a person's functioning. Take the woman who has agoraphobia. Her *behavior* changes when she has to quit her job because she thinks she is unable to ride the bus. Her *thinking* goes awry when she judges the risk she faces. The memory of past *feelings* of panic on the bus, when she was sure she would die, produces alterations in her *physiology* as her heart pounds, her head gets dizzy, and her hands sweat. Her behavior, thinking, emotions, and her body's physiological responses are all involved in her agoraphobia.

Evidence of these effects has guided research investigators who have tried to understand the causes of anxiety disorders. They have formed their theories by observing patients, listening carefully to what they say, and measuring their functioning in the laboratory. Scientists then go beyond these observations to test theories, either in the clinic or in scientific experiments. These experiments show that other aspects of anxiety and related disorders are not as clearly evident. Some of the most influential theories and bodies of research are described below.

Psychodynamic Theories

One possible cause of anxiety that is difficult for a nonspecialist to observe is psychological conflict arising from emotions and impulses that remain unconscious (outside of the person's awareness). Much of the theory proposed by Sigmund Freud early in this century assumes that such unconscious forces, mostly deriving from childhood, profoundly influence adult life, including abnormal anxious states. These influences, for the most part, are inferred from the memories and associations of patients who undergo intensive, prolonged therapy. Until the last two or three decades, Freud and the psychoanalytic investigators who revised his theories were the dominant force in explaining and treating anxiety-related conditions. Although now out of fashion in academic settings, the ideas of the psychoanalytic school have influenced thinking throughout society, especially in clinics where people are treated for mental health problems.

In the view of psychoanalysts, anxiety is a signal of danger—a danger that is not real and present, but, rather, is carried over from the memories and imaginations of childhood. Often, these dangers involve fantasies of loss of love (or actual separation from loved ones) or other fantasies that express guilt or sexually related events. When these fantasies are activated in adulthood—perhaps because something happens that the patient associates with the fantasies—they give rise to anxiety. The anxiety may be conscious or unconscious. In either case, it makes the person act defensively—that is, attempting to get away from the threat or, more often, to stop the fantasy from ever occurring by regulating or inhibiting the wishes that give rise to fantasies of danger. Because this defensive behavior relieves the anxiety, it tends to be repeated: it is, in other words, learned.

Modern psychodynamic research (that which focuses on mental conflicts) has put a great deal of emphasis on the anxiety that accompanies real or feared separation from a caretaker during childhood. Individuals who, as children, became extremely anxious whenever they were separated from their parents seem to be especially likely to develop agoraphobia later in life. Some 42 percent of agoraphobic patients report a history of childhood separation anxiety. This statistic suggests that agoraphobia may build on a foundation already present in early life or represent the aftermath of unresolved childhood separation anxiety.

In contemporary psychodynamic models, the person with agoraphobia avoids situations that symbolize or threaten separation from a loved one. This view explains why a death or other kind of loss may trigger agoraphobia. It also may explain why some agoraphobics can venture out when accompanied by a spouse, child, or friend.

Learning Theories

Psychoanalytic theory from Freud to the present day has given some role to learning as a necessity for the development of abnormal anxiety states. Another school of thought puts learning squarely at the center in its theory of anxiety. In the simplest learning model, an individual may learn fear through direct experience (e.g., being bitten by a snake) or indirectly by witnessing injury to someone else, by observing fear reactions of others, or by being warned of an object's dangers. More likely, however, the reaction is the result of an association between an unpleasant, fearful response and the chance presence of the object that later is viewed as threatening. As early as 1920, one experimental psychologist showed that a young boy could be trained to fear a harmless white rat if frightened by a loud noise every time the rat was nearby. Because the adult with a phobia seldom remembers such an event, the fear seems unreasonable.

Knowledge about learning also sheds light on the possible way in which agoraphobia develops. As with simple phobias, the person who first experiences panic attacks in the presence of a certain set of circumstances—alone in a crowd, for example—may learn to associate awful sensations of panic with all crowds. Repeating the experience, or anticipating it, may reproduce the feeling of threat. Avoiding crowds reduces the discomfort. Because the avoidance behavior is rewarded, the person is more likely to avoid crowds in the future. Avoidance also reduces the opportunity for the person to test whether crowds actually do cause panic. By foregoing this kind of potentially corrective experience, the person further strengthens the phobia.

Biological Theories

Observers studying anxiety, including Freud, have long predicted that the brain and the central nervous system would be found to be functioning abnormally in patients with serious anxiety disorders. Their predictions remained speculations, however, because they were limited by the methods and knowledge of their times. All that has changed. Because of recent technological advances, much of the research now being done on anxiety and related disorders focuses on the brain. Biological research workers also attempt to understand anxiety disorders by experimentally producing anxiety in human beings and other animals. Others look for physical symptoms that often accompany phobias or panic to see if they may play a role in causing the disorders.

The Brain and Central Nervous System

In light of what scientists would like to know about the role of the brain in anxiety disorders, this work has just begun. Research on neurotransmitters, the chemicals that carry messages from one nerve cell to another, has not found serious malfunctions associated with anxiety. But indirect measures suggest some abnormalities, particularly in the neurotransmitters norepinephrine, GABA, serotonin, and possibly adenosine.

Scientists are, however, still far from being able to say whether faulty brain function reflects the *cause* of anxiety disorders—some genetic fault coded into the person's hereditary apparatus, for example. Experts disagree about the meaning of some research findings. Much of the work, for example, has focused on the brain's processing of drugs that reduce anxiety. Such work suggests, but does not prove, how the brain functions during episodes of severe anxiety. Another problem so far has been that most research necessarily is confined to animals; whether the results apply to human beings is not certain. Pieces of the neuroscientific puzzle have been found, and they are beginning to fall into place.

Experimental "Anxiety"

Investigators have identified several substances over the past few years that can actually produce panic attacks in people who have already experienced them (but not in people who haven't). This line of evidence suggests that patients who are subject to panic attacks may be biologically different from other people. It also offers clues to just what those differences might be. The ability to induce panic attacks gives research investigators a powerful tool for understanding them.

The most thoroughly studied of these anxiety-producing chemicals is sodium lactate. The use of this substance to induce panic attacks is based on observation that some people who suffer extreme episodes of anxiety produce an excessive amount of the chemical lactate after routine exercise. For these people, exercise can actually set off a panic attack. Researchers have found that sodium lactate triggers panic attacks in a full 80 percent of patients with panic disorder, but in less than 20 percent of normal people. Lactate infusions may provide a means of suggesting which patients are biologically prone to panic attacks and thus apt to respond to drug treatments. It is unlikely, however, that lactate infusions will ever be a sure test.

Although less intensively studied, caffeine is another substance that can produce panic attacks in susceptible persons. Caffeine, of course, is common in coffee, tea, cola and other soft drinks, and many other foods such as chocolate. About half of panic disorder patients have panic experiences after consuming the caffeine equivalent to four or five cups of coffee. (Normal people also experience panic, but only after they ingest much higher amounts of caffeine.) Caffeine is thought to produce its effects by blocking the action of a brain chemical known as adenosine, a naturally occurring sedative. Clinical investigators have found that many people with panic attacks avoid caffeine after noticing that it causes attacks.

A Sampling of Other Biological Studies

Other types of biological research are also under way. One of the oldest experimental approaches tests physiological responses—for example, heart rate, blood pressure, sweating, or characteristics in the skin. Another type of research examines the role of hormones. But none of these studies has as yet been integrated with what is being learned from studies of the neurotransmitter systems in the brain.

Several studies have shown that patients suffering from agoraphobia and panic disorder have different physiological reactions to fear-producing stress than the average person has. Differences of this type may be present from birth and may explain why some individuals are more susceptible than are others to anxiety disorders.

Several years ago, a number of investigators reported that some agoraphobic patients have a mild heart condition known as mitral valve prolapse or MVP. Like agoraphobia itself, the condition tends to run in families. MVP can give rise to heart palpitations, which some experts believe might trigger panic attacks. It is also possible, however, that chronic anxiety and panic attacks may produce MVP or that both panic attacks and MVP may be symptoms of an underlying nervous system disorder. Finally, it still remains unclear whether there is *any* difference in the frequency of mitral valve prolapse in panic patients when compared to the general population.

Malfunctions in the thyroid gland have been reported in about one in ten patients who are prone to panic attacks. The relationship between these conditions, which can also cause heart palpitations, and panic is still in the early stages.

Because breathing difficulty is a hallmark of panic attacks, research scientists have recently become interested in hyperventilation, a condition marked by rapid breathing. The symptoms are similar to those experienced sometimes when blowing up a balloon: dizziness, inability to pay attention or concentrate, and tingling sensations around the mouth and fingers.

Anxiety as Heritage

The role of history—as recorded in our genes, passed on through our cultures, or learned in our families—is also under study. Barely under way are attempts to learn the relative contributions of nature and nurture to the development of phobias and panic disorder. Some investigators are studying families, because phobias and panic are more common in the relatives of patients than in the general population. Whether this tendency is inherited—passed on genetically— or learned by growing up or simply living close to other anxious people is not known, although some evidence suggests that the link is at least partly genetic.

Clues to what causes anxiety disorders also come from naturalistic observations of animals and human societies very unlike our own. Something like a phobia seems to occur in many animals. Some dogs who have never been touched by anything but a loving hand will cower and slink away at the sight of a broom. Their fear, as well as the common human fear of snakes, may hark back to some earlier stage in evolutionary development. In human societies, cultural differences seem to produce surprising variations in anxiety disorders—the age at which they begin, the course they follow, the symptoms, the distribution among different social groups, the source of anxiety, the experience of the emotion, and the consequences in the life of the sufferer.

Some fears are shared across cultures, suggesting that they enhanced the chance of surviving in the evolutionary history of the human race. Most phobias are directed toward a relatively small number of objects and situations, though there is no reason to believe that these items cause unpleasant experiences more frequently than many others. Phobic fear of truly dangerous electrical outlets, for example, is rare, while fear of seldom-encountered snakes and harmless insects is common. People in our culture are more likely to receive a shock from an outlet than a bite from a snake or one of these insects.

Scientists have sought to explain this paradox by speculating that humans may have an inborn predisposition to fear certain things. This so-called preparedness theory is consistent with the fact that most common phobias (darkness, animals, etc.) involve objects and situations that date from primitive times and were, in the distant past, serious sources of danger.

The Research in Sum

Despite all the research being done on the anxiety disorders—an activity that has accelerated in the last few years—none of the theories that are tested in the various types of studies is adequate to explain what causes phobias and panic. The explanation is probably not far off, however. As they are now propounded, theories about the causes of different types of anxiety disorders tend to cluster either around psychological and social factors or around biological factors. Simple phobias are usually explained in terms of early experience and learning, while agoraphobia and panic (and sometimes social phobia) are becoming increasingly understood as at least partially biological in origin. Most likely, all phobias and panic result from a mixture of influences, although that mixture probably changes with the type of phobia and individual differences among patients. Many theories reflect an implicit assumption that the more serious disorders, such as panic attacks and agoraphobia, are more likely to have a biological basis than the troubling, but less disabling, simple phobias.

Treatment

Even though causes of phobia and panic are not well understood, treatments for these disorders are often very effective. Therapists use a variety of techniques, their choice usually linked to their beliefs about the cause of the disorder. But, upon examination, it turns out that many of these techniques share a common feature: They all seem to require that patients confront the source of their discomfort. Some therapists ask their patients* to confront a feared situation in imagination, while others require a real-life confrontation. Some therapists define the source of fear as the external object or situation the patient identifies as fearful, while others find a deeper source within the patient—in the unconscious, in thoughts, or in physical sensations. Still another difference is that one therapist might set up an explicit program for confronting feared objects and situations, while another might use drugs or psychotherapy to prepare the patient to confront fearful situations in everyday life.

Psychotherapy

For the first two-thirds of this century, phobias, like other emotional disorders, were treated almost exclusively by psychoanalysis or related forms of psychotherapy. In psychoanalysis, unconscious conflict is seen as the source of anxiety.

The goal of therapy is to bring that conflict to light, analyze what it means to the patient, and substitute present-day realistic appraisals for fearful ones that are based on the limited understandings of childhood. Psychoanalysis techniques include free association (encouraging the patient to say whatever comes into his mind), analysis of dreams, and analysis of the relationship between the patient and the therapist. Other forms of psychotherapy are usually more directive in their techniques: instead of waiting for the patient's memories and feelings to emerge and drawing inferences from these patterns of association, some therapists actively try to provoke or suggest sources of conflict and direct their patients through "homework" assignments.

Unfortunately, psychoanalysis and related forms of psychotherapy prove disappointing in the treatment of phobias. Patients usually find the therapy helpful in resolving conflict, decreasing general anxiety, and identifying and modifying feelings and thoughts associated with panic attacks and phobic avoidance. But the phobic symptoms themselves often remain. Freud himself acknowledged the limitations of pure psychoanalysis in treating phobias (and anticipated the development of behavioral techniques), saying: "One can hardly ever master a phobia if one waits 'til the patient lets the analysis influence him to give it up. . . . One succeeds only when one can induce them through the influence of the analysis to go about alone and to struggle with their anxiety while they make the attempt."

Just such an approach has been found to be effective in helping phobic patients stop avoiding the thing they fear (see section on exposure therapy below). Many therapists find that such improvements are more lasting if patients undergo psychotherapy as well, either individually or in groups. By monitoring situations that seem to give rise to the panic attacks, for example, an agoraphobic can identify thoughts and feelings that are troublesome. The therapist can then help the patient to work out a course of action that might realistically change the source of distress and to give up the habitual style of avoiding it by retreat into phobic behavior. Therapists can also help the patient to become more assertive when involved in conflict with other people and train him in skills needed for other social situations. The support of a caring therapist may be crucial for long-term success of any treatment technique.

Early Behavioral Techniques

A landmark event in the development of treatment for phobias occurred with the publication of a book in 1958. In the book, Joseph Wolpe, a learning theorist, reported excellent results from treating adult phobic patients with a procedure called "systematic desensitization," which he had adapted from a technique developed in the 1920s for helping children overcome animal phobias. Systematic desensitization requires the client to learn formal, deep-muscle relaxation. It is up to the client also to rank situations related to the phobia that cause anxiety. An individual who fears snakes, for example, might place "holding a snake" at the top of the list of

---

* The term "patient," usually heard in medical settings, will be used here interchangeably with the term "client," more typically used by psychologists and social workers.

things that make him anxious and "viewing a caged snake from across the room" at the bottom of the list.

The client is then asked to imagine, in as much detail as possible, the least fear-provoking scene from his list. At the same time he is asked to relax as previously taught. By remaining comfortable while imagining the feared situation, the client may weaken the association between the situation and feelings of anxiety. Once the client has become comfortable imagining the least threatening situation, he moves up the list and masters each in turn.

Proponents of this method have claimed that facing a feared situation in imagination is as effective as confronting it in reality. But most therapists have found that there is a gap between fantasy and reality. In other words, once the client has desensitization treatment and undertakes to face the real object or situation, he is likely to have to move part of the way back down his list. For example, though he has learned to remain calm while holding an imaginary snake, he may at first be able to touch, but not to hold, a real snake. By practicing further in the real situation, however, he may eventually be able to fully master his fear.

Systematic desensitization was the first form of behavior therapy used to treat phobias. The late 1960s witnessed development of another, named "implosion," which soon came to be widely used in a modified form termed "imaginal flooding."

Flooding, like desensitization, involves the client's experiencing fear-provoking situations in his imagination. In other ways, flooding and desensitization are quite different. In flooding, the therapist, rather than the client, controls the time and content of the scenes to be imagined. He describes these scenes with great vividness, in a deliberate effort to make them as disturbing as possible. Also, the client is not instructed to relax; rather, the aim is for him to experience his fears and anxieties with maximum intensity, in the hope that by surviving "the worst," he can loosen the phobia's grip on him. The prolonged experience with these feared images is thought to help the client get used to them, so that they gradually lose their power to cause anxiety.

In the early days of implosive therapy and flooding, therapists included scenes referring to guessed-at unconscious conflicts believed to underlie the patient's phobias. But studies showed that not only were the horrifying scenes of implosion very disturbing to patients (sometimes causing nightmares), but also they did not make treatment any more effective than flooding alone. Thus, implosive techniques are no longer used.

A number of researchers have compared desensitization and flooding. They have found that the two forms of treatment are about equally effective: Both reduce phobic anxiety and behavior in people with simple phobias, but desensitization is not as effective as flooding for agoraphobia. Although not well studied, neither method appears to be very effective for social phobics.

Exposure Therapy

When behavior therapists observed that the exposure to the feared situation was the common ingredient in desensitization and flooding, they began to develop other techniques they hoped would be even more effective. While earlier methods were aimed at reducing anxiety so that clients could change their behavior (e.g., enter feared situations), the new techniques focused instead on altering behavior. Once behavior changed, the reasoning went, anxiety would diminish.

The underlying assumption is that phobic anxiety is maintained—it continues and may get more intense—when the person repeatedly avoids the object or situation that elicits the anxiety. Avoidance prevents him from "unlearning" the association between an object or situation and anxiety. Exposure to such situations, by contrast, gradually habituates the person to it—that is, he learns that no real danger is present. Gradually, the anxiety is extinguished. Some therapists believe that the more rapidly such exposure takes place, the more rapidly the phobia will be eliminated.

In treatment, the therapist explains this rationale to the client, outlines the procedure that will be followed, and helps him anticipate what his reactions are likely to be. The therapist assures the client that he will always be available to help the client cope with the sense of danger, and will be ready to stop the procedure at any time the client seems unable to tolerate the danger.

The client is then exposed to the object or situation he fears. Techniques differ in how gradually the person is made to encounter fearful objects and how long the exposure continues. In general, clients are asked to stay in the situation until their anxiety begins to diminish. With each session, they tolerate closer and longer confrontations with the threatening object or circumstance.

Such in vivo (in life) exposure has replaced methods that rely upon imagined danger. It is considered the treatment of choice for simple phobias. Most investigators also believe that it is the best available treatment for agoraphobia when accompanied by drug treatment (see below). Some therapists use exposure in imagination as a means of helping their clients confront feared situations in real life. There is some evidence that the effects of treatment may be more long-lasting when imagination-based exposure is used along with in vivo exposure, although not everyone needs both. Programs using in vivo exposure techniques have become the mainstay in the treatment of simple phobias and agoraphobia. Exposure does not seem to be as effective in treating social phobias, unless it is accompanied by training in specific social skills.

Cognitive Therapies

Several recently developed techniques that try to change the phobic's thought pattern may be used along with exposure. Most of these techniques have grown out of behavioral therapists' attempts to account for and change the persistent habits of thought that seem to bind people to their fears. One form of cognitive-behavioral treatment—"self-statement training"—teaches clients to become aware of such negative thought statements as, "I'll faint if I touch that," or, "I can't do it," and to replace them with positive coping statements like, "Of course, I *can* do it." Once the client has become familiar with this approach, he can use it to help himself through a behavioral treatment program.

Taking a completely different tack, therapists using "paradoxical intention" encourage clients to try to feel as anxious and panicky as possible. Clients are urged to exaggerate their symptoms, often with a note of humor. For example, a woman who is afraid she may faint or fall down might be instructed to "faint" on purpose and to warn those around her: "Stay out of my way. When I fall, I fall hard. I bet I'm the best fainter you've ever seen." Frequently, taking charge of the symptoms in this way diminishes their force. In fact, a client who is "trying" to faint, sweat, or tremble may find himself unable to do so.

Drug Therapy

Over the years, many drugs have been tried by phobic patients. Barbiturates provided little benefit. The newer class of drugs used to treat generalized anxiety, the benzodiazepines (such as Valium or Librium), do lessen the anticipatory anxiety that accompanies phobias, but do not generally block panic attacks. The exception is alprazolam, a modified benzodiazepine, which appears to be effective in moderate to high doses, although dependency is often an unavoidable side effect when the drug is taken for long periods of time.

Beginning in the early 1960s, however, it was discovered that certain antidepressants could prevent the unpredictable panic attacks characteristic of agoraphobia. The assumption is that once panic attacks no longer threaten the patient, the anxiety that accompanies anticipation of future panic attacks and the avoidance behavior will also diminish. The two types of drugs that have been most extensively tested and shown to be effective are the MAO inhibitors (for example, phenelzine) and tricyclic antidepressants (for example, imipramine). Although usually used to relieve depression, these drugs also produce antianxiety actions that are independent of their antidepressant effects. Anticipatory anxiety sometimes diminishes once panic attacks have stopped. Some patients respond at low dosages, but most appear to require amounts equal to that needed to reduce depression.

MAO inhibitors and tricyclic antidepressants do produce some unwanted side effects. Most of these side effects, such as drowsiness, gradually subside after the drug is taken for several weeks. MAO inhibitors require special caution, however. Patients taking these drugs must restrict their intake of certain foods, such as aged cheese, red wine, and other medications. Reactions between these substances and the MAO inhibitors can produce high blood pressure, severe headaches, and other side effects that in rare cases can be life-threatening. Despite these possible complications, the MAO inhibitors, when used judiciously, can produce remarkable improvements in patients prone to panic attacks.

Drug therapy for panic attacks is generally given for periods of 6 months to 1 year. Many patients can then manage well without drugs, although relapses requiring resumption of medication are common. The relative duration of success of various therapies is still a matter of controversy.

As noted, most antianxiety drugs are not thought to be effective in stopping panic attacks, although recent research suggests that in very high amounts they may be. The common tranquilizers, such as Valium and Librium, are sometimes also used to treat the generalized anxiety that accompanies phobias.

As noted earlier, a relatively new drug, alprazolam (Xanax), a type of benzodiazepine, has been found to block panic attacks quite dramatically within days after patients start taking it. This rapid response, along with many other positive features, may make alprazolam a useful drug for treating panic, although this use has not yet been approved by the U.S. Food and Drug Administration. Alprazolam has the disadvantage, however, of producing physical dependence and drowsiness in some patients. Seizures have also been reported when the drug is abruptly discontinued.

Another class of drugs, beta adrenergic blockers, has been found useful in treating some phobias, especially specific types of social phobias, such as public speaking phobia. These drugs, usually used to treat high blood pressure, may be used in patients who do not respond to other forms of treatment. There is some suggestion that they may be especially appropriate for patients who have such physical symptoms as trembling and heart palpitations. MAO inhibitors have also been demonstrated to be effective in the treatment of social phobias.

Nutrition

Solutions to the problem of phobias have also been sought in the realm of nutrition. Certainly, severely malnourished individuals are less able than others to cope with stress. And, patients who are subject to panic attacks have been found to be unusually sensitive to caffeine and may wish to gradually eliminate it from their diets. Otherwise, there is no reliable evidence that any special diet is likely to benefit most phobic patients.

Phobia Treatment Programs

Phobia treatment programs now exist in many parts of the United States. These programs use a variety of behavioral therapy techniques to help clients confront and overcome their fears. In addition, through these programs drugs may be recommended and prescribed for individuals likely to benefit from them.

In a typical program, phobic individuals work together in groups with a trained group leader. In some programs, family members and friends are also invited to attend the weekly meetings. Group sessions are used to teach attitudes and skills that are helpful in overcoming phobias. The client also has weekly practice sessions, either alone or in a group, with a therapist who is a mental health professional or a recovered phobic. During these sessions, the client uses his new coping skills in situations he would previously have avoided. With the therapist at his side, he gradually takes progressively more difficult steps toward his final goal. Setbacks are expected and viewed as opportunities for further practice and gain. Agoraphobic clients who are housebound sometimes begin their treatment in their own homes.

Although organized phobia treatment programs offer many advantages, they do not exist in all areas. Many individual therapists are experienced at working with phobic patients, and some will accompany their patients in fear-producing situations.

Referrals to treatment programs and therapists can be obtained by calling or writing to the local, regional, or state chapters of the American Psychological Association, the American Psychiatric Association, the National Association of Social Workers, the American Nurses Association, the American Association for Counseling and Development, and the Phobia Society of America. In addition, several books and tape cassettes offer self-treatment programs. Since the effectiveness of these programs has not been evaluated, referral to them in this pamphlet does not imply an endorsement by the National Institute of Mental Health.

A word of caution: Not every form of treatment is appropriate for every patient or client. Nor does every therapist or phobia program offer all forms of treatment—psychotherapy, behavior therapy, and medications. Often, a combination of these treatments is necessary. If you feel that you are not being helped by one clinic, program, or therapist, you may wish to seek help elsewhere.

Outcomes and Outlook

The outlook for people with phobias has improved greatly in the last two decades. People with simple phobias can often be relieved of their fears in a matter of weeks. People subject to panic attacks can usually find relief with antidepressant medication. Through the use of these drugs and exposure treatment, people with agoraphobia can be helped to venture out and face the threatening situations they have been avoiding. People with social phobias can be taught the social skills and helped somewhat with exposure therapy and medication. All can learn to understand their fears, and possibly solidify their progress, with the help of other therapies—group or individual psychotherapy or family therapy.

If you or someone you know has a phobia, don't bypass the chance for help. Because physical diseases sometimes mimic phobias, it is a good idea to consult a physician to make certain that symptoms don't mask a serious physical illness. Then find someone who is skilled in treating phobias. The odds are three to one that the treatment will succeed.

Glossary

Acrophobia. Fear of heights.

Aerophobia. Fear of flying.

Agoraphobia. Fear of open spaces.

Amathophobia. Fear of dust.

Apiphobia. Fear of bees.

Astrapophobia. Fear of lightning.

Batrachophobia. Fear of reptiles.

Blennophobia. Fear of slime.

Claustrophobia. Fear of enclosed spaces.

Cynophobia. Fear of dogs.

Decidophobia. Fear of making decisions.

Electrophobia. Fear of electricity.

Eremophoba. Fear of being alone.

Gamophobia. Fear of marriage.

Gatophobia. Fear of cats.

Gephyrophobia. Fear of crossing bridges.

Gynophobia. Fear of women.

Hydrophobia. Fear of water.

Kakorraphiaphobia. Fear of failure.

Katagelophobia. Fear of ridicule.

Keraunophobia. Fear of thunder.

Musophobia. Fear of mice.

Mysophobia. Fear of dirt, germs, or contamination.

Nyctophobia. Fear of night.

Ochlophobia. Fear of crowds.

Odynephobia. Fear of pain.

Ophidiophobia. Fear of snakes.

Pnigerophobia. Fear of smothering.

Pyrophobia. Fear of fire.

Scholionophobia. Fear of school.

Sciophobia. Fear of shadows.

Spheksophobia. Fear of wasps.

Technophobia. Fear of technology.

Thalassophobia. Fear of the ocean.

Topophobia. Fear of performing (stage fright).

Triskaidekaphoba. Fear of the number 13.

Tropophobia. Fear of moving or making changes.

For Further Information

Beck, A.T.; Emery, G.; and Greenberg, R.L. *Anxiety Disorders and Phobias—A Cognitive Perspective.* New York: Basic Books, 1985.

DuPont, R.L., ed. *Phobia: A Comprehensive Summary of Modern Treatments.* New York: Brunner/Mazel, 1982.

Ferber, L. Phobias and their vicissitudes. *Journal of the American Psychoanalytic Association.* 7:182, 1959.

Klein, D.F., and Rabkin, J.G., eds. *Anxiety: New Research and Changing Concepts.* New York: Raven Press, 1981.

Marks, I.M. *Cure and Care of Neuroses.* New York: Wiley, 1981.

Mavissakalian, M., and Barlow, D.H., eds. *Phobia: Psychological and Pharmacological Treatment.* New York: The Guilford Press, 1981.

Sheehan, D.V. *The Anxiety Disease.* New York: Charles Scribner's Sons, 1983.

Tuma, A.H., and Maser, J., eds. *Anxiety and the Anxiety Disorders.* Hillsdale, N.J.: Erlbaum, 1985.

Uhde, T.W., and Nemiah, J.C. Panic and generalized anxiety disorders. In *Comprehensive Textbook of Psychiatry,* 5th ed. Eds. H.I. Kaplan and B.J. Sadock, Baltimore: Williams and Wilkins, 1988.

VanPraag, H.M., ed. *Research in Neurosis.* New York: SP Medical and Scientific Books, 1978.

Weiss, E., ed. *Agoraphobia in the Light of Ego Psychology.* New York: Grune and Stratton, 1964.

Zitrin, C.M.; Klein, D.F.; Woerner, M.G.; and Ross, D.C. Treatment of phobias. I. Comparison of imipramine hydrochloride and placebo. *Archives of General Psychiatry,* 40:125, 1983.

This booklet was written by Bette Runck, science writer in the Science Communication Branch, Office of Scientific Information, National Institute of Mental Health (NIMH). An earlier version was done on contract for NIMH by Washington, D.C., science writer Elaine Blume. Drafts were reviewed, sometimes repeatedly, by many experts on phobia. The assistance of the following is gratefully acknowledged: Jack D. Maser, Ph.D., Barry Wolfe, Ph.D., Jack Blaine, M.D., Robert Prien, Ph.D., Barbara Scupi, M.S., Thomas W. Uhde, M.D., Robert M. Post, M.D., Jack D. Burke, Jr., M.D., and Jeffrey H. Boyd, M.D., all NIMH staff members; Donald F. Klein, M.D., and Michael R. Liebowitz, M.D., New York State Psychiatric Institute, New York City; Robert Michels, M.D., and Katherine Shear, M.D., the New York Hospital-Cornell University Medical Center, New York City; Peter A. Di Nardo, Ph.D., State University of New York, Oneonta, N.Y.; Michael J.

Kozak, Ph.D., Temple University School of Medicine, Philadelphia; and Bruce N. Cuthbert, Ph.D., University of Florida, Gainesville. Editorial assistance was provided by NIMH staff members Anne Cooley, Marilyn Sargent, Myrle Kahn, and Sherry Prestwich.

■ **Document Source:**
   U.S. Department of Health and Human Services, Public Health Service

Alcohol, Drug Abuse, and Mental Health Administration
National Institute of Mental Health
 5600 Fishers Ln., Rockville, MD 20857
 DHHS Publication No. (ADM) 89-1472
 Printed 1986. Reprinted 1989.

See also: Understanding Panic Disorder (page 303)

NEUROLOGICAL DISORDERS

■ ■ ■

ALZHEIMER'S DISEASE

What Is Alzheimer's?

"Alzheimer's disease" is the term used to describe a dementing disorder marked by certain brain changes, regardless of the age of onset. Alzheimer's disease is not a normal part of aging—it is not something that inevitably happens in later life. Rather, it is one of the dementing disorders, a group of brain diseases that lead to the loss of mental and physical functions. The disorder, whose cause is unknown, affects a small but significant percentage of older Americans. A very small minority of Alzheimer's patients are under 50 years of age. Most are over 65.

Alzheimer's disease is the exception, rather than the rule, in old age. Only 5 to 6 percent of older people are afflicted by Alzheimer's disease or a related dementia—but this means approximately 3 to 4 million Americans have one of these debilitating disorders. Research indicates that 1 percent of the population aged 65-74 has severe dementia, increasing to 7 percent of those aged 75-84 and to 25 percent of those 85 or older. At least half the people in U.S. nursing homes have Alzheimer's disease or a related disorder; in 1985, the annual cost of caring for individuals with Alzheimer's disease and related dementias in institutional and community settings was estimated between $24 billion and $48 billion for direct costs alone and is probably higher today. As our population ages and the number of Alzheimer's patients increases, costs of care will rise as well.

Although Alzheimer's disease is not curable or reversible, there are way to alleviate symptoms and suffering and to assist families. Not every person with this illness must necessarily move to a nursing home. Many thousands of patients—especially those in the early stages of the disease—are cared for by their families in the community. Indeed, one of the most important aspects of medical management is family education and family support services. When, or whether, to transfer a patient to a nursing home is a decision to be carefully considered by the family.

Who Gets Alzheimer's Disease?

The main risk factor for Alzheimer's disease is increased age. The rates of the disease increase markedly with advancing age, with 25 percent of people over 85 suffering from Alzheimer's or other severe dementia.

Some investigators, describing a family pattern of Alzheimer's disease, suggest that in some cases heredity may influence its development. A genetic basis has been identified through the discovery of a genetic marker on chromosome 21 for a small subgroup of families in which the disease has frequently occurred at relatively early ages (beginning before age 50). Some evidence points to chromosome 19 as implicated in certain other families that have frequently had the disease develop at later ages.

At the same time, data indicate that the likelihood that a close relative (sibling, child, or parent) of an afflicted individual will develop Alzheimer's disease is low. In most cases, such an individual's risk is only slightly higher than that of someone in the general population, where the lifetime risk is below 1 percent. And, of course, many disorders have a genetic potential that is never expressed—that is, despite being at risk for a certain illness, one might go through life without ever developing any symptom of the disease.

What to Expect When Someone Has Alzheimer's Disease

Mary Ellen's friends thought she was the perfect mother, wife, friend, and hostess. Her husband George, a prolific author, counted on her to edit his works and manage his schedule. He was the first to notice that she was no longer able to remember her good friends' names, her children's birthdays, or the details of her busy life. During social occasions, she could be seen sitting on the sidelines, answering politely but vaguely if spoken to, but never engaged in meaningful conversation. She was no longer able to go shopping or pay the household bills as she had done for the past 30 years. George was bewildered and could not understand what had happened to his close companion of so many years.

The onset of Alzheimer's disease is usually very slow and gradual, seldom occurring before age 65. Over time, however, it follows a progressively more serious course. Among the symptoms that typically develop, none is unique to Alzheimer's disease at its various stages. It is therefore essential for suspicious changes to be thoroughly evaluated before they become inappropriately or negligently labeled Alzheimer's disease.

Problems of memory, particularly recent or short-term memory, are common early in the course of the disease. For example, the individual may, on repeated occasions, forget to turn off the iron or may not recall which of the morning's medicines were taken. Mild personality changes, such as less spontaneity or a sense of apathy and a tendency to withdraw from social interactions, may occur early in the illness. As the disease progresses, problems in abstract thinking or in intellectual functioning develop. The individual may begin to have trouble with figures when working on bills, with understanding what is being read, or with organizing the day's work. Further disturbances in behavior and appearance may also be seen at this point, such as agitation, irritability, quarrelsomeness, and diminishing ability to dress appropriately.

Later in the course of the disorder, the affected individuals may become confused or disoriented about what month or year it is and be unable to describe accurately where they live or to name correctly a place being visited. Eventually they may wander, be unable to engage in conversation, seem inattentive and erratic in mood, appear uncooperative, lose bladder and bowel control, and, in extreme cases, become totally incapable of caring for themselves if the final stage is reached. Death then follows, perhaps from pneumonia or some other problem that occurs in severely deteriorated states of health. The average course of the disease from the time it is recognized to death is about 6 to 8 years, but it may range from under 2 to over 20 years. Those who develop the disorder later in life may die from other illnesses (such as heart disease) before Alzheimer's disease reaches its final and most serious stage.

Though the changes just described represent the general range of symptoms for Alzheimer's disease, the specific problems, along with the rate and severity of decline, can vary considerably with different individuals. Indeed, most persons with Alzheimer's disease can function at a reasonable level and remain at home far into the course of the disorder. Moreover, throughout much of the course of the illness individuals maintain the capacity for giving and receiving love, for sharing warm interpersonal relationships, and for participating in a variety of meaningful activities with family and friends.

A person with Alzheimer's disease may no longer be able to do math, but still be able to read a magazine with pleasure for months or years to come. Playing the piano might become too stressful in the face of increasing mistakes, but singing along with others may still be satisfying. The chess board may have to be put away, but one may still be able to play tennis. Thus, despite the many exasperating moments in the lives of Alzheimer patients and their families, many opportunities remain for positive interactions. Challenge, frustration, closeness, anger, warmth, sadness, and satisfaction may all be experienced by those who work to help the person with Alzheimer's disease cope as well as possible with the disease.

The reaction of an individual to the illness—his or her capacity to cope with it—also varies and may depend on such factors as lifelong personality patterns and the nature and severity of stress in the immediate environment. Depression, severe uneasiness, and paranoia or delusions may accompany

or result from the disease, but they can often be alleviated by appropriate treatments. Although there is no cure for Alzheimer's disease, treatments are available to alleviate many of the symptoms that cause suffering.

The Diagnosis of Alzheimer's Disease

Abnormal Brain Tissue Findings

1. Plaques and Tangles

Microscopic brain tissue changes have been described in Alzheimer's disease since Alois Alzheimer first reported them in 1906. The two principal changes are senile or neurotic plaques (chemical deposits consisting of degenerating nerve cells combined with a form of protein called beta amyloid) and neurofibrillary tangles (malformations within nerve cells). The brains of Alzheimer's disease patients of all ages reveal these findings on autopsy examination.

The plaques found in the brains of people with Alzheimer's disease appear to be made, in part, from protein molecules—amyloid precursor protein (APP)—that normally are essential components of the brain. Plaques are made when an enzyme snips APP apart at a specific place and then leaves the fragments—beta amyloid—in brain tissue where they come together in abnormal deposits. It has not as yet been definitely determined how neurofibrillary tangles are formed.

As research on Alzheimer's disease progresses, scientists are describing other abnormal anatomical and chemical changes associated with the disease. These include nerve cell degeneration in the brain's nucleus basalis of Meynert and reduced levels of the neurotransmitter acetylcholine in the brains of Alzheimer's disease victims. But from a practical standpoint, the "classical" plaque and tangle changes seen in the brain at autopsy typically suffice for a diagnosis of Alzheimer's disease. In fact, it is still only through the study of brain tissue from a person who was thought to have Alzheimer's disease that a definitive diagnosis of the disorder can be made.

2. Brain Scans

Computer-assisted tomography (CAT scan) changes become more evident as the disease progresses—not necessarily early on. Thus a CAT scan performed in the first stages of the disease cannot in itself be used to make a definitive diagnosis of Alzheimer's disease; its value is in helping to establish whether certain disorders (some reversible) that mimic Alzheimer's disease are present. Later on, CAT scans often reveal changes characteristic of Alzheimer's disease, namely an atrophied (shrunken) brain with widened sulci (tissue indentations) and enlarged cerebral ventricles (fluid-filled chambers).

Several new types of instrumentation are enabling researchers to learn even more about the brain. Both positron emission tomography (PET scan) and SPECT (single photon emission computerized tomography) can map regional cerebral blood flow, metabolic activity, and distribution of specific receptors, as well as integrity of the blood-brain barrier. These procedures may reveal abnormalities characteristic of Alzheimer's disease. Another method, magnetic resonance imaging (MRI), probes the brain by examining the interaction of the magnetic properties of atoms with an external magnetic field. MRI provides both structural and chemical information and distinguishes moving blood from static brain tissue (Taylor, 1990).

Clinical Features of Alzheimer's Disease

The "clinical" features of Alzheimer's disease, as opposed to the "tissue" changes, are threefold:

1. Dementia—significant loss of intellectual abilities such as memory capacity, severe enough to interfere with social or occupational functioning;
2. Insidious onset of symptoms—subtly progressive and irreversible course with documented deterioration over time;
3. Exclusion of all other specific causes of dementia by history, physical examination, laboratory tests, psychometric, and other studies.

Diagnosis By Exclusion

Based on these criteria, the clinical diagnosis of Alzheimer's disease has been referred to as "a diagnosis by exclusion," and one that can only be made in the face of clinical deterioration over time. There is no specific clinical test or finding that is unique to Alzheimer's disease. Hence, all disorders that can bring on similar symptoms must be systematically excluded or "ruled out." This explains why diagnostic workups of individuals where the question of Alzheimer's disease has been raised can be so frustrating to patient and family alike; they are not told that Alzheimer's disease has been specifically diagnosed, but that other possible diagnoses have been dismissed, leaving Alzheimer's disease as the likely diagnosis by the process of elimination.

Some scientists think that the results from biochemical research may lead to a diagnostic "marker" for certain persons evaluated for Alzheimer's disease. For example, research has discovered a protein, called Alzheimer's Disease Associated Protein (ADAP), in the autopsied brains of Alzheimer's patients, is mainly concentrated in the cortex covering the front and side sections of the brain regions involved in memory function. Researchers have found ADAP not only in brain tissue but also in spinal fluid. If they can perfect a test to detect the protein in the cerebrospinal fluid, or potentially even circulating in the blood, it may be possible to use this method of diagnosis on living patients.

Many scientists are working at developing other tests or procedures that may someday identify living persons with the disorder, perhaps even early in its course before behavioral changes become evident. Still, a reliable, specific diagnostic marker for Alzheimer's disease is not yet available.

Meanwhile, Alzheimer's disease is the most over diagnosed and misdiagnosed disorder of mental functioning in older adults. Part of the problem, already alluded to, is that many other disorders show symptoms that resemble those of Alzheimer's disease. The crucial difference, though, is that many of these disorders—unlike Alzheimer's disease—may be stopped, reversed, or cured with appropriate treatment. But

first they must be identified and not dismissed as Alzheimer's disease or senility.

Conditions that affect the brain and result in intellectual, behavioral, and psychological dysfunction are referred to as "organic mental disorders." These disorders represent a broad grouping of diseases and include Alzheimer's disease. Organic mental disorders that can cause clinical problems like those of Alzheimer's disease, but which might be reversible or controlled with proper diagnosis and treatment, include the following:

- ♦ **Side Effects of Medications:** Unusual reactions to medications, too much or too little of prescribed medications, combinations of medications which, when taken together, cause adverse side effects.
- ♦ **Substance Abuse:** Abuse of legal and/or illegal drugs, alcohol abuse.
- ♦ **Metabolic Disorders:** Thyroid problems, nutritional deficiencies, anemias, etc.
- ♦ **Circulatory Disorders:** Heart problems, strokes, etc.
- ♦ **Neurological Disorders:** Normal-pressure hydrocephalus, multiple sclerosis, etc.
- ♦ **Infections:** Especially viral or fungal infections of the brain.
- ♦ **Trauma:** Injuries to the head.
- ♦ **Toxic Factors:** Carbon monoxide, methyl alcohol, etc.
- ♦ **Tumors:** Any type within the skull—whether originating or metastasizing there.

In addition to organic mental disorders resulting from these diverse causes, other forms of mental dysfunction or mental health problems can also be confused with Alzheimer's disease. For example, severe forms of depression can cause problems with memory and concentration that initially may be indistinguishable from early symptoms of Alzheimer's disease. Sometimes these conditions, referred to as "pseudodementia," can be reversed. Other psychiatric problems can similarly masquerade as Alzheimer's disease, and, like depression, respond to treatment.

Of course, not all memory changes or complaints in later life signal Alzheimer's disease or mental disorder. Many memory changes are only temporary, such as those that occur with bereavement or any stressful situation that makes it difficult to concentrate. In fact, older people are often accused or accuse themselves of memory changes which are not really taking place. If a person in his thirties misplaces keys or a wallet, forgets the name of a neighbor, or calls one sibling by another's name, nobody gives it a second thought. But the same normal forgetfulness for people in their seventies may raise unjustifiable concern. On the other hand, serious memory difficulties should not be dismissed as an unavoidable part of normal aging. Since rigorous studies on intelligence in later life show that healthy people who stay intellectually active maintain a sharp mind throughout the life cycle, noticeable decline in older adults that interferes with functioning should be clinically explored for an underlying problem.

The Importance of a Comprehensive Clinical Evaluation

Because of the many other disorders that can be confused with Alzheimer's disease, a comprehensive clinical evaluation is essential to arrive at a correct diagnosis of symptoms that look like those of Alzheimer's disease. Such an assessment should include at least three major components—(1) a thorough general medical workup, (2) a neurological examination, and (3) a psychiatric evaluation that may include psychological or psychometric testing. The family physician can be consulted about the best way to get the necessary examinations.

> George tried to get Mary Ellen to see their family physician but she refused. Finally, he suggested that they both go in to have their blood pressure checked. The doctor was shocked at the deterioration in Mary Ellen's personality and scheduled a complete physical examination for her. He also made an appointment with a neurologist for further neurological examination, including a CAT scan. A psychiatrist working in the same office conducted a psychiatric evaluation. George helped by giving them many details of Mary Ellen's history. A tentative diagnosis of Alzheimer's disease was made, and George was instructed to bring Mary Ellen back in 6 months for further evaluation. George still hoped that Mary Ellen's condition was temporary and told no one of his distress. When their two daughters called, he always made excuses as to why their mother did not answer the telephone. He neglected his writing as more of his time was taken up with household tasks that Mary Ellen no longer even tried to do.

The Search for the Cause of Alzheimer's Disease

Alzheimer's disease has emerged as one of the great mysteries in modern day medicine, with a growing number of clues but still no answers as to its cause. The quest to uncover its cause has the air of a veritable whodunit saga. Though none of the leading theories about the genesis of Alzheimer's disease has resolved the mystery, each has led to certain intriguing findings that suggest further investigation is needed. It is important to examine these theories, not only to understand current thinking on Alzheimer's disease, but also to learn what popular ideas have provided to be incorrect. There have been at least five prominent theories about the cause of Alzheimer's disease.

Chemical Theories (Deficiencies and Toxic Excesses)

Biochemical Changes in Growth (Trophic) Factors: Much research is taking place in the examination of naturally occurring substances that may affect the nervous system and that may contribute to the dysfunction or death of brain cells in Alzheimer's. It is possible that one reason for nerve cell death in Alzheimer's patients is a decline in growth-promoting factors that maintain the functioning of brain cells, or, conversely, a spontaneous increase in factors that are toxic to brain cells.

A naturally occurring substance of interest is nerve growth factor (NGF). Experiments in aged rats indicate that specific nerve growth factors can stimulate the growth of new synaptic connections in the hippocampus and, as a result, restore some memory loss. Although there could be neurotoxic as well as growth-enhancing effects in the use of NGF, scientists are investigating methods of safely introducing NGF into the brain, possibly through the transplant of genetically engineered cells.

Other research is exploring whether changes or an imbalance in the metabolism of certain elements like calcium in brain cells may be part of the process by which the cells degenerate and die in Alzheimer's disease.

Chemical Deficiencies: One of the ways in which brain cells communicate with one another is through chemicals called neurotransmitters. Studies of Alzheimer's disease brains have uncovered diminished levels of various neurotransmitters that are thought to influence intellectual functioning and behavior. For example, reduced levels of the neurotransmitter acetylcholine (ACh) have been found in Alzheimer's disease. This finding has been coupled with observations that drugs whose side effects lower ACh levels in the brain can cause reversible memory problems. These findings have led to a number of drug studies employing pharmacologic agents to elevate ACh in patients. The treatments have included lecithin, choline, physostigmine, deprenyl, tacrine hydrochloride (THA), and others used alone or in different combinations with one another. The results of these experiments are difficult to interpret. In some of these studies, a few Alzheimer's disease patients seem to show minor improvement over a brief but not sustained period of time. Typically, any improvement may be on certain narrow test measures—and not usually on significant activities of daily living which would be more important to the person's family and physician.

Nonetheless, the researchers' enthusiasm is understandable, for they are dealing with the potential modifiability of underlying physiological phenomena that influence the Alzheimer's disease symptoms. The drugs they are studying now may not be the right ones, but they may point the way to the discovery of more effective pharmacologic agents. Of the drugs being studied, THA has received the most publicity. Students have indicated that THA appeared to have a slightly positive effect on patient functioning, but assessment by a skilled observer showed no overall improvement. These results recently led the Food and Drug Administration (FDA) to recommend further studies during which patients would take higher doses of the drug for longer periods of time. FDA has approved expanded access to THA for these studies under the investigational new drug (IND) program.

Toxic Chemical Excesses: Although some researchers have found increased levels of aluminum, mercury, or other metals in the brains of Alzheimer's disease victims, others have not. And while some investigators have hypothesized that aluminum may play a role in the genesis of Alzheimer's disease, most have regarded aluminum as an effect of the disorder rather than its cause. In other words, instead of aluminum's acting to induce brain tissue changes in Alzheimer's disease, it more likely accumulates in response to such changes. Research continues in an effort to better understand this phenomenon and to determine whether aluminum levels are a cause or a consequence of the disease, and, if the latter, whether they contribute further to the impairment already experienced.

The Genetic Theory

Genetic aspects of many diseases are confusing. For example, a disorder can occur more frequently in certain families than in others, but still not be genetic. Since family members living together are exposed to the same environment, they would all be at increased risk if an environmental toxin or infectious agent were the causative factor in a particular disease. Furthermore, a disorder can be congenital and not hereditary—that is, prenatal problems can cause developmental defects not brought on by heredity. And an illness can be hereditary but remain in a latent state if some other disease factor does not occur to trigger its onset.

Genetic interest in Alzheimer's disease was stirred by the discovery of an apparent Down syndrome in certain families. Also, when patients with Down syndrome survive into middle age, they typically develop dementia, and autopsies show findings in the brain indistinguishable from those that occur in Alzheimer's. Although a clear understanding of these findings remains elusive, it has led to efforts to identify a genetic marker for Alzheimer's disease on chromosome 21, because this is the same chromosome that is affected in Down syndrome.

Despite the identification of a genetic marker on chromosome 21 in that small number of families where Alzheimer's disease has occurred with unusual frequency, and the possible implication of chromosome 19 in certain other families, the extent of genetic and hereditary involvement in Alzheimer's disease remains unclear. There are a vast number of people affected with this disorder who are not part of a strong family pattern, and this has led some investigators to postulate that there may be a number of different subtypes of Alzheimer's disease, with different risk factors and causes.

The National Institute of Mental Health (NIMH) is supporting research to locate the genes that cause Alzheimer's disease, schizophrenia, and manic depression. Ten diagnostic centers, three of which study Alzheimer's, provide genetic material to a central gene bank. Scientists at the centers use identical diagnostic tests, chosen for their sensitivity and reliability, to select members of families whose blood is sent to the gene bank for processing, storage, and distribution. Participating families must have several members affected by one of the diseases. The centers studying Alzheimer's are: The Johns Hopkins University, Baltimore, Maryland; Massachusetts General Hospital, Boston, Massachusetts; and University of Alabama, Birmingham, Alabama.

The Autoimmune Theory

The body's immune system, which protects against potentially harmful foreign invaders, may erroneously begin to attack its own tissues, producing antibodies to its own essential cells. This is called an autoimmune response, and it may take place in the brain. Some scientists speculate that certain late life changes in aging neurons (the major nerve cells of the brain) might be triggering an autoimmune response that evokes symptoms of Alzheimer's disease in vulnerable individuals. Curiously, some antibrain antibodies have been identified in the brains of those with Alzheimer's disease. Their significance, though, is not known, especially since some antibrain antibodies have also been identified in aging brains without Alzheimer's disease. Moreover, even if changes are occurring in brain neurons to trigger an autoimmune response, what originally induces these brain cell changes is not known.

The Slow Virus Theory

Because a slow-acting virus has been identified as a cause of some brain disorders that closely resemble Alzheimer's disease (for example, Creutzfeldt-Jakob disease), a slow virus has been postulated in Alzheimer's disease. Various researchers have suggested that suspicious brain tissue changes in Alzheimer's disease victims may be caused by a virus. However, to date a virus has not been isolated from the brains of those with Alzheimer's disease, and no immune reaction has been found in the brains of Alzheimer's patients, comparable to that found in patients with other viral dementias. At present, the possibility of a viral cause of Alzheimer's cannot be either decisively eliminated or confirmed.

The Blood Vessel Theory

Defects in blood vessels supplying blood to the brain have been studied as a possible cause of Alzheimer's disease. Hardening of the brain's arteries, also known as cerebroarteriosclerosis, proved not to be a cause of Alzheimer's disease. Thus, the hyperbaric oxygen chamber treatment proved ineffective as a therapy for Alzheimer's.

Stroke, another blood vessel problem that most often occurs later in life, can cause symptoms like those of Alzheimer's disease. But this condition, called multi-infarct dementia, differs from Alzheimer's disease. More recently, the blood vessel theory has been expanded to hypothesize potential defects in the blood-brain barrier, a protective membrane-like mechanism that guards the brain from foreign bodies or toxic agents circulating in the bloodstream outside the brain.

There have been several reports of a possible association between serious head injuries involving a loss of consciousness and later onset of Alzheimer's disease. One theory as to why this connection might occur has to do with possible breaks in the blood-brain barrier as a result of these injuries to the brain.

The Treatment of Alzheimer's Disease

Two critical crossroads reached in the approach to treatment for Alzheimer's disease were (1) the recognition of Alzheimer's disease as a disorder distinct from the normal aging process; and (2) the realization that, in developing therapeutic and social interventions for a major illness or disability, the concept of care can be as important as that of cure. Moreover, in addition to the symptoms of Alzheimer's disease mentioned earlier, other symptoms and aggravating factors may compound the problem. Patient, environmental, and family stresses can converge to exaggerate patient dysfunction and family burden during the clinical course of Alzheimer's disease. Identifying these stresses and making appropriate changes can provide the foundation for more effective treatment and fewer everyday problems.

In the Alzheimer's disease patient, depression or delusions can aggravate dysfunction. These problems, which emerge during the course of the disorder in some individuals with Alzheimer's disease, compound memory impairment; they make the affected individual do worse than would be expected from the dementia alone—causing clinical conditions referred to as "excess disability" states. Depression by itself can mimic dementia—a condition that is sometimes termed pseudodementia. When combined with dementia, depression exacts yet greater incapacity and suffering in the Alzheimer's disease patient. Depression in Alzheimer's disease can be treated. Indeed this highlights one of the truly extraordinary phenomena that can be observed in Alzheimer's disease: By alleviating an excess disability state, actual clinical improvement can result—even though the underlying disease process is advancing. In other words, at a given point in time, the patient's symptoms can be reduced, suffering lowered, capacity to cope buttressed, with family burden eased as a further result. These are traditional goals of treatment for all illnesses.

Researchers in the NIMH Intramural program have developed and are testing a Dementia Mood Assessment Scale, designed to a rate mood in Alzheimer's patients. This scale tracks the mood states of the patients over the course of their illness and thus may be helpful in testing various antidepressant treatments.

The patient's immediate environment can also interfere with coping, adding to the level of impairment. Modifying the surroundings can reduce stresses imposed by environmental factors. There is the matter of safety, as in the need to protect the person from wandering toward a stairway and subsequently falling. There is the matter of lowering the individual's frustration level, such as by placing different cues in the immediate environment to combat memory loss and to reduce resulting stress and disorganization. There is the matter of finding the most protective but least restrictive setting for care which at some point may involve a move away from home to a nursing home or other care facility well equipped to deal with those who have Alzheimer's disease.

Stress on the family can take a toll on patient and caregiver alike. Caregivers are usually family members—either spouses or children—and are preponderantly wives and daughters. As time passes and the burden mounts, it not only places the mental health of family caregivers at risk, it also diminishes their ability to provide care to the Alzheimer's disease patient. Hence, assistance to the family as a whole must be considered.

As the disease progresses, families experience increasing anxiety and pain at seeing unsettling changes in a loved one, and they commonly feel guilt over not being able to do enough. The prevalence of reactive depression among family members in this situation is disturbingly high—caregivers are chronically stressed and are much more likely to suffer from depression than the average person. If caregivers have been forced to retire from positions outside the home, they feel progressively more isolated and no longer productive members of society.

An NIMH-funded study shows that caregivers not only have increased rates of infectious illness and depression, but often have suppressed immune systems. Another study of caregivers found depressed mood in 54 percent of caregivers and anger in 67 percent. Researchers hypothesize that the caregivers who hold in their anger may be at greater risk of cardiovascular disease.

The likelihood, intensity, and duration of depression among caregivers can all be lowered through available interventions. For example, to the extent that family members can offer emotional support to each other and perhaps seek professional consultation, they will be better prepared to help their loved one manage the illness and to recognize the limits of what they themselves can reasonably do.

> George and Mary Ellen's neighbors had become increasingly concerned as it was obvious something was very wrong. When they noticed that the newspaper had not been taken in one morning, two neighbors came over. When no one answered the door, they tried it, found it unlocked, and entered. George was lying on the floor near the telephone, and Mary Ellen was sitting at the piano trying to pick out a tune. The neighbors called an ambulance for George and then placed a long-distance call to one of his daughters. George, in the hospital suffering from a heart attack, for the first time shared with his children the events of the past months and realized that he must make plans for the future. One of his daughters stayed with him and Mary Ellen for 2 months after he left the hospital. She arranged for someone to come in once a week to clean the house. She also contacted Meals-on-Wheels to ensure nourishing meals for her parents. Through her parents' church, she enrolled Mary Ellen in a 5-day-a-week daycare program for the elderly. Each morning Mary Ellen was picked up by the daycare van and was brought back late in the afternoon. George, relieved of constant anxiety, recovered rapidly and began to catch up on his writing projects. Though he missed the social life they had once enjoyed with their friends, there were times when he and Mary Ellen still felt a close relationship. George now accepted the fact that someday Mary Ellen might have to enter a nursing home, but with the support of his family, friends, church, and community he would be able to deal with whatever came.

Since the components of the problem vary, so too should the focus, nature, and sources of interventions. Interventions should focus on the patient's symptoms, the affected individual's everyday environment, and the family support system. Specific interventions can involve support from the family, the help of a homemaker or other aide in the home, employment of behavioral therapies, and the use of medication. The sources for interventions can range from family support groups such as those available through the Alzheimer's Association (AA), to professional consultations for the patient and family with a mental health specialist, to a variety of community programs such as day or respite care. Information on what assistance is available in a given community can be gained by contacting the local Office on Aging, a community mental health center or local medical society, or a local chapter of the AA. In addition, every state has an agency on aging that provides information on services and programs.

Though Alzheimer's disease cannot at present be cured, reversed, or stopped in its progression, much can be done to help both the patient and the family live through the course of the illness with greater dignity and less discomfort. Toward this goal, appropriate clinical interventions and community services should be vigorously sought.

Hope for the Future through Research

While Alzheimer's disease remains a mystery, with its cause and cure not yet found, there is considerable excitement and hope about new findings that are unfolding in numerous research settings. The connecting pieces to the puzzle called Alzheimer's disease continue to be found. At the same time, there are more and more partners involved in the effort, with growing national and international interest. Government, industry, academia, and the volunteer sector are all becoming more and more active. Federal, state, community, corporate, and foundation support for new studies and better services are all on the rise.

The U.S. Department of Health and Human Services established a Departmental Task Force on Alzheimer's Disease, which first met in April 1983. This task force, later legislatively mandated as the Council on Alzheimer's Disease, is composed of representatives from the following agencies that have programs related to Alzheimer's disease: the National Institute of Mental Health, the National Institute on Aging, the National Institute of Neurological Disorders and Stroke, the National Institute of Allergy and Infectious Diseases, the National Center for Nursing Research, the Administration on Aging, the Agency for Health Care Policy and Research, the Health Care Financing Administration, the Health Resource and Services Administration, the National Center for Health Statistics, and the Department of Veterans Affairs. The council, which also includes both the Surgeon General and the Assistant Secretary for Planning and Evaluation as members, is chaired by the Assistant Secretary for Health. The council's recommendations are sent in an annual report to Congress.

In addition, a nonfederal Advisory Panel on Alzheimer's Disease was established by congressional action. The panel, which works closely with the council, consists of 15 national authorities on Alzheimer's disease selected for their depth and breadth of expertise in this area. The panel has issued three reports, for 1988–89, 1990, and 1991. The titles are in the reference list. The activities of both the council and the panel reflect the scope of concern and interest that is being focused by the federal government on Alzheimer's disease.

Glossary

Acetylcholine. A neurotransmitter found in reduced levels in the brains of Alzheimer's victims.

Amyloid precursor protein (APP). A normal, essential substance made by brain cells that contain beta amyloid. In Alzheimer's, APP is cut and releases beta amyloid. Beta amyloid then forms clumps called senile plaque.

Alzheimer's Disease Associated Protein (ADAP). A protein that seems to appear only in the tissue of people with Alzheimer's. It has been found in both the brain and spinal fluid.

Cortisol. The major natural glucocorticoid (GC) in humans. It is the primary stress hormone.

Dementia. Significant loss of intellectual abilities such as memory capacity, severe enough to interfere with social or occupational functioning.

Hippocampus. An area buried deep in the forebrain that helps regulate emotion and memory.

Multi-Infarct Dementia. Dementia brought on by a series of strokes.

Nerve Growth Factor. A substance that occurs naturally in the body and enhances the growth and survival of cholinergic nerves.

Neurotoxic. Poisonous to nerves or nerve tissue.

Nucleus basalis of Meynert. A small group of cholinergic nerve cells in the forebrain and connected to areas of the cerebral cortex.

Pseudodementia. A severe form of depression resulting from a progressive brain disorder in which cognitive changes mimic those of dementia.

References

Advisory Panel on Alzheimer's Disease. *Report of the Advisory Panel on Alzheimer's Disease.* DHHS Pub. No. (ADM) 89-1644, Washington, DC: Supt. of Docs., U.S. Govt. Print. Off., 1989. (Available from the Superintendent of Documents, Government Printing Office, Washington, DC 20402-9325, GPO S/N 017-024-01387-1, $2.25.)

Advisory Panel on Alzheimer's Disease. *Second Report of the Advisory Panel on Alzheimer's Disease, 1990.* DHHS Pub. No. (ADM) 91-1791, Washington, DC: Supt. of Docs., U.S. Govt. Print. Off., 1991. (Available from the Superintendent of Documents, Government Printing Office, Washington, DC 20402-9325, GPO S/N 017-024-01442-7, $3.00.)

Advisory Panel on Alzheimer's Disease. *Third Report of the Advisory Panel on Alzheimer's Disease, 1991.* DHHS Pub. No. (ADM) 92-1917, Washington, DC: Supt. of Docs., U.S. Govt. Print. Off., 1992. (Available from the Superintendent of Documents, Government Printing Office, Washington, DC 20402-9325, GPO S/N 017-024-01483-4, $3.50.)

Light, E., and Lebowitz, B.D. *Alzheimer's Disease Treatment and Family Stress: Directions for Research.* DHHS Pub. No. (ADM) 89-1569, Washington, DC: Supt. of Docs., U.S. Govt. Print. Off., 1989. (Available from the Superintendent of Documents, Government Printing Office, Washington, DC 20402-9325, GPO S/N 017-024-01365-0, $14.00.)

National Institute of Mental Health. *If You're Over 65 and Feeling Depressed . . . Treatment Brings New Hope.* DHHS Pub. No. (ADM) 90-1653, 1990. (Single copies available from Public Inquiries, NIMH, 5600 Fishers Lane, Room 15C-05, Rockville, MD 20857. Available in packages of 50 from the Superintendent of Documents, Government Printing Office, Washington, DC 20402-9325, GPO S/N 017-024-01376-5, $23.00 per package of 50.)

National Institute of Mental Health. *Plain Talk About Mutual Help Groups.* DHHS Pub. No. (ADM) 89-1138, 1989. (Single copies available from Public Inquiries, NIMH, 5600 Fishers Lane, Room 15C-05, Rockville, MD 20857.)

Taylor, Rob. Evolutions: Brain imaging, *The Journal of NIH Research,* May 1990, Vol. 2, p. 103.

U.S. Congress, Office of Technology Assessment. *Congressional Summary, Losing A Million Minds: Confronting the Tragedy of Alzheimer's Disease and Other Dementias,* OTA-BA-324, Washington, DC: Supt. of Docs., U.S. Govt. Print. Off., 1987.

U.S. Congress, Office of Technology Assessment. *Summary, Confused Minds, Burdened Families: Finding Help for People with Alzheimer's and Other Dementias,* OTA-BA-404, Washington, DC: Supt. of Docs., U.S. Govt. Print. Off., 1990.

Sources of Help

For a list of agencies that coordinate services for older Americans, providing information on services, programs, and opportunities see Appendix C.

This is the second revision of the brochure by Margaret Strock, staff member in the Information Resources and Inquiries Branch, Office of Scientific Information, National Institute of Mental Health (NIMH). Expert assistance was provided by Barry D. Lebowitz, Ph.D., George T. Niederehe, Ph.D., Jane L. Pearson, Ph.D., Benjamin Wolozin, M.D., Ph.D., and Trey Sunderland, M.D., NIMH staff members. Their help in assuring the accuracy of this pamphlet is gratefully acknowledged. An earlier version of the brochure was written by Gene D. Cohen, M.D., Ph.D., former Director of the NIMH Program on Aging, in 1987. It was printed as a cooperative public-private effort by the American Association for Geriatric Psychiatry.

■ **Document Source:**
U.S. Department of Health and Human Services, Public Health Service
National Institute of Mental Health
DHHS Publication No. (ADM) 92-1696
Printed 1990. Revised 1992

See also: Multi-Infarct Dementia (page 337)

NIDDK Fact Sheet

DIABETIC NEUROPATHY: THE NERVE DAMAGE OF DIABETES

What is diabetic neuropathy?

Diabetic neuropathy is a nerve disorder caused by diabetes. People who have had diabetes for years may experience numbness and sometimes pain in their hands, feet, and legs. Nerve damage caused by diabetes can also lead to problems with indigestion, diarrhea or constipation, dizziness, bladder infections, and impotence. In some cases, damaged nerves can strike suddenly, causing pain, weakness, and weight loss. Depression may follow. While some treatments are available, a great deal of research still needs to be done to understand how diabetes affects the nerves and to find better treatments for this complication.

How common is diabetic neuropathy?

Nerve problems can affect anybody with diabetes, but they are most common in people who have had diabetes more than 10 years. The majority of patients with neurological impairment due to diabetes do not have symptoms such as pain or numbness. However, some recent studies have reported that:

- 10 years after diagnosis, 30 percent of diabetes patients have symptoms or signs of diabetic neuropathy;
- 25 years after diagnosis, 40 percent of diabetes patients have symptoms or signs of neuropathy;
- 50 years after diagnosis, half of all diabetes patients have symptoms or signs of neuropathy.

Diabetic neuropathy appears to be more common in smokers, people over 40 years of age, and those who have had problems controlling the levels of glucose in their blood.

What causes diabetic neuropathy?

Scientists do not know how diabetic neuropathy occurs, but it is likely that several factors come into play. High blood glucose causes chemical changes in nerves, impairing their ability to transmit nerve signals. High blood glucose also damages blood vessels that carry oxygen and nutrients to the nerves. Also, inherited factors probably unrelated to diabetes may make some people more susceptible to nerve disease than others.

The study of the chemical changes that happen to nerves exposed to high blood glucose is a very active area of research. A normal substance called aldose reductase converts glucose to a type of sugar alcohol called sorbitol. Scientists have found that when tissues have a high level of glucose, sorbitol builds up and apparently damages the membranes lining body tissues.

Scientists have noted that in animals and humans with diabetes, nerves have less than normal amounts of a substance called myoinositol. It is thought that myoinositol plays a role in how nerve cells use energy to maintain the correct balance of salts. This balance is important to cells' ability to conduct nerve impulses.

Studies have also shown that proteins age more quickly when exposed to high glucose. This has the effect of weakening certain connective proteins called collagens, which line and support nerve tissue. While these changes occur with normal aging, high blood glucose speeds up the damage.

It is likely that all three processes are chemically linked. Scientists are studying how these changes occur, how they are connected, how they cause nerve damage, and how the damage can be prevented and treated.

What are the symptoms of diabetic neuropathy?

The symptoms of diabetic neuropathy vary a great deal. Some people notice no symptoms, while others are disabled by severe problems. Neuropathy may cause both pain and insensitivity to pain in the same person. Often, symptoms are slight at first, and since most nerve damage occurs over years, mild cases may go unnoticed for a long time. In some people, though, mainly those afflicted by mononeuropathy, the onset of pain may be sudden and severe.

Peripheral neuropathy

The most common type of neuropathy, peripheral neuropathy (also called "somatic neuropathy" or "distal sensory polyneuropathy"), can affect any of the nerves that transmit sensation throughout the body. However, the nerves of the limbs, and especially the feet, seem affected most often. Peripheral neuropathy usually involves nerves on both sides of the body. Some of the most common symptoms of this kind of neuropathy are:

- numbness or insensitivity to pain or temperature;
- tingling, burning, or prickling;
- sharp pains or cramps; and
- extreme sensitivity to touch, even very light touch.

These symptoms are often worse at night.

After years of peripheral neuropathy, the damage to nerves may result in loss of reflexes and muscle weakness. These, in turn, may cause:

◆ loss of balance and coordination;
◆ inability to raise the foot;
◆ curling of the toes or other foot problems.

Often the foot becomes wider and shorter, the gait changes, and foot ulcers appear as pressure is put on parts of the foot that are less protected.

Loss of sensation may occur without the warning signs of pain, numbness or tingling. As the damaged nerve grows less sensitive to pain, it is easy to overlook foot problems when they first happen. Injuries can easily become infected because the poor circulation caused by diabetes impedes healing. If an injury is not treated in time, the infection may lead to gangrene, sometimes requiring amputation of the limb. However, problems caused by minor injuries can usually be controlled if they are caught in time.

Autonomic neuropathy

Autonomic neuropathy (also called "visceral neuropathy") is usually found in people who already have peripheral neuropathy. Autonomic neuropathy affects the nerves that serve the heart and internal organs and produces changes in:

Urination and Sexual Response

Autonomic neuropathy most often affects the organs that control urination and reproduction. Nerve damage prevents the bladder from emptying completely, so bacteria grow more easily in the urinary tract (bladder or kidneys). When the nerves of the bladder are damaged, it may be difficult to control the bladder or to know when it is full.

The nerve damage and circulatory problems of diabetes can also lead to frequent vaginal infections and a gradual loss of sexual sensation or response in both men and women, although sex drive is unchanged. A man may be unable to have erections or may reach sexual climax without ejaculating normally.

Digestion

Autonomic neuropathy can also affect how food is digested. Nerve damage can cause the stomach to empty too slowly, a disorder called gastric stasis. When the condition is severe (gastroparesis), a person can have persistent nausea and vomiting, bloating, and loss of appetite. Blood glucose levels tend to fluctuate wildly.

If nerves in the esophagus are involved, swallowing may be difficult. Nerve damage to the bowels can cause constipation or frequent diarrhea, especially at night. Problems with the digestive system often lead to weight loss.

Cardiovascular System

Autonomic neuropathy least often affects the cardiovascular system, which controls the circulation of blood throughout the body. When it occurs, the nerve impulses from various parts of the body which signal the need for blood are not transmitted normally. As a result, blood pressure may drop sharply after sitting or standing, causing a person to feel dizzy or lightheaded, or even to faint (orthostatic hypotension).

Neuropathy that affects the cardiovascular system may also cause painless heart attacks and may raise the risk of a heart attack during general anesthesia. It can also hinder the body's normal response to low blood sugar or hypoglycemia.

Sweating and Salivation

Autonomic neuropathy can affect the nerves that control sweating and salivation. Sometimes, nerve damage interferes with the activity of the sweat glands, making it difficult to tolerate heat. Other times, it causes profuse sweating at night or while eating (gustatory sweating).

Mononeuropathy

Occasionally, diabetic neuropathy appears suddenly and affects specific nerves, most often in the torso, leg, or head. When mononeuropathy (including "multiplex neuropathy") occurs, it may cause:

◆ pain in the front of the thigh;
◆ severe pain in the lower back or pelvis;
◆ chest or abdominal pain sometimes mistaken for angina, heart attack, or appendicitis;
◆ aching behind the eye;
◆ inability to focus the eye;
◆ double vision;
◆ paralysis on one side of the face (Bell's palsy); or problems with hearing.

This kind of neuropathy is unpredictable and occurs most often in older people who have mild diabetes. Although mononeuropathy can be very painful, it tends to improve by itself after a period of weeks or months without causing long-term damage.

How do doctors diagnose diabetic neuropathy?

A doctor diagnoses neuropathy from symptoms and a physical exam. During the exam, the doctor may check muscle strength, reflexes, and sensitivity to position, vibration, temperature, and light touch. Sometimes special tests are used to help pinpoint the cause of symptoms and suggest treatment:

◆ *Ultrasound* employs sound waves too high to hear, which produce an image showing how well the bladder and other parts of the urinary tract are functioning.
◆ *Nerve conduction studies* check the flow of electrical current through a nerve. With this test, an image of the nerve impulse is projected on a screen as it transmits an electrical impulse. Impulses that seem slower or weaker than usual indicate possible damage to the nerve. This test allows the doctor to assess the condition of all of the nerves in the limb.
◆ *Electromyography (EMG)* is used to see how well muscles respond to electrical impulses transmitted by the nerves nearby. With an EMG, the electrical activity

of the muscle is displayed on screen. A response that is slower or weaker than usual suggests damage to the muscle. This test is often done at the same time as nerve conduction studies.

♦ *Nerve biopsy* involves removing a sample of nerve tissue, which is examined for damage. This test is most often used in research settings.

If your doctor suspects autonomic neuropathy, you may also be referred to a specialist in digestive disorders (gastroenterologist) for additional tests.

How is diabetic neuropathy usually treated?

Treatment aims at relieving discomfort and preventing further tissue damage. The first step is to bring blood sugar under control by diet and oral drugs or insulin injections, if needed. Although symptoms can sometimes worsen as blood sugar is brought under control with intensive treatment, careful long-term monitoring of blood sugar helps reverse the pain or loss of sensation that neuropathy can cause. Good control of blood sugar with diet and, if necessary, drug therapy may also help prevent or delay the onset of further problems.

Another important part of treatment involves special care of the feet, which are especially prone to problems. (See section under foot care.)

Relieving symptoms

A number of medications are used to relieve the symptoms of diabetic neuropathy:

♦ *Pain, burning, tingling, or numbness.* Your doctor may suggest an analgesic such as aspirin or acetaminophen; an anti-inflammatory drug containing ibuprofen; antidepressant medications such as amitriptyline, sometimes used with fluphenazine; or nerve medications such as carbamazepine or phenytoin sodium. Codeine is sometimes prescribed for short-term use to relieve severe pain.

Your doctor may also prescribe a therapy known as transcutaneous electronic nerve stimulation (TENS). In this treatment, small amounts of electricity block pain signals as they pass thorough a patient's skin. Other treatments include hypnosis, relaxation training, biofeedback, and acupuncture. Some people find that walking regularly or using elastic stockings helps relieve leg pain. Warm (not hot) baths, massage, or an analgesic ointment such as Ben Gay may also help.

♦ *Indigestion, belching, nausea or vomiting.* For patients with mild symptoms of slow stomach emptying, doctors suggest eating small, frequent meals and avoiding fats. Eating less fiber may also relieve symptoms. For patients with severe gastroparesis, the doctor may prescribe metoclopramide, which speeds digestion and relieves nausea. Other drugs that help regulate digestion or reduce stomach acid secretion may also be used. In each case, the potential benefits of these drugs need to be weighed against their side effects.

♦ *Diarrhea or other bowel problems.* Antibiotics or clonidine HCl, a drug used to treat high blood pressure, are sometimes prescribed. A wheat-free diet may also help bring relief since the gluten in flour sometimes causes diarrhea.

♦ *Urinary tract infections.* Your doctor may prescribe an antibiotic to clear up an infection and suggest drinking more fluids to prevent further infections. It is also a good idea to urinate at regular times (every 3 hours, for example) since you may not be able to tell when your bladder is full.

♦ *Lightheadedness, dizziness, or fainting.* Sitting or standing very slowly may help prevent these problems. Raising the head of your bed and wearing elastic stockings may also help. Increased salt in the diet and treatment with salt-retaining hormones such as fludrocortisone are other possible approaches. In research studies, drugs used to treat hypertension have increased blood pressure in some patients.

♦ *Muscle weakness or loss of coordination.* Physical therapy can often help strengthen muscles and improve coordination.

Sexual problems

The nerve and circulatory problems of diabetes can disrupt normal sexual function. After ruling out a hormonal cause of impotence, you doctor can advise you about the different methods available to treat impotence caused by neuropathy. Short-term solutions involve using a mechanical vacuum device or injecting a drug called a vasodilator into the penis before sex. Both methods raise blood flow to the penis, making it easier to have and maintain an erection. Surgical procedures, in which an inflatable or semi-rigid device is implanted in the penis, offer a more permanent solution. For some people, counseling may help relieve the stress caused by neuropathy and restore sexual function.

In women who feel their sexual life is not satisfactory, the role of diabetes and the solutions are less clear. Illness, vaginal or urinary infections, and anxiety about pregnancy complicated by diabetes can, for example, interfere with a woman's ability to enjoy intimacy. Infections can be reduced by good blood glucose control. Counseling may also help a woman identify and cope with sexual concerns.

Foot care

People with diabetes have to take special care of their feet. Since the nerves to the feet are the longest in the body, they are most often affected by neuropathy. At least 15 percent of all people with diabetes eventually have a foot ulcer, and 6 out of every 1,000 lose a limb to infection. However, doctors estimate that nearly three quarters of all amputations caused by neuropathy can be prevented with careful foot care.

Every day, you should check your feet and toes for any cuts, sores, bruises, bumps, or infections—using a mirror if necessary. Since diabetic neuropathy often causes numbness, you may be able to see injuries before you feel any discomfort. Also, poor circulation may cause infections to heal more slowly. To prevent foot problems from developing:

- Wash your feet daily, using warm water and a mild soap. (If you have neuropathy, you should test water temperature with your wrist.) Doctors do not advise soaking your feet for long periods since you may lose protective calluses. Dry your feet carefully with a soft towel, especially between toes.
- Cover your feet (except for the skin between the toes) with petroleum jelly, a lotion containing lanolin, or cold cream before putting on shoes and socks. The diabetic foot tends to sweat less than normal, leading to dry, cracked skin.
- Wear thick, soft socks, and avoid wearing slippery stockings, mended stockings, or stockings with seams.
- Wear shoes that fit your feet well and allow your toes to move. Break in new shoes gradually, wearing them for only an hour at a time. After years of neuropathy, as reflexes are lost, it is common for the feet to become wider and flatter. If you have problems finding shoes that fit well, ask your doctor to refer you to a specialist who can fit you with corrective shoes or inserts.
- Examine your shoes before putting them on to make sure they have no tears or sharp edges that might injure your feet.
- Cut your toenails straight across, but be careful not to leave any sharp corners that could cut the next toe.
- Use an emery board or a pumice stone to file away dead skin, but don't remove calluses, which act as protective padding. Don't try to cut off any growths yourself, and avoid using harsh chemicals such as wart remover on your feet.
- Don't take very hot baths and never go barefoot, even on the beach or by a pool.
- Wear socks if feet are cold at night—no heating pads or hot water bottles.
- Avoid sitting with your legs crossed. This can reduce the flow of blood to the feet.
- Ask your doctor to check your feet at every visit, and call your doctor if you notice that a sore isn't healing well.
- If you're not able to take care of your own feet, ask your doctor to recommend a podiatrist (specialist in the care and treatment of feet) who can help.

Some general hints

- If you smoke, try to stop since smoking makes circulatory problems worse and increases the risk of neuropathy and heart disease.
- Ask your doctor to suggest an exercise routine that's right for you. Many people who exercise regularly find the pain of neuropathy is less severe. Aside from helping you reach and maintain your ideal weight, exercise also improves the body's use of insulin, helps improve circulation, and strengthens muscles. Check with your doctor before starting exercise that can be hard on your feet, such as running or aerobics.
- Cut back on the amount of alcohol you drink. Recent research has indicated that as few as four drinks per week can worsen neuropathy.

Are there any experimental treatments for diabetic neuropathy?

Though still under study, new therapies may eventually prevent or reverse diabetic neuropathy. Extensive testing is required by the U.S. Food and Drug Administration to establish the safety and efficacy of drugs before they are approved for widespread use.

A new topical cream, capsaicin, is now in clinical trials and may prove to reduce the pain of neuropathy. Scientists believe that the ointment, a cayenne pepper extract, depletes the chemical that transmits pain signals to the brain.

Many doctors prescribe vitamin B1 because it appears to keep neuropathy from progressing, but there is no hard evidence of its benefits, and others feel it should not be prescribed. In addition, researchers are exploring treatment with another B vitamin called myoinositol. Early findings have shown that nerves in diabetic animals and humans have less than normal amounts of this substance. With supplements, myoinositol levels are increased in tissues of diabetic animals, but research is still needed to show any concrete, lasting benefits.

Another area of research concerns the drug amino guanidine. In animals, amino guanidine blocks cross-linking of proteins that occurs more quickly than normal in tissues exposed to high glucose. Very early clinical tests are under way to determine the effects of amino guanidine in humans.

One approach that appeared promising involved the use of aldose reductase inhibitors. These are a class of drugs that block the formation of the sugar alcohol sorbitol, which is thought to damage nerves. Scientists hoped these drugs would prevent and might even repair nerve damage. But so far, clinical trials have shown these drugs to have major side effects while improving neuropathy in only a small number of patients.

Future research

The National Institutes of Health (NIH) is an agency of the Public Health Service under the U.S. Department of Health and Human Services. Its mission is to improve human health through biomedical research. Several components of NIH—the National Institute of Diabetes and Digestive and Kidney Diseases, the National Institute of Neurological Disorders and Stroke, and the National Institute of Dental Research—conduct and support research on the nerve complications of diabetes. The knowledge gained from this research may one day offer a way to prevent or cure diabetic neuropathy and bring relief to millions of people.

Resources on diabetes

American Diabetes Association
National Service Center
1660 Duke Street
Alexandria, VA 22314
1-800-232-3472 or (703) 549-1500

A private, voluntary organization that fosters public awareness of diabetes and supports and promotes diabetes research. The American Diabetes Association has printed information on many aspects of diabetes, and local affiliates sponsor community programs. Local affiliates can be found in the telephone directory or through the national office.

American Dietetic Association
216 W. Jackson Boulevard
Chicago, IL 60606-6995
(312) 89900040
    A professional organization that can help someone locate a nutritionist in the community.

American Heart Association
7320 Greenville Avenue
Dallas, TX 75231
    A private, voluntary organization that has literature on heart disease and how to prevent it. Contact the local affiliate of the American Heart Association listed in telephone directories.

Juvenile Diabetes Foundation International
432 Park Avenue South
New York, NY 10016
1-800-223-1138
    A private, voluntary organization with an interest in insulin-dependent diabetes. Local affiliates are located across the country.

National Diabetes Information Clearinghouse
Box NDIC
9000 Rockville Pike
Bethesda, MD 20892
(301) 468-2162
    The National Diabetes Information Clearinghouse has a variety of publications for distribution to the public and to health professionals. The clearinghouse is a program of the National Institute of Diabetes and Digestive and Kidney Diseases, the lead federal agency in diabetes research.

Additional reading

For general information about diabetes:

Insulin-Dependent Diabetes, 1990. A booklet prepared by the National Institute of Diabetes and Digestive and Kidney Diseases. Single copies are free from the National Diabetes Information Clearinghouse.

Noninsulin-Dependent Diabetes, 1987. A booklet prepared by the National Institute of Diabetes and Digestive and Kidney Diseases. Single copies are free from the National Diabetes Information Clearinghouse.

Diabetes Dictionary, 1989. A booklet prepared by the National Institute of Diabetes and Digestive and Kidney Diseases. Single copies are free from the National Diabetes Information Clearinghouse.

For more information about diabetic neuropathy and diabetes research:

Albert, Leonard. "Restraining Pain: What's available for easing the pain of diabetic neuropathy." *Diabetes Forecast,* January 1988, pp. 39–41.

Bell, David and Clements, Jr., Rex, "Diabetes and the Digestive System." *Diabetes Forecast.* December 1987, pp. 43–46.

Cohen, Margo et al., Managing Diabetes Complications," *Patient Care,* December 15, 1988, pp. 28–39.

Diabetes Mellitus: Trans-NIH Research, NIDDK 1991. Single copies are free from the National Diabetes Information Clearinghouse.

Dyck, Peter James. "Aldose Reductase Inhibitors and Diabetic Neuropathy." *Diabetes Forecast,* May 1989, pp. 41–43.

Dyck, Peter James, "Resolvable Problems in Diabetic Neuropathy," *The Journal of NIH Research,* June 1990, pp. 57–62.

Gerding, Dale et al. "Problems in Diabetic Foot Care," *Patient Care,* August 15, 1988, pp. 102–18.

Haase, Gunter et al., "Neuropathy: Diabetic? Nutritional?," *Patient Care.* May 15, 1990, pp. 112–34.

Jaspan, Jonathan et al., "GI Complications of Diabetes," *Patient Care,* January 15, 1990, pp. 108–28.

"Report and Recommendations of the San Antonio Conference on Diabetic Neuropathy," sponsored by the American Diabetes Association

and the American Academy of Neurology, *Diabetes Care,* July/August 1988, pp. 592–97.

Vinik, Aaron and Mitchell, B. "Clinical Aspects of Diabetic Neuropathies," *Diabetes/Metabolism Reviews,* May 1988, pp. 223–53.

■ **Document Source:**
U.S. Department of Health and Human Services, Public Health Service
National Institutes of Health
National Institute of Diabetes and Digestive and Kidney Disease

See also: Diabetes Overview (page 110); Insulin-Dependent Diabetes (page 112); Noninsulin-Dependent Diabetes (page 116)

FACTS ABOUT NARCOLEPSY

Narcolepsy is a sleep disorder. The principal symptoms are excessive daytime sleepiness (EDS), cataplexy (loss of muscle tone), hallucinations, sleep paralysis, and disrupted night-time sleep. Doctors also diagnose narcolepsy by measuring how quickly the patient falls asleep, and how often rapid eye movements are present at or near the onset of sleep.

Excessive daytime sleepiness occurs every day, regardless of the amount of sleep obtained at night. EDS is usually experienced as a heightened sensitivity (sometimes an almost irresistible susceptibility) to becoming sleepy or falling asleep, especially in sleep-inducing situations. Patients describe the problem as sleepiness, tiredness, lack of energy, exhaustion, or a combination of these feelings, either continuously or at various times throughout the day. Sometimes sleepiness occurs so suddenly and with such overwhelming power that it is referred to as a "sleep attack." some patients have several "attacks" each day. When the attack occurs during the day, sleep usually lasts for less than 30 minutes, but sometimes the patient stays asleep for several hours.

Cataplexy is an abrupt loss of voluntary muscle tone, usually triggered by emotional arousal. Attacks can range in severity from a brief sensation of weakness to total physical collapse lasting several minutes. Hallucinations are intense, vivid, sometimes accompanied by frightening auditory, visual, and tactile sensations, and occur just on awakening or falling asleep. Occasionally they are extremely difficult to distinguish from reality. Sleep paralysis is a momentary inability to move when waking up or falling asleep. This condition can be terrifying, especially if it occurs with a frightening hallucination.

Scientists do not know what causes narcolepsy, but they think it may be due to a biochemical defect of the central nervous system. The disorder is often concentrated in families, and narcolepsy or a predisposition to it may be an inherited condition. Statistics on the prevalence of narcolepsy are hard to obtain. Recent estimates collected by the American Narcolepsy Association range from 100,000 to more than 250,000 cases in the United States alone.

Progress of Symptoms

Narcolepsy is a lifelong illness. There is no known cure and no report of lasting remission has been confirmed. Typically, symptoms (usually EDS) first become noticeable between the ages of 10 and 30. Symptoms are subtle at first, but become increasingly severe over the years.

Patients usually learn to pinpoint conditions likely to induce sleep or cataplexy, and they try either to avoid such conditions or, with proper medication, control the symptoms. Control is especially important when patients are driving or engaging in other potentially dangerous activities. Of itself, narcolepsy is not life-threatening and does not affect longevity.

Social Complications

The mild beginning symptoms of narcolepsy may cause no more than minor inconveniences. As they become increasingly severe, however, symptoms cause greater disruptions in patients' social and professional lives, and may become profoundly disabling. EDS often occurs at inopportune times—in the classroom, at business meetings, during a meal, or even in the middle of a conversation. Learning, for children and adults alike, may be hampered because the abilities to read, study, and concentrate are periodically (or in some cases continuously) impaired. Parents, teachers, spouses, and employers often mistake the patient's sleepiness for lack of interest, or misconstrue it as a sign of hostility, rejection, or laziness.

Cataplectic attacks commonly occur in situations involving perfectly normal emotions such as humor (hearing a joke, or especially telling a joke); competitiveness (bidding in a game of bridge); excitement (viewing, or especially participating in a sports event); and stress or self-assertion (asking for a pay raise). Patients' efforts to stave off cataplectic attacks by avoiding these emotions may greatly diminish the quality of their lives, and they may become severely restricted emotionally.

Diagnosis

Although symptoms are usually clear-cut, most patients have narcolepsy for 10 to 15 years before the disorder is correctly diagnosed. For one thing, patients may not suspect a medical disorder and usually do not seek help until symptoms become quite severe. Also, physicians often misdiagnose narcolepsy, mistaking the symptoms for those of other disorders, like depression. Sometimes the sleepiness is thought to be a side effect of medication. Cataplectic attacks also have been misdiagnosed as epileptic seizures, even though narcolepsy is *not* a form of epilepsy and requires different treatment. Narcolepsy can be confirmed or ruled out by a test (polysomnography) given in a sleep disorders clinic or laboratory under carefully controlled conditions.

Treatment

A clear understanding of recent developments in sleep disorders medicine is essential. Any physician in general practice can easily acquire this knowledge and provide narcolepsy patients with proper medical care.

Although there is no known cure for narcolepsy, several drugs help to control the symptoms. Stimulants are usually prescribed to treat EDS and sleep attacks, and certain antidepressants help control the cataplexy, sleep paralysis, and hallucinations. Narcolepsy symptoms vary from person to person, as does response to medications; also both symptoms and response are likely to change gradually over time. The proper choice of medication and dosage requires careful attention to the patient's needs and responses, and close cooperation between patient and physician. Medications used to treat narcolepsy usually have some undesirable side effects, in some cases serious enough to preclude drug treatment. However, for most patients medication is helpful.

Sleep habits are important for the patient with narcolepsy. Bedtimes should be regular, and nighttime sleep uninterrupted. Some patients find that naps at various intervals in the day help to offset excessive daytime sleepiness. A physician can work with the patient to establish the sleep schedule that is most effective and appropriate.

Research

Many research opportunities hold promise for people afflicted with narcolepsy. Basic research on how the brain regulates sleep is underway in several laboratories in the United States.

Animal models with naturally occurring symptoms identical to the human form of narcolepsy have been discovered. These models will enable scientists to probe brain anatomy, physiology, and biochemistry more extensively than is possible with human patients.

Of particular interest in narcolepsy is the brain chemical acetylcholine. This chemical regulates rapid eye movement (REM) sleep, the sleep state associated with dreaming. Natural events taking place during normal REM sleep parallel narcolepsy symptoms: the body becomes immobile as in sleep paralysis; muscle tone decreases as in cataplexy; and dreaming similar to hallucinations occurs. Narcoleptic sleep attacks are in fact the inappropriate appearance of REM sleep. Studies are underway to see whether acetylcholine is altered in narcolepsy.

Other biochemical studies center around norepinephrine and dopamine, the compounds responsible for maintaining wakefulness. Stimulants and antidepressants used to treat narcolepsy symptoms are thought to work by enhancing the effects of these compounds. Knowledge of how these drugs work to alter brain biochemistry may reveal the precise abnormality in narcolepsy and pave the way for developing more effective treatments. New drugs not yet ready for human use are being tested on the animal models.

The role of genetics in narcolepsy can be explored through data collected from family histories of patients and studies of breeding in colonies of narcolepsy animals. Information on narcolepsy's transmissibility and pattern of inheritance is essential for genetic counseling.

Two of the National Institutes of Health—the National Institute of Mental Health and the National Institute of Neurological Disorders and Stroke—support research in sleep disorders, including narcolepsy. This work is reported in the medical journal literature and at medical meetings. Patients and their families can keep up to date on research progress through the literature of the American Narcolepsy Association, described below.

Sources of Help and Information

The *American Narcolepsy Association (ANA)*, P.O. Box 1187, San Carlos, California 94070, is an independent non-profit corporation established in 1975 by persons afflicted with narcolepsy to help solve problems associated with narcolepsy and related chronic sleep disorders. The association encourages, supports and conducts research, and distributes free information about narcolepsy to patients, members of their families, the general public, and the medical profession. Free educational films and videotapes are made available to schools and civic groups to increase public awareness, understanding, and acceptance of the symptoms of narcolepsy. The ANA helps members form group self-help meetings, provides information about the locations of diagnostic facilities, and helps patients find physicians interested and skilled in treating sleep disorders. The association also publishes "The Eye Opener," a newsletter to inform members about ANA activities. All information and services are free.

The American Sleep Disorders Association (ASDA) was formed in 1975 to help ensure that the highest quality medical care is available at recognized centers having demonstrated expertise in evaluating and treating sleep disorders. Centers that meet the association's standards, as determined through on-site inspection by special ASDA committees, can be certified by the association. For information about certification standards or developmental assistance write: Office of the President, American Sleep Disorders Association, 604 Second Street, S.W., Rochester, Minnesota 55902. For a list of certified centers, write to the American Narcolepsy Association at the address given above.

■ **Document Source:**
U.S. Department of Health and Human Services, Public Health Services
National Institutes of Health
National Institute of Neurological Disorders and Stroke
NIH Publication No. 89-1637
Reprinted September 1989

See also: Sleep Disorders (page 298)

HUNTINGTON'S DISEASE RESEARCH HIGHLIGHTS

More than 100 years ago, Dr. George Huntington accurately described the disease that bears his name as ". . . coming on gradually but surely, increasing by degrees, and often occupying years in its development, until the hapless sufferer is but a quivering wreck of his former self." Huntington's disease (HD) is a devastating, progressive disorder of the brain that leads to uncontrolled movements, emotional instability, and loss of intellectual faculties.

Today, HD directly affects a total of about 25,000 people in the United States; at least 100,000 of their blood relatives live with constant uncertainty as they look for signs indicating that they, too, may have inherited the gene that will cause progressive disability and eventual death. The prevalence rate is probably understated because of misdiagnosis, and the number of deaths caused by HD is likely to be underreported.

HD results from genetically programmed degeneration of brain cells. Specifically affected early in the disease are cells of the basal ganglia, a structure deep in the center of the brain where movement is coordinated; later, cells of the brain's outer surface, or cortex, which control the functions of thought, perception, and memory, are attacked. The defective gene unleashes its destructive forces most often when persons are between the ages of 35 and 45, although, in some instances, those younger than 20 or older than 60 are not exempt from the dreaded onset of symptoms. An affected parent can pass HD along to his or her offspring, and each child of a parent has a 50 percent chance of inheriting the HD gene and developing the disease. How the flawed gene causes the brain to degenerate remains a mystery that scientists are seeking to solve.

The first signs of HD are subtle—a tic here, a twitch there, unexplained fluctuations of mood, an awareness of being more clumsy, depressed, or irritable than usual. There is slurring and slowing of speech. Diagnosis at this early stage, however, is particularly difficult, since symptoms may be indistinguishable from normal variations in mood and behavior or from changes induced by other causes.

During the 10- to 20-year span of the disease, a spectrum of progressively worsening symptoms appears and advances irreversibly, from uncontrollable muscle spasms to mental incompetence. Ultimately, HD confines people to wheelchair and bed, leaving them unaware of their surroundings. The long-endured emotional and financial burden to an HD patient's loved ones, some of whom may be at risk themselves and previewing their own futures, expands the tragedy. Yet there is substantial reason for hope that biomedical research will make this truly horrible disorder a thing of the past.

The National Institute of Neurological Disorders and Stroke (NINDS) is the federal government's focal point for research on HD. With NINDS support, investigators seek answers on a number of fronts using molecular biology, animal models, and modern brain imaging techniques.

Scientists Narrow Down Location of the Gene

Much exciting HD research is under way at the genetic level, as scientists zero in on a region near the tip of chromosome 4 where the HD gene is thought to lie. The process of isolating the responsible gene has been more arduous than anticipated, but scientists are confident of finding it. Once the gene is identified, scientists hope that the genetic defect can be elucidated and strategies developed to reduce its adverse effects.

In 1983, NINDS-supported researchers discovered the first genetic marker for HD, designated G-8, on chromosome 4. A marker is a segment of DNA that lies so close to a gene that the two are inherited together. Scientists use markers to identify the presence of a gene. The location of the first HD marker resulted in a presymptomatic test that is now 99 percent accurate.

The region on chromosome 4 which scientists believe contains the HD gene has been narrowed down to 2.5 million base pairs of DNA, still a relatively large region in molecular measurement. Investigators are concentrating on narrowing this region down to a more workable length. This entails finding a better marker—one much closer to the gene and found in many individuals. This marker will enable scientists to rule out large segments of DNA within the region, specifically those sections farthest away from the gene. In order to do this, investigators hope to find more individuals with recombination events—genetic combinations present in their parents—which will help rule out portions of the region or which are associated with the disease. This year, with the cooperation of HD families nationwide, NINDS-supported investigators have found unusual, promising recombination events and new markers within the region. Scientists have also been able to isolate several genetic segments, some of which are candidates for the HD gene.

NINDS-supported investigators are now studying these candidate genes by comparing postmortem brain specimens from HD-affected individuals and normal control specimens to see which genes are expressed—or which ones are active— in the brain. Differences in how the genes are expressed will tell scientists which of the HD candidate genes should be immediately sequenced and studied. This work depends on donated human brain tissue from the NINDS-supported Brain Tissue Resource Center of McLean Hospital in Belmont, Massachusetts, which has close affiliations with the NINDS-supported Huntington's Disease Research Center Without Walls at the Massachusetts General Hospital in Boston. Hundreds of scientists nationwide have requested tissue from the brain bank for their investigations.

Efforts to map and sequence the 2.5 million base pair region, including the genes that it contains, continue. Joining NINDS investigators are scientists funded by the Human Genome Project of the National Center for Human Genome Research. The center supports the development of mapping techniques to make the search easier and also funds a team of investigators at the University of California at San Francisco who are mapping the entire chromosome 4.

NINDS intramural scientist Dr. Craig Venter is using a new method to locate genes more quickly and efficiently than in the past. Dr. Venter is using expressed sequence tags (ESTs)—stretches of sequenced DNA taken from separate genes—much in the same way that police use fingerprints to identify suspects for a crime. Dr. Venter is using ESTs to sequence the HD gene region, and is supplying sequencing results to investigators working on isolating it.

In 1979, the NINDS established the Research Roster for Huntington's Disease at Indiana University in Indianapolis. The roster contains data on affected individuals, provides statistical and demographic data on large samplings of individuals, and serves as a liaison between investigators and specific HD families. The roster was an essential component in the identification of the G-8 and subsequently identified markers and continues to provide the DNA of many HD families to investigators involved in the search for the gene.

The lessons learned in identifying markers and tracking the elusive HD gene through analysis of blood and tissue samples have also been made possible by NINDS-supported yearly visits to the largest known HD kindred, living on Lake Maracaibo in Venezuela. The data on this large group, which now numbers 11,000, are stored in the Indiana University roster. Of continuing interest to investigators are twins, unaffected individuals who have affected offspring, and individuals who inherited two HD genes, one from each parent—a very rare occurrence elsewhere in the world.

NINDS support of research on other genetic neurological disorders is likely to shed light on possible mechanisms active in HD. For example, investigators recently found a new kind of genetic defect which causes a rare, progressive nerve disorder called Charcot-Marie-Tooth disease. This progressive, muscle-wasting disorder is caused by duplication of a small segment of DNA on chromosome 17. This is the first time that duplication of genes within a small part of chromosome has been shown to cause an illness. The study raises the possibility that HD and other inherited illness may be caused by gene duplication rather than by a defective gene.

Genetic Imprinting: Maternal and Paternal Factors Are Studied

It is an interesting and poorly understood fact that children who inherit the gene from their mothers develop HD later in life than children who inherit it from their fathers. How paternal or maternal factors alter the expression of particular genes in offspring is called genetic imprinting.

This year, NINDS investigators found further evidence of both a maternal factor which delays onset of the disease and a paternal factor which produces earlier onset. In one study, scientists found that those individuals who inherited HD from their grandfathers had a younger age of onset than those inheriting the disease from their grandmothers. A second hypothesis studied was whether early-onset mothers who inherited the disease from their fathers produced offspring who had older onset ages than the mothers themselves. The scientists found that the offsprings' ages of onset were on average 5.1 years older than their mothers', suggesting that their onset had been delayed by maternally transmitted factors. Similarly, fathers with a late onset of HD who inherited the disease from their mothers had offspring with earlier onset ages, by 6.3 years on average. The juvenile form of HD is thought to be a good example of the phenomenon of imprinting.

Research Focuses on Killer Gene Model

Although scientists know that certain brain cells die in HD, the cause of that death is still unknown. One idea suggests that the unknown killer is a toxic substance that seeks out and destroys specific nerve cells. Another hypothesis is that the HD gene may program brain cells to produce too much of a naturally occurring substance, resulting in nerve cell death.

NINDS-supported scientists have found a striking depression in the level of an enzyme found in the mitochondria of five HD patients studied, further suggesting that HD may be caused by a a mutation within mitochondrial DNA. Other scientists are developing methods to directly measure the mitochondrial energy process in HD postmortem tissue. It may well be that changes in mitochondria, the packets of enzymes within cells which are critical in energy metabolism, are an important part of the mechanism of programmed cell death in HD and other neurodegenerative disorders.

Excitatory amino acids are brain chemicals that play a crucial role in the transmission of nerve impulses. At high levels, some excitatory amino acids cause cell damage and are then known as excitotoxins. Excitotoxins kill nerve cells in the brain, and in animal models they produce the features of several different neurodegenerative disorders. NINDS scientists are exploring whether HD is caused by overproduction of an endogenous excitotoxin called quinolinic acid.

This year, a team of NINDS-supported investigators measured concentrations of quinolinic acid in the cerebrospinal fluid and postmortem tissue of both HD patients and normal control subjects. Concentrations tended to be lower in several areas of the basal ganglia of the HD brains, with significant reductions in three areas. While these findings do not support the hypothesis that an increase of quinolinic acid is responsible for the neurodegeneration in HD, why these reductions are present raises intriguing questions about quinolinic acid metabolism and is an area for further study.

Other NINDS scientists are studying the effects of quinolinic acid in rodents. By injecting the chemical into rats, investigators are finding that some types of neurons are more vulnerable to the chemical's destructive effects than are others. Scientists have found, however, that this pattern of vulnerability does not completely mimic HD. NINDS investigators have also found that large doses of quinolinic acid produce large lesions in the brain and that very low doses produce no lesions. Scientists are currently studying the effects of intermediate doses. NINDS investigators have also improved devices used to inject quinolinic acid in animal models, thus improving methods for studying the effects of this important brain chemical.

Other research supported by NINDS focuses on the production and storage of quinolinic acid in the brain. Scientists have found that brain cells can retain newly synthesized quinolinic acid for an extended period of time and that neuron-depleted tissue cannot store it. This finding is important for our understanding of how quinolinic acid is regulated and how it functions in the brain.

Another chemical present in the brain is basic fibroblast growth factor, or bFGF. This substance acts to protect the neurons of the striatum—part of the basal ganglia—from excitatory amino acid toxicity and enhances neuron survival. Little is known about its distribution in the striatum. This year, NINDS investigators found that although it may not be actively secreted from striatal neurons at all, bFGF markedly protects nerve cells exposed to quinolinic acid and helps them to survive.

Receptors are recognition sites in cells which cause a response in the body when stimulated by certain chemicals. Many scientists believe that the mechanism of action behind HD may involve overstimulation of a certain receptor in the brain, known as the NMDA receptor. A brain chemical called kynurenic acid protects the brain against overstimulation of the NMDA receptor, and a deficiency of kynurenic acid can contribute to neuronal degeneration.

This year, NINDS investigators studied the postmortem brains of 30 HD patients and 35 unaffected individuals and found a reduction of kynurenic acid in the HD brains. A separate NINDS-supported study found reduced kynurenic acid concentrations in six of eight regions of the cortex in HD brains, no difference in the cerebellum, and a small decrease in the caudate region of the basal ganglia.

Several NINDS studies are aimed at understanding the relationship of changes in receptor density and nerve cell loss in HD. Among these are studies to locate those receptors in the various parts of the basal ganglia in HD brains. By locating these receptors, investigators hope to learn which nerve cells are affected during the gradual progression of the disease and thereby produce the various symptoms associated with HD. NINDS-supported studies also suggest that different types of neurons are responsible for certain symptoms associated with different stages of HD. One type may control the initiation and completion of voluntary movements, while another controls the suppression of unwanted movements. As the disease progresses, clinical symptoms such as impaired eye movements, chorea, and rigidity and acinesia (impaired movement) begin to appear, each associated with a loss of a particular type of neuron.

NINDS-supported scientists continue to make progress in this area of research and recently isolated specific receptors in two parts of the basal ganglia, the substantia nigra and the striatum. A team of NINDS scientists is also collaborating with Dutch investigators who found neuronal losses in the hypothalamus in HD brains. Studies of how excitatory amino acid receptors are distributed in HD brains and in normal control brains are under way. This year, a team of scientists found dramatic losses of neurons in certain areas of the frontal cortex and the caudate, along with increased numbers of nerve cells called oligodendroglia.

Primates Serve as Model for HD

NINDS scientists at the Huntington's Disease Center Without Walls based at Massachusetts General Hospital in Boston are studying symptoms corresponding to HD in primates. As part of their study, investigators there are transplanting healthy cells into the damaged brains of monkeys and, for the first time, have shown that replacement of cells in a primate model can reduce these symptoms. Other studies with the primate model include investigations of how the brain chemical dopamine alters movement abnormalities similar to those seen in HD, and positron emission tomography (PET) imaging studies which visualize the damaged striatum.

Understanding Disease Progression Through Clinical Studies

Although there are presently no successful treatments for HD patients, scientists are pursuing clinical research studies which may one day lead to the development of new drugs to halt the disease's rate of progression.

In one study this year, NINDS investigators looked at 42 persons affected by HD to determine which factors are associated with the progression of the disease. The patients received a minimum of six neurological examinations and were followed up for at least 3 years. Men tended to have a slower disease progression than women, particularly those men who inherited HD from their mothers. Investigators also found that depression, tobacco and alcohol use, and treatment with two drugs, haloperidol and imipramine, were all unrelated to disease progression. In the study, slow progression was related to older age at onset and heavier weight at first examination. Investigators also confirmed previous findings that early onset in HD is related to rapid disease progression.

Yearly visits by NINDS grantees to the large extended kindred affected by HD in Venezuela continue to increase our understanding of how the disease strikes different individuals. This year, investigators concluded a 7-year (1981-1988) follow-up study of 593 symptomatic and at-risk persons. In this group, they found that the likelihood of developing HD within three years was 3 percent for those with normal first examinations, 23 percent for those with mildly abnormal first examinations, and 60 percent for those with highly abnormal first neurological examinations. The study suggests that there is not a distinct age of onset but rather a prolonged period of time during which symptoms unfold. The investigators also found that paternal or maternal inheritance did not appear to affect the rate of progression in the family members studied.

Role of PET in Diagnosing HD Studied

As geneticists work to locate the chromosomal defect responsible for HD, NINDS-supported scientists are using PET— the imaging partner of the biological sciences—to isolate where the genetic error ends up in the chemical systems of the body. PET visualizes abnormalities of metabolism or chemical abnormalities, and investigators hope to ascertain whether PET scans can reveal these abnormalities before clinical signs of the disease appear. The NINDS continues to support a number of studies which use PET scans to visualize the metabolic abnormalities of HD. The answer to the question of whether these abnormalities precede clinical signs of HD may result in the use of PET as a standard diagnostic tool for HD.

Scientists Look to the Future with Excitement and Hope

Investigators are optimistic that the damaging HD gene will be located so that its impact can be analyzed and neutralized. Identification of the gene will also mean individuals can be tested directly for the gene rather than for the marker, which requires data from other family members. Neurochemical analyses also hold promise that the element(s) causing brain damage can be identified. An array of approaches to characterize the onset of the disorder will help make diagnosis, modification of symptoms, and future treatment accurate and effective.

As reported above, the NINDS research program on Huntington's disease is exploring a host of genetic, biochemical, metabolic, and clinical leads. Results continue to accrue; the hope for developing meaningful methods of prevention and therapy is becoming more realistic.

■ Document Source:
National Institute of Neurological Disorders and Stroke
1992

MULTI-INFARCT DEMENTIA

Serious forgetfulness, mood swings, and other behavior changes are not a normal part of aging. Some of these changes are caused by problems that can be treated or corrected, like a poor diet or lack of sleep. Sometimes too many medicines cause these symptoms in older people. Feelings of loneliness, boredom, or depression also can cause a person to be forgetful. These problems are serious and should be treated. Often, though, they can be reversed.

Sometimes mental changes cannot be treated easily because they are caused by diseases that permanently damage brain cells. The term dementia is used to describe symptoms that are usually caused by changes in the normal activity of very sensitive brain cells. Dementia seriously interferes with a person's ability to carry out daily activities. Two common causes of dementia in older people are Alzheimer's disease and multi-infarct dementia.

Alzheimer's disease is the most common cause of dementia in older persons. Alzheimer's disease develops when nerve cells in the brain die. Symptoms begin slowly and become steadily worse. At this time, no one knows what causes the nerve cells to die, and there is no cure for the disease.

The second most common cause of dementia in older people is multi-infarct dementia. Multi-infarct dementia usually affects people between the ages of 60 and 75. Men are slightly more likely than women to have multi-infarct dementia. Multi-infarct dementia is caused by a series of strokes that damage or destroy brain tissue. A stroke occurs when blood cannot get to the brain. A blood clot or fatty deposits (called plaques) can block the vessels that supply blood to the brain, causing a stroke. A stroke also can happen when a blood vessel in the brain bursts. The main causes of strokes are untreated high blood pressure, high blood cholesterol, diabetes, and heart disease. Of these, the most important risk factor for multi-infarct dementia is high blood pressure. It is rare for a person without high blood pressure to develop multi-infarct dementia.

Symptoms

Symptoms that begin suddenly may be a sign of multi-infarct dementia. In addition to confusion and problems with recent memory, symptoms of multi-infarct dementia may include wandering or getting lost in familiar places; moving with rapid, shuffling steps; loss of bladder or bowel control (incontinence); emotional problems, such as laughing or crying inappropriately; difficulty following instructions; and problems handling money.

Multi-infarct dementia is often the result of a series of small strokes, called ministrokes or TIAs (transient ischemic attacks). The symptoms of a TIA often are very slight. They may include mild weakness in an arm or leg, slurred speech, and dizziness. The symptoms generally do not last for more than a few days. Several TIAs may occur before the person notices any symptoms of multi-infarct dementia. People with multi-infarct dementia may improve for short periods of time, then decline again upon having further strokes.

Diagnosis

People who show signs of dementia or who have a history of strokes should have a complete physical exam. The doctor will ask the patient and the family about the person's diet, medications, sleep patterns, personal habits, past strokes, and other medical problems. The doctor will ask about recent illnesses or stressful events like the death of someone close and problems at home or work that may account for the symptoms. To look for signs of stroke, the doctor will check for weakness or numbness in the arms or legs, difficulty with speech, or dizziness. To check for other health problems that could cause symptoms of dementia, the doctor may order office or laboratory tests. These tests may include a blood pressure reading, an electroencephalogram (EEG), a test of thyroid function, and blood tests.

The doctor also may ask for x-rays or special tests such as a computerized tomography (CT) scan or a magnetic resonance imaging (MRI) test. Both CT scans and MRI tests take pictures of sections of the brain. The pictures are then displayed on a computer screen to allow the doctor to see inside the brain. CT scans and MRI tests are painless and do not require surgery. Specialists called radiologists and neurologists interpret these tests. In addition, the doctor may send the patient to a psychologist or psychiatrist to test reasoning, learning ability, memory, and attention span.

Sometimes multi-infarct dementia is difficult to distinguish from Alzheimer's disease. It is possible for a person to have both multi-infarct dementia and Alzheimer's disease, making it hard for the doctor to diagnose either.

Treatment

While no treatment can reverse damage that has already been done, treatment to prevent additional strokes is very important. High blood pressure, the primary risk factor for multi-infarct dementia, can be treated successfully. Diabetes also is a treatable risk for stroke. To prevent additional strokes, doctors may prescribe medicines to control high blood pressure, high cholesterol, heart disease, and diabetes. They will counsel patients about good health habits such as exercising and avoiding smoking and drinking alcohol. The patient may require a special diet.

Doctors sometimes prescribe aspirin or other drugs to prevent clots from forming in the small blood vessels. Drugs also can be prescribed to relieve restlessness or depression or to help the patient sleep better. Sometimes doctors recommend a type of surgery known as carotid endarterectomy. This surgery is done to remove blockage in the carotid artery, the main blood vessel to the brain. Studies are under way to see how well this surgery works in treating patients with multi-infarct dementia. Some scientists also are studying drugs that increase the flow of blood to the brain.

Helping Someone with Multi-Infarct Dementia

Family members and friends can help someone with multi-infarct dementia cope with mental and physical problems. They can encourage patients to keep up their daily routines and regular social and physical activities. By talking with them about events and daily activities, family members can help patients use their mental abilities as much as possible. Some families find it helpful to use reminders such as lists, alarm clocks, and calendars to help the patient remember important times and events.

A person with multi-infarct dementia should be under the regular care of a doctor. If the patient has health problems such as diabetes, other specialists may be consulted as well.

Help and advice for home caregivers are available from a variety of sources, including nurses, family doctors, social workers, and physical and occupational therapists. Home health care and respite or day care services in some neighborhoods can provide much-needed relief to caregivers. A state or local health department, a local hospital, or the patient's doctor may be able to provide a telephone number to call for such services.

Support groups offer emotional support for family members caring for a person with dementia. A state or local health department, government agency on aging, or local hospital can provide information about support groups in the community.

The organizations listed below offer more information about some of the topics mentioned in this fact sheet.

Additional copies of this fact sheet and single copies of the *Age Pages* "Stroke Prevention and Treatment," "Memory Loss and Confusion in Old Age: It's Not What You Think," and "Depression: A Serious But Treatable Illness" are available from:

Alzheimer's Disease Education and Referral (ADEAR) Center
P.O. Box 8250
Silver Spring, MD 20907-8250
800-438-4380

A free information packet about multi-infarct dementia and information about support groups for families are available from:

Alzheimer's Association
919 North Michigan Avenue
Suite 1000
Chicago, IL 60611
800-272-3900

Information about stroke and current research on stroke-related conditions is available from:

National Institute of Neurological Disorders and Stroke
Building 31, Room 8A06
9000 Rockville Pike
Bethesda, MD 20892
301-496-5751

Information about stroke and support for stroke survivors and their families is available from:

National Stroke Association
Suite 240
300 East Hampden Avenue
Englewood, CO 80110
303-762-9922

Information about preventing stroke, including information about risk factors such as high blood pressure, high cholesterol, heart disease, and smoking, is available from:

National Heart, Lung, and Blood Information Center
P.O. Box 30105
Bethesda, MD 20824-0105
301-951-3260

Information about controlling diabetes, an important risk factor for stroke, is available from:

National Diabetes Information Clearinghouse
Box NDIC
9000 Rockville Pike
Bethesda, MD 20892
301-468-2162

Information about services and resources in your area, such as adult day care programs, transportation, and meal services, is available from:

Eldercare Locator Service
Administration on Aging
800-677-1116

■ **Document Source:**
   U.S. Department of Health and Human Services, Public Health Service
   National Institutes of Health
   National Institute on Aging
   NIH Publication No. 93-3433

See also: Alzheimer's Disease (page 321)

MULTIPLE SCLEROSIS

Introduction

Multiple sclerosis is a disease caused by inflammation and scarring of tissues in the brain and spinal cord. More specifically, the inflammation breaks down myelin, the white, fatty material that provides a thick sheath or covering for nerve fibers in the central nervous system. A healthy myelin sheath enables a nerve cell to send electrical impulses along its fiber at high velocity, a function critical for accomplishing such basic activities as walking, eating, or breathing.

As multiple sclerosis causes more and more of the sheath to be stripped away, a process called demyelination, electrical impulses proceed more and more slowly down the fiber. Depending on which nerves are affected, severe or mild disabilities can occur. If myelin in sensory nerves is lost, for example, a person may have an impaired sense of touch.

Multiple sclerosis gets its name because the demyelination is often followed by sclerosis, or hardening of nervous system tissue, usually at multiple sites. The sclerosis is the result of scar tissue forming in the central nervous system (a process called gliosis). In part because we can not determine in advance which nerve fibers will be affected in a particular patient—the disease can impair any part of the central nervous system—the severity of multiple sclerosis is often unpredictable. Some people may have mild problems, with no significant permanent disability. For others, multiple sclerosis means severe paralysis and confinement to a wheelchair. We

do know that the disease often strikes people in the prime of life, most commonly between the ages of 20 and 40, although some people do not develop multiple sclerosis until their forties or fifties. The disease strikes about twice as many women as men.

Symptoms

Although severe forms of multiple sclerosis can be devastating, the illness shortens a person's average life expectancy by only about five years. Common symptoms of the disease include fatigue and loss of strength. Patients often have increased muscle stiffness due to a condition known as spasticity, or muscle stiffness. There may be loss of sensation in the arms and legs, or an ever-present tingling sensation, like feeling pins and needles. People also may have facial pain. If multiple sclerosis has affected the cerebellum, a portion of the nervous system near the back of the brain, the patient may have poor coordination, loss of balance, or tremors.

If the optic nerve is involved, the patient may have blurred or reduced vision. Patients with demyelination of the brain stem, a region that controls eye movement, commonly have double vision, since each eye may no longer focus on the same object. If the illness has impaired the spinal cord, in addition to losing leg strength, the patient may lose bladder control, become constipated, or become impotent.

One common feature of multiple sclerosis is that many symptoms worsen when patients are exposed to heat. This is because elevated temperatures—whether from a hot bath, exercise, or exposure to the sun—further slow the conduction of electrical impulses in nerve fibers. Conversely, a cold bath can sometimes temporarily relieve symptoms or reduce some of the fatigue multiple sclerosis patients often feel.

Neurologists divide multiple sclerosis into two types. The first, known as exacerbating-remitting disease, is characterized by fluctuations in nerve function. Periods of deteriorating ability are followed by periods of recovery, although, as time passes, recovery often becomes less and less complete. The second form of the illness, chronic progressive disease, has more of a steady downhill course, typically without periods of temporary recovery. Frequently, people who initially have the fluctuating form of multiple sclerosis go on to develop the chronic form.

The Search for Causes

We do not yet know the cause of multiple sclerosis. Although there is considerable evidence that a virus may trigger the disease, researchers are still uncertain. Genetic factors and an imbalance in the immune system also may help predispose an individual to the illness.

Evidence for a Viral Link

The evidence for a viral or other environmental agent comes from many sources. First, multiple sclerosis is far more common in colder or temperate climates than in warmer climates. Within North America and Europe, there is a higher prevalence of the disease in the north than in the south. Studies of large immigrant populations suggest that people with multiple sclerosis were exposed to some environmental agent at a young age, possibly before age 15. The immigrant studies show that people who emigrated before age 15 had a prevalence of multiple sclerosis similar to that found in the region to which they moved. People who emigrated after age 15 had the same disease prevalence as found in the area from which they came.

Evidence for a virus as the environmental agent comes from studies of two epidemics of the disease in Iceland and Faroe Islands, the latter an area between Iceland and Scandinavia. Each year for about 20 years immediately following World War II, the incidence of the disease in these regions increased. Both regions were occupied by British troops during the war, and some investigators believe the troops may have inadvertently brought with them a still unknown virus or other disease-causing agent.

Viruses that may be linked to multiple sclerosis include the measles; mumps; rubella, the agent that causes German measles; and the monkey virus known as simian virus 5, or SV-5. Most recently, one of a trio of retroviruses collectively known as Human Immunodeficiency Lymphotropic Viruses (HTLVs) has been studied for possible association with the disease. Although the virus under investigation, HTLV-I, belongs to the same family of infectious agents as the AIDS virus (HTLV-III), there is no evidence that links AIDS with multiple sclerosis. HTLV-I, however, causes an inflammatory disease of the spinal cord that has many features, including demyelination, in common with multiple sclerosis. The spinal cord disease, found predominantly in the tropics and Japan, is called tropical spastic paraparesis. Thus, although the cause of multiple sclerosis remains unknown, we have discovered that a retrovirus causes a very similar illness. Such knowledge helps pave the way for better understanding and more effective treatment of multiple sclerosis.

Genetic Factors

People generally do not think of multiple sclerosis as an inherited disease, but its prevalence in families of patients with the disease runs somewhat higher than in the general population. For example, the prevalence of multiple sclerosis in the general population is about five to 10 cases per 10,000 people (.05 to .1 percent). But in a family with one member who has the illness, the chance of a brother or sister developing multiple sclerosis is about 20 times higher (1 to 2 percent). One could argue that the increased incidence could be due to either genetic factors or an environmental agent since family members share the same environment. But evidence from studies of twins suggests a strong genetic influence. Fraternal (nonidentical) twins had the same higher prevalence for multiple sclerosis as brothers and sisters who were not twins. But if one of a pair of identical twins had the illness, researchers found that the other twin had a far higher likelihood, about a 25 to 50 percent chance, of also developing multiple sclerosis. Because identical twins have the same genes, one or more genetic factors appear important for developing the illness.

Indeed, researchers have found genetic markers associated with the disease—proteins more commonly found in immune system and other cells of people with multiple sclerosis than in the general population. Work has focused on certain classes of proteins found on the surface of white blood cells called leukocytes. Scientists have detected one particular human leukocyte-associated protein, known as HLA-DQN1, in about 90 percent of people with multiple sclerosis. (In contrast, about 70 percent of people in the general population have this protein.) Another protein, HLA-DR2, has been identified in about 60 percent of people with multiple sclerosis, but only in about 18 to 20 percent of the general population. In addition, some forms of another leukocyte protein, known as the T-cell receptor molecule, also appear more prevalent among multiple sclerosis patients than in the general population. Finding more than one genetic marker indicates that more than one gene may be needed to trigger onset of the illness.

The Autoimmune Connection

We also have evidence that a defect in the immune system may predispose an individual to multiple sclerosis. Normally, the immune system fights off infections from foreign invaders such as bacteria or viruses. But in some diseases, for reasons that remain unknown, the immune system attacks the body's own tissues, a reaction known as an autoimmune response. Some studies suggest an autoimmune reaction might cause multiple sclerosis. This research focuses on an animal disease, known as experimental allergic encephalomyelitis, or EAE, that causes demyelination and inflammation similar to that seen in multiple sclerosis. Scientists have induced EAE in animals by making them allergic to a myelin protein called myelin basic protein. The allergy causes the animals' immune systems to attack the nervous system and induce a disease highly similar to multiple sclerosis, without injecting a virus or other infectious agent.

Other studies indicate an imbalance between certain cells in the immune system may set the stage for an autoimmune response that could result in multiple sclerosis. To understand the imbalance requires a bit of explanation about some of the key players in the immune system. Certain white blood cells, called B-cells because they originate in the bone marrow, can transform into plasma cells, which then make antibodies. But the B-cells usually need help from other immune system cells, called helper T-cells, in order to efficiently make the antibodies.

The collaboration between B-cells and helper T-cells is regulated by several factors, including suppressor T-cells. Such regulation is critical because otherwise the collaboration between B-cells and helper T-cells would continue even when antibodies are no longer needed. Without the suppressor T-cells to stop them, the helper T-cells and B-cells could make antibodies against a person's own body tissues. Moreover, studies indicate that multiple sclerosis patients may have impaired function of suppressor T-cells, possibly triggering an immune system attack against body tissue the system normally protects: central nervous system myelin.

Drug studies provide further evidence for an autoimmune role in causing multiple sclerosis. In clinical trials, several drugs that suppress the immune system have been more effective in treating the disease than drugs that boost immune function.

In actuality, a combination of all three effects described above—infection by a virus, genetic factors, and an autoimmune reaction—may explain the occurrence of multiple sclerosis. Some researchers believe that if a viral infection in a genetically susceptible person occurs at a particularly vulnerable time in the development of the immune system, probably in the early teenage years, it could trigger an autoimmune response. This may happen, for example, if proteins on a virus resemble those proteins belonging to body tissue. If the body's immune system has trouble distinguishing between the viral proteins and its own, it may attack both. Scientists speculate that years later such an autoimmune reaction might develop into multiple sclerosis.

Treatment

There are two basic strategies for treating multiple sclerosis. One regimen attempts to reduce the underlying inflammation and the presumed impaired immune attack against the nervous system. The other strategy emphasizes relief of symptoms.

Treating the Causes of Inflammation and Immune System Dysfunction

The choice of drugs to reduce inflammation depends on the type of multiple sclerosis. For people with exacerbating-remitting multiple sclerosis, the more mild form of the illness, physicians often prescribe a pituitary hormone known as adrenocorticotrophic hormone, or ACTH. This hormone stimulates the adrenal glands to produce cortisol and certain other steroids that reduce inflammation. Alternatively, synthetic steroids, such as prednisone or methylprednisolone, may be given to lower inflammation in the nervous system.

Other agents that might more effectively reduce inflammation are under study. Preliminary research indicates that alpha and beta interferon may be of benefit, and ongoing studies seek to determine the optimum dose of these naturally occurring substances. Another promising drug for people with relatively mild multiple sclerosis is copolymer-I. A small study suggests that the drug can help people who take it for an extended period. Unlike many other drugs used to treat multiple sclerosis, copolymer-I appears to have few side effects. A larger, multicenter, controlled study of the drug is underway.

People who have chronic progressive multiple sclerosis, the more severe form of the illness, are much more difficult to treat. Drugs for this illness tend to be stronger immunosuppressive agents and carry more serious side effects. Neurologists debate whether these drugs should be used at all. Some believe that the risks of using these drugs far outweigh their benefits. Others believe that they should treat multiple sclerosis aggressively, even if it means using a drug that can only temporarily stop the disease from getting worse until a better, safer treatment comes along. One of the better known drugs that falls into this category is cyclophosphamide, or Cytoxan.

Data indicate that only about a third of people who receive the drug show improvement; another one-third remain stable, neither improving or deteriorating; and one-third deteriorate at about the same rate that would be expected if they did not take the drug.

Another experimental treatment for severe and milder forms of multiple sclerosis is plasma exchange, or plasmapheresis. In this procedure, blood is removed from the body and the plasma portion is discarded before the red and white blood cells are returned. The strategy behind this treatment is that plasmapheresis may remove harmful antibodies or other harmful substances circulating in the blood that may damage the nervous system. A large, multicenter study underway in Canada may determine the effectiveness of the treatment.

Another procedure recently tested in multiple sclerosis patients is total lymphoid radiation. This treatment, which involves radiation of the immune system, has been used successfully for 20 years in treating early stages of a cancer called Hodgkin's disease. Preliminary studies at the Medical College of New Jersey suggest that the treatment may help stabilize people with chronic progressive multiple sclerosis for as long as three to four years. A larger clinical trial is planned.

Monoclonal antibodies are one of the more promising experimental therapies for multiple sclerosis, and one which you will be hearing more about in the next few years. Monoclonal antibodies are pure antibodies that can be generated in huge quantities in animals, usually mice. And unlike drugs that suppress the entire immune system, causing unwanted side effects, these antibodies can be directed against specific cells believed to damage the nervous system in multiple sclerosis patients. Various clinical trials are underway or being planned to evaluate monoclonal antibodies directed against all T-cells, against helper T-cells, or against the subset of activated T-cells. Activated T-cells, as opposed to resting cells, are believed to mediate damage to the nervous system in people with multiple sclerosis. Researchers at Stanford University plan to test monoclonal antibodies against HLA-DR2, the genetic marker discussed above. Future studies also are likely to examine the ability to block certain T-cell receptor molecules that may be common in tissue damaged by multiple sclerosis.

Treating Symptoms

We are generally more successful at treating symptoms than the root causes of multiple sclerosis. The drug baclofen (Lioresal) treats such symptoms as painful spasms and stiffness. Another anti-spastic drug, dantrolen (Dantrium), is effective but can cause serious liver damage. Two drugs can reduce fatigue in multiple sclerosis patients: amantadine (Symmetrel) and semoline (Cylert).

The inability to control bladder function is a distressing problem that leaves many people with multiple sclerosis ashamed to leave home. The drug Ditropan helps control bladder function. Constipation, another symptom frequently seen in patients, can be treated with several compounds. A first treatment might be Metamucil alone or in combination with a stool softener such as Colace or Surfak. If these do not work, Milk of Magnesia, Dulcolax or several other agents may be prescribed. An enema may be needed to keep the constipation from causing serious damage.

Facial pain and other painful syndromes can be treated with anticonvulsive medications such as carbamazepine (Tegretol), phenytoin sodium (Dilantin) or Valproic Acid (Depakote). Elavil, originally manufactured as an antidepressant, also helps treat pain originating in the nervous system, as in multiple sclerosis. As a last resort, if severe pain persists and interferes with such basic functions as speaking or chewing, some people may have a section of the nerve surgically removed or blocked. People who undergo this procedure will have numbness over part of much of the face. A surgeon can first reversibly block the nerve to give the patient an idea of the numbness that will be produced. For some, the loss of feeling may be as disturbing as the pain they had before surgery.

Exercise can cause problems for people with multiple sclerosis because the resulting overheating can make neurological symptoms worse. But because cold temperatures increase the velocity of electrical impulses in nerves, which are slowed in multiple sclerosis, exercising in cold water may temporarily help relieve symptoms of multiple sclerosis. The ability to dissipate heat in cold water, combined with the buoyancy that people have in water, allows patients to maintain fitness without suffering the side effects of overheating they would experience if they exercised in more conventional ways. In addition, an experimental drug, 4-aminopyridine, appears to increase the velocity of impulses in demyelinated nerves. This and/or related drugs are expected to become generally available to treat multiple sclerosis during the next few years.

Physical medicine and rehabilitation are important complements to drug therapy for multiple sclerosis. Physical therapists work with the patient on developing strength, coordination, balance, and stamina to perform activities without tiring. Occupational therapists concentrate more on coping with daily living and have introduced several devices that help people function more easily, for example, with dressing and eating. One of the most useful innovations is the motor scooter, a vehicle that has allowed people to maintain their jobs long after they would have had to retire on disability. The device is useful not only for people who can no longer walk, but also for ambulatory people who tire easily due to the disease.

In addition, vocational rehabilitation has taken on greater emphasis. People who can no longer physically perform their jobs can learn new skills in an increasing number of vocational programs, including many sponsored by local chapters of the Multiple Sclerosis Society.

Conclusion

All of these various forms of therapy—established and experimental drug treatments, physical therapy, occupational therapy, and new mechanical devices—have helped to promote a much greater degree of independence among people with multiple sclerosis. Increasingly, people with this disease are leading happier, fuller, and more productive lives. The large number of clinical trials and research studies underway promises to offer even more effective treatments for multiple sclerosis in the future.

Questions and Answers

Q. Do nutritional factors play a role in the disease? Can improved nutrition arrest or reverse multiple sclerosis?
A. We have no evidence that nutritional deficiencies have anything to do with causing the disease. There is little evidence to suggest that a particular diet or a nutritional supplement can help treat multiple sclerosis. However, relatively few scientific studies have been conducted on nutrition and multiple sclerosis. Most of the recommendations various people make regarding nutritional therapy are based on unproven theories. Almost none of the dietary therapies have been evaluated in standard, double-blind, controlled studies.

Q. Is there any correlation between memory disturbances in Alzheimer disease and multiple sclerosis?
A. We are becoming more aware these days that people with multiple sclerosis may have some impaired cognitive function, including some memory disturbance. For most people with the illness, it is not a severe problem. Memory impairment is a relatively new area of investigation in multiple sclerosis, and the Multiple Sclerosis Society recently has begun funding this research.

Q. Is multiple sclerosis contagious? Can I catch the disease from working near or living with someone who has it?
A. Although a virus may be associated with multiple sclerosis, there is no evidence that people with the disease can transmit the illness to healthy individuals. Sexual or other intimate contact with a person that has multiple sclerosis does not appear to increase one's chances of getting the disease. For instance, spouses of patients with multiple sclerosis do not have an increased incidence of the illness.

Q. What affect does pregnancy have on someone with multiple sclerosis?

A. On average, women with multiple sclerosis tend to have fewer symptoms of the disease during pregnancy. But in the year following pregnancy, symptoms often worsen. Symptoms usually return to pre-pregnancy levels during the second year after pregnancy, but some women who have very severe disease during that first year will not recover fully. They may develop severe, permanent impairment after pregnancy, although often the persistent symptoms may not be as bad as those experienced during the first year after pregnancy.

■ Document Source:
   U.S. Department of Health and Human Services, Public Health Service
   National Institutes of Health
   Warren Grant Magnuson Clinical Center, Clinical Center Communications
   NIH Publication No. 90-3015
   August 1990

NUTRITION AND WEIGHT LOSS

■ ■ ■

A Reprint from FDA Consumer Magazine

AN FDA GUIDE TO DIETING

by Ruth Papazian

Like millions of her fellow Americans, talk show host Oprah Winfrey has known the thrill of weight loss and the agony of watching the pounds creep back on. Some three years after losing 67 pounds on a liquid formula diet, Oprah lost her battle to stay a size 10 and has sworn off dieting forever.

Considering that weight-loss programs, pills and potions typically slim the wallet but not the dieter, Oprah may be on to something. And, with research pointing to genetic and metabolic differences between stout and slim people, obesity experts are now debating whether dieting can achieve permanent weight loss.

Defining Obesity

Obesity is associated with such health problems as diabetes, gallstones, hypertension, and heart disease. Obesity is also linked to colorectal cancer and to breast, uterine and ovarian cancer in women and prostate cancer in men. But how many extra pounds does it take before a person crosses the line from overweight to obese? It depends on whom you ask: The definition of obesity is currently in a state of flux.

Traditionally, obesity was defined as 20 percent or more above an optimal weight for height derived from actuarial statistics that correlated with lowest death rates. Now, some health experts say that the weight-for-height yardstick is both imprecise and overly restrictive.

Recent research suggests that more important than the amount of extra weight a person carries is where it is located. "Rather than weight-for-height, obesity should be defined in terms of waist-to-hip ratio," says C. Wayne Callaway, M.D., associate clinical professor of medicine at George Washington University in Washington, D.C., and a leading authority on obesity.

Waist-to-hip ratio can be calculated by dividing the number of inches around the waistline by the circumference of the hips. For example, someone who has a 27-inch waist and 38-inch hips would have a ratio of 0.71. A woman whose ratio is 0.8 or higher would be at high risk of weight-related health problems, as would a man whose ratio is 0.95 or above.

Numerous studies show that fat in the hips and thighs is less health-threatening than abdominal fat. While other fat cells empty directly into general circulation, the fatty acid contents of abdominal fat cells go straight to the liver, by way of the portil vein, before being circulated to the muscles. This process interferes with the liver's ability to clear insulin from the bloodstream. As blood levels of insulin increase, muscles and other cells become insulin-resistant, and blood glucose levels rise as a result. In response, the pancreas cranks out more insulin, prompting the autonomic nervous system (which controls heart rate, blood pressure, and other vital signs) to produce norepinephrine, an adrenalin-like chemical that raises blood pressure. This sets the stage for the development of diabetes, hypertension, and heart problems.

Callaway also points out that weight tables do not take age-related weight gain into account (as people age, fat cells become less metabolically active, so one can weigh more and still be healthy) and "arbitrarily" assign lower weights to women at a given height than to men. "There is no evidence showing that women live longer if they weigh less than men of equal stature," he says.

To be a more useful indicator of health risks, experts advocate broadening the definition of obesity to meet three criteria: weight for age and height rather than for gender and height, waist-to-hip ratio, and presence of such weight-related health problems as hypertension.

Food or Fate?

As researchers try to figure out why some people get fat and others don't, it is becoming increasingly apparent that obesity has a variety of causes—heredity, environment, metabolism, and level of physical activity—and, therefore, no single "cure."

Adipose tissue (fat cells) stores energy in the form of fat to meet the body's energy needs when other sources, such as glucose, are unavailable or depleted.

The body has an almost limitless capacity to store fat. Not only can each fat cell balloon to more than 10 times its original size, but should the available cells get filled to the brim, new ones will propagate. As the body stores more fat, weight and girth increase.

A number of studies have shown that genetics may be the most important determinant of how much you weigh. Some people are more prone to weight gain than others even when caloric intake is the same, according to a study of 12 pairs of identical male twins aged 19 to 27 conducted at Quebec's Laval University and reported in the May 24, 1990, issue of the *New England Journal of Medicine*. After eating an extra 1,000 calories six days a week for 100 days, some of the twins gained 9 pounds apiece while others gained as much as 29 pounds each—in some twin pairs, the extra calories were stored as fat while others used up the excess calories by building muscle tissue. The twins in each pair gained the same amount of weight and in the same places, suggesting that as-yet unidentified genetic factors influence the amount of weight gain and its distribution.

> *Research indicates that obesity may be linked to the proportion of fat in the diet rather than to the amount of calories consumed.*

The same issue of the *New England Journal of Medicine* also reported on a study comparing the body mass of 673 pairs of identical and fraternal Swedish twins who had been raised together or apart to determine how much influence heredity had over obesity (identical twins have the exact same genetic makeup whereas fraternal twins do not; twins who were raised together were subject to the same environmental influences while those who were raised apart were not). Even if they had grown up together, the fraternal twins were less likely than the identical twins to share a similar pattern of body weight whereas identical twins—even when raised apart—did not vary significantly in weight. The researchers concluded that genetic factors, apart from diet or lifestyle, strongly influence how much a person weighs.

Previously, researchers at the University of Iowa found evidence of a recessive obesity gene (the child needs one copy of the gene from each parent to have the tendency towards overweight). A study of 277 schoolchildren and their families showed a pattern of obesity that followed the classic model for recessive inheritance.

However, it is likely that a number of genetic mechanisms exert influence on weight, among them genes that dictate metabolism and appetite. One that is being investigated actively is the gene that codes for lipoprotein lipase (LPL), an enzyme produced by fat cells to help store calories as fat. If too much LPL is produced, the body will be especially efficient at storing calories.

LPL is partly controlled by reproductive hormones (estrogen in women, testosterone in men), so gender-based differences in the activity of the enzyme also factor into obesity. In women, fat cells in the hips, thighs and breasts secrete LPL, while in men the enzyme is produced by fat cells in the midriff region. Fat cells in the abdominal area release their contents for quick energy, while fat in the thighs and buttocks are used for long-term energy storage. Thus, a man can often pare his paunch more readily than a woman can shed her saddlebags.

LPL also makes it easier to regain lost weight, according to a study conducted at Cedars-Sinai Medical Center in Los Angeles and reported in the April 12, 1990, issue of the *New England Journal of Medicine*. Nine people who lost an average of 90 pounds had their LPL levels measured before dieting and after maintaining their new weights for three months. The researchers found that levels of the enzyme rose after weight loss, and that the fatter the person was to start with, the higher the LPL levels were—as though the body was fighting to regain the weight. They believe that weight loss activated the gene producing the enzyme. This may be one reason why it is easier for a dieter to regain lost weight than for someone who has never been obese to put weight on.

Set for Life?

This study supports the much-debated "set point" theory, which holds that inner mechanisms set a person's weight at a predetermined level and if anything is done to change the weight, the body will adjust to restore fat content to the set point.

"I regard body temperature, which stays around 98.6 degrees F, to be a set point. Weight doesn't have a set point in that sense," says Xavier Pi-Sunyer, M.D., director of the Obesity Research Center at St. Luke's-Roosevelt Hospital Center in New York.

If there is a set point for weight, it generally seems to move in one direction—that is, the body will not make adjustments to counteract a large weight gain but will fight efforts to lose the weight. "When a person gains weight and stays at that weight a while, the body will defend that weight. It becomes the new 'set point'," explains Pi-Sunyer.

Aside from the action of LPL, the body uses other adaptive mechanisms when food intake is reduced. To cite just two of them: Dieting depresses the metabolic rate so that calories are burned more slowly, and as fat cells shrink, they become more responsive to the action of insulin and do not release their contents as readily.

"The body is very good at defending itself from the danger of underweight, but is not really equipped to handle overweight. Throughout the ages, people have not had a problem with having too much to eat. That's a modern problem," says Pi-Sunyer.

Though a definitive study has yet to be done in humans showing that weight gain becomes more likely after each successive diet (the so-called "yo-yo" syndrome), the Cedars-Sinai study strengthens this controversial hypothesis. However, in order to show conclusively that weight loss gets harder each time a person loses and regains weight, the subjects in the Cedars-Sinai study would have to be followed through several cycles of weight gain and loss to determine whether LPL levels kept rising after each diet.

Repeatedly losing and gaining weight may have other health consequences, according to a report in the June 27, 1991, *New England Journal of Medicine*. American and Swedish researchers analyzed weight fluctuations and later health problems over a period of 32 years in more than 3,000 women and men who participated in the Framingham (Mass.) Health Study. The researchers said that people who repeatedly lose and regain weight appear to have an overall higher death rate and to be at greater risk of heart disease and some cancers than those whose weight remains stable (even if overweight) or steadily increases.

Are All Calories Created Equal?

"The body will do what it was programmed to do even if that's not what you want it to do," notes Callaway. For this reason, restricting food intake to 1,000 or 1,200 calories in order to lose weight is "doomed to failure," he says. "For many people, going on one more diet isn't going to solve a weight problem in the long run."

Even well-established weight-loss programs are not individualized enough to account for genetics, past dieting attempts, and a person's activity level, he says.

While Pi-Sunyer agrees that putting everyone on the same prepackaged weight-loss regimen can be counterproductive, he believes that restricting caloric intake is an important weight-control tool. "You can easily cut caloric intake just by restricting the amount of fat and sugar you eat. This might be the only adjustment a moderately overweight person would need to make in order to lose weight."

Research indicates that obesity may be linked to the proportion of fat in the diet rather than to the amount of calories consumed, according to a survey of the diets and exercise habits of 107 men and 109 women reported in the September 1990 issue of *American Journal of Clinical Nutrition*. Researchers at Indiana University in Bloomington found that overweight subjects got 35 percent of their calories from fat and 46 percent from carbohydrates, compared to 29 percent of calories from fat and 53 percent from carbohydrates for their slender counterparts. A recent University of Vermont study suggests that limiting fat intake to about 20 percent of total calories enabled chronically obese patients who failed to lose weight on a variety of reducing programs to lose an average of 20 to 30 pounds over the course of a year.

Scientists used to think that all calories were created equal. That is, whether it came from fat, carbohydrates or protein, a calorie produced a certain amount of heat when the body burned it to fuel metabolic processes. Thus, according to "The Dieter's Law of Thermodynamics," mashed potatoes and milkshakes were no more culpable in promoting weight gain than pasta and peas—as long as caloric intake was limited to 1,000 or some other magic number.

Alas, further research has shown this to be an illusion. Calories from carbohydrates, fat and protein are used differently by the body. Virtually all fat calories are immediately stored in fat cells. Carbohydrates and protein are converted into glucose for fuel, with only those calories in excess of the body's energy needs being stored.

Compounding the problem, a gram of fat has 9 calories while an equal amount of carbohydrates or protein has 4. "For the same number of calories, a person can have a much bigger serving of a food that is primarily carbohydrate as one that is high in fat," observes Walter Glinsmann, M.D., associate director for clinical nutrition at the Food and Drug Administration's Center for Food Safety and Applied Nutrition. For instance, a 6.5-ounce baked potato has the same number of calories as 1.5 ounces of potato chips (about 225).

The type of fat in the diet is important as well. Currently, the National Cholesterol Education Program recommends that the diet be limited to 30 percent of calories from fat, with no more than 10 percent of those coming from saturated fats. "Unsaturated fats are precursors of such biologically active molecules as prostaglandins, which are involved in a variety of body processes, including blood pressure regulation and immune system function. Various types of fat have different roles in health maintenance and disease risk," says Glinsmann.

Exercise the Key

Rather than severely restricting caloric intake and depressing metabolic activity as a result, weight-loss specialists now advise moderate exercise as a means of achieving weight control. "A person not only burns calories while exercising, but if he or she is eating an adequate amount of food, calories will continue to be burned at a higher rate for up to several hours afterward," says Callaway.

"For most people, cutting fat intake and adding moderate exercise can work as well as a commercial weight control program," says Pi-Sunyer. Exercisers are also more likely than sedentary people to keep weight off, whether they use a "do-it-yourself" diet or attend a program.

Unfortunately, weight maintenance is a universal failing of all weight-loss programs, regardless of how expensive or well-established. "If you're going to evaluate weight-loss success, you can't just look at the number of pounds lost. You have to look at long-term weight maintenance," says Callaway.

"Diet programs make money on the weight-loss phase, not the weight maintenance phase. At the time when people need the most help in controlling their weight, many programs cut them off," says Pi-Sunyer. By various estimates, as many as 85 percent of dieters put the weight back on within two years after weight loss.

"Perhaps weight-loss programs should be less focused on weight control and more focused on identifying individual risk factors and dietary patterns associated with obesity, and to modify them where possible," suggests Glinsmann.

"Obesity is not yet well understood," concedes Pi-Sunyer, "and all we can do right now is to tell people to exercise and to cut down on fat intake." However, while genetic predisposition towards obesity can be mitigated by exercise and sensible eating habits, some people will have to work a lot harder at keeping weight at optimal levels than others. "It's like jazz—there's a theme and rhythm and you've got to work within that framework, but you can improvise," says Callaway.

Product Bans and Controversies

In the wake of last year's House Committee on Small Business hearings on the $33 billion weight-loss industry, FDA and the Federal Trade Commission separately announced investigations into the safety and efficacy of diet pills and programs, and how they are promoted in advertising. FDA also moved to pull dangerous or ineffective products off store shelves.

In the fall of 1990, FDA proposed a ban on 111 ingredients in over-the-counter (OTC) diet products, including amino acids, cellulose, grapefruit extract, and kelp. The agency had given manufacturers of these products an opportunity to provide data from clinical tests showing they were effective in promoting weight loss, but did not receive adequate information to support advertising claims, according to William Gilbertson, Pharm.D., director of FDA's OTC Drug Review Program. "Many of these ingredients had been marketed before 1962 [when an amendment to the 1938 Food, Drug, and Cosmetic Act was passed requiring drugs not only to be safe, but also effective] and had never been evaluated for efficacy," Gilbertson explains.

He says that manufacturers wanting to market weight-loss drugs using the banned ingredients will have to get prior FDA approval—which means filing a new drug application and supplying data from clinical tests to support claims.

FDA also recalled Cal-Ban 3000, a heavily advertised diet pill containing guar gum (a vegetable gum that swells when it absorbs moisture, providing a feeling of fullness, according to advertising claims) after receiving a number of consumer complaints of adverse reactions. In a number of cases, the tablet caused gastric or esophageal obstruction, and one person died as a result of complications following surgery to remove the mass of gum blocking his throat.

The most widely used ingredient in OTC diet pills, phenylpropanolamine hydrochloride (PPA), an appetite suppressant that is chemically related to amphetamines, has been the subject of a decade-long medical dispute. Though clinical tests yielded conflicting results (often due to defects in study design), an FDA panel concluded in 1982 that enough data existed to support the efficacy of PPA in curbing the appetite to qualify it as an OTC weight-loss aid. However, a controversy developed over PPA's safety. The drug can cause small elevations of blood pressure at recommended doses, and there are a few reports of marked blood pressure elevation and intracranial bleeding associated with its use. Whether such events are truly drug-related and can occur at recommended doses is the subject of debate.

In May, FDA held a public meeting to explore such issues as whether PPA can cause such central nervous system damage as stroke when taken at (or over) the recommended dosage, whether the drug poses a health hazard to teenagers, and whether PPA is especially hazardous to those with eating disorders.

For its part, FTC has begun to look into advertising claims of 14 diet programs. "We are concerned with programs that go beyond promising weight loss and claim to be able to keep the weight off," says Richard Kelly, assistant director of FTC's division of service industry practices. Additionally, FTC is looking into whether diet companies are touting the safety of their programs while playing down such health risks as the development of gallstones or loss of muscle tissue. Kelly expects the FTC investigation to be completed by the end of the year.

FTC also monitors advertising claims for diet aids on an ongoing basis and takes legal action to get companies to stop making unfounded claims. Among the agency's recent targets: Fat-Magnet, a pill that claimed to break up into thousands of tiny "fat-attracting" particles that "flush" fat from the body, and Fibre Trim, a high-fiber supplement that its manufacturer claimed could aid in weight reduction.

FDA's ban of ineffective diet drugs could make future FTC action easier. "The FDA says these products are not efficacious, which is a good piece of evidence to have when we go to trial," says Judy Wilkenfeld, assistant director of FTC's advertising practices division.

Consumers can get a list of ineffective diet aids by writing to: FDA, HFE-20, 5600 Fishers Lane, Rockville, MD 20857.

Ruth Papazian is a freelance writer in New York City specializing in health and medicine.

■ Document Source:
   U.S. Department of Health and Human Services, Public Health Service
   Food and Drug Administration, HFI-40, Rockville, MD 20857.
   DHHS Publication No. (FDA) 92-1188
   October 1991

NUTRITION AND YOUR HEALTH: DIETARY GUIDELINES FOR AMERICANS

What should Americans eat to stay healthy?

These guidelines help answer this question. They are advice for healthy Americans ages 2 years and over—not for younger children and infants, whose dietary needs differ. The guidelines reflect recommendations of nutrition authorities who agree that enough is known about diet's effect on health to encourage certain dietary practices by Americans.

Many American diets have too many calories and too much fat (especially saturated fat), cholesterol, and sodium. They also have too little complex carbohydrates and fiber. Such diets are one cause of America's high rates of obesity and of certain diseases—heart disease, high blood pressure, stroke, diabetes, and some forms of cancer. The exact role of diet in some of these is still being studied.

Diseases caused by vitamin and mineral deficiencies are rare in this country. But some people do not get recommended amounts of a few nutrients, especially calcium and iron.

Food alone cannot make you healthy. Good health also depends on your heredity, your environment, and the health care you get. Your lifestyle is also important to your health— how much you exercise and whether you smoke, drink alcoholic beverages to excess, or abuse drugs, for example. But a diet based on these guidelines can help you keep healthy and may improve your health.

The first two guidelines form the framework for the diet: "Eat a variety of foods" for the nutrients you need and for energy (calories) to "Maintain healthy weight." The next two guidelines stress the need for many Americans to change their diets to be lower in fat, especially saturated fat, and higher in complex carbohydrates and fiber. Other guidelines suggest only moderate use of sugars, salt, and, if used at all, alcoholic beverages.

These guidelines call for moderation—avoiding extremes in diet. Both eating too much and eating too little can be harmful. Also, be cautious of diets based on the belief that a food or supplement alone can cure or prevent disease.

Dietary Guidelines for Americans

♦ **Eat a variety of foods**
♦ **Maintain healthy weight**
♦ **Choose a diet low in fat, saturated fat, and cholesterol**
♦ **Choose a diet with plenty of vegetables, fruits, and grain products**
♦ **Use sugars only in moderation**
♦ **Use salt and sodium only in moderation**
♦ **If you drink alcoholic beverages, do so in moderation.**

Your good health may depend on your learning more about yourself. Are you at your healthy weight? Are your blood pressure and your blood cholesterol levels too high? If so, diet or medicine your doctor prescribes may help reduce them. Generally, the sooner a problem is found, the easier it is to treat.

The foods Americans have to choose from are varied, plentiful, and safe to eat. These guidelines can help you choose a diet that is both healthful and enjoyable.

Read on for more about each guideline—what it means, how it is important to health, brief "advice for today," and some tips on using the guideline.

Eat a Variety of Foods

You need more than 40 different nutrients for good health. Essential nutrients include vitamins, minerals, amino acids from protein, certain fatty acids from fat, and sources of calories (protein, carbohydrates, and fat).

These nutrients should come from a variety of foods, not from a few highly fortified foods or supplements. Any food that supplies calories and nutrients can be part of a nutritious diet. The content of the total diet over a day or more is what counts.

Many foods are good sources of several nutrients. For example, vegetables and fruits are important for vitamins A and C, folic acid, minerals, and fiber. Breads and cereals supply B vitamins, iron, and protein; whole-grain types are also good sources of fiber. Milk provides protein, B vitamins, vitamins A and D, calcium, and phosphorus. Meat, poultry, and fish provide protein, B vitamins, iron, and zinc.

No single food can supply all nutrients in the amounts you need. For example, milk supplies calcium but little iron; meat supplies iron but little calcium. To have a nutritious diet, you must eat a variety of foods.

One way to assure variety—and with it, an enjoyable and nutritious diet—is to choose foods each day from five major food groups (see box). Individuals who do not eat foods from one or more of the food groups may want to contact a dietitian for help in planning how to meet nutritional needs.

People who are inactive or are trying to lose weight may eat little food. They need to take special care to choose lower calorie, nutrient-rich foods from the five major food groups. They also need to eat less of foods high in calories and low in essential nutrients, such as fats and oils, sugars, and alcoholic beverages.

Diets of some groups of people are notably low in some nutrients. Many women and adolescent girls need to eat more calcium-rich foods, such as milk and milk products, to get the calcium they need for healthy bones throughout life. Young children, teenage girls, and women of childbearing age must take care to eat enough iron-rich foods such as lean meats; dry beans; and whole-grain and iron-enriched breads, cereals, and other grain products.

A Daily Food Guide

Eat a variety of foods daily, choosing different foods from each group. Most people should have at least the lower number of servings suggested from each food group. Some people may need more because of their body size and activity level. Young children should have a variety of foods but may need small servings.

Food group	Suggested servings
Vegetables	3-5 servings
Fruits	2-4 servings
Breads, cereals, rice, and pasta	6-11 servings
Milk, yogurt, and cheese	2-3 servings
Meats, poultry, fish, dry beans and peas, eggs, and nuts	2-3 servings

Supplements of some nutrients taken regularly in large amounts can be harmful. Vitamin and mineral supplements at or below the Recommended Dietary Allowances (RDA) are safe, but are rarely needed if you eat a variety of foods. Here are exceptions in which your doctor may recommend a supplement:

♦ Pregnant women often need an iron supplement. Some other women in their childbearing years may also need an iron supplement to help replace iron lost in menstrual bleeding.

♦ Certain women who are pregnant or breast-feeding may need a supplement to meet their increased requirements for some nutrients.

♦ People who are unable to be active and eat little food may need supplements.

♦ People, especially older people, who take medicines that interact with nutrients may need supplements.

Advice for today: Get the many nutrients your body needs by choosing different foods you enjoy eating from these five groups daily: vegetables, fruits, grain products, milk and milk products, and meats and meat alternatives.

Maintain Healthy Weight

If you are too fat or too thin, your chances of developing health problems are increased.

Being too fat is common in the United States. It is linked with high blood pressure, heart disease, stroke, the most common type of diabetes, certain cancers, and other types of illness.

Being too thin is a less common problem. It occurs with anorexia nervosa and is linked with osteoporosis in women and greater risk of early death in both women and men.

Whether your weight is "healthy" depends on how much of your weight is fat, where in your body the fat is located, and whether you have weight-related medical problems, such as high blood pressure, or a family history of such problems.

Suggested Weights for Adults		
Height[1]	Weight in pounds[2]	
	19 to 34 years	35 years and over
5'0"	[3]97-128	108-138
5'1"	101-132	111-143
5'2"	104-137	115-148
5'3"	107-141	119-152
5'4"	111-146	122-157
5'5"	114-150	126-162
5'6"	118-155	130-167
5'7"	121-160	134-172
5'8"	125-164	138-178
5'9"	129-169	142-183
5'10"	132-174	146-188
5'11"	136-179	151-194
6'0"	140-184	155-199
6'1"	144-189	159-205
6'2"	148-195	164-210
6'3"	152-200	168-216
6'4"	156-205	173-222
6'5"	160-211	177-228
6'6"	164-216	182-234

[1] Without shoes.
[2] Without clothes.
[3] The higher weights in the ranges generally apply to men, who tend to have more muscle and bone; the lower weights more often apply to women, who have less muscle and bone.
Document Source: Derived from National Research Council, 1989.

What is a healthy weight for you? There is no exact answer right now. Researchers are trying to develop more precise ways to describe healthy weight. In the meantime, you can use the guidelines suggested below to help judge if your weight is healthy.

See if your weight is within the range suggested in the table for persons of your age and height. The table shows higher weights for people 35 years and above than for younger adults. This is because recent research suggests that people can be a little heavier as they grow older without added risk to health. Just how much heavier is not yet clear. The weight ranges given in the table are likely to change based on research under way.

Ranges of weights are given in the table because people of the same height may have equal amounts of body fat but differ in muscle and bone. The higher weights in the ranges are suggested for people with more muscle and bone.

Weights above the range are believed to be unhealthy for most people. Weights slightly below the range may be healthy for some small-boned people but are sometimes linked to health problems, especially if sudden weight loss has occurred.

Research also suggests that, for adults, body shape as well as weight is important to health. Excess fat in the abdomen is believed to be of greater health risk than that in the hips and thighs. There are several ways to check body shape. Some require the help of a doctor; others you can do yourself.

A look at your profile in the mirror may be enough to make it clear that you have too much fat in the abdomen. Or you can check your body shape this way:

- Measure around your waist near your navel while you stand relaxed, not pulling in your stomach.
- Measure around your hips, over the buttocks, where they are largest.
- Divide the waist measure by the hips measure to get your waist-to-hip ratio. Research in adults suggests that ratios close to or above one are linked with greater risk for several diseases. However, ratios have not been defined for all populations or age groups.

If your weight is within the range in the table, if your waist-to-hip ratio does not place you at risk, and if you have no medical problem for which your doctor advises you to gain or lose weight, there appears to be no health advantage to changing your weight. If you do not meet all of these conditions, or if you are not sure, you may want to talk to your doctor about how your weight might affect your health and what you should do about it.

Heredity plays a role in body size and shape as do exercise and what you eat. Some people seem to be able to eat more than others and still maintain a good body size and shape.

No one plan for losing weight is best for everyone. If you are not physically active, regular exercise may help you lose weight and keep it off. If you eat too much, decreasing your calorie intake may help. However, getting enough of some nutrients is difficult in diets of 1,200 calories or less. Long-term success usually depends upon new and better lifelong habits of both exercise and eating.

Do not try to lose weight too fast. A steady loss of 1/2 to 1 pound a week until you reach your goal is generally safe. Avoid crash weight-loss diets that severely restrict the variety of foods or the calories you can have.

Avoid other extreme approaches to losing weight. These include inducing vomiting and using medications such as laxatives, amphetamines, and diuretics. Such approaches are not appropriate for losing weight and can be dangerous.

You probably do not need to try to lose weight if your weight is already below the suggested range in the table and if you are otherwise healthy. If you lose weight suddenly or for unknown reasons, see a doctor. Unexplained weight loss may be an early clue to a health problem.

Children need calories to grow and develop normally; weight-reducing diets are usually not recommended for them. Overweight children may need special help in choosing physical activities they enjoy and nutritious diets with adequate but not excessive calories.

Advice for today: Check to see if you are at a healthy weight. If not, set reasonable weight goals and try for long-term success through better habits of eating and exercise. Have children's heights and weights checked regularly by a doctor.

Choose a Diet Low in Fat, Saturated Fat, and Cholesterol

Most health authorities recommend an American diet with less fat, saturated fat, and cholesterol. Populations like ours with diets high in fat have more obesity and certain types of cancer. The higher levels of saturated fat and cholesterol in our diets are linked to our increased risk for heart disease.

A diet low in fat makes it easier for you to include the variety of foods you need for nutrients without exceeding your calorie needs because fat contains over twice the calories of an equal amount of carbohydrates or protein.

To Increase Calorie Expenditure—Be More Physically Active.		
Activity	Calories expended per hour[1]	
	Man[2]	Woman[2]
Sitting quietly	100	80
Standing quietly	120	95
Light activity: Cleaning house Office work Playing baseball Playing golf	300	240
Moderate activity: Walking briskly (3.5 mph) Gardening Cycling (5.5 mph) Dancing Playing basketball	460	370
Strenuous activity: Jogging (9 min./ mile) Playing football Swimming	730	580
Very strenuous activity: Running (7 min/ mile) Racquetball, Skiing	920	740

[1] May vary depending on environmental conditions.
[2] Healthy man, 175 lbs; healthy woman, 140 lbs
Document Source: Derived from McArdle, et al., *Exercise Physiology,* 1986.

A diet low in saturated fat and cholesterol can help maintain a desirable level of blood cholesterol. For adults this level is below 200 mg/dl. As blood cholesterol increases above this level, greater risk for heart disease occurs. Risk can also be increased by high blood pressure, cigarette smoking, diabetes, a family history of premature heart disease, obesity, and being a male.

The way diet affects blood cholesterol varies among individuals. However, blood cholesterol does increase in most people when they eat a diet high in saturated fat and cholesterol and excessive in calories. Of these, dietary saturated fat has the greatest effect; dietary cholesterol has less.

Suggested goals for fats in American diets are as follows:

Total fat. An amount that provides 30 percent or less of calories is suggested. Thus, the upper limit on the grams of fat in your diet depends on the calories you need. For example, at 2,000 calories per day, your suggested upper limit is 600 calories from fat (2,000 x .30). This is equal to 67 grams of fat (600 divided by 9, the number of calories each gram of fat provides).

Saturated fat. An amount that provides less than 10 percent of calories (less than 22 grams at 2,000 calories per

day) is suggested. All fats contain both saturated and unsaturated fat (fatty acids). The fats in animal products are the main sources of saturated fat in most diets, with tropical oils (coconut, palm kernel, and palm oils) and hydrogenated fats providing smaller amounts.

Cholesterol. Animal products are the source of all dietary cholesterol. Eating less fat from animal sources will help lower cholesterol as well as total fat and saturated fat in your diet.

These goals for fats are not for children under 2 years, who have special dietary needs. As children begin to eat with the family, usually at about 2 years of age or older, they should be encouraged to choose diets that are lower in fat and saturated fat and that provide the calories and nutrients they need for normal growth. Older children and adults with established food habits may need to change their diets gradually toward the goals.

These goals for fats apply to the diet over several days, not to a single meal or food. Some foods that contain fat, saturated fat, and cholesterol, such as meats, milk, cheese, and eggs, also contain high-quality protein and are our best sources of certain vitamins and minerals. Lowfat choices of these foods are lean meat and lowfat milk and cheeses.

To Decrease Calorie Intake—
Eat a variety of foods that is low in calories and high in nutrients:
♦ Eat less fat and fatty foods.
♦ Eat more fruits, vegetables, and breads and cereals— without fats and sugars added in preparation and at the table.
♦ Eat less sugars and sweets.
♦ Drink little or no alcoholic beverages. Eat smaller portions; limit second helpings.

Advice for today: Have your blood cholesterol level checked, preferably by a doctor. If it is high, follow the doctor's advice about diet and, if necessary, medication. If it is at the desirable level, help keep it that way with a diet low in fat, saturated fat, and cholesterol: Eat plenty of vegetables, fruits, and grain products; choose lean meats, fish, poultry without skin, and lowfat dairy products most of the time; and use fats and oils sparingly.

Choose a Diet with Plenty of Vegetables, Fruits, and Grain Products

This guideline recommends that adults eat at least three servings of vegetables and two servings of fruits daily. It recommends at least six servings of grain products, such as breads, cereals, pasta, and rice, with an emphasis on whole grains. Children should also be encouraged to eat plenty of these foods.

Vegetables, fruits, and grain products are important parts of the varied diet discussed in the first guideline. They are emphasized in this guideline especially for their complex carbohydrates, dietary fiber, and other food components linked to good health.

For a Diet Low in Fat, Saturated Fat, and Cholesterol

Fats and oils

♦ Use fats and oils sparingly in cooking.

♦ Use small amounts of salad dressings and spreads, such as butter, margarine, and mayonnaise. One tablespoon of most of these spreads provides 10 to 11 grams of fat.

♦ Choose liquid vegetable oils most often because they are lower in saturated fat.

♦ Check labels on foods to see how much fat and saturated fat are in a serving.

Meat, poultry, fish, dry beans, and eggs

♦ Have two or three servings, with a daily total of about 6 ounces. Three ounces of cooked lean beef or chicken without skin—the size of a deck of cards—provides about 6 grams of fat.

♦ Trim fat from meat; take skin off poultry.

♦ Have cooked dry beans and peas instead of meat occasionally.

♦ Moderate the use of egg yolks and organ meats.

Milk and milk products

♦ Have two or three servings daily. (Count as a serving: 1 cup of milk or yogurt or about 1-1/2 ounces of cheese.)

♦ Choose skim or lowfat milk and fat-free or lowfat yogurt and cheese most of the time. One cup of skim milk has only a trace of fat, 1 cup of 2-percent-fat milk has 5 grams of fat, and 1 cup of whole milk has 8 grams of fat.

For a Diet with Plenty of Vegetables, Fruits, and Grain Products, Have Daily—

Three of more servings of various vegetables.
(Count as a serving: 1 cup of raw leafy greens, 1/2 cup of other kinds)

♦ Have dark-green leafy and deep-yellow vegetables often.

♦ Eat dry beans and peas often. (Count 1/2 cup of cooked dry beans or peas as a serving of vegetables or as 1 ounce of the meat group.)

♦ Also eat starchy vegetables, such as potatoes and corn.

Two or more servings of various fruits.
(Count as a serving: 1 medium apple, orange, or banana; 1/2 cup of small diced fruit; 3/4 cup of juice)

♦ Have citrus fruits or juices, melons, or berries regularly.

♦ Choose fruits as desserts and fruit juices as beverages.

Six or more servings of grain products (breads, cereals, pasta, and rice)
(Count as a serving: 1 slice of bread; 1/2 bun, bagel, or english muffin; 1 ounce of dry ready-to-eat cereal; 1/2 cup of cooked cereal, rice, or pasta)

♦ Eat products from a variety of grains, such as wheat, rice, oats, and corn.

♦ Have several servings of whole-grain breads and cereals daily.

Vegetables, fruits, and grain products are generally low in calories if fats and sugars are used sparingly in their preparation and at the table.

These foods are generally low in fats. By choosing the suggested amounts of them, you are likely to increase carbohydrates and decrease fats in your diet, as health authorities suggest. You will also get more dietary fiber.

Complex carbohydrates, such as starches, are in breads, cereals, pasta, rice, dry beans and peas, and other vegetables, such as potatoes and corn. Dietary fiber—a part of plant foods—is in whole-grain breads and cereals, dry beans and peas, vegetables, and fruits. It is best to eat a variety of these fiber-rich foods because they differ in the kinds of fiber they contain.

Eating foods with fiber is important for proper bowel function and can reduce symptoms of chronic constipation, diverticular disease, and hemorrhoids. Populations like ours with diets low in dietary fiber and complex carbohydrates and high in fat, especially saturated fat, tend to have more heart disease, obesity, and some cancers. Just how dietary fiber is involved is not yet clear.

Some of the benefit from a higher fiber diet may be from the food that provides the fiber, not from fiber alone. For this reason, it's best to get fiber from foods rather than from supplements. In addition, excessive use of fiber supplements is associated with greater risk for intestinal problems and lower absorption of some minerals.

Advice for today: Eat more vegetables, including dry beans and peas; fruits; and breads, cereals, pasta, and rice. Increase your fiber intake by eating more of a variety of foods that contain fiber naturally.

Use Sugars Only in Moderation

Americans eat sugars in many forms. Sugars provide calories and most people like their taste. Some serve as natural preservatives, thickeners, and baking aids in foods. This guideline cautions about eating sugars in large amounts and about frequent snacks of foods containing sugars and starches.

Sugars and many foods that contain them in large amounts supply calories but are limited in nutrients. Thus, they should be used in moderation by most healthy people and sparingly by people with low calorie needs. For very active people with high calorie needs, sugars can be an additional source of calories.

Both sugars and starches—which break down into sugars—can contribute to tooth decay. Sugars and starches are in many foods that also supply nutrients—milk; fruits; some vegetables; and breads, cereals, and other foods with sugars and starches as ingredients. The more often these foods—even small amounts—are eaten and the longer they are in the mouth before teeth are brushed, the greater the risk for tooth decay. Thus, eating such foods as frequent between-meal snacks may be more harmful to teeth than having them at meals.

Regular daily brushing with a fluoride toothpaste helps reduce tooth decay by getting fluoride to the teeth. Fluoridated water or other sources of fluoride that a doctor or dentist suggests are especially important for children whose unerupted teeth are forming and growing.

Diets high in sugars have not been shown to cause diabetes. The most common type of diabetes occurs in overweight adults, and avoiding sugars alone will not correct overweight.

Advice for today: Use sugars in moderate amounts—sparingly if your calorie needs are low. Avoid excessive snacking and brush and floss your teeth regularly.

What Is Meant By "Sugars"?

table sugar (sucrose)	honey
brown sugar	syrup
raw sugar	corn sweetener
glucose (dextrose)	high-fructose corn syrup
fructose	molasses
maltose	fruit juice concentrate
lactose	

Read food labels. A food is likely to be high in sugars if its ingredient list shows one of the above first or second or if it shows several of them.

For Healthier Teeth and Gums—

- Moderate the use of foods containing sugars and starches between meals.
- Brush and floss teeth regularly.
- Use a fluoride toothpaste.
- Ask your dentist or doctor about the need for supplemental fluoride, especially for children.
- Do not use a nursing bottle with any beverage other than water as a pacifier.

Use Salt and Sodium Only in Moderation

Table salt contains sodium and chloride—both are essential in the diet. However, most Americans eat more salt and sodium than they need. Food and beverages containing salt provide most of the sodium in our diets, much of it added during processing and manufacturing.

In populations with diets low in salt, high blood pressure is less common than in populations with diets high in salt. Other factors that affect blood pressure are heredity, obesity, and excessive drinking of alcoholic beverages.

In the United States, about one in three adults has high blood pressure. If these people restrict their salt and sodium, usually their blood pressure will fall.

Some people who do not have high blood pressure may reduce their risk of getting it by eating a diet with less salt and other sources of sodium. At present there is no way to predict who might develop high blood pressure and who will benefit from reducing dietary salt and sodium. However, it is wise for most people to eat less salt and sodium because they need much less than they eat and reduction will benefit those people whose blood pressure rises with salt intake.

Advice for today: Have your blood pressure checked. If it is high, consult a doctor about diet and medication. If it is normal, help keep it that way: maintain a healthy weight, exercise regularly, and try to use less salt and sodium. (Normal blood pressure for adults: systolic less than 140 mmHg and diastolic less than 85 mmHg.)

To Moderate Use of Salt and Sodium—

- Use salt sparingly, if at all, in cooking and at the table.
- When planning meals, consider that—
  - fresh and plain frozen vegetables prepared without salt are lower in sodium than canned ones.
  - cereals, pasta, and rice cooked without salt are lower in sodium than ready-to-eat cereals.
  - milk and yogurt are lower in sodium than most cheeses.
  - fresh meat, poultry, and fish are lower in sodium than most canned and processed ones.
  - most frozen dinners and combination dishes, packaged mixes, canned soups, and salad dressings contain a considerable amount of sodium. So do condiments, such as soy and other sauces, pickles, olives, catsup, and mustard.
- Use salted snacks, such as chips, crackers, pretzels, and nuts, sparingly.
- Check labels for the amount of sodium in foods. Choose those lower in sodium most of the time.

If You Drink Alcoholic Beverages, Do So in Moderation

Alcoholic beverages supply calories but little or no nutrients. Drinking them has no net health benefit, is linked with many health problems, is the cause of many accidents, and can lead to addiction. Their consumption is not recommended. If adults elect to drink alcoholic beverages, they should consume them in moderate amounts.

Some people should **not** drink alcoholic beverages:

- **Women who are pregnant or trying to conceive.** Major birth defects have been attributed to heavy drinking by the mother while pregnant. Women who are pregnant or trying to conceive should not drink alcoholic beverages. However, there is no conclusive evidence that an occasional drink is harmful.
- **Individuals who plan to drive or engage in other activities that require attention or skill.** Most people retain some alcohol in the blood 3 to 5 hours after even moderate drinking.
- **Individuals using medicines, even over-the-counter kinds.** Alcohol may affect the benefits or toxicity of medicines. Also, some medicines may increase blood alcohol levels or increase alcohol's adverse effect on the brain.
- **Individuals who cannot keep their drinking moderate.** This is a special concern for recovering alcoholics and people whose family members have alcohol problems.
- **Children and adolescents.** Use of alcoholic beverages by children and adolescents involves risks to health and other serious problems.

Heavy drinkers are often malnourished because of low food intake and poor absorption of nutrients by the body. Too much alcohol may cause cirrhosis of the liver, inflammation of the pancreas, damage to the brain and heart, and increased risk for many cancers.

Some studies have suggested that moderate drinking is linked to lower risk for heart attacks. However, drinking is also linked to higher risk for high blood pressure and hemorrhagic stroke.

Advice for today: If you drink alcoholic beverages, do so in moderation; and don't drive.

What's Moderate Drinking?

Women: No more than 1 drink a day
Men: No more than 2 drinks a day
Count as a drink:
- 12 ounces of regular beer
- 5 ounces of wine
- 1-1/2 ounces of distilled spirits (80 proof)

Some of the Scientific Basis for These Guidelines

- The Surgeon General's Report on Nutrition and Health. 1988. Public Health Service, U.S. Department of Health and Human Services.
- Diet and Health: Implications for Reducing Chronic Disease Risk. 1989. National Research Council, National Academy of Sciences.
- Recommended Dietary Allowances, 10th Ed. 1989. National Research Council, National Academy of Sciences.

Information on How to Put the Guidelines into Practice

Contact the Human Nutrition Information Service, USDA, Room 325-A, 6505 Belcrest Road, Hyattsville, MD 20782, for how to order:

- The USDA Food Guide in "Preparing Foods and Planning Menus Using the Dietary Guidelines." HG-232-8, 1989.
- "Dietary Guidelines and Your Diet." HG-232-1 through - 11, 1986 and 1989. Bulletins on eating right the Dietary Guidelines way.
- "Nutritive Value of Foods," HG-72. 1985.

Contact the National Institutes of Health, Room 10 A 24, Building 31, Bethesda, MD 20892, for this and other bulletins:

- "Eating for Life." NIH Publication No. 88-3000, 1988.

Contact your county extension home economist (Cooperative Extension System) or a nutrition professional in your local Public Health Department, hospital, American Red Cross, dietetic association, diabetes association, heart association, or cancer society.

Acknowledgments: The U.S. Department of Agriculture and the U.S. Department of Health and Human Services acknowledge the recommendations of the Dietary Guidelines Advisory Committee—the basis for this edition. The Committee consisted of Malden C. Nesheim, Ph.D. (chairman); Lewis A. Barness, M.D.; Peggy R. Borum, Ph.D.; C. Wayne Callaway, M.D.; John C. LaRosa, M.D.; Charles S. Lieber, M.D.; John A. Milner, Ph.D.; Rebecca M. Mullis, Ph.D., and Barbara O. Schneeman, Ph.D.

■ **Document Source:**
U.S. Department of Health and Human Services, Public Health Service
U.S. Department of Agriculture
Home and Garden Bulletin No. 232
Revised November 1990

See also: An FDA Guide to Dieting (page 343)

SKIN DISEASES AND DISORDERS

■ ■ ■

FEVER BLISTERS AND CANKER SORES

Fever blisters and canker sores are two of the most common disorders of the mouth, causing discomfort and annoyance to millions of Americans. Both cause small sores to develop in or around the mouth, and often are confused with each other. Canker sores, however, occur only *inside* the mouth—on the tongue and the inside linings of the cheeks, lips and throat. Fever blisters, also called cold sores, usually occur *outside* the mouth—on the lips, chin, cheeks or in the nostrils. When fever blisters do occur inside the mouth, it is usually on the gums or the roof of the mouth. Inside the mouth, fever blisters are smaller than canker sores, heal more quickly, and often begin as a blister.

Both canker sores and fever blisters have plagued mankind for thousands of years. Scientists at the National Institute of Dental Research, one of the federal government's National Institutes of Health, are seeking ways to better control and ultimately prevent these and other oral disorders.

Fever Blisters

In ancient Rome, an epidemic of fever blisters prompted Emperor Tiberius to ban kissing in public ceremonies. Today fever blisters still occur in epidemic proportions. About 100 million epidodes of recurrent fever blisters occur yearly in the United States alone. An estimated 45 to 80 percent of adults and children in this country have had at least one bout with the blisters.

What causes fever blisters?

Fever blisters are caused by a contagious virus called herpes simplex. There are two types of herpes simplex virus. Type 1 usually causes oral herpes, or fever blisters. Type 2 usually causes genital herpes. Although both type 1 and type 2 viruses can infect oral tissues, more than 95 percent of recurrent fever blister outbreaks are caused by the type 1 virus.

Herpes simplex virus is highly contagious when fever blisters are present, and the virus frequently is spread by kissing. Children often become infected by contact with parents, siblings or other close relatives who have fever blisters.

A child can spread the virus by rubbing his or her cold sore and then touching other children. About 10 percent of oral herpes infections in adults result from oral-genital sex with a person who has active genital herpes (type 2). These infections, however, usually do not result in repeat bouts of fever blisters.

Most people infected with the type 1 herpes simplex virus became infected before they were 10 years old. The virus usually invades the moist membrane cells of the lips, throat or mouth. In most people, the initial infection causes no symptoms. About 15 percent of patients, however, develop many fluid-filled blisters inside and outside the mouth 3 to 5 days after they are infected with the virus. These may be accompanied by fever, swollen neck glands and general aches. The blisters tend to merge and then collapse. Often a yellowish crust forms over the sores, which usually heal without scarring within 2 weeks.

The herpes virus, however, stays in the body. Once a person is infected with oral herpes, the virus remains in a nerve located near the cheek-bone. It may stay permanently inactive in this site, or it may occasionally travel down the nerve to the skin surface, causing a recurrence of fever blisters. Recurring blisters usually erupt at the outside edge of the lip or the edge of the nostril, but can also occur on the chin, cheeks, or inside the mouth.

The symptoms of recurrent fever blister attacks usually are less severe than those experienced by some people after an initial infection. Recurrences appear to be less frequent after age 35. Many people who have recurring fever blisters feel itching, tingling or burning in the lip 1 to 3 days before the blister appears.

What causes a recurrence of fever blisters?

Several factors weaken the body's defenses and trigger an outbreak of herpes. These include emotional stress, fever, illness, injury and exposure to sunlight. Many women have recurrences only during menstruation. One study indicates that susceptibility to herpes recurrences is inherited. Research is under way to discover exactly how the triggering factors interact with the immune system and the virus to prompt a recurrence of fever blisters.

What are the treatments for fever blisters?

Currently there is no cure for fever blisters. Some medications can relieve some of the pain and discomfort associated with the sores, however. These include ointments that numb the blisters, antibiotics that control secondary bacterial infections, and ointments that soften the crusts of the sores.

Is there a vaccine for fever blisters?

Currently there is no vaccine for herpes simplex virus available to the public. Many research laboratories, however, are working on this approach to preventing fever blisters. For example, scientists at the National Institute of Dental Research and the National Institute of Allergy and Infectious Diseases have developed a promising experimental herpes vaccine. In tests on laboratory mice, the vaccine has prevented the herpes simplex virus from infecting the animals and establishing itself in the nerves.

Although these findings are encouraging, the scientists must complete more animal studies on the safety and effectiveness of the vaccine before a decision can be made whether to test it in humans. The vaccine would be useful only for those not already infected with herpes simplex virus.

What can the patient do?

If fever blisters erupt, keep them clean and dry to prevent bacterial infections. Eat a soft, bland diet to avoid irritating the sores and surrounding sensitive areas. Be careful not to touch the sores and spread the virus to new sites, such as the eyes or genitals. To make sure you do not infect others, avoid kissing them or touching the sores and then touching another person.

There is good news for people whose fever blister outbreaks are triggered by sunlight. Scientists at the National Institute of Dental Research have confirmed that sunscreen on the lips can prevent sun-induced recurrences of herpes. They recommend applying the sunscreen before going outside and reapplying it frequently during sun exposure. The researchers used a sunblock with a protection factor of 15 in their studies.

Little is known about how to prevent recurrences of fever blisters triggered by factors other than sunlight. People whose cold sores appear in response to stress should try to avoid stressful situations. Some investigators have suggested adding lysine to the diet or eliminating foods such as nuts, chocolate, seeds or gelatin. These measures have not, however, been proven effective in controlled studies.

What research is being done?

Researchers are working on several approaches to preventing or treating fever blisters. As mentioned earlier, they are trying to develop a vaccine against herpes simplex virus. Several laboratories are developing and testing antiviral drugs designed to hamper or prevent fever blister outbreaks. Researchers also are trying to develop ointments that make it easier for antiviral drugs to penetrate the skin.

Acyclovir is an antiviral drug that prevents the herpes simplex virus from multiplying. The U.S. Food and Drug Administration has approved the drug for use in treating genital herpes, and is considering its approval for use in treating oral herpes. Researchers have found that acyclovir *taken in pill form* reduces the symptoms and frequency of fever blister recurrences in some patients. In one study, 50 percent of patients who took four acyclovir pills daily for 4 months had no fever blister outbreaks. Before taking the drug, they had an average of one recurrence every 2 months. In separate studies, pills taken at the onset of symptoms or acyclovir cream applied to the blisters or to areas of the lip that tingled or itched were found to be only minimally effective. The long-term effects of daily oral doses of acyclovir are not known, nor are the effects the drug might have on an unborn child.

Basic research on how the immune system interacts with herpes simplex viruses may lead to new therapies for fever blisters. The immune system uses a wide array of cells and chemicals to defend the body against infections. Scientists are trying to identify the immune components that prevent recurrent attacks of oral herpes.

Scientists are also trying to determine the precise form and location of the inactive herpes virus in nerve cells. This information might allow them to design antiviral drugs that can attack the herpes virus while it lies dormant in nerves.

In addition, researchers are trying to understand how sunlight, skin injury and stress can trigger recurrences of fever blisters. They hope to develop methods for blocking reactivation of the virus.

Canker Sores

Recurrent canker sores afflict about 20 percent of the general population. The medical term for the sores is aphthous stomatitis.

Canker sores are usually found on the movable parts of the mouth such as the tongue or the inside linings of the lips and cheeks. They begin as small oval or round reddish swellings, which usually burst within a day. The ruptured sores are covered by a thin white or yellow membrane and edged by a red halo. Generally, they heal within 2 weeks. Canker sores range in size from an eighth of an inch wide in mild cases to more than an inch wide in severe cases. Severe canker sores may leave scars. Fever is rare, and the sores are rarely associated with other diseases. Usually a person will have only one or a few canker sores at a time.

Most people have their first bout with canker sores between the ages of 10 and 20. Children as young as 2, however, may develop the condition. The frequency of canker sore recurrences varies considerably. Some people have only one or two episodes a year, while others may have a continuous series of canker sores.

What causes canker sores?

The cause of canker sores is not well understood. More than one cause is likely, even for individual patients. Canker sores do not appear to be caused by viruses or bacteria, although an allergy to a type of bacterium commonly found in the mouth may trigger them in some people. The sores may be an allergic reaction to certain foods. In addition, there is research suggesting that canker sores may be caused by a faulty immune system that uses the body's defenses against disease to attack and destroy the normal cells of the mouth or tongue.

British studies show that, in about 20 percent of patients, canker sores are due partly to nutritional deficiencies, especially lack of vitamin B12, folic acid and iron. Similar studies performed in the United States, however, have not confirmed this finding. In a small percentage of patients, canker sores occur with gastrointestinal problems, such as an inability to digest certain cereals. In these patients, canker sores appear to be part of a generalized disorder of the digestive tract.

Female sex hormones apparently play a role in causing canker sores. Many women have bouts of the sores only during certain phases of their menstrual cycles. Most women experience improvement or remission of their canker sores during pregnancy. Researchers have used hormone therapy successfully in clinical studies to treat some women.

Both emotional stress and injury to the mouth can trigger outbreaks of canker sores, but these factors probably do not cause the disorder.

Who is susceptible?

Women are more likely than men to have recurrent canker sores. Genetic studies show that susceptibility to recurrent outbreaks of the sores is inherited in some patients. This partially explains why the disorder is often shared by family members.

What are the treatments for canker sores?

Most doctors recommend that patients who have frequent bouts of canker sores undergo blood and allergy tests to determine if their sores are caused by a nutritional deficiency, an allergy or some other preventable cause. Vitamins and other nutritional supplements often prevent recurrences or reduce the severity of canker sores in patients with a nutritional deficiency. Patients with food allergies can reduce the frequency of canker sores by avoiding those foods.

There are several treatments for reducing the pain and duration of canker sores for patients whose outbreaks cannot be prevented. These include numbing ointments such as benzocaine, which are available in drug stores without a prescription. Anti-inflammatory steroid mouth rinses or gels can be prescribed for patients with severe sores.

Mouth rinses containing the antibiotic tetracycline may reduce the unpleasant symptoms of canker sores and speed healing by preventing bacterial infections in the sores. Clinical studies at the National Institute of Dental Research have shown that rinsing the mouth with tetracycline several times a day usually relieves pain in 24 hours and allows complete healing in 5 to 7 days. The U.S. Food and Drug Administration warns, however, that tetracycline given to pregnant women and young children can permanently stain youngsters' teeth. Both steroid and tetracycline treatments require a prescription and care of a dentist or physician.

Patients with severe recurrent canker sores may need to take steroid or other immunosuppressant drugs orally. These potent drugs can cause many undesirable side effects, and should be used only under the close supervision of a dentist or physician.

What can the patient do?

If you have canker sores, avoid abrasive foods such as potato chips that can stick in the cheek or gum and aggravate the sores. Take care when brushing your teeth not to stab the gums or cheek with a toothbrush bristle. Avoid acidic and spicy foods. Canker sores are not contagious, so patients do not have to worry about spreading them to other people.

What research is being done?

Researchers are trying to identify the malfunctions in patients' immune systems that make them susceptible to recurrent bouts of canker sores. By analyzing the blood of people with and without canker sores, scientists have found several differences in immune function between the two groups. Whether these differences cause canker sores is not yet known.

Researchers also are developing and testing new drugs designed to treat canker sores. Most of these drugs alter the patients' immune function. Although some of the drugs appear to be effective in treating canker sores in some patients, the data are still inconclusive. Until these drugs are proven to be absolutely safe and effective, they will not be available for general use.

■ Document Source:
U.S. Department of Health and Human Services, Public Health Service
National Institutes of Health
National Institute of Dental Research
Bethesda, Maryland 20892
NIH Publication No. 92-247
Revised July 1992

CancerFax from the National Cancer Institute
KAPOSI'S SARCOMA

Description

What is Kaposi's Sarcoma?

Kaposi's sarcoma (KS) is a disease in which cancer (malignant) cells are found in the tissues under the skin or mucous membranes that line the mouth, nose, and anus. KS causes red or purple patches (lesions) on the skin and/or mucous membranes and spreads to other organs in the body, such as the lungs, liver, or intestinal tract.

Until the early 1980s, Kaposi's sarcoma was a very rare disease that was found mainly in older men, patients who had organ transplants, or African men. With the acquired immunodeficiency syndrome (AIDS) epidemic in the early 1980s, doctors began to notice more cases of Kaposi's sarcoma in Africa and in gay men with AIDS. Kaposi's sarcoma usually spreads more quickly in these patients.

If you have signs of KS, your doctor will examine your skin and lymph nodes carefully (lymph nodes are small bean-shaped structures that are found throughout the body;

they produce and store infection-fighting cells). Your doctor also may order other tests to see if you have other diseases.

Your chance of recovery (prognosis) depends on what type of Kaposi's sarcoma you have, your age, your general health, and whether or not you have AIDS.

Stage Explanation

Stages of Kaposi's sarcoma

There is no accepted staging system for Kaposi's sarcoma. Patients are grouped depending on which type of Kaposi's sarcoma they have. There are four types of Kaposi's sarcoma:

Classic
Classic Kaposi's sarcoma usually occurs in older men of Jewish, Italian, or Mediterranean heritage. This type of Kaposi's sarcoma progresses slowly, sometimes over 10 to 15 years. As the disease gets worse, the lower legs may swell and the blood may not be able to flow properly. After some time, the disease may spread to other organs. Many patients with classic Kaposi's sarcoma may develop another type of cancer later on in their lives.

Immunosuppressive treatment related
Kaposi's sarcoma may occur in people who are taking drugs to make their immune systems weaker (immunosuppressants). The immune system helps the body fight off infection. People who have had an organ transplant (such as a liver or kidney transplant) have to take drugs to prevent their immune system from attacking the new organ.

Epidemic
Kaposi's sarcoma in patients who have acquired immunodeficiency syndrome (AIDS) is called epidemic Kaposi's sarcoma. AIDS is caused by a virus called the human immunodeficiency virus (HIV), which attacks and weakens the immune system. Infections and other diseases can then invade the body, and the immune system cannot fight against them. Kaposi's sarcoma in people with AIDS usually spreads more quickly than other kinds of Kaposi's sarcoma and often is found in many parts of the body.

Recurrent
Recurrent disease means that the KS has come back (recurred) after it has been treated. It may come back in the area where it first started or in another part of the body.

Treatment Options Overview

How Kaposi's Sarcoma Is Treated

There are treatments for all patients with Kaposi's sarcoma. Four kinds of treatment are used:

surgery (taking out the cancer)
chemotherapy (using drugs to kill cancer cells)
radiation therapy (using high-dose x-rays to kill cancer cells)

biological therapy (using the body's immune system to fight cancer).

Radiation therapy is a common treatment for Kaposi's sarcoma. Radiation therapy uses high-dose x-rays or other high-energy rays to kill cancer cells and shrink tumors. Radiation for Kaposi's sarcoma comes from a machine outside the body (external beam radiation therapy).

Surgery means taking out the cancer. Your doctor may remove the cancer using one of the following:

- Local excision cuts out the lesion and some of the tissue around it.
- Electrodesiccation and curettage burns the lesion and removes it with a sharp instrument.
- Cryotherapy freezes the tumor and kills it.

Chemotherapy uses drugs to kill cancer cells. Chemotherapy may be taken by pill, or it may be put into the body by a needle in a vein or muscle. Chemotherapy is called a systemic treatment because the drug enters the bloodstream, travels through the body, and can kill cancer cells outside the original site. Chemotherapy for Kaposi's sarcoma also may be injected into the lesion (intralesional chemotherapy).

Biological therapy tries to get your own body to fight cancer. It uses materials made by your own body or made in a laboratory to boost, direct, or restore your body's natural defenses against disease. Biological therapy is sometimes called biological response modifier (BRM) therapy or immunotherapy.

Treatment by Stage

Treatment for Kaposi's sarcoma depends on the type of Kaposi's sarcoma you have, your age, and your general health.

You may receive treatment that is considered standard based on its effectiveness in a number of patients in past studies, or you may choose to go into a clinical trial. Not all patients are cured with standard therapy and some standard treatments may have more side effects than are desired. For these reasons, clinical trials are designed to find better ways to treat cancer patients and are based on the most up-to-date information. Clinical trials are going on in most parts of the country for most stages of Kaposi's sarcoma. If you want more information, call the Cancer Information Service at 1-800-4-CANCER (1-800-422-6237).

Treatment options: Classic Kaposi's sarcoma
Your treatment may be one of the following:
1. Radiation therapy.
2. Local excision.
3. Systemic or intralesional chemotherapy.
4. Chemotherapy plus radiation therapy.

Treatment options: Immunosuppressive treatment related Kaposi's sarcoma
Depending on your condition, the cancer may be controlled if you stop taking immunosuppressive drugs. If you cannot stop taking the drugs or if this does not work, your treatment may be one of the following:

1. Radiation therapy.

2. A clinical trial of chemotherapy.

Treatment options: Epidemic Kaposi's sarcoma

Your treatment may be one of the following:

1. Surgery (local excision, electrodesiccation and cu-rettage, or cryotherapy).
2. Intralesional chemotherapy.
3. Systemic chemotherapy. Clinical trials are testing new drugs and drug combinations.
4. A clinical trial of biological therapy.

Treatment options: Recurrent Kaposi's sarcoma

Treatment for recurrent Kaposi's sarcoma depends on your type of Kaposi's sarcoma, your general health, and your response to earlier treatments. You may want to take part in a clinical trial.

To learn more about Kaposi's sarcoma, call the National Cancer Institute's Cancer Information Service at 1-800-4-CANCER (1-800-422-6237). By dialing this toll-free number, you can speak with someone who can answer your questions.

If you have AIDS, you can get information about services for AIDS patients by calling the AIDS hotline at 1-800-342-AIDS (1-800-342-2437). Additional information on clinical trials for AIDS patients can be obtained by calling the AIDS Clinical Trials Information Service at 1-800-TRI-ALS-A (1-800-874-2572) or by writing to the service at the following address:

AIDS Clinical Trials Information Service
P.O. Box 6421
Rockville, MD 20850

■ **Document Source:**
  National Cancer Institute
  Building 31, Room 10A24 9000 Rockville Pike, Bethesda, MD
  20892
  PDQ 208/01271
  02/01/94

See also: Caring for Someone with AIDS (page 1); Skin Cancer (page 359)

PREVENTING PRESSURE ULCERS: A PATIENT'S GUIDE

Purpose of this booklet

Pressure ulcers are serious problems that can lead to pain, a longer stay in the hospital or nursing home, and slower recovery from health problems. Anyone who must stay in a bed, chair, or wheelchair because of illness or injury can get pressure ulcers.

Fortunately, most pressure ulcers can be prevented, and when pressure ulcers do form, they do not have to get worse. This booklet describes where pressure ulcers form and how to tell if you are at risk of getting a pressure ulcer. It also lists steps to take to prevent them or keep them from getting worse, and suggests how to work effectively with your health care team.

What are pressure ulcers?

A pressure ulcer is an injury usually caused by unrelieved pressure that damages the skin and underlying tissue. Pressure ulcers are also called bed sores and range in severity from mild (minor skin reddening) to severe (deep craters down to muscle and bone).

Unrelieved pressure on the skin squeezes tiny blood vessels, which supply the skin with nutrients and oxygen. When skin is starved of nutrients and oxygen for too long, the tissue dies and a pressure ulcer forms. Skin reddening that disappears after pressure is removed is normal and not a pressure ulcer.

Other factors cause pressure ulcers too. If a person slides down in the bed or chair, blood vessels can stretch or bend and cause pressure ulcers. Even slight rubbing or friction on the skin may cause minor pressure ulcers.

Where pressure ulcers form

Pressure ulcers form where bone causes the greatest force on the skin and tissue and squeezes them against an outside surface. This may be where bony parts of the body press against other body parts, a mattress, or a chair. In persons who must stay in bed, most pressure ulcers form on the lower back below the waist (sacrum), the hip bone (trochanter), and on the heels. In people in chairs or wheelchairs, the exact spot where pressure ulcers form depends on the sitting position. Pressure ulcers can also form on the knees, ankles, shoulder blades, back of the head, and spine.

Nerves normally "tell" the body when to move to relieve pressure on the skin. Persons in bed who are unable to move may get pressure ulcers after as little as 1-2 hours. Persons who sit in chairs and who cannot move can get pressure ulcers in even less time because the force on the skin is greater.

Your risk

Confinement to bed or a chair, being unable to move, loss of bowel or bladder control, poor nutrition, and lowered mental awareness are "risk factors" that increase your chance of getting pressure ulcers. Your risk results from the number and seriousness of the risk factors that apply to you.

1. *Bed or chair confinement.* If you must stay in bed, a chair, or a wheelchair, the risk of getting a pressure ulcer can be high.
2. *Inability to move.* If you cannot change positions without help, you are at great risk. Persons who are in a coma or who are paralyzed or who have a hip fracture are at special risk. Risks of getting pressure ulcers are lower when persons can move by themselves.
3. *Loss of bowel or bladder control.* If you cannot keep your skin free of urine, stool, or perspiration, you have a higher risk. These sources of moisture may irritate the skin.
4. *Poor nutrition.* If you cannot eat a balanced diet, your skin may not be properly nourished. Pres-

sure ulcers are more likely to form when skin is not healthy.

5. *Lowered mental awareness.* When mental awareness is lowered, a person cannot act to prevent pressure ulcers. Mental awareness can be affected by health problems, medications, or anesthesia.

Fortunately, you can lower your risk. Following the steps in this booklet can help you and your health care provider to reduce your risk of pressure ulcers.

Key steps

The following steps for prevention are based on research, professional judgment, and practice. These steps can also keep pressure ulcers from getting worse. Some steps apply to all prevention efforts; others apply only in specific conditions. It may help to talk to a nurse or doctor about which steps are right for you.

Take care of your skin

Your skin should be inspected at least once a day. Pay special attention to any reddened areas that remain after you have changed positions and the pressure has been relieved. This inspection can be done by yourself or your caregiver. A mirror can help when looking at hard-to-see areas. Pay special attention to pressure points shown on page 2. The goal is to find and correct problems before pressure ulcers form.

Your skin should be cleaned as soon as it is soiled. A soft cloth or sponge should be used to reduce injury to skin.

Take a bath when needed for comfort or cleanliness. If a daily bath or shower is preferred or necessary, additional measures should be taken to minimize irritation and prevent dry skin. When bathing or showering, warm (not hot) water and a mild soap should be used.

To prevent dry skin:

♦ Use creams or oils on your skin.
♦ Avoid cold or dry air.

Minimize moisture from urine or stool, perspiration, or wound drainage. Often urine leaks can be treated. To obtain a copy of *Managing Urinary Incontinence: A Patient's Guide,* call 1-800-358-9295 or write to the AHCPR Publications Clearinghouse, P.O. Box 8547, Silver Spring, MD 20907.

When moisture cannot be controlled:

♦ Pads or briefs that absorb urine and have a quick drying surface that keeps moisture away from the skin should be used.
♦ A cream or ointment to protect skin from urine, stool, or wound drainage may be helpful.

Protect your skin from injury

Avoid massage of your skin over bony parts of the body. Massage may squeeze and damage the tissue under the skin and make you more likely to get pressure ulcers.

Limit pressure over bony parts by changing positions or having your caregiver change your position.

♦ If you are in bed, your position should be changed at least every 2 hours.
♦ If you are in a chair, your position should be changed at least every hour. *(If you are able to shift your own weight, you should do so every 15 minutes while sitting.)*

Reduce friction (rubbing) by making sure you are lifted, rather than dragged, during repositioning. Friction can rub off the top layer of skin and damage blood vessels under the skin. You may be able to help by holding on to a trapeze hanging from an overhead frame. If nurses or others are helping to lift you, bed sheets or lifters can be used. A thin film of corn starch can be used on the skin to help reduce damage from friction.

Avoid use of donut-shape (ring) cushions. Donut-shape cushions can increase your risk of getting a pressure ulcer by reducing blood flow and causing tissue to swell.

If you are confined to bed:

♦ A special mattress that contains foam, air, gel, or water helps to prevent pressure ulcers. The cost and effectiveness of these products vary greatly. Talk to your health care provider about the best mattress for you.
♦ The head of the bed should be raised as little and for as short a time as possible if consistent with medical conditions and other restrictions. When the head of the bed is raised more than 30 degrees, your skin may slide over the bed surface, damaging skin and tiny blood vessels.
♦ Pillows or wedges should be used to keep knees or ankles from touching each other.
♦ Avoid lying directly on your hip bone (trochanter) when lying on your side. Also, a position that spreads weight and pressure more evenly should be chosen—pillows may also help.
♦ If you are completely immobile, pillows should be put under your legs from midcalf to ankle to keep heels off the bed. **Never** place pillows behind the knee.

If you are in a chair or wheelchair:

♦ Foam, gel, or air cushions should be used to relieve pressure. Ask your health care provider which is best for you. Avoid donut-shape cushions because they reduce blood flow and cause tissue to swell, which can increase your risk of getting a pressure ulcer.
♦ Avoid sitting without moving or being moved.
♦ Good posture and comfort are important.

Eat well

Eat a balanced diet. Protein and calories are very important. Healthy skin is less likely to be damaged.

If you are unable to eat a normal diet, talk to your health care provider about nutritional supplements that may be desirable.

Improve your ability to move

A rehabilitation program can help some persons regain movement and independence.

Be active in your care

This booklet tells how to reduce your risk of getting pressure ulcers. Not all steps apply to every person at risk. The best program for preventing pressure ulcers will consider what you want and be based on your condition.

Be sure you:

♦ Ask questions.
♦ Explain your needs, wants, and concerns.
♦ Understand what and why things are being done.
♦ Know what is best for you. Talk about what you can do to help prevent pressure ulcers—at home, in the hospital, or in the nursing home.

You can help to prevent most pressure ulcers. The extra effort can mean better health.

Additional resources

National and international organizations provide a variety of resources for people concerned with pressure ulcers.

International Association of Enterostomal Therapy
(Will refer patients to local Enterostomal Therapy Nurses)
27241 La Paz Road, Suite 121
Laguna Niguel, CA 92656
714-476-0268

National Pressure Ulcer Advisory Panel
(Offers information for caregivers, families providing care at home, and others)
SUNY at Buffalo
Beck Hall
3435 Main Street
Buffalo, NY 14214
716-831-2143

For more information

The information in this booklet was taken from the *Clinical Practice Guideline* on *Pressure Ulcers in Adults: Prediction and Prevention*. The guideline was developed by an expert panel of doctors, nurses, other health care providers, and a consumer representative, and it was sponsored by the Agency for Health Care Policy and Research. Other guidelines on common health problems are being developed and will be released in the near future. For more information about the guidelines or to receive more copies of this booklet, call toll free 1-800-358-9295 or write to:

Agency for Health Care Policy and Research
Publications Clearinghouse
P.O. Box 8547
Silver Spring, MD 20907

■ **Document Source:**
    U.S. Department of Health and Human Services, Public Health Service
    Agency for Health Care Policy and Research

Executive Office Center, Suite 501, 2101 East Jefferson Street, Rockville, MD 20852
AHCPR Publication No. 92-0048
May 1992

CancerFax from the National Cancer Institute
SKIN CANCER

Description

What Is Skin Cancer?

Skin cancer is a disease in which cancer (malignant) cells are found in the outer layers of your skin. Your skin protects your body against heat, light, infection, and injury. It also stores water, fat, and vitamin D.

The skin has two main layers and several kinds of cells. The top layer of skin is called the epidermis. It contains three kinds of cells: flat, scaly cells on the surface called squamous cells; round cells called basal cells; and cells called melanocytes, which give your skin its color.

The inner layer of skin is called the dermis. This layer is thicker, and contains blood vessels, nerves, and sweat glands. The hair on your skin also grows from tiny pockets in the dermis, called follicles. The dermis makes sweat, which helps to cool your body, and oils that keep your skin from drying out.

There are several types of cancer that start in the skin. The most common are basal cell cancer and squamous cell cancer, which are covered in this PDQ patient information statement. These types of skin cancer are called nonmelanoma skin cancer. Melanoma is a type of skin cancer that starts in the melanocytes. It is not as common as basal cell or squamous cell skin cancer, but it is much more serious. See the patient information statement on melanoma for information on the treatment of that type of cancer.

Skin cancer is more common in people with light colored skin who have spent a lot of time in the sunlight. Skin cancer can occur anywhere on your body, but it is most common in places that have been exposed to more sunlight, such as your face, neck, hands, and arms.

Skin cancer can look many different ways. The most common sign of skin cancer is a change on the skin, such as a growth or a sore that won't heal. Sometimes there may be a small lump. This lump can be smooth, shiny and waxy looking, or it can be red or reddish brown. Skin cancer may also appear as a flat red spot that is rough or scaly. Not all changes in your skin are cancer, but you should see your doctor if you notice changes in your skin.

Like most cancers, skin cancer is best treated when it is found (diagnosed) early. If you have a spot or lump on your skin, your doctor may remove the growth and look at the tissue under a microscope. This is called a biopsy. A biopsy can usually be done in your doctor's office. Before the biopsy, you will be given a local anesthetic to numb the area for a short period of time.

Most nonmelanoma skin cancers can be cured. Your chance of recovery (prognosis) and choice of treatment depend on the type of skin cancer you have and how far it has spread.

Other kinds of cancer that may affect the skin include cutaneous T-cell lymphoma, a cancer of the lymph system, and Kaposi's sarcoma. See the patient information statements on cutaneous T-cell lymphoma or Kaposi's sarcoma for treatment of these cancers. Cancers that start in other parts of the body may also spread (metastasize) to the skin.

Stage Explanation

Types of Skin Cancer

Once skin cancer is found, more tests may be done to see if the cancer has spread. This is called staging. Your doctor needs to know the stage and type of your skin cancer to plan treatment. The following types are used to plan treatment:

Basal cell cancer
Basal cell cancer is the most common type of nonmelanoma skin cancer. It usually occurs on areas of your skin that have been in the sun. Often this cancer appears as a small raised bump that has a smooth, pearly appearance. Another type looks like a scar, and it is firm to the touch. Basal cell cancers may spread to tissues around the cancer, but it usually does not spread to other parts of the body.

Squamous cell carcinoma
Squamous cell tumors also occur on areas of your skin that have been in the sun, often on the top of the nose, forehead, lower lip, and hands. They may also appear on areas of your skin that have been burned, exposed to chemicals, or had x-ray therapy. Often this cancer appears as a firm red bump. Sometimes the tumor may feel scaly or bleed or develop a crust. Squamous cell tumors may spread to the lymph nodes in the area (lymph nodes are small bean-shaped structures that are found throughout the body; they produce and store infection-fighting cells).

Actinic keratosis
Actinic keratosis is a skin condition that is not cancer, but can change into basal cell or squamous cell skin cancer in some people. It appears as rough, red or brown, scaly patches on the skin, usually in areas that have been exposed to the sun.

Recurrent
Recurrent disease means that the cancer has come back (recurred) after it has been treated.

Treatment Options Overview

How Skin Cancer Is Treated

There are treatments for all patients with skin cancer. Three kinds of treatments are used:

surgery (taking out the cancer)
chemotherapy (using drugs to kill cancer cells)
radiation therapy (using x-rays to kill cancer cells).

Biological therapy (using your body's immune system to fight cancer) is being tested in clinical trials.

Many skin cancers are treated by doctors who treat skin diseases (dermatologists). Often, the cancer can be treated in your doctor's office.

Surgery is the most common treatment for skin cancer. Your doctor may remove the cancer using one of the following:

- ♦ Electrodesiccation and curettage burns the lesion and removes it with a sharp instrument.
- ♦ Cryosurgery freezes the tumor and kills it.
- ♦ Simple excision cuts the cancer from your skin along with some of the healthy tissue around it.
- ♦ Micrographic surgery removes the cancer and as little normal tissue as possible. During this surgery, the doctor removes the cancer and then uses a microscope to look at the cancerous area to make sure no cancer cells remain.
- ♦ Laser therapy uses a narrow beam of light to remove cancer cells.

Surgery may leave a scar on your skin. Depending on the size of the cancer, skin may be taken from another part of your body and put on the area where the cancer was removed. This is called a skin graft. New ways of doing surgery and grafting may reduce scarring.

Radiation therapy uses x-rays to kill cancer cells and shrink tumors. Radiation therapy for skin cancer comes from a machine outside the body (external radiation therapy).

Chemotherapy uses drugs to kill cancer cells. In treating skin cancer, chemotherapy is often given as a cream or lotion placed on the skin to kill cancer cells (topical chemotherapy). Chemotherapy may also be taken by pill, or it may be put into the body by a needle in a vein or muscle. Chemotherapy given in this way is called a systemic treatment because the drug enters the bloodstream, travels through the body, and can kill cancer cells outside the skin. Systemic chemotherapy is being tested in clinical trials.

Biological therapy tries to get your own body to fight cancer. It uses materials made by your own body or made in a laboratory to boost, direct, or restore your body's natural defenses against disease. Biological therapy is sometimes called biological response modifier (BRM) therapy or immunotherapy.

Photodynamic therapy uses a certain type of light and a special chemical to kill cancer cells.

Treatment by Type

Treatment for skin cancer depends on the type and stage of your disease, your age, and your overall health.

You may receive treatment that is considered standard based on its effectiveness in a number of patients in past studies, or you may choose to go into a clinical trial. Not all patients are cured with standard therapy and some standard treatments may have more side effects than are desired. For these reasons, clinical trials are designed to find better ways to treat cancer patients and are based on the most up-to-date information. Clinical trials are going on in some parts of the country for patients with skin cancer. If you want more information, call the Cancer Information Service at 1-800-4-CANCER (1-800-422-6237).

Treatment options: Basal cell carcinoma of the skin

Your treatment may be one of the following:

1. Micrographic surgery.
2. Simple excision.
3. Electrodesiccation and curettage.
4. Cryosurgery.
5. Radiation therapy.
6. Laser therapy.
7. Topical chemotherapy.
8. Clinical trials of chemoprevention.
9. Clinical trials of biological therapy.
10. Photodynamic therapy.

It is important to have your skin examined regularly so the cancer can be treated if it comes back (recurs).

Treatment options: Squamous cell carcinoma of the skin

Your treatment may be one of the following:

1. Micrographic surgery.
2. Simple excision.
3. Electrodesiccation and curettage.
4. Cryosurgery.
5. Radiation therapy.
6. Topical chemotherapy.
7. Laser therapy.
8. Clinical trials of biological therapy with or without chemoprevention.

It is important to have your skin examined regularly so the cancer can be treated if it comes back (recurs).

Treatment options: Actinic keratosis

Your treatment may be one of the following:

1. Topical chemotherapy.
2. Cryosurgery.
3. Electrodesiccation and curettage.
4. Removing the top layer of skin with a special machine (dermabrasion).
5. Shaving the very top layer of skin (shave excision).
6. Laser therapy.

Treatment options: Recurrent skin cancer

Your treatment may consist of any of the previous treatments, or a combination of treatments.

To learn more about skin cancer, call the National Cancer Institute's Cancer Information Service at 1-800-4-CANCER (1-800-422-6237). By dialing this toll-free number, you can speak with someone who can answer your questions.

■ Document Source:
National Cancer Institute
   Building 31, Room 10A24, 9000 Rockville Pike, Bethesda, MD
      20892
   PDQ 208/01228
   02/01/94

See also: Kaposi's Sarcoma (page 355); What You Need to Know About Melanoma (page 361)

WHAT YOU NEED TO KNOW ABOUT MELANOMA

The National Cancer Institute (NCI) has prepared this booklet to help patients and their families better understand melanoma. We also hope it will encourage all readers to learn more about this disease. The information presented here—on the symptoms, diagnosis, and treatment of melanoma and on living with cancer—is intended to add to information from doctors, nurses, and other members of the medical team.

Our knowledge about melanoma is increasing. Research sponsored by the NCI and by other groups is leading to better diagnosis and treatment of this disease. For up-to-date information on this subject, call the NCI-supported Cancer Information Service (CIS) toll-free at 1-800-4-CANCER.

Throughout this booklet, words that may be new to readers are printed in *italics*. Definitions of these and other terms related to melanoma can be found in the "Medical Terms" section. For some words, a "sounds-like" spelling is also given.

Other NCI publications about cancer, its treatment, and living with the disease are also listed.

The Skin

Weighing about 6 pounds, the skin is the body's largest organ. It protects us against heat, light, injury, and infection. It helps regulate body temperature and stores water, fat, and vitamin D. It is made up of two main layers: the outer *epidermis* and the inner *dermis*.

The epidermis (outer layer of skin) is mostly made up of flat, scale-like cells called *squamous cells*. Under the squamous cells are round cells called *basal cells*. The deepest part of the epidermis also contains *melanocytes*. These cells produce *melanin*, which gives the skin its color.

The dermis (inner layer of skin) contains blood and lymph vessels, hair *follicles*, and glands. These glands produce sweat, which helps regulate body temperature, and *sebum*, an oily substance that helps keep the skin from drying out. Sweat and sebum reach the skin's surface through tiny openings called pores.

What Is Cancer?

Cancer is a group of more than 100 diseases. Although each kind differs from the others in many ways, every cancer is a disease of some of the body's cells.

Healthy cells that make up the body's tissues grow, divide, and replace themselves in an orderly way. This process keeps the body in good repair. Sometimes, however, certain cells lose the ability to limit and direct their growth. They divide too rapidly and grow without any order. Too many cells are produced, and *tumors* begin to form. Tumors can be *benign* or *malignant*.

♦ Benign tumors are not cancer. They do not spread to other parts of the body and are seldom a threat to life. Often, benign tumors can be removed by surgery, and they are not likely to return.

♦ Malignant tumors are cancer. They can invade and destroy nearby healthy tissues and organs. Cancer cells also can spread, or *metastasize*, to other parts of the body and form new tumors.

Cancer that develops in melanocytes (the pigment cells) is called melanoma. It may also be called cutaneous melanoma or malignant melanoma. (Another type of melanoma develops in the eye. It is called ocular melanoma and is not discussed in this booklet.)

Melanoma is a very serious disease because it may spread to other parts of the body through the *lymphatic system*. This system is made up of a network of thin tubes that branch, like blood vessels, into all the tissues of the body. Cancer cells break off from the primary tumor and are carried along by *lymph*, a colorless, watery fluid that contains infection-fighting cells. Along this network of vessels are groups of small, bean-shaped organs called *lymph nodes*. Clusters of lymph nodes are found in the underarms, groin, neck, and abdomen. Surgeons often remove lymph nodes to find out whether they contain cancer cells. Melanoma also can spread through the bloodstream.

Two other types of skin cancer, basal cell cancer and squamous cell cancer, are much more common. These skin cancers are less serious than melanoma because they rarely spread. (More information about basal cell and squamous cell cancers of the skin can be found in the booklet called *What You Need To Know About Skin Cancer.*)

Symptoms

Often, the first sign of melanoma is a change in the size, shape, or color of a mole. A normal mole is a brown, tan, or black spot on the skin. It can be flat or raised, and its shape can be round or oval. Usually, moles are small—less than the size of a pencil eraser. A mole may be present at birth, or it may appear later on—usually in the first 10 years of a person's life. Most moles fade away in older people.

Most people have between 10 and 30 moles on their body. The vast majority of these moles are perfectly harmless. However, a change in a mole is a sign that you should see your doctor. Thinking of "ABCD" can help you remember the signs of melanoma:

♦ **A**symmetry—The shape of one half does not match the other.
♦ **B**order—The edges are ragged, notched, or blurred.
♦ **C**olor—The color is uneven. Shades of black, brown, or tan are present. Areas of white, red, or blue may be seen.
♦ **D**iameter—There is a change in size.

Other signs of melanoma may include scaling, oozing, or bleeding of a mole or a change in the way a mole feels; it may become hard, lumpy, itchy, swollen, or tender. Melanoma may also appear like a new mole on the body.

Detection and Diagnosis

Detection

Melanoma in men occurs most often on the trunk (the area between the shoulders and hips) or head and neck. In women, melanoma is often found on the arms and lower legs. It is found most often in people with fair skin. Blacks and people with dark skin are more likely to have melanomas on the palms of the hands and the soles of the feet.

Any health problem should be diagnosed and treated as early as possible, and this is especially true for melanoma. The earlier melanoma is detected, the better a person's chances for a full recovery. People should check their skin regularly for new growths or other changes.

New growths or any changes in moles should be reported to the doctor without delay. Anyone who has already had melanoma should be especially sure to have regular medical exams so that the doctor can check to see that it hasn't returned.

In some families, individuals have unusual moles called *dysplastic nevi*, which may turn into melanoma much more frequently than do normal moles. People with dysplastic nevi may have more than 100 moles. These people are at increased risk of developing melanoma and should have regular checkups to detect problems early. More information about the causes of and risk factors for melanoma can be found in the NCI booklets *Research Report: Melanoma and Dysplastic Nevi.*

Diagnosis

Because melanoma can spread, it is important for the doctor to find out as early as possible whether a suspicious-looking area is cancer. The sooner melanoma is found, the sooner the doctor can begin treatment to control the disease.

A *biopsy* is the only way to make a definite diagnosis. For this test, the doctor removes part or all of the growth. This can usually be done in the doctor's office using local anesthesia. To check for cancer cells, the tissue is examined under a microscope by a *pathologist* or a *dermatologist*.

If melanoma is found, the doctor needs to determine the extent, or stage, of the disease. The stage of the disease is based on the thickness of the tumor, the depth of skin penetration, and whether the cancer has spread (metastasized) to nearby lymph nodes or distant parts of the body. Staging is important in planning treatment.

Treating Melanoma

The doctor considers a number of factors to determine the best treatment for melanoma. Among these are the location, size, and depth of the tumor. In addition, the doctor considers where the cancer may have spread, as well as the age and general health of the patient.

Treatment Planning

Before starting treatment, the patient might want a second doctor to review the diagnosis and suggested treatment. If so, there are a number of ways to get a second opinion:

- The patient's doctor can discuss the case with other physicians who treat melanoma. Names of doctors and information on cancer treatment are available from the NCI's database called PDQ (Physician Data Query). Many of these doctors conduct clinical trials—studies of new treatments—and have a special interest in melanoma.
- Patients and their doctors can get names of other doctors to consult from a local medical society, a nearby hospital or medical school, or the *Directory of Medical Specialists*, a book available in many public libraries.
- The Cancer Information Service, at 1-800-4-CANCER, may also be able to help patients locate a doctor to consult for a second opinion.

Methods of Treating Melanoma

Most patients with melanoma are treated with surgery. Usually, the doctor removes the melanoma and an area of tissue around it. Sometimes, a skin graft may be needed. For this procedure, the doctor uses a piece of skin from another part of the body to replace the skin that was removed. Although doctors try to cause as little scarring as possible, surgery to remove melanomas, with or without skin grafts, may leave some scars.

Patients with melanoma that is deep or has spread face a high risk of having the disease recur after surgery. To improve the outlook for these patients, research is under way using chemotherapy (treatment with anticancer drugs) following surgery. This is known as *adjuvant therapy*.

Chemotherapy is usually a *systemic treatment*. The anticancer drugs are given in different ways: some are given by mouth; others are injected into a muscle or a blood vessel. The drugs enter the bloodstream and reach cells all over the body.

However, if melanoma occurs on an arm or leg, chemotherapy may be given with a technique called *perfusion*. For this treatment, drugs are put directly into the bloodstream of the affected limb. In this way, more of the drug reaches the tumor.

Because current drugs and drug combinations are not very effective against advanced melanoma, researchers continue to study new treatments. One new area of study is *biotherapy*, a type of cancer treatment that uses natural and man-made substances to stimulate or restore the body's immune system to fight disease more effectively. Interleukin-2 and interferon are two forms of biotherapy used to treat melanoma.

Occasionally, *radiation therapy* may be used. Radiation therapy uses high-powered x-rays to destroy the ability of cancer cells to grow and multiply. This treatment (also called x-ray therapy, radiotherapy, cobalt treatment, or irradiation) is most commonly used to control pain.

Side Effects of Treatment

Loss of appetite can be a serious problem for patients. Researchers are learning that patients who eat well can handle the side effects of treatment better. Therefore, nutrition is an important part of the treatment plan. Eating well means getting enough calories to prevent weight loss and having enough protein to build and repair the skin, hair, muscles, and organs. Many patients find that having several small meals and snacks throughout the day is easier than trying to eat three large meals.

The side effects that patients have during cancer therapy vary from person to person. They may even be different from one treatment to the next. Doctors try to plan treatment to keep side effects to a minimum, and, fortunately, most side effects are temporary. Doctors, nurses, and dietitians can explain the side effects of cancer treatment and suggest ways to deal with them. Further information about cancer treatment and coping with side effects is given in the NCI publications *Chemotherapy and You, Radiation Therapy and You,* and *Eating Hints*.

Followup Care

Because melanoma patients are at an increased risk for developing additional melanomas, they should be examined by a physician regularly. Depending on the size and extent of the original growth, followup exams may include x-rays. For patients who have many moles, the doctor may take photographs of the skin to help find unusual changes. Patients should also examine themselves often (keeping in mind the "ABCD" guidelines), visit the doctor for regular checkups, and follow their doctor's instructions on how to reduce their chance of developing melanoma again.

Adjusting to the Disease

When people have cancer, life can change for them and for the people who care about them. These changes in daily life can be difficult to handle. When someone finds out he or she has cancer, a number of different and sometimes confusing emotions may arise.

At times, patients and family members may be frightened, angry, or depressed. Their feelings may vary from hope to despair or from courage to fear. Patients usually are better able to cope with their emotions if they can talk openly about their illness and their feelings with family members and friends.

Concerns about the future—as well as about medical tests, treatment, a hospital stay, and medical bills—are common. Talking with doctors, nurses, or other members of the health care team may help to ease these concerns. Patients can ask questions about their disease and its treatment and can take an active part in decisions about their medical care. Often, patients and family members find it helpful to write down questions for the doctor as they think of them. Taking notes during visits to the doctor also can help them remember what was said. Patients should ask the doctor to repeat or explain anything that is not clear.

Patients have many important questions to ask about cancer, and their doctor is the best person to provide answers. Most people ask what kind of cancer they have, how it can be treated, and how successful the treatment is likely to be. The following are some other questions that patients might want to ask the doctor:

- What are my treatment choices?
- What are the benefits of treatment?
- What are the risks and side effects of treatment?
- Will there be a scar?

♦ Can I keep working?
♦ Will I need to change my normal activities?
♦ How can I protect myself from getting melanoma again?
♦ How often do I need checkups?

The patient's doctor is the best person to give advice about working or limiting other activities. If it is hard to talk with the doctor about feelings and other very personal matters, patients may find it helpful to talk with others who are facing similar problems. This kind of help is available through support groups, such as those described in the next section. A mental health counselor or a member of the clergy can also offer emotional support.

Living with any serious illness can be difficult and challenging. The public library is a good source of books and articles on living with cancer. Also, cancer patients and their families can find helpful suggestions in the NCI booklet called *Taking Time*.

Support for Cancer Patients

Adapting to the changes that are brought on by cancer is easier for patients and those who care about them when they have helpful information and support services. Often, the social service office at the hospital or clinic can suggest local and national agencies that will help with emotional support, financial aid, transportation, home care, or rehabilitation.

The American Cancer Society (ACS), for example, is a nonprofit organization that offers a variety of services to patients and their families. Local ACS offices are listed in the telephone book.

Information about other programs and services is available through the Cancer Information Service (CIS), whose toll-free telephone number is 1-800-4-CANCER.

What the Future Holds

There are more than 5 million Americans living today who have had some type of cancer. The outlook for a person with early melanoma is good; over 70 percent are cured. Researchers continue to look for better ways to treat advanced melanoma, and the possibility of controlling this disease is improving.

Doctors often talk about "surviving" cancer, or they may use the word *"remission"* rather than "cure." Even though many patients recover completely, doctors use these terms because the disease can show up again at a later time. Patients are naturally concerned about their future and often try to use statistics they have read or heard to figure out their own chances of being cured. It is important to remember, however, that statistics are an average based on the experience of large numbers of people, and no two cancer patients are alike. Only the doctor who takes care of a patient knows enough about the case to discuss that person's *prognosis*.

The Promise of Cancer Research

Scientists at hospitals and medical centers throughout the country are studying the possible causes of melanoma and how the disease might be prevented. In addition, they are exploring new methods of treatment.

Cause and Prevention

Studies show that the number of cases of melanoma is increasing and that melanoma affects all age groups. Researchers are trying to learn which people are more likely to get the disease and what aspects of our surroundings and lifestyles may cause it. They are looking at occupation, heredity, and the difference in skin sensitivity to sunlight to see whether these factors relate to the development of melanoma.

We know that ultraviolet (UV) radiation from the sun is a risk factor that increases the chance of getting melanoma. People with red or blond hair, blue eyes, and fair skin that freckles are more likely to develop this disease. Blacks get melanoma less often than do whites, probably because they have more melanin in their skin to protect them. The risk for melanoma is also increased for people with dysplastic nevi, or a family history of melanoma, or those with very large moles.

The risk of developing melanoma is also affected by where a person lives. People who live in areas that get high levels of UV radiation from the sun are more likely to get the disease. In the United States, for example, melanoma is more common in Texas than it is in Minnesota, where the sun is not as strong. Worldwide, the highest rates of melanoma are found in Australia.

Protective clothing, such as hats and long sleeves, can block out the sun's harmful rays. Also, lotions or creams that contain sunscreens help protect the skin. Sunscreens often contain *para-aminobenzoic acid* (PABA) and are rated in strength according to an SPF (sun protection factor), which ranges from 2 to 15 and higher. The higher the number on the label, the greater the protection a sunscreen provides, meaning that more of the sun's harmful rays will be blocked out.

People can reduce their risk of developing melanoma by:

♦ Avoiding or limiting sunlight exposure during noontime hours (11 a.m. to 1 p.m.).
♦ Limiting exposure to sunlight during early childhood.
♦ Gradually building up exposure to sunlight.

Advances in Treatment

Researchers are studying new treatments for melanoma. When a new treatment method shows promise, the method is used to treat cancer patients in *clinical trials*. These trials are designed to answer scientific questions and to find out whether a promising new treatment is both safe and effective. Patients who take part in research make an important contribution to medical science and may have the first chance to benefit from improved treatment methods.

Patients with melanoma are encouraged to consider participating in a trial and should discuss this possibility with their doctor. *What Are Clinical Trials All About?* is an NCI publication for patients who may be interested in participating in clinical research.

The NCI's PDQ (Physician Data Query) database helps doctors across the country learn about these trials. A doctor can obtain information from PDQ by using an office computer or the services of a medical library. Most Cancer Information Service (CIS) offices provide PDQ searches and can tell doctors how to obtain regular access to the database. Information about current research is also available to patients and the public through the CIS.

Medical Terms

Adjuvant therapy (AD-joo-vant THER-a-pee). Treatment given to kill undetected cancer cells that may remain in the body after surgery.

Basal cells (BAY-sal). Small, round cells found in the lower part, or base, of the epidermis.

Benign (bee-NINE). Noncancerous; does not spread to other parts of the body.

Biopsy (BY-op-see). The removal and microscopic examination of a sample of tissue to see whether cancer cells are present.

Biotherapy (by-o-THER-a-pee). Treatment that uses natural and man-made substances that can stimulate or restore the body's immune system to fight disease more effectively. Also called immunotherapy.

Cancer. A general term for more than 100 diseases that are characterized by uncontrolled, abnormal growth of cells. Cancer cells can spread through the bloodstream and lymphatic system.

Chemotherapy (kee-mo-THER-a-pee). Treatment with anticancer drugs.

Clinical trials. Studies conducted with cancer patients, usually to evaluate a new treatment. Each study is designed to answer scientific questions and to find better ways to treat patients.

Dermatologist (der-ma-TOL-o-jist). A doctor who specializes in the diagnosis and treatment of skin problems.

Dermis (DER-mis). The lower or inner layer of the two main layers that make up the skin.

Dysplastic nevi (dis-PLAS-tik NEE-vi). Unusual moles that may occur in greater numbers than normal moles and that may turn into melanoma.

Epidermis (ep-i-DER-mis). The outer surface layer of the skin that contains both squamous and basal cells.

Follicles (FAHL-i-kulz). Shafts through which hair grows.

Groin. The area where the thigh meets the hip.

Lymph (limf). The almost colorless fluid that bathes body cells and contains cells that help fight infection.

Lymph nodes. Small, bean-shaped structures that act as filters, collecting bacteria or cancer cells.

Lymphatic system (lim-FAT-ik). The lymph nodes, spleen, and thymus—which produce and store infection-fighting cells—and the network that carries lymph fluid.

Malignant (ma-LIG-nant). Cancerous (see Cancer).

Melanin (MEL-a-nin). The pigment of the skin. The amount of this substance accounts for the color of the skin.

Melanocytes (me-LAN-o-sites). Cells in the skin that form and contain pigment called melanin.

Metastasize (me-TAS-ta-size). To spread from one part of the body to another. When cancer cells metastasize and cause secondary tumors, the cells in the metastatic tumor are like those in the original tumor.

Nevus (NEE-vus). Medical term for mole.

Para-aminobenzoic acid (PAR-a-am-EE-no-BEN-zo-ik). A chemical used in sunscreen products; also called PABA. It helps protect the skin from the harmful rays of the sun.

Pathologist (pa-THOL-o-jist). A specialist who diagnoses disease by studying how tissues and cells look under a microscope.

Perfusion (per-FYOO-zhun). A special technique used to give chemotherapy. Anticancer drugs are added to the blood of an affected limb. In this way, a larger dose reaches the tumor.

Prognosis (prog-NO-sis). The probable outcome of a disease; the prospect of recovery.

Radiation therapy (ray-dee-AY-shun THER-a-pee). The use of high-energy waves to treat disease. Sources of radiation include x-ray, cobalt, and radium.

Remission. The temporary or permanent disappearance of the signs and symptoms of disease.

Risk factor. A substance or condition that increases an individual's chances of getting a particular type of cancer.

Sebum (SEB-bum). An oily substance produced by glands in the skin.

Squamous cells (SKWAY-mus). Flat cells that look like fish scales and make up most of the epidermis.

Stage. The extent of disease.

Systemic treatment (sis-TEM-ik). Treatment that reaches and affects cells all over the body.

Tumors. Abnormal masses of tissue that result from excessive cell division. Tumors perform no useful function. They may be either benign (not cancer) or malignant (cancer).

Resources

General information about cancer is widely available. Some helpful resources and publications are listed below. You may wish to check your local library and to contact support groups in your community.

Cancer Information Service
1-800-4-CANCER

The NCI-supported Cancer Information Service (CIS) is a nationwide telephone service that responds to inquiries from cancer patients and their families, health care professionals, and the public. Information specialists can provide information and publications on all aspects of cancer. They also may know about cancer-related services in local areas. Spanish-speaking CIS staff members are available. By dialing the CIS number, you will be connected to the CIS office serving your area.

American Cancer Society
1599 Clifton Road, NE
Atlanta, GA 30329
(404) 320-3333

The ACS is a national voluntary organization that offers a wide range of services to patients and their families and carries out programs of research and education. Additional information about these activities can be obtained from the national headquarters or a local chapter (listed in the telephone book under American Cancer Society).

Skin Cancer Foundation
245 Fifth Avenue
New York, NY 10016
(212) 725-5176

This nonprofit organization provides a wide variety of publications on the diagnosis and treatment of skin cancers. Send a stamped, self-addressed envelope to receive published materials. The Skin Cancer Foundation also publishes *Sun and Skin News* and *The Skin Cancer Foundation Journal*, which have nontechnical articles on the prevention and treatment of melanoma and other cancers that begin in the skin.

American Academy of Dermatology
1567 Maple Avenue
Evanston, IL 60201
(312) 869-3954

The American Academy of Dermatology (AAD) is a professional organization of specialists who diagnose and treat skin problems. The AAD provides a publication on melanoma for the general public. Patients may receive referrals to dermatologists by calling 1-800-238-2300.

American Society of Plastic and Reconstructive Surgeons
444 East Algonquin Road
Arlington Heights, IL 60005
1-800-635-0635

The American Society of Plastic and Reconstructive Surgeons (ASPRS) offers names of board-certified plastic surgeons in a patient's area. The ASPRS also sends information on various surgical procedures.

For Further Information

The following printed materials may be helpful to cancer patients, their families, and others. They are available free of charge by calling 1-800-4-CANCER or writing:

Office of Cancer Communications
National Cancer Institute
Building 31, Room 10A24
Bethesda, MD 20892

♦ *About Dysplastic Nevi*
♦ *Advanced Cancer: Living Each Day*
♦ *Answers to Your Questions About Metastatic Cancer*
♦ *Chemotherapy and You*
♦ *Eating Hints*
♦ *Good News, Better News, Best News: Cancer Prevention*
♦ *Questions and Answers About Pain Control*
♦ *Radiation Therapy and You*
♦ *Research Report: Melanoma*
♦ *Taking Time: Support for People with Cancer and the People Who Care About Them*
♦ *What Are Clinical Trials All About?*
♦ *What You Need To Know About Skin Cancer*
♦ *When Cancer Recurs: Meeting the Challenge Again*

■ **Document Source:**
U.S. Department of Health and Human Services, Public Health Service
National Institutes of Health
National Cancer Institute
NIH Publication No. 90-1563
Revised September 1988. Reprinted June 1990

See also: Chemotherapy and You: A Guide to Self-Help During Treatment (page 40); Radiation Therapy and You: A Guide to Self-Help During Treatment (page 56); Skin Cancer (page 359); What Are Clinical Trials All About? A Booklet for Patients with Cancer (page 68)

UROGENITAL SYSTEM DISORDERS

■ ■ ■

CancerFax from the National Cancer Institute
BLADDER CANCER

Description

What Is Cancer of the Bladder?

Bladder cancer is a disease in which cancer (malignant) cells are found in the bladder. The bladder is a hollow organ in the lower part of the abdomen that stores urine. It is shaped like a small balloon, and it has a muscular wall that allows it to get larger and smaller. Urine is the liquid waste that is made by the kidneys when they clean the blood. The urine passes from the two kidneys into the bladder through two tubes called ureters. When the bladder is emptied during urination, the urine goes from the bladder to the outside of the body through another tube called the urethra.

Like most cancers, cancer of the bladder is best treated when it is found (diagnosed) early. You should see your doctor if you have any of the following: blood in the urine (urine that looks bright red or rusty), pain when you urinate, passing urine often, or feeling like you need to urinate but nothing comes out.

If you have symptoms, your doctor may use several tests to see if you have cancer of the bladder. Your urine may be sent to a laboratory for tests to see if any cancer cells are present. Your doctor may also do an internal examination by inserting gloved fingers into the vagina and/or rectum to feel for lumps. Your doctor may then order a special x-ray called an intravenous pyelogram (IVP). For this x-ray, a special dye containing iodine is given to you by a needle in a vein. The dye then goes into the urine, making the bladder easier to see on the x-rays. Your may feel warm as the dye is given to you.

Your doctor may also look directly into the bladder with a thin, lighted tube called a cystoscope. The cystoscope is inserted into the bladder through the urethra. If tissue that is not normal is found, your doctor will need to cut out a small piece of this tissue and look at it under the microscope to see if there are any cancer cells. This is called a biopsy. Other special x-rays may also be done to help diagnose cancer of the bladder.

Your chance of recovery (prognosis) and choice of treatment depend on the stage of your cancer (whether it is just in the lining of the bladder or has spread to other places in the body) and your general state of health.

Stage Explanation

Stages of Cancer of the Bladder

Once cancer of the bladder has been diagnosed, more tests will be done to find out if cancer cells have spread to other parts of the body (staging). Your doctor needs to know the stage of your disease to plan treatment. The following stages are used for cancer of the bladder:

Stage 0 or carcinoma in situ
Stage 0 is very early cancer. The cancer is found only on the inner lining of the bladder. After the cancer is taken out, no swelling or lumps are felt during an internal examination.

Stage I
Cancer cells have spread a little deeper into the inner lining of the bladder but have not spread to the muscular wall of the bladder.

Stage II
Cancer cells have spread to the inside lining of the muscles lining the bladder.

Stage III
Cancer cells have spread throughout the muscular wall of the bladder, and/or to the layer of tissue surrounding the bladder. Your doctor may feel swelling or lumps after you have had an operation to take out the cancer.

Stage IV
Cancer cells have spread to the nearby reproductive organs or to the lymph nodes in the area. (Lymph nodes are small, bean-shaped structures that are found throughout the body; they produce and store infection-fighting cells.) The cancer may have also spread to lymph nodes and other places far away from the bladder.

Recurrent
Recurrent disease means that the cancer has come back (recurred) after it has been treated. It may come back in the original place or in another part of the body.

Treatment Options Overview

How Cancer of the Bladder Is Treated

There are treatments for all patients with cancer of the bladder. Four kinds of treatment are used:

surgery (taking out the cancer in an operation)
radiation therapy (using high-dose x-rays or other high-
    energy rays to kill cancer cells and shrink tumors)
chemotherapy (using drugs to kill cancer cells)
biological therapy (using the body's immune system to
    fight cancer).

A new type of treatment called photodynamic therapy is being tested in clinical trials.

Surgery is a common treatment for cancer of the bladder. Your doctor may take out the cancer using one of the following operations:

♦ Transurethral resection is an operation that uses a cystoscope inserted into the bladder through the urethra. The doctor then uses a tool with a small wire loop on the end to remove the cancer or to burn the tumor away with high-energy electricity (fulguration).

♦ Segmental cystectomy is an operation to take out the part of the bladder where the cancer is found. Because bladder cancer often occurs in more than one part of the bladder, this operation is used only in selected cases where the cancer is in one area.

♦ Cystectomy is an operation to take out the bladder.

♦ Radical cystectomy is an operation to take out the bladder and the tissue around it. In women, the uterus, ovaries, fallopian tubes, part of the vagina, and urethra are also removed. In men, the prostate and the glands that produce fluid that is part of the semen (seminal vesicles) are also removed, and the urethra may be removed as well. The lymph nodes in the pelvis may also be taken out (pelvic lymph node dissection).

♦ Urinary diversion is an operation to make a way for urine to pass out of the body so that it does not go through the bladder. It is used to relieve bladder symptoms when the tumor has spread.

If your bladder is removed, your doctor will need to make a new way for you to store and pass urine. There are several ways to do this. Sometimes your doctor will use part of the small intestine to make a tube through which urine can pass out of the body through an opening (stoma) on the outside of the body. This is sometimes called an ostomy or urostomy. If you have an ostomy, you will need to wear a special bag to collect urine. This special bag, which sticks to the skin around the stoma with a special glue, can be thrown away after it is used. This bag does not show under clothing and most people take care of these bags themselves. Your doctor may also use part of your small intestine to make a new storage pouch (a continent reservoir) inside the body where the urine can collect. You would then need to use a tube (catheter) to drain the urine through the stoma. Even newer methods use a part of the small intestine to make a new storage pouch that is connected to the remaining part of the urethra if it has not been removed. Urine then passes out of the body through the urethra, and a stoma is not necessary.

Chemotherapy uses drugs to kill cancer cells. Chemotherapy may be taken by pill, or it may be put in the body through a needle in a vein or muscle. Chemotherapy is called a systemic treatment because the drug enters the bloodstream, travels through the body, and can kill cancer cells outside the bladder. Chemotherapy may also be given in a fluid that is put into the bladder through a tube going through the urethra (intravesical chemotherapy).

If your doctor removes all the cancer that can be seen at the time of the operation, you may be given chemotherapy after surgery to kill any cancer cells that are left. Chemotherapy given after an operation to a person who has no cancer cells that can be seen is called adjuvant chemotherapy. For bladder cancer, chemotherapy is sometimes given before surgery to try to improve results or to preserve the bladder. Chemotherapy given in this manner is called neoadjuvant chemotherapy. Neoadjuvant chemotherapy is being carefully studied in a clinical trial sponsored by the National Cancer Institute.

Radiation therapy uses high-energy x-rays to kill cancer cells and shrink tumors. Radiation may come from a machine outside the body (external radiation therapy) or from putting materials that produce radiation (radioisotopes) through thin plastic tubes in the area where the cancer cells are found (internal radiation therapy).

Biological therapy tries to get your own body to fight cancer. It uses materials made by your own body or made in a laboratory to boost, direct, or restore your body's natural defenses against disease. Biological therapy is sometimes called biological response modifier (BRM) therapy or immunotherapy.

Photodynamic therapy is a new type of treatment that uses special drugs and light to kill cancer cells. A drug that makes cancer cells more sensitive to light is put into the bladder and a special light is used to shine on the bladder. This therapy is being studied for early stages of bladder cancer.

Treatment by Stage

Treatment of cancer of the bladder depends on the stage of your disease, the type of your disease, your age, and your overall condition.

You may receive treatment that is considered standard based on its effectiveness in a number of patients in past studies, or you may choose to go into a clinical trial. Not all patients are cured with standard therapy and some standard treatments may have more side effects than are desired. For these reasons, clinical trials are designed to find better ways to treat cancer patients and are based on the most up-to-date information. Clinical trials are going on in most parts of the country for most stages of cancer of the bladder. If you want more information, call the Cancer Information Service at 1-800-4-CANCER (1-800-422-6237).

Treatment options: Stage 0 bladder cancer
Your treatment may be one of the following:
1. Removal of the cancer using a cystoscope inserted through the urethra to cut out the tumor and burn away any remaining cancer cells (transurethral resection with fulguration).

2. Transurethral resection with fulguration followed by intravesical chemotherapy or biological therapy.
3. Surgery to remove part of the bladder (segmental cystectomy).
4. Intravesical chemotherapy or intravesical biological therapy alone. Clinical trials are evaluating new agents to be given this way.
5. Surgery to remove the whole bladder and organs around it (radical cystectomy).
6. A clinical trial of photodynamic therapy.

Treatment options: Stage I bladder cancer

Your treatment may be one of the following:
1. Removal of the cancer using a cystoscope inserted through the urethra to cut out the tumor and burn away any remaining cancer cells (transurethral resection with fulguration).
2. Transurethral resection and fulguration followed by intravesical chemotherapy or biological therapy.
3. Intravesical chemotherapy or biological therapy alone.
4. Surgery to remove part of the bladder (segmental cystectomy).
5. Internal radiation therapy with or without external beam radiation therapy.
6. Surgery to remove the whole bladder and organs around it (radical cystectomy).
7. A clinical trial of agents to prevent cancer.
8. A clinical trial of intravesical therapy.

Treatment options: Stage II bladder cancer

Your treatment may be one of the following:
1. Surgery to remove the whole bladder and the organs around it (radical cystectomy). The lymph nodes in the pelvis may also be removed (lymph node dissection).
2. External beam radiation therapy alone.
3. Internal radiation therapy before or after external beam radiation therapy.
4. Internal radiation therapy alone.
5. Removal of the cancer using a cystoscope inserted through the urethra to cut out the tumor and burn away any remaining cancer cells (transurethral resection with fulguration).
6. Surgery to remove part of the bladder (segmental cystectomy).
7. Clinical trials of systemic chemotherapy before cystectomy (neoadjuvant chemotherapy) or after cystectomy (adjuvant chemotherapy).
8. A clinical trial of systemic chemotherapy plus radiation therapy.

Treatment options: Stage III bladder cancer

Your treatment may be one of the following:
1. Radical cystectomy. The lymph nodes in the pelvis may also be removed (pelvic lymph node dissection).
2. External radiation therapy.
3. External beam and internal radiation therapy.

4. Surgery to remove part of the bladder (segmental cystectomy).
5. Internal radiation therapy.
6. External beam radiation and chemotherapy.
7. A clinical trial of systemic chemotherapy before cystectomy (neoadjuvant chemotherapy) or after cystectomy (adjuvant chemotherapy).
8. A clinical trial of chemotherapy and radiotherapy to allow you to keep your bladder.

Treatment options: Stage IV bladder cancer

If you have stage IV cancer that has spread to nearby tissue or lymph nodes, but not to other parts of the body, your treatment may be one of the following:
1. Radical cystectomy.
2. External beam radiation therapy.
3. Surgery to make a way for urine to flow out of the body so that it does not go into the bladder (urinary diversion), to reduce symptoms.
4. Surgery to remove the bladder (cystectomy) to relieve symptoms.
5. Systemic chemotherapy by itself or in addition to surgery.
6. A clinical trial of systemic chemotherapy before cystectomy (neoadjuvant chemotherapy) or after cystectomy (adjuvant chemotherapy).
7. A clinical trial of chemotherapy and radiation therapy to allow you to keep your bladder.

If the cancer is found in lymph nodes or other places far away from the bladder, your treatment may be one of the following:

1. External beam radiation therapy.
2. Surgery to make a way for urine to pass out of the body without going through the bladder (urinary diversion), to reduce symptoms.
3. Surgery to remove the bladder (cystectomy) and to make a urinary diversion to reduce symptoms.
4. Systemic chemotherapy alone or in addition to surgery.
5. A clinical trial of chemotherapy.

Treatment options: Recurrent bladder cancer

If your cancer comes back only in the bladder, you may receive surgery, chemotherapy, or radiation therapy, depending on what treatment you received when you first got your cancer. If your cancer comes back following surgery to remove all of the bladder, you may receive chemotherapy. You may also choose to participate in a clinical trial.

To learn more about cancer of the bladder, call the National Cancer Institute's Cancer Information Service at 1-800-4-CANCER (1-800-422-6237). By dialing this toll-free number, you can speak with someone who can answer your questions.

■ Document Source:
National Cancer Institute
Building 31, Room 10A24, 9000 Rockville Pike, Bethesda, MD 20892
PDQ 208/01206
02/01/94

See also: Chemotherapy and You: A Guide to Self-Help During Treatment (page 40); Radiation Therapy and You: A Guide to Self-Help During Treatment (page 56)

END-STAGE RENAL DISEASE: CHOOSING A TREATMENT THAT'S RIGHT FOR YOU

Introduction

This booklet is for people whose kidneys fail to work. This condition is called end-stage renal disease (ESRD).

Today, there are new and better treatments for ESRD that replace the work of healthy kidneys. By learning about your treatment choices, you can work with your doctor to pick the one that's best for you. No matter which type of treatment you choose, there will be some changes in your life. But with the help of your health care team, family, and friends, you may be able to lead a full, active life.

This booklet describes the choices for treatment: hemodialysis, peritoneal dialysis, and kidney transplantation. It gives the pros and cons of each. It also discusses diet and paying for treatment. It gives tips for working with your doctor, nurses, and others who make up your health care team. It provides a list of groups that offer information and services to kidney patients. It also lists magazines, books, and brochures that you can read for more information about treatment.

You and your doctor will work together to choose a treatment that's best for you. This booklet can help you make that choice.

When Your Kidneys Fail

Healthy kidneys clean the blood by filtering out extra water and wastes. They also make hormones that keep your bones strong and blood healthy. When both of your kidneys fail, your body holds fluid. Your blood pressure rises. Harmful wastes build up in your body. Your body doesn't make enough red blood cells. When this happens, you need treatment to replace the work of your failed kidneys.

Hemodialysis

Purpose

Hemodialysis is a procedure that cleans and filters your blood. It rids your body of harmful wastes and extra salt and fluids. It also controls blood pressure and helps your body keep the proper balance of chemicals such as potassium, sodium, and chloride.

How It Works

Hemodialysis uses a dialyzer, or special filter, to clean your blood. The dialyzer connects to a machine. During treatment, your blood travels through tubes into the dialyzer. The dialyzer filters out wastes and extra fluids. Then the newly cleaned blood flows through another set of tubes and back into your body.

Getting Ready

Before your first treatment, an access to your bloodstream must be made. The access provides a way for blood to be carried from your body to the dialysis machine and then back into your body. The access can be internal (inside the body—usually under your skin) or external (outside the body).

Who Performs It

Hemodialysis can be done at home or at a center. At a center, nurses or trained technicians perform the treatment. At home, you perform hemodialysis with the help of a family member or friend. If you decide to do home dialysis, you and your partner will receive special training.

The Time It Takes

Hemodialysis usually is done three times a week. Each treatment lasts from 2 to 4 hours. During treatment, you can read, write, sleep, talk, or watch TV.

Possible Complications

Side effects can be caused by rapid changes in your body's fluid and chemical balance during treatment. Muscle cramps and hypotension are two common side effects. Hypotension, a sudden drop in blood pressure, can make you feel weak, dizzy, or sick to your stomach.

It usually takes a few months to adjust to hemodialysis. You can avoid many of the side effects if you follow the proper diet and take your medicines as directed. You should always report side effects to your doctor. They often can be treated quickly and easily.

Your Diet

Hemodialysis and a proper diet help reduce the wastes that build up in your blood. A dietitian can help you plan meals according to your doctor's orders. When choosing foods, you should remember to:

♦ Eat balanced amounts of foods high in protein such as meat and chicken. Animal protein is better used by your body than the protein found in vegetables and grains.

♦ Watch the amount of potassium you eat. Potassium is a mineral found in salt substitutes, some fruits, vegetables, milk, chocolate, and nuts. Too much or too little potassium can be harmful to your heart.

♦ Limit how much you drink. Fluids build up quickly in your body when your kidneys aren't working. Too much fluid makes your tissues swell. It also can cause high blood pressure and heart trouble.

♦ Avoid salt. Salty foods make you thirsty and cause your body to hold water.

♦ Limit foods such as milk, cheese, nuts, dried beans, and soft drinks. These foods contain the mineral phosphorus. Too much phosphorus in your blood causes calcium to be pulled from your bones. Calcium helps keep bones strong and healthy. To prevent bone problems, your doctor may give you special medicines. You must take these medicines everyday as directed.

Pros and Cons

Each person responds differently to similar situations. What may be a negative factor for one person may be positive for another. However, in general, the following are pros and cons for each type of hemodialysis.

In-Center Hemodialysis

Pros

- You have trained professionals with you at all times.
- You can get to know other patients.

Cons

- Treatments are scheduled by the center.
- You must travel to the center for treatment.

Home Hemodialysis

Pros

- You can do it at the hours you choose. (*But you still must do it as often as your doctor orders.*)
- You don't have to travel to a center.
- You gain a sense of independence and control over your treatment.

Cons

- Helping with treatments may be stressful to your family.
- You need training.
- You need space for storing the machine and supplies at home.

Working With Your Health Care Team

Questions you may want to ask:

- Is hemodialysis the best treatment choice for me? Why or why not?
- If I am treated at a center, can I go to the center of my choice?
- What does hemodialysis feel like? Does it hurt?
- What is self-care dialysis?
- How long does it take to learn home hemodialysis? Who will train my partner and me?
- What kind of blood access is best for me?
- As a hemodialysis patient, will I be able to keep working? Can I have treatments at night if I plan to keep working?
- How much should I exercise?
- Who will be on my health care team? How can they help me?

- Who can I talk with about sexuality, family problems, or money concerns?
- How/where can I talk to other people who have faced this decision?

Peritoneal Dialysis

Purpose

Peritoneal dialysis is another procedure that replaces the work of your kidneys. It removes extra water, wastes, and chemicals from your body. This type of dialysis uses the lining of your abdomen to filter your blood. This lining is called the peritoneal membrane.

How It Works

A cleansing solution, called dialysate, travels through a special tube into your abdomen. Fluid, wastes, and chemicals pass from tiny blood vessels in the peritoneal membrane into the dialysate. After several hours, the dialysate gets drained from your abdomen, taking the wastes from your blood with it. Then you fill your abdomen with fresh dialysate and the cleaning process begins again.

Getting Ready

Before your first treatment, a surgeon places a small, soft tube called a catheter into your abdomen. This catheter always stays there. It helps transport the dialysate to and from your peritoneal membrane.

Types of Peritoneal Dialysis

There are three types of peritoneal dialysis.

1. **Continuous Ambulatory Peritoneal Dialysis (CAPD).** CAPD is the most common type of peritoneal dialysis. It needs no machine. It can be done in any clean, well-lit place. With CAPD, your blood is always being cleaned. The dialysate passes from a plastic bag through the catheter and into your abdomen. The dialysate stays in your abdomen with the catheter sealed. After several hours, you drain the solution back into the bag. Then you refill your abdomen with fresh solution through the same catheter. Now the cleaning process begins again. While the solution is in your body, you may fold the empty plastic bag and hide it under your clothes, around your waist, or in a pocket.
2. **Continuous Cyclic Peritoneal Dialysis (CCPD).** CCPD is like CAPD except that a machine, which connects to your catheter, automatically fills and drains the dialysate from your abdomen. The machine does this at night while you sleep.
3. **Intermittent Peritoneal Dialysis (IPD).** IPD uses the same type of machine as CCPD to add and drain the dialysate. IPD can be done at home, but it's usually done in the hospital. IPD treatments take longer than CCPD.

Who Performs It

CAPD is a form of self-treatment. It needs no machine and no partner. However, with IPD and CCPD, you need a machine and the help of a partner (family member, friend, or health professional).

The Time It Takes

With CAPD, the dialysate stays in your abdomen for about 4 to 6 hours. The process of draining the dialysate and replacing fresh solution takes 30 to 40 minutes. Most people change the solution four times a day.

With CCPD, treatments last from 10 to 12 hours every night.

With IPD, treatments are done several times a week, for a total of 36 to 42 hours per week. Sessions may last up to 24 hours.

Possible Complications

Peritonitis, or infection of the peritoneum, can occur if the opening where the catheter enters your body gets infected. You can also get it if there is a problem connecting or disconnecting the catheter from the bags. Peritonitis can make you feel sick. It can cause a fever and stomach pain.

To avoid peritonitis, you must be careful to follow the procedure exactly. You must know the early signs of peritonitis. Look for reddening or swelling around the catheter. You should also note if your dialysate looks cloudy. It is important to report these signs to your doctor so that the peritonitis can be treated quickly to avoid serious problems.

Your Diet

Diet for peritoneal dialysis is slightly different than diet for hemodialysis.

- You may be able to have more salt and fluids.
- You may eat more protein.
- You may have different potassium restrictions.
- You may need to cut back on the number of calories you eat. This limitation is because the sugar in the dialysate may cause you to gain weight.

Pros and Cons

There are pros and cons to each type of peritoneal dialysis.

CAPD

Pros

- You can perform treatment alone.
- You can do it at times you choose.
- You can do it in many locations.
- You don't need a machine.

Cons

- It disrupts your daily schedule.

CCPD

Pros

- You can do it at night, mainly while you sleep.

Cons

- You need a machine and help from a partner.

IPD

Pros

- Health professionals usually perform treatments.

Cons

- You may need to go to a hospital.
- It takes a lot of time.
- You need a machine.

Working with Your Health Care Team

Questions you may want to ask:

- Is peritoneal dialysis the best treatment choice for me? Why or why not? Which type?
- How long will it take me to learn peritoneal dialysis?
- What does peritoneal dialysis feel like? Does it hurt?
- How will peritoneal dialysis affect my blood pressure?
- How do I know if I have peritonitis? How is peritonitis treated?
- As a peritoneal dialysis patient, will I be able to continue working?
- How much should I exercise?
- Who will be on my health care team? How can they help me?
- Who can I talk with about sexuality, finances, or family concerns?
- How/where can I talk to other people who have faced this decision?

Dialysis Is Not a Cure

Hemodialysis and peritoneal dialysis are treatments that try to replace your failed kidneys. These treatments help you feel better and live longer, but they are not cures for ESRD. While patients with ESRD are now living longer than ever, ESRD can cause problems over the years. Some problems are bone disease, high blood pressure, nerve damage, and anemia (having too few red blood cells). Although these problems won't go away with dialysis, doctors now have new and better ways to treat or prevent them. You should discuss these treatments with your doctor.

Kidney Transplantation

Purpose

Kidney transplantation is a procedure that places a healthy kidney from another person into your body. This one new kidney does all the work that your two failed kidneys cannot do.

How It Works

A surgeon places the new kidney inside your body between your upper thigh and abdomen. The surgeon connects the artery and vein of the new kidney to your artery and vein. Your blood flows through the new kidney and makes urine, just like your own kidneys did when they were healthy. The new kidney may start working right away or may take up to a few weeks to make urine. Your own kidneys are left where they are, unless they are causing infection or high blood pressure.

Getting Ready

You may receive a kidney from a member of your family. This kind of donor is called a living-related donor. You may receive a kidney from a person who has recently died. This type of donor is called a cadaver donor. Sometimes a spouse or very close friend may donate a kidney. This kind of donor is called a living-unrelated donor.

It is very important for the donor's blood and tissues to closely match yours. This match will help prevent your body's immune system from fighting off, or rejecting, the new kidney. A lab will do special tests on blood cells to find out if your body will accept the new kidney.

The Time It Takes

The time it takes to get a kidney varies. There are not enough cadaver donors for every person who needs a transplant. Because of this, you must be placed on a waiting list to receive a cadaver donor kidney. However, if a relative gives you a kidney, the transplant operation can be done sooner.

The surgery takes from 3 to 6 hours. The usual hospital stay may last from 10 to 14 days. After you leave the hospital, you will go to the clinic for regular followup visits.

If a relative or close friend gives you a kidney, he or she will probably stay in the hospital for one week or less.

Possible Complications

Transplantation is not a cure. There is always a chance that your body will reject your new kidney, no matter how good the match. The chance of your body accepting the new kidney depends on your age, race, and medical condition.

Normally, 75 to 80 percent of transplants from cadaver donors are working one year after surgery. However, transplants from living relatives often work better than transplants from cadaver donors. This fact is because they are usually a closer match.

Your doctor will give you special drugs to help prevent rejection. These are called immunosuppressants. You will need to take these drugs every day for the rest of your life. Sometimes these drugs cannot stop your body from rejecting the new kidney. If this happens, you will go back to some form of dialysis and possibly wait for another transplant.

Treatment with these drugs may cause side effects. The most serious is that they weaken your immune system, making it easier for you to get infections. Some drugs also cause changes in how you look. Your face may get fuller. You may gain weight or develop acne or facial hair. Not all patients have these problems, and makeup and diet can help.

Some of these drugs may cause problems such as cataracts, extra stomach acid, and hip disease. In a smaller number of patients, these drugs also may cause liver or kidney damage when used for a long period of time.

Your Diet

Diet for transplant patients is less limiting than it is for dialysis patients. You may still have to cut back on some foods, though. Your diet probably will change as your medicines, blood values, weight, and blood pressure change.

- You may need to count calories. Your medicine may give you a bigger appetite and cause you to gain weight.
- You may have to limit eating salty foods. Your medications may cause salt to be held in your body, leading to high blood pressure.
- You may need to eat less protein. Some medications cause a higher level of wastes to build up in your bloodstream.

Pros and Cons

There are pros and cons to kidney transplantation.

Pros

- It works like a normal kidney.
- It helps you feel healthier.
- You have fewer diet restrictions.
- There's no need for dialysis.

Cons

- It requires major surgery.
- You may need to wait for a donor.
- One transplant may not last a lifetime. Your body may reject the new kidney.
- You will have to take drugs for the rest of your life.

Working with Your Health Care Team

Questions you may want to ask:

- Is transplantation the best treatment choice for me? Why or why not?
- What are my chances of having a successful transplant?
- How do I find out if a family member or friend can donate?
- What are the risks to a family member or friend if he or she donates?
- If a family member or friend doesn't donate, how do I get placed on a waiting list for a kidney? How long will I have to wait?
- What are the symptoms of rejection?
- Who will be on my health care team? How can they help me?
- Who can I talk to about sexuality, finances, or family concerns?

◆ How/where can I talk to other people who have faced this decision?

Conclusion

It's not always easy to decide which type of treatment is best for you. Your decision depends on your medical condition, lifestyle, and personal likes and dislikes. Discuss the pros and cons of each with your health care team. If you start one form of treatment and decide you'd like to try another, talk it over with your doctor. The key is to learn as much as you can about your choices. With that knowledge, you and your doctor will choose a treatment that suits you best.

Paying for Treatment

Treatment for ESRD is expensive, but the federal government helps pay for much of the cost. Often, private insurance or state programs pay the rest.

Medicare

Medicare pays for 80 percent of the cost of your dialysis treatments or transplant, no matter how old you are. To qualify,

◆ you must have worked long enough to be insured under Social Security (or be the child of someone who has) or
◆ you already must be receiving Social Security benefits.

You should apply for Medicare as soon as possible after beginning dialysis. Often, a social worker at your hospital or dialysis center will help you apply.

Private Insurance

Private insurance often pays for the entire cost of treatment. Or it may pay for the 20 percent that Medicare does not cover. Private insurance also may pay for your prescription drugs.

Medicaid

Medicaid is a state program. Your income must be below a certain level to receive Medicaid funds. Medicaid may pay for your treatments if you cannot receive Medicare. In some states, it also pays the 20 percent that Medicare does not cover. It also may pay for some of your medicines. To apply for Medicaid, talk with your social worker or contact your local health department.

Veterans Administration (VA) Benefits

If you are a veteran, the VA can help pay for treatment. Contact your local VA office for more information.

Social Security Income (SSI) and Social Security Disability Income (SSDI)

These benefits are available from the Social Security Administration. They assist you with the costs of daily living.

To find out if you qualify, talk to your social worker or call your local Social Security office.

Organizations That Can Help

There are several groups that offer information and services to kidney patients. You may wish to contact the following:

American Kidney Fund
Suite 1010
6110 Executive Boulevard
Rockville, MD 20852
(800) 638-8299

American Association of Kidney Patients
Suite LL1
1 Davis Boulevard
Tampa, FL 33606
(813) 251-0725

National Kidney Foundation, Inc.
30 East 33rd Street
New York, NY 10016
(800) 622-9010

National Kidney and Urologic Diseases Information Clearinghouse
Box NKUDIC
9000 Rockville Pike
Bethesda, MD 20892
(301) 654-4415

Additional Reading

If you would like to learn more about ESRD and its treatment, you may be interested in reading:

Your New Life With Dialysis—A Patient Guide for Physical and Psychological Adjustment
Edith T. Oberley, M.A., and Terry D. Oberley, M.D., Ph.D. Fourth edition, 1991
Charles C. Thomas Publishers
2600 South First Street
Springfield, IL 62794-9265

Understanding Kidney Transplantation
Edith T. Oberley, M.A., and Neal R. Glass, M.D., F.A.C.S.
Charles C. Thomas Publishers, 1987
2600 South First Street
Springfield, IL 62794-9265

Kidney Disease: A Guide for Patients and Their Families
American Kidney Fund
Suite 1010
6110 Executive Boulevard
Rockville, MD 20852
(800) 638-8299

National Kidney Foundation Patient Education Brochures
Includes information on treatment, diet, work, and exercise.
National Kidney Foundation, Inc.
30 East 33rd Street
New York, NY 10016
(800) 622-9010

Medicare Coverage of Kidney Dialysis and Kidney Transplant Services: A Supplement to Your Medicare Handbook
Publication Number HCFA-02183
U.S. Department of Health and Human Services
Health Care Financing Administration
Suite 500
1331 H Street, NW
Washington, DC 20005
(301) 966-7843

Renalife Magazine
American Association of Kidney Patients (AAKP)
Suite LL1

1 Davis Boulevard
Tampa, FL 33606
(813) 251-0725
Published quarterly.

Family Focus Newsletter
National Kidney Foundation, Inc.
30 East 33rd Street
New York, NY 10016
(800) 622-9010

For Patients Only Magazine
Suite 400
20335 Ventura Boulevard
Woodland Hills, CA 91364
(818) 704-5555
Published six times per year.

■ Document Source:
U.S. Department of Health and Human Services, Public Health Service
National Institutes of Health
National Institute of Diabetes, and Digestive and Kidney Diseases
NIH Publication No. 93-2412
July 1993

CancerFax from the National Cancer Institute

PROSTATE CANCER

Description

What Is Cancer of the Prostate?

Cancer of the prostate, a common form of cancer, is a disease in which cancer (malignant) cells are found in the prostate. The prostate is one of the male sex glands and is located just below the bladder (the organ that collects and empties urine) and in front of the rectum (the lower part of the intestine). The prostate is about the size of a walnut. It surrounds part of the urethra, the tube that carries urine from the bladder to the outside of the body. The prostate makes fluid that becomes part of the semen, the white fluid that contains sperm.

Cancer of the prostate is found mainly in older men. As you get older, your prostate may get bigger and block the urethra or bladder, which can cause you to have difficulty urinating or may interfere with sexual functions. This condition is called benign prostatic hyperplasia (BPH), and although it is not cancer, you may need surgery to correct it. The symptoms of BPH or of other problems in the prostate may be similar to symptoms for prostate cancer.

Like most cancers, the chance for cure for cancer of the prostate is greatest when the cancer is diagnosed and treated when it is small (at an early stage). You should see a doctor if you have any of the following: weak or interrupted flow of urine, urinating often (especially at night), difficulty urinating, pain or burning when you urinate, blood in the urine, or nagging pain in the back, hips, or pelvis. Often there are no symptoms of early cancer of the prostate. To examine you, usually your doctor will insert a gloved finger into the rectum (a rectal exam) to feel for lumps in the prostate. A special test called an ultrasound, which uses sound waves to make a picture of your bladder, may also be done.

If your doctor feels anything that is not normal, he or she may need to take cells from your prostate and look at them under a microscope. Your doctor will usually do this by putting a needle into the prostate to remove some cells. To get to your prostate, your doctor may put the needle through the rectum or through the space between the scrotum and the anus (the perineum). This is called a fine needle aspiration or a needle biopsy.

Your chance of recovery (prognosis) and choice of treatment depend on the stage of your cancer (whether it is just in the prostate or has spread to other places in the body) and your general state of health.

Stage Explanation

Stages of Cancer of the Prostate

Once cancer of the prostate has been found (diagnosed), more tests will be done to find out if cancer cells have spread from the prostate to tissues around it or to other parts of the body. This is called "staging." Your doctor needs to know the stage of your disease to plan treatment. The following stages are used for cancer of the prostate:

Stage A
Prostate cancer at this stage cannot be felt and causes no symptoms. The cancer is only in the prostate and usually is found accidentally when surgery is done for other reasons, such as for BPH.

Stage A1: cancer cells are found in only one area of the prostate

Stage A2: cancer cells are found in many areas of the prostate

Stage B
The tumor can be felt in the prostate during a rectal exam, but the cancer cells are found only in the prostate gland.

Stage C
Cancer cells have spread outside the covering (capsule) of the prostate to tissues around the prostate. The glands that produce semen (the seminal vesicles) may have cancer in them.

Stage D
Cancer cells have spread (metastasized) to lymph nodes or to organs and tissues far away from the prostate.

Stage D1: cancer cells have spread to lymph nodes near the prostate (Lymph nodes are small, bean-shaped structures that are found throughout the body. They produce and store infection-fighting cells.)

Stage D2: cancer cells have spread to lymph nodes far from the prostate or to other parts of the body, such as the bone, liver, or lungs

Recurrent
Recurrent disease means that the cancer has come back (recurred) after it has been treated. It may come back in the prostate or in another part of the body.

Treatment Options Overview

How Cancer of the Prostate Is Treated

There are treatments for all patients with cancer of the prostate. Three kinds of treatment are commonly used:

> surgery (taking out the cancer)
> radiation therapy (using high-dose x-rays or other high-energy rays to kill cancer cells)
> hormone therapy (using hormones to stop cancer cells from growing).

Surgery is a common treatment for cancer of the prostate. Your doctor may take out the cancer using one of the following operations:

Radical prostatectomy removes the prostate and some of the tissue around it. Your doctor may do the surgery by cutting into the space between the scrotum and the anus (the perineum) in an operation called a perineal prostatectomy or by cutting into the lower abdomen in an operation called a retropubic prostatectomy. Radical prostatectomy is done only if the cancer has not spread outside the prostate. Often before the prostatectomy is done, your doctor will do surgery to take out lymph nodes in the pelvis to see if they contain cancer. This is called a pelvic lymph node dissection. If the lymph nodes contain cancer, usually your doctor will not do a prostatectomy, and may or may not recommend other therapy at this time. Impotence can occur in men treated with surgery.

Transurethral resection cuts cancer from the prostate using a tool with a small wire loop on the end that is put into the prostate through the urethra. This operation is sometimes done to relieve symptoms caused by the tumor before other treatment or in men who cannot have a radical prostatectomy because of age or other illness.

Cryosurgery is a type of surgery that kills the cancer by freezing it.

Radiation therapy uses high-energy x-rays to kill cancer cells and shrink tumors. Radiation may come from a machine outside the body (external radiation therapy) or from putting materials that produce radiation (radioisotopes) through thin plastic tubes in the area where the cancer cells are found (internal radiation therapy). Impotence may occur in men treated with radiation therapy.

Hormone therapy uses hormones to stop cancer cells from growing. Hormone therapy for prostate cancer can take several forms. Male hormones (especially testosterone) can help prostate cancer grow. To stop the cancer from growing, female hormones or drugs that decrease the amount of male hormones made may be given. Sometimes an operation to remove the testicles (orchiectomy) is done to stop the testicles from making testosterone. This treatment is usually used in men with advanced prostate cancer. Growth of breast tissue is a common side effect of therapy with female hormones (estrogens); hot flashes can occur after orchiectomy and other hormone therapies.

Chemotherapy uses drugs to kill cancer cells. Chemotherapy may be taken by pill, or it may be put into the body by a needle in the vein or muscle. Chemotherapy is called a systemic treatment because the drug enters the bloodstream, travels through the body, and can kill cancer cells outside the prostate. To date, chemotherapy has not had significant value in treating prostate cancer, but clinical trials are in progress to find more effective drugs.

Treatment by Stage

Treatment of cancer of the prostate depends on the stage of your disease, your age, and your overall condition. If you do not have any symptoms, your doctor may follow you closely without any treatment if you are older, if you have another more serious illness, or if your tumor cells appear only slightly abnormal.

You may receive treatment that is considered standard based on its effectiveness in a number of patients in past studies, or you may choose to go into a clinical trial. Not all patients are cured with standard therapy and some standard treatments may have more side effects than are desired. For these reasons, clinical trials are designed to find better ways to treat cancer patients and are based on the most up-to-date information. Clinical trials are going on in most parts of the country for most stages of cancer of the prostate. If you want more information, call the Cancer Information Service at 1-800-4-CANCER (1-800-422-6237).

Treatment options: Stage A prostate cancer
Your treatment depends on whether you have stage A1 or stage A2 prostate cancer.

If you have stage A1 cancer and you are older, your doctor may follow you closely without any treatment. Your doctor may choose this option for you because your cancer is not causing any symptoms or other problems and may be growing slowly. If you are younger, you may have surgery to remove the prostate and the tissue around it (radical prostatectomy) or external radiation therapy.

If you have stage A2 cancer, your treatment may be one of the following:
1. External radiation therapy.
2. Surgery to remove the prostate and the tissue around it (radical prostatectomy), with or without new techniques to preserve the nerves necessary for an erection as well as preventing leakage of urine from the bladder (nerve sparing technique). Usually some of the lymph nodes in the pelvis are also removed (pelvic lymph node dissection). Radiation therapy may be given after surgery in some cases.
3. A clinical trial of internal radiation therapy, often in addition to pelvic lymph node dissection.
4. If you are older or have another more serious illness, your doctor may follow you closely without treatment.
5. A clinical trial of cryosurgery.
6. A clinical trial of external radiation therapy using new techniques to protect your normal tissues from radiation.

Treatment options: Stage B prostate cancer
Your treatment may be one of the following:
1. Surgery to remove the prostate and the tissue around it (radical prostatectomy), with or without techniques to preserve the nerves necessary for an erection as well as preventing leakage of urine from the bladder (nerve sparing technique).

Usually some of the lymph nodes in the pelvis are also removed (pelvic lymph node dissection). Radiation therapy may be given following surgery.

2. External radiation therapy. Clinical trials are testing new types of radiation.

3. A clinical trial of internal radiation therapy, often in addition to pelvic lymph node dissection.

4. If you are older or have another more serious illness, your doctor may follow you closely without treatment. Your doctor may choose this option for you because your cancer is not causing any symptoms or other problems and may be growing slowly.

5. A clinical trial of external radiation therapy using new techniques to protect your normal tissues from the radiation.

6. A clinical trial of cryosurgery.

Treatment options: Stage C prostate cancer

Your treatment may be one of the following:

1. External radiation therapy. Clinical trials are testing new types of radiation.

2. Surgery to remove the prostate and the tissue around it (radical prostatectomy). Usually some of the lymph nodes in the pelvis are also removed (pelvic lymph node dissection). Radiation therapy may be given following surgery.

3. If you are older or have another more serious illness, your doctor may follow you closely without treatment. Your doctor may choose this option for you because your cancer is not causing any symptoms or other problems and may be growing slowly.

4. A clinical trial of internal radiation therapy, often in addition to pelvic lymph node dissection.

If you are unable to have surgery or radiation therapy, your doctor may give you treatments to relieve symptoms such as problems urinating. In this case, your treatment may be one of the following:

1. Radiation therapy to relieve symptoms.

2. Surgery to cut the cancer from the prostate using a tool with a small wire loop on the end that is put into the prostate through the urethra (transurethral resection).

3. Hormone therapy.

Treatment options: Stage D prostate cancer

Your treatment depends on whether you have stage D1 or stage D2 prostate cancer.

If you have stage D1 cancer, your treatment may be one of the following:

1. External radiation therapy. Clinical trials are testing new forms of radiation. Hormone therapy may be given in addition to radiation.

2. Clinical trials of surgery to remove the prostate and the tissue around it (radical prostatectomy) and surgery to remove the testicles (orchiectomy).

3. If you are older or have another more serious illness, your doctor may follow you closely without treatment. Your doctor may choose this option for you because your cancer is not caus-

ing any symptoms or other problems and may be growing slowly.

4. A clinical trial of hormone therapy

If you have stage D2 disease, your treatment may be one of the following:

1. Hormone therapy.

2. External beam radiation therapy to relieve symptoms.

3. Surgery to cut the cancer from the prostate using a tool with a small wire loop on the end that is put into the prostate through the urethra (transurethral resection) to relieve symptoms.

4. Your doctor may follow you closely and wait until you develop symptoms before giving you treatment.

5. Clinical trials of chemotherapy, radiation therapy, or surgery.

Treatment options: Recurrent prostate cancer

Your treatment depends on many things, including what treatment you had before. If you had surgery to remove the prostate (prostatectomy) and the cancer comes back in only a small area, you may receive radiation therapy. If the disease has spread to other parts of the body, you will probably receive hormone therapy. Radiation therapy may be given to relieve symptoms, such as bone pain. You may also choose to take part in a clinical trial of chemotherapy.

To learn more about cancer of the prostate, call the National Cancer Institute's Cancer Information Service at 1-800-4-CANCER (1-800-422-6237). By dialing this toll-free number, you can speak with someone who can answer your questions.

■ Document Source:
National Cancer Institute
  Building 31, Room 10A24, 9000 Rockville Pike, Bethesda, MD 20892
  PDQ 208/01229
  02/01/94

See also: Radiation Therapy and You: A Guide to Self-Help During Treatment (page 56)

CancerFax from the National Cancer Institute

RENAL CELL CANCER

Description

What Is Renal Cell Cancer?

Renal cell cancer (also called cancer of the kidney or renal adenocarcinoma) is a disease in which cancer (malignant) cells are found in certain tissues of the kidney. Renal cell cancer is one of the less common kinds of cancer. It occurs more often in men than in women.

The kidneys are a "matched" pair of organs found on either side of your backbone. The kidneys of an adult are about 5 inches long and 3 inches wide and are shaped like a kidney bean. Inside each kidney are tiny tubules that filter and clean your blood, taking out waste products, and making urine. The urine made by the kidneys passes through a tube called a ureter into the bladder where it is held until it is passed from your body. Renal cell cancer is a cancer of the lining of the tubules in the kidney. If you have cancer in the part of the kidney that collects urine and drains it to the ureters (the renal pelvis) or if you have cancer in the ureters, refer to the PDQ patient information statement on transitional cell cancer of the renal pelvis and ureter.

Like most cancers, renal cell cancer is best treated when it is found (diagnosed) early. You should see your doctor if you have one or more of the following: blood in your urine, a lump (mass) in your abdomen, or a pain in your side that doesn't go away. If you have cancer of the kidney, you may also feel very tired or have loss of appetite, weight loss without dieting, and anemia (too few red blood cells).

If you have signs of cancer, your doctor will usually feel your abdomen for lumps. Your doctor may order a special x-ray called an intravenous pyelogram (IVP). During this test, a dye containing iodine is injected into your bloodstream. This allows your doctor to see the kidney more clearly on the x-ray. Your doctor may also do an ultrasound, which uses sound waves to find tumors, or a special x-ray called a CT scan to look for lumps in the kidney. A special scan called magnetic resonance imaging (MRI), which uses magnetic waves to find tumors, may also be done.

Your chance of recovery (prognosis) and choice of treatment depend on the stage of your cancer (whether it is just in the kidney or has spread to other places in the body) and your general state of health.

Stage Explanation

Stages of Renal Cell Cancer

Once renal cell cancer has been found, more tests will be done to find out if cancer cells have spread to other parts of the body. This is called staging. Your doctor needs to know the stage of your disease to plan treatment. The following stages are used for renal cell cancer:

Stage I
Cancer is found only in the kidney.

Stage II
Cancer has spread to the fat around the kidney, but the cancer has not spread beyond this to the capsule that contains the kidney.

Stage III
Cancer has spread to the main blood vessel that carries clean blood from the kidney (renal vein), to the blood vessel that carries blood from the lower part of the body to the heart (inferior vena cava), or to lymph nodes around the kidney. (Lymph nodes are small, bean-shaped structures that are found throughout the body; they produce and store infection-fighting cells.)

Stage IV
Cancer has spread to nearby organs such as the bowel or pancreas or has spread to other places in the body such as the lungs.

Recurrent
Recurrent disease means that the cancer has come back (recurred) after it has been treated. It may come back in the original area or in another part of the body.

Treatment Options Overview

How Renal Cell Cancer Is Treated

There are treatments for most patients with renal cell cancer. Five kinds of treatment are used:

surgery (taking out the cancer in an operation)
chemotherapy (using drugs to kill cancer cells)
radiation therapy (using high-dose x-rays or other high-energy rays to kill cancer cells)
hormone therapy (using hormones to stop cancer cells from growing)
biological therapy (using your body's immune system to fight cancer).

Surgery is a common treatment for renal cell cancer. Your doctor may take out the cancer using one of the following:

♦ Partial nephrectomy removes the cancer and part of the kidney around the cancer. This is usually done only in special cases, such as when the other kidney is damaged or has already been removed.
♦ Simple nephrectomy removes the whole kidney. The kidney on the other side of the body can take over filtering the blood.
♦ Radical nephrectomy removes the kidney with the tissues around it. Some lymph nodes in the area may also be removed.

Chemotherapy uses drugs to kill cancer cells. Chemotherapy may be taken by pill, or it may be put into the body by a needle in a vein or muscle. Chemotherapy is called a systemic treatment because the drugs enter the bloodstream, travel through the body, and can kill cancer cells throughout the body.

Radiation therapy uses x-rays or other high-energy rays to kill cancer cells and shrink tumors. Radiation may come from a machine outside the body (external radiation therapy) or from putting materials that contain radiation through thin plastic tubes (internal radiation therapy) in the area where the cancer cells are found. Radiation can be used alone or before or after surgery and/or chemotherapy.

Hormone therapy uses hormones (taken by pill or injected with a needle) to stop cancer cells from growing.

Biological therapy tries to get your own body to fight cancer. It uses materials made by your own body or made in a laboratory to boost, direct, or restore your body's natural defenses against disease. Biological therapy is sometimes called biological response modifier (BRM) therapy or immunotherapy.

Sometimes a special treatment called arterial embolization is used to treat renal cell cancer. A narrow tube (catheter) is used to inject small pieces of a special gelatin sponge into the main blood vessel that flows into the kidney to block the blood cells that feed the tumor. This prevents the cancer cells from getting oxygen or other substances they need to grow.

Treatment by Stage

Treatments for renal cell cancer depend on the type and stage of your disease, your age, and your general health.

You may receive treatment that is considered standard based on its effectiveness in a number of patients in past studies, or you may choose to go into a clinical trial. Not all patients are cured with standard therapy and some standard treatments may have more side effects than are desired. For these reasons, clinical trials are designed to find better ways to treat cancer patients and are based on the most up-to-date information. Clinical trials are going on in most parts of the country for most stages of renal cell cancer. If you want more information, call the Cancer Information Service at 1-800-4-CANCER (1-800-422-6237).

Treatment options: Stage I renal cell cancer
Your treatment may be one of the following:
1. Surgery to remove the kidney and the tissues around it (radical nephrectomy). Lymph nodes in the area may also be removed.
2. Surgery to remove only the kidney (simple nephrectomy).
3. Surgery to remove the part of the kidney where the cancer is found (partial nephrectomy).
4. External beam radiation therapy to relieve symptoms in patients who cannot have surgery.
5. Injection of small pieces of a special gelatin sponge into the main artery that flows to the kidney to block blood flow to the cancer cells (arterial embolization). This is usually done only in patients who cannot have surgery.

Treatment options: Stage II renal cell cancer
Your treatment may be one of the following:
1. Surgery to remove the kidney and the tissues around it (radical nephrectomy). Lymph nodes in the area may also be removed.
2. External beam radiation therapy before or after radical nephrectomy.
3. Surgery to remove the part of the kidney where the cancer is found (partial nephrectomy).
4. External beam radiation therapy to relieve symptoms in patients who cannot have surgery.
5. Injection of small pieces of a special gelatin sponge into the main artery that flows to the kidney to block blood flow to the cancer cells (arterial embolization). This is usually done only in patients who cannot have surgery.

Treatment options: Stage III renal cell cancer
Your treatment may be one of the following:
1. Surgery to remove the kidney and the tissues around it (radical nephrectomy). Lymph nodes in the area may also be removed. If the cancer has spread to the main blood vessels that carry blood to and from the kidney (the renal vein or vena cava), part of the blood vessel may also be removed.
2. Injection of small pieces of a special gelatin sponge into the main artery that flows to the kidney to block blood flow to the cancer cells (arterial em-

bolization). This may be followed by radical nephrectomy.
3. External beam radiation therapy to relieve symptoms.
4. Surgery to remove the kidney (simple or radical nephrectomy) to relieve symptoms.
5. A clinical trial of external beam radiation therapy to relieve symptoms.

Treatment options: Stage IV renal cell cancer
Your treatment may be one of the following:
1. Biological therapy.
2. External radiation therapy to relieve symptoms.
3. Surgery to remove the kidney (nephrectomy) to relieve symptoms.
4. If cancer has spread only to the area around the kidney, surgery to remove the kidney and the tissue around it (radical nephrectomy). If the cancer has spread to a limited area, surgery to remove the cancer where it has spread (metastasized) in addition to radical nephrectomy.

Treatment options: Recurrent renal cell cancer
Your treatment may be one of the following:
1. If cancer has spread only to one or a few areas in the body, surgery to remove the cancer.
2. Radiation therapy to relieve symptoms.
3. Biological therapy.
4. Chemotherapy.

To learn more about renal cell cancer, call the National Cancer Institute's Cancer Information Service at 1-800-4-CANCER (1-800-422-6237). By dialing this toll-free number, you can speak with someone who can answer your questions.

■ Document Source:
National Cancer Institute
   Building 31, Room 10A24, 9000 Rockville Pike, Bethesda, MD
   20892
   PDQ 208/01070
   02/01/94

See also: Chemotherapy and You: A Guide to Self-Help During Treatment (page 40); Radiation Therapy and You: A Guide to Self-Help During Treatment (page 56)

TREATING YOUR ENLARGED PROSTATE

Purpose of this booklet

This booklet can help you understand benign prostatic hyperplasia (BPH) and how it can be treated. BPH is an enlarged but otherwise normal prostate. It is common in older men and may cause no problems at all. If you want or need to choose a treatment, however, this booklet describes both benefits and risks of all treatments.

What is your prostate?

The prostate makes some of the milky fluid (semen) that carries sperm. The gland is the size of a walnut and is found just below the bladder, which stores urine. The prostate wraps around a tube (the urethra) that carries urine from the bladder out through the tip of the penis.

During a man's orgasm (sexual climax), muscles squeeze the prostate's fluid into the urethra. Sperm, which are made in the testicles, also go into the urethra during orgasm. The milky fluid carries the sperm through the penis during orgasm.

Understanding the problem

What is BPH?

BPH means that the prostate gland has grown larger than normal.

BPH is not cancer and does not cause cancer.

"Benign" means the cells are not cancerous. "Hyperplasia" means there are more cells than normal.

BPH results from growing older and cannot be prevented. Your chances of having prostate trouble increase as you age. BPH is common in men over age 50. More than half of all men over age 60 have BPH. By age 80, about 8 out of 10 men have it.

BPH does not always cause problems. Fewer than half of all men with BPH ever show any symptoms of the disease. And only some men with symptoms will need treatment.

What are the symptoms of BPH?

The most common symptom of BPH is trouble urinating. Many men with BPH have no bothersome symptoms. But BPH may cause some men to have problems urinating. Below is a list of symptoms that you may have:

- ♦ I feel that I have not completely emptied my bladder after I stop urinating.
- ♦ I urinate often.
- ♦ I stop and start when I urinate.
- ♦ I have a strong and sudden desire to urinate that is hard to delay.
- ♦ My urine stream is weak.
- ♦ I need to push or strain to start the urine stream.
- ♦ I often wake up at night to urinate.

What causes symptoms?

As the prostate grows in BPH, it squeezes the urethra (urinary tube). This narrows the tube and can cause problems with urination. Sometimes with BPH you can also have urinary infection or bleeding.

In the early stages of BPH, the bladder muscle can still force urine through the narrowed urethra by squeezing harder. But if the blockage continues, the bladder muscle gets stronger, thicker, and more sensitive. The result is a stronger need to urinate.

In some cases, you may have trouble forcing urine through the urethra.

This means the bladder cannot empty completely. Some men may find that they suddenly cannot urinate (a condition called acute urinary retention). Over time, a few men might have bladder or kidney problems or both.

Sometimes BPH causes infection of the urinary tract. This can cause burning or pain when you urinate. The urinary tract is the path that urine takes as it leaves the body. The tract includes the kidneys, ureters, bladder, and urethra.

When should you see a doctor?

If you have symptoms that bother you, see a doctor. He or she can find out if BPH—or another disease—is the cause. If you do have BPH, your doctor can also see if it has caused other problems.

How is BPH diagnosed?

During your visit, the doctor will most likely:

- ♦ **Give you a list of questions** about your symptoms. These questions are important. Your answers will help the doctor decide if your symptoms are mild, moderate, or severe.
- ♦ **Take your medical history.** Your doctor will ask you about past and current medical problems.
- ♦ **Examine your prostate** gland by inserting a gloved, lubricated finger into your rectum.
- ♦ **Do a physical exam** to see if other medical problems may be causing your symptoms.
- ♦ **Check your urine** for blood or signs of infection (a urinalysis).
- ♦ **Test your blood** to see if the prostate has affected your kidneys. Your doctor may also recommend a blood test to help detect prostate cancer.

These tests are not painful or costly. They are done to help confirm that you have BPH and to find any problems it has caused. But tests used to diagnose your condition cannot predict if BPH will cause problems later if not treated now.

Your doctor may also recommend other tests. They may help find if BPH has affected your bladder or kidneys and make sure your problems are not caused by cancer. These tests may help some patients but not everyone:

- ♦ **Uroflowmetry** measures how fast your urine flows and how much you pass. This test can help find how much the urine is blocked.
- ♦ **Residual urine measurement** shows how much urine is left in your bladder after you urinate. This test can help find how much your bladder has been affected by BPH. The test can be done several ways. You and your doctor should talk about the method used.
- ♦ **Pressure-flow studies** measure the pressure in your bladder as you urinate. Some doctors feel this test is the best way to find out how much your urine is blocked. The test can help most if results of other tests are confusing or if your doctor thinks you have bladder problems. In the test, a small tube called a catheter is inserted into the penis, through the urethra, and into the

bladder. The test may cause discomfort for a short time. In a few men, it may cause a urinary tract infection.

◆ **Prostate-specific antigen (PSA)** is a blood test that can help find prostate cancer. BPH does not cause cancer. But some men do have BPH and cancer at the same time.

The PSA test is not always accurate. PSA test results can suggest cancer in BPH patients who do not have prostate cancer. The results can also sometimes suggest no cancer in men who do have cancer.

Not all doctors agree that being tested for PSA levels lowers a patient's chance of dying from prostate cancer. Each man with BPH is different. You and your doctor may want to discuss this test.

Your doctor may also suggest other tests such as x-rays, cystoscopy, and ultrasound. Many men do not need these tests. They are costly and not very helpful for most men with BPH. Also, cystoscopy and x-rays can cause discomfort or problems for some men. But the tests can help patients with some BPH problems or men with other problems such as blood in the urine.

◆ Cystoscopy lets the doctor look directly at the prostate and bladder. This test helps the doctor find the best method in men who choose invasive treatments (such as surgery). In cystoscopy, a small tube is inserted into the penis, through the urethra, and into the bladder. Some men may have discomfort during and after the test. A few may get urinary infections or blood in the urine; a few may not be able to urinate for a short time after the test.

◆ An x-ray called a urogram lets the doctor see blockage in the urinary tract. A dye injected into a vein makes the urine show up on the x-ray. Some men are allergic to the dye.

◆ Ultrasound lets the doctor see the prostate, kidneys, and bladder without a catheter or x-rays. A probe put on the skin sends sound waves (ultrasound) into the body. The echoes result in pictures of the prostate, kidneys, or bladder on a TV screen. This test is not harmful or painful. A special probe put in the rectum can give a better view of the prostate when the doctor wants to check for prostate cancer.

When should BPH be treated?

BPH needs to be treated only if:
◆ The symptoms are severe enough to bother you.
◆ Your urinary tract is seriously affected.

An enlarged prostate alone is not reason enough to get treatment. Your prostate may not get bigger than it is now, and your symptoms may not get worse.

Ask yourself how much your symptoms really bother you:
◆ Do they keep you from doing the things you enjoy, such as fishing or going to sports events?
◆ Would you be a lot happier or do more if the symptoms went away?
◆ Do you want treatment now?

◆ Are you willing to accept some risks to try to get rid of your symptoms?
◆ Do you understand the risks?

Your answers to these questions can help you choose a treatment that is right for you.

What are your treatment choices?

Currently, the five ways of treating BPH are:
◆ Watchful waiting.
◆ Alpha blocker drug treatment.
◆ Finasteride drug treatment.
◆ Balloon dilation.
◆ Surgery.

Surgery will do the best job of relieving your urinary symptoms, but it also has more risk than the other treatments. Unless you have a serious complication of BPH that makes surgery the only good choice, you can choose from a range of treatments. Which one you choose—if any—depends on how much your symptoms bother you. Your choice also depends on how much risk you are willing to take to improve your symptoms. You and your doctor will decide together.

Watchful waiting

If you have BPH but are not bothered by your symptoms, you and your doctor may decide on a program of "watchful waiting." Watchful waiting is not an active treatment like taking medicine or having surgery. It means getting regular exams—about once a year—to see if your BPH is getting worse or causing problems. At these exams, your doctor will ask about any problems you have. He or she may also order some simple tests to see if your BPH is causing kidney or bladder problems.

A small number of men in watchful waiting become unable to urinate at all. Some also get infections or bleed, or their bladder or kidneys are damaged. But such major problems are uncommon.

Your doctor may suggest some tips to help control your symptoms. One is to drink fewer liquids before going to bed. Another is not to take over-the-counter cold and sinus medicines with decongestants, which can make a prostate condition worse.

Without treatment, BPH symptoms may get better, stay the same, or get worse. If your symptoms become a problem, talk to your doctor about treatment choices.

Alpha blocker drug treatment

Alpha blocker drugs are taken by mouth, usually once or twice a day. The drugs help relax muscles in the prostate, and some men will notice that their urinary symptoms get better.

During the first 3 or 4 weeks, the doctor may see you regularly to make sure everything is okay. The doctor will check your symptoms and see if the medicine's dosage (how much you take and how often) is right for you. After that, you will visit the doctor from time to time to have your symptoms checked and prescription refilled. There is no evidence that alpha blockers reduce the rate of BPH complications or the need for future surgery.

Side effects can include headaches or feeling dizzy, light-headed, or tired. Low blood pressure is also possible. Because alpha blocker treatment for BPH is new, doctors do not know its long-term benefits and risks.

Alpha blockers include doxazosin (Cardura), prazosin (Minipress), and terazosin (Hytrin). Hytrin is the only alpha blocker now approved for BPH treatment by the Food and Drug Administration.

Finasteride drug treatment

Finasteride (Proscar) is taken by mouth once a day. It can cause the prostate to shrink, and some men will notice that their urinary symptoms get better. It may take 6 months or more before you notice the full benefit of finasteride. You still need to see your doctor on a regular basis while you take this drug. There is no evidence that finasteride reduces the rate of BPH complications or the need for future surgery.

Finasteride drug treatment is new, and doctors do not know its long-term benefits and risks. Also, finasteride lowers the blood level of prostate-specific antigen. Doctors do not know if this affects the ability of the PSA test to detect prostate cancer.

Side effects of finasteride include less interest in having sex, problems getting an erection, and problems with ejaculation.

Balloon dilation

Balloon dilation is done in the operating room in a hospital or doctor's office. After the patient gets anesthesia (medicine to reduce pain), the doctor inserts a catheter (plastic tube) into the penis. The catheter goes through the urethra and into the bladder. The catheter has a limp balloon at the end.

The doctor inflates the balloon to stretch the urethra where it has been squeezed by the prostate. In some patients, this can allow urine to flow more easily.

Balloon dilation can cause bleeding or infection. It can also make patients unable to urinate for a time. If there are no problems, you may go home the same day. Some patients have to stay overnight at the hospital.

Balloon dilation is a fairly new treatment for BPH, and doctors do not know all its long-term benefits and risks. In many patients, this treatment seems to work for only a short time.

Surgery

Because surgery has been used for many years to treat BPH, its benefits and risks are fairly well known. Compared with other treatments, surgery has the best chance for relief of BPH symptoms. Although surgery is also most likely to cause major problems, most men who undergo surgery have no major problems.

By itself, an enlarged prostate does not mean you need surgery. An enlarged prostate may not become larger. Also, no operation for BPH lowers the chance of getting prostate cancer in the future.

Surgery is almost always recommended for men with certain problems caused by BPH. These include:

♦ Not being able to urinate at all.
♦ Urine backup into the kidneys that damages the kidneys.
♦ Frequent urine infection.
♦ Major bleeding through the urethra caused by BPH.
♦ Stones in the bladder.

If you do not have any of these serious problems, but you are bothered by your BPH, you may still want to consider surgery.

There are three types of surgery for BPH:

♦ Transurethral resection of the prostate (TURP).
♦ Transurethral incision of the prostate (TUIP).
♦ Open prostatectomy.

TURP is the most common. It is a proven way to treat BPH effectively. TURP relieves symptoms by reducing pressure on the urethra.

After the patient gets anesthesia, the doctor inserts a special instrument into the urethra through the penis. No skin needs to be cut. The doctor then removes part of the inside of the prostate.

After TURP, patients usually need to wear a catheter (a tube in the penis for draining urine) for 2-3 days and stay in the hospital for about 3 days. Most patients find that their symptoms improve quickly after TURP. These men do well for many years.

TUIP may be used when the prostate is not enlarged as much. In TUIP, tissue is not removed. Instead, an instrument is passed through the urethra to make one or two small cuts in the prostate. These cuts reduce the prostate's pressure on the urethra, making it easier to urinate. TUIP may have less risk than TURP in certain cases.

Open prostatectomy may be used if the prostate is very large. In this procedure, an incision is made in the lower abdomen to remove part of the inside of the prostate.

Surgery for BPH improves symptoms in most patients, but some symptoms may remain. For example, the bladder might be weak because of blockage. This means there still could be problems urinating even after prostate tissue is removed.

New treatments

New treatments for BPH appear every year. Examples are laser surgery, microwave thermal therapy, prostatic stents, and new drugs. Use of a laser is still surgery, and doctors do not yet know if its benefits and risks are higher or lower than standard surgery.

There is not yet enough information about these treatments to include them in this booklet. If your doctor suggests a treatment not discussed here, ask for the same type of information on risks and benefits given below for other treatments.

What are the benefits and risks?

Each treatment may improve your symptoms. But each treatment has different chances of success. All treatments, even watchful waiting, have some risks.

Ask your doctor these questions about each treatment:

- ♦ What is my chance of getting better?
- ♦ How much better will I get?
- ♦ What are the chances that the treatment will cause problems?
- ♦ How long will the treatment work?

Both benefits and risks are given below for each treatment. This can help you and your doctor make the best choice for you.

But even with TURP, your chances for improvement are somewhat uncertain. This is because doctors do not know the exact chances that each patient's symptoms will improve. In general, the worse your symptoms are before treatment, the more they will improve if the treatment works. The success of TUIP and open prostatectomy is similar to TURP.

Most of the time, treatments do not cause problems. Most problems are not serious, but some are. TURP can cause serious problems such as urinary infection, bleeding that requires transfusion, or blocked urine flow. Few patients have these serious problems after surgery (see Balance Sheet for benefits and risks).

For patients taking alpha blocker drugs, the most common side effects are feeling dizzy and tired and having headaches.

With finasteride, about 5 out of 100 patients have some kind of sexual problem such as a lower sex drive or trouble getting an erection.

With watchful waiting, there is no active treatment and no added chance of problems right away. But over time, the BPH itself can cause symptoms to grow worse or cause other problems. Only TURP clearly reduces that risk. Doctors do not know if alpha blocker drugs, finasteride, or balloon dilation lower the risk of future BPH problems.

The average age of men diagnosed with BPH is 67. The chances that a 67-year-old man might die from any cause are about 8 out of 1,000 in a 3-month period. There is a greater chance (although small) of dying up to 3 months after TURP—about 15 out of 1,000 patients. If you are healthy, your chance of dying after TURP is lower.

Some BPH treatments can make it hard to control urine, leading to leakage (urinary incontinence). Over time, BPH itself can cause incontinence. Also, men treated with alpha blocker drugs, finasteride, or balloon dilation may have some risk of incontinence from BPH in the future.

Although it is rare, some men have severe uncontrollable incontinence after treatment. About 7 to 14 out of 1,000 men have this problem after TURP. Men in a program of watchful waiting have no immediate risk of uncontrollable incontinence.

The chance of needing surgery in the future differs for each treatment. Some men who at first choose watchful waiting or nonsurgical treatment may later decide to have surgery to relieve bothersome symptoms. Also, some men who have surgery may need to have surgery again. One reason is that the prostate may grow back. Another is that a scar may form and block the urinary tract.

Within 8 years after TURP, 5 to 15 out of every 100 men will need another operation. Doctors are uncertain if treatment

with alpha blocker drugs, finasteride, or balloon dilation lowers the chance that surgery will be needed in the future.

Figure 1 shows the chance of becoming impotent (not being able to get an erection) because of BPH treatment. Each year, about 2 out of every 100 men 67 years old will become impotent without BPH treatment.

Figure 1. Chance of Impotence (Loss of Erection)	
Treatment	*Risk*
Watchful waiting	Probably no added risk
Alpha blocker drugs	
Finasteride	4 out of 100 men. Impotence may end when drug is stopped.
Balloon dilation	Unknown
TURP	For most, 5-10 out of 100 men; may be higher in men with sexual problems before surgery.

There is probably no added risk of impotence with watchful waiting and alpha blocker drugs. Finasteride has a small added risk of impotence, but the problem should stop when the drug is stopped. The risk with balloon dilation is unknown, but probably low. With TURP, the risk of impotence ranges from 3 to 35 out of 100 patients. If your erections are normal before surgery, however, the risk of impotence after surgery may be no higher than with watchful waiting.

Figure 2 shows about how many days you can expect to lose from work or from what you normally do over the first year. Time at the doctor's office and in the hospital is included.

Figure 2. Loss of Work and Activity Time, First Year	
Treatment	*Days*
Watchful waiting*	1
Alpha blocker drugs*	3.5
Finasteride*	2
Balloon dilation	4
TURP	7-21
*Mainly from visits to the doctor's office.	

One other problem—retrograde ejaculation—can result. It is common with surgery and rare with alpha blocker drug treatment. Retrograde ejaculation means that during sexual climax, semen flows back into the bladder rather than out of the penis.

Men with this problem may not be able to father children. But it does not affect the ability to get an erection or have sex, and it does not cause any other problems. You may want to talk to your doctor about retrograde ejaculation.

Between 40 and 70 out of 100 patients have this problem after surgery. About 7 out of 100 patients have the problem while taking alpha blocker drugs. Retrograde ejaculation does not occur with watchful waiting or finasteride. Some men who take finasteride do notice that they make less semen.

The Balance Sheet lists the benefits and risks for each treatment. You can use this table to compare treatments. For example, treatment with either alpha blocker drugs or TURP can result in problems, but some are minor and others are serious.

Balance Sheet: Outcomes of BPH Treatments

Benefit or risk	Watchful waiting	Alpha blocker	Finasteride	Balloon dilation	TURP
Chance of symptoms improving	31-55%	59-86%	54-78%	37-76%	75-96%
Amount of symptom improvement	Unknown; probably less than other treatments	51%	31%	51%	85%
Chance of immediate harms or complications as a result of surgical treatment				2-10% (includes complications during dilation: bleeding, infection, temporary inability to urinate)	5-31% (includes complications during surgery: bleeding, infection, temporary inability to urinate)
Chance of harms or complications as a result of conservative treatment	1-5% (problems from progression of BPH)	3-43% (includes dizziness, lightheadedness, low blood pressure, and tiredness)	14-19% (mainly sexual problems)		
Chance of dying within 3 months after treatment	Probably no added risk. The chance of dying for a 67-year-old man is 8 out of 1,000 in a 3-month period.			Unknown; probably less than TURP	0.5-3.3%
Chance of uncontrollable urinary leakage as a result of treatment	0	0	0	None reported	0.7-1.4%
Chance of experiencing inability to get an erection (impotence) as a result of treatment	About 2% (1/50) of men 67 years old become impotent per year. Long-term data on alpha blockers are not available.	2.5-5.3%		Unknown but probably uncommon	3-5% (uncommon in men functioning entirely normally before surgery)
Estimated number of days lost from work or usual activities during first year of treatment	1	3.5	2	4	7.21

What is the next step?

Before choosing a treatment, ask yourself these two important questions:

1. If my BPH is not likely to cause me serious harm, do I want any treatment other than watchful waiting?
2. If I do want treatment, which is best for me based on the benefits and risks of each?

No matter what you decide, talk it over with your doctor. Take this booklet with you to your visits. Ask questions. Together, you and your doctor can choose the treatment best for you.

Learning more about BPH

Several national groups can provide more information on BPH and its treatment. They include:

Prostate Health Council
American Foundation for Urologic Disease, Inc.
300 West Pratt Street
Baltimore, MD 21201
(800) 242-2383

National Kidney and Urologic Diseases Information Clearinghouse
Box NKUDIC
Bethesda, MD 20892
(301) 468-6345

For more information

The information in this booklet was based on the *Benign Prostatic Hyperplasia: Diagnosis and Treatment. Clinical Practice Guideline.* The guideline was developed by an expert panel sponsored by the Agency for Health Care Policy and Research (AHCPR), an agency of the U.S. Public Health Service. Other guidelines on common health problems are available, and more are being developed to be released in the near future.

For more information on guidelines and to receive additional copies of this booklet, call toll free (800) 358-9295 or write to:

AHCPR Publications Clearinghouse
P.O. Box 8547
Silver Spring, MD 20907

■ **Document Source:**
U.S. Department of Health and Human Services, Public Health Service
Agency for Health Care Policy and Research
Executive Office Center, Suite 501, 2101 East Jefferson Street, Rockville, MD 20852
AHCPR Publication No. 94-0584
February 1994

URINARY INCONTINENCE IN ADULTS: A PATIENT'S GUIDE

How Your Body Makes, Stores, and Releases Urine

When you eat and drink, your body absorbs the liquid. The kidneys filter out waste products from the body fluids and make urine.

Urine travels down tubes called ureters into a muscular sac called the urinary bladder, which stores the urine.

When you are ready to go to the bathroom, your brain tells your system to relax.

Urine travels out of your bladder through a tube called the urethra. You release urine by relaxing the urethral sphincter and contracting the bladder muscles. The urethral sphincter is a group of muscles that tightens to hold urine in and loosens to let it out.

Purpose of This Booklet

Many people lose urine when they don't want to. When this happens enough to be a problem, it is called urinary incontinence.

Urinary incontinence is very common. But some people are too embarrassed to get help. The good news is that millions of men and women are being successfully treated and cured.

Reading this booklet will help you. But it is important to tell your health care provider (such as a doctor or nurse) about the problem. You may even want to bring this booklet with you to help you talk about your incontinence.

Causes of Urinary Incontinence

Urinary incontinence is not a natural part of aging. It can happen at any age, and can be caused by many physical conditions. Many causes of incontinence are temporary and can be managed with simple treatment. Some causes of temporary incontinence are:

- Urinary tract infection
- Vaginal infection or irritation
- Constipation
- Effects of medicine

Incontinence can be caused by other conditions that are not temporary. Other causes of incontinence are:

- Weakness of muscles that hold the bladder in place
- Weakness of the bladder itself
- Weakness of the urethral sphincter muscles
- Overactive bladder muscles
- Blocked urethra (can be from prostate enlargement)
- Hormone imbalance in women
- Neurologic disorders
- Immobility (not being able to move around)

In almost every case, these conditions can be treated. Your health care provider will help to find the exact cause of your incontinence.

Types of Incontinence

There are also many different types of incontinence. Some people have more than one type of incontinence. You should be able to identify the type of incontinence you have by comparing it to the list below.

Urge Incontinence

People with urge incontinence lose urine as soon as they feel a strong need to go to the bathroom. If you have urge incontinence you may leak urine:

- When you can't get to the bathroom quickly enough
- When you drink even a small amount of liquid, or when you hear or touch running water

You may also . . .
- Go to the bathroom very often; for example, every two hours during the day and night. You may even wet the bed

Stress Incontinence

People with stress incontinence lose urine when they exercise or move in a certain way. If you have stress incontinence, you may leak urine:

- When you sneeze, cough, or laugh
- When you get up from a chair or get out of bed
- When you walk or do other exercise

You may also . . .
- Go to the bathroom often during the day to avoid accidents

Overflow Incontinence

People with overflow incontinence may feel that they never completely empty their bladder. If you have overflow incontinence, you may:

- Often lose small amounts of urine during the day and night
- Get up often during the night to go to the bathroom
- Often feel as if you have to empty your bladder but can't
- Pass only a small amount of urine but feel as if your bladder is still partly full
- Spend a long time at the toilet, but produce only a weak, dribbling stream of urine

Some people with overflow incontinence do not have the feeling of fullness, but they lose urine day and night.

Finding the Cause of Urinary Incontinence

Once you tell your health care provider about the problem, finding the cause of your urinary incontinence is the next step.

Your health care provider will talk with you about your medical history and urinary habits. You probably will have a physical examination and urine tests. You may have other tests, as well. These tests will help find the exact cause of your incontinence and the best treatment for you. The table at the end of this booklet lists some of the tests you may be asked to take.

Treating Urinary Incontinence

Once the type and cause of your urinary incontinence is known, treatment can begin. Urinary incontinence is treated in one or more of three ways: behavioral techniques, medication, and surgery.

Behavioral Techniques

Behavioral techniques teach you ways to control your own bladder and sphincter muscles. They are very simple and work well for certain types of urinary incontinence. Two types of behavioral techniques are commonly used—*bladder training* and *pelvic muscle exercises.* You may also be asked to change the amount of liquid that you drink. You may be asked to drink more or less water depending on your bladder problem.

Bladder training is used for urge incontinence, and may also be used for stress incontinence. Both men and women can benefit from bladder training. People learn different ways to control the urge to urinate. Distraction (thinking about other things) is just one example. A technique called prompted voiding—urinating on a schedule—is also used. This technique has been quite successful in controlling incontinence in nursing home patients.

Pelvic muscle exercises called Kegel exercises are used for stress incontinence. The Kegel exercises help to strengthen weak muscles around the bladder.

Medication

Some people need to take medicine to treat conditions that cause urinary incontinence. The most common types of medicine treat infection, replace hormones, stop abnormal bladder muscle contractions, or tighten sphincter muscles. You will be told if you need medication and how and when to take it.

Surgery

Surgery is sometimes needed to help treat the cause of incontinence. Surgery can be used to:

♦ Return the bladder neck to its proper position in women with stress incontinence
♦ Remove tissue that is causing a blockage
♦ Replace or support severely weakened pelvic muscles
♦ Enlarge a small bladder to hold more urine

There are many different surgical procedures that may be used to treat incontinence. The type of operation you may need depends on the type and cause of your incontinence. Your doctor will discuss the specific procedure you might need.

Be sure to ask questions so that you fully understand the procedure.

Some other products can be used to help manage incontinence. These include pads and catheters. Catheters are used when a person cannot urinate. A catheter is a tube that is placed in the bladder to drain urine into a bag outside the body. The catheter usually is left inside the bladder, but some catheters are not left in. They are put in and taken out of the bladder as needed to empty it every few hours. Condom catheters (mostly used in men) attach to the outside of the body and are not placed directly in the bladder. Specially designed pads are available to help men and women with incontinence.

Catheters and pads are not the first and only treatment for incontinence. They should only be used to make other treatments more effective or when other treatments have failed.

What to Do Next

Your health care provider will tell you about the type of incontinence you have and will recommend a treatment. While you are being treated, be sure to:

♦ Ask questions
♦ Follow instructions
♦ Take all of your medicine
♦ Report side effects of your medicine, if any
♦ Report any changes, good and bad, to your health care provider

. . . and remember, incontinence is not a natural part of aging. In most cases, it can be successfully treated and reversed.

Common Tests Used to Diagnose Urinary Incontinence	
Name of test	**Purpose**
Blood tests	Examines blood for levels of various chemicals.
Cystoscopy	Looks for abnormalities in bladder and lower urinary tract. It works by inserting a small tube into the bladder * that has a telescope for the doctor to look through.
Post-void residual (PVR) measurement	Measures how much urine is left in the bladder after urinating by placing a small soft tube into the bladder or by using ultrasound (sound waves).
Stress test	Looks for urine loss when stress is put on bladder muscles usually by coughing, lifting, or exercise.
Urinalysis	Examines urine for signs of infection, blood, or other abnormality.
Urodynamic testing	Examines bladder and urethral sphincter function (may involve inserting a small tube into the bladder; x-rays also can be used to see the bladder).

* Because you may be uncomfortable during this part of the test, you may be given some medication to help relax you.

Risks and Benefits of Treatment

Three types of treatment are recommended for urinary incontinence:

- ◆ Behavioral techniques
- ◆ Medicine
- ◆ Surgery

How well each of these treatments works depends on the cause of the incontinence and, in some cases, patient effort. The risks and benefits described below are based on current medical knowledge and expert opinion. How well a treatment works may also depend on the individual patient. A treatment that works for one patient may not be as effective for another patient. Therefore, it is important to talk with a health care provider about treatment choices.

Behavioral techniques. Between 54 and 95 percent of persons using behavioral treatment show significant improvement in their incontinence. Between 12 and 16 percent of persons are cured. There are no risks for this type of treatment.

Medicine. As much as 77 percent of patients who need medicine to treat their incontinence show significant improvement, and 44 percent are cured. As with most drugs, there is a risk of having a side effect. If you are taking medicine for other conditions, the drugs could react with each other. Therefore, it is important to work with the health care provider and report all of your medicines and any side effects as soon as they happen.

Surgery. Approximately 78 to 92 percent of patients who need surgery to treat their incontinence are cured. With any surgery there is a possibility of a risk or complication. It is important to discuss these risks with your surgeon.

Coping with Incontinence

Several national organizations help people with urinary incontinence. They may be able to put you in touch with local groups that can give you more information, ideas, and emotional support in coping with urinary incontinence.

Alliance for Aging Research
(Information on bladder training program)
2021 K Street, N.W.
Suite 305
Washington, DC 20006

Help for Incontinent People
P.O. Box 544
Union, SC 29379
(803) 579-7900

Simon Foundation for Continence
Box 835
Wilmette, IL 60091
(800) 23-SIMON

For Further Information

The information in this booklet was taken from the *Clinical Practice Guideline on Urinary Incontinence in Adults*. The guideline was developed by an expert panel of doctors, nurses, other health care providers, and consumers sponsored by the Agency for Health Care Policy and Research. Other guidelines on common health problems are being developed and will be released in the near future. For more information about the guidelines or to receive additional copies of this booklet, contact:

Agency for Health Care Policy and Research
Publications Clearinghouse
Post Office Box 8547
Silver Spring, MD 20907
(800) 358-9295, (301) 495-3453

■ **Document Source:**
Department of Health and Human Services, Public Health Service
Agency for Health Care Policy and Research
Executive Office Center, 2101 East Jefferson Street, Suite 501
    Rockville, MD 20852
Publication No. AHCPR 92-0040

URINARY TRACT INFECTION IN ADULTS

Infections of the urinary tract are common—only respiratory infections occur more often. Each year, urinary tract infections (UTI's) account for about 8 million doctor visits. Women are especially prone to UTI's for reasons that are poorly understood. One woman in five develops a UTI during her lifetime.

The urinary system consists of the kidneys, ureters, bladder, and urethra. The key players in the system are the kidneys, a pair of purplish-brown organs located below the ribs toward the middle of the back. The kidneys remove liquid waste from the blood in the form of urine, keep a stable balance of salts and other substances in the blood, and produce a hormone that aids the formation of red blood cells. Narrow tubes called ureters carry urine from the kidneys to the bladder, a triangle-shaped chamber in the lower abdomen. Urine is stored in the bladder and emptied through the urethra.

The average adult passes about a quart and a half of urine each day. The amount of urine varies, depending on the fluids and foods a person consumes. The volume formed at night is about half that formed in the daytime.

Causes

Normal urine is sterile. It contains fluids, salts, and waste products, but it is free of bacteria, viruses, and fungi. An infection occurs when microorganisms, usually bacteria from the digestive tract, cling to the opening of the urethra and begin to multiply. Most infections arise from one type of bacteria, Escherichia coli (E. coli), which normally live in the colon.

In most cases, bacteria first begin growing in the urethra. An infection limited to the urethra is called urethritis. From there bacteria often move on to the bladder, causing a bladder infection (cystitis). If the infection is not treated promptly, bacteria may then go up the ureters to infect the kidneys (pyelonephritis).

Microorganisms called chlamydia and mycoplasma may also cause UTI's in both men and women, but these infections tend to remain limited to the urethra and reproductive system.

Unlike E. coli, chlamydia and mycoplasma may be sexually transmitted, and infections require treatment of both partners.

The urinary system is structured in a way that helps ward off infection. The ureters and bladder normally prevent urine from backing up toward the kidneys, and the flow of urine from the bladder helps wash bacteria out of the body. In men, the prostate gland produces secretions that slow bacterial growth. In both sexes, immune defenses also prevent infection. Despite these safeguards, though, infections still occur.

Who Is at Risk

Some people are more prone to getting a UTI than others. Any abnormality of the urinary tract that obstructs the flow of urine (a kidney stone, for example) sets the stage for an infection. An enlarged prostate gland also can slow the flow of urine, thus raising the risk of infection.

A common source of infection is catheters, or tubes, placed in the bladder. A person who cannot void, is unconscious or critically ill, often needs a catheter that stays in place for a long time. Some people, especially the elderly or those with nervous system disorders who lose bladder control, may need a catheter for life. Bacteria on the catheter can infect the bladder, so hospital staff take special care to keep the catheter sterile and remove it as soon as possible.

People with diabetes have a higher risk of a UTI because of changes of the immune system. Any disorder that suppresses the immune system raises the risk of a urinary infection.

UTI's may occur in infants who are born with abnormalities of the urinary tract, which sometimes need to be corrected with surgery. UTI's are rarely seen in boys and young men. In women, though, the rate of UTI's gradually increases with age. Scientists are not sure why women have more urinary infections than men. One factor may be that a woman's urethra is short, allowing bacteria quick access to the bladder. Also, a woman's urethral opening is near sources of bacteria from the anus and vagina. For many women, sexual intercourse seems to trigger an infection, although the reasons for this linkage are unclear.

According to several studies, women who use a diaphragm are more likely to develop a UTI than women who use other forms of birth control. Recently, researchers found that women whose partners use a condom with spermicidal foam also tend to have growth of E. coli bacteria in the vagina.

Recurrent Infections

Many women suffer from frequent UTI's. Nearly 20 percent of women who have a UTI will have another, and 30 percent of those will have yet another. Of the last group, 80 percent will have recurrences.

Usually, the latest infection stems from a strain or type of bacteria that is different from the infection before it, indicating a separate infection. (Even when several UTI's in a row are due to E. coli, slight differences in the bacteria indicate distinct infections.)

Research funded by the National Institutes of Health (NIH) suggests that one factor behind recurrent UTI's may be the ability of bacteria to attach to cells lining the urinary tract.

A recent NIH-funded study has also shown that women with recurrent UTI's tend to have certain blood types. Some scientists speculate that women with these blood types are more prone to UTI's because the cells lining the vagina and urethra may allow bacteria to attach more easily. Further research will show whether this association is sound and proves useful in identifying women at high risk for UTI's.

Infections in Pregnancy

Pregnant women seem no more prone to UTI's than other women. However, when a UTI does occur, it is more likely to travel to the kidneys. According to some reports, about 2 to 4 percent of pregnant women develop a urinary infection. Scientists think that hormonal changes and shifts in the position of the urinary tract during pregnancy make it easier for bacteria to travel up the ureters to the kidneys. For this reason, many doctors recommend periodic testing of urine.

Symptoms

Not everyone with a UTI has symptoms, but most people get at least some. These may include a frequent urge to urinate and a painful, burning feeling in the area of the bladder or urethra during urination. It is not unusual to feel bad all over—tired, shaky, washed out—and to feel pain even when not urinating. Often, women feel an uncomfortable pressure above the pubic bone, and some men experience a fullness in the rectum. It is common for a person with a urinary infection to complain that, despite the urge to urinate, only a small amount of urine is passed. The urine itself may look milky or cloudy, even reddish if blood is present. A fever may mean that the infection has reached the kidneys. Other symptoms of a kidney infection include pain in the back or side below the ribs, nausea, or vomiting.

In children, symptoms of a urinary infection may be overlooked or attributed to another disorder. A UTI should be considered when a child or infant seems irritable, is not eating normally, has an unexplained fever that does not go away, has incontinence or loose bowels, or is not thriving. The child should be seen by a doctor if there are any questions about these symptoms, especially if there is a change in the child's urinary pattern.

Diagnosis

To find out whether you have a UTI, your doctor will test a sample of urine for pus and bacteria. You will be asked to give a "clean catch" urine sample by washing the genital area and collecting a "midstream" sample of urine in a sterile container. (This method of collecting urine helps prevent bacteria around the genital area from getting into the sample and confusing the test results.) Usually, the sample is sent to a laboratory, although some doctors' offices are equipped to do the testing.

In the urinalysis test, the urine is examined for white and red blood cells and bacteria. Then the bacteria are grown in a culture and tested against different antibiotics to see which drug best destroys the bacteria. This last step is called a sensitivity test.

Some microbes, like chlamydia and mycoplasma, can only be detected with special bacterial cultures. A doctor suspects one of these infections when a person has symptoms of a UTI and pus in the urine, but a standard culture fails to grow any bacteria.

When an infection does not clear up with treatment and is traced to the same strain of bacteria, the doctor will order a test that makes images of the urinary tract. One of these tests is an intravenous pyelogram (IVP), which gives x-ray images of the bladder, kidneys, and ureters. An opaque dye visible on x-ray film is injected into a vein, and a series of x-rays are taken. The film shows an outline of the urinary tract, revealing even small changes in the structure of the tract.

If you have recurrent infections, your doctor also may recommend an ultrasound exam, which gives pictures from the echo patterns of soundwaves bounced back from internal organs. Another useful test is cystoscopy. A cystoscope is an instrument made of a hollow tube with several lenses and a light source, which allows the doctor to see inside the bladder from the urethra.

Treatment

UTI's are treated with antibacterial drugs. The choice of drug and length of treatment depends on the patient's history and the urine tests that identify the offending bacteria. The sensitivity test is especially useful in helping the doctor select the most effective drug. The drugs most often used to treat routine, uncomplicated UTI's are trimethoprim (Trimpex), trimethoprim/sufamethoxazole (Bactrim, Septra, Cotrim), amoxicillin (Amoxil, Trimox, Wymox), nitrofurantoin (Macrodantin, Furadantin), and ampicillin.

Often, a UTI can be cured with 1 or 2 days of treatment if the infection is not complicated by an obstruction or nervous system disorder. Still, many doctors ask their patients to take antibiotics for a week or two to assure that the infection has been cured. Single-dose treatment is not recommended for some groups of patients, for example, those who have delayed treatment or have signs of a kidney infection, patients with diabetes or structural abnormalities, or men who have prostate infections. Longer treatment is also needed by patients with infections caused by mycoplasma or chlamydia, which are usually treated with tetracycline, trimethoprim/sulfamethoxazole (TMP/SMZ), or doxycycline. A followup urinalysis helps to confirm that the urinary tract is infection-free. It is important to take the full course of treatment because symptoms may disappear before the infection is fully cleared.

Severely ill patients with kidney infections may be hospitalized until they can take fluids and needed drugs on their own. Kidney infections generally require several weeks of antibiotic treatment. Researchers at the University of Washington found that 2-week therapy with TMP/SMZ was as effective as 6 weeks of treatment with the same drug in women with kidney infections that did not involve an obstruction or nervous system disorder. In such cases, kidney infections rarely lead to kidney damage or kidney failure unless they go untreated.

Various drugs are available to relieve the pain of a UTI. A heating pad or a warm bath may also help. Most doctors suggest that drinking plenty of water helps cleanse the urinary tract of bacteria. For the time being, it is best to avoid coffee, alcohol, and spicy foods. (And one of the best things a smoker can do for his or her bladder is to quit smoking. Smoking is the major known cause of bladder cancer.)

Recurrent Infection in Women

About 4 out of 5 women who have a UTI get another in 18 months. Many women have them even more often. A woman who has frequent recurrences (three or more a year) should ask her doctor about one of the following treatment options:

- ◆ Take low doses of an antibiotic such as TMP/SMZ or nitrofurantoin daily for 6 months or longer. (If taken at bedtime, the drug remains in the bladder longer and may be more effective.) NIH-supported research at the University of Washington has shown this therapy to be effective without causing serious side effects.
- ◆ Take a single dose of an antibiotic after sexual intercourse.
- ◆ Take a short course (1 or 2 days) of antibiotics when symptoms appear.

Dipsticks that change color when an infection is present are now available without prescription. The strips detect nitrite, which is formed when bacteria change nitrate in the urine to nitrite. The test can detect about 90 percent of UTI's and may be useful for women who have recurrent infections.

Doctors suggest some additional steps that a woman can take on her own to avoid an infection:

- ◆ Drink plenty of water every day. Some doctors suggest drinking cranberry juice, which in large amounts inhibits the growth of some bacteria by acidifying the urine. Vitamin C (ascorbic acid) supplements have the same effect.
- ◆ Urinate when you feel the need; don't resist the urge to urinate;
- ◆ Wipe from front to back to prevent bacteria around the anus from entering the vagina or urethra;
- ◆ Take showers instead of tub baths;
- ◆ Cleanse the genital area before sexual intercourse;
- ◆ Empty the bladder shortly before and after sexual intercourse; and
- ◆ Avoid using feminine hygiene sprays and scented douches, which may irritate the urethra.

Infections in Pregnancy

A pregnant woman who develops a UTI should be treated promptly to avoid premature delivery of her baby and other risks such as high blood pressure. Some antibiotics are not safe to take during pregnancy. In selecting the best treatment, doctors consider various factors such as the drug's effectiveness, the stage of pregnancy, the mother's health, and potential effects on the fetus.

Complicated Infections

Curing infections that stem from a urinary obstruction or nervous system disorder depends on finding and correcting the underlying problem, sometimes with surgery. If the root cause goes untreated, this group of patients is at risk of kidney damage. Also, such infections tend to arise from a wider range of bacteria, and sometimes from more than one type of bacteria at a time.

UTI's are unusual in men. They usually stem from an obstruction—for example, a urinary stone or enlarged prostate—or a medical procedure involving a catheter. The first step is to identify the infecting organism and the drugs to which it is sensitive. Usually, doctors recommend lengthier therapy in men than in women, in part to prevent infection of the prostate gland. Prostate infections (prostatitis) are harder to cure because antibiotics are unable to penetrate infected prostate tissue effectively. For this reason, men with prostatitis often need long-term treatment with a carefully selected antibiotic.

Research in Urinary System Disorders

The NIH conducts and supports a variety of research in diseases of the kidney and urinary tract. The knowledge gained from these studies is advancing scientific understanding of why UTI's develop and is leading to improved methods of diagnosing, treating, and preventing infections.

The National Institute of Diabetes and Digestive and Kidney Diseases, part of the NIH, has established six research centers around the country with the goal of reducing the major causes of kidney and urinary tract diseases through innovative research. The lead researchers, their institutions, and research focus are listed on the following pages.

George M. O'Brien Kidney and Urological Research Centers

Barry M. Brenner, M.D.
Division of Nephrology
Brigham and Women's Hospital
75 Francis Street
Boston, Massachusetts 02115
(617) 732-5850
Kidney Disease of Diabetes Mellitus, Kidney Transplant Rejection

Roger C. Wiggins, M.D.
Division of Nephrology
University of Michigan
3914 Taubman Center
1500 East Medical Center Drive
Ann Arbor, Michigan 48109-0364
(313) 936-5645
Glomerulonephritis

Harry R. Jacobson, M.D.
Vanderbilt University School of Medicine
53223 Medical Center North
21st Avenue, South
Nashville, Tennessee 37232-2732
(615) 322-4794
Progressive Glomerular Sclerosis, Kidney Transplant Rejection

David G. Warnock, M.D.
Division of Nephrology
University of Alabama at Birmingham
Room 647 THT, UAB Station
Birmingham, Alabama 35294
(205) 934-3585
Effects of High Blood Pressure on the Kidney, Glomerulonephritis, Interstitial Nephritis

Ahmad Elbadawi, M.D.
SUNY Upstate Center
750 East Adams Street
Syracuse, New York 13210
(315) 464-5737
Urinary Tract Obstruction

John T. Grayhack, M.D.
Department of Urology
Northwestern University Medical School
303 East Chicago Avenue
Chicago, Illinois 60611
(312) 908-8145
Prostate Enlargement

Suggestions for Additional Reading

The following materials can be found in medical libraries, many college and university libraries, and through interlibrary loan in most public libraries.

Corriere, Joseph N. Jr. et al., "Cystitis: Evolving Standard of Care," *Patient Care*, Feb. 29, 1988, pp. 33-47.

Fowler, Jackson E. Jr., "Urinary Tract Infections in Women," *Urologic Clinics of North America*, Nov. 1986, pp. 673-683.

Gillenwater, Jay Y. et al., eds. *Adult and Pediatric Urology*, vol. 1. Chicago: Yearbook Medical Publishers, 1987.

Goldman, Peggy L. et al., "Evaluating Dysuria in the Era of STDs," *Patient Care*, January 15, 1991, pp. 51-69.

Hooton, Thomas M. et al., "Escherichia coli Bacteriuria and Contraceptive Method," *Journal of the American Medical Association*, January 2, 1991, pp. 64-69.

Krieger, John N., "Complications and Treatment of Urinary Tract Infections During Pregnancy," *Urologic Clinics of North America*, Nov. 1986, pp. 685-693.

Kunin, Calvin M. *Detection, Prevention and Management of Urinary Tract Infections*, 4th edition. Philadelphia: Lea and Febiger, 1987.

Prostate Enlargement: Benign Prostatic Hyperplasia. A patient education booklet prepared by the National Institute of Diabetes and Digestive and Kidney Diseases, NIH, 1991.

Sheinfeld, Joel et al., "Association of the Lewis Blood-Group Phenotype with Recurrent Urinary Tract Infections in Women, *New England Journal of Medicine*, March 23, 1989, pp. 773-776.

Spencer, Julia R., and Schaeffer, Anthony J., "Pediatric Urinary Tract Infections," *Urologic Clinics of North America*, Nov. 1986, pp. 661-672.

Stamm, Walter E. et al., "Acute Renal Infection in Women: Treatment with Trimethoprim-Sulfamethoxazole or Ampicillin for Two or Six Weeks: A Randomized Trial," *Annals of Internal Medicine*, March 1987, pp. 341-345.

Stapleton, Ann et al., "Postcoital Antimicrobial Prophylaxis for Recurrent Urinary Tract Infection: a randomized, double-blind, placebo-controlled trial," *Journal of the American Medical Association*, August 8, 1990, pp. 703-706.

Walsh, Patrick C. et al., eds. *Campbell's Urology*, vol 1. 5th edition. Philadelphia: W.B. Saunders, 1986.

Additional Information

The NIDDK sponsors the National Kidney and Urologic Diseases Information Clearinghouse, which collects and produces information about kidney and urinary tract disorders for health professionals and the public. For information about kidney and urinary tract disorders, contact the National Kidney and Urologic Diseases Information Clearinghouse, Box NKUDIC, 9000 Rockville Pike, Bethesda, MD 20892, telephone (301) 468-6345.

■ Document Source:
  U.S. Department of Health and Human Services, Public Health Service
  National Institutes of Health
  National Institute of Diabetes, and Digestive and Kidney Diseases
  NIH Publication No. 91-2097
  Revised September 1991

WHAT YOU NEED TO KNOW ABOUT TESTICULAR CANCER

The National Cancer Institute (NCI) has prepared this booklet to help patients and their families better understand and deal with testicular cancer. We also hope it will encourage all readers to learn more about this disease. The information presented here on the symptoms, diagnosis and treatment of testicular cancer and on living with the disease is intended to add to information from doctors, nurses, and other members of the medical team.

Throughout this booklet, words that may be new to readers are printed in *italics*. Definitions of these words and other terms related to testicular cancer are listed in the "Medical Terms" section. For some words, a "sounds-like" spelling is also given.

Research sponsored by NCI and other groups has led to better methods of diagnosing and treating this disease. Most men with testicular cancer can now be cured, and continuing research offers hope that in the future even more people with this disease will be treated successfully. Our knowledge about testicular cancer continues to increase. For up-to-date information, call the NCI-supported Cancer Information Service (CIS) at 1-800-4-CANCER (1-800-422-6237).

Other NCI publications about cancer, its treatment, and living with the disease, and the NCI-supported Cancer Information Service are also listed.

The Testicles

The testicles (also called testes or gonads) are the male sex glands. They are located behind the penis in a pouch of skin called the *scrotum*. The testicles produce and store sperm, and they are also the body's main source of male *hormones*. These hormones control the development of the reproductive organs and other male characteristics, such as body and facial hair, low voice, and wide shoulders.

What Is Cancer?

Cancer is a group of more than 100 diseases. Although each kind differs from the others in many ways, every type of cancer is a disease of some of the body's cells.

Healthy cells that make up the body's tissues grow, divide, and replace themselves in an orderly way. This process keeps the body in good repair.

Sometimes, however, some cells lose the ability to limit and direct their growth. They grow too rapidly and without any order. Too much tissue is produced, and *tumors* are formed. Tumors can be either *benign* or *malignant*.

- Benign tumors are not cancer. They do not spread to other parts of the body and are seldom a threat to life. Benign tumors can often be removed by surgery, and they are not likely to return.
- Malignant tumors are cancer. They can invade and destroy nearby healthy tissues and organs. Also, cancer cells can spread, or *metastasize*, to other parts of the body and form new tumors.

Cancer that develops in a testicle is called testicular cancer. When testicular cancer spreads, the cancer cells are carried by blood or by *lymph*, an almost colorless fluid produced by tissues all over the body. The fluid passes through *lymph nodes*, which filter out bacteria and other abnormal substances such as cancer cells. Surgeons often remove the lymph nodes deep in the abdomen to learn whether testicular cancer cells have spread.

Symptoms

Testicular cancer is one of the most common cancers in young men between the ages of 15 and 34. But the disease also occurs in other age groups, so all men should be aware of its symptoms.

Most testicular cancers are found by men themselves, by accident or when doing testicular self-examination (TSE). The testicles are smooth, oval-shaped, and rather firm. Men who examine themselves regularly become familiar with the way their testicles normally feel. Any changes in the way they feel from month to month should be reported to a doctor. (Detailed TSE instructions are on page 395.)

Testicular cancer can cause a number of symptoms. Listed below are warning signs that men should watch for:

- A lump in either testicle;
- Any enlargement of a testicle;
- A feeling of heaviness in the scrotum;
- A dull ache in the lower abdomen or the *groin;*
- A sudden collection of fluid in the scrotum;
- Pain or discomfort in a testicle or in the scrotum;
- Enlargement or tenderness of the breasts.

These symptoms are not sure signs of cancer. They can also be caused by other conditions. However, it is important to see a doctor if any of these symptoms lasts as long as 2 weeks. Any illness should be diagnosed and treated as soon as possible. Early diagnosis of testicular cancer is especially important because the sooner cancer is found and treated, the better a man's chance for complete recovery.

Diagnosing Testicular Cancer

When a man's symptoms suggest that there might be cancer in a testicle, the doctor will ask about his personal and family medical history and do a complete physical exam. In addition to checking general signs of health (temperature, pulse, blood pressure, and so on), the doctor will carefully examine the scrotum. Also, the patient will usually have a chest x-ray and blood and urine tests. If the physical exam and lab tests do not show an infection or another disorder, the doctor is likely to suspect cancer because most tumors in the testicles are cancer.

The only sure way to know whether cancer is present is for a *pathologist* to examine a sample of tissue under a microscope. To obtain the tissue, the affected testicle is removed through the groin. This operation is called *inguinal orchiectomy.* The surgeon does *not* cut through the scrotum and does *not* remove just a part of the testicle because, if the problem is cancer, cutting through the outer layer of the testicle might cause local spread of the disease.

The most common types of testicular cancer are *seminoma* and *nonseminoma.*

- Seminomas make up about 40 percent of all cases.
- Nonseminomas are actually a group of cancers. They include choriocarcinoma, embryonal carcinoma, teratoma, and yolk sac tumors.

Each of these two major types of testicular cancer grows and spreads differently—and they are treated differently.

Treating the Disease

Testicular cancer is almost always curable if it is found early. This disease responds well to treatment, even if it has spread to other parts of the body.

Staging

If a man has testicular cancer, it is important to find out the extent, or stage, of the disease (whether it has spread from the testicle to other parts of the body). *Staging* procedures include a thorough physical exam, blood tests, x-rays and scans, and, in some cases, additional surgery.

- Most patients have *computed tomography,* also called CT or CAT scan, which is a series of x-rays of various sections of the body. Some have *intravenous pyelography* (IVP), x-rays used with a special dye to outline the urinary system. Some doctors recommend *lymphangiography,* x-rays taken with a special dye that outlines the lymph system in the abdomen. *Ultrasonography,* which creates a picture from the echoes of high-frequency sound waves bounced off internal organs, also may be useful.
- Special lab tests can reveal certain substances in the blood. These substances are called *tumor markers* because they often are found in abnormal amounts in patients with some types of cancer. The levels of specific tumor markers in the blood can help the doctor determine what type of testicular cancer the patient has. (Tumor markers used to help diagnose testicular cancer are defined in the glossary.)
- Surgery may be recommended to remove the lymph nodes deep in the abdomen. A pathologist then examines the nodes to see whether they contain cancer cells. For patients with nonseminoma, removing the nodes helps stop the spread of their disease. Seminoma patients do not need this surgery because cancer cells in

their lymph nodes can be destroyed with *radiation therapy.*

Planning Treatment

Decisions about treatment for testicular cancer are complex. Sometimes it is helpful to have more than one doctor's advice. Before starting treatment, the patient might want a second opinion about the diagnosis and treatment plan. It may take a week or two to arrange to see another doctor. This short delay will not make treatment less effective. There are a number of ways to find a doctor for a second opinion:

- The patient's doctor may be able to suggest a doctor who has a special interest in testicular cancer.
- The Cancer Information Service, at 1-800-4-CANCER, can tell callers about cancer centers and other NCI-supported programs in their area.
- Patients can get the names of doctors from their local medical society, a nearby hospital, or a medical school.

Methods of Treating Testicular Cancer

Testicular cancer can be treated with surgery, radiation therapy, and *chemotherapy.* The doctor may use just one method or a combination. Often, the patient is referred to medical centers that specialize in testicular cancer treatment.

Surgery. In most cases, surgery is done to remove the testicle. Sometimes it also is necessary to remove lymph nodes in the abdomen. In addition, tumors that have spread to other parts of the body may be partly or entirely removed by surgery.

Radiation therapy. In radiation therapy (also called x-ray therapy, radiotherapy, cobalt treatment, or irradiation), high-energy rays are used to damage cancer cells and stop their growth. Like surgery, radiation therapy is a *local treatment;* it affects only the cells in the treated area. The patient usually receives radiation therapy as an outpatient.

Seminomas are highly sensitive to radiation. Following surgery, men with seminomas generally have radiation therapy to their abdominal lymph nodes.

Nonseminomas are somewhat less sensitive to radiation. Patients with this type of cancer usually have other types of treatment.

Chemotherapy. The use of drugs to treat cancer is called chemotherapy. Anticancer drugs are recommended when there are signs that the cancer has spread. Also, chemotherapy is sometimes used when the doctor suspects that undetected cancer cells remain in the body after surgery or irradiation. The use of anticancer drugs following surgery for early stage cancer is known as adjuvant therapy.

Chemotherapy may be given by mouth or by injection into a muscle or a blood vessel. Chemotherapy is a *systemic treatment*—the drugs enter the bloodstream and reach cells all over the body. Depending on the specific drugs and the patient's general condition, chemotherapy may be taken as an outpatient—at the hospital, at the doctor's office, or at home. Sometimes, however, the person must be hospitalized for a time, so the effects of the treatment can be watched.

Side Effects of Treatment

The treatments used against cancer must be very powerful. That's why patients may have some unpleasant side effects.

Many men worry that losing one testicle will affect their ability to have sexual intercourse or make them *sterile*. But a man with one healthy testicle can still have a normal erection and produce sperm. Therefore, an operation to remove just one testicle does not make a patient impotent and seldom interferes with *fertility*. Men can also have an artificial testicle, called a *prosthesis,* placed in the scrotum. The implant has the weight and feel of a normal testicle.

Surgery to remove the lymph nodes does not change a man's ability to have an erection or an orgasm, but the operation can cause sterility because it interferes with *ejaculation*. Some men recover the ability to ejaculate without treatment; others may be helped by medication. Patients should talk with the doctor about the possibility of removing the lymph nodes using a special surgical technique that may protect the ability to ejaculate.

Radiation therapy affects both normal and cancerous cells, but normal cells are able to recover. Having treatments 5 days a week for several weeks spreads out the total dose of radiation and gives the patient weekend rest breaks. Nevertheless, the body must work very hard during radiation therapy to repair the tissues injured by the treatment. Patients may feel unusually tired, and they should try to rest as much as possible. Radiation therapy does not change the ability to have sex. Radiation therapy does, however, interfere with sperm production. Usually the effect is temporary, and most patients regain their fertility within a matter of months.

Other unpleasant effects of radiation therapy include diarrhea, nausea, and vomiting. These problems can usually be controlled with medication. Also, there may be skin reactions in the area being treated, and it is important to treat the skin gently. Lotions and creams should not be used on these areas without the doctor's advice.

Chemotherapy causes side effects because it damages not only cancer cells, but other rapidly growing cells as well. Often anticancer drugs are given in cycles; treatment periods alternate with rest periods. The side effects of chemotherapy depend on the specific drugs that are given and the response of the individual patient. These drugs commonly affect hair cells, blood-forming cells, and cells that line the digestive tract. As a result, they may cause various problems, including hair loss, lowered resistance to infection, loss of appetite, nausea and vomiting, and mouth sores. Most men who receive chemotherapy for testicular cancer can continue to function sexually, although some anticancer drugs interfere with sperm production. Although this effect is permanent for some patients, many recover their fertility later on.

Loss of appetite can be a serious problem for patients receiving radiation therapy or chemotherapy. Researchers are learning that patients who eat well are better able to withstand the side effects of their treatment. Therefore, good nutrition is important. Eating well means getting enough calories to prevent weight loss and having enough protein to build and repair skin, hair, muscles, and organs. Many patients find that having several small meals and snacks throughout the day is easier than trying to eat three large meals.

The side effects of cancer therapy vary from person to person and may even be different from one treatment to the next. Patients may find that they are less interested in sexual activity if they are tired or feel ill. Doctors try to plan treatment to keep problems to a minimum, and fortunately, most side effects are temporary. Doctors, nurses, and dietitians can explain the side effects of cancer treatment and suggest ways to deal with them. Helpful information about cancer treatment and coping with side effects is given in the NCI publications *Radiation Therapy and You, Chemotherapy and You,* and *Eating Hints.*

Followup Care

Regular followup exams are very important for anyone treated for testicular cancer. The doctor will continue to watch the patient closely for several years to be sure the cancer is completely gone. If the cancer does recur, it is very important for the doctor to detect it right away and start additional treatment.

Followup care may vary for different types and stages of testicular cancer. Generally, patients are checked and have blood tests to measure tumor marker levels every month for the first 2 years after treatment. They also have regular x-rays and scans. After that, checkups may be needed just once or twice a year. Testicular cancer seldom recurs after a patient has been free of the disease for 3 years.

Patients who have been treated for cancer in one testicle have about a 1 percent chance of developing cancer in the remaining one. If cancer does arise in the second testicle, it is nearly always a new disease rather than a metastastis from the first tumor. Patients should be checked regularly by their doctor and should continue to do testicular self-examination every month. Any unusual symptoms should be reported to the doctor without delay. As with the patient's first cancer, the earlier a new tumor is detected and treated, the greater the chance of cure.

Adjusting to the Disease

When people have cancer, life can change—for them and for the people who care about them. These changes in daily life can be difficult to handle. When a man learns that he has testicular cancer, it's natural to have many different and sometimes confusing emotions.

At times, patients and family members may be frightened, angry, or depressed. Their feelings may vary from hope to despair or from courage to fear. Patients are usually better able to handle these feelings if they talk about their illness and share their feelings with family members and friends.

Concerns about the future—as well as about medical tests and treatments, hospital stays, medical bills, and sexuality—are common. Talking with doctors, nurses, or other members of the health care team may help ease fear and confusion. Patients should ask questions about their disease and its treatment and take an active part in decisions about their medical care. Patients and family members often find it helpful to write down questions as they think of them to prepare for the next visit to the doctor. Taking notes during talks with the doctor can be a useful aid to memory. Patients should ask the doctor to repeat or explain anything that is not clear.

Most people want to know what kind of cancer they have, how it can be treated, and how successful the treatment is likely to be. The following are some other questions patients might want to ask the doctor:

♦ What are the expected benefits of treatment?
♦ What are the risks and side effects of treatment?
♦ Will my sex life change?
♦ Will I be able to father children?
♦ Is it possible to keep working during treatment?
♦ Will changes in my normal daily activities be required?
♦ How often are checkups needed?

The patient's doctor is the best person to answer questions and give advice about working or other activities. If it is hard to talk with the doctor about feelings and other very personal matters, patients may find it helpful to talk with others facing similar problems. This kind of help is available through support groups, such as those described in the next section. If the patient or his family finds that emotional problems become too hard to handle, a mental health counselor may be able to help.

The public library is a good source of books and articles on living with cancer. Also, cancer patients and their families and friends can find helpful suggestions in the NCI booklets listed at the end of this booklet.

Support for Cancer Patients

Adapting to the changes that are brought about by having cancer is easier for patients and those who care about them when they have helpful information and support services. Often, the social service office at the hospital or clinic can suggest local and national agencies that will help with emotional support, financial aid, transportation, home care, or rehabilitation.

The American Cancer Society (ACS), for example, is a nonprofit organization that offers a variety of services to patients and their families. Local ACS offices are listed in the telephone directory.

Information about other programs and services for cancer patients and their families is available through the Cancer Information Service (CIS), whose toll-free telephone number is 1-800-4-CANCER.

What the Future Holds

More than 8 million Americans living today have had some type of cancer. The outlook for men with testicular cancer is excellent. Because researchers have found better ways to diagnose and treat this disease, the chance of recovering has improved dramatically. Today, a large majority of testicular cancer patients are cured by their initial treatment, and many of those who have a recurrence can be cured too.

The Promise of Cancer Research

Scientists at hospitals and medical centers throughout the United States are studying testicular cancer. They are working toward a better understanding of its causes, prevention, diagnosis, and treatment.

Cause and Prevention

Researchers study patterns of cancer in the population to discover whether some people are more likely than others to get certain cancers. If they can learn what causes the disease, they may be able to suggest ways to prevent it.

Although any man can get testicular cancer, the disease is rare. It accounts for only about 1 percent of all cancers in American men. Although most other cancers affect mostly older people, testicular cancer usually occurs in young men. It is more common in white men than in black.

We know that testicular cancer is *not* contagious. No one can "catch" it from another person. However, doctors do not know exactly what causes this disease. They can seldom explain why one person gets it while another doesn't, but research does show that some men are more likely to develop testicular cancer. For example, the risk is higher than average for boys born with their testicles in the lower abdomen rather than in the scrotum. The cancer risk for boys with this condition (called undescended testicles or *cryptorchidism*) is increased if the problem is not corrected in early childhood. Research has also shown that testicular cancer is sometimes linked to certain other rare conditions in which the testicles do not develop normally.

Some men whose mothers took a hormone called DES (diethylstilbestrol) during pregnancy to prevent miscarriage have testicular abnormalities. But scientist do not know whether prenatal exposure to DES (or any other female hormone) increases the risk of testicular cancer.

Some patients with testicular cancer have a history of injury to the scrotum. But no one knows whether such an injury can actually cause cancer. Many doctors think such an injury simply calls attention to a tumor that was already growing.

Detection and Diagnosis

Every man can help himself by doing testicular self-examination (TSE) every month, by getting regular checkups that include a testicular exam, and by seeing a doctor promptly if he notices any symptoms of testicular disease.

Researchers are looking for additional tumor markers that may be present in abnormal amounts in the blood or urine of a person with very early testicular cancer. If such markers are found, it might be possible to detect testicular cancer even before any symptoms are noticed. Several such markers have been studied, and research is continuing.

Treatment

Researchers are looking for treatment methods that are more effective and easier for patients to tolerate. They are studying new drugs and drug combinations, varied doses, and different treatment schedules.

How to Do Testicular Self-Examination (TSE)

Men can improve their chance of finding a tumor by performing a simple procedure called testicular self-examination (TSE) once a month.

TSE should be performed after a warm bath or shower. The heat relaxes the scrotum, making it easier to find anything unusual. The procedure itself is simple and takes only a few minutes:

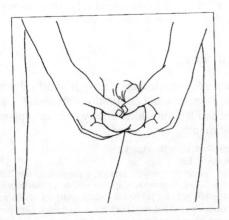

- ♦ Stand in front of a mirror. Look for any swelling on the skin of the scrotum.
- ♦ Examine each testicle with both hands. The index and middle fingers should be placed under the testicle while the thumbs are placed on the top. Gently roll the testicle between the thumbs and fingers. It's normal for one testicle to be larger than the other.

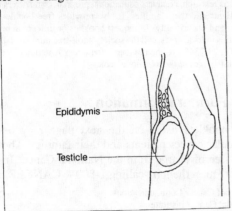

Epididymis

Testicle

- • Find the epididymis (the soft, tubelike structure at the back of the testicle that collects and carries the sperm). Do not mistake the epididymis for an abnormal lump.

If you find a lump, contact your doctor right away. Most lumps are found on the sides of the testicle, but some appear on the front. Remember that testicular cancer is highly curable, especially when treated promptly.

Testicular self-examination performed regularly is an important health habit, but it cannot substitute for a physician's examination. Your doctor should check your testicles when you have a physical exam. You also can ask your doctor to teach you how to do TSE.

When research shows that a new treatment method has promise, the method is used to treat cancer patients in *clinical trials*. These trials are designed to answer scientific questions and find out whether a new approach is both safe and effective. Patients who take part in research make an important contribution to medical science and may have the first chance to benefit from improved treatment methods.

Patients with testicular cancer are encouraged to consider participating in a trial and should discuss this option with their doctor. The NCI booklet *What Are Clinical Trials All About?* is for patients who may be interested in taking part in clinical research.

One way to learn about clinical trials is through PDQ, a computerized resource of cancer treatment information. Developed by NCI, PDQ contains an up-to-date list of trials all over the country. Doctors can obtain an access code and use a personal computer to get PDQ information, or they can use the services of a medical library. Also, the Cancer Information Service, at 1-800-4-CANCER, can provide PDQ information to doctors, patients, and the public.

There is much yet to learn about what causes testicular cancer and how it might be prevented. Our understanding is growing, and as new knowledge is gained, we hope that fewer men will develop the disease. At the same time, better methods of detection and treatment already have contributed to greatly increased survival rates for men with testicular cancer. The remarkable improvements in dealing with this disease may, in fact, lead the way in other types of cancer.

Medical Terms

Adjuvant therapy (AD-ju-vant THER-a-pee). Treatment given in addition to the primary treatment.

Androgen (AN-dro-jin). A hormone that promotes the development and maintenance of male sex characteristics.

Benign tumor (bee-NINE). A noncancerous growth that does not spread to other parts of the body.

Biopsy (BY-op-see). The removal and examination of a sample of tissue with a microscope to see whether cancer cells are present.

Cancer. A general term for more than 100 diseases in which there is an uncontrolled, abnormal growth of cells. Cancer cells can spread through the bloodstream and lymphatic system to other parts of the body.

Chemotherapy (Kee-mo-THER-a-pee). Treatment with anticancer drugs.

Clinical trial. A study conducted with cancer patients to evaluate a new treatment. Each study is designed to answer scientific questions and to find better ways to help patients.

Computed tomography (tom-OG-rah-fee). An x-ray procedure that uses a computer to produce a detailed picture of a cross-section of the body; also called CT scan or CAT scan.

Cryptorchidism (kript-OR-kid-izm). A condition in which one or both testicles fail to move from the abdomen, where they develop before birth, into the scrotum; also called undescended testicles.

Ejaculation (ee-jak-yoo-LAY-shun). The sudden, forceful discharge of semen.

Fertility (fer-TIL-i-tee). The ability to father children.

Groin. The area where the thigh joins the abdomen.

Hormones. Chemicals produced by certain glands in the body.

Impotent (IM-po-tent). Unable to have and maintain an erection.

Inguinal orchiectomy (In-gwin-al or-kee-EK-to-mee). Surgery to remove the testicle through the groin.

Intravenous pyelography (in-tra-VEE-nus py-LOG-ra-fee). X-ray study of the kidneys and urinary tract. Structures are made visible by the injection of a substance that blocks x-rays. Also called IVP.

Local treatment. Treatment that affects the tumor and the area close to it.

Lymph (limf). A nearly colorless fluid that bathes body tissues and contains cells that help the body fight infection.

Lymph nodes. Small bean-shaped structures located throughout the body along the channels of the lymphatic system: also called lymph glands. Nodes filter circulating lymph and trap bacteria or cancer cells that may travel through the lymphatic system.

Lymphangiography (limf-an-jee-OG-ra-fee). X-ray study of lymph nodes and lymph vessels made visible by the injection of a special dye.

Lymphatic system (lim-FAT-ik). The tissues and organs—including the bone marrow, spleen, thymus, and lymph nodes—that produce and store cells that fight infection and the network of channels that carry lymph.

Malignant (ma-LIG-nant). Cancerous (see *Cancer*).

Metastasize (me-TAS-ta-size). To spread from one part of the body to another. When cancer cells metastasize and cause secondary tumors, the cells in the metastatic tumor are like those in the original cancer.

Nonseminoma (non-sem-i-NO-ma). A classification of testicular cancers that arise in specialized sex cells called germ cells. Nonseminomas include embryonal carcinoma, teratoma, choriocarcinoma, and yolk sac tumor.

Oncologist (on-KOL-s-jist). A doctor who specializes in treating cancer.

Orchiectomy (or-kee-EK-to-mee). Surgery to remove a testicle.

Pathologist (path-OL-o-jist). A doctor who specializes in the diagnosis of disease by studying cells and tissues removed from the body.

Prognosis (prog-NO-sis). The probable outcome of a disease; the prospect of recovery.

Prosthesis (pros-THEE-sis). An artificial replacement for a missing body part.

Radiation therapy (ray-dee-AY-shun THER-a-pee). Treatment with high-energy radiation from x-rays or other sources of radiation.

Scrotum (SKRO-tum). The pouch of skin that contains the testicles.

Seminoma (sem-in-O-ma). A type of testicular cancer that arises from sex cells, or germ cells, at a very early stage in their development.

Staging. The process of learning whether cancer has spread from its original site to another part of the body.

Sterile. Unable to father children because of a reduced sperm count.

Systemic treatment (sis-TEM-ik). Treatment that reaches and affects cells all over the body.

Tumor. An abnormal mass of tissue.

Tumor marker. A substance detectable in the blood or urine that suggests the presence of cancer. Examples are alphafetoprotein (AFP), human chorionic gonadotropin, and lactate dehydrogenase (LDH).

Ultrasonography (UL-tra-suh-NOG-ra-fee). A diagnostic technique in which high-frequency sound waves are bounced off tissues inside the body and converts the echoes into pictures. Tissues of different densities reflect sound waves differently.

Urologist (yur-OL-o-jist). A doctor who specializes in diseases of the urinary organs in females and the urinary and sex organs in males.

X-ray. High-energy radiation used in low doses to diagnose cancer and in high doses to treat the disease.

Resources

General information about cancer is widely available. Some helpful resources and publications are listed below. Others may be available at a local library or from support groups in the community.

Cancer Information Service (CIS)
1-800-4-CANCER

The Cancer Information Service, a program of the National Cancer Institute, provides nationwide telephone service for cancer patients and their families and friends, the public, and health care professionals. The staff can answer questions and can send booklets about cancer. They also know about local resources and services. One toll-free number, 1-800-4-CANCER (1-800-422-6237), connects callers all over the country with the office that serves their area. Spanish-speaking staff members are available.

American Cancer Society (ACS)
1599 Clifton Road, N.E.
Atlanta, GA 30329
1-800-ACS-2345

The American Cancer Society is a voluntary organization with a national office (at above address) and local units all over the country. It supports research, conducts educational programs, and offers many services to patients and their families. It also provides free booklets on testicular cancer and on sexuality. To request booklets or to learn about services and activities in local areas, call the society's toll-free number, 1-800-ACS-2345 (1-800-227-2345), or the number listed under American Cancer Society in the white pages of the telephone book.

For Further Information

The booklets listed on the next page may be helpful to testicular cancer patients and their families. They are available free of charge from the National Cancer Institute. You may request them by calling 1-800-4-CANCER or writing:

Office of Cancer Communications
National Cancer Institute
Building 31, Room 10A24
Bethesda, MD 20892

Booklets About Cancer Treatment

- ♦ *Chemotherapy and You: A Guide to Self-Help During Treatment*
- ♦ *Eating Hints: Recipes and Tips for Better Nutrition During Cancer Treatment*
- ♦ *Questions and Answers About Pain Control* (also available from the American Cancer Society)
- ♦ *Radiation Therapy and You: A Guide to Self-Help During Treatment*
- ♦ *What Are Clinical Trials All About?*

Booklets About Living with Cancer

- ♦ *Taking Time: Support for People With Cancer and the People Who Care About Them*

♦ *Facing Forward: A Guide for Cancer Survivors*
♦ *When Cancer Recurs: Meeting the Challenge Again*
♦ *Advanced Cancer: Living Each Day*

■ **Document Source:**
U.S Department of Health and Human Services, Public Health Service
National Institutes of Health
National Cancer Institute

NIH Publication No. 93-1565
Revised July 1992. Printed November 1992

See also: Chemotherapy and You: A Guide to Self-Help During Treatment (page 40); Radiation Therapy and You: A Guide to Self-Help During Treatment (page 56); What Are Clinical Trials All About? A Booklet for Patients with Cancer (page 68)

WOMEN'S HEALTH

■ ■ ■

BREAST BIOPSY: WHAT YOU SHOULD KNOW

You have a lump or some other change in your breast. Most breast lumps or other changes are *not* cancer. However, to be sure, your doctor tells you that a biopsy must be done.

A biopsy is minor surgery to take out all or part of a breast lump or the tissue in question. A doctor called a pathologist looks at the biopsy tissue under a microscope to see if cancer is present. A biopsy is the only way to know for sure if a breast change is benign (not cancer) or malignant (cancer).

This booklet will give you the facts you need to make decisions about your biopsy. It contains information that can help you to:

♦ Prepare for your biopsy.
♦ Learn what happens during a biopsy.
♦ Review your treatment choices if cancer is found.
♦ Understand the terms used when talking about breast cancer.

Although this booklet has a lot of information, every woman's case is different. Be sure to ask your doctor and nurse what *your* care will involve. You also may want to share this booklet with family and friends who have questions.

Before Your Biopsy

It's important to discuss your biopsy with doctors, nurses, and other members of your health care team so that you can take an active part in your care. Talking with other women who have had a biopsy will also help you understand the procedure.

You will have many important questions, and your doctor is the best person to answer them. Most women want to know what the biopsy will be like and what will happen if they have cancer. It's often helpful to write down questions as you think of them.

To help you remember what the doctor says, you may want to take a family member or friend with you. Many women also find taking notes useful while talking with their doctor. Ask the doctor to explain anything that is not clear.

Here are some questions you may want to ask:

♦ What type of biopsy will I have?
♦ How long will the biopsy take?
♦ Will I be put to sleep?
♦ Can I eat or drink before the biopsy?
♦ Will the biopsy leave a scar?
♦ How soon will I know if I have cancer?
♦ If I do have cancer, what other tests will need to be done?
♦ What are my treatment choices if I have cancer, and how soon will treatment start?

What Happens During a Biopsy?

You have a choice between two procedures for your biopsy. The most common is the two-step procedure. For this procedure, the biopsy is done first. Then if cancer is found, treatment begins a week or two later. Some women choose a one-step procedure. When this is used, the woman is treated immediately if cancer is found. This section explains each of these procedures.

Two-Step Procedure

Most women have biopsies in the hospital outpatient or "same day surgery" department. They usually do not need to stay overnight. Your doctor or nurse will tell you if you may eat or drink before surgery. At the hospital, you will have some routine tests such as blood and urine tests, a chest x-ray, and an EKG (electrocardiogram), which records the activity of your heart. These tests tell your doctor about your general health. Sometimes these tests are done a few days before the biopsy.

You will be asked to sign a paper called an "informed consent form." It explains what the doctor is going to do and gives your permission for the procedure. If you do not understand this form, be sure to ask the doctor or nurse to explain it to you.

When it is time for the biopsy, you will be taken to the operating room. You will be given local or general anesthesia. For local anesthesia, the doctor injects some medicine in the breast so you won't feel anything as the lump is removed. For general anesthesia, you will be put to sleep for a short time while the doctor removes the suspicious tissue. The doctor often removes all of the lump or area in question (excisional biopsy). This type of biopsy usually takes about an hour.

The pathologist then checks the tissue to see if it is cancer. Using a procedure called a frozen section, the pathologist looks at thin slices of frozen tissue under a microscope. It takes just a few minutes and is a quick way of telling if cancer is present. If the lump is very small or if a more detailed study is needed, the pathologist looks at the tissue using a procedure called a permanent section. The results of this test are usually known in a few days. From the permanent section the doctor can tell the type of breast cancer and learn other information that may be needed to plan treatment.

If the biopsy shows cancer and enough tissue is available, the pathologist does more tests called hormone receptor assays. These tests tell whether the cancer needs the female hormones, estrogen and progesterone, to grow. Doctors do hormone receptor assays at the time of the biopsy because the tissue needed for these tests may be hard to get later on. This information is important to help the doctor decide how the cancer should be treated.

After the biopsy, you will be taken to your room or the outpatient care area. Most women have very little discomfort after a biopsy. If you have general anesthesia, you will probably be sleepy and want to rest. Depending on how you feel, you will be ready to go home 2 to 3 hours after the biopsy. It's best for a family member or friend to take you home. Before leaving the hospital, you will get instructions on how to take care of the incision. If you have any questions, ask your doctor or nurse.

You should be able to return to your normal routine within a day or two. However, for the next week or so your breast may be sore and slightly bruised. Also, the incision may feel firm for 3 to 4 months.

You may be told the results of your biopsy before you leave the hospital. However, the results from a permanent section will take a few days. If you have cancer, your doctor will talk with you about treatment options. Treatment for breast cancer usually begins within a couple of weeks after the biopsy. This gives you time to:

♦ Learn about treatment options and breast reconstruction.
♦ Get another medical opinion.
♦ Have tests that tell if the cancer has spread to other parts of the body.
♦ Prepare yourself emotionally.
♦ Make personal and work arrangements.

A short delay between the biopsy and treatment will not reduce the chances that your treatment will be successful.

Biopsy Methods

Your doctor can use several biopsy methods to remove tissue for the pathologist to examine. The choice depends on such things as the size and location of the lump or suspicious area and your general health. Ask your doctor which of these methods will be used for your biopsy:

♦ *Aspiration*. The use of a needle and syringe to try to drain the lump. If the lump is a cyst (a fluid-filled sac that is not cancer), removing the fluid will collapse it. No other treatment will be needed.

♦ *Fine-Needle Aspiration*. The use of a thin needle and syringe to collect cell clumps or single cells from the lump.
♦ *Needle Biopsy*. The removal of a small piece of breast tissue using a needle that has a special cutting edge; also called a core needle biopsy.

  If cancer is not found using fine-needle aspiration or needle biopsy, the doctor will most likely do an excisional or incisional biopsy. The doctor uses these tests to make sure cancer cells were not missed by the needle.

♦ *Excisional Biopsy*. The removal of all of the lump. Used most often, it is the current "standard" procedure for small (less than about an inch in diameter) lumps. Also called a lumpectomy.
♦ *Incisional Biopsy*. The removal of part of the lump. This method may be used if the breast lump is large.
♦ *Mammographic Localization With Biopsy*. Used when a breast change can be seen on a mammogram (an x-ray of the breast) but cannot be felt. In this procedure, the doctor uses the mammogram as a guide for placing small needles (needle localization) at the site of the breast change. Sometimes dye is used instead of needles to mark the site. The suspicious tissue then can be removed for examination by the pathologist.

One-Step Procedure

After talking about treatment choices with their doctor, some women choose the one-step procedure. This means they have a mastectomy immediately if their biopsy shows cancer. If you have a one-step procedure, you probably will go to the hospital the night before your biopsy. Some routine tests such as blood and urine tests, a chest x-ray, and an EKG are usually done to tell the doctor about your general health.

You also will be asked to sign a consent form that gives your doctor permission to do more surgery if the biopsy shows cancer. If you do not know what treatment is planned, be sure to ask your doctor or nurse to explain it to you. Shortly before your surgery, you will be given some medicine to help you relax. Then you will be taken to the operating room where the anesthesiologist will put you to sleep. The surgeon will remove the suspicious tissue and send it to the pathologist. The pathologist will check for cancer by looking at frozen sections of the tissue. If the tissue is not cancer, the biopsy will take about an hour. You will probably be able to go home later that same day or the next day.

If cancer is found, the doctor will remove part or all of the breast at that time. You will need to stay in the hospital for 3 to 5 days after this surgery.

Awaiting the Diagnosis

Many women who have had a breast biopsy say that bringing their suspicions of breast cancer to the doctor was one of the most difficult experiences of their lives. When you find a lump or breast change, you may find it very hard to go to your doctor. You may be afraid just waiting for your appointment. Once you go to your doctor, you will probably have to wait for test results. You also may have to wait for an appointment with another doctor for a second opinion or referral. The waiting may be hard because you don't know what you may have to cope with or how to plan for the future. These feelings are common for women facing the possibility of breast cancer.

You may not have all of these problems, and you may have your own way of coping with them. Throughout this stressful time, seek support from your friends and loved ones who can help you.

Uncertainty

Not knowing what the future holds can cause a great deal of emotional stress. This is especially true for a woman about to have a breast biopsy. You may feel better if you:

♦ Talk about your fears and concerns. It is very important for you to be open about your feelings with those people who are close to you. Openness can set the tone for continued sharing. This is a good time to talk frankly with family and friends. Don't hide your hurt or pain— share it. Don't hesitate to seek out professionals such as psychologists, social workers, or members of the clergy to help you deal with your anxiety or anger.

♦ Think through how you might deal with a diagnosis of cancer and what plans you'd make. Learn about your treatment options. Think about your needs—for example, who will care for your children or who can fill in for you at work. Find the best medical facility and kind of care that are available to you. Talk to others who have gone through similar things and learn from their experiences.

Fear of Cancer

Cancer is frightening, but it can often be treated successfully. More than 5 million Americans who have been treated for cancer are considered cured. If you need to have treatment, you may have to change your daily activities temporarily, but most cancer patients return to their usual lifestyle. Many women who have been treated for breast cancer say that they found new sources of strength within themselves to cope with the emotional demands they faced.

Fear of Loss

If you think you may have breast cancer, of course you are concerned about possibly losing a breast. You may be worried about sex and how your partner may react. If you have a mastectomy, you (and your partner) may be depressed or have other feelings similar to those associated with other losses. Coping with loss is different for each woman. However, recognizing and talking about your feelings—such as anger, frustration, sadness, and fear—can help. These feelings lessen with time. You may even find that your relationships with loved ones are stronger than before.

If You Need Treatment

Knowing about your options for breast cancer treatment will help you take an active part in your health care. You can learn more about the various treatments for breast cancer in the National Cancer Institute (NCI) booklet *Breast Cancer: Understanding Treatment Options*.

Mastectomy

Mastectomy is surgery to remove the breast. It is the most common treatment for breast cancer. There are several types of mastectomy; each removes a different amount of tissue. Most women have a **modified radical mastectomy**. During this operation, the doctor removes the breast, the lymph nodes under the arm, and the lining over the chest muscles. A pathologist checks the lymph nodes to see if they contain cancer cells. The NCI booklet *Mastectomy: A Treatment for Breast Cancer* provides more information about this treatment.

Many women who have a mastectomy choose to have breast reconstruction. For some women this can be done at the same time as the mastectomy. Some doctors prefer to wait 6 months or a year after surgery before doing reconstruction. You can decide about reconstruction months or even years after surgery. For more information about this procedure, you may want to read the NCI booklet *Breast Reconstruction: A Matter of Choice*.

Lumpectomy with Radiation Therapy

Lumpectomy followed by radiation therapy is a treatment choice for women who are diagnosed with early stage breast cancer. Research has shown that lumpectomy with radiation is as effective as mastectomy in treating early stage breast cancer.

In this procedure, the doctor removes the breast lump and, a few days later, the lymph nodes under the arm. About 2 weeks after lymph node surgery, treatment with external radiation begins and continues for 5 to 6 weeks. When these treatments end, an extra "boost" of radiation is usually given to the area where the tumor was located. You can learn more about radiation therapy in the NCI booklets *Radiation Therapy: A Treatment for Early Stage Breast Cancer* and *Radiation Therapy and You: A Guide to Self-Help During Treatment*.

Adjuvant Therapy

For women with early stage breast cancer, chemotherapy or hormone therapy should be considered after surgery and/or radiation. Called adjuvant therapy, it kills cancer cells that may still be in the body. It is used to prevent breast cancer from coming back or to delay its return. The choice between chemotherapy or hormone therapy depends on the patient's age, menopausal status, the results of the hormone receptor assays, and other factors. More information about adjuvant therapy is found in the NCI booklet *Adjuvant Therapy: Facts for Women With Breast Cancer*.

Chemotherapy

Chemotherapy is the use of anticancer drugs to kill cancer cells. To treat breast cancer, the doctor usually uses a combination of two or more drugs. Anticancer drugs may be given by mouth or injected into a muscle or vein. Chemotherapy is given in cycles: a treatment period followed by a rest period, then another series of treatments, and so on.

Hormone Therapy

Hormone therapy (also called antihormone therapy) keeps cancer cells from getting the hormones they need to grow. Drugs may be given to change the way hormones work. Or, surgery may be done to remove organs (such as the ovaries) that make hormones.

Clinical Trials

If your biopsy shows that you have breast cancer, you may want to think about entering a clinical trial. Clinical trials are carefully designed research studies to test new and promising cancer treatments. By taking part in a trial, you may be among the first patients to benefit from new treatment. Patients participate in clinical trials only if they choose to, and they are free to leave the trial at any time. Learning as much as you can about the various treatment options for breast cancer may help you decide if a clinical trial is right for you. To learn more about clinical trials, see the NCI booklet *What Are Clinical Trials All About?*

Resources for Patients and Families

General information about cancer is widely available. Some of the resources and publications listed below might be helpful to you. You may also wish to see what the local library has to offer and contact support groups in your community. You don't have to be an active member of these groups to use their information.

Cancer Information Service

The NCI-supported Cancer Information Service (CIS) is a nationwide telephone service that answers questions from cancer patients and their families, health care professionals, and the public. Information specialists can provide information and publications on all aspects of cancer. They also may know about cancer-related services in local areas.

By dialing 1-800-4-CANCER (1-800-422-6237), you will reach a CIS office serving your area. A trained staff member can answer your questions and listen to your concerns. Spanish-speaking staff members are available.

Physician Data Query

People who have cancer, those who care about them, and doctors need up-to-date and accurate information about cancer treatment. To help these people, NCI developed PDQ (Physician Data Query). This computer database gives quick and easy access to:

♦ State-of-the-art treatment information for both patients and doctors.
♦ Information about clinical trials (research studies) that are open to patients and that test new and promising cancer treatments.
♦ Names of organizations and doctors involved in caring for people with cancer.

To use PDQ, doctors may use an office computer or the services of a medical library. By calling the CIS at 1-800-4-CANCER, doctors and patients can get PDQ information and learn how to use this system.

NCI Publications

You may also want to read some NCI booklets and fact sheets that discuss various aspects of cancer, cancer treatment, and patient concerns. Available free of charge, the publications may be ordered by calling the CIS at 1-800-4-CANCER or by writing to the National Cancer Institute, Building 31, Room 10A24, Bethesda, Maryland 20892. The following booklets might be especially helpful:

♦ *Breast Exams: What You Should Know*
♦ *Questions and Answers About Breast Lumps*
♦ *What You Need to Know About Breast Cancer*
♦ *Breast Cancer: Understanding Treatment Options*
♦ *Mastectomy: A Treatment for Breast Cancer*
♦ *Radiation Therapy: A Treatment for Early Stage Breast Cancer*
♦ *Adjuvant Therapy: Facts for Women With Breast Cancer*
♦ *Breast Reconstruction: A Matter of Choice*
♦ *Taking Time: Support for People With Cancer and the People Who Care About Them*

Support Programs and Organizations

Health professionals and patients alike have learned the value of mutual support among patients. When someone who has a serious illness feels frightened or depressed, it often helps to talk about those feelings with another person who has been through the same experience. This can help patients get practical information, understand their feelings, and develop their own ways of handling their problems. Families and other people who are close to someone with a serious illness also can use this type of help.

The American Cancer Society
The American Cancer Society (ACS) is a nonprofit organization that offers a variety of services to patients and their families. Their Reach to Recovery program provides special help for breast cancer patients. Trained volunteers, who have had breast cancer themselves, visit patients at the doctor's request. These volunteers provide emotional support to women before and after treatment. They also share their experiences with breast cancer treatment, breast reconstruction, and rehabilitation. Reach to Recovery also provides family members with information to help them better understand some of the problems the patients may have. The ACS also conducts a wide variety of support groups. To find an ACS chapter near you, check your local telephone book or contact the national office at this address and telephone number:

American Cancer Society
National Headquarters
1599 Clifton Road, NE
Atlanta, GA 30329
(404) 320-3333

ENCORE
ENCORE (Encouragement, Normalcy, Counseling, Opportunity, Reaching Out, Energies Revived), sponsored by the national YWCA, is a program to help breast cancer patients after surgery. The program includes exercise to music, water exercises, and a discussion period. A woman may join a group the third week after surgery, with her doctor's permission. For more information, check with your local YWCA listed in the telephone book.

National Alliance of Breast Cancer Organizations
You may also wish to contact the National Alliance of Breast Cancer Organizations (NABCO). The NABCO is a nonprofit organization that provides breast cancer patients with information to help them make decisions

about treatment. This organization also can help you find a local support group. Contact NABCO at this address and telephone number:

National Alliance of Breast Cancer Organizations
1180 Avenue of the Americas
New York, New York 10036
(212) 719-0154

Glossary

Adjuvant therapy. Treatment given in addition to the primary treatment (surgery or radiation). For breast cancer, thermotherapy or hormone therapy is used.

Anesthesia. Loss of feeling or sensation so that the patient does not feel pain.

Anesthesiologist. A doctor who specializes in giving anesthesia.

Aspiration. Removal of fluid or tissue by suction through a needle.

Benign tumor. A growth that is not cancer; it will not spread to other parts of the body.

Biopsy. Removal of a sample of tissue that is looked at under a microscope to see if cancer cells are present.

Cancer. Term for more than 100 diseases that have uncontrolled, abnormal growth of cells. Cancer cells may invade and destroy healthy tissues and spread through the bloodstream and lymphatic system to other parts of the body.

Chemotherapy. Treatment with drugs to kill cancer cells.

Clinical trials. Studies of new medical treatments. Studies answer scientific questions and lead to better ways to treat patients.

Cyst. An abnormal sac or capsule within a tissue or an organ that is filled with fluid or semisolid substance. Cysts are not cancer.

Early stage breast cancer. Breast cancer that has not spread beyond the breast and underarm lymph nodes to other parts of the body.

Estrogen. A female hormone that some types of breast cancer cells need to grow.

External radiation. Radiation therapy that uses a machine located outside the body to aim high-energy rays at the cancer.

Frozen section. A thin slice of frozen biopsy tissue that is looked at under a microscope; a quick way to prepare biopsy tissue so that it can be examined to see if cancer is present.

Hormone receptor assays. Tests that are done on breast cancer cells to tell if they need hormones to grow and if hormone therapy would be useful.

Hormones. Chemicals produced by certain glands in the body.

Hormone therapy. Cancer treatment that blocks, removes, or adds hormones to keep cancer cells from growing; sometimes called *antihormone therapy*.

Incision. A cut into tissue made by a surgeon.

Lumpectomy. Surgery that removes only the breast lump or cancerous tissue. Lumpectomy is usually followed by removal of the underarm lymph nodes and radiation therapy.

Lymph nodes. Small, bean-shaped organs that filter harmful bacteria. Nodes are found throughout the body in places such as the neck, underarm, and groin. Also called lymph glands.

Malignant. Cancerous (see *Cancer*).

Mammogram. An x-ray of the breast. It can show cancer even before it can be felt.

Mastectomy. Surgery to remove the breast.

One-step procedure. Biopsy and surgical treatment done at the same time that cancer is found.

Pathologist. A doctor who identifies diseases by studying cells and tissues under a microscope.

Permanent section. Thin slices of biopsy tissue that are mounted on slides and looked at under a microscope. A permanent section takes several days to prepare. It tells doctors if the tissue is cancer, the type of cancer it is, and other information that helps to plan treatment.

Progesterone. A female hormone that some breast cancer cells may need to grow.

Radiation therapy. Use of high-energy rays from x-rays or other sources to kill cancer cells.

Two-step procedure. Biopsy and treatment done in two stages, usually a week or two apart.

X-ray. A type of radiation that is used at low levels to diagnose disease or in its high-energy form to treat cancer.

■ **Document Source:**
   U.S. Department of Health and Human Services, Public Health Service
   National Institutes of Health
   National Cancer Institute
   NIH Publication No. 90-657
   Revised December 1989. Printed July 1990

See also: Mastectomy: A Treatment for Breast Cancer (page 428); Radiation Therapy: A Treatment for Early Stage Breast Cancer (page 438); Radiation Therapy and You: A Guide to Self-Help During Treatment (page 56); What Are Clinical Trials All About? A Booklet for Patients with Cancer (page 68)

CancerFax from the National Cancer Institute
BREAST CANCER

Description

What Is Breast Cancer?

Breast cancer, a common cancer in women, is a disease in which cancer (malignant) cells are found in the tissues of the breast. Each breast has 15 to 20 sections called lobes, which have many smaller sections called lobules. The lobes and lobules are connected by thin tubes called ducts. The most common type of breast cancer is ductal cancer. It is found in the cells of the ducts. Cancer that begins in the lobes or lobules is called lobular carcinoma. Lobular carcinoma is more often found in both breasts than other types of breast cancer. Inflammatory breast cancer is an uncommon type of breast cancer. In this disease, the breast is warm, red, and swollen.

Like most cancers, breast cancer is best treated when it is found (diagnosed) early. You should feel your breasts each month to find any lumps or thick spots in your breasts (see the last section of this statement for more information on breast self-examination). You should see your doctor if you notice changes in your breast. Women over the age of 50 should also have a special x-ray called a mammogram, which can find tumors that are too small to feel. Check with your doctor on how often you should have this x-ray.

If you have a lump in your breast, your doctor may need to cut out a small piece and look at it under the microscope to see if there are any cancer cells. This is called a biopsy. Sometimes the biopsy is done by inserting a needle into the breast and drawing out some of the tissue. If the biopsy shows that there is cancer, it is important that certain tests (called estrogen and progesterone receptor tests) be done on the cancer cells.

Estrogen and progesterone receptor tests can tell whether hormones affect how the cancer grows. They can also give information about the chances of the tumor coming back (recurring). The results help your doctor decide whether to use hormone therapy to stop the cancer from growing. Tissue from the tumor needs to be taken to the laboratory for estrogen and progesterone tests at the time of biopsy because it may be hard to get enough cancer cells later on.

Your chance of recovery (prognosis) and choice of treatment depend on the stage of your cancer (whether it is just in the breast or has spread to other places in the body), the type of breast cancer, certain characteristics of the cancer cells, and your age, menopausal status (whether or not you still have periods), and general state of health.

Stage Explanation

Stages of Breast Cancer

Once breast cancer has been found, more tests will be done to find out if the cancer has spread from the breast to other parts of the body. This is called staging. Your doctor needs to know the stage of your disease to plan treatment. The following stages are used for breast cancer:

Breast cancer in situ
About 15-20% of breast cancers are very early cancers. They are sometimes called carcinoma in situ (found only in the duct area). Other terms for this type of breast cancer are intraductal carcinoma or ductal carcinoma in situ and lobular carcinoma in situ. Lobular carcinoma in situ is found on some occasions when a biopsy is done for another lump or abnormality found on the mammogram. It is not cancer. Patients with this condition have a 25% chance of developing breast cancer in either breast in the next 25 years.

Stage I
The cancer is no bigger than 2 centimeters (about 1 inch) and has not spread outside the breast.

Stage II
Any of the following may be true:

- The cancer is no bigger than 2 centimeters but has spread to the lymph nodes under the arm (the axillary lymph nodes).
- The cancer is between 2 and 5 centimeters (from 1 to 2 inches). The cancer may or may not have spread to the lymph nodes under the arm.
- The cancer is bigger than 5 centimeters (larger than 2 inches), but has not spread to the lymph nodes under the arm.

Stage III
Stage III is divided into stages IIIA and IIIB.

Stage IIIA is defined by either of the following:

- The cancer is smaller than 5 centimeters and has spread to the lymph nodes under the arm, which have grown into each other or into other structures and are attached to them.
- The cancer is bigger than 5 centimeters and has spread to the lymph nodes under the arm.

Stage IIIB is defined by either of the following:

- The cancer has spread to tissues near the breast (chest wall, including the ribs and the muscles in the chest).
- The cancer has spread to lymph nodes near the collarbone.

Stage IV
The cancer has spread to other organs of the body, most often the bones, lungs, liver, or brain.

Inflammatory breast cancer
Inflammatory breast cancer is a special class of breast cancer that is rare. The breast looks as if it is inflamed because of its red appearance and warmth. The skin may show signs of ridges and wheals or it may have a pitted appearance. It tends to spread quickly.

Recurrent
Recurrent disease means that the cancer has come back (recurred) after it has been treated. It may come back in the breast, in the soft tissues of the chest (the chest wall), or in another part of the body.

Treatment Options Overview

How Breast Cancer Is Treated

There are treatments for all patients with breast cancer. Four types of treatment are used:

surgery (taking out the cancer in an operation)
radiation therapy (using high-dose x-rays to kill cancer cells)
chemotherapy (using drugs to kill cancer cells)
hormone therapy (using hormones to stop the cells from growing).

Biological therapy (using your body's immune system to fight cancer) and bone marrow transplantation are being tested in clinical trials.

Surgery has a role in the treatment of most patients with breast cancer. It is used to take out the cancer from the breasts. Usually, some of the lymph nodes under the arm are also taken out and looked at under the microscope to see if there are any cancer cells.

A number of different operations are used:

- Lumpectomy (sometimes called excisional biopsy) takes out just the lump in the breast. It is usually followed by radiation therapy to the part of the breast that remains. Most doctors also take out some of the lymph nodes under the arm.
- Partial or segmental mastectomy takes out the cancer, some of the breast tissue around it, and the lining over

the chest muscle. Usually some of the lymph nodes under the arm are taken out. In most cases, radiation therapy follows.

♦ Total or simple mastectomy removes the whole breast. Sometimes lymph nodes under the arm are also taken out.

♦ Modified radical mastectomy takes the breast, some of the lymph nodes under the arm, and the lining over the chest muscles (but leaves the muscles). This is the most common operation for breast cancer.

♦ Radical mastectomy (also called the Halsted radical mastectomy) takes the breast, chest muscles, and all of the lymph nodes under the arm. This was the main operation for many years, but is used now only when the tumor has spread to the chest muscles.

If you are going to have a mastectomy, you may want to think about having breast reconstruction (making a new breast). It may be done at the time of the mastectomy or at some future time. The breast may be made with your own tissue, or by using implants. Different types of implants can be used. Recently, the Food and Drug Administration (FDA) asked that breast implants filled with silicone gel not be used until the FDA can determine their safety. However, saline-filled breast implants, which contain saltwater rather than silicone gel, may be used.

Radiation therapy uses high-energy x-rays to kill cancer cells and shrink tumors. Radiation may come from a machine outside the body (external radiation therapy) or from putting materials that produce radiation (radioisotopes) through thin plastic tubes in the area where the cancer cells are found (internal radiation therapy).

Chemotherapy uses drugs to kill cancer cells. Chemotherapy may be taken by mouth or it may be put into the body by a needle in a vein or muscle. Chemotherapy is called a systemic treatment because the drugs enter the bloodstream, travel through the body, and can kill cancer cells outside the breast area.

Hormone therapy is used to stop the hormones in the body that help cancer grow. This may be done by using drugs that change the way hormones work or by surgery that takes out organs that make hormones, such as the ovaries. Hormone therapy can act on cells all over the body and, at higher doses, may increase your chance of getting cancer of the uterus; you should report any uterine bleeding other than your menstrual period to your doctor.

If your doctor removes all the cancer that can be seen at the time of the operation, you may be given radiation therapy, chemotherapy, or hormone therapy after surgery to kill any cancer cells that are left. Therapy given after an operation when there are no cancer cells that can be seen is called adjuvant therapy.

Biological therapy tries to get your own body to fight cancer. It uses materials made by your own body or made in a laboratory to boost, direct, or restore your body's natural defenses against disease. Biological therapy is sometimes called biological response modifier (BRM) therapy or immunotherapy.

Bone marrow transplantation is a newer type of treatment. Sometimes breast cancer becomes resistant to treatment with radiation therapy or chemotherapy. Very high doses of chemotherapy may then be used to treat the cancer. Because the high doses of chemotherapy can destroy your bone marrow, marrow is taken from your bones before treatment. The marrow is then frozen and you are given high-dose chemotherapy with or without radiation therapy to treat the cancer. The marrow you had taken out is then thawed and given to you through a needle in a vein to replace the marrow that was destroyed. This type of transplant is called an autologous transplant. If the marrow you are given is taken from another person, the transplant is called an allogeneic transplant.

Treatment by Stage

Treatment for breast cancer depends on the type and stage of your disease, your age and menopausal status, and your overall health.

You may receive treatment that is considered standard based on its effectiveness in a number of patients in past studies, or you may choose to go into a clinical trial. Not all patients are cured with standard therapy and some standard treatments may have more side effects than are desired. For these reasons, clinical trials are designed to find better ways to treat cancer patients and are based on the most up-to-date information. Clinical trials are going on in most parts of the country for all stages of breast cancer. If you want more information, call the Cancer Information Service at 1-800-4-CANCER (1-800-422-6237).

Treatment options: Breast cancer in situ
Your treatment depends on whether you have ductal carcinoma in situ or lobular carcinoma in situ. Since it is difficult to distinguish between these two possibilities, it is helpful to have your biopsy preparations (slides) observed through the microscope by pathologists at a major cancer center or at the Armed Forces Institute of Pathology in Washington, DC.

If you have ductal carcinoma in situ, your treatment may be one of the following:
1. Surgery to remove the whole breast (total mastectomy).
2. Surgery to remove only the cancer (lumpectomy) followed by radiation therapy.

Rarely, some of the lymph nodes under the arm may also be removed during the above surgeries. Surgery to remove the cancer and part of the breast (partial or segmental mastectomy) without follow-up radiation is under study.

If you have lobular carcinoma in situ (LCIS), you have a marker for a higher risk of an invasive cancer in both breasts; about a 25% chancer over 25 years. Therefore, LCIS is not breast cancer. Many women with LCIS never develop breast cancer. The treatment options for LCIS are varied and quite controversial. Your treatment may be one of the following:
1. Biopsy to remove the LSIC followed by regular examinations and mammograms to make sure you don't develop invasive cancer. A large clinical trial is testing hormone therapy with the drug tamoxifen to see whether it can prevent cancer from occurring again. You can call the Cancer Information Service for more information (1-800-4-CANCER).

2. Surgery to remove one or both breasts (total mastectomy). Lymph nodes under the arm may or may not be taken out.

Treatment options: Stage I breast cancer
Your treatment may be one of the following:
1. Surgery to remove only the cancer and some surrounding breast tissue (lumpectomy) followed by radiation therapy. Some of the lymph nodes under the arm are also removed. This treatment provides identical long-term cure rates as those from mastectomy. Your doctor's recommendation on which procedure to have is based on tumor size and location and its appearance on mammogram.
2. Surgery to remove part of the breast (partial or segmental mastectomy) and some of the lymph nodes under the arm followed by radiation therapy. This treatment provides identical long-term cure rates as those from mastectomy. Your doctor's recommendation on which procedure to have is based on tumor size and location and its appearance on mammogram.
3. Surgery to remove the whole breast (total mastectomy) or the whole breast and the lining over the chest muscles (modified radical mastectomy). Some of the lymph nodes under the arm are also taken out.

Chemotherapy or hormone therapy may be given in addition to the treatments listed above. Clinical trials are testing new chemotherapy drugs, combinations of drugs, and new ways of giving chemotherapy.

Treatment options: Stage II breast cancer
Your treatment may be one of the following:
1. Surgery to remove only the cancer and some surrounding breast tissue (lumpectomy) followed by radiation therapy. Some of the lymph nodes under the arm are also removed. This treatment provides identical long-term cure rates as those from mastectomy. Your doctor's recommendation on which procedure to have is based on tumor size and location and its appearance on mammogram.
2. Surgery to remove part of the breast (partial or segmental mastectomy) and some of the lymph nodes under the arm. Radiation therapy is given following surgery. This treatment provides identical long-term cure rates as those from mastectomy. Your doctor's recommendation on which procedure to have is based on tumor size and location and its appearance on mammogram.
3. Surgery to remove the whole breast (total mastectomy) or the whole breast and the lining over the chest muscles (modified radical mastectomy). Some of the lymph nodes under the arm are also taken out.
4. Surgery to remove the whole breast, the chest muscles, and the lymph nodes under the arm (radical mastectomy). This operation is used only in special situations.

Following surgery, chemotherapy and/or hormonal therapy may be given. Clinical trials are testing new chemotherapy and hormonal drugs, new drug combinations, and new ways of giving chemotherapy. Clinical trials are also testing no chemotherapy or hormonal therapy for certain patients. In some cases, adjuvant radiation therapy may be given to the chest following mastectomy to reduce the risk of recurrence.

Treatment options: Stage III breast cancer
Stage III breast cancer is further divided into stage IIIA (can be operated on) and IIIB (cannot be operated on, and includes inflammatory breast cancer).

If you have stage IIIA cancer, your treatment may be one of the following:
1. Surgery to remove the whole breast and the lining over the chest muscles (modified radical mastectomy). Some of the lymph nodes under the arm are also taken out.
2. Surgery to remove the whole breast, the chest muscles, and the lymph nodes under the arm (radical mastectomy).

Radiation therapy is given before or after surgery. Chemotherapy with or without hormone therapy is also given following surgery. Clinical trials are testing new chemotherapy and hormonal drugs, new drug combinations, new ways of giving chemotherapy, and breast preservation. If you have stage IIIB cancer, your treatment will probably be biopsy followed by radiation therapy to the breast and the lymph nodes. A mastectomy may be done following radiation therapy. Chemotherapy or hormonal therapy may be given before or after surgery and radiation therapy. Clinical trials are testing new chemotherapy drugs and biological therapy, new drug combinations, and new ways of giving chemotherapy.

Treatment options: Stage IV breast cancer
Your treatment will probably be biopsy followed by radiation therapy or mastectomy. Hormonal therapy or chemotherapy will probably also be given. Clinical trials are testing new chemotherapy and hormonal drugs and new combinations of drugs.

Treatment options: Inflammatory breast cancer
Your treatment will probably be a combination of chemotherapy, hormonal therapy, and radiation therapy, maybe followed by surgery to remove the breast. The treatment is usually similar to that for stage IIIB or IV breast cancer.

Treatment options: Recurrent breast cancer
Breast cancer that comes back (recurs) can often be treated, but usually cannot be cured when the breast cancer recurs in another part of the body. Some patients with recurrence in the breast can be cured, however. Your choice of treatment depends on hormone receptor levels, the kind of treatment you had before, the length of time from first treatment to when the cancer came back, where the cancer recurred, whether you still have menstrual periods, and other factors.

Your treatment may be one of the following:
1. For the small group of patients whose cancer has come back only in one place, surgery and/or radiation therapy.

2. Radiation therapy to help relieve pain due to the spread of the cancer to the bones and other places.
3. Chemotherapy or hormonal therapy.
4. A clinical trial of new chemotherapy drugs, new hormonal drugs, biological therapy, or bone marrow transplantation.

To learn more about breast cancer, call the National Cancer Institute's Cancer Information Service at 1-800-4-CANCER (1-800-422-6237). By dialing this toll-free number, you can speak with someone who can answer your questions.

For more information on breast implants, you can write to the FDA at this address:

Breast Implants
Food and Drug Administration
HFE-88
Rockville, MD 20857

The FDA also has a hotline number to answer questions about silicone gel-filled breast implants. You can call 1-800-532-4440, Monday through Friday, 9 am to 7 pm Eastern standard time.

■ **Document Source:**
National Cancer Institute
Building 31, Room 10A24, 9000 Rockville Pike, Bethesda, MD 20892
PDQ 208/00013
02/01/94

See also: Breast Biopsy: What You Should Know (page 398); Breast Cancer: Understanding Treatment Options (page 406); Mastectomy: A Treatment for Breast Cancer (page 428); Radiation Therapy: A Treatment for Early Stage Breast Cancer (page 438)

BREAST CANCER: UNDERSTANDING TREATMENT OPTIONS

As recently as a decade ago, most doctors considered removal of the breast the only treatment for breast cancer. The most common procedure was a radical **mastectomy,*** the removal of the entire breast, the chest muscles under the breast, and the underarm lymph nodes. Breast cancer treatment almost always caused women serious physical and emotional trauma. Many women feared the treatment as much as the disease.

Today, radical mastectomies are rarely done. There has been much progress in the early identification and treatment of breast cancer. Beginning with the time a breast lump is found, women have a number of treatment options. As developments occur, doctors are continuing to learn about the advantages and disadvantages of these different treatments. Because of the different stages at which breast cancer is diagnosed, there is no one treatment that is best for all women.

If you discover a lump in your breast or if your doctor suspects you have breast cancer, now is the time to learn about the various treatments available, as well as their risks and benefits. This booklet will help you get started.

The options available to you will depend on a number of factors, including the type of tumor, the extent of the disease at the time of diagnosis, your age, and your medical history. But your personal feelings about the treatment, your self-image, and your lifestyle will also be important considerations in your doctor's assessment and recommendations. You and your doctor should discuss these treatment methods and how they apply to your situation.

Right now, you may be asking yourself, "Why me?" Cancer has suddenly intruded on your life and threatened your health and well-being. You don't have to lose control of your personal health, however. You can continue to take care of yourself by working in partnership with the health care professionals responsible for your treatment and safe recovery. By becoming informed, asking questions, and participating in treatment decisions, you can have a positive influence on your own well-being.

Biopsy: Learning If You Have Breast Cancer

If you have noticed a lump or other change in your breast, your doctor may recommend several tests to determine if you have cancer. After taking your medical history and performing a manual breast exam, your doctor may recommend a breast x-ray or mammogram. If the lump is suspected to be a cyst, your doctor may use a needle to drain fluid from the lump. Another test is a **biopsy**, in which tissue is removed and examined under a microscope by a pathologist. Part or all of the lump is removed under local or general **anesthesia**. Biopsy is the only certain way to diagnose breast cancer.

During the biopsy procedure, the surgeon removes the suspicious tissue and sends it to the pathology department to be analyzed. The pathologist will examine the tissue to see if it is **benign** or **malignant**. If it is malignant, the pathologist will try to identify the type of cancer cells present, how fast they reproduce, if the blood vessels or lymph system contains cancer cells, and if the cancer's growth is affected by hormones. All of this information allows your doctor to determine the best treatment for you.

There are two ways that a pathologist prepares the tissue for examination—a "frozen section," which is a quick procedure that takes about 30 minutes, and a "permanent section," which takes a day or two. The frozen section is a quick way of determining whether or not cancer is present. The permanent section is the most accurate method.

The Frozen Section

The frozen section is done while the patient is in the operating room; the surgeon does not continue the operation until the pathologist reports the results from the frozen section.

* Boldface words are defined in the glossary

In the frozen section, the pathologist cuts thin slices of tissue and fast-freezes them to be able to look quickly at the tissue. The disadvantage of the frozen section is that the freezing process distorts the cells and the method is not always accurate.

The Permanent Section

The permanent section takes longer than a frozen section—usually a day or two. In this process, the tissue is treated by a series of chemical solutions that give a high-quality slide. The advantage of this process is that it is more accurate and allows the pathologist to make a more correct diagnosis. Permanent sections are always performed, even if a frozen section is done too.

If your lump is cancer, estrogen and progesterone receptor assay tests may be performed. These tests will determine if hormone treatment may benefit you.

Other diagnostic procedures may be performed including special blood tests, additional x-rays, radioisotope scans, and/or computerized body scans.

There are two basic options for having a biopsy: the one-step and the two-step procedures.

One-Step Procedure

In this procedure, biopsy, diagnosis of cancer, and breast removal are completed in a single operation. With this procedure, you and your doctor must agree before surgery that your breast will be removed if the lump is cancerous. Your doctor will explain the full details of a mastectomy (surgical removal of the breast) before biopsy—even though the lump may not be cancerous. In the past, the one-step procedure was thought to be the best way to treat breast cancer. However, studies have shown that treatment can safely follow a biopsy by a week or two—even if the lump is cancerous.

Two-Step Procedure

This method involves biopsy on one day; then, if the lump is cancerous, the treatment takes place within a couple of weeks. In many cases, the biopsy can be done on an outpatient basis, and it may be possible to perform the biopsy under local, rather than general, anesthesia. The short time between biopsy and treatment (which will not reduce the chances for success) allows time to examine the permanent section slides, to perform additional tests to determine the extent of the disease, to discuss treatment options, to gain another medical opinion, to make home and work arrangements, and to prepare emotionally for the treatment.

If you are going to have a biopsy, discuss these procedures with your doctor. The two of you can decide which option is best for you. Additional information about biopsy can be found in *Breast Biopsy: What You Should Know*, another National Cancer Institute booklet.

Breast Surgery

Mastectomy is the medical term for surgical removal of the breast. It refers to a number of different operations, ranging from those that remove the breast, chest muscles, and under-arm **lymph nodes**, to those that remove only the breast. Other kinds of surgery remove only the breast lump.

The different types of breast surgery are described below. Based on the size and location of the lump, your doctor will recommend the type of surgery that offers you the best chance of successful treatment.

Most medical and surgical procedures carry some risk. The risk may be small or serious, frequent or rare. Because there is such a wide range of potential risks and benefits from the various treatments for the different stages and kinds of breast cancer, you should discuss with your doctor the particular benefits and risks of the treatment methods suitable for you.

Radical Mastectomy

This type of surgery removes the breast, the chest muscles, all of the underarm lymph nodes, and some additional fat and skin. It is also called a "Halsted radical" (after the surgeon who developed the procedure). A radical mastectomy was the standard treatment for breast cancer for more than 70 years and is still used today for some women.

- *Advantages*—Cancer can be completely removed if it has not spread beyond the breast or nearby tissue. Examination of the lymph nodes provides information that is important in planning future treatment.
- *Disadvantages*—Removes the entire breast and chest muscles, and leaves a long scar and a hollow chest area. May cause **lymphedema** (swelling of the arm), some loss of muscle power in the arm, restricted shoulder motion, and some numbness and discomfort. Breast reconstruction is also more difficult.

Modified Radical Mastectomy

This procedure removes the breast, the underarm lymph nodes, and the lining over the chest muscles. Sometimes the smaller of the two chest muscles is also removed. This procedure is also called "total mastectomy with axillary (or underarm) dissection" and today is the most common treatment of early stage breast cancer.

- *Advantages*—Keeps the chest muscle and the muscle strength of the arm. Swelling is less likely, and when it occurs it is milder than the swelling that can occur after a radical mastectomy. Leaves a better appearance than the radical. Survival rates are the same as for the radical mastectomy when cancer is treated in its early stages. Breast reconstruction is easier and can be planned before surgery.
- *Disadvantages*—The breast is removed. In some cases, there may be swelling of the arm because of the removal of the lymph nodes.

Total or Simple Mastectomy

This type of surgery removes only the breast. Sometimes a few of the underarm lymph nodes closest to the breast are removed to see if the cancer has spread beyond the breast. It may be followed by radiation therapy.

♦ *Advantages*—Chest muscles are not removed and arm strength is not diminished. Most or all of the underarm lymph nodes remain, so the risk of swelling of the arm is greatly reduced. Breast reconstruction is easier.

♦ *Disadvantages*—The breast is removed. If cancer has spread to the underarm lymph nodes, it may remain undiscovered.

Partial or Segmental Mastectomy

This procedure removes the tumor plus a wedge of normal tissue surrounding it, including some skin and the lining of the chest muscle below the tumor. It is followed by radiation therapy. Many surgeons also remove some or all of the underarm lymph nodes to check for possible spread of cancer.

♦ *Advantages*—If a woman is large-breasted, most of the breast is preserved. There is little possibility of loss of muscle strength or arm swelling.

♦ *Disadvantages*—If a woman has small- or medium-sized breasts, this procedure will noticeably change the breast's shape. There is a possibility of arm swelling.

Lumpectomy

Lumpectomy removes only the breast lump and is followed by radiation therapy. Many surgeons also remove and test some of the underarm lymph nodes for possible spread of cancer.

♦ *Advantages*—The breast is not removed.

♦ *Disadvantages*—Small-breasted women with large lumps may have a significant change in breast shape. Scar tissue from the treatment may make it more difficult to examine the breast later. There is a possibility of arm swelling.

For more information, contact the National Cancer Institute for a copy of *Mastectomy: A Treatment for Breast Cancer*.

A Word About Breast Reconstruction

As you consider mastectomy as a treatment option, you should be aware of breast reconstruction, a way to recreate the breast's shape after a natural breast has been removed. This procedure is gaining in popularity, although many women are still unaware of it.

Today, almost any woman who has had a mastectomy can have her breast reconstructed. Successful reconstruction is no longer hampered by radiation-damaged, thin, or tight skin, or the absence of chest muscles.

Reconstruction is not for everyone, however. And it may not be right for you. After mastectomy, many women prefer to wear artificial breast forms inside their brassieres.

Both a general surgeon and a plastic surgeon may help you decide whether to have breast reconstruction. If possible, you should discuss breast reconstruction before your surgery because the position of the incision may affect the reconstruction procedure. However, many women consider the option of reconstruction only after surgery.

For more information on breast reconstruction, contact the National Cancer Institute for a copy of *Breast Reconstruction: A Matter of Choice*.

Radiation Therapy

Radiation therapy as primary treatment is a promising technique for women who have early stage breast cancer. This procedure allows a woman to keep her breast and involves lumpectomy followed by radiation (x-ray) treatment.

Once a biopsy has been done and breast cancer has been diagnosed, radiation treatment usually involves the following steps:

♦ Surgery to remove some or all of the underarm lymph nodes to see if the cancer has spread beyond the breast;

♦ External radiation therapy to the breast and surrounding area; and

♦ "Booster" radiation therapy to the biopsy site.

For external radiation therapy, a machine beams x-rays to the breast and possibly the underarm lymph nodes. The usual schedule for radiation therapy is 5 days a week for about 5 weeks. In some instances, a "booster" or concentrated dose of radiation may be given to the area where the cancer was located. This can be done with an electron beam or internally with an implant of radioactive materials.

If you are having radiation therapy as primary treatment for early stage breast cancer, it should be done by a qualified, board-certified radiation therapist who is experienced in this form of treatment.

♦ *Advantages*—The breast is not removed. Lumpectomy with radiation therapy as a primary treatment for breast cancer currently appears to be as effective as mastectomy for treating early stage breast cancer. Because this is a new treatment procedure, researchers are continuing to collect information on long-term results. Usually there is not much deformity of surrounding tissues. This skin usually regains a normal appearance after treatment is completed.

♦ *Disadvantages*—A full course of treatment requires short daily visits to the hospital as an outpatient for about 5 weeks, as well as hospitalization for a few days if implant radiation therapy is used. Treatment may produce a skin reaction like a sunburn, and may cause tiredness. Itching or peeling of the skin may also occur. Radiation therapy can sometimes cause a temporary decrease in white blood cell count, which may increase the risk of infection.

For detailed information about radiation therapy, contact the National Cancer Institute for a copy of *Radiation Therapy: A Treatment for Early Stage Breast Cancer*.

Adjuvant Therapy

Recent studies have shown that women with early stage breast cancer may benefit from adjuvant (additional) therapy following primary treatment (mastectomy or lumpectomy with radiation therapy). These studies indicate that many breast cancer patients whose underarm lymph nodes show no sign of cancer (known as node negative) may benefit from **chemotherapy** or hormonal therapy after primary treatment. (These findings do not apply to women with preinvasive or *in situ* breast cancer.)

Until now, women whose underarm lymph nodes were free of cancer usually received no additional therapy because they have a relatively good chance of surviving the disease after primary treatment. But scientists know that cancer may return in about 30 percent of these women. Adjuvant therapy may prevent or delay the return of cancer.

Based on these findings, the National Cancer Institute has alerted doctors to consider using adjuvant therapy for their node negative breast cancer patients. Although there is strong evidence of the benefits of adjuvant therapy, there also are certain risks and expenses. Therefore, each woman should discuss her treatment options with her doctor.

The Breast Cancer Treatment Team

During your treatment you are likely to meet several health professionals who will perform the various tests and treatments your doctor recommends. It may be difficult at first to talk with them about your illness and your feelings about treatment. But each of them can offer information to help you feel more at ease. By talking with the professionals who care for you, you will come to understand more about cancer and its treatment and be better able to cope.

These are some of the specialists you may meet or hear about:

- *Anesthesiologist*—A doctor who administers drugs or gases to put you to sleep before surgery.
- *Clinical nurse specialist*—A nurse with special knowledge in a particular area, such as postoperative care or radiation therapy.
- *Medical oncologist*—A doctor who administers anti-cancer drugs or chemotherapy.
- *Pathologist*—A doctor who examines tissue removed by biopsy to see if the tissue is cancer.
- *Personal physician*—Your doctor, who will be responsible for coordinating your treatment and working with you to ensure that treatment is satisfactory. Your personal physician may be a surgeon, radiation oncologist, medical oncologist, or family physician.
- *Physical therapist*—A specialist who helps in rehabilitation after surgery by using exercise, heat, light, and massage.
- *Plastic surgeon*—A doctor who specializes in rehabilitative and cosmetic surgery. Plastic surgeons perform breast reconstruction.
- *Radiation oncologist*—A doctor who supervises radiation therapy.
- *Radiation therapy technologist*—A specially trained technician who helps the radiation oncologist give external radiation treatments.
- *Surgeon*—A doctor who performs surgery, such as biopsy and mastectomy.

Informed Consent: When Surgery is Recommended

When surgery is recommended, most health care facilities require patients to sign a form stating their willingness to permit diagnosis and medical treatment. This certifies that you understand what procedures will be done and that you have consented to have them performed.

Before consenting to any course of treatment, ask your doctor for information on:

- The recommended procedure;
- Its purpose;
- Risks and side effects associated with it;
- Likely consequences with and without treatment;
- Other available alternatives; and
- Advantages and disadvantages of one treatment over another.

You are likely to discover that your anxiety over treatment decreases as your understanding of breast cancer and its treatment increases.

Making Decisions About Treatment

Important decisions are always hard to make, particularly when they concern your health.

However, there are a number of things you can do to make decisions about breast cancer treatment easier. One is gathering information. You can:

- *Talk with your doctor*. There are a number of treatments that may be used for breast cancer. To make sure you will be comfortable with your decision to have a particular treatment, you may want to get another medical opinion.
- *Gather additional information from published reports*. Many articles and books have been written about breast cancer for patients and professionals. There is also much information available about cancer in general. Some recommended reading materials are listed at the back of this booklet. Others are available at local libraries and may be available through local offices of the American Cancer Society.
- *Call the Cancer Information Service (CIS)*. This program, sponsored by the National Cancer Institute, is available to answer questions about cancer from the public, cancer patients and their families, and health professionals. Call this toll-free number and you will automatically be connected to the CIS office serving your area: 1-800-4-CANCER. Spanish-speaking CIS staff members are also available.
- *Ask your doctor to consult PDQ*. The National Cancer Institute has developed PDQ (Physician Data Query), a computerized database designed to give doctors quick and easy access to the latest treatment information for most types of cancer; descriptions of clinical trials that are open for patient entry; and names of organizations and physicians involved in cancer care. To access PDQ, a doctor may use an office computer with a telephone hookup and a PDQ access code or the services of a

medical library with online searching capability. Cancer Information Service offices provide free PDQ searches and can tell doctors how to get regular access. Patients may ask their doctor to use PDQ or may call 1-800-4-CANCER themselves.

Some of the other things you might want to do before making a final decision about various treatments are:

♦ *Discuss them with friends or relatives*. Although you and your doctor are in the best position to evaluate treatment options, it sometimes helps to discuss your feelings with others whose judgment you respect. Often, close friends and relatives can provide insights that can help your own thinking.

♦ *Talk with other women who have had breast cancer*. Many women who have been treated for breast cancer are willing to share their experiences. Your local American Cancer Society (ACS) office may be able to direct you to such women through its Reach to Recovery program. This program, which works through volunteers who have had breast cancer, helps women meet the physical, emotional, and cosmetic needs of their disease and its treatment. Some ACS offices have volunteer visitors who have had a mastectomy, breast reconstruction, radiation, or chemotherapy. Sometimes they are able to meet with women before surgery. Contact your local ACS office for more information.

Remember that you have time to consider options. Except in rare cases, breast cancer patients do not need to be rushed to the hospital for treatment as soon as the disease is diagnosed. Most women have time to learn more about available options, make arrangements at medical facilities where treatments will be given, and organize home and work lives before beginning treatment. A long delay, however, is not advisable because it may interfere with the success of your treatment.

Glossary

Anesthesia. Loss of feeling or sensation resulting from the administration of drugs or gases.

Benign. Not cancerous.

Biopsy. Removal of a sample of tissue to see if cancer cells are present.

Chemotherapy. Treatment with drugs to destroy cancer cells. Most often used to supplement surgery or radiation therapy.

Lymph nodes. Part of the lymph system that removes wastes from body tissue and carries the fluids that help the body fight infection. Lymph nodes in the underarm are those most likely to be invaded by cancer cells and are therefore often removed during breast cancer surgery.

Lymphedema. Swelling in the patient's arm caused by excess fluid that collects when the lymph nodes and vessels are removed during surgery or damaged by x-ray. The patient's arm and hand become more prone to infection.

Malignant. Cancerous.

Mastectomy. Surgical removal of the breast.

Pectoral muscles. Muscles that overlay the chest wall and help to support the breasts.

Other NCI Breast Cancer Patient Education Booklets

For free copies of other booklets in the Breast Cancer Patient Education Series, call the Cancer Information Service or write to the Office of Cancer Communications, National Cancer Institute, Building 31, Room 10A24, Bethesda, MD 20892.

♦ *Breast Exams: What You Should Know*
♦ *Questions and Answers About Breast Lumps*
♦ *Breast Biopsy: What You Should Know*
♦ *Mastectomy: A Treatment for Breast Cancer*
♦ *Radiation Therapy: A Treatment for Early Stage Breast Cancer*
♦ *Adjuvant Therapy: Facts for Women With Breast Cancer*
♦ *Breast Reconstruction: A Matter of Choice*
♦ *After Breast Cancer: A Guide to Followup Care*
♦ *When Cancer Recurs: Meeting the Challenge Again*
♦ *Advanced Cancer: Living Each Day*

■ Document Source:
U.S. Department of Health and Human Services, Public Health Service
National Institutes of Health
National Cancer Institute
NIH Publication No. 91-2675
Revised June 1990. Printed December 1990

See also: Breast Biopsy: What You Should Know (page 398); Breast Cancer (page 402); Mastectomy: A Treatment for Breast Cancer (page 428); Radiation Therapy: A Treatment for Early Stage Breast Cancer (page 438)

CancerFax from the National Cancer Institute
CERVICAL CANCER

Description

What Is Cancer of the Cervix?

Cancer of the cervix, a common kind of cancer in women, is a disease in which cancer (malignant) cells are found in the tissues of the cervix. The cervix is the opening of the uterus (womb). The uterus is the hollow, pear-shaped organ where a baby develops. The cervix connects the uterus to the vagina (birth canal).

Cancer of the cervix usually grows slowly over a period of time. Before cancer cells are found on the cervix, the tissues of the cervix go through changes in which cells that are not normal begin to appear (known as dysplasia). A Pap smear will usually find these cells. Later, cancer cells start to grow and spread more deeply into the cervix and to surrounding areas.

Since there are usually no symptoms associated with cancer of the cervix, you must be sure your doctor does a series of tests to look for it. The first of these is a Pap smear, using a piece of cotton, a brush, or a small wooden stick to gently scrape the outside of the cervix in order to pick up cells. You may feel some pressure, but you usually do not feel pain.

If cells that are not normal are found, your doctor will need to cut a sample of tissue (called a biopsy) from the cervix and look at it under a microscope to see if there are any cancer cells. A biopsy that needs only a small amount of tissue may be done in your doctor's office. If your doctor needs to take a larger, cone-shaped piece of tissue (conization), you may need to go to the hospital.

Your prognosis (chance of recovery) and choice of treatment depend on the stage of your cancer (whether it is just in the cervix or has spread to other places) and your general state of health.

Stage Explanation

Stages of Cancer of the Cervix

Once cancer of the cervix is found (diagnosed), more tests will be done to find out if cancer cells have spread to other parts of the body (staging). Your doctor needs to know the stage of your disease to plan treatment. The following stages are used for cancer of the cervix:

Stage 0 or carcinoma in situ
Stage 0 cervical cancer is very early cancer. The cancer is found only in the first layer of cells of the lining of the cervix.

Stage I
Cancer is found throughout the cervix, but has not spread nearby.
  stage IA: a very small amount of cancer is found deeper in the tissues of the cervix
  stage IB: a larger amount of cancer is in the tissues of the cervix

Stage II
Cancer has spread to nearby areas, but is still inside the pelvic area.
  stage IIA: cancer has spread beyond the cervix to the upper two-thirds of the vagina
  stage IIB: cancer has spread to the tissue around the cervix

Stage III
Cancer has spread throughout the pelvic area. Cancer cells may have spread to the bones of the pelvis and/or gone into the lower part of the vagina. The cells also may have spread to block the tubes that connect the kidneys to the bladder (the ureters).

Stage IV
Cancer has spread to other parts of the body.
  stage IVA: cancer has spread to the bladder or rectum (organs close to the cervix)
  stage IVB: cancer has spread to faraway organs such as the lungs

Recurrent
Recurrent disease means that the cancer has come back (recurred) after it has been treated. It may come back in the cervix or in another place.

Treatment Options Overview

How Cancer of the Cervix Is Treated

There are treatments for all patients with cancer of the cervix. Three kinds of treatment are used:

surgery (taking out the cancer in an operation)
radiation therapy (using high-dose x-rays or other high-energy rays to kill cancer cells)
chemotherapy (using drugs to kill cancer cells).

Your doctor may use one of several types of surgery for very early cancer of the cervix:

♦ Cryosurgery kills the cancer by freezing it.
♦ Diathermy kills the cancer by heat from electrical or magnetic currents.
♦ Laser surgery uses a narrow beam of intense light to kill cancer cells

Your doctor may also take out the cancer using one of these operations:
♦ Conization means taking out a cone-shaped piece of tissue where the cancer is found. Conization may be used to take out a piece of tissue for biopsy, but it can also be used to treat early cancers of the cervix.
♦ Hysterectomy is an operation in which the uterus and cervix are taken out along with the cancer. If the uterus is taken out through the vagina, the operation is called a vaginal hysterectomy. If the uterus is taken out through a cut (incision) in your abdomen, the operation is called a total abdominal hysterectomy. Sometimes the ovaries and fallopian tubes are also removed, which is called a bilateral salpingo-oophorectomy.
♦ A radical hysterectomy is an operation in which the cervix, uterus, and part of the vagina are removed. Lymph nodes in the area may also be removed (this is called lymph node dissection). (Lymph nodes are small bean-shaped structures that are found throughout the body. They produce and store cells that fight infection).
♦ If the cancer has spread outside the cervix or the female organs, your doctor may take out the lower colon, rectum, or bladder (depending on where the cancer has spread) along with the cervix, uterus, and vagina. This is called an exenteration. You may need plastic surgery to make an artificial vagina after this operation.

Radiation therapy uses x-rays or other high-energy rays to kill cancer cells and shrink tumors. Radiation may come from a machine outside the body (external radiation) or from putting materials that produce radiation (radioisotopes) through thin plastic tubes in the area where the cancer cells are found (internal radiation). Radiation may be used alone or in addition to surgery.

Chemotherapy uses drugs to kill cancer cells. Chemotherapy may be taken by pill, or it may be put into the body by a needle in a vein. Chemotherapy is called a systemic treatment because the drugs enter the bloodstream, travel through the body, and can kill cancer cells outside the cervix.

Treatment by Stage

Treatments for cancer of the cervix depend on the stage of your disease, the size of your tumor, your age, your overall condition, and your desire to have children.

You may receive treatment that is considered standard based on its effectiveness in a number of patients in past studies, or you may choose to go into a clinical trial. Not all patients are cured with standard therapy and some standard treatments may have more side effects than are desired. For these reasons, clinical trials are designed to find better ways to treat cancer patients and are based on the most up-to-date information. Clinical trials are going on in most parts of the country for most stages of cancer of the cervix. If you wish to know more about clinical trials, call the Cancer Information Service at 1-800-4-CANCER (1-800-422-6237).

Treatment options: Stage 0 cervical cancer
Your treatment may be one of the following:
1. Cryosurgery.
2. Laser surgery.
3. Diathermy.
4. Conization.
5. Surgery to remove the cancer, cervix, and uterus (total abdominal or vaginal hysterectomy) for those women who cannot or no longer want to have children.

Treatment options: Stage I cervical cancer
Treatment may by one of the following:
   For stage IA cancer:
1. Surgery to remove the cancer, uterus, and cervix (total abdominal hysterectomy). The ovaries may also be taken out (bilateral salpingo-oophorectomy), but are usually not removed in younger women.
2. Internal radiation therapy.
3. Conization.

   For stage IB cancer:
1. Internal and external radiation therapy combined.
2. Surgery to remove the cancer, the uterus and cervix, ovaries, and part of the vagina (radical hysterectomy) along with the lymph nodes in the pelvic area (lymph node dissection).
3. Radical hysterectomy and lymph node dissection followed by radiation therapy.

Treatment options: Stage II cervical cancer
Your treatment may be one of the following:
   For stage IIA cancer:
1. Internal and external radiation therapy combined.
2. Surgery to remove the cancer, the uterus and cervix, ovaries, and part of the vagina (radical hysterectomy) along with the lymph nodes in the pelvic area (lymph node dissection).
3. Radiation therapy followed by surgery.
4. Clinical trials of radical hysterectomy and lymph node dissection followed by radiation therapy.

   For stage IIB cancer:
1. Internal and external radiation therapy combined.

2. Clinical trials of radiation therapy plus chemotherapy.
3. Clinical trials of surgery to determine your stage of disease with removal of lymph nodes thought to contain cancer followed by external radiation therapy.

Treatment options: Stage III cervical cancer
Your treatment may be one of the following:
1. Internal and external radiation therapy combined.
2. Radiation therapy plus chemotherapy.
3. Clinical trials of surgery to determine your stage of disease with removal of lymph nodes thought to contain cancer followed by external radiation therapy.

Treatment options: Stage IV cervical cancer
Your treatment may be one of the following:
   For stage IVA cancer:
1. Internal and external radiation therapy combined.
2. Surgery to take out the lower colon, rectum, or bladder (depending on where the cancer has spread) along with the cervix, uterus, and vagina (exenteration).
3. Radiation therapy plus chemotherapy.
4. Clinical trials of surgery to determine your stage of disease followed by external radiation therapy.

   For stage IVB cancer:
1. Radiation therapy to relieve symptoms such as pain.
2. Systemic chemotherapy.

Treatment options: Recurrent cervical cancer
If the cancer has come back (recurred) in the pelvis, your treatment may be one of the following:
1. Surgery to take out the lower colon, rectum, or bladder (depending on where the cancer has spread) along with the cervix, uterus, and vagina (exenteration).
2. Radiation therapy and chemotherapy.

If the cancer has come back outside of the pelvis, you may choose to go into a clinical trial of systemic chemotherapy. To learn more about cancer of the cervix, call the National Cancer Institute's Cancer Information Service at 1-800-4-CANCER (1-800-422-6237). By dialing this toll-free number, you can speak with someone who can answer your questions.

■ Document Source:
National Cancer Institute
Building 31, Room 10A24, 9000 Rockville Pike, Bethesda, MD 20892
PDQ 208/00103
02/01/94

See also: Chemotherapy and You: A Guide to Self-Help During Treatment (page 40); The Controversial Pap Test: It Could Save Your Life (page 417); Radiation Therapy and You: A Guide to Self-Help During Treatment (page 56)

CHOOSING A TREATMENT FOR UTERINE FIBROIDS

by Eleanor Mayfield

Uterine fibroids, one of the most common noncancerous gynecological conditions occurring in reproductive-age women, are estimated to affect more than 1 out of 5 women under 50 and account for 3 out of every 10 hysterectomies performed annually in the United States.

A fibroid, or myoma, is a noncancerous mass of muscle and connective tissue in the uterus (womb). No one knows what causes fibroids, but scientists believe their growth may be stimulated by the female sex hormone estrogen.

"A fibroid can be as small as a pinhead or as large as a watermelon," says Gene Williams, M.D., a medical officer in the obstetrics and gynecological devices branch of FDA's Center for Devices and Radiological Health. "It can cause no symptoms or a lot of symptoms. To the woman who has one, a fibroid may feel like a rock-hard bulge in the lower abdomen."

Every year, about 175,000 American women—most of them 35 to 55—undergo hysterectomy, or surgical removal of the uterus, as treatment for fibroids. According to American College of Obstetricians and Gynecologists guidelines, a fibroid that makes a woman's uterus bigger than it would be at 12 weeks of pregnancy, even if the woman is suffering no other symptoms, is an indication for a hysterectomy.

However, the practice of routinely recommending hysterectomy for fibroids has come under increasing scrutiny from both consumer organizations and doctors concerned about the high rate of hysterectomy in the United States. By age 60, more than a third of American women have had a hysterectomy, a rate higher than in any other Western country.

Blue Cross/Blue Shield of Illinois, in a study of all the hysterectomies performed in the state between 1987 and 1989, concluded that one-third were unnecessary. Most of the unnecessary surgeries, the insurer found, were performed for fibroids and other benign (noncancerous) conditions.

Fibroid Types

Fibroids are classified by their position in the uterus. Intramural fibroids, the most common type, grow inside the uterine wall. Subserous or subserosal fibroids grow outward from the uterine wall into the abdominal cavity. Submucous fibroids grow inward from the uterine wall, taking up space within the uterus itself. This type of fibroid is the most likely to cause symptoms of heavy, prolonged menstrual bleeding. A fibroid can be as big as 20 centimeters (nearly 8 inches) in diameter and can weigh more than 20 pounds.

Small fibroids usually cause few if any symptoms. But, as a fibroid grows larger, it may press on the bladder and the ureters, the pair of tubes that connect the bladder to the kidneys. Pressure on the bladder can cause urinary frequency; pressure on the ureters can lead to kidney and urinary tract infections. Fibroids can sometimes be a cause of miscarriages and infertility.

A woman with a moderate-to-large fibroid may also notice a protruding stomach and a sensation of heaviness in the abdomen. For many women, the most distressing symptom is prolonged, heavy bleeding at the time of their menstrual periods, as well as spotty vaginal bleeding outside of the normal menstrual cycle. Women who lose too much blood may become anemic.

Sometimes a fibroid develops a thin stalk "like a balloon on a string," says David Barad, M.D., head of reproductive endocrinology at New York's Montefiore Medical Center. This is called a pedunculated fibroid. In some cases, the stalk can become twisted, cutting off its own blood supply, and causing severe pain.

Fibroids tend to grow in spurts, with periods of rapid growth punctuated by periods of no or very slow growth. As a woman approaches menopause, a fibroid may begin to grow rapidly. After menopause, however, fibroids stop growing and may start to shrink.

Options Increase

New medications and less-invasive surgeries have made more treatment options available to women whose fibroids cause them problems. A number of doctors interviewed for this article say the most important consideration in treating a fibroid should be how the patient feels about her condition and what level of intervention she is comfortable with.

"The physician should look objectively at the patient's symptoms, inform her of the treatment choices, and give her the autonomy to decide what she wants to do," says Barad.

"There are probably hundreds of thousands of women who have fibroids on their uteruses that don't need to have anything done to them. At the other end of the spectrum, if a woman who has completed her family has a large fibroid that is causing distressing symptoms—like painful cramps, heavy menstrual bleeding, and anemia—she would be a candidate for hysterectomy."

In the March 1993 issue of the *American Journal of Obstetrics and Gynecology,* Andrew J. Friedman, M.D., and Susan T. Haas, M.D., of Harvard Medical School, write that the recommendation for surgery when fibroids make a woman's uterus larger than a 12-week pregnancy is based on three main concerns:

♦ Ovarian cancer might go undetected because the presence of a fibroid makes it difficult for the doctor to feel the ovaries during a pelvic examination.

♦ A rapidly growing fibroid may signal uterine cancer.

♦ A growing fibroid may produce more debilitating symptoms and add to the risks of surgery later on.

Friedman and Haas, advocating a less aggressive approach to fibroid treatment, respond to these concerns this way:

♦ The development of ultrasound (the use of high-frequency sound waves to produce an image of a part of the body) makes it possible to look at a woman's ovaries even when a fibroid prevents a manual examination. In any case, ovarian cancer is rare before age 50, and most hysterectomies for fibroids are done on women ages 35 to 44.

♦ Ultrasound and magnetic resonance imaging can be used to screen for uterine cancer, also rare in women under 50.

♦ Studies of hysterectomies done because of fibroids have not shown that removing a larger uterus poses a greater risk of surgical complications. "Watchful waiting" and treatment of problematic symptoms with medication or minimally invasive surgery may be just as effective as hysterectomy.

Exploring Drug Therapy

Many doctors prescribe drugs chemically similar to gonadotropin releasing hormone (GnRH) to treat fibroids. GnRH, produced by the pituitary gland, stimulates the production of estrogen. The drugs, known as GnRH analogs, block release of the hormone, thereby preventing the production of estrogen. These drugs, which include leuprolide (Lupron), nafarelin (Synarel), and goserelin (Zoladex), are approved by FDA to treat endometriosis in women and prostate cancer in men. Although FDA has not approved these drugs for treatment of fibroids, as with other approved medications, doctors may prescribe them if in their professional judgment a patient will benefit from them.

"Placing a woman on these drugs creates a false menopause," says Lisa Rarick, M.D., a medical officer in the division of metabolism and endocrine drug products of FDA's Center for Drug Evaluation and Research. "Her periods stop. The lack of estrogen usually causes the fibroid to shrink, just as they do after natural menopause. Sometimes other symptoms, such as pressure or pain, can be relieved by the shrinkage."

Side effects of GnRH analogs include many of the symptoms experienced by women during menopause: "hot flashes," vaginal dryness, and bone loss. Because of these side effects, the drugs are not approved for use for longer than six months. And once the medication is stopped, the fibroid usually starts to grow again.

Some gynecologists are now experimenting with combining GnRH analogs with hormone replacement therapy to "add back" lost estrogen. "This is not generally accepted clinical use as yet," says Barad. "We don't know that simply adding back estrogen will address all the safety considerations of long-term use of GnRH analogs."

Barad and others have found a useful role for GnRH analogs as preoperative therapy to shrink fibroids and stop heavy bleeding. "Both anesthesia and surgery are easier and safer if you can first make the fibroid smaller and stop the heavy bleeding so the patient isn't anemic," says Barad.

The drug danazol (Danocrine), which is chemically similar to the male sex hormone testosterone, may also be prescribed to stem heavy menstrual bleeding caused by a fibroid. Like the GnRH analogs, danazol is approved for treatment of endometriosis but not for treatment of fibroids. Its main side effect is to increase male characteristics, such as facial hair and deepening of the voice; however, not all patients experience this side effect.

New Surgical Techniques

The development of endoscopes, lasers, and electrosurgical devices has led to new, less-invasive surgical techniques to remove fibroids. An endoscope is a thin fiberoptic tube that surgeons insert into the body. It can transmit an image to a television-like screen. Specialized endoscopes for viewing the abdominal cavity are called laparoscopes. Endoscopes designed to view the inside of the uterus are known as hysteroscopes. A laser is a device that uses a thin, intense light beam to "cut" or vaporize tissue, while electrosurgery or electrocautery devices use electricity to destroy tissue by applying heat.

One Woman's Decision

In 1983, Diane Trent (not her real name), 42, began experiencing pain on the left side of her abdomen during her monthly period. Then she began to have extremely heavy periods lasting as long as two weeks. She went to see her gynecologist, who performed a pelvic examination and told her she had a fibroid in her uterus. The doctor recommended a hysterectomy.

Trent requested an ultrasound examination, which showed that the fibroid was about 7 centimeters (2-3/4 inches) in diameter. She decided she only wanted to undergo a hysterectomy as a last resort and asked her doctor if there was a less drastic option.

In response, the gynecologist performed an endometrial biopsy, which showed no cancer, and a dilation and curettage (D&C), a procedure that involves dilating the cervix (neck of the womb) and scraping the uterine lining. The D&C stemmed Trent's heavy bleeding for a while. But after a few months the problem recurred. At times, she says, the bleeding "was so disabling that I couldn't go to work." Because the fibroid was pressing on her bladder, she had to urinate frequently.

Many women in Trent's situation would have opted for a hysterectomy. Instead, Trent consulted a reproductive endocrinologist, who agreed to monitor the fibroid's growth.

After three years, it had grown to 10 centimeters (4 inches) in diameter—about the size of a grapefruit. Her new doctor now recommended a hysterectomy.

"My feeling was that this was not life threatening and I didn't know what the long-term outcome of surgery would be," Trent says. "I decided I would rather put up with some discomfort that I knew would go away eventually." So she found another specialist who was willing to continue monitoring the fibroid.

The mass did not enlarge during the next five to six years. Trent is now 52. Since she reached menopause about two years ago, the fibroid has shrunk slightly. She continues to have an ultrasound examination every year. Her doctor says the fibroid should keep shrinking slowly, but it will never disappear completely.

Lisa Rarick, M.D., a medical officer in FDA's Center for Drug Evaluation and Research, says Trent's experience illustrates that the "best" treatment for a fibroid may be what the patient is most comfortable with.

"The issue is whether you can live with the symptoms. It's very individual. It depends how uncomfortable you are and how you feel about having surgery."

E.M.

These devices can be combined in several ways to perform a variety of procedures. Some devices combine the visualization and surgical functions in one instrument, such as the hysteroscopic resectoscope, which consists of a hysteroscope with an electrosurgery device built into it. This device is often used to remove submucous fibroids, the type most likely to cause symptoms of heavy menstrual bleeding.

The most appropriate procedure for each patient will depend on factors such as the size and position of the fibroid, the severity of symptoms, and future child-bearing plans. Hysterectomy, by removing the uterus, makes it impossible to become pregnant or carry a baby.

Endometrial ablation, in which an electrosurgical device is used to remove the lining of the womb, may be recommended if a woman's major fibroid-related symptom is heavy, debilitating menstrual bleeding. This procedure also makes pregnancy impossible.

Myomectomy, or surgical removal of a fibroid leaving the uterus in place, may be an alternative to hysterectomy, particularly for women who still want to have children. In determining whether to recommend a myomectomy, a doctor will take into consideration the woman's overall health as well as the number and location of the fibroids, says Grant Bagley, M.D., of FDA's Office of Health Affairs.

"A myomectomy can be a very simple procedure or it can be very complicated," says Bagley. "A thorough discussion is needed with each patient as to whether their particular case will be difficult."

According to Barad of Montefiore, myomectomies can result in higher than average blood loss and scarring of the uterus that can adversely affect a woman's chances of becoming pregnant. "The operation you are performing to preserve reproductive potential may actually have the opposite effect." However, Bagley says newer techniques can be used to limit blood loss and preserve fertility.

If the fibroid is approachable from inside the uterus, a myomectomy may be performed using a hysteroscope. This procedure may be done in a physician's office if the fibroids are small. In some cases, patients can resume normal work and leisure activities within about a week.

A woman who has discomfort and heavy menstrual bleeding caused by a large fibroid, and who does not want to become pregnant, may opt to have a hysterectomy. A traditional abdominal hysterectomy is major surgery, requiring a four to five-day hospital stay and a recuperation period of about six weeks.

Women with relatively smaller fibroids may be able to have a vaginal hysterectomy instead. In this procedure, the uterus is removed through the vagina, thereby avoiding a large abdominal incision. Some doctors will prescribe GnRH analogs for several months before surgery to try to shrink the woman's uterus so that a vaginal hysterectomy can be performed instead of an abdominal one. In some cases, a vaginal hysterectomy is done with the assistance of a laparoscope. Most patients will have a shorter hospital stay and recovery period for a vaginal hysterectomy than for an abdominal procedure.

Physicians differ in their approach to the treatment of fibroids, Rarick points out. "Some will only do hysterectomies. Others will do everything they can to preserve the uterus."

And Williams advises: "Patients need to ask questions and be aware of all their options."

Eleanor Mayfield is a writer in Silver Spring, Md.

■ **Document Source:**
U.S. Department of Health and Human Services, Public Health Service
Food and Drug Administration
FDA Consumer
November 1993

See also: Ovarian Epithelial Cancer (page 436); What You Need to Know About Cancer of the Uterus (page 470)

CONTROLLING 'YEAST' INFECTIONS

by Amy Roffmann New

Intense itching is usually the hallmark of a vaginal yeast infection. Once a woman has experienced it, she's not likely to forget it.

Nearly 75 percent of all women will have at least one such infection in their lifetime. Many are plagued by recurring yeast infection, which are most frequent between the ages of 16 and 35.

Yeast is a term for single-celled fungi. The technical name for the variety of fungus often present in the human body is candida, and the technical name for infections caused by these fungi is candidiasis. Such infections occur not only in the vagina, but also in other parts of the body in both sexes.

In December 1990, the Food and Drug Administration approved the over-the-counter (nonprescription) sale of the first of several products for treating vaginal yeast infections in women previously diagnosed by their doctors as having them.

A woman who has had one vaginal yeast infection can usually recognize its symptoms if it recurs. And a woman who has had several infections has no doubt about what's wrong when the next yeast infection starts.

There are several symptoms, but, according to Michael Spence, M.D., director of the Public Health and Preventive Medicine Program at Hahnemann University in Philadelphia, "If a woman does not itch, it's unlikely that she has a yeast infection."

Another symptom is a thick, mostly odorless discharge. But this can be misleading because, according to Spence, "Discharge in and of itself is not diagnostic. If you have a white discharge with an intense irritating itch, you may have an infection. Unfortunately, many women will, in response to increased estrogen at mid-cycle and the increased production of cervical mucus, develop a white, curdy discharge. That is not a yeast infection."

While not all women experience the following symptoms of a vaginal yeast infection, it's possible to have: vaginal soreness or irritation, a rash on the vulva around the vagina, pain or discomfort during intercourse, abdominal pain, soreness of the vulva or vagina, burning during urination, and even vaginal bleeding in some cases in addition to itching and discharge.

> Women who get vaginal yeast infections may want to limit their use of pantyhose and other tight garb, and instead wear loose, natural-fiber clothing.

Causes of Yeast Infection

Candidiasis is caused by one of four varieties of candida: *Candida albicans, Candida glabrata, Candida tropicalis,* and *Candida krusei.* By far the most common—causing nearly 80 percent of vaginal yeast infections—is *Candida albicans.*

Most people have these organisms in the genital or intestinal tract to some degree at various times. It's the overgrowth of the fungus that causes problems.

According to Spence, there are a number of causes of the uncontrolled growth, usually related to some type of immune suppression. Sometimes there's been a significant change in diet. Other times it's due to use of antibiotics to treat another infection, such as strep throat or acne.

Broad-spectrum antibiotics such as penicillin or tetracycline can kill or suppress helpful bacteria in the genital tract, allowing yeast to grow unchecked, according to Philip Mead, M.D., Professor of Obstetrics and Gynecology at the University of Vermont College of Medicine.

It's even possible that an underlying disorder, like diabetes, is the root cause of the infection. "Whenever you see a fungal infection in a woman, these are the things that come immediately to mind," says Spence.

When physicians see recurrent yeast infections without another cause, they have to wonder about HIV disease. Because HIV (the virus that leads to AIDS) involves a lowering of the immune system, it could significantly impair a woman's ability to combat yeast, says Spence.

"Yeast infections can be passed back and forth between partners in unprotected intercourse, but because yeast is frequently present anyway, a sexual partner is more likely to pick up the infection if his or her immune system is also depressed," says Mead.

Immunity can become depressed by a number of factors besides HIV infection. Illness or infection of any kind weakens the immune system. Physical or mental stress can also wreak havoc, leaving the immune system less able to combat yeast infections. Lack of sleep, poor nutrition, and taking any medication, including birth control pills, can upset the body's balance, allowing yeast to thrive. Pregnant women also have a tendency to have more yeast infections, as the immune system becomes temporarily altered by hormonal surges.

Diagnosis

Diagnosing vaginal yeast infections can be tricky, especially at first. Several other disorders, including inflammation of the cervix or sexually transmitted diseases such as trichomoniasis (a parasitic infection) or herpes, can have similar symptoms.

According to Mead, clinical diagnosis of yeast infections starts with a slide of vaginal secretions examined under the microscope. "Those slides [can be] very specific. If you see the yeast organisms, you can assume that's the diagnosis."

(Slides are actually examined for a particular stage of the fungus form called mycelia. While yeast is a commonly present form of fungus, mycelia is the variation of the fungus type that can grow out of control and cause infection problems.)

It's possible to have a yeast infection that doesn't show up in the limited examination of a single slide smear. Mead says that if a woman has a negative slide smear, but still has significant symptoms, her physician is likely to order a culture.

For example, there is one variety of candida—*Candida glabrata*—that causes symptoms but does not characteristically show up under the microscope. For that, a culture may be necessary. "A culture is more sensitive," says Mead. "It should pick up virtually anything."

While studies have shown that women are able to correctly identify recurring vaginal yeast infections most of the time, there is still some concern about misdiagnosing and mistreating other problems that may mimic symptoms. Through package and product labeling of products sold without prescription, FDA and pharmaceutical companies are working to make sure that women with an infection that differs even slightly from the symptoms of a previous yeast infection return to their doctors.

OTC Availability—With Warnings

Until 1990, drugs to treat vaginal yeast infections were available only by prescription. In December 1990, after receiving the advice of a number of experts, FDA gave Schering-Plough Health Care the go-ahead to market and sell over-the-counter its antifungal medication Gyne-Lotrimin, a brand name for clotrimazole. It has been joined by several other products that are either clotrimazole or another antifungal, miconazole nitrate. (The first miconazole nitrate drug to be allowed to be sold OTC for vaginal yeast infections was Advanced Care Products' Monistat 7.)

Both clotrimazole and miconazole nitrate are from the same antifungal drug family and work very similarly by breaking down the cell wall of the yeast organism, causing it to dissolve completely.

The products are supplied in one of two ways: as vaginal inserts or suppositories or as a cream with a special applicator. Both formulations are for use at bedtime every night for seven nights.

While most women note improvement within just a few days, it's important to finish the seven-day treatment to make sure all of the troublemaking fungus has been disabled. Women who don't see rapid improvement of their symptoms are likely to have a problem other than a vaginal yeast infection.

"The benefit [of OTC sale of these products] is that they are readily available for women to purchase without having to go to a physician," says Joseph Winfield, M.D., a medical officer in FDA's anti-infective drugs division. Ready availability of OTC treatments means that women no longer have to suffer while waiting for an appointment, or rearrange work and family life to find time to go to the doctor's office for a recurrent infection.

"Vaginal candidiasis is a rather common occurrence," says Winfield. "It doesn't present any life-threatening condition to the individual [with an infection] and it's okay to treat over the counter—but only for women [who] have had an infection diagnosed by a physician previously. As those same symptoms recur, they should be able to treat themselves."

In October 1992, FDA required additions to printed information accompanying OTC products for vaginal yeast infections. One significant addition to the patient package insert was a notice that recurrent vaginal yeast infections, especially those that do not clear up easily with proper treatment, may also be the result of serious medical conditions, including HIV infection. The labeling also says: *If you experience vaginal yeast infections frequently (they recur within a two-month period) or if you have vaginal yeast infections that do not clear up easily with proper treatment, you should see your doctor promptly to determine the cause and to receive proper medical care.*

"While it is true that women who are HIV-infected are much more likely to have chronic vaginal yeast infections." says Mead. "most women with recurrent vaginal yeast infections aren't HIV-positive [HIV-infected]."

Other Yeast Infections

Even though vaginal yeast infections are the most common type of candida infections, there are other ways in which yeast can cause problems.

Thrush is the name given to an oral yeast infection. It is most often seen in infants or in people with severely suppressed immune systems—as in AIDS. Its symptoms are painful sores in the mouth and throat that appear as creamy white patches and reveal red sores when scraped. Left untreated, thrush may spread to the throat and esophagus. (Other infections can cause similar symptoms, so anyone with these symptoms should have their condition accurately diagnosed by a health professional.)

Other candida infections can occur nearly anywhere on the body where there is a skin fold: under the arms, under the breasts, between the toes. The skin around the fingernails can be affected.

Candida infections have been reported in women who wear artificial fingernails. Fungal infections can start in the space between the artificial and natural nail if they become separated. The nails may become discolored by infection and may require drug treatment.

The drugs used to treat these other candida infections are similar, but not always identical to those used for vaginal yeast infections. Most of the treatments are from the "azole" drug family (clotrimazole, fluconazole). Some drugs are oral medications, although those are most often used only for stubborn or persistent infections. A fairly new drug (approved by FDA in January 1990), fluconazole is effective in a single dose by tablet or intravenous injection, but is most often used only in serious fungal infections, such as those in persons with HIV disease.

It's important to note that over-the-counter products for vaginal yeast infections are not appropriate for other types of fungal infections. Those products are only for the uses stated on the package. For any other yeast infection, see your doctor.

A.R.N.

In addition to the HIV notice, the following warnings also appear on information accompanying the products:

♦ Do not use if you have abdominal pain, fever, or foul-smelling vaginal discharge. You may have a condition that is more serious than a yeast infection. Contact your doctor immediately.

♦ Do not use if this is your first experience with vaginal itch and discomfort. See your doctor.

♦ If there is no improvement within three days, you may have a condition other than a yeast infection. Stop using this product and see your doctor.

♦ If symptoms recur within a two-month period, contact your doctor.

♦ Do not use during pregnancy except under the advice and supervision of a doctor.

♦ This medication is for vaginal yeast infections only. It is not for use in the mouth or the eyes. If accidentally swallowed, seek professional assistance or contact a Poison Control Center immediately.

♦ Keep this and all other drugs out of the reach of children. This product is not to be used in children less than 12 years of age.

Prevention

In general, candida likes warm, moist places. It's not possible to prevent every yeast infection, but a few simple steps can help reduce the number of infections women get.

Wear loose, natural-fiber clothing and underwear with a cotton crotch. As much as possible, avoid pantyhose, tights or leggings, nylon underwear, and tight jeans. Limit the use of deodorant tampons and feminine hygiene products if you feel an infection beginning, as they can interfere with the helpful bacteria in the vagina. Keep genitals dry after bathing or swimming (don't stay in a wet swimsuit for hours).

Seasonal changes can affect the likelihood of getting an infection, too. During high-heat, high-humidity periods, it's easier to get a yeast infection. Heavy winter clothing, which prevents easy release of perspiration and moisture, can also spell trouble.

Amy Roffmann New is a writer in Chandler, Ariz.

■ Document Source:
U.S. Department of Health and Human Services, Public Health Service
Food and Drug Administration
FDA Consumer
December 1993

A Reprint from FDA Consumer Magazine

THE CONTROVERSIAL PAP TEST: IT COULD SAVE YOUR LIFE

---

by Ellen Hale

Sixty-five years ago, George Papanicolaou, M.D., observed that cervical cancer could be detected by studying cells taken from a woman's genital tract. His finding was put to use 25 years later with the development of the Pap test, named after him.

In the decades since then, the Pap test has become a routine part of gynecologic examinations and one of the most widely used procedures for detecting cancer. The American Cancer Society credits the Pap smear—so called because cells are "smeared" on a glass slide—and regular gynecologic check-ups with cutting deaths from cervical cancer by 70 percent over the last 40 years. Although 6,000 women will die from it this year, four decades ago cervical cancer claimed the lives of 20,000 American women annually. For years, Pap test results have reassured millions of women that they are either free of cervical cancer or it has been detected at an early stage, with a high probability of cure.

Recently, though, the Pap test has been surrounded by controversy. Reports suggest that 10 to 40 percent of cervical cancers or the cell abnormalities that precede them may be missed because of sloppy laboratory work or poor tissue sampling. The reports have prompted medical organizations and the federal government to investigate quality control in Pap testing and propose stricter standards to ensure more reliable test results for cervical cancer and other diseases and conditions.

Meanwhile, researchers are trying to devise more accurate ways to detect the early signs of cervical cancer and to zero in on who is at risk for it. At the same time, health and medical groups once at odds over guidelines for cervical cancer screening have joined forces to develop unified recommendations for how often women should have a Pap test.

The Best Screening Tool for Cancer

"For all the problems that have come to the forefront, the Pap smear is still by far the best screening tool we have for any cancer," says William Creasman, M.D., professor and head of the Department of Obstetrics and Gynecology at the University of South Carolina and head of the cancer screening task force of the American College of Obstetricians and Gynecologists.

The American Cancer Society estimates that in 1989, 47,000 American women will be diagnosed with uterine cancer. Of these, 13,000 will be found to have cancer of the cervix—the neck of the uterus, which opens into the vagina. The remaining 34,000 women will be diagnosed with cancer of the body of the uterus or of the endometrium, its lining.

Cervical cancer develops slowly over years, and when caught early is very curable. In the very earliest stages of cervical cancer, cells on the surface of the cervix change in structure—a condition known as dysplasia. Dysplasia is most often treated by cryosurgery (freezing) or laser therapy. In some cases, however, effective treatment calls for surgical excision of the lesion or hysterectomy—surgical removal of the entire uterus.

In the next step, abnormal cells develop into a localized cancer ("carcinoma *in situ*"). Carcinoma *in situ* is virtually 100 percent curable by surgery—either conization, in which a cone of tissue surrounding the cancer is removed, or a total hysterectomy. The choice of procedure often depends on whether the woman wants to have children. For patients diagnosed early but with more invasive cancer, the survival rate is from 80 to 90 percent, and treatment involves radiation, hysterectomy or both. The five-year survival rate for all cervical cancer patients is 66 percent, according to the American Cancer Society, which implies that some cases are not being found and treated early.

Properly done, the Pap test is highly effective in detecting abnormal cervical cells before they become cancerous. (It is only about 50 percent effective in detecting endometrial cancer. Because endometrial cancer afflicts mostly middle-aged or older women, the American Cancer Society recommends that women at risk of this disease have tissue samples taken (curretage) at menopause. Their risk factors include infertility, obesity, failure to ovulate, and prolonged estrogen therapy.)

A Labor-Intensive Test

The accuracy of the Pap test depends on meticulous care in each of its steps, from cell collection, preparation, and staining on the slide to the interpretation of each specimen.

The test is a "uniquely labor intensive complex process" compared with other medical and laboratory tests, and its outcome "depends entirely on human judgment," states Leonard G. Koss, M.D., pathologist at the Albert Einstein College of Medicine, the Bronx, N.Y., in a recent issue of the *Journal of the American Medical Association*. Improperly done, the value of the test is "seriously compromised," notes the American Medical Association in a recent report on quality control in Pap testing.

The Pap smear is a seemingly easy procedure. A hollow tube-like instrument called a speculum is inserted into the vagina to spread the walls and expose the cervix. Then a cotton-tipped swab, wooden spatula, or cervical brush is used to collect cells from the opening of the cervix and its inner and outer surfaces. The cells are quickly pressed on a glass slide and "fixed" to prevent them from drying and changing appearance.

The doctor or nurse must take important information about the patient, such as age and obstetric and gynecologic history, which is forwarded along with the slide to the testing laboratory. There the sample is examined under a microscope by specially trained technologists who search for abnormalities among the 50,000 to 300,000 cells on each slide. Any suspicious slides are sent on to a pathologist.

In the past, Pap smear diagnoses were often reported as a class number, one through five. In 1988, a workshop sponsored by the National Cancer Institute developed a new format called the "Bethesda System," which uses descriptive terms for reporting Pap smear results. Cytopathology laboratories are encouraged to use such descriptive diagnoses in order to improve communication with the physician and patient.

Koss estimates that from 10 to 20 percent of Pap smears are inadequate from the first step. "It is generally assumed that obtaining a cervical smear is an easily executed, clinically simple procedure," says Koss. "This is not true."

Some practitioners don't do it properly—either not collecting enough cells, collecting them from the wrong place, or fixing them improperly on the slide—and so a flawed sample is sent for screening. And some laboratories, perhaps fearful of losing the physician's business, do not reject poor samples, according to Creasman.

Screening of the samples may be inadequate, too. In November 1987, the *Wall Street Journal* reported that some so-called "Pap mills" around the country screen smears much too quickly and in haphazard ways that may fail to reveal abnormalities. The *Journal's* report set off congressional and professional reviews of the quality control of medical testing and prompted legislation to tighten regulations of laboratories that do Pap screening.

Koss estimates that each smear requires at least five minutes of study. The American Society of Cytotechnology suggests that no technologist screen more than 12,000 cases annually—or 50 to 100 slides a day. (A case may consist of one or two slides.) Yet, the *Wall Street Journal* reported laboratories in which individual workers screened as many as 35,000 slides in a single year.

New Quality Control Regulations

The American College of Obstetricians and Gynecologists believes that up to 40 percent of Pap smears may fail to disclose cancer or the cellular abnormalities that can lead to it. As many as half of those errors may result from inadequate sampling; the rest are apparently caused by shortcomings in the laboratories.

Currently, the federal Centers for Disease Control requires that cytology laboratories engaged in interstate commerce (and thus subject to federal regulation) must rescreen 10 percent of negative Pap smears as a means of quality control. New York state licenses laboratories only after a mandatory examination of the cytotechnologists. A California law forbids that state's cytotechnologists from screening more than 75 slides a day.

And Congress last year amended the 20-year-old Clinical Laboratory Improvement Act to require quality standards for the estimated 12,000 labs receiving Medicare and Medicaid funding or engaging in interstate commerce. Congress also ordered the Health Care Financing Administration (HCFA) to regulate doctors' office laboratories that examine Pap smears.

In effect, HCFA officials say, the new rules will cover nearly all commercial laboratories and should go a long way toward improving cervical cancer detection. Among the requirements: proficiency testing for examiners and laboratories and a ceiling on the number of slides to be screened by each technician.

Out of the controversy comes hope for greater survival. Increased attention to quality control, a new consensus on Pap test guidelines, and research on who is at risk and how testing can be improved could eventually lower deaths from cervical cancer still further. "We certainly could knock the incidence of invasive disease down to a greater degree," says Creasman. "But we'll never get rid of it entirely because some women won't get Pap smears or won't get them done when they should."

Who Should Be Tested—How Often?

For years, women and their doctors have been confused about how often Pap testing should be done because health organi-

zations made different recommendations. Last year, seven medical, professional and scientific organizations announced new uniform guidelines for Pap testing.

The organizations, including the American Cancer Society and the American College of Obstetricians and Gynecologists (ACOG), determined that all women who are or have been sexually active or are over 18 should have an annual Pap test and pelvic examination. After three consecutive normal results, they said, the test could be done less often—if the woman and her doctor agree. However, the groups advised that all women at high risk for cervical cancer should have annual Pap tests.

If possible, the best time to have a Pap smear taken is 10 to 14 days after the first day of the last menstrual period. Women should avoid using vaginal douches or lubricants for 48 hours before the examination.

U.S. Cervical Cancer Mortality Rate 1950-1985 (Per 100,000 women)							
1950	1955	1960	1965	1970	1975	1980	1985
9.9	9.3	8.1	6.9	5.1	3.9	3.1	2.7

Rates age-adjusted to 1970
Document Source: Surveillance, Epidemiology and End Results Program, National Cancer Institute.

Who Is at High Risk?

Studies show that women who become sexually active early in their teen years, who have multiple sex partners, who have their first child before the age of 20, and who have many pregnancies are at higher than average risk. Also at higher risk are women whose sex partners have other partners.

The risk of cervical cancer is much lower in women in monogamous relationships, and studies indicate that the disease occurs much less often in celibate women. But recent studies show that half of all married women and from 70 to 80 percent of married men have had multiple sex partners. About half of all teenagers have had more than one sexual partner by the time they reach 16, according to ACOG. In effect, then, the consortium of medical groups recommends that nearly all women who are sexually active have annual Pap tests regardless of age, according to Creasman.

"If a woman is in any of these high-risk groups she should have annual Pap tests and cervical exams," says George Morley, M.D., the president of ACOG. "To do any less is to play Russian roulette with her life. The annual Pap test will be her early warning system to protect her health and perhaps her life."

Women whose mothers took the hormone diethylstilbestrol (DES) during pregnancy are at a higher risk of a rare form of vaginal cancer, which may be detected by a Pap test. Prescribed in the late 1940s and 1950s to prevent miscarriage, DES is no longer given for that purpose.

Some specialists estimate that most women who develop cervical cancer are infected with HPV. The incidence of HPV-caused genital warts has been increasing dramatically the last few years, suggesting an eventual increase in cervical cancer. Although a link between cervical cancer and herpes virus type 2 has also been suggested, it is far less certain than that between HPV and the disease.

In a study reported earlier this year in the *Journal of the American Medical Association,* University of Utah scientists noted another possible risk factor for cervical cancer: passive or active smoking. The researchers found that women who don't smoke but who are exposed to cigarette smoke for three hours or more a day were nearly three times more likely to get the disease. Women who smoke are more than three times as likely to get the disease. The Utah study has not yet been duplicated.

In the past, some doctors have suggested that women over 60 or 65 need not get Pap tests, but the new guidelines have no such cutoff. After three years of negative tests, older women, like younger ones, should discuss with their doctors how often they should have a Pap test.

Creasman also recommends that women who have had hysterectomies for treatment of a malignant cervical lesion should have an annual Pap test to make sure that the tumor has not recurred. If the hysterectomy was for a benign lesion, the risk is much lower and testing can be done every two to three years, he says.

Most important, say experts, is that every woman should discuss her risks with her physician and the two of them then should decide how often she should be tested.

Where goes that smear?

Until better tests for cervical cancer come along and new federal guidelines controlling quality of laboratory testing are in place, William Creasman, M.D., head of the cancer screening task force for the American College of Obstetricians and Gynecologists, says women should question their physicians closely about Pap testing. He recommends the following:

♦ Ask where your specimen will be sent. Is the laboratory certified by a professional organization like the College of American Pathologists? If the lab does testing for Medicare- or Medicaid-funded patients, chances are it is accredited.

♦ Is the lab near your doctor? A doctor and laboratory that are close geographically are probably more likely to communicate. Also, if a lab is far away, it suggests that specimens are being sent that far to save money—not a good practice when your life is at stake.

The most important thing to remember, say experts, is that cervical cancer is one of the most curable of all cancers because the cellular changes that lead to it are slow to develop and can be detected by a Pap test.

E.H.

Pap Test Saves Lives

Some instances of precancerous cell changes are missed in Pap tests because changes in the cells are too slight for technologists to detect. Several companies are now working on tests that detect the human papilloma virus in cervical tissue before precancerous lesions develop. The first such test, called Virapap, was approved by the Food and Drug Administration in January 1989 for use in high-risk women as an adjunct to the Pap smear.

Efforts are also under way to find better ways of reading the Pap smear. One technique involves using a computerized microscope to measure dye absorbed by cells—a potential clue to cancer or the cellular changes that precede it.

Still, Creasman believes there is nothing on the immediate horizon that will replace the Pap test. "We've been waiting for years to get a computer to do it . . . and we're still waiting."

Says ACOG President Morley: "Our main defense against death from the disease is prevention. We can prevent death through early detection. We detect the disease through regular pelvic examinations and Pap tests. The earlier we detect it, the greater the chances for cure."

It may not be perfect, but the Pap test saves lives.

Ellen Hale is a free-lance writer in Washington, D.C.

■ Document Source:
U.S. Department of Health and Human Services, Public Health Service
Food and Drug Administration
Office of Public Affairs, 5600 Fishers Lane, Rockville, MD 20857
DHHS Publication No. (FDA) 90-1159
Reprinted September 1989

See also: Cervical Cancer (page xxx)

CancerFax from the National Cancer Institute

ENDOMETRIAL CANCER

Description

What Is Cancer of the Endometrium?

Cancer of the endometrium, a common kind of cancer in women, is a disease in which cancer (malignant) cells are found in the lining of the uterus (endometrium). The uterus is the hollow, pear-shaped organ where a baby grows. Cancer of the endometrium is different from cancer of the muscle of the uterus, which is called sarcoma of the uterus. Refer to the PDQ statement on sarcoma of the uterus for treatment of that disease.

Like most cancers, cancer of the endometrium is best treated when it is found (diagnosed) early. You should see a doctor if you have any of the following problems: bleeding or discharge not related to your periods (menstruation), difficult or painful urination, pain during intercourse, and pain in the pelvic area.

Your doctor may use several tests to see if you have cancer, usually beginning with an internal (pelvic) exam. During the exam, your doctor will feel for any lumps or changes in the shape of the uterus. Your doctor will then do a Pap test, using a piece of cotton, a brush, or a small wooden stick to scrape gently the outside of the cervix (opening of the uterus) and vagina to pick up cells.

Because cancer of the endometrium begins inside the uterus, it does not usually show up on the Pap test. For this reason, your doctor may also do a dilation and curettage (D and C) or similar test to remove pieces of the lining of the uterus. During a D and C, the opening of the cervix is stretched with a spoon-shaped instrument and the walls of the uterus are scraped gently to remove any growths. This tissue is then checked for cancer cells.

Your chance of recovery (prognosis) and choice of treatment depend on the stage of your cancer (whether it is just in the endometrium or has spread to other parts of the uterus or other parts of the body) and your general state of health. If you have early stage cancer, your prognosis may also depend on whether female hormones (progesterones) affect the growth of the cancer.

Stage Explanation

Stages of Cancer of the Endometrium

Once cancer of the endometrium has been found, more tests will be done to find out if the cancer has spread from the endometrium to other parts of the body (staging). Your doctor needs to know the stage of your disease to plan treatment. The following stages are used for cancer of the endometrium:

Stage 0 or carcinoma in situ
Stage 0 cancer of the endometrium is a very early cancer. The cancer is found inside the uterus only and is in only the surface layer of the endometrium.

Stage I
Cancer is found only in the main part of the uterus (it is not found in the cervix).

Stage II
Cancer cells have spread to the cervix.

Stage III
Cancer cells have spread outside the uterus but have not spread outside the pelvis.

Stage IV
Cancer cells have spread beyond the pelvis, to other body parts, or into the lining of the bladder (the sac which holds urine) or rectum.

Recurrent
Recurrent disease means the cancer has come back (recurred) after it has been treated.

Treatment Options Overview

How Cancer of the Endometrium Is Treated

There are treatments for all patients with cancer of the endometrium. Four kinds of treatment are used:

surgery (taking out the cancer in an operation)
radiation therapy (using high-dose x-rays or other high-energy rays to kill cancer cells and shrink tumors)
chemotherapy (using drugs to kill cancer cells)
hormone therapy (using female hormones to kill cancer cells).

Surgery is the most common treatment for cancer of the endometrium. Your doctor may take out the cancer using one of the following operations:

♦ Total abdominal hysterectomy and bilateral salpingo-oophorectomy, taking out the uterus, fallopian tubes, and ovaries through a cut in the abdomen. Lymph nodes in the pelvis may also be taken out (lymph node dissection). (The lymph nodes are small, bean-shaped structures that are found throughout the body. They produce and store infection-fighting cells, but may contain cancer cells.)
♦ Radical hysterectomy, taking out the cervix, uterus, fallopian tubes, ovaries, and part of the vagina. Lymph nodes in the area may also be taken out (lymph node dissection).

Radiation therapy uses high-dose x-rays to kill cancer cells and shrink tumors. Radiation may come from a machine outside the body (external radiation) or from putting materials that produce radiation (radioisotopes) through thin plastic tubes into the area where the cancer cells are found (internal radiation). Radiation may be used alone or before or after surgery.

Chemotherapy uses drugs to kill cancer cells. Chemotherapy may be taken by pill, or it may be put into the body by a needle in the vein. Chemotherapy is called a systemic treatment because the drugs enter the bloodstream, travel through the body, and can kill cancer cells outside the uterus.

Hormone therapy uses hormones, usually taken by pill, to kill cancer cells.

Treatment by Stage

Treatment for cancer of the endometrium depends on the stage of your disease, the type of disease, your age, and your overall condition.

You may receive treatment that is considered standard based on its effectiveness in a number of patients in past studies, or you may choose to go into a clinical trial. Not all patients are cured with standard therapy and some standard treatments may have more side effects than are desired. For these reasons, clinical trials are designed to find better ways to treat cancer patients and are based on the most up-to-date information. Clinical trials are going on in most parts of the country for most stages of cancer of the endometrium. If you want more information, call the Cancer Information Service at 1-800-4-CANCER (1-800-422-6237).

Treatment options: Stage 0 endometrial cancer
Your treatment may be one of the following:
1. Dilation and curettage (D and C) followed by hormone therapy. Your doctor may tell you not to take any more medicine that contains estrogen.
2. Hysterectomy.

Treatment options: Stage I endometrial cancer
Your treatment may be one of the following:
1. Surgery to remove the uterus and both ovaries and fallopian tubes (total abdominal hysterectomy and bilateral salpingo-oophorectomy) with removal of some of the lymph nodes in the pelvis and abdomen to see if they contain cancer.
2. Total abdominal hysterectomy and bilateral salpingo-oophorectomy with removal of some of the lymph nodes in the pelvis and abdomen to

see if they contain cancer, followed by radiation therapy to the pelvis.

3. Clinical trials of radiation and/or chemotherapy following surgery.
4. Radiation therapy alone for selected patients.

Treatment options: Stage II endometrial cancer

Your treatment may be one of the following:

1. Total abdominal hysterectomy, bilateral salpingo-oophorectomy, and removal of some of the lymph nodes in the pelvis and abdomen to see if they contain cancer, followed by radiation therapy.
2. Internal and external beam radiation therapy followed by surgery to remove the uterus and both ovaries and fallopian tubes (total abdominal hysterectomy and bilateral salpingo-oophorectomy). Some of the lymph nodes in the pelvis and abdomen are also removed to see if they contain cancer.
3. Surgery to remove the cervix, uterus, fallopian tubes, ovaries, and part of the vagina (radical hysterectomy). Lymph nodes in the area may also be taken out (lymph node dissection).

Treatment options: Stage III endometrial cancer

Your treatment may be one of the following:

1. Surgery to remove the cervix, uterus, fallopian tubes, ovaries, and part of the vagina (radical hysterectomy). Lymph nodes in the area may also be taken out (lymph node dissection). Surgery is usually followed by radiation therapy.
2. Internal and external beam radiation therapy.
3. Hormone therapy.

Treatment options: Stage IV endometrial cancer

Your treatment may be one of the following:

1. Internal and external beam radiation therapy.
2. Hormone therapy.
3. Clinical trials of chemotherapy.

Treatment options: Recurrent endometrial cancer

If your cancer has come back, your treatment may be one of the following:

1. Radiation therapy to relieve symptoms, such as pain, nausea, and abnormal bowel functions.
2. Hormone therapy.
3. Clinical trials of chemotherapy.

To learn more about cancer of the endometrium, call the National Cancer Institute's Cancer Information Service at 1-800-4-CANCER (1-800-422-6237). By dialing this toll-free number, you can speak with someone who can answer your questions.

■ Document Source:
  National Cancer Institute
  Building 31, Room 10A24, 9000 Rockville Pike, Bethesda, MD 20892
  PDQ 208/01176
  02/01/94

See also: Chemotherapy and You: A Guide to Self-Help During Treatment (page 40); Radiation Therapy and You: A Guide to Self-Help During Treatment (page 56); What You Need to Know About Cancer of the Uterus (page 470)

FACTS ABOUT CESAREAN CHILDBIRTH

Cesarean childbirth, an operation to deliver a baby through an incision in the abdomen, can be traced back through history to Egypt in 3000 B.C. The procedure's name comes from a set of Roman laws, *Lex Caesare,* which in 715 B.C. mandated surgical removal of an unborn fetus upon death of the mother.

Until recent decades the operation usually had been used as a last resort because of a high rate of maternal complications and death. But with the availability of antibiotics to fight infection and the development of modern surgical techniques, the once high maternal mortality rate has dropped dramatically. As a result, the cesarean childbirth rate has increased dramatically. From 1970 to 1980, the number of cesareans in the U.S. more than tripled, increasing from 5 percent of all births to 16.5 percent. In some localities the rate is much higher.

This startling increase has become a matter of national concern. In the fall of 1980, the National Institute of Child Health and Human Development convened a panel to gather information and develop a draft report on the subject. This report formed the basis for a three-day conference held to examine the issues related to cesarean childbirth, reach general agreement and make recommendations to guide practicing physicians. This "consensus development" panel, made up of leading scientists, practicing physicians and consumers, produced a 540-page final report which is highlighted in this fact sheet.

Basically, the panel concluded that the rising cesarean birth rate can be stopped and perhaps reversed, without sacrificing continued improvements in the quality and success of pregnancy care.

What is cesarean childbirth?

A major operation, each cesarean actually involves a series of separate incisions in the mother. The skin, underlying muscles and abdomen are opened first and then the uterus is opened allowing removal of the infant.

There are two main types of cesarean operations, each named according to the location and direction of the uterine incision:

- cervical—a transverse (horizontal) or vertical incision in the lower uterus, and
- classical—a vertical incision in the main body of the uterus.

Today, the low *transverse cervical* incision is used almost exclusively. It has the lowest incidence of hemorrhage during surgery as well as the least chance of rupturing in later pregnancies. Sometimes, because of fetal size (very large or very small) or position problems (breech or transverse), a *low vertical* cesarean may be performed.

In the *classical* operation, a vertical incision allows a greater opening and is used for fetal size or position problems and in some emergency situations. This approach involves more bleeding in surgery and a higher risk of abdominal infection. Although any uterine incision may rupture during a subsequent labor, the classical is more likely to do so and more likely to result in death for the mother and fetus than a cervical incision.

Why have cesarean rates increased?

Many factors account for rising cesarean birth rates. By the 1960's, increasing emphasis was being placed on the health of the fetus. With declining birth rates and couples having fewer children, even greater attention was given to improving the outcome of pregnancy, and infant survival in general. The nation's infant mortality rate began to be seen as an international yardstick on the quality of health care.

At the same time, advances in medical care combined to make maternal death from cesarean childbirth a rare occurrence. The safer the procedure became, the easier it was to decide to perform the operation. As a safe alternative to normal delivery, the cesarean became a practical way to try to improve the outcome of difficult pregnancies.

Studies suggesting the benefit of cesarean birth in dealing with various pregnancy complications also led to more cesareans. Obstetricians came to favor surgery in pregnancies with difficult deliveries that formerly would have required the use of forceps. The diagnosis of "dystocia," a catch-all term meaning difficult labor, was made more frequently and handled more often with the cesarean operation. Fetal distress during labor—a condition often resulting in a cesarean—was more apt to be detected with the introduction of electronic fetal monitoring. Increasingly, physicians used the cesarean method to deliver infants in the breech position prior to birth, adding still further to the rising cesarean rate.

Another important contributing factor was the rising number of repeat cesareans. As the number of women having their first cesarean increased, the long-held tenet "once a cesarean, always a cesarean" led to a rapid increase in the number of repeat cesarean births.

What is the current medical thinking about repeat cesarean deliveries?

Having had a prior cesarean delivery is one of the two major reasons women have the operation today. (The other is the diagnosis of dystocia.) The consensus development panel found that the rate of repeat cesareans is likely to increase further if present trends continue. Currently more than 98 percent of women in the U.S. who have had a cesarean undergo a repeat cesarean for subsequent pregnancies.

This practice was begun in the late 1900s to avoid the risk of uterine scar rupture and hemorrhage during labor. At that time the classical cesarean incision was most widely used and the cesarean birth rate was extremely low.

Physicians now know that the classical, low vertical and "inverted T" incisions have a higher rate of rupture than the low transverse incision now in general use. The low transverse cervical cesarean also has been shown to result in fewer cases of lasting health disorders or death among mothers and infants. Today, many women who had earlier low transverse cesareans safely deliver subsequent children vaginally.

In studying the issue, the consensus panel found that the risk of maternal death in a repeat cesarean is two times that of a vaginal delivery. In addition, the maternal mortality rate for repeat cesareans has not fallen since 1970. The group concluded that the practice of routine repeat cesarean birth is open to question, and that labor and vaginal delivery after a previous low *transverse cervical* cesarean birth are of low risk to the mother and child in properly selected cases.

The panel recommended that:

♦ In hospitals with appropriate facilities, services and staff for prompt emergency cesarean birth, some women who have had a previous low transverse cervical cesarean may safely be allowed a trial of labor and vaginal delivery.

♦ The present practice of repeat cesareans should continue for patients who have had previous cesareans with classical, inverted T or low vertical incisions, or for whom there is no record of the type of incision.

♦ In hospitals without appropriate facilities, services and staff, the risk of labor for women having had a previous cesarean may exceed the risk to mother and infant from a properly timed, elective repeat cesarean birth. To allow patients to make an informed decision, they should be told in advance about the limits of the institution's capabilities and the availability of other institutions offering this service.

♦ More adequate information should be compiled on the risks and benefits of trying labor in patients with previous low transverse cervical incisions.

♦ Institutions offering labor trials following low transverse cesareans should develop guidelines for managing those labors.

♦ Patient education on initial and repeat cesarean birth should continue throughout pregnancy as an important part of patient participation in making decisions about the delivery.

What if the baby is in the breech position prior to birth?

There is a continuing trend to use the cesarean method to deliver a "breech baby"—a fetus positioned in the womb to be born in some way other than the normal head first manner. Nationally, the proportion of breech positioned infants delivered by cesarean rose from about 12 percent in 1970 to 60 percent in 1978.

Breech positioning involves higher risks for the mother and child, regardless of whether the delivery is vaginal or cesarean. Cesareans are being selected more often in these cases to try to improve the outcome in the face of the increased risks. But the consensus group found scientific data in this area generally inadequate to make firm conclusions about the desirability of one approach over the other.

Most clinical reviews suggest that the cesarean may involve less risk for the premature breech infant, but this may not be true for term breech babies. Several studies indicate that vaginal delivery of the uncomplicated term breech infant is preferable because an elective cesarean birth involves risk of significant complications for the mother and little or no decrease in the risk of infant death.

Deciding which method of delivery to use in these situations involves considering many factors. These include maternal pelvic size, size of the fetus, the type of breech position and the experience of the physician with vaginal breech delivery.

In general, the consensus panel concluded that the cesarean presents a lower risk to the infant than a vaginal delivery when a breech fetus is 8 pounds or larger, when a fetus is in a complete or footling breech position or when a fetus is breech with marked hyperextension of the head.

The group recommended that vaginal delivery of term breech babies should remain an acceptable choice when the following conditions exist:

♦ anticipated fetal weight of less than 8 pounds;
♦ normal pelvic dimensions and structure in the mother;
♦ frank breech positioning without hyperextended head; and
♦ delivery by a physician experienced in vaginal breech delivery.

What is the most common, single reason for performing a cesarean?

Dystocia is a catch-all medical term covering a broad range of problems which can complicate labor. The consensus group found that this diagnosis was the largest contributor to the overall rise in the cesarean rate, accounting for 30 percent of all cesareans.

Included under the dystocia, or difficult labor, diagnosis are the following three basic types of problems which may impede labor:

♦ abnormalities of the mother's birth canal, such as a small pelvis;
♦ abnormalities in the position of the fetus, including breech position or large fetal size; and
♦ abnormalities in the forces of labor, including infrequent or weak uterine contractions.

The first two categories are well-defined areas. The physician usually recognizes size or position problems early; guidelines for appropriate obstetrical action are available; and the effects of the various approaches for mother and infant are reasonably well known.

The consensus panel agreed that the last category—forces of labor—is most in need of scrutiny and offers an opportunity for moderating the cesarean rate. Generally, this diagnosis occurs with low-risk infants of normal weight and size. Studies have not shown that infants in this group are better off with either cesarean or vaginal deliveries, although the maternal mortality rate for dystocia in 1978 was 41.9

deaths per 100,000 cesarean births compared with 11.1 deaths per 100,000 vaginal births.

The panel concluded that in handling a difficult or slowly progressing labor without fetal distress, a physician should consider various options before performing a cesarean. These include having the patient rest or walk around, sedating the patient or stimulating labor with a drug called oxytocin.

The panel recommended that because the diagnosis of dystocia is poorly defined and so prominent in increasing the cesarean rate, practice review boards in hospitals should include dystocia cases when conducting reviews. The panel also stressed the need for more research on the factors affecting the progress of labor.

Has the use of electronic fetal monitoring led to more cesareans?

Another diagnosis accounting for the rise in cesarean birth rates is fetal distress. Occurring during labor, this problem can result in various complications, the most serious being fetal brain damage because of oxygen deprivation.

The use of electronic fetal monitoring techniques has led to an increase in the diagnosis of fetal distress but not necessarily to the increase in cesarean deliveries, according to the consensus panel.

Because current data are insufficient on the possible risks or benefits of handling this condition with either cesarean or vaginal deliveries, the panel recommended studies to gather information on the outcomes of births involving fetal distress and development of new techniques to improve the accuracy of the diagnosis. These steps, the panel said, may be expected to improve fetal outcome and lower cesarean birth rates.

Are there other medical conditions which would necessitate a cesarean?

Because of a need for early delivery, certain medical problems in either the mother or fetus can lead to cesarean birth. Examples include maternal diabetes, pregnancy-induced hypertension, vaginal herpes infection, and erythroblastosis fetalis, a blood disease related to the Rh factor in the mother. This entire group, however, contributes only a small part of the cesarean birth rate increases.

The consensus panel said that in some of these situations vaginal birth would be a safe alternative if a more effective method of stimulating labor before term was available. The panel recommended research to develop such methods.

What are the benefits of the cesarean method?

There are certain times when conditions in the mother or infant make cesarean delivery the method of first choice. By providing an alternate route of delivery, the procedure offers great benefit in situations when a vaginal delivery carries a high risk of complications and death.

A cesarean is usually used when an expectant mother has diabetes mellitus. Such women have a high risk of having stillborns late in pregnancy. In these cases, a slightly early cesarean helps prevent this occurrence.

The cesarean can also be a lifesaving procedure when the following conditions are present:

- ♦ Placenta previa—when the placenta blocks the infant from being born.
- ♦ Abruptio placentae—when the placenta prematurely separates from the uterine wall and hemorrhage occurs.
- ♦ Obstructed labor—which can occur with a fetus in the shoulder breech, or any other abnormal position.
- ♦ Ruptured uterus.
- ♦ Presence of weak uterine scars from previous surgery or cesarean.
- ♦ Fetus too large for the mother's birth canal.
- ♦ Rapid toxemia—a condition in which high blood pressure can lead to convulsions in late pregnancy.
- ♦ Vaginal herpes infection—which could infect an infant being born vaginally, and lead to its eventual death.
- ♦ Pelvic tumors—which obstruct the birth canal and weaken the uterine wall.
- ♦ Absence of effective uterine contractions after labor has begun.
- ♦ Prolapse of the umbilical cord—when the cord is pushed out ahead of the infant, compressing the cord and cutting off blood flow.

What are the maternal risks in cesarean childbirth?

The risks of any medical procedure are determined by examining the related mortality statistics showing death rates and morbidity figures showing complications, injuries or disorders linked to the event. These vary from hospital to hospital and from locale to locale.

Although maternal death during childbirth is extremely uncommon, national figures show cesarean birth carries up to four times the risk of death compared to a vaginal delivery. The maternal mortality rate for vaginal delivery in 1978 was about 10 deaths per 100,000 births. For cesareans, the rate was about 41 deaths per 100,000 births. (In some cases, maternal deaths indicated in these figures were caused by illness rather than the surgery.)

The morbidity rates associated with cesarean births are higher than with vaginal delivery. Because major surgery is involved, the chance of infection and complication is greater. The most common are endometritis (an inflammation of tissue lining the uterus) and urinary tract or incision infections.

Does cesarean childbirth require special anesthesia?

The use of anesthesia during childbirth is unique because it requires attention to the infant about to be born as well as the mother. Although rare, anesthesia-related maternal deaths continue to occur. Most, however, are potentially avoidable.

There are three major anesthetic techniques for cesarean birth. Spinal anesthesia is widely used, although the use of lumbar epidural anesthesia is increasing. Both are considered "regional" anesthesia because they deaden pain in only part of the body without putting the patient to sleep. General anesthesia, which renders the patient unconscious, is often used in an emergency situation and with women who object to the spinal or epidural approach.

The consensus panel recommended that the types of anesthesia available should be discussed among the patient, obstetrician and anesthesiologist. Each approach has advantages and disadvantages. If possible, the report recommends, the patient should have the option of receiving regional instead of general anesthesia.

Are there risks to the infant?

Infants delivered with elective cesarean surgery, especially if it is performed before the onset of labor, appear to have a greater risk of respiratory distress syndrome (RDS). This condition, in which the infant's lungs are not fully mature, may result if an error is made in estimating the age of the developing fetus. Under these circumstances, an infant—who otherwise would have been healthy if allowed to develop fully—encounters the problems of prematurity when removed too soon by cesarean. These include RDS and other lung disorders, feeding problems and various complications which in some cases require a long hospital stay.

Measures and techniques to assess the maturity of the fetus and the degree of lung development are readily available in the United States. The consensus report stressed the need for improving physician and patient education about the safe and effective use of these techniques in planning for elective cesarean delivery. Respiratory distress is unlikely to be a problem, regardless of the type of delivery, if the infant is born at or near term.

What are the psychological effects of cesarean childbirth?

Other factors must be taken into consideration when weighing the prospects of a cesarean. Although there has been only limited research on the psychological effects on parents following a cesarean birth, it is clear that surgery is an increased psychological and physical burden compared to vaginal delivery. In limited followup studies of infants, there has been no evidence of an adverse psychologic effect on infants born by cesarean.

In some hospitals, family-centered maternity care has been extended to cesarean deliveries. The presence of the father in the operating room and the closer contact between the mother and newborn in this approach appear to improve the cesarean process.

The consensus panel recommended strengthening the information exchange and education of prospective parents about the overall cesarean experience. They urged hospitals to allow fathers in the operating room when possible and to avoid routinely separating the newborn from its parents immediately following delivery.

For more information

Single free copies of the following publications are available by writing to NICHD, P.O. Box 2911, Washington, D.C. 20040.

Cesarean Childbirth is the 540-page final report of the consensus development task force. The report contains evidence gathered by the panel, as well as findings and recommendations. Ask for NIH Publication No. 82-2067.

"Cesarean Childbirth Consensus Statement" is a ten-page summary of the questions examined at the three-day Consensus Development Conference held September 22-24, 1980. The summary contains the specific findings and recommendations of the panel.

The "Facts About" series is prepared by the Office of Research Reporting at the National Institute of Child Health and Human Development. The Institute, one of the federal government's National Institutes of Health, conducts and supports research on the various processes that determine the health of children, adults, families and populations. For more copies of this fact sheet or others in the series, write to NICHD, P.O. Box 29111, Washington, D.C. 20040.

Other publications in this series:

♦ *Facts About Anorexia Nervosa*
♦ *Facts About Childhood Hyperactivity*
♦ *Facts About Down Syndrome*
♦ *Facts About Dyslexia*
♦ *Facts About Dysmenorrhea and Premenstrual Syndrome*
♦ *Facts About Oral Contraceptives*
♦ *Facts About Precocious Puberty*
♦ *Facts About Pregnancy and Smoking*
♦ *Facts About Premature Birth*
♦ *Facts About Vasectomy Safety*

■ Document Source:
U.S. Department of Health and Human Services, Public Health Service
National Institutes of Health
National Institute of Child Health and Human Development

FACTS ABOUT ENDOMETRIOSIS

Endometriosis is a common, yet poorly understood disease. It can strike women of any socioeconomic class, age, or race. It is estimated that between 10 and 20 percent of American women of childbearing age have endometriosis. While some women with endometriosis may have severe pelvic pain, others who have the condition have no symptoms. Nothing about endometriosis is simple, and there are no absolute cures. The disease can affect a woman's whole existence—her ability to work, her ability to reproduce, and her relationships with her mate, her child, and everyone around her.

The National Institute of Child Health and Human Development (NICHD), part of the federal government's National Institutes of Health (NIH), conducts and supports research on the various processes that determine the health of children, adults, families, and populations. As part of NICHD's mandate in the reproductive sciences, NICHD has established a Reproductive Medicine Network linking several institutions across the country. While this cooperative effort focuses on other important issues such as infertility and various male and female reproductive disorders, developing an optimal treatment for endometriosis is one of its primary goals.

What is endometriosis?

The name endometriosis comes from the word "endometrium," the tissue that lines the inside of the uterus. If a woman is not pregnant this tissue builds up and is shed each month. It is discharged as menstrual flow at the end of each cycle. In endometriosis, tissue that looks and acts like endometrial tissue is found outside the uterus, usually inside the abdominal cavity.

Endometrial tissue residing outside the uterus responds to the menstrual cycle in a way that is similar to the way endometrium usually responds in the uterus. At the end of every cycle, when hormones cause the uterus to shed its endometrial lining, endometrial tissue growing outside the uterus will break apart and bleed. However, unlike menstrual fluid from the uterus, which is discharged from the body during menstruation, blood from the misplaced tissue has no place to go. Tissues surrounding the area of endometriosis may become inflamed or swollen. The inflammation may produce scar tissue around the area of endometriosis. These endometrial tissue sites may develop into what are called "lesions," "implants," "nodules," or "growths."

Endometriosis is most often found in the ovaries, on the fallopian tubes, and the ligaments supporting the uterus, in the internal area between the vagina and rectum, on the outer surface of the uterus, and on the lining of the pelvic cavity. Infrequently, endometrial growths are found on the intestines or in the rectum, on the bladder, vagina, cervix, and vulva (external genitals), or in abdominal surgery scars. Very rarely, endometrial growths have been found outside the abdomen, in the thigh, arm, or lung.

Physicians may use stages to describe the severity of endometriosis. Endometrial implants that are small and not widespread are considered minimal or mild endometriosis. Moderate endometriosis means that larger implants or more extensive scar tissue is present. Severe endometriosis is used to describe large implants and extensive scar tissue.

What are the symptoms?

Most commonly, the symptoms of endometriosis start years after menstrual periods begin. Over the years, the symptoms tend to gradually increase as the endometriosis areas increase in size. After menopause, the abnormal implants shrink away and the symptoms subside.

The most common symptom is pain, especially excessive menstrual cramps (dysmenorrhea) which may be felt in the abdomen or lower back or pain during or after sexual activity (dyspareunia). Infertility occurs in about 30 to 40 percent of women with endometriosis. Rarely, the irritation caused by endometrial implants may progress into infection or abscesses causing pain independent of the menstrual cycle. Endometrial patches may also be tender to touch or pressure, and intestinal pain may also result from endometrial patches on the walls of the colon or intestine.

The amount of pain is not always related to the severity of the disease—some women with severe endometriosis have no pain; while others with just a few small growths have incapacitating pain.

Endometrial cancer is very rarely associated with endometriosis, occurring in less than 1 percent of women who have the disease. When it does occur, it is usually found in more advanced patches of endometriosis in older women and the long-term outlook in these unusual cases is reasonably good.

How is endometriosis related to fertility problems?

Severe endometriosis with extensive scarring and organ damage may affect fertility. It is considered one of the three major causes of female infertility. However, unsuspected or mild endometriosis is a common finding among infertile women and how this type of endometriosis affects fertility is still not clear. While the pregnancy rates for patients with endometriosis remain lower than those of the general population, most patients with endometriosis do not experience fertility problems.

What is the cause of endometriosis?

The cause of endometriosis is still unknown. One theory is that during menstruation some of the menstrual tissue backs up through the fallopian tubes into the abdomen, where it implants and grows. Another theory suggests that endometriosis may be a genetic process or that certain families may have predisposing factors to endometriosis. In the latter view, endometriosis is seen as the tissue development process gone awry.

Whatever the cause of endometriosis, its progression is influenced by various stimulating factors such as hormones or growth factors. In this regard, NICHD investigators are studying the role of the immune system in activating cells that may secrete factors which, in turn, stimulate endometriosis.

In addition to these new hypotheses, investigators are continuing to look into previous theories that endometriosis is a disease influenced by delayed childbearing. Since the hormones made by the placenta during pregnancy prevent ovulation, the progress of endometriosis is slowed or stopped during pregnancy and the total number of lifetime cycles is reduced for a woman who had multiple pregnancies.

How is endometriosis diagnosed?

Diagnosis of endometriosis begins with a gynecologist evaluating the patient's medical history. A complete physical exam, including a pelvic examination, is also necessary. However, diagnosis of endometriosis is only complete when proven by a laparoscopy, a minor surgical procedure in which a laparoscope (a tube with a light in it) is inserted into a small incision in the abdomen. The laparoscope is moved around the abdomen, which has been distended with carbon dioxide gas to make the organs easier to see. The surgeon can then check the condition of the abdominal organs and see the endometrial implants.

The laparoscopy will show the locations, extent, and size of the growths and will help the patient and her doctor make better-informed decisions about treatment.

What is the treatment?

While the treatment for endometriosis has varied over the years, doctors now agree that if the symptoms are mild, no further treatment other than medication for pain may be needed. For those patients with mild or minimal endometriosis who wish to become pregnant, doctors are advising that, depending on the age of the patient and the amount of pain associated with the disease, the best course of action is to have a trial period of unprotected intercourse for 6 months to 1 year. If pregnancy does not occur within that time, then further treatment may be needed.

For patients not seeking a pregnancy where treatment specific for the management of endometriosis is required and a definitive diagnosis of endometriosis by laparoscopy has been made, a physician may suggest hormone suppression treatment. Since this therapy shuts off ovulation, women being treated for endometriosis will not get pregnant during such therapy, although some may elect to become pregnant shortly after therapy is stopped.

Hormone treatment is most effective when the implants are small. The doctor may prescribe a weak synthetic male hormone called Danazol, a synthetic progestin alone, or a combination of estrogen and progestin such as oral contraceptives.

Danazol has become a more common treatment choice than either progestin or the birth control pill. Disease symptoms are improved for 80 to 90 percent of the patients taking Danazol, and the size and the extent of implants are also reduced. While side effects with Danazol treatment are not uncommon (e.g., acne, hot flashes, or fluid retention), most of them are relatively mild and stop when treatment is stopped. Overall, pregnancy rates following this therapy depend on the severity of the disease. However, some recent studies have shown that with mild to minimal endometriosis, Danazol alone does not improve pregnancy rates.

It is important to remember that Danazol treatment is unsafe if there is any chance that a woman is pregnant. A fetus accidentally exposed to this drug may develop abnormally. For this same reason, although pregnancy is not likely while a woman is taking this drug, careful use of a barrier birth control method such as a diaphragm or condom is essential during this treatment.

Another type of hormone treatment is a synthetic pituitary hormone blocker called gonadotropin-releasing hormone agonist, or GnRH agonist. This treatment stops ovarian hormone production by blocking pituitary gland hormones that normally stimulate ovarian cycles.

These hormones are currently being tested using different methods of administration. One such treatment involves a drug that is administered as a nasal spray twice daily for 6 months and works by suppressing production of estrogen, which controls the growth of the endometrial tissue. Other treatments being developed in this category include daily or monthly hormone injections. One concern is the loss of bone mineral which occurs with this type of hormone therapy. This may limit the duration and frequency of this type of treatment.

While pregnancy rates for women with fertility problems resulting from endometriosis are fairly good with no therapy and with only a trial waiting period, there may be women who need more aggressive treatment. Those women who are older and who feel the need to become pregnant more quickly or those women who have severe physical changes due to the disease, may consider surgical treatment. Also, women who are not interested in pregnancy, but who have severe, debilitating pain, may also consider surgery.

Conservative surgery attempts to remove the diseased tissue without risking damage to healthy surrounding tissue. This surgery is called laparotomy and is performed in a hospital under anesthesia. Pregnancy rates are highest during the first year after surgery, as recurrences of endometriosis are fairly common. The specifics of the surgery should be discussed with a doctor.

Some patients may need more radical surgery to correct the damage caused by untreated endometriosis. Hysterectomy and removal of the ovaries may be the only treatment possible if the ovaries are badly damaged. In some cases, hysterectomy alone without the removal of the ovaries may be reasonable.

New surgical treatments are being developed that further utilize the laparoscope instead of full abdominal surgery. During routine laparoscopy, the surgeon can cauterize small areas of endometriosis. Other evolving techniques include using a laser during laparoscopy to vaporize abnormal tissue. This involves a shorter recovery time. Laparoscopy treatment is possible, however, only if the surgeon can see pelvic structures clearly through the laparoscope. These newer techniques should be performed by surgeons specializing in such delicate procedures. Although these techniques are promising, more study is needed to determine if they yield results comparable to conventional surgical management.

Where to look for answers. . .

Because endometriosis affects each woman differently, it is essential that the patient maintains a good, clear, honest communication with her doctor. For the single truth about endometriosis is that there are no clear-cut, universal answers.

If pregnancy is an issue, then age may affect the treatment plan. If it is not an issue, then treatment decisions will depend primarily on the severity of symptoms.

Because these decisions can be difficult and confusing, there are organizations that provide information and offer support and help to those who are affected by this disease.

Endometriosis Association
8585 North 76th Place
Milwaukee, Wisconsin 53223
(414) 355-2200

The American College of Obstetricians and Gynecologists
409 12th Street, SW
Washington, DC 20024-2188
(202) 638-5577

American Fertility Society
2140-11th Avenue South
Suite 200
Birmingham, Alabama 35205-2800
(205) 933-8494

■ Document Source:
   U.S. Department of Health and Human Services, Public Health Service
   National Institutes of Health
   National Institute of Child Health and Human Development
   NIH Publication No. 91-2413

MASTECTOMY: A TREATMENT FOR BREAST CANCER

You've been diagnosed as having breast cancer and your doctor has recommended a **mastectomy***. If you're like most women, you probably have many concerns about this treatment for breast cancer.

Surgery of any kind is a frightening experience, but surgery for breast cancer raises special concerns. You may be wondering if the surgery will cure your cancer, how you'll feel after surgery—and how you're going to look.

It's not unusual to think about these things. More than 100,000 women in the United States will have mastectomies this year. Each of them will have personal concerns about the impact of the surgery on her life.

This booklet is designed to ease some of your fears by letting you know what to expect—from the time you enter the hospital to your recovery at home. It may also help the special people in your life who are concerned about your well-being.

Over the years, mastectomy has proven to be an effective treatment for breast cancer. Today, doctors may choose from a range of procedures depending on the extent of the disease at the time of diagnosis, the patient's medical history, her age, the type of tumor, and other factors. You can feel confident that your doctor is taking steps to see that you can continue to lead an active and full life.

Though breast surgery and recovery will cause you to take time out from your normal routine, it need not cause a permanent change in your lifestyle. Like hundreds of other women who have had mastectomies, you can plan to continue doing the things you enjoy—whether it's working, raising a family, maintaining your home and personal relationships, or pursuing other interests.

---

* Boldface words are defined in the glossary.

Informed Consent: When Surgery Is Recommended

When surgery is recommended, most health care facilities now require patients to sign a form stating their willingness to permit diagnosis and medical treatment. This is to certify that you understand what procedures will be done and have consented to have them performed.

Consent to surgical or other treatment is only meaningful if given by a patient who has had an opportunity to learn about recommended alternatives and to evaluate them. Before consenting to any course of treatment, be sure your doctor lets you know:

- The recommended procedure;
- Its purpose;
- Risks and side effects associated with it;
- Likely consequences with and without treatment;
- Other available alternatives; and
- Advantages and disadvantages of one treatment over another.

Even if you want your doctor to assume full responsibility for all decision making, you are likely to discover that your concerns about treatment decrease as your understanding of breast cancer and its treatment increases.

Types of Surgery

Mastectomy is the most common treatment for breast cancer today. As recently as 15 years ago, many doctors considered radical mastectomy the only procedure. It removed the entire breast, the chest muscles under the breast, and all underarm **lymph nodes,** leaving a hollow chest area. Many women feared the treatment as much as the disease.

Thanks to medical advances, there is now a wide range of effective procedures that may be used, depending on the individual case. In addition to the radical mastectomy, also called a "Halsted radical," surgical options include:

- *Modified radical mastectomy*—Removes the breast and the underarm lymph nodes and the lining over the chest muscles. Sometimes the smaller of the two chest muscles is also removed. This procedure is also called a "total mastectomy with axillary (or underarm) dissection" and today is the most common treatment of early stage breast cancer.

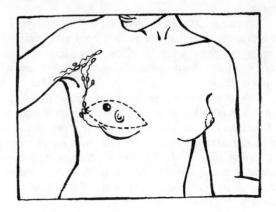

- Total or simple mastectomy—Removes only the breast. Sometimes a few of the underarm lymph nodes closest to the breast are removed to see if the cancer has spread beyond the breast. May be followed by radiation therapy.

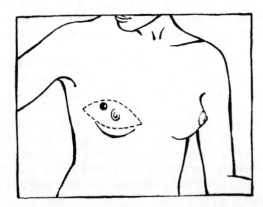

- *Partial or segmental mastectomy*—Removes the tumor plus a wedge of normal tissue surrounding it, including some skin and the lining of the chest muscle below the tumor. It is followed by radiation therapy. Many surgeons also remove some or all of the underarm lymph nodes to check for possible spread of cancer.

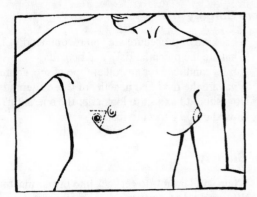

- *Lumpectomy*—Removes the breast lump and is followed by radiation therapy. Many surgeons also remove and test some of the underarm lymph nodes.

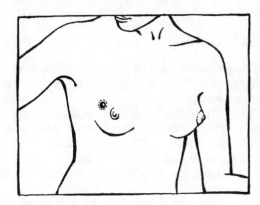

A Word About Breast Reconstruction

Since you are about to have breast surgery, you should be aware of breast reconstruction, a way to recreate a breast shape after a natural breast has been removed. Though this procedure is gaining in popularity, many women are still unaware of it.

Some women have reconstruction at the same time as their mastectomies; others have it done several months or even years later. Almost any woman who has had a mastectomy can have her breast reconstructed. Successful reconstruction is not hampered by radiation-damaged, thin, or tight skin, or the absence of chest muscles.

Reconstruction isn't for everyone, however. And it may not be right for you. After mastectomy, many women prefer to wear an artificial breast form, called a **prosthesis,** inside their brassieres.

Both a general surgeon and a plastic surgeon can help you decide whether to have breast reconstruction. If possible, this should be discussed before your surgery because the position of the incision may affect the reconstruction procedure. However, many women consider breast reconstruction only after surgery.

For more information on breast reconstruction, contact the National Cancer Institute for a copy of *Breast Reconstruction: A Matter of Choice.*

Questions to Ask Your Doctor

Before Surgery

♦ What kind of procedure are you recommending?
♦ What are the potential risks and benefits?
♦ Am I a candidate for any other type of procedure?
♦ What are the risks and benefits of those alternatives?
♦ How should I expect to look after the operation?
♦ How should I expect to feel?

After Surgery

♦ When will I be able to get back into my normal routine?
♦ What can I do to ensure a safe recovery?
♦ What problems, if any, should I report to you?
♦ What type of exercises should I do?
♦ How frequently should I see you for a checkup?

In the Hospital

Hospital procedures and policies vary, but there are a number of things you probably can expect to have happen when you check in for surgery.

You will probably be admitted the afternoon before your operation so that some routine tests, such as blood and urine tests and a chest x-ray, can be performed. Shortly before the operation, the surgical area (breast and underarm) will be shaved, and you may be given some medicine to help you relax.

When it is time for surgery, you will be taken to the operating room and an anesthesiologist will put you to sleep. Electrocardiogram sensors will be attached to your arms and legs with adhesive pads to check your heart rate during surgery. The surgical area will be cleaned and sterile sheets will be draped over your body, except for the area around the operation. Depending on the procedure, surgery will take between 2 and 4 hours.

Recovery

When you awaken from surgery, you will be in the recovery room. Your breast area will be bandaged and a tube will be in place at the surgical site to drain away any fluid that may accumulate. Your throat may be sore from the tube that was placed in it to carry air to your lungs during surgery. You may also feel a little nauseated and have a dry mouth—common side effects of **anesthesia.**

You will spend an hour or so in the recovery room. Oxygen will be available in case you need it to ease your breathing. Wires may be taped to your chest to measure your heartbeat. An **intravenous** (IV) tube will be inserted into a vein in your arm to give fluid, nourishment, or medication after surgery. The IV will probably be removed after you begin to drink and eat.

It's common to feel drowsy for several hours after surgery. You may also feel some discomfort in your breast area. Some women experience numbness, tingling, or pain in the chest, shoulder area, upper arm, or armpit. Others feel pain in the breast that was removed. Doctors are not sure why this "phantom pain" occurs, but it does exist; it's not imaginary. If you are in pain, ask for medication to relieve it.

After Surgery

After you return to your room, a nurse will frequently check your temperature, pulse, blood pressure, and bandage. The nurse will ask you to turn, cough, and breathe deeply to keep your lungs clear after the anesthesia. You may also be encouraged to move your feet and legs to improve your blood circulation. Although each woman reacts to surgery differently, you will probably discover that by the next day you will be able to drink some juice or broth and, with help, to sit up in bed and walk from your bed to a chair in your room. Your doctor will probably encourage you to walk around and eat solid food as soon as possible.

You will be taking sponge baths for a few days after surgery until your incision starts to heal. Before you leave the hospital, ask the doctor or nurse for instructions on taking care of your incision. When you have permission to bathe or shower, do so gently and pat, don't rub, the area of your incision.

The average stay in the hospital is 7 to 10 days. Before you leave, the tube that drains fluid from your incision will be removed. Some of your stitches may also be removed before you leave the hospital. The remaining stitches will be taken out within 1 to 3 weeks at the doctor's office or clinic.

With your doctor's permission, a Reach to Recovery volunteer may visit you in the hospital. Reach to Recovery is an American Cancer Society program that brings volunteers who have had mastectomies together with breast cancer patients. A volunteer will be able to discuss with you any concerns you may have about coping with your mastectomy. She may also give you a lightweight, fiber-filled or cotton breast form to fasten inside your bra, robe, or nightgown while you are recuperating.

Exercising After Mastectomy

Exercising will help you ease the tension in your arm and shoulder and will hasten your recovery. You will probably be able to begin exercising within a few days of your operation. Your doctor, nurse, or physical therapist can show you what exercises to do. The key is to exercise only to the point of pulling or pain—don't push yourself.

Ask your doctor if you might begin with these few simple movements:

- Lie in bed with your arm at your side. Raise your arm straight up and back trying to touch the headboard.
- Raise your shoulders. Rotate them forward, down, and back in a circular motion to loosen your chest, shoulders, and upper back muscles.
- Lying in bed, clasp your hands behind your head and push your elbows into the mattress.
- With your elbow bent and your arm at a 90 degree angle to your body, rotate your shoulder forward until the forearm is down and then backward until it is up.
- With your arm raised, clench and unclench your fist.
- Breathe deeply.
- Rotate your chin to the left and right. Cock your head sideways.

In addition to exercises such as these, many communities offer swimming, exercise, and dance classes specifically for breast cancer patients.

Precautions

A problem that may arise after treatment is swelling of the arm on the side of the mastectomy. Called **lymphedema,** this condition is caused by the loss of underarm lymph nodes and their connecting vessels. Because the lymph nodes have been removed, circulation of lymph fluid is slowed, making it harder for your body to fight infection. You should take special care of your arm to prevent infection. (If you have had breasts removed, ask your doctor about any special precautions.)

Follow these simple rules:

- Avoid burns while cooking or smoking;
- Avoid sunburns;
- Have all injections, vaccinations, blood samples, and blood pressure tests done on the other arm whenever possible;
- Use an electric razor with a narrow head for underarm shaving to reduce the risk of nicks or scratches;
- Carry heavy packages or handbags on the other arm;
- Wash cuts promptly, treat them with antibacterial medication, and cover them with a sterile dressing; check often for redness, soreness, or other signs of infection;
- Never cut cuticles; use hand cream or lotion instead;
- Wear watches or jewelry loosely, if at all, on the operated arm;
- Wear protective gloves when gardening and when using strong detergents, etc.;
- Use a thimble when sewing;
- Avoid harsh chemicals and abrasive compounds;
- Use insect repellent to avoid bites and stings; and
- Avoid elastic cuffs on blouses and nightgowns.

Call your doctor at once if your arm becomes red, swollen, or feels hot. In the meantime, try to keep your arm over your head and periodically pump your fist.

Though you should be cautious, it's also important to use your arm normally—don't favor it or keep it dependent.

Recovering at Home

After breast surgery, there are a number of steps you can take to ensure a safe physical recovery. Your physical health will not be your only concern, however. A mastectomy often has a dramatic emotional impact as well.

Taking Care of Yourself

Once you are home, you should continue to exercise until you have regained the full use of your arm. As you increase your exercise and daily activities, be careful not to overdo. Take clues from your body; rest before you become overly tired.

To keep your skin soft and to promote healing, you may want to massage your incision gently with cocoa butter or vitamin E cream. As time goes by and the incision begins to heal, the redness, bruising, and swelling will disappear. As you are healing, be sure to watch for any signs of infection such as swelling, inflammation, tenderness, or drainage. If you see any of these signs or develop a fever, call your doctor.

Although each woman recovers from a mastectomy at her own rate, you will probably discover that within 2 to 3 weeks after surgery you will be doing most of the things you have always done. Within about 6 weeks you will be able to resume your normal activities. Over time the numbness under your arm will decrease, but total feeling may not return for a long time.

Adjusting Emotionally

After you've had a mastectomy, you'll have a lot of things on your mind. You may think about the fact that you've just been treated for a serious disease. You've had an operation that has changed your appearance, perhaps your self-image. You might wonder how the mastectomy will affect your lifestyle and your personal relationships. You might even be unsure how to act toward your family and friends.

Though every woman reacts to mastectomy differently, these types of concerns are common. Just as you will be taking action to help yourself physically recover from treatment, you can take steps to ease your emotional adjustment as well.

Expressing your feelings to your doctor and the people you love can be important emotional medicine. If you try to handle your problems alone, everyone will lose. You will lose chances to express yourself, your family and friends will lose opportunities to share your difficulties and help you work through them, and your doctor may not understand what you need to fully recover.

Remember, your family and close friends can be your strongest supporters. But chances are, they aren't quite sure how they can show their support. You can help them by being open and honest about the way you feel.

Others Are Willing To Help

In addition to talking with your doctor, your nurse, and the people closest to you, you may also want to talk with other women who have had similar experiences.

As described earlier, Reach to Recovery is an American Cancer Society program designed to help patients meet the physical, emotional, and cosmetic needs related to breast cancer and its treatment. Women who have had mastectomies volunteer to participate in the program by sharing their experiences with others. All volunteers are carefully selected and trained.

If your doctor authorizes a visit from a Reach to Recovery volunteer, she will contact you about an appointment while you are in the hospital or shortly after you go home. When you get together, she'll bring a kit containing a temporary breast form and information for husbands, children, other loved ones, and friends. She'll be prepared to discuss all aspects of mastectomy, including your personal concerns. Programs vary from city to city, so contact your local American Cancer Society chapter for more information.

ENCORE is a national YWCA discussion and exercise program for women who have had breast cancer. This once-a-week, 90-minute program consists of floor and swimming pool exercise sessions and group discussions. Contact your local YWCA for more information about ENCORE.

If informal approaches to dealing with your feelings don't work, consider professional help. Psychiatrists, psychologists, social workers, nurses, and religious counselors can help you adjust.

Intimacy

Whether you are single or married, you are likely to wonder how your mastectomy will affect your intimate relationships. Your partner will also have concerns. You can help each other by expressing them.

Intimate relationships are built on mutual love, trust, attraction, shared interests, common experiences, and a host of other feelings. A mastectomy will not necessarily change these feelings. What it may change is some of the physical aspects of love-making—what's pleasurable to you and what's not. It may also temporarily affect your partner's and your attitude toward intimacy.

After mastectomy you will still be the person your partner has come to love and enjoy. You can bring new closeness to your relationship by talking about the changes in your body, accepting them, and reaffirming your joy of being alive and being together.

At first, there may be some awkward moments. It may be helpful to let your partner see your body soon after surgery to decrease the anxiety both of you feel. Sometimes a partner is afraid that touching a mastectomy incision will hurt you. Let your partner know what's comfortable to you and what's not.

Sometimes a partner assumes that you will not be ready for sex for some time after surgery. Women often interpret this waiting as rejection. You may prevent this potential problem by letting your partner know when you feel ready for sex, that you still need your partner, and that it is important for you to know that your partner still finds you attractive and desirable.

Helping Children Cope

Children react to illness in a variety of ways. Some feel angry at their mothers for becoming ill. Others are frightened. Still others worry that they might have caused the illness.

Although you may be tempted to protect your children by not telling them about your operation or the disease that caused it, it's usually better to be honest. Even young children sense when something is wrong. Preschool children often feel deserted when their mother goes to the hospital. And if she returns feeling weak or depressed, they may become frightened. Adolescents sometimes suddenly change their behavior because they fear their mother's illness will keep them from maintaining the independence they have begun to enjoy. If you can avoid imposing too much responsibility on your teenage children, and if you share some of your feelings with them, you may be able to keep their problems to a minimum.

It is a good idea to tell your children the truth as simply and positively as possible. Be careful not to burden them with any more information than is necessary. Encourage their questions, and answer those questions honestly. You will probably find that talking helps your children to accept your illness and the temporary disruption it causes. A booklet that may be helpful to you is called *When Some In Your Family Has Cancer*. It is written for young people who have a parent or sibling with cancer and is available from the National Cancer Institute.

Common Questions About Breast Surgery

Q. Is breast surgery dangerous?
A. Doctors have been performing mastectomies for many years and are continuing to improve their techniques. There are risks associated with any kind of surgery, however. Risk depends on a lot of things, including your age, your medical history, your response to anesthesia, and your general health. After considering these factors, your doctor will recommend the type of surgery that will offer you the most benefit with the least amount of risk.

Q. How frequently should I plan to see a doctor after a mastectomy?
A. Your surgeon will tell you when to schedule your first postoperative exam. The two of you will then decide whether you should continue to make regular visits to the surgeon, or to a medical oncologist, an internist, a gynecologist, or a family practitioner. Most doctors believe that women treated for breast cancer should have professional exams every 3 to 6 months for the first 3 years after surgery. More information on followup exams, possible signs of recurrence, and taking care of yourself can be found in *After Breast Cancer: A Guide to Followup Care*, another booklet available from the National Cancer Institute.

Q. What is chemotherapy and when is it used?
A. Chemotherapy is the use of drugs to treat cancer. (Remember, a mastectomy treats only the cancer in the breast.) Anticancer drugs are used to reach areas of the body where cancer

cells may be hiding, and to destroy them before they multiply and hurt the normal cells and organs. More information on this supplementary treatment can be found in *Chemotherapy and You: A Guide to Self-Help During Treatment* and *Adjuvant Therapy: Facts for Women With Breast Cancer,* both of which are available from the National Cancer Institute.

Breast Self-Examination

After a mastectomy, breast self-examination (BSE) should be part of your routine. You will want to examine your natural breast and the surgical site once a month to note any changes in the way they look or feel. Though you may have been doing self-exams before your surgery, you will have to re-learn what's considered "normal" for you now. About half the women who have mastectomies report that their remaining breast becomes larger. For a step-by-step guide for performing a BSE, see page 454.

Shopping for a Permanent Prosthesis

Ask your doctor when it's appropriate for you to shop for a permanent breast form. You can probably begin shopping as soon as you're feeling strong and the swelling and tenderness are gone from the incision. If you are planning to have breast reconstruction, you may want a prosthesis before it's time for your surgery.

Breast forms are available in many shapes and sizes. Some prostheses feel like plastic bags, some are rubbery, some feel very much like skin. They may be covered with a soft fabric, polyurethane, or a silicone envelope, and they may be filled with foam rubber, water, air, chemical gel, polyethylene materials, polyurethane foam, silicone gel, or ceramic particles. Like natural breasts, prostheses vary in weight, and their consistency varies from very soft and pliable to relatively firm. Some brands have models specifically for the right or left side; some are made with a modified nipple and can be worn with or without a bra. Custom-made forms, which adhere to the chest wall and closely match the remaining breast, are also available.

Small prostheses, sometimes called equalizers, are available for women who have had lumpectomies or segmental mastectomies. Women whose reconstructive surgery does not replace the nipple or whose breast form does not have a nipple may choose a nipple prosthesis. Extremely lightweight forms are available to wear in a nightgown or with leisure clothes.

When selecting your prosthesis you'll also need to find a properly fitting bra that will hold the breast form in place. You may be able to wear the same bra you have always worn if it fits well and does not have underwires. Special post-mastectomy bras are available—they are built up to cover a larger area of the chest and have wider straps and pockets inside the cup to hold the prosthesis. You can sew a pocket into your swimsuit and your standard bras to keep the breast form in place.

Breast prostheses are sold in surgical supply stores, in lingerie and corset shops, and in the underwear departments of large department stores. Many stores that sell breast forms also carry lingerie and sportswear specially designed for women who have had mastectomies. Look in the *Yellow Pages* under "Brassieres" or "Surgical Appliances." Reach to Recovery volunteers can often provide information on types of permanent prostheses and a list of where they are available locally.

Before you go out to try various breast forms, you should call ahead and see if the supplier has a professional fitter to meet with you. More than a dozen different breast forms are on the market, and the only way to find the best one for you is to try them on. Your breast form should feel comfortable, have a natural contour and consistency, and remain in place when you move. It may feel heavy at first, but you will get used to the extra weight. Ask the fitter if the form absorbs perspiration or other chemicals from the skin and how to clean and care for your prosthesis. Most prostheses are guaranteed for 1 to 5 years.

Prices for breast forms range from $7 to $265. Custom-made forms are more expensive. The expense is covered, at least partly, by most medical insurance policies. A written prescription from your doctor will help ensure payment. If your insurance does not cover a prosthesis, you may be able to deduct the cost as a medical expense on your income tax.

If you want some emotional support when you shop, ask your partner or a good friend to go with you. Wear a form-fitting blouse or sweater so you can see how the form will make you look.

The most important thing to do is shop around. It's worth your time to find a prosthesis that feels comfortable and keeps you looking your best.

Glossary

Anesthesia. Entire or partial loss of feeling from the giving of drugs or gases.

Intravenous (IV). Being within or entering by way of the veins.

Lymph nodes. Part of the lymphatic system that removes wastes from body tissue and carries fluids that help the body fight infection.

Lymphedema. Swelling of the arm on the mastectomy side.

Mastectomy. Surgical removal of the breast.

Prosthesis. An artificial breast form (or any artificial replacement for a body part).

For More Information

The Cancer Information Service (CIS) is a nationwide toll-free telephone program sponsored by the National Cancer Institute. Trained information specialists are available to answer questions about cancer from the public, cancer patients and their families, and health professionals. By calling the following toll-free number, you will be automatically connected to the CIS office serving your area: 1-800-4-CANCER. Spanish-speaking CIS staff members are also available.

The National Cancer Institute has developed PDQ (Physician Data Query), a computerized database designed to give doctors quick and easy access to:

♦ The latest treatment information for most types of cancer.

♦ Descriptions of clinical trials that are open for patient entry.
♦ Names of organizations and physicians involved in cancer care.

To get access to PDQ, a doctor can use an office computer with a telephone hookup and a PDQ access code or the services of a medical library with online searching capability. Cancer Information Service offices (1-800-4-CANCER) provide free PDQ searches and can tell doctors how to get regular access to the database. Patients may ask their doctor to use PDQ or may call 1-800-4-CANCER themselves. Information specialists at this toll-free number use a variety of sources, including PDQ, to answer questions about cancer prevention, diagnosis, and treatment.

For a copy of the following booklets or other information about cancer, call the Cancer Information Service or write to the Office of Cancer Communications, National Cancer Institute, Building 31, Room 10A24, Bethesda, MD 20892.

♦ *Breast Exams: What You Should Know*
♦ *Questions and Answers About Breast Lumps*
♦ *Breast Biopsy: What You Should Know*
♦ *Breast Cancer: Understanding Treatment Options*
♦ *Radiation Therapy: A Treatment for Early Stage Breast Cancer*
♦ *Adjuvant Therapy: Facts for Women With Breast Cancer*
♦ *Breast Reconstruction: A Matter of Choice*
♦ *After Breast Cancer: A Guide to Followup Care*
♦ *When Cancer Recurs: Meeting the Challenge Again*
♦ *Advanced Cancer: Living Each Day*
♦ *When Someone In Your Family Has Cancer*

■ **Document Source:**
U.S. Department of Health and Human Services, Public Health Service
National Institutes of Health
National Cancer Institute
NIH Publication No. 91-658
Revised June 1990. Printed December 1990

See also: Breast Cancer (page 402); Breast Cancer: Understanding Treatment Options (page 406)

OSTEOPOROSIS

A major health problem, osteoporosis or "porous bone," affects an estimated 20 million Americans. This bone loss disease is most common in the elderly and in postmenopausal women. The loss of bone mass places extra stress on the thin, fragile bone structure that remains causing bones to be susceptible to fracture. Osteoporosis is estimated to cause 1.3 million bone fractures a year in people over 45 years of age. Moreover, in 1985, the national estimated cost of osteoporotic fractures was estimated to be $7 billion a year.

Osteoporosis-related fractures can occur in any of the bones, but the main fractures occur in the vertebral spinal column, the wrist, and the hip. In the spinal column, loss of bone mass starts in women during their 50s and 60s. A simple action like bending forward can be enough to cause a "crush fracture," or spinal compression fracture. These vertebral fractures cause loss of height and a humped back, or a "dowager's hump."

Wrist fractures called a "Colles fracture" also commonly occur among women with osteoporosis. Typically, the fracture occurs when a woman falls and uses her hand to break the fall; this results in a broken wrist.

Fractures of the hip are the most severe. They are associated with more death, more disability, and higher medical costs than all other osteoporotic fractures combined. Twelve to 20 percent of older people with hip fractures die within a year after the fracture. Of the survivors, only a few return to the full level of activities that they enjoyed before the hip fracture.

Risk Factors

Many risk factors for osteoporosis have been identified. They include:

♦ *age.* The chief risk factor for this disease is age; the likelihood of developing osteoporosis increases progressively as we grow older.
♦ *being a woman.* Osteoporosis is estimated to be six to eight times more common in women than in men. In early adult life women develop less bone mass than men do. Even more critical is that for years after menopause, women lose bone mass much more rapidly because of a reduction in their production of estrogen.
♦ *early menopause.* The chances of developing osteoporosis increase during early menopause or surgical menopause (after removal of the ovaries), which causes a sudden significant drop in estrogen.
♦ *being caucasian.* White women are at higher risk than black women, and white men are at higher risk than black men. In general, blacks have 10 percent greater bone mass than whites do.
♦ *a consistently low calcium intake.*
♦ *lack of weight-bearing exercise.* The significant loss of bone mass in our astronauts who spend considerable time in the weightless environment of outer space dramatically demonstrates the importance of weight-bearing exercise.
♦ *being underweight.*
♦ *a family history of osteoporosis.*
♦ *smoking cigarettes.* The concentration of estrogen in the bloodstream is lowered by cigarette smoking.
♦ *excessive use of cortisone-like drugs such as prednisone.*

Symptoms

Osteoporosis is a silent disease. Usually, it develops for many years until the bones become so weak that a minor injury can cause the bones to fracture. Detection of bone loss with ordinary x-rays does not show up until a person has lost 30 percent of their bone density.

Several techniques for early detection of bone loss have been developed in recent years. In one technique, photon absorptiometry, a machine measures how much the rays like x-rays penetrate the bone (measuring how dense the bones are). Another very useful technique is computerized tomography (CT), which uses x-rays that yield a three-dimensional image.

Bone Growth and Loss

Bone continues to grow and develop throughout childhood and adolescense. During a person's twenties, bone growth increases by 15 percent. Peak bone mass, when the bones are most dense and strong, occurs at 30 to 35 years of age. After this time bone mass gradually diminishes and the bones become less dense.

There is a great need to understand how bone grows and diminishes. By studying the cellular processes responsible for bone growth, researchers hope to discover new treatments for osteoporosis. There is much active and promising research in this area.

Treatment and Prevention

Scientists now know that a leading cause of osteoporosis in women is postmenopausal estrogen deficiency. They have discovered that estrogen not only slows bone loss but also prevents bone fractures if given when a woman's production of estrogen drops. It is important that the hormone be given during or shortly after menopause because estrogen given years later is of less value. Women who have gone through menopause, and especially those with an early or surgical menopause, should discuss the benefits and risks of estrogen replacement therapy with their physicians.

Another benefit of estrogen therapy is its positive effect on the cardiovascular system. Estrogen reduces cholesterol and the concentration of other lipids (fats) in the bloodstream associated with heart disease. For women on estrogen therapy, the risk of developing endometrial cancer increases from one per 1,000 women to about four per 1,000 women. Fortunately, endometrial cancer is easy to detect and is highly curable. In fact, the death rate from endometrial cancer is lower than the death rate for osteoporotic hip fracture.

One side effect women on estrogen replacement therapy may experience is periodic bleeding. This is because estrogen therapy causes the lining of the uterus to build up. Estrogen usually is prescribed for 20 days, then the hormone is stopped for the remaining 10 days. The lining of the uterus is shed during the days off estrogen.

Progestogen, another female hormone, given in combination with estrogen may help reduce the risk of endometrial cancer. Women in the menopausal period are encouraged to discuss estrogen or progestogen therapy with their doctors.

Calcium Intake

The average American consumes about 450 to 550 milligrams of calcium a day. Experts recommend that both men and women take at least 1,000 milligrams of calcium daily. This is the amount of calcium contained in three eight-ounce glasses of milk. Other sources of calcium include yogurt, cheese, salmon, canned sardines, oysters, shrimp, dried beans, and dark green vegetables such as broccoli, turnip greens, and kale.

People who do not meet their daily requirements of calcium through their diet are encouraged to take a daily supplement of calcium such as calcium carbonate, calcium lactate, calcium gluconate, or calcium citrate. Older men and women should increase their calcium intake up to 1,200 to 1,500 milligrams a day, or about four to five glasses of milk, because calcium absorption from the digestive tract is reduced in the elderly.

Exercise

Research has shown clearly that inactivity leads to bone loss. Studies revealed that astronauts in space lost a great deal of bone from lack of exercise against gravity. A program of moderate weight-bearing exercise three to four hours a week, such as brisk walking, running, tennis, or aerobic dance, is recommended. Swimming is not as valuable because it is not a weight-bearing exercise.

Experimental Treatments

Several promising treatments for osteoporosis are being investigated. Calcitonin, a new drug approved by the Food and Drug Administration in 1984, slows the breakdown of bone. Calcitonin, produced naturally in the body, is a hormone produced by the thyroid gland. The synthetic form is given by daily injection and is expensive. Recently, a less expensive nasal spray of calcitonin has been developed.

Scientists also are studying fluoride combined with calcium for osteoporosis. Still experimental, flouride is promising in that it has been shown to increase bone mass. Some people experience side effects including nausea, vomiting, diarrhea, and pain in their lower extremities. Fluoride compounds currently are available for treatment in Germany and France. However, more research is needed before this treatment can be proven to be both safe and effective.

Research Direction

This booklet has described the steps to be taken to protect the bones. Recent studies on nutrition is one new area of research. Clinicians know that by taking calcium at the right time in life there is hope of preventing bone loss. Researchers also know more about exercise as a method of preventing osteoporosis.

Until recently, there were no clues as to how the hormone, estrogen, prevented osteoporosis. Now investigators have reported the discovery of estrogen receptors on bone. New methods might be harnessed to treat osteoporosis. Through continued research, there is hope for future treatments of osteoporosis.

■ **Document Source:**
U.S. Department of Health and Human Services, Public Health Service
National Institutes of Health
National Institute of Arthritis and Musculoskeletal and Skin Diseases

NIH Publication No. 89-2893
April 1989

CancerFax from the National Cancer Institute
OVARIAN EPITHELIAL CANCER

Description

What Is Cancer of the Ovary?

Cancer of the ovary, a common cancer in women, is a disease in which cancer (malignant) cells are found in the ovary. The ovary is a small organ in the pelvis that makes female hormones and holds egg cells that can develop into a baby. There are two ovaries: one located on the left side of the uterus (the hollow, pear-shaped organ where a baby grows) and one located on the right. This PDQ statement has information on cancer that occurs in the lining (epithelium) of the ovary. Cancer that is found in the egg-making cells in the ovary is called a germ cell tumor of the ovary, and is explained in a separate PDQ patient information statement.

Like most cancers, cancer of the ovary is best treated when it is found (diagnosed) early. You should see a doctor if you have any of the following problems: abdominal swelling or bloating, discomfort in the lower part of your abdomen, feeling full after a light meal, nausea or vomiting, not feeling hungry, gas, indigestion, losing weight, constant need to go to the bathroom, diarrhea or constipation, or bleeding that is not part of your periods (menstruation). If your female relatives by birth, especially your mother, sister, or daughter, have had ovarian cancer, you have a greater chance of getting it and should see your doctor regularly to be checked.

Your chance of recovery (prognosis) and choice of treatment depend on your age, your general state of health, the type and size of your tumor, and the stage of your cancer.

Cancer of the ovary can be hard to find early. Often there are no symptoms in the very early stages, and many women have cancer that has spread to other parts of the body when it is found. Because cancer of the ovary may spread to the sac inside the abdomen that holds the intestines, uterus, and ovaries (peritoneum), many women with cancer of the ovary may have fluid inside the peritoneum (called ascites), which causes swelling of the abdomen. If the cancer has spread to the muscle under the lung that controls breathing (the diaphragm), fluid may build up under the lungs and cause shortness of breath.

Your doctor will use several tests to see if you have cancer, usually beginning by giving you an internal (pelvic) exam. Your doctor may feel for lumps or changes in the shape of the pelvic organs. A Pap test may also be done, using a piece of cotton, a small wooden stick, or brush to scrape gently the outside of the cervix (opening of the uterus) and the vagina to pick up cells. Because the ovaries are above the cervix, this cancer does not usually show on the Pap test. Blood and urine tests and an ultrasound exam may be done. During the ultrasound exam, sound waves are used to find tumors.

Stage Explanation

Stages of Cancer of the Ovary

Once cancer of the ovary has been found, more tests will be done to find out if the cancer has spread to other parts of the body (staging). Unless your doctor is sure the cancer has spread from the ovaries to other parts of the body, an operation called a laparotomy will be done to help stage your cancer. Your doctor must cut into your abdomen and carefully look at all the organs to see if they contain cancer. During the operation your doctor will cut out small pieces of tissue (biopsy) so they can be looked at under a microscope to see whether they contain cancer. Usually your doctor will remove the cancer and other organs that contain cancer during the laparotomy (see section on How Cancer of the Ovary is Treated). Your doctor needs to know the stage of your disease to plan further treatment. The following stages are used for cancer of the ovary:

Stage I
Cancer is found only in one or both of the ovaries.

Stage II
Cancer is found in one or both ovaries and/or has spread to the uterus, and/or the fallopian tubes (the pathway used by the egg to get from the ovary to the uterus), and/or other body parts within the pelvis.

Stage III
Cancer is found in one or both ovaries and has spread to lymph nodes or to other body parts inside the abdomen, such as the surface of the liver or intestine. (Lymph nodes are small bean-shaped structures that are found throughout the body. They produce and store infection-fighting cells.)

Stage IV
Cancer is found in one or both ovaries and has spread outside the abdomen or has spread to the inside of the liver.

Recurrent or refractory
Recurrent disease means that the cancer has come back (recurred) after it has been treated. It may come back in the ovary that is left or in another place. Refractory disease means the cancer did not respond to the initial therapy.

Treatment Options Overview

How Cancer of the Ovary Is Treated

There are treatments for all patients with cancer of the ovary. Three kinds of treatments are used:

surgery (taking out the cancer in an operation)
radiation therapy (using high-energy x-rays to kill cancer cells)
chemotherapy (using drugs to kill cancer cells).

Surgery is the most common treatment for cancer of the ovary. Your doctor may take out the cancer in an operation called a total abdominal hysterectomy and bilateral salpingo-oophorectomy. In this operation, the ovaries, fallopian tubes, and uterus are taken out. Your doctor may also take out the area of tissue that stretches from the stomach to the nearby organs in the abdomen in an operation called an omentectomy. If only one ovary is taken out along with the fallopian tube on the same side of the body, the operation is called a unilateral salpingo-oophorectomy. Tumor debulking means taking out as much of the cancer as possible.

Radiation therapy uses high-energy x-rays to kill cancer cells and shrink tumors. Radiation may come from a machine outside the body (external beam radiation therapy) or it may be put directly into the sac that lines the abdomen (peritoneum) in a liquid that is radioactive (intraperitoneal radiation).

Chemotherapy uses drugs to kill cancer cells. It may be taken by pill or put into the body by a needle in a vein. Chemotherapy is called a systemic treatment because the drugs enter the bloodstream, travel through the body, and kill cancer cells outside the ovaries. Chemotherapy can also be given by a needle put through the abdominal wall into the peritoneum (intraperitoneally).

Treatment by Stage

Treatment for cancer of the ovary depends on the stage of your disease, the type of disease, your age, and your overall condition.

You may receive treatment that is considered standard based on its effectiveness in a number of patients in past studies, or you may choose to go into a clinical trial. Not all patients are cured with standard therapy and some standard treatments may have more side effects than are desired. For these reasons, clinical trials are designed to find better ways to treat cancer patients and are based on the most up-to-date information. Clinical trials are going on in most parts of the country for most stages of cancer of the ovary. If you want more information, call the Cancer Information Service at 1-800-4-CANCER (1-800-422-6237).

Treatment options: Stage I ovarian epithelial cancer
Your treatment may be one of the following:
1. Surgery to remove the cancer, both ovaries, the fallopian tubes, uterus, and part of the tissue that stretches from the stomach to nearby organs in the abdomen (omentum). This is called a total abdominal hysterectomy and bilateral salpingo-oophorectomy with omentectomy. During surgery, samples of lymph nodes and other tissues in the pelvis and abdomen are cut out (biopsied) and checked for cancer.
2. Surgery to remove the ovary in which the cancer is found and the fallopian tube on the same side of the body (unilateral salpingo-oophorectomy), in selected patients who wish to have children at a later time. Lymph nodes and other tissues in the pelvis and abdomen are biopsied during surgery.
3. Total abdominal hysterectomy and bilateral salpingo-oophorectomy with omentectomy and biopsy of lymph nodes and other tissues in the pelvis and abdomen, followed by intraperitoneal radiation therapy.
4. Total abdominal hysterectomy and bilateral salpingo-oophorectomy with omentectomy and biopsy of lymph nodes and other tissues in the

pelvis and abdomen, followed by systemic chemotherapy.
5. Total abdominal hysterectomy and bilateral salpingo-oophorectomy with omentectomy and biopsy of lymph nodes and other tissues in the pelvis and abdomen, followed by external beam radiation therapy to the abdomen and pelvis.

Treatment options: Stage II ovarian epithelial cancer
Your treatment will probably be surgery to remove both ovaries, both fallopian tubes, the uterus, and as much of the cancer as possible (total abdominal hysterectomy and bilateral salpingo-oophorectomy with tumor debulking). During the surgery, samples of lymph nodes and other tissues in the pelvis and abdomen are cut out (biopsied) and checked for cancer. After the operation, your treatment may be one of the following:
1. Systemic chemotherapy. Clinical trials are testing new drugs and combinations of drugs.
2. External beam radiation therapy to the abdomen and pelvis.
3. Intraperitoneal radiation therapy when only a small amount of tumor is found.

Treatment options: Stage III ovarian epithelial cancer.
Your treatment will probably be surgery to remove both ovaries, both fallopian tubes, the uterus, and as much of the cancer as possible (total abdominal hysterectomy and bilateral salpingo-oophorectomy with tumor debulking). During the surgery, samples of lymph nodes and other tissues in the pelvis and abdomen are cut out (biopsied) and checked for cancer. After the operation, your treatment may be one of the following:
1. Systemic chemotherapy. Clinical trials are testing new drugs and combinations of drugs.
2. External beam radiation therapy to the abdomen and pelvis.
3. Clinical trials of intraperitoneal chemotherapy.

Your doctor may operate again to look for any remaining cancer.

Treatment: Stage IV ovarian epithelial cancer
Your treatment will probably be surgery to remove as much of the cancer as possible (tumor debulking), followed by one of the following:
1. Systemic chemotherapy. Clinical trials are testing new drugs and combinations of drugs.
2. Clinical trials of intraperitoneal chemotherapy if the cancer has not spread outside the abdomen.

Treatment options: Recurrent ovarian epithelial cancer
If the cancer comes back, your treatment may be one of the following:
1. Surgery to relieve symptoms.
2. Systemic chemotherapy. Clinical trials are testing new drugs and combinations of drugs.
3. Clinical trials of intraperitoneal chemotherapy.

To learn more about cancer of the ovary, call the National Cancer Institute's Cancer Information Service at 1-800-4-CANCER (1-800-422-6237). By dialing this toll-free number, you can speak with someone who can answer your questions.

■ Document Source:
   National Cancer Institute
     Building 31, Room 10A24, 9000 Rockville Pike, Bethesda, MD
       20892
     POQ 208/00950
     02/01/94

See also: Chemotherapy and You: A Guide to Self-Help During Treatment (page 40); Radiation Therapy and You: A Guide to Self-Help During Treatment (page 56)

RADIATION THERAPY: A TREATMENT FOR EARLY STAGE BREAST CANCER

Radiation therapy as primary treatment for breast cancer is a promising technique for women who have early stage breast cancer. This procedure, which allows a woman to keep her breast, involves removing the lump or cancerous tissue from the breast (**lumpectomy***) and some or all of the underarm **lymph nodes.** The breast is then treated with radiation (x-ray).

During the last 20 years, considerable experience has been gained with this form of treatment. Research comparing this treatment with the traditional surgical approach, **mastectomy,** is continuing. Preliminary research results are encouraging, though data on the long-term effects are still being collected. At present, the survival rates for women with early stage breast cancer who are treated with radiation therapy seem to be equal to those for women treated by mastectomy.

This booklet describes the procedures used in radiation therapy and tells you what to expect—from the beginning of your treatment to your recovery at home. After reading this booklet and discussing it with your doctor, you may want to talk with another woman who has had radiation therapy to treat her breast cancer. She may have some practical advice and be able to answer some of your questions.

Informed Consent: When Treatment Is Recommended

When treatment is recommended, most health care facilities now require patients to sign a form stating their willingness to proceed. This is to certify that you understand what procedures will be done and have consented to have them performed.

Consent to treatment is only meaningful if given by a patient who has had an opportunity to learn about recommended alternatives and to evaluate them. Before consenting to any course of treatment, be sure your doctor lets you know:

- ♦ The recommended procedure;
- ♦ Its purpose;
- ♦ Risks and side effects associated with it;
- ♦ Likely consequences with and without treatment;
- ♦ Other available alternatives; and
- ♦ Advantages and disadvantages of one treatment over another.

Even if you want your doctor to assume full responsibility for all decision making, you are likely to discover that your concerns about treatment decrease as your understanding of breast cancer and its treatment increases.

Questions To Ask Your Doctor

Before Radiation Therapy

- ♦ What kind of procedure are you recommending?
- ♦ What are the potential risks and benefits?
- ♦ Am I a candidate for any other type of procedure?
- ♦ What are the risks and benefits of those alternatives?
- ♦ How should I expect to look after the treatment?
- ♦ How should I expect to feel?

After Radiation Therapy

- ♦ When will I be able to get back into my normal routine?
- ♦ What can I do to ensure a safe recovery?
- ♦ What problems, if any, should I report to you?
- ♦ What type of exercises should I do?
- ♦ How frequently should I see you for a checkup?

Treatment Steps

Once the lump has been removed and breast cancer has been diagnosed, radiation treatment usually involves the following steps:

- ♦ Surgery to remove some or all of the underarm lymph nodes;
- ♦ External radiation therapy to the breast and surrounding area; and
- ♦ "Booster" radiation therapy to the biopsy site.

Lymph Node Surgery

Before radiation therapy begins, some or all of the underarm lymph nodes are usually removed to determine if the cancer has spread beyond the breast. If all of the lymph nodes are removed, the surgery is called **axillary dissection;** if only some of the lymph nodes are removed, it is called **axillary sampling.** Other tests such as bone and liver scans may also be done to provide your doctor with valuable information needed to plan further treatment. This process is known as "staging" the disease.

---

* Boldface words are defined in the glossary.

Hospital procedures and policies vary, but there are a number of things you can probably expect to have happen when you check in for lymph node surgery.

In the Hospital. You will probably be admitted the afternoon before your surgery so that some routine tests, such as blood and urine tests and a chest x-ray, can be performed. Shortly before the operation, the surgical area (underarm) will be shaved, and you may be given some medication to help you relax.

When it is time for your surgery, you will be taken to the operating room and an **anesthesiologist** will put you to sleep. Electrocardiogram sensors will be attached to your arms and legs with adhesive pads to monitor your heart rate during surgery. The surgical area will be cleaned, and sterile sheets will be draped over your body, except for the area around the operation. An axillary dissection usually takes several hours; an axillary sampling, about an hour.

When you awaken from surgery, you will be in the recovery room. Your underarm area will be bandaged, and a tube may be in place at the surgical site to drain any fluid that may accumulate. Your throat may be sore from the tube that was placed in it to carry air to your lungs during surgery. You may also feel a little nauseated and have a dry mouth—these are common side effects of anesthesia.

You will spend an hour or so in the recovery room. Oxygen will be available in case you need it to ease your breathing. Wires may be taped to your chest to measure your heartbeat. An intravenous (IV) tube will be in a vein in your arm to give fluid, nourishment, or medication after surgery. The IV tube will probably be removed after you begin to drink and eat.

It's common to feel drowsy for several hours after surgery. You may feel some discomfort under your arm; some women experience numbness, tingling, or pain in the chest, shoulder area, and upper arm. Your doctor will prescribe medication to relieve any discomfort you may have following your surgery. The numbness under your arm will decrease gradually, but total feeling may not return for a long time.

After you return to your room, a nurse will check your temperature, pulse, blood pressure, and bandage. She will ask you to turn, cough, and breathe deeply to keep your lungs clear after the anesthesia. You may also be encouraged to move your feet and legs to improve your blood circulation. Although each woman reacts to surgery differently, you will probably discover that by the next day you will be able to sit up in bed and walk from your bed to a chair in your room. Your doctor will probably encourage you to walk around and eat solid food as soon as possible.

After Surgery. At first you will have to be careful not to move your arm too much. But by the second or third day, you may be ready to begin exercises to ease the tension in your arm and shoulder. Women who have axillary sampling usually recover their arm motion fairly quickly because their surgery is not as extensive as axillary dissection.

You will be taking sponge baths for a few days after surgery until your incision starts to heal. Before you leave the hospital, ask the doctor or nurse for instructions on taking care of your incision. When you have permission to bathe or shower, do so gently and pat, don't rub, the area of your incision.

The average stay in the hospital for an axillary dissection is 7 to 10 days, and 2 to 4 days for an axillary sampling. Before you leave, the tube that drains fluid from your incision will be removed. Your stitches will be taken out in 1 to 3 weeks at the doctor's office or clinic.

Once you are home, you should continue to exercise until you have regained the full use of your arm. As you increase your exercise and begin to renew your daily activities, you must be careful not to overexert yourself. Take clues from your body; rest before you become tired.

To keep your skin soft and to promote healing, you may want to massage your incision gently with cocoa butter or vitamin E cream. As time goes by, the redness, bruising, and swelling will disappear. But you should watch for any signs of infection such as inflammation, tenderness, or drainage. If you develop any of these signs or a fever, call your doctor. Although each woman recovers from surgery at her own rate, most women are ready for the next part of their treatment, radiation therapy, about 1 or 2 weeks after their lymph node surgery.

Exercising After Surgery. Exercising will help you ease the tension in your arm and shoulder and will hasten your recovery. It is especially important for women who have had an axillary dissection. You will probably be able to begin exercising within a few days of your operation. Your doctor, nurse, or physical therapist can show you what exercises to do.

Ask your doctor if you might begin with these few simple movements:

- Lie in bed with your arm at your side. Raise your arm straight up and back, trying to touch the headboard behind you.
- Raise your shoulders. Rotate them forward, down, and back in a circular motion to loosen your chest, shoulder, and upper back muscles.
- Lying in bed, clasp your hands behind your head and push your elbows into the mattress.
- With your elbow bent and your arm at a 90 degree angle to your body, rotate your shoulder forward until the forearm is down and then backward until it is up.
- With your arm raised, clench and unclench your fist.
- Breathe deeply.
- Rotate your chin to the left and right. Cock your head sideways.

The key is to exercise only to the point of pulling or pain—don't push yourself.

External Radiation Therapy

During this procedure, high-energy x-rays are aimed at the breast and sometimes at nearby areas that still contain some lymph nodes, such as under the arm (if only a "sampling" was done), above the collarbone, and along the breastbone. The goal of radiation therapy is to destroy any cancer cells that may still remain in the breast or surrounding lymph node areas.

These high-energy x-rays are delivered by a linear accelerator or a cobalt machine. The difference between the two machines is simply that the beams are produced by different energy sources.

Often, a patient's first visit to the radiation department takes 1 to 2 hours and doesn't involve any treatments. You will probably talk with the radiation therapist, a physician with special training in the use of radiation, who will review your records and decide the best way to proceed with your treatment.

You will probably also meet the technician who delivers the treatment, and the radiation therapy nurse, who works closely with the doctor and can answer any questions you have about treatment, potential side effects, and what you can do about them.

During the first visit, ink lines or small tattoo marks will be drawn on your skin around the treatment area to mark exactly where to aim the radiation. The marks are generally made with permanent ink, and you should not attempt to wash them off until treatment is completed. These marks ensure that the area treated is the same every day. Many women wear old under-clothes during treatment because the marking may stain clothing.

The radiation therapist will consult with the dosimetrist, who computes the dosages of radiation. The standard treatment for early stage breast cancer is almost always 4,400 to 5,000 **rads** (radiation absorbed dose). A rad refers to the amount of radiation that is absorbed by the breast tissue.

Your actual number of treatments will depend on the total dose you need. Usually, treatments are given 5 days a week, Monday through Friday, for about 5 weeks. To protect normal tissue, it is better to give a little radiation each day than to give a lot of radiation all at once. A single treatment takes about 20 to 25 minutes. Only a few minutes of this time are of exposure to radiation; most of the time is spent putting the patient in position. Most people continue to work or pursue other activities throughout the treatment period.

It is very important to have all your treatments. However, if you have to miss a treatment, it can be made up. If you do not finish the full course, you may not have gotten enough radiation to destroy the cancer cells.

For more information about what to expect during radiation therapy, contact the National Cancer Institute for a copy of *Radiation Therapy and You: A Guide to Self-Help During Treatment.*

"Booster" Radiation Therapy

About 1 or 2 weeks after the external radiation therapy has been completed, nearly all women will receive a concentrated "booster" dose of radiation to the area where the breast lump was located.

This treatment may be done either externally, using an electron beam, or internally, using an implant of radioactive material. The electron beam "booster" is delivered by a type of linear accelerator machine similar to the one used in external radiation therapy. The treatment procedure is also similar to that of external radiation therapy, with the patient coming to the hospital daily for 5 to 10 days. If you have this type of booster treatment, you may notice an increase in skin redness at the site of the electron beam treatments—this is normal.

The implant procedure requires a short hospital stay of 2 to 3 days. Thin plastic tubes are threaded through the breast tissue where the original lump was removed. This may be done using either a local or general anesthesia. The number and location of the tubes depend on the size and location of the tumor that was removed. The doctor may take an x-ray of your breast after inserting the tubes to make sure they are in the correct position. When you return to your hospital room, radioactive seeds (usually iridium) will be inserted into the tubes. The implant will remain in your breast for 2 to 3 days, during which time it will deliver approximately 2,000 rads to the surrounding tissue.

While the implant is in place, you will stay in a private room because the implant emits small amounts of radiation, which may be a possible risk to those who come in close contact with you. For that reason, visitors and the nursing staff will have to limit their time with you.

You may notice some breast sensitivity around the area of the implant, especially if you move around a lot, but you should not have much pain or other discomfort. If you are uncomfortable, ask your nurse for some pain medication. You'll be free to move around your room, sit and read, do needlework or write letters.

The implant will be removed in your room, without anesthesia. The process feels very much like having stitches taken out. Once it is removed there is no risk of radiation exposure to others and you can usually go home.

Side Effects of Radiation Therapy

During Treatment

Many women feel mildly to moderately tired during radiation therapy, especially as treatments progress. Treatment for cancer can be stressful and the daily trips to the hospital take a lot of energy. Try to rest as much as you can and plan your activities at levels that are comfortable for you. Don't push yourself. It is especially important to eat properly while you are having radiation treatments, because your body needs wholesome food to restore its strength and to repair injured cells. It's also important for you to maintain your weight. Even if you are overweight, do not try to lose weight until you have finished all of your treatments.

The skin around the treated area may begin to look reddened, irritated, tanned, or sunburned. In some women the skin becomes quite dry; in others it becomes very moist, especially under the breast fold. These side effects are most likely to occur toward the end of treatment.

Be gentle with your skin. Try not to irritate it. Don't use perfumed or deodorant soaps, ointments, or anything besides lukewarm water and plain soap (such as Ivory) on your breast. Some women wear soft cotton bras, without wiring, or go braless whenever possible. Some like to wear a soft T-shirt or other loose clothing.

Your doctor and nurse will be watching you closely as treatment progresses. Be sure to mention any side effects you may have.

After Treatment

You may notice other changes in your breast due to the radiation therapy and changes may continue for 6 to 12 months after treatment. As the redness goes away, you will notice a slight darkening of the skin—as when a sunburn fades to a suntan. The pores may be enlarged and more noticeable.

You may have some change in skin sensitivity—some women report increased sensation, others have decreased feeling. The skin and the fatty tissue of the breast may feel thicker, and you may notice that your breast is firmer than it was before your radiation treatment. Some older women have said that their breast feels and looks as it did when they were in their twenties. Others report a change in the size of the treated breast—it may become larger because of fluid buildup or smaller because of development of fibrous tissue, but many women have little or no change at all.

After 10 to 12 months, you should notice few additional changes caused by the radiation therapy. If changes in size, shape, appearance, or texture occur after this time, report them to your doctor at once.

Precautions

A problem that may arise after treatment for breast cancer is swelling of the arm on the side of the treatment. This condition, called **lymphedema,** is caused by the loss or damage of underarm lymph nodes and their connecting vessels. It occurs because circulation of lymph fluid is slowed in the arm, making it harder to fight infection. You should take special care of your arm to prevent infection.

Follow these simple rules:

♦ Avoid burns while cooking or smoking;
♦ Avoid sunburns;
♦ Have all injections, vaccinations, blood samples, and blood pressure tests done on the other arm whenever possible;
♦ Use an electric razor with a narrow head for underarm shaving to reduce the risk of nicks or scratches;
♦ Carry heavy packages or handbags on the other arm;
♦ Wash cuts promptly, treat them with antibacterial medication, and cover them with a sterile dressing; check often for redness, soreness, or other signs of infection;
♦ Never cut cuticles; use hand cream or lotion;
♦ Wear watches or jewelry loosely, if at all, on the operated arm;
♦ Wear protective gloves when gardening and when using strong detergents, etc.;
♦ Use a thimble when sewing;
♦ Avoid harsh chemicals and abrasive compounds;
♦ Use insect repellent to avoid bites and stings; and
♦ Avoid elastic cuffs on blouses and nightgowns.

Call your doctor at once if your arm becomes red, swollen, or feels hot. In the meantime, put your arm over your head and alternately squeeze and relax your fist.

Though you should be cautious, it's also important to use your arm normally—don't favor it or keep it dependent.

Common Questions About Radiation Therapy

Q. Will radiation affect my normal cells?
A. Radiation is a strong treatment for cancer and can sometimes affect normal cells. However, normal cells are not as sensitive to radiation and will usually recover when treatment is finished.

Q. Will anything be done to protect me from excess radiation?
A. The x-ray machine with which you'll be treated has special protections built in to limit your radiation to the specific area outlined. If needed, other areas of your body will be covered by special lead shields.

Q. What will radiation feel like during the treatment?
A. Radiation treatment is like having a regular x-ray; most patients feel no sensation. You may feel warmth or a tingling, but you're not likely to feel any pain or discomfort.

Q. Will I be radioactive after treatments?
A. No. The treatment beam is the only thing that is radioactive when you receive external radiation therapy. Neither your normal tissues nor the cancerous tissues are radioactive during or after treatment. If you have a radiation implant, small amounts of radiation will be emitted. However, once the implant is removed, you are no longer radioactive.

Q. What will my breast look like after treatment?
A. There is no way to predict the cosmetic outcome of this type of treatment for a particular woman. The extent of the initial surgery, the size of the breast, the type of incision, and the effects of radiation on the skin are all factors. However, the breast usually looks quite normal and most women are pleased that they chose this breast-saving treatment.

Q. What is chemotherapy and when is it used?
A. Chemotherapy is the use of drugs to destroy cancer cells. Anticancer drugs are used to reach areas of the body where cancer cells may be hiding, and to eliminate them before they multiply and hurt the normal cells and organs. More information on this supplementary treatment can be found in *Chemotherapy and You: A Guide to Self-Help During Treatment* and *Adjuvant Therapy: Facts for Women With Breast Cancer,* both of which are available from the National Cancer Institute.

Q. How frequently should I plan to see a doctor after radiation therapy treatment?
A. Your doctor will tell you when to schedule your first post-treatment exam. The two of you will then decide whether you should continue to make regular visits to him or her or to a medical oncologist, an internist, a gynecologist, or a family practitioner. Most doctors believe that women treated for breast cancer should have professional exams every 3 to 6 months for the first 3 years after surgery. More information on followup exams, possible signs of recurrence, and taking care of yourself can be found in *After Breast Cancer: A Guide to Followup Care,* another booklet available from the National Cancer Institute.

Adjusting Emotionally

After you have completed treatment, you'll have a lot of things on your mind. You may think about the fact that you've just been treated for a serious disease and hope this treatment will control your cancer forever. Breast cancer often has a dramatic emotional impact and you may be wondering how it will affect your lifestyle and your personal relationships. You might even be unsure how to act toward your family and friends.

Although every woman reacts to breast cancer differently, these types of concerns are common. Just as you will be taking action to help yourself physically recover from treatment, you can take steps to ease your emotional adjustment as well.

Expressing your feelings to your doctor and the people you love can be important emotional medicine. If you try to handle your problems alone, everyone will lose: you will lose chances to express yourself, your family and friends will lose opportunities to share your difficulties and help you work through them, and your doctor may not understand what you need to fully recover.

Remember, your family and close friends can be your strongest supporters. But chances are, they aren't quite sure how they can show their support. You can help them by being open and honest about the way you feel.

If informal approaches to dealing with your feelings don't work, consider professional help. Psychiatrists, psychologists, social workers, nurses, and religious counselors can help your emotional adjustment.

Others Are Willing to Help

You may also want to talk with other women who have had similar experiences. Reach to Recovery is an American Cancer Society program designed to help breast cancer patients meet the physical, emotional, and cosmetic needs related to cancer and its treatment. Women who have had radiation therapy to treat their breast cancer volunteer to participate in the program by providing practical information and sharing their experiences with others. All volunteers are carefully selected and trained.

Programs vary from city to city. Call your local American Cancer Society unit for more information or contact departments of radiation therapy at major medical centers.

Intimacy

Whether you are single or married, you are likely to wonder how your treatment for breast cancer will affect your intimate relationships. Your partner will also have concerns. You can help each other by expressing them.

Intimate relationships are built on mutual love, trust, attraction, shared interests, common experiences, and a host of other feelings. Breast cancer treatment will not necessarily change these feelings. What it may change is some of the physical aspects of lovemaking—what's pleasurable to you and what's not. It may also temporarily affect your partner's and your attitudes toward intimacy.

Because fatigue often is associated with radiation treatment, you may need additional rest. You can continue to enjoy an intimate relationship by planning special time to spend alone with your partner.

Sometimes a partner is afraid that touching the treated breast will hurt you. Let your partner know what's comfortable to you and what's not. You can bring new closeness to your relationship by talking about your treatment and the way you feel.

Helping Children Cope

Children react to illness in a variety of ways. Some feel angry at their mothers for becoming ill. Others are frightened. Still others worry that they might have caused the illness.

Although you may be tempted to protect your children by not telling them about your disease and its treatment, it's usually better to be honest. Even young children sense when something is wrong. Preschool children often feel deserted when their mother goes to the hospital. And if she returns feeling weak or depressed, they may become frightened. Teenagers sometimes suddenly change their behavior because they fear their mother's illness will keep them from maintaining the independence they have begun to enjoy. If you can avoid imposing too much responsibility on your teenage children, and if you share some of your feelings with them, you may be able to keep their problems to a minimum.

It is a good idea to tell your children the truth as simply and positively as possible. Be careful not to burden them with any more information than is necessary. Encourage their questions, and answer those questions honestly. You will probably find that talking helps your children to accept your illness and the temporary disruption it causes.

Breast Self-Examination

After radiation therapy, breast self-examination (BSE) should continue to be part of your routine. You will want to examine your breasts and your scar (if you had the lymph nodes removed) once a month to note any changes in the way they look or feel. Though you may have been doing BSE before your treatment, you will have to relearn what's considered "normal" for you now.

If you menstruate, the best time to do BSE is 2 or 3 days after your period ends, when your breasts are least likely to be tender or swollen. If you no longer menstruate, pick a day, such as the first day of the month, to do BSE. See page 454 for an example of how to perform a BSE.

For More Information

The Cancer Information Service (CIS) is a nationwide toll-free telephone program sponsored by the National Cancer Institute. Trained information specialists are available to answer questions about cancer from the public, cancer patients and their families, and health professionals. By calling the following toll-free number, you will be automatically connected to the CIS office serving your area: 1-800-4-CANCER. Spanish speaking staff members are also available.

The National Cancer Institute also has developed PDQ (Physician Data Query), a computerized database designed to give doctors quick and easy access to:

♦ The latest treatment information for most types of cancer.

♦ Descriptions of clinical trials that are open for patient entry.

♦ Names of organizations and physicians involved in cancer care.

To get access to PDQ, a doctor can use an office computer with a telephone hookup and a PDQ access code or the services of a medical library with online searching capability. Most Cancer Information Service offices (1-800-4-CANCER) provide physicians with free PDQ searches and can tell doctors how to get regular access to the database. Patients may ask their doctor to use PDQ or may call 1-800-4-CANCER themselves. Information specialists at this toll-free number use a variety of sources, including PDQ, to answer questions about cancer prevention, diagnosis, and treatment.

Glossary

Anesthesiologist. A doctor who administers drugs or gases to put a patient to sleep before surgery.

Axillary dissection. Removal of all the underarm lymph nodes.

Axillary sampling. Removal of some of the underarm lymph nodes.

Chemotherapy. Treatment with drugs to destroy cancer cells. Most often used to supplement surgery or radiation therapy.

Lumpectomy. Surgical removal of the lump or cancerous tissue from the breast and some or all of the underarm lymph nodes. Also sometimes called "local excision" or "tylectomy."

Lymph nodes. Part of the lymphatic system that removes wastes from body tissue and carries fluids that help the body fight infection.

Lymphedema. Swelling in the arm caused by excess fluid that collects when the lymph nodes and vessels are removed during surgery or damaged by radiation therapy.

Mastectomy. Surgical removal of the breast.

Rad. Stands for "radiation absorbed dose." A unit of measurement for radiation therapy.

Other NCI Breast Cancer Patient Education Booklets

For free copies of other booklets in the Breast Cancer Patient Education Series, call the Cancer Information Service or write to the Office of Cancer Communications, National Cancer Institute, Building 31, Room 10A24, Bethesda, MD 20892.

♦ *Breast Exams: What You Should Know*
♦ *Questions and Answers About Breast Lumps*
♦ *Breast Biopsy: What You Should Know*
♦ *Breast Cancer: Understanding Treatment Options*
♦ *Mastectomy: A Treatment for Breast Cancer*
♦ *Adjuvant Therapy: Facts for Women With Breast Cancer*
♦ *Breast Reconstruction: A Matter of Choice*
♦ *After Breast Cancer: A Guide to Followup Care*
♦ *When Cancer Recurs: Meeting the Challenge Again*
♦ *Advanced Cancer: Living Each Day*

■ **Document Source:**
   U.S. Department of Health and Human Services, Public Health Service
   National Institutes of Health
   National Cancer Institute
   NIH Publication No. 91-659
   Reprinted November 1990

See also: Breast Cancer (page 402); Breast Cancer: Understanding Treatment Options (page 406); Chemotherapy and You: A Guide to Self-Help During Treatment (page 40); Radiation Therapy and You: A Guide to Self-Help During Treatment (page 56)

UNDERSTANDING BREAST CHANGES: A HEALTH GUIDE FOR ALL WOMEN

Breast cancer is hard to ignore. It is the most common form of cancer among American women, and almost everyone knows at least one person—aunt, coworker, neighbor, childhood friend, sister-in-law—who has been treated for it.

Understandably, women are concerned about getting breast cancer. This concern prompts all women to watch for breast changes. Breast changes are common and, even though the great majority are benign, they can be worrisome.

This booklet is designed to help you with these concerns. It describes screening practices that will help you monitor the health of your breasts, explains the various types of breast changes that women experience, and outlines methods that doctors use to distinguish between benign changes and cancer. It reviews factors that can increase a woman's cancer risk and reports on current approaches to breast cancer prevention.

We hope that you will find the information in this booklet helpful. Information is a powerful ally in maintaining good health. Keep in mind as you read, however, that for information to make an impact on your life, you must be willing to translate it into action. It is up to you to assume an active role in managing your good health.

Breast Cancer: Status Report

This year in the United States an estimated 182,000 women will learn they have breast cancer. Two-thirds of the cases of breast cancer occur in older women, but it affects younger women too (and about 900 men a year).

More women are getting breast cancer, but no one yet knows all the reasons why. Some of the increase can be traced to better ways of recognizing cancer and greater efforts to detect cancers in an early stage. Some of it may be the result of changes in the way we live—postponing motherhood, taking replacement hormones and oral contraceptives, eating high-fat foods, or drinking more alcohol.

The encouraging news is that, more and more, breast cancer is being detected early, while the tumor is limited to the breast and very small. Currently, two-thirds of newly diagnosed breast cancers show no signs that the cancer has spread beyond the breast, and a quarter of the cancers are smaller than one-third of an inch.

With prompt and appropriate treatment, the outlook for women with breast cancer is good. Moreover, when a cancer is detected while it is still small, a woman may have the option of choosing a treatment that preserves her breast.

The Key: Early Detection

The key to finding breast cancer is early detection, and the key to early detection is **screening:** looking for cancer in women who have no symptoms of disease. The National Cancer Institute (along with a dozen other major health organizations) suggests a three-part program for early detection. The three steps, based on a partnership between a woman and her physician, are:

Mammography
Breast examination by a doctor or nurse
Breast self-examination

Used together, and on a regular basis, a breast exam by a doctor or nurse and mammography offer the best chance of finding breast cancer early. Studies have shown that having regular mammograms along with breast exams by a doctor or nurse can reduce deaths from breast cancer by a third or more. In addition, all women should perform breast self-examinations each month.

Mammography

A mammogram is an x-ray of the breast. Mammography can find a lump as much as 2 years before it can be felt.

Cancers that are found on mammograms but that cannot be felt (nonpalpable cancers) are smaller than cancers that can be felt, and they may not have spread. The vast majority of cancers that are too small to be felt and have not spread are curable.

On the other hand, mammography is not foolproof. Some breast changes, including lumps that can be felt, do not show up on a mammogram. Changes can be especially difficult to spot in the dense, glandular breasts of younger women. This is why women of all ages should have their breasts examined every year by a physician.

Mammography is a simple procedure. The standard screening exam includes two views of each breast, one from above and one angled from the side. A registered technologist positions the breast between two flat plastic plates. The two plates are then pressed together. The idea is to flatten the breast as much as possible; spreading the tissue out makes any abnormal details easier to spot with a minimum of radiation. The technologist steps from the room and takes the x-ray, then returns and repeats the procedure for the next view.

The pressure from the plates can be uncomfortable, or even slightly painful. It helps to remember that each x-ray takes just a few moments—and that it could save your life. It also helps to schedule mammography just after your period, when your breasts are least likely to be tender.

Although some women are concerned about radiation exposure, the risk of any harm is extremely small. First of all, the doses of radiation used for mammography are very low. Specialized mammography facilities have experienced personnel as well as modern equipment that is custom-designed for mammograms. The combination of good technology and expertise makes it possible to obtain good quality x-ray images with very low doses of radiation. (See "More Info: Choosing a Mammography Facility.")

> **A lump should never be ignored just because it is not visible on a mammogram.**

Women should be further reassured to know that any effect of radiation on the breasts decreases sharply with age. Studies of women exposed to large doses of radiation in years past (for instance, in the course of treatment for tuberculosis) show that breast cancer developed more commonly only among those who had been young—often in their early teens—at the time they received the radiation.

The exact amount of radiation needed for a specific mammogram will depend on several factors. For instance, breasts that are large or dense will require higher doses to get a clear image. Federal mammography guidelines limit the radiation used for two views of one breast to 1 rad. (A "rad" is a unit of measurement that stands for radiation absorbed dose.) In practice, most mammograms deliver just a small fraction of this amount.

Reading a Mammogram

The mammogram is first checked by the technologist and then read by a diagnostic radiologist, a doctor who specializes in interpreting x-rays. The radiologist looks for unusual shadows, masses, distortions, special patterns of tissue density, and differences between the two breasts. The shape of a mass can be important too. A growth that is benign (noncancerous), such as a cyst, looks smooth and round and has a clearly defined edge. Breast cancer, in contrast, often has an irregular outline with finger-like extensions.

Many mammograms show nontransparent white specks. These are calcium deposits known as **calcifications.**

Macrocalcifications are coarse calcium deposits. They are usually found in women over 50 and are often seen in both breasts. Macrocalcifications are most likely due to aging or old injuries or inflammations, and they are typically associated with benign conditions.

Microcalcifications are tiny flecks of calcium found in an area of rapidly dividing cells. Clusters of numerous microcalcifications in one area can be an early sign of a localized form of breast cancer called ductal carcinoma in situ. About half of the cancers found by mammography are detected as clusters of microcalcifications.

The radiologist will report the findings from your mammogram directly to you or to your doctor, who will contact you with the results. If you need further tests or examinations, your doctor will let you know. If you don't get a report, call and ask for the results.

Your mammograms constitute an irreplaceable part of your health history. Being able to compare earlier mammograms with new x-rays helps your doctor evaluate areas that look suspicious. If you move, ask your radiologist for your films and hand-carry them to your new physician, so they can be kept with your file.

Mammography and Breast Implants

A woman who has had breast implants should continue to have mammograms. (A woman who has had an implant following breast cancer surgery should ask her doctor whether a mammogram is still necessary.) However, the woman should inform the technologist and radiologist beforehand and make sure they are experienced in x-raying patients with breast implants.

Because silicone implants are not transparent on x-ray, they can block a clear view of the tissues behind them. This is especially true if the implant has been placed in front of, rather than beneath, the chest muscles.

Experienced technologists and radiologists know how to take special care when compressing the breasts to avoid the danger of rupturing the implant. They can also use special techniques to detect abnormalities, sliding the implant backward against the chest wall, and pulling the breast tissue over and in front of it. Interpreting the mammogram can also be difficult, especially if scar tissue has formed around the implant or if silicone has leaked into nearby breast tissues.

Choosing a Mammography Facility

You can go many places to get a mammogram—breast clinics, radiology departments of hospitals, mobile vans, private radiology practices, doctors' offices. Your doctor can arrange for a mammogram for you, or you can schedule the appointment yourself.

It is important to choose a facility carefully, however, because quality can vary widely from one place to another. One good way to tell if a facility measures up is to find out if it is accredited by the American College of Radiology (ACR).

Facilities accredited by the ACR have their equipment, personnel, and procedures evaluated and approved. To be accredited, facilities must have doctors and other staff members who have been specially trained to perform and interpret breast x-rays. They also must have equipment capable of producing high-quality mammograms with the lowest possible amount of radiation exposure. And they must perform mammography regularly and frequently.

To find out if a facility is ACR-accredited, you can ask to see its ACR certificate, or you can call the Cancer Information Service at 1-800-4-CANCER (1-800-422-6237).

The ACR program is voluntary, and not all high-quality facilities have yet been accredited. If you are considering a facility that is not ACR-accredited, you will want to be sure that your mammogram will be taken with the proper equipment and that the people who take the x-rays and those who check them are properly trained.

The following questions will help you in making your selection. Don't hesitate to call and ask these questions before you make an appointment. A qualified facility should have staff able to answer your questions easily. Choose one whose staff answer "yes" to all of them.

Q. Does the facility use machines specifically designed for mammography?

A. These are called "dedicated" mammography machines. You should not choose a facility that x-rays the breast with a machine used to take x-rays of the bones and other parts of the body.

Q. Is the person who takes the mammograms a registered technologist?

A. Mammographic technologists are trained to position the breast correctly to get a good image. They should be certified by the American Registry of Radiological Technologists or be licensed by the state.

Q. Is the radiologist who reads the mammograms specifically trained to do so?

A. The mammograms should be read by a board-certified radiologist who has taken special courses in mammography.

Q. Are mammograms a regular part of the facility's practice?

A. Studies have shown that facilities performing large numbers of mammograms are likely to comply with many quality standards. The ACR suggests choosing a facility that performs at least 10 mammograms each week.

Q. Is the mammography machine calibrated at least once a year?

A. The machine should be checked by a radiological physicist and adjusted as necessary to be sure that its measurements and doses are correct.

In addition to quality, another important consideration is cost. Most mammograms cost between $50 and $150. More than 40 states now have laws requiring health insurance companies to reimburse all or part of the cost of screening mammograms; check with your insurance company. For women 65 and older, the federal Medicare program pays some of the cost for screening mammography once every 2 years.

Some health service agencies and some employers provide mammograms free, or at low cost. Low cost does not mean low quality, however. A large government survey found that some of the facilities charging the lowest fees (often because they deal in large volumes) were among the best in terms of complying with high-quality standards.

Your doctor, local health department, clinic, or chapter of the American Cancer Society, as well as the Cancer Information Service, may be able to direct you to low-cost programs in your area.

Getting a Regular Mammogram

More women are getting mammograms. A 1992 survey found that the number of women who obtained a mammogram in the preceding year doubled between 1987 and 1990, from 17 to 33 percent. However, many women are not having mammograms and breast examinations at regular intervals. Sadly, those least likely to have regular exams include those at highest risk, women aged 60 and older.

The reason women most frequently give for having—or not having—a mammogram is whether or not the doctor suggested it. Although surveys show that more physicians are routinely advising mammography, some physicians fail to do so—some because they forget, some because they assume that another doctor has done so. If your doctor doesn't suggest mammography, it will be up to you to raise the issue.

Common Myths About Mammography

1. If my doctor doesn't recommend a mammogram, I don't need one.
Don't wait for him to bring it up. Tell him or her that you want to discuss mammography.
2. I'll be exposed to too much radiation.
The reality is, the radiation exposure from today's quality mammography equipment is minimal. It is far more dangerous not to find breast cancer at its earliest stage than to be exposed to a low dose of radiation.
3. My mother and my grandmother never had breast cancer, so I don't need to worry about it.
The reality is, if you're a woman, and getting older, you are at risk for breast cancer. Eighty percent of the women who get breast cancer have no family history of the disease. A woman whose mother, sister, or daughter had breast cancer should talk to her doctor about getting checked more often. But all women, once they reach age 40, need to get regular mammograms.
4. I don't need to have a mammogram unless I feel a lump or have symptoms of breast cancer.
The reality is, screening mammograms are for women with no lumps or other symptoms. The best time to find breast cancer is before you can feel it.

Other Techniques for Detecting Breast Cancer

Currently, mammography and breast exams by the doctor or nurse are the most common and useful techniques for finding breast cancer early. Other methods such as ultrasound may be helpful in narrowing the diagnosis for women who have suspicious breast changes. However, no other method is yet effective for screening women with no symptoms, and most of them are used primarily in research programs.

Ultrasound works by sending high-frequency sound waves into the breast. The pattern of echoes from these sound waves is converted into an image, called a sonogram, of the breast's interior. Ultrasound, which is painless and harmless, is especially good in distinguishing between tumors, which are solid, and cysts, which are filled with fluid. Sonograms of the breast can also be helpful in evaluating some lumps that can be felt but are hard to see on mammography, especially in the dense breasts of young women. Unlike mammography, ultrasound cannot detect the microcalcifications that sometimes indicate cancer, nor does it pick up small tumors.

Computed tomography, or CT scanning, uses a computer to organize the information from multiple x-ray views and constructs a cross-sectional image of the body. CT is sometimes helpful in locating breast lesions that are difficult to pinpoint with mammography or ultrasound—for instance, a tumor that is so close to the chest wall that it shows up in only one mammographic view.

Several even newer techniques for imaging the breast are in the research stage. These include **Magnetic Resonance Imaging,** or MRI, which relies on magnetic fields and radio waves to produce a likeness of body tissues, and **Positron Emission Tomography (PET scanning),** which can identify tissues that are abnormally active. **Laser beam scanning** shines a powerful laser beam through the breast while a special camera on the far side of the breast records the image.

Research is also under way to develop laboratory tests that could be used to detect cancer in blood samples. **Tumor markers** are substances produced either by tumors or by the body in response to tumors. Elevated blood levels of certain biomarkers can be helpful in confirming a diagnosis or watching for tumor recurrence. However, because most biomarkers can be elevated even in some healthy people, they are not yet practical for screening for breast cancer.

Someday it may be possible to identify **genetic changes** that predispose women to breast cancer. At present, this type of testing is limited to certain rare families whose members are inclined to develop breast cancer at an early age and who have cells that carry an inherited genetic mutation.

A Physical Breast Exam Is a Must

As important as requesting regular mammograms for the early detection of breast cancer, is getting periodic breast exams by a doctor or nurse. You may find it convenient to schedule this exam during your routine physical. If a breast exam is not part of your regular checkup, you should ask to have it done. The examiner will look at your breasts while you are sitting and while you are lying down. You may be asked to raise your arms over your head or let them hang by your sides, or to press your hands against your hips. The examiner checks each breast carefully for changes in the skin, such as dimpling, scaling, or puckering, or any discharge from the nipples, or any difference in appearance, either size or shape. The next step is **palpation:** Using the pads of the fingers to feel for lumps, the examiner will systematically inspect the entire breast, the underarm, and even the collarbone area, first on one side, then on the other.

A lump is generally the size of a pea before a skilled examiner can detect it. Lumps that are soft, round, smooth, and movable tend not to be cancerous. An irregular, hard lump that feels firmly anchored within the breast tissue is more likely to be a cancer. However, these are general guidelines, not hard and fast rules.

A breast exam by a doctor or nurse can find some cancers missed by mammography, even very small ones. In addition to the skill and carefulness of the examiner, the success of a breast exam can be influenced by your monthly cycle, by the size of your breast, as well as by the size and location of the lump itself. Lumps are harder to find in a large breast.

Breast Self-Exam (BSE)

Screening for breast cancer begins at home. Women of all ages should make it a habit to examine their breasts once a month. It is a fact that most women with breast cancer find their own tumors, often accidentally. Women who practice BSE find tumors at an earlier stage, while they are smaller and before they have spread.

A major goal of regular BSE is to let you become familiar with the feel of your own breasts. Then, if a change occurs, you will be quick to recognize it.

Breasts come in all sizes and shapes, just as women do. A woman's breasts change over her lifetime too. The shape, size, and feel of your breasts will be influenced by monthly menstrual cycles, childbirth, breast-feeding, birth control pills or hormone replacement therapy, menopause, weight changes, and age.

When you do BSE, you are looking for a lump or an unusual thickening that feels different from the rest of your breast. Many women say that BSE can be confusing because their breasts always feel lumpy. The key to doing BSE effectively is to learn what is normal for you. This means practicing BSE regularly. In fact, some doctors and nurses recommend that, for the first month, you do BSE every day so that you really get to know the "topography" of your own breasts.

The best time to do BSE is 2 or 3 days after the end of your period, when your breasts are least likely to be tender or swollen. A woman who is no longer menstruating may find it helpful to pick a particular day that is easy to remember, such as the first of the month.

At the end of this brochure is a guide that takes you through a breast self-exam step by step. In addition, you can get a better understanding of the procedure by reviewing it with your doctor. Following your breast exam, ask the doctor to guide you through a BSE and to explain what you are feeling in your breasts. This can ensure that you are doing BSE correctly and thoroughly and make you more confident examining your breasts each month.

About Breast Lumps and Other Breast Changes

A woman practicing BSE can encounter a broad variety of benign breast conditions. These include normal changes that occur during the menstrual cycle as well as several types of benign lumps. What they have in common is that they are **not** cancer. Even among breast lumps that warrant a biopsy, some 80 percent prove to be benign.

Each breast has 15 to 20 sections, called lobes, each with many smaller lobules. The lobules end in dozens of tiny bulbs that can produce milk. The lobes, lobules, and bulbs are all linked by thin tubes called ducts. These ducts lead to the nipple in the center of a dark area of skin called the areola. Fat fills the spaces between lobules and ducts. There are no muscles in the breasts, but muscles lie under each breast and cover the ribs.

These normal features can sometimes make the breasts feel lumpy, especially in women who are thin or who have small breasts.

In addition, from the time a girl begins to menstruate, her breasts undergo regular changes each month. Many doctors believe that nearly all breasts develop some lasting changes, beginning when the woman is about 30. Eventually, about half of all women will experience symptoms such as lumps, pain, or nipple discharge. Generally these disappear with menopause.

Some studies show that the chances of developing benign breast changes are higher for a woman who has never had children, has irregular menstrual cycles, or has a family history of breast cancer. Benign breast conditions are less common among women who take birth control pills or who are overweight. Because they usually involve the glandular tissues of the breast, benign breast conditions are more of a problem for women of child-bearing age, who have more glandular breasts.

Generalized Breast Lumpiness

One common type of benign breast change is a **generalized breast lumpiness.** This condition is known by several names, including **fibrocystic changes** and **benign breast disease.** Such lumpiness, which is sometimes described as "ropy" or "granular," can often be felt in the area around the nipple and areola and in the upper outer part of the breast. Such lumpiness may become more obvious as a woman approaches middle age and the milk-producing glandular tissue of her breasts increasingly gives way to soft, fatty tissue. Unless she is taking replacement hormones, this type of lumpiness generally disappears for good after menopause.

The menstrual cycle also brings change. Many women experience swelling, tenderness, and pain before and sometimes during their periods. At the same time, one or more lumps or a feeling of increased lumpiness may develop, because of extra fluid collecting in the breast tissue. These lumps normally go away by the end of the period.

During pregnancy, the milk-producing glands become swollen and the breasts may feel lumpier than usual. It can be difficult to examine your breasts when you are pregnant, but you should continue to do so; although not common, breast cancer has been diagnosed during pregnancy. If you have a question about the way your breasts feel, talk to your doctor.

Benign breast conditions also include several types of distinct, solitary lumps. Such lumps, which can appear at any time, may be large or small, soft or rubbery, fluid-filled or solid.

Cysts are fluid-filled sacs. They occur most often in women 35 to 50 years of age, and they often enlarge and become tender and painful just before the menstrual period. They are usually found in both breasts. Some cysts are so small they cannot be felt; rarely, they may be several inches across. Cysts are usually treated by observation or by fine-needle aspiration. Cysts show up clearly on ultrasound. (See "Aspirating a Cyst.")

Fibroadenomas are solid and round benign tumors that are made up of both structural (fibro) and glandular (adenoma) tissues. Usually these lumps are painless, and usually they are found by the woman herself. They feel rubbery and can easily be moved around. Fibroadenomas are the most common type of tumors in women in their late teens and early twenties, and they occur twice as often in African-American women as in other American women.

Fibroadenomas have a typically benign appearance on mammography (smooth, round masses with a clearly defined edge), and they can sometimes be diagnosed with fine needle aspiration. Although fibroadenomas do not become malignant, they can enlarge with pregnancy and breast-feeding. Most surgeons believe that it is a good idea to remove fibroadenomas to make sure they are benign.

Fat necrosis is the name given to painless, round and firm lumps formed by damaged and disintegrating fatty tissues. This condition typically occurs in obese women with very large breasts. It often develops in response to a bruise or blow to the breast, even though the woman may not remember the specific injury. Sometimes the skin around the lumps looks red or bruised. Fat necrosis can easily be mistaken for cancer, so such lumps are removed in a surgical biopsy (See "Biopsy.")

Sclerosing adenosis is a benign condition involving the excessive growth of tissues in the breast's lobules. It frequently causes breast pain. Usually the changes are microscopic, but adenosis can produce lumps, and it can show up on mammography, often as calcifications. Short of biopsy, adenosis can be difficult to distinguish from cancer. The usual approach is surgical biopsy, which furnishes both diagnosis and treatment.

Some benign breast conditions produce **a discharge from the nipple.** Since the breast is a gland, secretions from the nipple of a mature woman are not unusual, nor even necessarily a sign of disease. For example, small amounts of discharge commonly occur in women taking birth control pills or certain other medications, including sedatives and tranquilizers. If the discharge is being caused by a disease, the disease is more likely to be benign than cancerous.

Nipple discharges come in a variety of colors and textures. A milky discharge can be traced to many causes, including thyroid malfunction and oral contraceptives or other drugs. Women with generalized breast lumpiness may have a sticky discharge that is brown or green.

The doctor will take a sample of the discharge and send it to a laboratory to be analyzed. Benign sticky discharges are treated chiefly by keeping the nipple clean. A discharge caused by infection may require antibiotics.

One of the most common sources of a bloody or sticky discharge is an **intraductal papilloma**, a small wartlike growth that projects into breast ducts near the nipple. Any slight bump or bruise in the area of the nipple can cause the papilloma to bleed. Single (solitary) intraductal papillomas usually affect women nearing menopause. If the discharge becomes bothersome, the diseased duct can be removed surgically without damaging the appearance of the breast. Multiple intraductal papillomas, in contrast, are more common in younger women. They often occur in both breasts and are more likely to be associated with a lump than with nipple discharge. Multiple intraductal papillomas, or any papillomas associated with a lump, need to be removed.

Some benign breast conditions are characterized by **infections and/or inflammation.**

Mastitis (sometimes called "postpartum mastitis") is an infection most often seen in women who are breast-feeding. A duct may become blocked, allowing milk to pool, causing inflammation and setting the stage for infection by bacteria. The breast appears red and feels warm, tender, and lumpy.

In its earlier stages, mastitis can be cured by antibiotics. If a pus-containing abscess forms, it will need to be drained or surgically removed.

Mammary duct ectasia is a disease of women nearing menopause. Ducts beneath the nipple become inflamed and can become clogged. Mammary duct ectasia can become painful, and it can produce a thick and sticky discharge that is grey to green in color. Treatment consists of warm compresses, antibiotics, and, if necessary, surgery to remove the duct.

Benign Breast Conditions and the Risk of Breast Cancer

Most benign breast changes do not increase a woman's risk of getting cancer. Recent studies show that only certain very specific types of microscopic changes put a woman at higher risk. These changes feature excessive cell growth, or hyperplasia.

Approximately 70 percent of the women who have a biopsy showing a benign condition have **no** evidence of hyperplasia. *These women are at little increased risk of breast cancer.*

About 25 percent of the benign breast biopsies show signs of hyperplasia, including conditions such as intraductal papilloma and sclerosing adenosis. Hyperplasia slightly increases the risk of developing breast cancer.

The remaining 5 percent of benign breast biopsies reveal both excessive cell growth—hyperplasia—and cells that are abnormal—atypia. A diagnosis of **atypical hyperplasia**, as it is called, *moderately* increases breast cancer risk.

When You Find a Lump

If you discover a lump in one breast, either during breast self-examination or by chance, examine the other breast. If both breasts feel the same, the lumpiness is probably normal. You should, however, mention it to your doctor at your next visit.

But if the lump is something new or unusual and does not go away after your menstrual period, it is time to call your doctor. The same is true if you discover a discharge from the nipple or skin changes such as dimpling or puckering. If you do not have a doctor of your own, your local medical society may be able to help you find a doctor in your area.

You should not let fear delay you. It's natural to be concerned if you find a lump in your breast. But it's important to remember that four-fifths of all biopsied breast lumps are benign, which means no cancer is present. The sooner any problem is diagnosed, the sooner you can take care of it.

Clinical Evaluation

No matter how your breast lump was discovered, the doctor will want to begin with your "history": What symptoms do you have and how long have you had them? What is your age, menstrual status, general health? Are you pregnant? Are you taking any medications? How many children do you have? Do you have any relatives with benign breast conditions or breast cancer? Have you previously been diagnosed with benign breast changes?

The doctor will then carefully examine your breasts and will probably schedule you for mammography. If you have a symptom suggestive of breast cancer, whether it was found through BSE, the annual exam, or by chance, you should not hesitate to have a mammogram if your doctor recommends it.

Mammography for diagnosis, as distinct from mammography for screening women who have no symptoms, is designed to obtain as much information as possible about an existing change. This may be either a lump that can be felt or an abnormality discovered on a screening mammogram. Diagnostic mammography may include additional views or use special techniques to magnify a suspicious area or to eliminate shadows produced by overlapping layers of normal breast tissue. The doctor will want to compare the diagnostic mammograms with any previous mammograms. If the lump appears to be a cyst, your doctor may ask you to have a sonogram (ultrasound study).

Aspirating a Cyst

When a cyst is suspected, some doctors proceed directly with **aspiration.** This procedure, which uses a very thin needle and a syringe, takes only a few minutes and can be done in the doctor's office. The procedure is not usually painful, since most of the nerves in the breast are in the skin.

Holding the lump steady, the doctor inserts the needle and attempts to draw out any fluid. If the lump is indeed a cyst, removing the fluid will cause the cyst to collapse and the lump to disappear. Unless the cyst reappears in the next week or two, no other treatment is needed. If the cyst reappears at a later date, it can simply be drained again.

If the lump turns out to be solid, it may be possible to use the needle to suck out some clumps of cells, which can then be sent to a laboratory for further testing. (Cysts are so rarely associated with cancer that the fluid removed from a cyst is not usually tested unless it is bloody or the woman is older than 55 years of age.)

Biopsy

The only certain way to learn whether a breast lump or mammographic abnormality is cancerous is a biopsy: Tissue is removed by a surgeon or other specialist and examined under a microscope by a pathologist. The pathologist is a physician who specializes in identifying tissue changes that are characteristic of disease, including cancer.

Tissue samples for biopsy can be obtained either with surgery or with needles. The choice of biopsy technique depends on such things as the nature and location of the lump as well as the woman's general health.

Surgical biopsies can be either excisional or incisional.

An **excisional biopsy** removes the lump or the suspicious area in its entirety. Excision is currently the standard procedure for biopsying lumps that are smaller than an inch or so in diameter. In effect it is similar to a "lumpectomy," surgery to remove the lump and a margin of surrounding tissue, which is often used (in combination with radiotherapy) as the basic treatment for early breast cancer.

An excisional biopsy is typically performed in the outpatient department of a hospital. A local anesthetic is injected into the woman's breast, and perhaps she is given a tranquilizer. The surgeon makes an incision along the contour of the breast and removes the lump along with a small margin of normal tissue. Because no skin is removed, the biopsy scar is usually small. The procedure typically takes less than an hour. After spending an hour or two in the recovery room, the woman goes home the same day.

An **incisional biopsy** removes only a portion of the tumor (by slicing into or incising it) for the pathologist to examine. Incisional biopsies are generally reserved for tumors that are larger. They too are usually performed under local anesthesia, with the woman going home the same day.

Whether or not a surgical biopsy will change the shape of your breast depends partly on the size of the lump and where it is located in the breast as well as how much of a "margin" of healthy tissue the surgeon feels it is wise to

remove. You should talk with your doctor beforehand so you understand just how extensive the surgery will be and what the result is going to look like.

Needle biopsies can be performed with either a very fine needle or a cutting needle large enough to remove a small nugget of tissue.

Fine-needle aspiration, as noted above, uses a fine-gauge needle and syringe, either to remove fluid from a cyst or clusters of cells from a solid mass. Accurate fine-needle aspiration biopsy of a solid mass takes great skill, gained through experience with hundreds of cases.

Core needle biopsy uses a somewhat larger needle with a special cutting edge. The needle is inserted, under local anesthesia, through a small incision in the skin, and a small core of tissue is removed. This technique may not work well for lumps that are very hard or very small. Core needle biopsy may cause some bruising, but rarely leaves a scar, and the procedure is over in a matter of minutes.

At some institutions with extensive experience, aspiration biopsy is considered as reliable as surgical biopsy, trusted to confirm the malignancy of a clinically suspicious mass or, alternatively, to support a benign diagnosis for a breast lump that appears noncancerous. Should the needle biopsy results be uncertain, the diagnosis is pursued with a surgical biopsy. At some institutions, doctors prefer to verify all aspiration biopsy results with a surgical biopsy before proceeding with treatment.

Localization biopsy (also known as needle localization) is a procedure that uses mammography to locate and biopsy breast abnormalities that can be seen on a mammogram but cannot be felt (nonpalpable abnormalities). Localization can be used in conjunction with surgical biopsy, fine needle aspiration, or core needle biopsy.

For a surgical biopsy, the radiologist relocates the abnormality on a mammogram (or a sonogram) just prior to surgery. Using the mammogram as a guide, the radiologist inserts a fine needle or wire so the tip rests in the suspect area—typically, an area of microcalcifications. (The breast may look bizarre with a needle sticking out of it, but the procedure is remarkably pain free.) The needle is anchored with a gauze bandage, and a second mammogram is taken to confirm that the needle is on target.

The woman, along with her mammograms, goes to the operating room, where the surgeon locates and cuts out the needle-targeted area. The more precisely the needle is placed, the less tissue needs to be removed.

Sometimes the surgeon will be able to feel the lump during surgery. In other cases, especially where the mammogram showed only microcalcifications, the mass can be neither seen nor felt. To make sure the surgical specimen in fact contains the abnormality, it is x-rayed on the spot. If this **specimen x-ray** fails to show the mass or the calcifications, the surgeon is able to remove additional tissue.

Stereotactic localization biopsy is a newer approach that relies on a three-dimensional x-ray to guide the needle biopsy of a nonpalpable mass. With one type of equipment, the patient lies face down on an examining table with a hole in it that allows the breast to hang through; the x-ray machine and the maneuverable needle "gun" are set up underneath. Alternatively, specialized stereotactic equipment can be attached to a standard mammography machine.

The breast is x-rayed from two different angles and a computer plots the exact position of the suspicious area. (Because only a small area of the breast is exposed to the radiation, the doses are similar to those from standard mammography.) Once the target is clearly identified, the radiologist positions the gun and advances the biopsy needle into the lesion.

Tissue Studies

The cells or tissue removed through needle or surgical biopsy are promptly sent (along with the x-ray of the specimen, if one was made) to the pathology laboratory. If the excised lump is large enough, the pathologist can take a preliminary look by quick-freezing a small portion of the tissue sample, making it hard enough to slice into razor-thin sections that can be examined under the microscope. A "frozen section" provides an immediate if provisional diagnosis, and the surgeon may be able to give you the result before you go home.

A frozen section is not 100 percent guaranteed, however. A more thorough assessment will take a few days longer, while the pathologist processes "permanent sections" of tissue that can be examined in greater detail.

When the biopsy specimen is small—as is often the case when the abnormality consists of mammographic calcifications only—many doctors prefer to forego a frozen section so the tiny specimen can be analyzed in its entirety.

The pathologist looks for abnormal cell shapes and unusual growth patterns. In many cases the diagnosis will be clear-cut. However, the distinctions between benign and cancerous can be subtle, and even experts don't always agree. When in doubt, pathologists readily consult their colleagues. If there is any question about the results of your biopsy, you will want to make sure your slides have been reviewed by more than one pathologist.

Deciding To Biopsy

Not every lump or mammographic change merits a biopsy. Nearly all mammographic masses that look smooth and clearly outlined, for instance, are benign. Your physician needs to thoughtfully weigh the findings from your physical examination and mammogram along with your background and your medical history in forming her or his recommendation.

Although benign lumps *do not* turn into cancer, cancerous lumps can develop near benign lumps and can be hidden on a mammogram. Even if you have had a benign lump removed in the past, you cannot be sure any new lump is also benign.

In some instances the doctor may suggest watching the suspicious area for a month or two. Because many lumps are caused by normal hormonal changes, this waiting period may provide additional information.

Similarly, if the changes on your mammogram show all the hallmarks of benign disease, your doctor may advise waiting a few months and then taking another mammogram, to be followed by additional mammograms over the next 3 years. If you choose this option, however, you must be strongly committed to regular followup.

If you feel uncomfortable about waiting, express your concerns to your doctor. You may also want to get a second opinion, perhaps from a breast specialist or surgeon. Many cities have breast clinics where you can get a second opinion.

Biopsy: One Step or Two

Not too many years ago, all women undergoing surgery for breast symptoms had a "one-step" procedure: If the surgical biopsy showed cancer, the surgeon proceeded immediately with mastectomy. The woman went into surgery not knowing if she had cancer, and woke up not knowing if her breasts were intact.

Today a woman facing biopsy has a broader range of options. In most cases, biopsy and diagnosis will be separated from any further treatment by an interval of several days or weeks. Such a "two-step" procedure does not adversely affect outcome, and it provides several benefits. It allows time for the tissue sample to be examined in detail and, if cancer is found, it gives the woman time to adjust to the diagnosis. She can review her treatment options, seek a second opinion, receive counseling, and arrange her schedule.

Some women nonetheless prefer a one-step procedure. They have decided beforehand that, if the surgical biopsy and frozen section show cancer, they want to go ahead with surgery, either mastectomy or breast-conserving surgery and axillary dissection (removal of the underarm lymph nodes). If, on the other hand, the lump proves to be benign, the incision will be closed; the procedure will have taken less than an hour, and the woman may go home the same day or the next day.

A one-step procedure avoids the physical and psychological stress, as well as the costs in time and money, of two rounds of surgery and anesthesia—a particularly important consideration for women who are ill or frail. Women who have clinical signs of cancer can find the wait between biopsy and surgery emotionally draining, and they may be relieved to have a one-step procedure to take care of the problem as quickly as possible.

No single solution is right for everyone. Each woman should consult with her doctors and her family, weigh the alternatives, and decide what approach is appropriate. Being involved in the decision-making process gives a woman a sense of control over her body and her life.

Factors That Increase the Risk of Breast Cancer

Simply being a woman and getting older puts you at risk for developing breast cancer. The older you are, the greater your chance of getting breast cancer. The breast cancer incidence rate, per 100,000 women per year, is 222 for women age 40 to 64; for women older than 65, it climbs to 435.

Risk is also increased for older women who have a family history of breast cancer. The mothers, daughters, and sisters of women with breast cancer, especially if the relative developed this cancer at a young age, are two to five times more likely to develop breast cancer themselves than are women without a family history. Women who themselves have already had cancer in one breast also run an increased risk of developing cancer in the other breast.

To a lesser extent, risk is influenced by various aspects of a woman's reproductive history. Risk is increased for women who began menstruating earlier (before age 12, compared to after 15), had their first child later (after age 30, compared to before 20) or were never pregnant, or completed menopause later (after age 55 compared to women who had their ovaries removed—a "surgical menopause"—at age 45).

Risk is also increased for women who are overweight, especially those who carry excess fat in the upper body—abdomen, shoulders, nape of the neck. As noted above, risk is increased moderately for women who have the benign breast changes known as atypical hyperplasia.

Many aspects of the American lifestyle are suspected of possibly influencing the growing incidence of breast cancer. Current research is looking into the roles of obesity, hormones, and fat metabolism; the risks and benefits of postmenopausal hormone replacement therapy; the impact of taking oral contraceptives at an early age and for many years; alcohol use; and diet. Caffeine, on the other hand, appears to have no influence on the incidence of breast cancer.

It is important to keep in mind that these factors that increase cancer risk—**risk factors**—do not necessarily cause cancer; they are merely associations. Having one or more does not mean that you are certain or even likely to develop breast cancer. Even among women with a strong family history—both a mother and a sister or two sisters, one of whom developed breast cancer in both breasts or before menopause—three-fourths will not develop breast cancer.

Prevention Research

Many of the factors that influence your chances of developing breast cancer—your age, a family history of breast cancer, the age at which you began to menstruate—are beyond your control. Others, however, present opportunities for change, and several large research trials are looking at possibilities for "intervention."

The Breast Cancer Prevention Trial is a randomized study of **tamoxifen,** a drug that has been widely used in the treatment of women with breast cancer. Because tamoxifen has been found to markedly reduce the occurrence of new cancers in the opposite breast of women who have already had breast cancer, it is now being tried as a preventive in healthy women at increased risk for breast cancer because they are 60 or older or are younger but have combinations of other risk factors. (Tamoxifen also appears to offer protection against heart attacks and osteoporosis.)

Dietary **"chemoprevention"** is being tested in Italy, where women who have already been treated for breast cancer are taking 4-HPR, a synthetic form of vitamin A, in hopes of preventing cancer from developing in the opposite breast. Other researchers are investigating the protective potential of several other vitamins, including C and E as well as beta-carotene, the form of vitamin A found in fruits and vegetables. Yet other scientists are checking out naturally occurring chemicals, called phytochemicals, found in common fruits, vegetables, and other edible plants, in hopes of finding cancer-fighting substances that can be extracted, purified, and added to our diets.

Diet itself is another target of prevention research. In the Women's Health Initiative, a project of the National Institutes of Health, 70,000 women over 50 are being enrolled in a series of clinical trials to measure the effectiveness of a low-fat diet (less than 20 percent of calories from fat) and calcium plus vitamin D supplements, along with hormone replacement therapy, in combatting heart disease and osteoporosis as well as cancer. Another large trial evaluating a low-fat diet in high-risk women is under way in Canada.

A much more drastic approach to breast cancer prevention is surgery to remove both breasts. Such a procedure, known as **prophylactic mastectomy,** is sometimes chosen by women with a very high risk for breast cancer—for instance, having a mother and one or more sisters with bilateral premenopausal breast cancer, plus a diagnosis of atypical hyperplasia and a history of several breast biopsies.

Unless a woman finds that anxiety is undermining the quality of her life, she is usually counseled not to choose this physically and psychologically draining surgery. The vast majority of breasts removed prophylactically show no signs of cancer. Moreover, since even an ordinary ("total") mastectomy can leave a small amount of breast tissue behind, it cannot guarantee the woman will remain cancer-free. The preferred approach for most high-risk women is careful surveillance with clinical breast exams and mammography once or twice a year. Also, monthly breast self-examinations are performed.

If you are considering a prophylactic mastectomy, with or without subsequent breast reconstruction, you will want to get a second opinion, preferably from a breast specialist. There is seldom reason to rush your decision. Many doctors advise a woman to give herself several months to weigh the options.

Preventive Steps

Whether your risk of breast cancer is low or high, there are some preventive steps you can take:

You can follow early detection practices. Request mammograms—every 1-2 years if you are age 40 or older, and every year if age 50 or older; get yearly breast exams by a doctor or nurse; and perform monthly breast self-exams.

If your risk is elevated, you can enroll in one of the prevention trials; for information, call the Cancer Information Service at 1-800-4-CANCER.

In making decisions about hormone-containing drugs, you can consult your doctor about your personal situation and carefully weigh any potential risks against the benefits. You can stay informed as new research findings become available.

You can lose excess weight, eat a balanced diet that provides a good variety of nutrients and plenty of fiber, limit dietary fat, and drink alcohol only in moderation. These are "good health" measures that make sense for everyone.

Questions to Ask Your Doctor

We hope that this booklet has answered many of your questions about breast changes and the early detection of breast cancer. However, no booklet can take the place of talking directly with your doctor. Take any questions you have to your doctor. If you don't understand the answer, ask her or him to explain further.

Many women find it helpful to write down their questions ahead of time. The following list contains some of the most common questions that women have. You may have others. Jot them down as you think of them and take the list with you when you see your doctor.

- ♦ Do I need to have a mammogram? How often? Or if not, why not?
- ♦ How often should I schedule appointments with you?
- ♦ Will you teach me how to do BSE and check to see that I'm doing it properly?
- ♦ What should I watch for when I do BSE?
- ♦ How can I distinguish lumps from the normal parts of my breast?
- ♦ What kind of lumps do I have?
- ♦ Do you think I need to have a biopsy? If not, why not?
- ♦ Is there anything in my background that indicates I should have mammograms more often than is usually recommended?

Glossary

Abscess. A pocket of pus that forms as the body's defenses attempt to wall off infection-causing germs.

Adenocarcinoma. A cancer that develops in gland-forming tissue. Most breast cancers are adenocarcinomas.

Anesthetics. Drugs or gases that produce complete or partial loss of feeling or sensation. Local anesthetics numb a specific (local) part of the body. General anesthetics produce a state of unconsciousness and eliminate pain sensation throughout the body.

Areola. The colored tissue that encircles the nipple.

Aspiration. Removing fluid from a cyst or cells from a mass, using a needle and syringe.

Atypical hyperplasia. Cells that are both abnormal (atypical) and increased in number. Benign microscopic breast changes known as atypical hyperplasia moderately increase a woman's risk of developing breast cancer.

Benign. Not cancerous; cannot invade neighboring tissues or spread to other parts of the body.

Benign breast conditions. Noncancerous changes in the breast. Benign breast conditions can cause pain, lumpiness, nipple discharge, and other problems.

Biopsy. The removal of a sample of tissue or cells for examination under a microscope for purposes of diagnosis.

Breast self-exam (BSE). A method for checking one's own breasts for changes in the way they look or the way they feel.

Calcifications. Small deposits of calcium in tissue, which are visible on mammograms.

Cancer. A general name for more than 100 diseases in which abnormal cells grow out of control. Cancer cells can invade and destroy healthy tissues, and they can spread through the bloodstream and the lymphatic system to other parts of the body.

Carcinoma. Cancer that begins in tissues lining or covering the surfaces (epithelial tissues) of organs, glands, or other body structures. Most cancers are carcinomas. (See Adenocarcinoma.)

Carcinoma in situ. Cancer that is confined to the cells where it began, and has not spread into surrounding tissues. (See Noninvasive cancer.)

Chemoprevention. The use of drugs or vitamins to prevent cancer in people who have precancerous conditions or a high risk of cancer, or to prevent the recurrence of cancer in people who already have been treated for it.

Computed tomography (CT) scanning. An imaging technique that uses a computer to organize the information from multiple x-ray views and construct a cross-sectional image of areas inside the body.

Core needle biopsy. The use of a small cutting needle to remove a core of tissue for microscopic examination.

Cyclic breast changes. Normal tissue changes that occur in response to the changing levels of female hormone during the menstrual cycle. Cyclic breast changes can produce swelling, tenderness, and pain.

Cyst. Fluid-filled sac. Breast cysts are benign.

Diagnostic mammography. The use of mammography to evaluate the breasts of a woman who has symptoms of disease, such as a lump, or whose screening mammogram shows an abnormality.

Duct. A channel that carries body fluids. Breast ducts transport milk from the breast's lobules out to the nipple.

Emission tomography. A technique that uses emissions from radioactive tracers to construct images of the distribution of the tracers in the human body.

Estrogen. A female hormone. Estrogen is involved in breast development and may help some types of breast cancer to grow.

Excisional biopsy. The surgical removal (excision) of an abnormal area of tissue, usually along with a margin of healthy tissue, for microscopic examination. Excisional biopsies in the breast remove the entire lump.

Fat necrosis. Lumps of fatty material that form in response to a bruise or blow to the breast (or surgery or radiation therapy).

Fibroadenoma. Benign breast tumor made up of both structural (fibro) and glandular (adenoma) tissues.

Fibrocystic disease. See Generalized breast lumpiness.

Fine-needle aspiration. The use of a slender needle to remove fluid from a cyst or clusters of cells from a solid lump.

Frozen section. A sliver of frozen biopsy tissue. A frozen section provides a quick preliminary diagnosis but is not 100 percent reliable.

Generalized breast lumpiness. Breast irregularities and lumpiness, commonplace and noncancerous. Sometimes called "fibrocystic disease" or "benign breast disease."

Genetic change. An alteration in a section of a chromosome.

Hormone replacement therapy. Hormone-containing medications taken to offset the symptoms and other effects of the hormone loss that accompanies menopause.

Hormones. Chemicals produced by various glands in the body, which produce specific effects on specific target organs and tissues.

Hyperplasia. Excessive growth of cells. Several types of benign breast conditions involve hyperplasia.

Incisional biopsy. The surgical removal of a portion of an abnormal area of tissue, by cutting into (incising) it, for microscopic examination.

Infection. Invasion of body tissues by microorganisms such as bacteria and viruses.

Inflammation. The body's protective response to injury (including infection). Inflammation is marked by heat, redness, swelling, pain, and loss of function.

Intraductal papilloma. A small wartlike growth that projects into a breast duct.

Invasive cancer. Cancer that spreads into and destroys nearby tissues.

Laser scanning. A technique using laser beams and camera imaging to scan the body's tissue.

Lobes, lobules, bulbs. Each of the breast's 15 to 20 lobes branches into smaller lobules, and each lobule ends in scores of tiny bulbs. The bulbs produce milk which is carried by ducts to the nipple.

Localization biopsy. The use of mammography to locate tissue containing an abnormality that can be detected only on mammograms, so it can be removed for microscopic examination.

Lymphatic system. The tissues and organs that produce, store, and transport cells that fight infection and disease.

Macrocalcifications. Coarse calcium deposits typically associated with benign breast conditions.

Malignant. Cancerous. Can invade surrounding tissues and spread to other parts of the body.

Mammary duct ectasia. A benign breast condition in which ducts beneath the nipple become dilated and sometimes inflamed, and which can cause pain and nipple discharge.

Mammogram. An x-ray of the breast.

Mastitis. Infection of the breast. Mastitis is most often seen in nursing mothers.

Menopause. The time when a woman's monthly menstrual periods cease. Menopause is sometimes called the "change of life."

Menstruation. The monthly discharge, during a woman's reproductive years, of blood and tissues from the uterus.

Metastasis. The spread of cancer, through the bloodstream or the lymphatic system, from one part of the body to another.

Microcalcification. A small deposit of calcium in the breast, which can show up on a mammogram. Certain patterns of microcalcifications are sometimes a sign of breast cancer.

MRI (Magnetic Resonance Imaging). A technique that uses a powerful magnet linked to a computer to create detailed pictures of areas inside the body.

Needle biopsy. Use of a needle to extract cells or bits of tissue for microscopic examination.

Nipple discharge. Fluid coming from the nipple.

Noninvasive cancer. A growth made up of cells that are cancerous in appearance, but which has not spread into neighboring tissues. Noninvasive breast cancers are known as ductal carcinoma in situ and lobular carcinoma in situ.

Nonpalpable breast abnormalities. Changes in breast tissue that can be seen on mammograms but which cannot be felt.

One-step procedure. Biopsy and surgical treatment combined into a single operation.

Palpation. Use of the fingers to press body surfaces, to feel tissues and organs underneath. Palpating the breast for lumps is a cornerstone of physical breast examination and BSE.

Pathologist. A doctor who diagnoses disease by studying cells and tissues under a microscope.

Permanent section. Biopsy tissue specially prepared and mounted on slides so that it can be examined under a microscope by a pathologist.

Prophylactic mastectomy. Surgery to remove a breast that is not known to contain breast cancer for the purpose of eliminating cancer risk.

Rad. A unit of measure for radiation. It stands for radiation absorbed dose.

Radiation. Energy carried by waves or by streams of particles. Various forms of radiation can be used in low doses to diagnose disease and in high doses to treat disease. (See X-rays.)

Radiologist. A doctor with special training in the use of x-rays (and related technologies such as ultrasound) to image body tissues and to treat disease.

Recurrence. Reappearance of cancer at the same site (local recurrence), near the original site (regional recurrence), or in other areas of the body (metastasis).

Risk factors. Conditions or agents that increase a person's chances of getting cancer. Risk factors do not necessarily cause cancer; rather, they are indicators, statistically associated with an increase in risk.

Sclerosing adenosis. A benign breast disease that involves the excessive growth of tissues in the breast's lobules.

Screening. Looking for signs of disease such as cancer in people who are symptom-free.

Sonogram. The image produced by ultrasound.

Specimen x-ray. An x-ray of tissue that has been surgically removed (surgical specimen).

Stereotactic localization. A technique that employs three-dimensional x-ray to pinpoint a specific target area. It is used in conjunction with needle biopsy of nonpalpable breast abnormalities.

Surgical biopsy. See Excisional biopsy and Incisional biopsy.

Tamoxifen. A hormonally related drug that has been used to treat breast cancer and is being tested as a possible preventive.

Tumor. An abnormal growth of tissue. Tumors may be either benign or cancerous.

Tumor markers. Substance in blood or other body fluids that may serve as indicators for the presence of cancer.

Two-step procedure. Biopsy and treatment done in two stages, usually a week or two apart.

Ultrasound. The use of sound waves to produce images of body tissues.

X-rays. A high-energy form of radiation. X-rays form an image of body structures by traveling through the body and striking a sheet of film. Breast x-rays are called mammograms.

Other Resources

Information about cancer is available from the sources listed below. You may wish to check for additional information at your local library or bookstore and from support groups in your community.

Cancer Information Service (CIS)

1-800-4-CANCER

The Cancer Information Service, a program of the National Cancer Institute (NCI), provides a nationwide telephone service for cancer patients and their families and friends, the public, and health care professionals. The staff can answer questions and can send booklets about cancer. They also may know about local resources and services. One toll-free number, 1-800-4-CANCER (1-800-422-6237), connects callers with the office that serves their area. Spanish-speaking staff members are available.

PDQ

People who have cancer, their families, and doctors who care for cancer patients need up-to-date and accurate information about cancer treatment. To meet these needs, NCI developed PDQ. This computer database gives quick and easy access to: state-of-the-art treatment information for both patients and doctors; screening guidelines; a list of approved mammography facilities; information about clinical trials (research studies) that are open to patients and that test new and promising cancer trials; and names of organizations and doctors involved in caring for people with cancer.

To use PDQ, doctors may use an office computer or the services of a medical library. By calling CIS at 1-800-4-CANCER, doctors and patients can get PDQ information and learn how to use this system.

American Cancer Society (ACS)

1599 Clifton Road, N.E.
Atlanta, GA 30329
1-800-ACS-2345

The American Cancer Society is a voluntary organization with a national office (at the above address) and local units all over the country. It supports research, conducts educational programs, and offers many services to patients and their families. To obtain information about services and activities in local areas, call the society's toll-free number, 1-800-ACS-2345 (1-800-227-2345), or the number listed under "American Cancer Society" in the white pages of the telephone book.

■ **Document Source:**
 National Institutes of Health
 National Cancer Institute
 NIH Publication No. 93-3536
 Printed April 1993

See also: Breast Biopsy: What You Should Know (page 398); Breast Cancer (page 402); Breast Cancer: Understanding Treatment Options (page 406); Radiation Therapy: A Treatment for Early Stage Breast Cancer (page 438)

Breast Self-Examination (BSE)

Here is one way to do BSE:

1. Stand before a mirror. Check both breasts for anything unusual. Look for a discharge from the nipples, puckering, dimpling, or scaling of the skin.

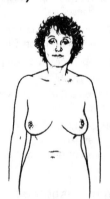

The next two steps are done to check for any change in the shape or contour of your breasts. As you do them, you should be able to feel your chest muscles tighten.

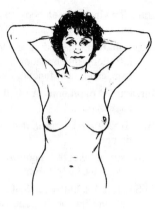

2. Watching closely in the mirror, clasp your hands behind your head and press your hands forward.

3. Next, press your hands firmly on your hips and bow slightly toward the mirror as you pull your shoulders and elbows forward.

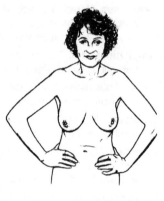

Some women do the next part of the exam in the shower. Your fingers will glide easily over soapy skin, so you can concentrate on feeling for changes inside the breast.

4. Raise your left arm. Use three or four fingers of your right hand to feel your left breast firmly, carefully, and thoroughly. Beginning at the outer edge, press the flat part of your fingers in small circles, moving the circles slowly around the breast. Gradually work toward the nipple. Be sure to cover the whole breast. Pay special attention to the area between the breast and the underarm, including the underarm area itself. Feel for any unusual lump or mass under the skin.

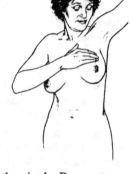

5. Gently squeeze the nipple and look for a discharge. (If you have any discharge during the month—whether or not it is during BSE—see your doctor.) Repeat the exam on your right breast.

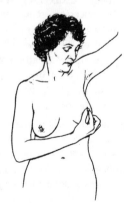

6. Steps 4 and 5 should be repeated lying down. Lie flat on your back, with your left arm over your head and a pillow or folded towel under your left shoulder. This position flattens the breast and makes it easier to check it. Use the same circular motion described above. Repeat on your right breast.

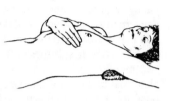

UNDERSTANDING GESTATIONAL DIABETES: A PRACTICAL GUIDE TO A HEALTHY PREGNANCY

Approximately 3 to 5 percent of all pregnant women in the United States are diagnosed as having gestational diabetes. These women and their families have many questions about this disorder. Some of the most frequently asked questions are: What is gestational diabetes and how did I get it? How does it differ from other kinds of diabetes? Will it hurt my baby? Will my baby have diabetes? What can I do to control gestational diabetes? Will I need a special diet? Will gestational diabetes change the way or the time my baby is delivered? Will I have diabetes in the future?

This brochure will address these and many other questions about diet, exercise, measurement of blood sugar levels, and general medical and obstetric care of women with gestational diabetes. It must be emphasized that these are general guidelines and only your health care professional(s) can tailor a program specific to your needs. You should feel free to discuss any concerns you have with your doctor or other health care provider, as no one knows more about you and the condition of your pregnancy.

What is gestational diabetes and what causes it?

Diabetes (actual name is diabetes mellitus) of any kind is a disorder that prevents the body from using food properly. Normally, the body gets its major source of energy from glucose, a simple sugar that comes from foods high in simple carbohydrates (e.g., table sugar or other sweeteners such as honey, molasses, jams, and jellies, soft drinks, and cookies), or from the breakdown of complex carbohydrates such as starches (e.g., bread, potatoes, and pasta). After sugars and starches are digested in the stomach, they enter the blood stream in the form of glucose.* The glucose in the blood stream becomes a potential source of energy for the entire body, similar to the way in which gasoline in a service station pump is a potential source of energy for your car. But, just as someone must pump the gas into the car, the body requires some assistance to get glucose from the bloodstream to the muscles and other tissues of the body. In the body, that assistance comes from a hormone called insulin. Insulin is manufactured by the pancreas, a gland that lies behind the stomach. Without insulin, glucose cannot get into the cells of the body where it is used as fuel. Instead, glucose accumulates in the blood to high levels and is excreted or "spilled" into the urine through the kidneys.

When the pancreas of a child or young adult produces little or no insulin we call this condition juvenile-onset diabetes or Type I diabetes (insulin-dependent). This is not the type of diabetes you have. Unlike women with Type I diabetes, women with gestational diabetes have plenty of insulin. In fact, they usually have more insulin in their blood than women who are not pregnant. However, the effect of their insulin is partially blocked by a variety of other hormones made in the placenta, a condition often called insulin resistance.

The placenta performs the task of supplying the growing fetus with nutrients and water from the mother's circulation. It also produces a variety of hormones vital to the preservation of the pregnancy. Ironically, several of these hormones such as estrogen, cortisol, and human placental lactogen (HPL) have a blocking effect on insulin, a "contra-insulin" effect. This contra-insulin effect usually begins about midway (20 to 24 weeks) through pregnancy. The larger the placenta grows, the more these hormones are produced, and the greater the insulin resistance becomes. In most women the pancreas is able to make additional insulin to overcome the insulin resistance. When the pancreas makes all the insulin it can and there still isn't enough to overcome the effect of the placenta's hormones, gestational diabetes results. If we could somehow remove all the placenta's hormones from the mother's blood, the condition would be remedied. This, in fact, usually happens following delivery.

How does gestational diabetes differ from other types of diabetes?

There are several different types of diabetes. Gestational diabetes begins during pregnancy and disappears following delivery. Another type is referred to as juvenile-onset diabetes (in children) or Type I (in young adults). These individuals usually develop their disease before age 20. People with Type I diabetes must take insulin by injection every day. Approximately 10 percent of all people with diabetes have Type I (also called insulin-dependent diabetes).

Type II diabetes or noninsulin-dependent diabetes (formerly called adult-onset diabetes) is also characterized by

---

* For the purpose of this brochure the words sugar and glucose are used synonymously.

high blood sugar levels, but these patients are often obese and usually lack the classic symptoms (fatigue, thirst, frequent urination, and sudden weight loss) associated with Type I diabetes. Many of these individuals can control their blood sugar levels by following a careful diet and exercise program, by losing excess weight, or by taking oral medication. Some, but not all, need insulin. People with Type II diabetes account for roughly 90 percent of all diabetics.

Who is at risk for developing gestational diabetes and how is it detected?

Any woman might develop gestational diabetes during pregnancy. Some of the factors associated with women who have an increased risk are obesity; a family history of diabetes; having given birth previously to a very large infant, a still-birth, or a child with a birth defect; or having too much amniotic fluid (polyhydramnios). Also, women who are older than 25 are at greater risk than younger individuals. Although a history of sugar in the urine is often included in the list of risk factors, this is not a reliable indicator of who will develop diabetes during pregnancy. Some pregnant women with perfectly normal blood sugar levels will occasionally have sugar detected in their urine.

The Council on Diabetes in Pregnancy of the American Diabetes Association strongly recommends that all pregnant women be screened for gestational diabetes. Several methods of screening exist. The most common is the 50-gram glucose screening test. No special preparation is necessary for this test, and there is no need to fast before the test. The test is performed by giving 50 grams of a glucose drink and then measuring the blood sugar level 1-hour later. A woman with a blood sugar level of less than 140 milligrams per deciliter (mg/dl) at 1-hour is presumed not to have gestational diabetes and requires no further testing. If the blood sugar level is greater than 140 mg/dl the test is considered abnormal or "positive." Not all women with a positive screening test have diabetes. Consequently, a 3-hour glucose tolerance test must be performed to establish the diagnosis of gestational diabetes.

If your physician determines that you should take the complete 3-hour glucose tolerance test, you will be asked to follow some special instructions in preparation for the test. For 3 days before the test, eat a diet that contains at least 150 grams of carbohydrates each day. This can be accomplished by including one cup of pasta, two servings of fruit, four slices of bread, and three glasses of milk every day. For 10 to 14 hours before the test you should not eat and not drink anything but water. The test is usually done in the morning in your physician's office or in a laboratory. First, a blood sample will be drawn to measure your fasting blood sugar level. Then you will be asked to drink a full bottle of a glucose drink (100 grams). This glucose drink is extremely sweet and occasionally makes some people feel nauseated. Finally, blood samples will be drawn every hour for 3 hours after the glucose drink has been consumed. The normal values for this test are shown below.

If two or more of your blood sugar levels are higher than the diagnostic criteria, you have gestational diabetes. This testing is usually performed at the end of the second trimester

or the beginning of the third trimester (between the 24th and 28th weeks of pregnancy) when insulin resistance usually begins. If you had gestational diabetes in a previous pregnancy or there is some reason why your physician is unusually concerned about your risk of developing gestational diabetes, you may be asked to take the 50-gram glucose screening test as early as the first trimester (before the 13th week). Remember, merely having sugar in your urine or even having an abnormal blood sugar on the 50-gram glucose screening test does not necessarily mean you have gestational diabetes. The 3-hour glucose tolerance test must be abnormal before the diagnosis is made.

3-Hour Glucose Tolerance Test for Gestational Diabetes		
	Diagnostic Criteria *Blood Glucose Level*	**Normal Mean Values** *Blood Glucose Level*
Fasting	105 mg/dl	80 mg/dl
1 hour	190 mg/dl	120 mg/dl
2 hour	165 mg/dl	105 mg/dl
3 hour	145 mg/dl	90 mg/dl

From 752 Unselected Pregnancies
Document Source: O'Sullivan, J.B. Establishing Criteria for Gestational Diabetes. *Diabetes Care* 3:437-439, 1980.

How does gestational diabetes affect pregnancy and will it hurt my baby?

The complications of gestational diabetes are manageable and preventable. The key to prevention is careful control of blood sugar levels just as soon as the diagnosis of gestational diabetes is made.

You should be reassured that there are certain things gestational diabetes does not usually cause. Unlike Type I diabetes, gestational diabetes generally does not cause birth defects. For the most part, birth defects originate sometime during the first trimester (before the 13th week) of pregnancy. The insulin resistance from the contra-insulin hormones produced by the placenta does not usually occur until approximately the 24th week. Therefore, women with gestational diabetes generally have normal blood sugar levels during the critical first trimester.

One of the major problems a woman with gestational diabetes faces is a condition the baby may develop called "macrosomia." Macrosomia means "large body" and refers to a baby that is considerably larger than normal. All of the nutrients the fetus receives come directly from the mother's blood. If the maternal blood has too much glucose, the pancreas of the fetus senses the high glucose levels and produces more insulin in an attempt to use the glucose. The fetus converts the extra glucose to fat. Even when the mother has gestational diabetes, the fetus is able to produce all the insulin it needs. The combination of high blood glucose levels from the mother and high insulin levels in the fetus results in large deposits of fat which causes the fetus to grow excessively large, a condition known as macrosomia. Occasionally, the baby grows too large to be delivered through the vagina and a cesarean delivery becomes necessary. The obstetrician can often determine if the fetus is macrosomic by doing a physical examination. However, in many cases a special test called an ultrasound is used to measure the size of the fetus. This and other special tests will be discussed later.

In addition to macrosomia, gestational diabetes increases the risk of hypoglycemia (low blood sugar) in the baby immediately after delivery. This problem occurs if the mother's blood sugar levels have been consistently high causing the fetus to have a high level of insulin in its circulation. After delivery the baby continues to have a high insulin level, but it no longer has the high level of sugar from its mother, resulting in the newborn's blood sugar level becoming very low. Your baby's blood sugar level will be checked in the newborn nursery and if the level is too low, it may be necessary to give the baby glucose intravenously. Infants of mothers with gestational diabetes are also vulnerable to several other chemical imbalances such as low serum calcium and low serum magnesium levels.

All of these are manageable and preventable problems. The key to prevention is careful control of blood sugar levels in the mother just as soon as the diagnosis of gestational diabetes is made. By maintaining normal blood sugar levels, it is less likely that a fetus will develop macrosomia, hypoglycemia, or other chemical abnormalities.

What can be done to reduce problems associated with gestational diabetes?

In addition to your obstetrician, there are other health professionals who specialize in the management of diabetes during pregnancy including internists or diabetologists, registered dietitians, qualified nutritionists, and diabetes educators. Your doctor may recommend that you see one or more of these specialists during your pregnancy. In addition, a neonatologist (a doctor who specializes in the care of newborn infants) should also be called in to manage any complications the baby might develop after delivery.

One of the essential components in the care of a woman with gestational diabetes is a diet specifically tailored to provide adequate nutrition to meet the needs of the mother and the growing fetus. At the same time the diet has to be planned in such a way as to keep blood glucose levels in the normal range (60 to 120 mg/dl). Specific details about diet during pregnancy are discussed later.

An obstetrician, diabetes educator, or other health care practitioner can teach you how to measure your own blood glucose levels at home to see if levels remain in an acceptable range on the prescribed diet. The ability of patients to determine their own blood sugar levels with easy-to-use equipment represents a major milestone in the management of diabetes, especially during pregnancy. The technique called "self blood glucose monitoring" (discussed in detail later) allows you to check your blood sugar levels at home or at work without costly and time-consuming visits to your doctor. The values of your blood sugar levels also determine if you need to begin insulin therapy sometime during pregnancy. Short of frequent trips to a laboratory, this is the only way to see if blood glucose levels remain under good control.

What is self blood glucose monitoring?

Once you are diagnosed as having gestational diabetes, you and your health care providers will want to know more about your day-to-day blood sugar levels. It is important to know how your exercise habits and eating patterns affect your blood sugars. Also, as your pregnancy progresses, the placenta will release more of the hormones that work against insulin. Testing your blood sugar level at important times during the day will help determine if proper diet and weight gain have kept blood sugar levels normal or if extra insulin is needed to help keep the fetus protected.

Self blood glucose monitoring is done by using a special device to obtain a drop of your blood and test it for your blood sugar level. Your doctor or other health care provide will explain the procedure to you. Make sure that you are shown how to do the testing before attempting it on your own. Some items you may use to monitor your blood sugar levels are:

Lancet—a disposable, sharp needle-like sticker for pricking the finger to obtain a drop of blood.
Lancet device—a spring-loaded finger sticking device.
Test strip—a chemically treated strip to which a drop of blood is applied.
Color chart—a chart used to compare against the color on the test strip for blood sugar level.
Glucose meter—a device which "reads" the test strip and gives you a digital number value.

Your health care provider can advise you where to obtain the self-monitoring equipment in your area. You may want to inquire if any places rent or loan glucose meters, since it is likely you won't be needing it after your baby is born.

How often and when should I test?

You may need to test your blood several times a day. Generally, these times are fasting (first thing in the morning before you eat) and 2 hours after each meal. Occasionally, you may be asked to test more frequently during the day or at night. As each person is an individual, your health care provider can advise the schedule best for you.

How should I record my test results?

Most manufacturers of glucose testing products provide a record diary, although some health care providers may have their own version.

You should record any test result immediately because it's easy to forget what the reading was during the course of a busy day. You should always have this diary with you when you visit your doctor or other health care provider or when you contact them by phone. These results are very important in making decisions about your health care.

Are there any other tests I should know about?

In addition to blood testing, you may be asked to check your urine for ketones. Ketones are by-products of the breakdown of fat and may be found in the blood and urine as a result of inadequate insulin or from inadequate calories in your diet. Although it is not known whether or not small amounts of ketones can harm the fetus, when large amounts of ketones are present they are accompanied by a blood condition, acidosis, which is known to harm the fetus. To be on the safe side, you should watch for them in your urine and report any positive results to your doctor.

How do I test for ketones?

To test the urine for ketones, you can use a test strip similar to the one used for testing your blood. This test strip has a special chemically treated pad to detect ketones in the urine. Testing is done by passing the test strip through the stream of urine or dipping the strip in and out of urine in a container. As your pregnancy progresses, you might find it easier to use the container method. All test strips are disposable and can be used only once. This applies to blood sugar test strips also. You cannot use your blood sugar test strips for urine testing, and you cannot use your urine ketone test strips for blood sugar testing.

When do I test for ketones?

Overnight is the longest fasting period, so you should test your urine first thing in the morning every day and any time your blood sugar level goes over 240 mg/dl on the blood glucose test. It is also important to test if you become ill and are eating less food than normal. Your health care provider can advise what's best for you.

Is it ever necessary to take insulin?

Yes, despite careful attention to diet some women's blood sugars do not stay within an acceptable range. A pregnant woman free of gestational diabetes rarely has a blood glucose level that exceeds 100 mg/dl in the morning before breakfast (fasting) or 2 hours after a meal. The optimum goal for a gestational diabetic is blood sugar levels that are the same as those of a woman without diabetes.

There is no absolute blood sugar level that necessitates beginning insulin injections. However, many physicians begin insulin if the fasting sugar exceeds 105 mg/dl or if the level 2 hours after a meal exceeds 120 mg/dl on two separate occasions. Blood sugar levels measured by you at home will help your doctor know when it is necessary to begin insulin. The ability to perform self blood glucose monitoring has made it possible to begin insulin therapy at the earliest sign of high sugar levels, thereby preventing the fetus from being exposed to high levels of glucose from the mother's blood.

Will my baby be healthy?

The ultimate concern of any expectant mother is, "Will my baby be all right?" There is an array of simple, safe tests used to assess the condition of the fetus before birth and these can be particularly valuable during a pregnancy complicated by gestational diabetes. Tests that may be given during your pregnancy include:

Ultrasound. Ultrasound uses short pulses of high-frequency, low-intensity sound waves to create images. Unlike x-rays, there is no radiation exposure to the fetus. First used during World War II to detect enemy submarines below the surface of the water, ultrasound has since been used safely in obstetrics. Occasionally, the date of your last menstrual period is not sufficient to determine a due date. Ultrasound can provide an accurate gestational age and due date that may be very important if it is necessary to induce labor early or perform a cesarean delivery. Ultrasound can also be used to determine the position of the placenta if it is necessary to perform an amniocentesis (another test discussed later).

Fetal movement records. Recording fetal movement is a test you can do by yourself to help determine the condition of the baby. Fetal activity is generally a reassuring sign of well-being. Women are often asked to count fetal movements regularly during the last trimester of pregnancy. You may be asked to set aside specific times to lie down on your back or side and count the number of times the baby moves or kicks. Three or more movements in a 2-hour period is considered normal. Contact your obstetrician if you feel fewer than three movements to determine if other tests are needed.

Fetal monitoring. Modern instruments make it possible to monitor the baby's heart rate before delivery. Currently, there are two types of fetal monitors—internal and external. The internal monitor consists of a small wire electrode attached directly to the scalp of the fetus after the membranes have ruptured. The external monitor uses transducers secured to the mother's abdomen by an elastic belt. One transducer records the baby's heart rate by a sensitive microphone called a doppler. The other transducer measures the firmness of the abdomen during a contraction of the uterus. It is a crude measure of the strength and frequency of contractions. Fetal monitoring is the basis for the nonstress test and the oxytocin challenge test described below.

Nonstress test. The "nonstress" test refers to the fact that no medication is given to the mother to cause movement of the fetus or contraction of the uterus. It is often used to confirm the well-being of the fetus based on the principle that a healthy fetus will demonstrate an acceleration in its heart rate following movement. Fetal activity may be spontaneous or induced by external manipulation such as rubbing the mother's abdomen or making a loud noise above the abdomen with a special device. When movement of the fetus is noted, a recording of the fetal heart rate is made. If the heart rate goes up, the test is normal. If the heart rate does not accelerate, the fetus may merely be "sleeping"; if, after stimulation, the fetus still does not react, it may be necessary to perform a "stress test" (oxytocin challenge test).

Stress test (oxytocin challenge test). Labor represents a stress to the fetus. Every time the uterus contracts, the fetus is momentarily deprived of its usual blood supply and oxygen. This is not a problem for most babies. However, some babies are not healthy enough to handle the stress and demonstrate an abnormal heart rate pattern. This test is often done if the non-stress test is abnormal. It involves giving the hormone oxytocin (secreted by every mother when normal labor begins) to the mother to stimulate uterine contractions. The contractions are a challenge to the baby, similar to the challenge of normal labor. If the baby's heart rate slows down rather than speeds up after a contraction, the baby may be in jeopardy. The stress test is considered more accurate than the non-stress test. Nevertheless, it is not 100 percent foolproof and your obstetrician may want to repeat it on another occasion to ensure its accuracy. Most women describe this test as mildly uncomfortable but not painful.

Amniocentesis. Amniocentesis is a method of removing a small amount of fluid from the amniotic sac for analysis. Either the fluid itself or the cells shed by the fetus into the fluid can be studied. In mid-pregnancy the cells in amniotic fluid can be analyzed for genetic abnormalities such as Down syndrome. Many women over the age of 35 have amniocentesis for just this reason. Another important use for amniocentesis late in pregnancy is to study the fluid itself to determine if the lungs of the fetus are mature and able to withstand early delivery. This information can be very important in deciding the best time for a woman with Type I diabetes to deliver. It is not done as frequently to women with gestational diabetes.

Amniocentesis can be performed in an obstetrician's office or on an outpatient basis in a hospital. For genetic testing, amniocentesis is usually performed around the 16th week when the placenta and fetus can be located easily with ultrasound and a needle can be inserted safely into the amniotic sac. The overall complication rate for amniocentesis is less than 1 percent. The risk is even lower during the third trimester when the amniotic sac is larger and easily identifiable.

Does gestational diabetes affect labor and delivery?

Most women with gestational diabetes can complete pregnancy and begin labor naturally. Any pregnant woman has a slight chance (about 5 percent) of developing preeclampsia (toxemia), a sudden onset of high blood pressure associated with protein in the urine, occurring late in pregnancy. If preeclampsia develops, your obstetrician may recommend an early delivery. When an early delivery is anticipated, an amniocentesis is usually performed to assess the maturity of the baby's lungs.

Gestational diabetes, by itself, is not an indication to perform a cesarean delivery, but sometimes there are other reasons your doctor may elect to do a cesarean. For example, the baby may be too large (macrosomic) to deliver vaginally, or the baby may be in distress and unable to withstand vaginal delivery. You should discuss the various possibilities for delivery with your obstetrician so there are no surprises.

Careful control of blood sugar levels remains important even during labor. If a mother's blood sugar level becomes elevated during labor, the baby's blood sugar level will also become elevated. High blood sugars in the mother produce high insulin levels in the baby. Immediately after delivery high insulin levels in the baby can drive its blood sugar level very low since it will no longer have the high sugar concentration from its mother's blood.

Women whose gestational diabetes does not require that they take insulin during their pregnancy, will not need to take insulin during their labor or delivery. On the other hand, a women who does require insulin during pregnancy may be given insulin by injection on the morning labor begins, or in some instances, it may be given intravenously throughout labor. For most women with gestational diabetes there is no need for insulin after the baby is born and blood sugar level returns to normal immediately. The reason for this sudden return to normal lies in the fact that when the placenta is removed the hormones it was producing (which caused the insulin resistance) are also removed. Thus, the mother's insulin is permitted to work normally without resistance. Your doctor may want to check your blood sugar level the next morning, but it will most likely be normal.

Should I expect my baby to have any problems?

One of the most frequently asked questions is, "Will my baby have diabetes?" Almost universally the answer is no. However, the baby is at risk for developing Type II diabetes later in life, and of having other problems related to gestational diabetes, such as hypoglycemia (low blood sugar) mentioned earlier. If your blood sugars were not elevated during the 24 hours before delivery, there is a good chance that hypoglycemia will not be a problem for your baby. Nevertheless, a neonatologist (a doctor who specializes in the care of newborn infants) or other doctor should check your baby's blood sugar level and give extra glucose if necessary.

Another problem that may develop in the infant of a mother with gestational diabetes is jaundice. Jaundice occurs when extra red blood cells in the baby's circulation are destroyed, releasing a substance called bilirubin. Bilirubin is a pigment that causes a yellow discoloration of the skin (jaundice). A minor degree of jaundice is common in many newborns. However, the presence of large amounts of bilirubin in the baby's system can be harmful and requires placing the baby under special lights which help get rid of the pigment. In extreme cases, blood transfusions may be necessary.

Will I develop diabetes in the future?

For most women gestational diabetes disappears immediately after delivery. However, you should have your blood sugars checked after your baby is born to make sure your levels have returned to normal. Women who had gestational diabetes during one pregnancy are at greater risk of developing it in a subsequent pregnancy. It is important that you have appropriate screening tests for gestational diabetes during future pregnancies as early as the first trimester.

Pregnancy is a kind of "stress test" that often predicts future diabetic problems. In one large study more than one-half of all women who had gestational diabetes developed overt Type II diabetes within 15 years of pregnancy. Because of the risk of developing Type II diabetes in the future, you should have your blood sugar level checked when you see your doctor for your routine check-ups. There is a good chance you will be able to reduce the risk of developing diabetes later in life by maintaining an ideal body weight and exercising regularly.

Why is a special diet recommended?

A nutritionally balanced diet is always essential to maintaining a healthy mother and successful pregnancy. The foods you choose become the nutrient building blocks for the growth of the fetus. For a woman with gestational diabetes, proper diet alone often keeps blood sugar levels in the normal range and is generally the first step to follow before resorting to insulin injections. Careful attention should be paid to the total calories eaten daily, to avoid foods which increase blood sugar levels, and to emphasize the use of foods which help the body maintain a normal blood sugar. A registered dietitian is the best person to help you with meal planning to meet your individual needs. Your physician can help you find a dietitian if this service is not a part of his or her office or clinic. Your local chapter of the American Dietetic Association or the American Diabetes Association can also help you locate a registered dietitian.

How much weight should I gain?

Of all questions asked by pregnant women, this is the most common. The answer is particularly important for women with gestational diabetes. The weight that you gain is a rough indication of how much nutrition is available to the fetus for growth. An inadequate weight gain may result in a small baby who lacks protective calorie reserves at birth. This baby may have more illness during the first year of life. An excessive weight gain during pregnancy, however, has an insulin-resistant effect, just like the hormones produced by the placenta, and will make your blood sugar level higher.

The "optimal" weight to gain depends on the weight that you are before becoming pregnant. Your pre-pregnancy weight is also a rough indication of how well-nourished you are before becoming pregnant. If you are at a desirable weight for your body size before you become pregnant, a weight gain of 24 to 27 pounds is recommended. If you are approximately 20 pounds or more above your desirable weight before pregnancy, a weight gain of 24 pounds is recommended. Many overweight women, however, have healthy babies and gain only 20 pounds. If you become pregnant when you are underweight, you need to gain more weight during the pregnancy to give your baby the extra nutrition he or she needs for the first year. You should gain 28 to 36 pounds, depending on how underweight you are before becoming pregnant. The table below shows whether your pre-pregnancy weight is considered underweight, normal weight, or overweight. Your nutrition advisor or health care provider can recommend an appropriate weight gain. How your weight gain is distributed is illustrated below.

Total recommended weight gain is often not as helpful as a weekly rate of gain. Most women gain 3 to 5 pounds during the first trimester (first 3 months) of pregnancy. During the second and third trimesters, a good rate of weight gain is about three-quarters of a pound to one pound per week. Gaining too much weight (2 or more pounds per week) results in putting on too much body fat. This extra body fat produces an insulin-resistant effect which requires the body to produce more insulin to keep blood sugar levels normal. An inability to produce more insulin, as in gestational diabetes, causes

your blood sugar levels to rise above acceptable levels. If weight gain has been excessive, often limiting weight gain to approximately three-quarters of a pound per week (3 pounds per month) can return blood sugar levels to normal. Fetal growth and development depend on proper nourishment and will be placed at risk by drastically reducing calories. However, you can limit weight gain by cutting back on excessive calories and by eating a nutritionally sound diet that meets your needs and the needs of your baby. Remember that dieting and severely cutting back on weight gain may increase the risk of delivering prematurely. If blood sugar levels continue to go up and you are not gaining excessive weight or eating improperly, the safest therapy for the well-being of the fetus is insulin.

Pre-Pregnancy Weight			
Pre-pregnancy weight for height. Use this chart to determine if your pre-pregnancy weight is normal, underweight, or overweight.			
Height without Shoes	*Underweight If You Weighed This or Less*	*Normal Weight Range**	*Overweight If You Weighed This or More*
4'10"	88	89-108	109
4'11"	91	92-112	113
5'	94	95-115	116
5'1"	99	100-121	122
5'2"	104	105-127	128
5'3"	108	109-132	133
5'4"	113	114-138	139
5'5"	118	119-144	145
5'6"	123	124-150	151
5'7"	127	128-155	156
5'8"	132	133-161	162
5'9"	137	138-167	168
5'10"	142	143-173	174
5'11"	146	147-178	179
6'	151	152-184	185
* Normal weight for "thin-boned" women will be closer to the lower end of this range. For "big-boned" women, it will be closer to the higher end. Reprinted with permission from: Judith E. Brown. *Nutrition for Your Pregnancy*. University of Minnesota Press, 1983.			

Occasionally, your weight may go up rapidly in the last trimester (after 28 weeks) and you may notice an increase in water retention, such as swelling in the feet, fingers, and face. If there is any question as to whether the rapid weight gain is due to eating too many calories or too much water retention, keeping records of how much food you eat and your exercise patterns at this time will be very helpful. By examining your food and exercise record sheet, your nutrition advisor can help you determine which is causing the rapid weight gain. In addition, by examining your legs and body for signs of fluid retention, your physician can help you to determine the cause of your weight gain. If your weight gain is due to water retention, cutting back drastically on calories may actually cause more fluid retention. Bed rest and resting on your side will help you to lose the build-up of fluid. Limit your intake of salt (sodium chloride) and very salty foods, as they tend to contribute to water retention.

```
┌─────────────────────────────────────────────┐
│        Distribution of Weight Gain During     │
│                   Pregnancy                   │
│                                               │
│                Weight in Pounds               │
│                                               │
│   7.5-8.5      Fetus                          │
│   7.5          Stores of Fat & Protein        │
│   4.0          Blood                          │
│   2.7          Tissue Fluids                  │
│   2.0          Uterus                         │
│   1.8          Amniotic Fluid                 │
│   1.5          Placenta & Umbilical Cord      │
│   1.0          Breasts                        │
│   28-29.0 Pounds                              │
└─────────────────────────────────────────────┘
```

Marked fluid retention when combined with an increase in blood pressure and possibly protein in the urine are the symptoms of preeclampsia. This is a disorder of pregnancy that can be harmful to both the mother and baby. Inform your obstetrician of any rapid weight gain, especially if you are eating moderately and gaining more than 2 pounds per week. Should you develop preeclampsia, be especially careful to eat a well-balanced diet with adequate calories.

After being diagnosed as having gestational diabetes, many women notice a slower weight gain as they start cutting the various sources of sugar out of their diet. This seems to be harmless and lasts only 1 or 2 weeks. It may be that sweets were contributing a substantial amount of calories to the diet.

How should I eat during my pregnancy?

As with any pregnancy, it is important to eat the proper foods to meet the nutritional needs of the mother and fetus. An additional goal for women with gestational diabetes is to maintain a proper diet to keep blood sugars as normal as possible.

The daily need for calories increases by 300 calories during the second and third trimesters of pregnancy. If non-pregnant calorie intake was 1,800 calories per day and weight gain was maintained, a calorie intake of 2,100 calories per day is usual from 14 weeks until delivery. This is the equivalent of an additional 8 ounce glass of 2% milk and one-half of a sandwich (1 slice of bread, approximately 1 ounce of meat, and 1 teaspoon of margarine, mayonnaise, etc.) per day. The need for protein also increases during pregnancy. Make sure your diet includes foods high in protein, but not high in fat. Most vitamins and minerals are also needed in larger amounts during pregnancy. This can be attained by increasing dairy products, especially those low in fat, and making sure you include whole grain cereals and breads, as well as fruits and vegetables in your diet each day. To make sure you get enough folate (a B vitamin critical during pregnancy) and iron, your obstetrician will probably recommend a prenatal vitamin. Prenatal vitamins do not replace a good diet; they merely help you to get the nutrients you need. To absorb the most iron from your prenatal vitamin, take it at night before going to bed, or in the morning on an empty stomach.

The Daily Food Guide serves as a guideline for food sources that provide important vitamins and minerals, as well as carbohydrates, protein, and fiber during pregnancy. The recommended minimal servings per day appear in parentheses after each food group listed. This guide emphasizes foods that are low in fat and in sugar (discussed later).

The food guide is divided into six groups: milk and milk products; meat, poultry, fish, and meat substitutes; breads, cereals, and other starches; fruits; vegetables; and fats. Each group provides its own combination of vitamins, minerals, and other nutrients which play an important part in nutrition during pregnancy. Omitting the foods from one group will leave your diet inadequate in other nutrients. Plan your meals using a variety of foods within each food group, in the amounts recommended, and you'll be most likely to get all the vitamins, minerals, and other nutrients the fetus needs for growth and development.

Other nutritional and non-nutritional considerations:

Alcohol. There is no known safe level of alcohol to allow during pregnancy. Daily heavy alcohol intake causes severe defects in development of the body and brain of the fetus, called Fetal Alcohol Syndrome. Even moderate drinking is associated with delayed fetal growth, spontaneous abortions, and lowered birth weight in babies. The Surgeon General's office warns: "Women who are pregnant or even considering pregnancy should avoid alcohol completely and should be aware of the alcohol content of food and drugs."

Salt. Salt restriction is no longer routinely advised during pregnancy. Recent research shows that during pregnancy the body needs salt to help provide the proper fluid balance. Your health care provider may recommend that you use salt in moderation.

Caffeine. Studies conflict on the potential danger of caffeine to the fetus. Caffeine is found primarily in coffee, tea, and some sodas. Moderation is recommended. Talk to your doctor or other health professional about the maximum amount of caffeine recommended.

Caffeine Comparisons		
Food	*Serving*	*Amount of Caffeine*
Regular coffee	8 oz.	80-200 mg.
Instant coffee	8 oz.	60-100 mg.
Decaffeinated coffee	8 oz.	3-5 mg.
Tea	8 oz.	60-65 mg.
Carbonated drinks e.g., colas	12 oz.	30-65 mg.
Hot chocolate	8 oz.	13 mg.

Megavitamins. Megavitamins are defined as 10 times the Recommended Dietary Allowance* of vitamins and minerals and are not recommended for pregnant women. Although it

---

* Dietary allowances established by the National Academy of Sciences—National Research Council.

Daily Food Guide (Each item equals one serving)

Milk and Milk Products *(4 Servings Per Day)*	1 cup milk, skim or low-fat 1/3 cup powdered non-fat milk 1 cup reconstituted powdered non-fat milk 1 1/2 oz. low-fat cheese* (no more than 6 grams of fat per ounce) 1 cup low-fat yogurt**	(high protein calcium, vitamin D)
Meat, Poultry, Fish, and Meat Substitutes *(5-6 Servings Per Day)*	1 oz. cooked poultry, fish, or lean meat (beef, lamb, pork) 1 tbsp. peanut butter 1 egg 1/4 cup low-fat cottage cheese 1/2 cup cooked dried beans or lentils	(high protein, B vitamins, iron)
Breads, Cereals, and Other Starches *(5-6 Servings Per Day)*	1 slice whole grain bread 5 crackers 1 muffin, biscuit, pancake, or waffle 3/4 cup dry cereal, unsweetened 1/2 cup pasta (macaroni, spaghetti), rice, mashed potatoes, or cooked cereal 1/3 cup sweet potatoes or yams 1/2 cup cooked dried beans or lentils 1/2 bagel, 1/2 english muffin, or 1/2 flour tortilla 1 small baked potato 2 taco shells	(high complex carbohydrates) (emphasize whole grains, or use fortified or enriched) (a good source of protein, B-vitamins, fiber and minerals)
Fruit *(2 servings per day)*	1/2 cup fresh fruit, 1/2 banana, or 1 medium-sized fruit (apple, orange) 1/2 cup orange, grapefruit, or other juice fortified with vitamin C 1/2 medium-sized grapefruit 1 cup strawberries 1/2 cup fresh apricots, nectarines, purple plums, cantaloup, or 4 halves dried apricots (vitamin A source)	(fresh fruit provides fiber) (include one vitamin C source daily)
Vegetables*** *(2 servings per day)*	1/2 cup cooked or 1 cup raw: broccoli, spinach, carrots, (vitamin A source) 1/3 cup mixed vegetables	(include good vitamin A sources at least every other day)
Fats	1 tsp. butter or margarine 1 tsp. oil or mayonnaise 1 tbsp. regular salad dressing 2 tbsp. low-calorie salad dressing 1/4 cup nuts or seeds	

* 1 oz. low-fat cheese can also be used a 1 serving from the Meat, Poultry, Fish, and Meat Substitutes group if sufficient calcium is already being provided from 4 servings.

**This refers to plain yogurt. Commercially fruited yogurt contains a lot of added sugar.

***Starchy vegetables such as corn, peas, and potatoes are included in Breads, Cereals and Other Starches list.

is possible to get all of the necessary nutrients from food alone, your doctor may prescribe some prenatal vitamins and minerals. If taken regularly, along with a balanced diet, you will be getting all the vitamins and minerals needed during your pregnancy.

Smoking. Research has shown without question that smoking during pregnancy increases the risk of fetal death and preterm delivery, impairs fetal growth, and can lead to low birth weight. It is best to stop smoking entirely and permanently, or at the very least, to cut back drastically on the number of cigarettes you smoke.

What food patterns help keep blood sugar levels normal?

The following outlines food patterns which help to keep blood sugar levels within an acceptable range.

Avoid sugar and foods high in sugar. Most women with gestational diabetes, just like those without diabetes, have a desire for something sweet in their diet. In pregnant women, sugar is rapidly absorbed into the blood and requires a larger release of insulin to maintain normal blood sugar levels. Without the larger release of insulin, blood sugar levels will increase excessively when you eat sugar-containing foods.

There are many forms of sugar such as table sugar, honey, brown sugar, corn syrup, maple syrup, turbinado sugar, high fructose corn syrup, and molasses. Generally, food that ends in "ose" is a sugar (e.g., sucrose, dextrose, and glucose).

Foods that usually contain high amounts of sugar include pies, cakes, cookies, ice cream, candy, soft drinks, fruit drinks, fruit packed in syrup, commercially fruited yogurt, jams, jelly, doughnuts, and sweet rolls. Many of these foods are high in fat as well.

Be sure to check the list of ingredients on food products. Ingredients are listed in order of amount. If an ingredient is first on the list, it is present in the highest amount. If some type of sugar is listed first, second, or third on the list of ingredients, the product should be avoided. If sugar is further down, fourth, fifth, or sixth, it probably will not cause your blood sugar levels to go up excessively.

Fruit juices should only be taken with a meal and limited to 6 ounces. Tomato juice is a good choice because it is low in sugar. Six ounces of most other juice (apple, grapefruit, orange) with no sugar added still contain approximately 4 to 5 teaspoons of sugar. However, these do not contain much of the fiber of a piece of fruit which normally would act to slow the absorption of sugar into the blood. If you drink juice frequently to quench your thirst during the day, a high blood sugar level may result. Use only whole fruit for snacks.

To help with the occasional sweet tooth that we all have, artificial sweeteners may be used in foods. Aspartame has been extensively tested for safety. Use during pregnancy has been approved by the Food and Drug Administration and by the American Medical Association's Review Board. However, aspartame has not been tested for long-term safety and has not been on the market very long. It may be best to avoid its use until more tests have been done.

Saccharin is not advised during pregnancy. Likewise, use of mannitol, xylitol, sorbitol, or other artificial sweeteners is not recommended until further research is done.

Fructose is a special type of sugar that is slowly absorbed into the system. A small amount of fructose can be used if your blood sugar levels are within normal range. However, fructose still has 4 calories per gram, as much as table sugar. High fructose corn syrup is part fructose and part corn syrup, making it very similar to table sugar in composition. It will raise blood sugar levels and should definitely be avoided.

Emphasize the use of complex carbohydrates. These include vegetables, cereal, grains, beans, peas, and other starchy foods. A well-balanced diet with plenty of fiber provided by vegetables, dried beans, cereals, and other starchy foods decreases the amount of insulin your body needs to keep blood sugars within a normal range. Anything that decreases the need for insulin is beneficial. The American Diabetes Association recommends that at least one-half of your calories come from complex carbohydrates. Starchy foods include pasta, rice, grains, cereals, crackers, bread, potatoes, dried beans, peas, and legumes. Also, contrary to popular belief, carbohydrates are not highly fattening when eaten in moderate amounts and without the rich sauces and toppings often added.

Emphasize foods high in dietary fiber. Fiber is the edible portion of foods of plant origin that is not digested (e.g., skins, membranes, seeds, bran). Foods with a high fiber content include whole grain cereals and breads, fruits, vegetables, and legumes (dried peas and beans). Fiber aids digestion and helps prevent constipation. The fiber found in fruits, vegetables, and legumes also helps keep your blood sugar level from becoming too high without requiring extra insulin.

Keep your diet low in fat. Some fat is needed to help with the absorption of certain vitamins and to provide the essential fatty acids necessary for fetal growth. A diet which is high in fat causes the insulin to react in a less efficient manner, necessitating more insulin to keep blood sugar levels within normal range. Foods high in saturated fats such as fatty meats, butter, bacon, cream (light, coffee, sour cream, etc.), and whole milk cheeses are likely to be high in total fat. Most foods with saturated fat are also high in cholesterol because they are fats from animal origin. However, foods such as crackers made with coconut, palm, or palm kernel oil can be high in saturated fats as well. Read labels carefully. Unsaturated fats are found in foods such as fish, margarine and vegetable oils. Keep your use of salad dressings to a minimum and whenever possible use those prepared with olive oil. To help keep the diet lower in fat, avoid adding extra fats such as rich sauces and creamy desserts, and bake or broil foods instead of frying them. Replacing fatty foods with those high in complex carbohydrates is also helpful.

Include a bedtime snack that is a good source of protein and complex carbohydrates. Women with gestational diabetes have a tendency toward lower than normal blood sugar levels during the night. This causes the body to increase its utilization of fats as a fuel source. As fat is used, ketones (discussed later) are produced as a by-product of the breakdown of fats, and in large amounts, may be harmful to the fetus. This can be prevented by having a bedtime snack that provides protein and complex carbohydrates such as starchy foods. Starch will stabilize your blood sugar level in the early night, while protein acts as a long-acting stabilizer. Examples of a bedtime snack are:

1 oz. American-processed cheese + 5 crackers
1/2 chicken sandwich on whole wheat bread
3 cups unbuttered popcorn + 1/4 cup nuts

If you need to take insulin, a bedtime snack is critical and you should not omit it. When taken by injection, insulin acts to lower blood sugar level, even during the night when meals are not eaten. A bedtime snack is protective against low blood sugars while sleeping or upon arising. If a bedtime snack causes heartburn, sleep with your head raised on pillows, and be careful that you are not eating too large a bedtime snack.

How do I plan meals?

A registered dietitian or qualified nutritionist can help you plan a meal pattern that is right for you. Most women with gestational diabetes need three meals and a bedtime snack each day. It is unwise for anyone who is pregnant to go long periods of time (greater than 5 hours) without eating, as this will produce ketones. Extra snacks are necessary if your schedule results in a long time between meals. Blood sugars will be easier to keep in the normal range if meal times and amounts (total calories) are evenly spaced. It's more likely that a higher blood sugar will result if the majority of calories are eaten at dinner, than if they are distributed more evenly throughout the day. If insulin injections prove necessary, the time at which meals are eaten and the amounts eaten should be approximately the same from day to day. Do not skip meals and snacks, as this often results in hypoglycemia (low blood sugar), which may be harmful to the fetus and makes you feel irritable, shaky, or may result in a headache.

Sample Menu—2000 Calories

This diet is planned for women whose normal non-pregnant weight should be 130-135 lbs. For women who weigh less than 130 before pregnancy, the diet should contain fewer calories. Women who are overweight are at higher risk for gestational diabetes. Your health care provider can discuss this and help you make necessary changes.

BREAKFAST

1/2 grapefruit
3/4 cup oatmeal, cooked
1 tsp. raisins
1 cup 2% milk
1 whole wheat English muffin
1 tsp. margarine

LUNCH

Salad with:
      1 cup romaine lettuce
      1/2 cup kidney beans, cooked
      1/2 fresh tomato
1 oz. part skim mozzarella cheese
2 tbsp. low-calorie Italian dressing
1 bran muffin
1/2 cup cantaloupe chunks

AFTERNOON SNACK

2 rice cakes
6 oz. low-fat yogurt, plain
1/2 cup blueberries

DINNER

3/4 cup vegetable soup with 1/4 cup cooked barley
3 oz. chicken, without skin
1 baked potato
1/2 cup cooked broccoli
1 piece whole wheat bread
1 tbsp. margarine
1 fresh peach

BEDTIME SNACK

1 apple
2 cups popcorn, plain
1/4 cup peanuts

What can be done to slow weight gain during pregnancy?

Gaining too much weight during pregnancy will make blood sugar levels higher than normal for women with gestational diabetes. Yet, for many pregnant women it is very difficult to gain weight slowly and still get all of the recommended nutrients. Luckily, fat, which is high in calories (9 calories per gram), is needed in only small amounts during pregnancy. Carbohydrates and protein, in contrast to fat, provide only 4 calories per gram. To cut calories without depriving the fetus of any necessary nutritional factors, it is best to avoid fats and fatty foods.

- ♦ Avoid high-fat meats. Choose lean cuts of beef, pork, and lamb. Emphasize more fish and poultry (without the skin).
- ♦ Avoid frying meat, fish, or poultry in added oil, shortening, or lard. Bake, broil, or roast instead.
- ♦ Avoid foods fried in oil such as chips, french fries, and doughnuts. Substitute pretzels, unbuttered popcorn, or breadsticks instead.
- ♦ Avoid using cream sauces and butter sauces, as well as salt pork for seasoning on vegetables. Season with herbs instead.
- ♦ Avoid using the fat drippings from meat or poultry for gravy. Use broth or bouillon instead and thicken with cornstarch.
- ♦ Avoid using mayonnaise or oil for salads. Use vinegar, lemon juice, or low-calorie salad dressings instead.

To help reduce calories choose low-fat dairy products. During pregnancy you need 1200 mg calcium daily to build the fetal skeleton without drawing from maternal calcium stores. Table 7 points out foods in which the calcium content is almost the same, yet the calories are not due to the difference in fat content.

The difference between 600 calories and 340 calories is only 260 calories and may seem insignificant. Yet, if your diet is cut by 260 calories daily for 1 week, your weight gain slows down by approximately 1/2 pound per week. In other words, instead of gaining 1-1/2 pound per week you will only gain 1 pound per week.

If cheese is a part of your daily diet, use low-fat cheeses such as low-fat cottage cheese, Neufchatel, mozzarella, farmers, and pot cheese. Avoid using cream cheese, as it has little protein and most of its calories come from fat.

Even though pregnancy can be a very hectic time, with little time for meal preparation, eat less and less often at "fast food" restaurants. Studies have shown that some foods from fast food restaurants average 40 to 60 percent of their calories from fat, and are quite high in calories*. For example, chicken and fish that are coated with batter and deep-fried in fat may contain more fat and calories than a hamburger or roast beef sandwich.

---

* *Fast Food Facts: Nutritive and Exchange Values for Fast Food Restaurants.* Marion J. Franz, International Diabetes Center, Minneapolis, Minnesota, 1987. 54 pp.

Calorie Comparisons	
Food	*Calories*
4-8 oz. glasses whole milk	600
4-8 oz. glasses 2% milk	480
4-8 oz. glasses skim milk	340
2-8 oz. glasses whole milk plus 3 oz. American processed cheese	600
2-8 oz. glasses 2% milk plus 3 oz. American processed cheese	540
2-8 oz. glasses skim milk plus 3 oz. American processed cheese	470

Go lightly when using butter and margarine. Adding only an extra three pats of butter or margarine (same calories) daily could add an extra pound of weight gain next month. It may be better to emphasize the use of foods rich in complex carbohydrates that don't use butter, margarine, or cream sauce to make them palatable. Many people find rice, noodles, and spaghetti tasty without a lot of butter. Use a variety of spices and herbs (such as curry, garlic, and parsley) to flavor rice and tomato sauce to flavor pasta without additional fats.

It is also a good idea to eat small amounts frequently, thereby keeping the edge off your appetite. This will assist your "self-control" in avoiding large portions of food that you should not have. Avoid skipping meals or trying to cut back drastically on breakfast or lunch. It will leave you too hungry for the next meal to exercise any control. Your doctor or dietitian can help you determine how you can cut extra calories.

You may find it helpful to keep food records of what you eat, as most of us tend to forget or not realize the extent of our snacking. Recording everything you eat or drink tends to be a sobering and instructive experience.

Be careful to maintain a weight gain of at least 1/2 pound per week, over several weeks, if you are in the second trimester (14 weeks or more of gestation). Cutting back more than this may increase the risk of having a low-birth-weight infant.

Is breast-feeding recommended?

Breast-feeding is strongly encouraged. For most women this represents the easiest way back to pre-pregnancy weight after delivery. The body draws on the calories stored during the first part of pregnancy to use in milk production. Approximately 800 calories per day are used during the first 3 months of milk production, and even more during the next 3 months. By 6 weeks after delivery, women who breast-feed usually have lost 4 pounds more than women who bottle-feed. This can be a very important factor, as it is strongly recommended that women with gestational diabetes return to their desirable body weight 4 to 5 months postpartum. As previously mentioned, maintaining a weight appropriate for your height and frame may reduce the risk of developing diabetes later in life.

In addition, breast-feeding has many advantages for your baby. Protection from infection and allergies are transferred to the baby through breast milk. This milk is also easier to digest than formula, and its minerals are better absorbed than those in formula.

Should I exercise?

A daily exercise program is an important part of a healthy pregnancy. Daily exercise helps you feel better and reduces stress. In addition, being physically fit protects against back pain, and maintains muscle tone, strength, and endurance. For women with gestational diabetes, exercise is especially important.

- ♦ Regular exercise increases the efficiency or potency of your body's own insulin. This may allow you to keep your blood sugar levels in the normal range while using less insulin.
- ♦ Moderate exercise also helps blunt your appetite, helping you to keep your weight gain down to normal levels. Maintaining the correct weight gain is very important in preventing high blood sugar levels.

Talk with your doctor about what exercise program is right for you. Your doctor can advise you about limitations, warning signs, and any special considerations. Generally, you can continue any exercise program or sport you participated in prior to pregnancy. Use caution, however, and avoid sports or exercises where you might fall, or that involve jolting. Pre-pregnancy bicycling, jogging, and cross-country skiing are good exercises to continue during pregnancy. If you plan to start an exercise program during pregnancy, talk to your doctor before beginning and start slowly. Vigorous walking is good for women who need to start exercising and have not been active before pregnancy.

Exercising frequently, 4 to 5 days per week, is necessary to get the "blood sugar lowering" advantages of an exercise program. Don't omit a warm-up period of 5 to 10 minutes and a cool-down period of 5 to 10 minutes. Always stop exercising if you feel pain, dizziness, shortness of breath, faintness, palpitations, back or pelvic pain, or experience vaginal bleeding. Also, avoid vigorous exercise in hot, humid weather or if you have a fever. It is important to prevent dehydration during exercise, especially during pregnancy. The American College of Obstetricians and Gynecologists (ACOG) recommends drinking fluids prior to and after exercise, and if necessary, during the activity to prevent dehydration.

An ACOG report*, issued in 1985, warned that target heart rates for pregnant and postpartum women should be set approximately 25 to 30 percent lower than rates for non-pregnant women. It may be that exercising too vigorously will direct blood flow away from the uterus and fetus. ACOG recommends that pregnant women measure their heart rate during activity and that maternal heart rate not exceed 140 beats per minute.

---

* *Home Exercise Program: Exercise During Pregnancy and the Postnatal Period.* American College of Obstetricians and Gynecologists. May 1985, 6 pp.

If you need to be on insulin during your pregnancy, take a few precautions. Because both insulin and exercise lower blood sugar levels, the combination can result in hypoglycemia or low blood sugar. You need to be aware that this is a potential problem, and you should be familiar with the symptoms of hypoglycemia (confusion, extreme hunger, blurry vision, shakiness, sweating). When exercising, take along sugar in the form of hard, sugar-sweetened candies just in case your blood sugar becomes too low. When on insulin, you should always carry some form of sugar for potential episodes of hypoglycemia.

It may be necessary for you to eat small snacks between meals if the exercise results in low blood sugar levels.

◆ One serving of fruit will keep blood sugars normal for most short-term activities (approximately 30 minutes).
◆ One serving of fruit plus a serving of starch will be enough for activities that last longer (60 minutes or more).

If you exercise right after a meal, eat the snack after the exercise. If the exercise is 2 hours or more after a meal, eat the snack before the exercise.

What happens if diet and exercise fail to control my blood sugars?

If your blood sugars tend to go over the acceptable levels (105 mg/dl or below for fasting, 120 mg/dl or below 2 hours after a meal) you may need to take insulin injections. Insulin is a protein and would be digested like any other protein in food if it were given orally. The needles used to inject insulin are extremely fine, so there is little discomfort. If insulin injections are necessary, you will be taught how to fill the syringe and how to do the injections yourself.

Your physician will calculate the amount of insulin needed to keep blood sugar levels within the normal range. It is very likely that the amount or dosage of insulin needed to keep your levels of blood sugar normal will increase as your pregnancy advances. This does not mean your gestational diabetes is getting worse. As any healthy pregnancy progresses, the placenta will grow and produce progressively higher levels of contra-insulin hormones. As a result you will likely need to inject more insulin to overcome their effect. Some women may even require two injections each day. This does not imply anything about the severity of the problem or the outcome of the pregnancy. The goal is to maintain normal blood sugar levels with whatever dosage of insulin is needed.

Can my blood sugar level go too low, and if so, what do I do?

Occasionally, your blood sugar level may get too low if you are taking insulin. This can happen if you delay a meal or exercise more than usual, especially at the time your insulin is working at its peak. This low blood sugar is called "hypoglycemia" or an "insulin reaction." This is a medical emergency and should be promptly treated, never ignored.

The symptoms of insulin reaction vary from sweating, shakiness, or dizziness to feeling faint, disoriented, or a tin-gling sensation. Remember, if you take insulin injections, you need to keep some form of sugar-sweetened candy in your purse, at home, at work, and in your car. In case of an episode of hypoglycemia, you will be prepared to treat it immediately. Be sure to eat something more substantial afterward. Also, report any insulin reactions or high blood sugar levels to your doctor right away in case an adjustment in your treatment needs to be made.

As you can see from reading this booklet, extra care, work, and commitment on the part of you and your spouse or partner are required to provide the special medical care necessary. Don't worry if you occasionally go off your diet or miss a planned exercise program. Your doctor and other health care professionals will work along with you to make sure you receive the specialized care that has resulted in dramatically improved pregnancy outcome.

An ounce of prevention is worth a pound of cure! Eat as directed. Exercise as directed. Monitor as directed. Do these things and you are doing your part toward a happy, healthy pregnancy.

Glossary

Carbohydates. A type of food, usually from plants versus animals. Carbohydrates include simple carbohydrates (sugar, fruit) and complex carbohydrates (vegetables, starches). One of three nutrients that supply calories to the body. (See fat and protein.)

Diabetes mellitus. A disorder that prevents the body from converting digested food into the energy needed for daily activities.

Fat. One of three nutrients that supply calories to the body. Included are vegetable oil, lard, margarine, butter, shortening, mayonnaise, and salad dressing. (See carbohydrates and protein.)

Gestational diabetes. A form of diabetes which begins during pregnancy and usually disappears following delivery.

Glucose tolerance test. A blood test used to make the diagnosis of diabetes, including gestational diabetes. After drinking a liquid containing 100 grams of glucose, blood is drawn every hour for 3 hours. Two or more abnormally elevated blood sugar levels indicate gestational diabetes.

Health care providers. Health care professionals who specialize in the management of certain conditions. In the case of gestational diabetes, the health care providers may include an obstetrician, an internist, a diabetologist, a registered dietitian, a qualified nutritionist, a diabetes educator, and a neonatologist.

Hormone. A chemical substance produced within the body which has a "regulatory" effect on the activity of a certain tissue in the body. Estrogen, cortisol, and human placental lactogen are hormones produced by the placenta which cause changes in the mother's body to prepare her for the pregnancy and birth. These hormones also have a contra-insulin effect.

Hypoglycemia. A condition where the blood sugar is lower than normal. This is a dangerous condition and should be avoided or treated rapidly.

Insulin. A hormone manufactured by the pancreas. Insulin helps glucose leave the blood and enter the muscles and other tissues of the body.

Insulin-resistance. A partial blocking of the effect of insulin. This interference can be caused by hormones produced by the placenta or by excessive weight gain.

Ketone. A break-down product of fat that accumulates in the blood as a result of inadequate insulin or inadequate calorie intake.

Legumes. Beans, peas, and lentils which supply fiber and nutrients and are high in vegetable protein.

Macrosomia. A term meaning "large body." This refers to a baby that is considerably larger than normal. This condition occurs when the mother's blood sugar levels have been higher than normal during the pregnancy. This is a preventable complication of gestational diabetes.

Nutrients. Proteins, carbohydrates, fats, vitamins, and minerals. These are provided by food and are necessary for growth and the maintenance of life.

Pancreas. A long gland that lies behind the stomach. The pancreas manufactures insulin and digestive enzymes.

Placenta. A special tissue that joins the mother and fetus. It provides hormones necessary for a successful pregnancy, and supplies the fetus with water and nutrients (food) from the mother's blood.

Protein. A substance found in many parts of the body that helps the body to resist disease. Protein often, but not always, comes from animal products. High protein foods include meat, poultry, fish, eggs, hard cheese, cottage cheese, yogurt, and milk. Non-animal sources of protein are nuts and seeds, peanut butter, legumes, whole grains, and tofu. One of three nutrients that supply calories to the body. (See carbohydrates and fat.)

Recommended Dietary Allowances. Recommendations for daily intake of specific nutrients for groups of healthy individuals. There is a specific recommendation for pregnant and for lactating women. These recommendations are set by the Food and Nutrition Board of the National Research Council of the National Academy of Science.

Self (or home) blood glucose monitoring. A process by which blood sugars can be determined at home by pricking the finger, putting a drop of blood on a chemically treated test strip, and comparing the color changes to a chart.

Trimester. A period of 3 months. Pregnancy is divided into three trimesters. The first trimester is 0-13 weeks gestation. The second trimester is 14-26 weeks gestation. The third trimester is 27 weeks gestation until birth.

■ **Document Source:**
U.S. Department of Health and Human Services, Public Health Service
National Institutes of Health
National Institute of Child Health and Human Development
NIH Publication No. 93-2788
Reprinted February 1993

See also: Diabetes Overview (page 110); Insulin-Dependent Diabetes (page 112); Noninsulin-Dependent Diabetes (page 116)

VAGINITIS: IMPORTANT INFORMATION FOR YOUR GOOD HEALTH

Vaginitis is a medical term that is used to refer to *any* infection or inflammation of the vagina. The symptoms of vaginitis are common and most women will have at least one form of vaginitis in their lifetime. Even though vaginitis is so common, many women know little about it.

The term "yeast infection" is what most women think of when they hear the word vaginitis. However, a yeast infection is only *one kind* of vaginal infection. Vaginitis can be caused by several different organisms, sometimes at the same time, as well as by hormonal changes, allergies, or irritations.

Because vaginitis can have many causes, it is important to see your doctor or other health care professional so that the proper cause can be identified and the correct treatment can be prescribed. Once started, the medication should be used exactly according to your doctor's instructions in order to cure the vaginitis. The symptoms may go away before you finish the medication. Even so, you should complete the therapy to help ensure a cure.

Vaginitis can sometimes be a sign of other health problems. Knowing more about the signs and symptoms of this common condition will help you and your health care provider make a proper diagnosis.

What is vaginitis?

"Vaginitis" is a word that is used to describe disorders that cause infection or inflammation ("itis" means inflammation) of the vagina. Vulvovaginitis refers to inflammation of both the vagina and vulva (the external female genitals). These conditions can result from an infection caused by organisms such as bacteria, yeast, or viruses, as well as by irritations from chemicals in creams, sprays, or even clothing that are in contact with this area. In some cases, vaginitis results from organisms that are passed between sexual partners.

How do I know if I have vaginitis?

The common symptoms of vaginitis are itching, burning, and vaginal discharge that is different from your normal secretions. The itching and burning can be inside the vagina or on the skin or vulva just outside the vagina. Discomfort during urination or sexual intercourse may also occur. If everyone with vaginitis had these symptoms, then the diagnosis would be fairly simple. However, it is important to realize that as many as 4 out of every 10 women with vaginitis may not have these typical symptoms. Frequently, a routine gynecologic exam will confirm vaginitis even if symptoms are not present. This is one reason why it is important to have a gynecologic exam at least every 2 years.

Is vaginal discharge normal?

A woman's vagina normally produces a discharge that is usually described as clear or slightly cloudy, nonirritating, and odor-free. During the normal menstrual cycle the amount and consistency of discharge vary. At one time of the month there may be a small amount of a very thin or watery discharge and at another time, a more extensive, thicker discharge may appear. All of these descriptions could be considered normal.

A vaginal discharge that has an odor or that is irritating is usually an abnormal discharge. The irritation might be itching or burning or both. The burning could feel like a bladder infection. The itching may be present at any time of the day but it is often most bothersome at night. Both of these symptoms are usually made worse by sexual intercourse. It is important to see a doctor or clinician if there has been a *change* in the amount, appearance, or smell of the discharge.

What are the most common types of vaginitis?

The six most common types of vaginitis are:

- *Candida* or "yeast" vaginitis
- Bacterial vaginosis
- *Trichomoniasis* vaginitis
- *Chlamydia* vaginitis
- Viral vaginitis
- Noninfectious vaginitis

Although each of these causes of vaginal infection can have different symptoms, it is not always easy for a patient to figure out which type of vaginitis she has; in fact, diagnosis can even be tricky for an experienced clinician. Part of the problem is that sometimes more than one type of vaginitis can be present at the same time. Often vaginitis is present without any symptoms at all.

To help you better understand these six major causes of vaginitis, let's look briefly at each one of them and how they are treated.

What are *Candida* or "yeast" infections?

Yeast infections of the vagina are what most women think of when they hear the term "vaginitis." They are caused by one of the many species of fungus called *Candida*. *Candida* normally live in small numbers in the vagina as well as in the mouth and digestive tract of both men and women.

Yeast infections produce a thick, white vaginal discharge with the consistency of cottage cheese. Although the discharge can be somewhat watery, it is odorless. Yeast infections usually cause the vagina and the vulva to be very itchy and red.

Risk Factors for Vaginal Candida Infections

- Recent Course of Antibiotics
- Uncontrolled Diabetes
- Pregnancy
- High Estrogen Contraceptives
- Immunosuppression
- Thyroid or Endocrine Disorders
- Corticosteroid Therapy

Since yeast is normal in a woman's vagina, what makes it cause an infection? Usually this happens when a change in the delicate balance in a woman's system occurs. For example, a woman may take an antibiotic to treat a urinary tract infection and the antibiotic kills her "friendly" bacteria that normally keep the yeast in balance; as a result the yeast overgrows and causes the infection. Other factors which can upset the delicate balance include pregnancy which changes hormone levels and diabetes which allows too much sugar in the urine and vagina.

What is bacterial vaginosis?

Although "yeast" is the name most women know, bacterial vaginosis is actually the most common vaginal infection in women of reproductive age. Bacterial vaginosis will often cause a vaginal discharge. The discharge is usually thin and milky and is described as having a "fishy" odor. This odor may become more noticeable after intercourse. Redness or itching of the vagina are not common symptoms of bacterial vaginosis. It is important to note that many women with bacterial vaginosis have no symptoms at all and the vaginitis is only discovered during a routine gynecologic exam. Bacterial vaginosis is caused by a combination of several bacteria. These bacteria seem to overgrow much the same way as *Candida* will when the vaginal balance is upset. The exact reason for this overgrowth is not known. Since bacterial vaginosis is caused by bacteria, not by yeast, it is easy to see that different methods are needed to treat the different infections. A medicine that is appropriate for yeast is not effective against the bacteria that causes bacterial vaginosis.

What are *trichomoniasis, chlamydia,* and viral vaginitis?

Trichomonias, commonly called "trich" (pronounced "trick"), is caused by a tiny single-celled organism known as a "protozoa." When this organism infects the vagina it can cause a frothy, greenish-yellow discharge. Often this discharge will have a foul smell. Women with trichomonal vaginitis may complain of itching and soreness of the vagina and vulva, as well as burning during urination. In addition, there can be discomfort in the lower abdomen and vaginal pain with intercourse. These symptoms may be worse after the menstrual period. Many women, however, do not develop any symptoms. It is important to understand that this type of vaginitis can be transmitted through sexual intercourse. For treatment to be effective, the sexual partner must be treated at the same time as the patient.

Another primarily sexually transmitted form of vaginitis is caused by the germ known as *Chlamydia*. Unfortunately, most women do not have symptoms. This makes diagnosis difficult. A vaginal discharge is sometimes present with this infection but not always. More often a woman might experience light bleeding especially after intercourse. She may have pain in the lower abdomen and pelvis. Chlamydial vaginitis is most common in young women (18 to 35 years) who have multiple sexual partners. If you fit this description, you should request screening for *Chlamydia* during your annual checkup. The best "treatment" for *Chlamydia* is prevention. Use of a condom will decrease your risk of contracting not only *Chlamydia*, but other sexually transmitted diseases as well.

Viruses are a common cause of vaginitis. One form caused by the *herpes simplex virus* (HSV) is often just called "herpes" infection. These infections are also spread by sexual intimacy. The primary symptom of herpes vaginitis is pain associated with lesions or "sores." These sores are usually visible on the vulva or the vagina but occasionally are inside the vagina and can only be seen during a gynecologic exam. Outbreaks of HSV are often associated with stress or emotional upheaval.

Another source of viral vaginal infection is the human papillomavirus (HPV). HPV can also be transmitted by sexual intercourse. This virus can cause painful warts to grow in the vagina, rectum, vulva, or groin. These warts are usually white to gray in color, but they may be pink or purple. However, visible warts are not always present and the virus may only be detected when a Pap smear is abnormal.

> *Many of the germs that cause vaginitis can be spread between men and women during sexual intercourse. Use of a barrier contraceptive such as a condom can help reduce your risk of contracting these and more serious germs such as the human immunodeficiency virus (HIV) which can lead to AIDS.*

What is noninfectious vaginitis?

Occasionally, a woman can have itching, burning, and even a vaginal discharge without having an infection. The most common cause is an allergic reaction or irritation from vaginal sprays, douches, or spermicidal products. The skin around the vagina can also be sensitive to perfumed soaps, detergents, and fabric softeners.

Another noninfectious form of vaginitis results from a decrease in hormones because of menopause or because of surgery that removes the ovaries. In this form, the vagina becomes dry or "atrophic." The woman may notice pain, especially with sexual intercourse, as well as vaginal itching and burning.

How do you treat vaginitis?

The key to proper treatment of vaginitis is proper diagnosis. This is not always easy since the same symptoms can exist in different forms of vaginitis. You can greatly assist your health care practitioner by paying close attention to exactly which symptoms you have and when they occur, along with a description of the color, consistency, amount, and smell of any abnormal discharge. Do *not* douche before your office or clinic visit; it will make accurate testing difficult or impossible.

Because different types of vaginitis have different causes, the treatment needs to be *specific* to the type of vaginitis present. When a woman has had a yeast infection diagnosed by her doctor, she is usually treated with a prescription for a vaginal cream or suppositories. If the infection clears up for some period of time but then the *exact same* symptoms occur again, a woman can obtain, with her doctor or pharmacist's advice, a vaginal cream or suppository without a prescription that can completely treat the infection. The important thing to understand is that this medication may only cure the most common types of *Candida* associated with vaginal yeast infections and will not cure other yeast infections or any other type of vaginitis. If you are not absolutely sure, see your doctor. You may save the expense of buying the wrong medication and avoid delay in treating your type of vaginitis.

When obtaining these over-the-counter medicines, be sure to read all of the instructions completely before using the product. Be sure to use all of the medicine and don't stop just because your symptoms have gone away.

Be sure to see your health care practitioner if:
♦ All of the symptoms do not go away completely.
♦ The symptoms return immediately or shortly after you finish treatment.
♦ You have any other serious medical problems such as diabetes.
♦ You might be pregnant.

Other forms of infectious vaginitis are caused by organisms that need to be treated with oral medication and/or a vaginal cream prescribed by your doctor. Products available without a prescription will probably not be effective. As with all medicine, it is important to follow your doctor's instructions as well as the instructions that come with the medication. Do not stop taking the medicine when your symptoms go away. Do not be embarrassed to ask your doctor or health care practitioner questions. Good questions to ask include: Is it okay to douche while on this vaginal cream? Should you abstain from sexual intercourse during treatment? Should your sexual partner(s) be treated at the same time? Will the medication for this vaginitis agree with your other medication(s)? Should you continue the vaginal cream or suppositories during your period? Do you need to be reexamined and if so, when?

"Noninfectious" vaginitis is treated by changing the probable cause. If you have recently changed your soap or laundry detergent or have added a fabric softener, you might consider stopping the new product to see if the symptoms remain. The same instruction would apply to a new vaginal spray, douche, sanitary napkin, or tampon. If the vaginitis is due to hormonal changes, estrogen may be prescribed to help reduce symptoms.

How can I prevent vaginitis?

There are certain things that you can do to decrease the chance of getting vaginitis. If you suffer from yeast infections, it is usually helpful to avoid garments that hold in heat and moisture. The wearing of nylon panties, pantyhose without a cotton panel, and tight jeans can lead to yeast infections. Good hygiene is also important. Many doctors have found that if a woman eats yogurt that contains active cultures (read the label) she will get fewer infections.

Because they can cause vaginal irritation, most doctors do not recommend vaginal sprays or heavily perfumed soaps for cleansing this area. Likewise, repeated douching may cause irritation or, more importantly, may hide a vaginal infection.

Safe sexual practices can help prevent the passing of diseases between partners. The use of condoms is particularly important.

If you are approaching menopause, have had your ovaries removed, or have low levels of estrogen for any reason, discuss with your doctor the use of hormone pills or creams to keep the vagina lubricated and healthy.

Summary

♦ "Vaginitis" is a medical term that describes an infection or irritation of the vagina and/or vulva by yeast, bacteria, viruses, other organisms, or chemical irritants.

♦ When present, symptoms of different types of vaginitis overlap which can make diagnosis difficult. In addition, more than one cause of vaginitis can be present at the same time in the same woman.

♦ Proper diagnosis by your doctor or health care practitioner is the key to proper treatment. Yeast, bacteria, viruses, and other organisms each require a specific type of therapy. Use of the wrong medication will not help and will only delay proper treatment.

♦ All vaginitis is not caused by yeast. The use of a nonprescription medication or other treatment may make the proper diagnosis more difficult if yeast is not the cause of the infection.

♦ Some forms of vaginitis are sexually transmitted and can co-exist with other more serious sexually transmitted diseases. The proper use of condoms can be helpful in preventing some forms of vaginitis.

♦ Follow complete instructions in treating your vaginal infection. If symptoms do not clear completely or if they reoccur, see your doctor or health care practitioner for further instructions.

> *Good health habits are important! Have a complete gynecologic exam, including a Pap smear at least every 2 years. If you have multiple sexual partners, you should request screening for sexually transmitted diseases.*

■ **Document Source:**
U.S. Department of Health and Human Services, Public Health Service
National Institutes of Health
National Institute of Child Health and Human Development
NIH Pub. No. 93-3512
July 1993

WHAT YOU NEED TO KNOW ABOUT CANCER OF THE UTERUS

Each year, more than 32,000 women in the United States find out they have cancer of the uterus. The National Cancer Institute (NCI) has written this booklet to help these women and their families and friends better understand this disease. We also hope others will read it to learn more about this type of cancer.

This booklet describes the symptoms, diagnosis, and treatment of cancer of the uterus. Other NCI booklets about cancer, its treatment, and living with the disease are listed at the end of this booklet. We know that booklets like these cannot answer every question you may have. They cannot take the place of talks with doctors, nurses, and other members of the health care team, but we hope our booklets will help with those talks.

Throughout this booklet, words that may be new to readers are printed in *italics*. Definitions of these and other terms related to uterine cancer are listed in the "Medical Terms" section. For some words, a "sounds-like" spelling is also given.

Our knowledge about cancer of the uterus keeps increasing. For up-to-date information, call the NCI-supported Cancer Information Service (CIS) at 1-800-4-CANCER (1-800-422-6237).

The Uterus

The *uterus* (womb) is a hollow, pear-shaped organ located in a woman's lower abdomen between the *bladder* and the *rectum*. The narrow, lower portion of the uterus is the *cervix*; the broader, upper part is the *corpus*. The corpus is made up of two layers of tissue.

In women of childbearing age, the inner layer of the uterus (*endometrium*) goes through a series of monthly changes known as the menstrual cycle. Each month, endometrial tissue grows and thickens in preparation to receive a fertilized egg. Menstruation occurs when this tissue is not used and passes out through the *vagina*. The outer layer of the corpus (*myometrium*) is a muscle that expands during pregnancy to hold the growing *fetus*. Because most uterine *cancer* develops in the endometrium, cancer of the uterus also is called endometrial cancer. (Information about cancer of the cervix is found in the NCI booklet *What You Need To Know About Cancer of the Cervix.*)

What Is Cancer?

Cancer is a group of more than 100 diseases. Cancer occurs when cells become abnormal and divide without control or order.

The organs of the body are made up of many kinds of cells. Cells normally divide in an orderly way to produce more cells only when they are needed. This process helps keep the body healthy.

If cells divide when new cells are not needed, they form too much *tissue*. The mass of extra tissue, called a *tumor*, can be *benign* or *malignant*.

Benign Tumors

Benign tumors are not cancer. They do not spread to other parts of the body and are seldom a threat to life. Several types of benign tumors occur in the uterus. In some cases, these growths do not need to be treated. Sometimes, however, benign tumors must be removed by *surgery*. Once removed, these tumors are not likely to return.

Fibroids are benign tumors in the uterus that are found most often in women over 35 years of age. Although single fibroid tumors do occur, multiple tumors are more common. Symptoms of fibroids depend on the size and location of the tumors and may include irregular bleeding, vaginal discharge, and frequent urination. When fibroids press against nearby organs and cause pain, surgery may be recommended. Often, however, fibroids do not cause symptoms and do not need to be treated, although they should be checked often. When a woman stops having menstrual periods (*menopause*), fibroids may become smaller, and sometimes they disappear.

Another benign condition of the uterus is *endometriosis*. In this condition, tissue that looks and acts like endometrial tissue begins to grow in unusual places, such as on the surface of the *ovaries*, on the outside of the uterus, and in other tissues in the abdomen. Endometriosis is most common in women in their thirties and forties. This condition causes painful menstrual periods and abnormal bleeding; sometimes, it causes infertility. Some patients with endometriosis are treated with medication, and some are treated with surgery.

Hyperplasia is an increase in the number of normal cells lining the uterus. Although this condition is not cancer, it may develop into cancer in some women. The most common symptoms of hyperplasia are heavy menstrual periods and bleeding between periods. Treatment depends on the extent of the condition (mild, moderate, or severe) and on the age of the patient. Young women usually are treated with female hormones, and the endometrial tissue is checked often. Hyperplasia in women near or after menopause may be treated with hormones if the condition is not severe. Surgery to remove the uterus is the usual treatment for severe cases.

Malignant Tumors

Malignant tumors are cancer. They invade and destroy nearby healthy tissues and organs. Cancer cells also can *metastasize*, or spread, to other parts of the body and form new tumors. When cancer of the uterus spreads, it may travel through the bloodstream or *lymphatic system*. Cancer cells can be carried along by blood or *lymph*, an almost colorless fluid discharged by tissues into the lymphatic system. *Lymph nodes* scattered along this system filter bacteria and abnormal substances such as cancer cells. For this reason, surgeons often remove pelvic lymph nodes to learn whether they contain cancer cells.

Because uterine cancer can spread, it is important for the doctor to find out as early as possible if a tumor is present and whether it is benign or malignant. As soon as a diagnosis is made, the doctor can begin treatment.

Symptoms

Abnormal bleeding after menopause is the most common symptom of cancer of the uterus. Bleeding may begin as a watery, blood-streaked discharge. Later, the discharge may contain more blood.

Cancer of the uterus does not often occur before menopause, but it does occur around the time menopause begins. The reappearance of bleeding should not be considered simply part of menopause; it should always be checked by a doctor.

Abnormal bleeding is not always a sign of cancer. It is important for a woman to see her doctor, however, because that is the only way to find out what the problem is. Any illness should be diagnosed and treated as soon as possible, but early diagnosis is especially important for cancer of the uterus.

Diagnosing Cancer of the Uterus

When symptoms suggest uterine cancer, the doctor asks a woman about her medical history and conducts a thorough exam. In addition to checking general signs of health (temperature, pulse, blood pressure, and so on), the doctor usually performs one or more of the following exams:

- ♦ Pelvic exam. The doctor thoroughly examines the uterus, vagina, ovaries, bladder, and rectum (*pelvic exam*). The doctor feels these organs for any abnormality in their shape or size. A speculum is used to widen the opening of the vagina so that the doctor can look at the upper portion of the vagina and the cervix.
- ♦ Biopsy. For a *biopsy*, the doctor surgically removes a small amount of uterine tissue, which is examined under a microscope by a *pathologist*.
- ♦ D and C. In a *D and C*, the doctor dilates (widens) the cervix and inserts a curette (a small spoon-shaped instrument) to remove pieces of the lining of the uterus. A sample of the uterine lining also can be removed by applying suction through a slender tube (called suction curettage). The tissue is examined for evidence of cancer.
- ♦ Pap smear. The *Pap smear* is often used to detect cancer of the cervix. While it is sometimes done for cancer of the uterus, it is not a reliable test for uterine cancer because it cannot always detect abnormal cells from the endometrium.

If cancer cells are found, doctors use other tests to find out whether the disease has spread from the uterus to other parts of the body. These procedures include blood tests and a chest x-ray. For some patients, special x-rays are needed. For example, *computed tomography* (also called CT or CAT scan) is used to take a series of x-rays of various sections of the abdomen. Doctors may also use *ultrasound* to view organs inside the body. In this procedure, high-frequency sound waves are bounced off internal organs, and the echoes can be seen on a screen that resembles a television. Patients also may have special exams of the bladder, colon, and rectum.

Treating Cancer of the Uterus

The doctor considers a number of factors to determine the best treatment for cancer of the uterus. Among these factors are the stage of the disease, the growth rate of the cancer, and the age and general health of the woman.

Planning Treatment

Decisions about treatment for uterine cancer are complex. Before starting treatment, the patient might want a second opinion about the diagnosis and the treatment plan. It may take a week or two to arrange to see another doctor. This short delay will not make treatment less effective.

There are a number of ways to find a doctor for a second opinion:

- ♦ The patient's doctor may refer her to a specialist who treats uterine cancer.
- ♦ The Cancer Information Service, at 1-800-4-CANCER, can tell callers about cancer centers and other NCI-supported programs in their area.

◆ Patients can get the names of doctors from their local medical society, a nearby hospital, or a medical school.

Methods of Treating Uterine Cancer

Surgery, radiation therapy, hormone therapy, or *chemotherapy* may be used to treat uterine cancer. Radiation therapy (also called x-ray therapy, radiotherapy, or irradiation) uses high-energy rays to kill cancer cells. Radiation may be given from a machine located outside the body (external radiation therapy), or radioactive material may be placed inside the body (internal radiation therapy). In hormone therapy, female hormones are used to stop the growth of cancer cells. Chemotherapy is the use of drugs to treat cancer. Often, a combination of these methods is used. In some cases, the patient is referred to specialists in the different kinds of cancer treatment.

In its early stage, cancer of the uterus usually is treated with surgery. The uterus and cervix are removed (*hysterectomy*), as well as the fallopian tubes and ovaries (*salpingo-oophorectomy*). Some doctors recommend radiation therapy before surgery to shrink the cancer. Others prefer to evaluate the patient carefully during surgery and recommend radiation therapy after surgery for patient whose tumors appear likely to recur. A combination of external and internal radiation therapy often is used. If the cancer has spread extensively or has recurred after treatment, the doctor may recommend a female hormone (progesterone) or chemotherapy.

Side Effects of Treatment

It is rarely possible to limit the effects of cancer treatment so that only cancer cells are destroyed. Normal, healthy cells may be damaged at the same time. That's why the treatment often causes side effects.

Hysterectomy is major surgery. After the operation, the hospital stay usually lasts about 1 week. For several days after surgery, patients may have problems emptying their bladder and having normal bowel movements. The lower abdomen will be sore. Normal activities, including sexual intercourse, usually can be resumed in 4 to 8 weeks.

Women who have their uterus removed no longer have menstrual periods. When the ovaries are not removed, women do not have symptoms of menopause (change of life) because their ovaries still produce hormones. If the ovaries are removed or damaged by radiation therapy, menopause occurs. Hot flashes or other symptoms of menopause caused by treatment may be more severe than those of natural menopause.

Sexual desire and the ability to have intercourse usually are not affected by hysterectomy. However, many women have an emotionally difficult time after a hysterectomy. They may have feelings of deep emotional loss because they are no longer able to become pregnant.

Radiation therapy destroys the ability of cells to grow and divide. Both normal and diseased cells are affected, but most normal cells are able to recover quickly. Patients usually receive external radiation therapy as an outpatient. Treatments are given 5 days a week for several weeks. This schedule helps to protect healthy tissues by spreading out the total dose of radiation.

Internal radiation therapy puts the radiation as close as possible to the site of the cancer, while sparing most of the healthy tissues around it. This type of radiation therapy requires a short hospital stay. A radiation implant, a capsule containing radioactive material, is inserted through the vagina into the uterus. The implant usually is left in place 2 or 3 days.

During radiation therapy, patients may notice a number of side effects, which usually disappear when treatment is completed. Patients may have skin reactions (redness or dryness) in the area being treated, and they may be unusually tired. Some may have diarrhea and frequent and uncomfortable urination. Treatment can also cause dryness, itching, and burning in the vagina. Intercourse may be painful, and some women are advised not to have intercourse at this time. Most women can resume sexual activity within a few weeks after treatment ends.

Hormones occur naturally in the body; their purpose is to regulate the growth of specific cells or organs. In cancer treatment, hormones are sometimes used to stop the growth of cancer cells. Hormones travel through the bloodstream to all parts of the body, affecting cancer cells far from the original tumor. Hormone therapy usually causes few side effects.

Anticancer drugs also travel through the bloodstream to almost every area of the body. Drugs used to treat cancer may be given in different ways: some are given by mouth; others are injected into a muscle, a vein, or an artery. Chemotherapy is most often given in cycles—a treatment period, followed by a recovery period, then another treatment period, and so on.

Depending on the drugs that the doctor orders, the patient may need to stay in the hospital for a few days so that the effects of the drugs can be watched. Often, the patient receives treatment as an outpatient at the hospital, at a clinic, at the doctor's office, or at home.

The side effects of chemotherapy depend on the drugs given and the individual response of the patient. Chemotherapy commonly affects hair cells, blood-forming cells, and cells lining the digestive tract. As a result, patients may have side effects such as hair loss, lowered blood counts, nausea, or vomiting. Most side effects go away during the recovery period or after treatment is over.

Loss of appetite can be a serious problem for patients receiving radiation therapy or chemotherapy. Researchers are learning that patients who eat well are often better able to withstand the side effects of treatment. Therefore, nutrition is important. Eating well means getting enough calories to prevent weight loss and having enough protein in the diet to build and repair skin, hair, muscles, and organs. Many patients find that eating several small meals throughout the day is easier than eating three large meals.

The side effects that patients have during cancer therapy vary from person to person and may even be different from one treatment to the next. Doctors try to plan treatment to keep problems to a minimum, and fortunately, most side effects are temporary. Doctors, nurses, and dietitians can explain the side effects of cancer treatment and suggest ways to deal with them. Further information about cancer treatment and side effects is given in the NCI publications *Radiation Therapy and You, Chemotherapy and You,* and *Eating Hints.*

Followup Care

Regular followup exams are very important for any woman who has been treated for cancer of the uterus. The doctor will want to watch the patient closely for several years to be sure that the cancer has not returned. In general, followup examinations include a pelvic exam, a chest x-ray, and laboratory tests.

Adjusting to the Disease

When people have cancer, life can change for them and for the people who care about them. These changes in daily life can be difficult to handle. When a woman finds out she has uterine cancer, a number of different and sometimes confusing emotions may appear.

At times, patients and family members may feel depressed, angry, or frightened. At other times, feelings may vary from hope to despair or from courage to fear. Patients usually are better able to cope with their emotions if they can talk openly about their illness and their feelings with family members and friends.

Concerns about the future, as well as about medical tests, treatments, hospital stays, and medical bills, often arise. Talking to doctors, nurses, or other members of the health care team may help to ease fear and confusion. Patients can ask questions about their disease and its treatment and can take an active part in decisions about their medical care. Patients and family members often find it helpful to write down questions for the doctor as they think of them. Taking notes during visits to the doctor also can help patients remember what was said. Patients should ask the doctor to repeat or explain more fully anything that is not clear.

Patients have many important questions to ask about cancer, and their doctor is the best person to provide answers. Most people ask what kind of cancer they have, how it can be treated, and how successful the treatment is likely to be. The following are some other questions that patients might want to ask the doctor:

◆ What are the expected benefits of treatment?
◆ What are the risks and side effects of treatment?
◆ Will changes in my normal activities be required?
◆ Is it possible to keep working?
◆ How often are checkups needed?

Many women become concerned, especially after surgery and radiation therapy, that the changes to their bodies will affect how other people feel about them. They may worry about working, caring for their family, or about how cancer and its treatment will affect their sex life. Usually, as the patient recovers, the changes to her body become more accepted. With love and support, patients gradually feel reassured that they are just as appreciated as before.

The patient's doctor is the best person to give advice about working or other activities, but it may be hard to talk to the doctor about feelings and other very personal matters. Many patients find it helpful to talk with others who are facing similar problems. This kind of help is available through cancer-related support groups, such as those described in the next section. If the emotional problems of the patient or family become too hard to handle, a mental health counselor may be able to help.

Living with any serious disease is a difficult challenge. The public library is a good source of books and articles on living with cancer.

Support for Cancer Patients

Adapting to the changes brought about by having cancer is easier for both patients and their families when they get helpful information and support services. Often, the hospital or clinic social service office can suggest local and national agencies that will help with rehabilitation, emotional support, financial aid, transportation, or home care. The American Cancer Society (ACS), for example, is a nonprofit organization that offers a variety of services to patients and their families. Local offices of the ACS are listed in the telephone book.

Information about other resources and services is available through the Cancer Information Service at 1-800-4-CANCER.

What the Future Holds

There are more than 8 million Americans living today who have had some type of cancer. Many are women who have had cancer of the uterus. The outlook for women with very early cancer of the uterus is excellent; nearly all patients with this condition can be cured. The chances of controlling advanced disease are improving as researchers continue to look for better ways to treat this disease.

Doctors often talk about "surviving" cancer, or they may use the word "remission" rather than "cure." Even though many patients recover completely, doctors use these terms because cancer of the uterus may show up again at a later time. Patients are naturally concerned about their future and often try to use statistics they have read or heard about to figure out their own chances of being cured. It is important to remember that statistics describe an average of large numbers of people, and no two cancer patients are alike. The outlook for a particular patient depends on the type and stage of her disease, her age and general health, her response to treatment, and other variables.

The Promise of Cancer Research

Scientists at hospitals and medical centers throughout the country are studying the possible causes of uterine cancer and how the disease might be prevented. In addition, they are researching new methods of treatment.

Cause and Prevention

Researchers study patterns of cancer in the population to discover which people are more likely to get certain cancers and what aspects of our surroundings and lifestyles may cause cancer.

Cancer of the uterus occurs most often in women between the ages of 55 and 70. This disease accounts for about 6 percent of all cancers in women. Research shows that some women are more likely than others to develop cancer of the uterus. These women are said to be "at risk." Obese women, women who have few or no children, women who began menstruating at a young age, those who had a late menopause, and women of high socioeconomic status are at increased risk of developing this disease. It appears that most of the risk factors for cancer of the uterus are related to hormones, especially excess estrogen.

Studies have shown that women taking estrogen replacement therapy (ERT) for menopausal symptoms have two to eight times greater risk of developing uterine cancer than women who do not take estrogens. The risk increases after 2 to 4 years of use and seems to be greatest when large doses are taken for long periods of time. A woman who takes ERT after her uterus has been removed is in no danger of developing uterine cancer. Many doctors now believe that using a combination of estrogen and progestin (another female hormone) for replacement therapy decreases the risk of cancer of the uterus. It is especially important for all women taking replacement therapy to be checked regularly for any signs of cancer. Unusual bleeding should be reported to the doctor at once.

Recent evidence shows that the use of birth control pills may decrease the risk of developing uterine cancer. Women who use a combination pill (containing both estrogen and progestin in each pill) for at least 1 year have only half the risk of endometrial cancer as women who use other types of birth control pills or none. The longer a woman takes the combination pill, the more this protection increases.

Treatment

Scientists continue to study new treatments for cancer of the uterus, including new drugs, drug combinations, and combinations of radiation therapy and chemotherapy. Scientists are studying these methods closely to learn whether they can be of value in future treatment.

When laboratory research shows that a new treatment method has promise, the method is used to treat cancer patients in clinical trials. These trials are designed to answer scientific questions and to find out if a promising new treatment is both safe and effective. They are done with the cooperation of cancer patients. Patients who take part in clinical trials make an important contribution to medical science and may have the first chance to benefit from improved treatment methods. Any woman with uterine cancer may consider participating in a trial and should discuss her interest with her doctor. (Such studies are the subject of *What Are Clinical Trials All About?*, an NCI publication for patients who may be interested in participating in clinical research.)

One way to learn about clinical trials is through PDQ, a computerized resource of information about cancer. Developed by NCI, PDQ contains an up-to-date list of trials all over the country. Doctors can obtain an access code and use a personal computer to get PDQ information, or they can use the services of a medical library. Also, the Cancer Information Service, at 1-800-4-CANCER, can provide PDQ information to doctors, patients, and the public.

Medical Terms

Benign tumor (bee-NINE). A noncancerous growth that does not invade nearby tissue or spread to other parts of the body.

Biopsy (BY-op-see). The removal and microscopic examination of a sample of tissue to see if cancer cells are present.

Bladder. The hollow organ that stores urine.

Cancer. A general term for more than 100 diseases that are characterized by uncontrolled, abnormal growth of cells. Cancer cells can invade nearby tissue and can spread through the bloodstream and lymphatic system to other parts of the body.

Carcinoma (kar-sin-O-ma). Cancer that begins in the tissues lining or covering an organ.

Cervix (SER-viks). The lower, narrow end of the uterus.

Chemotherapy (kee-mo-THER-a-pee). Treatment with anticancer drugs.

Clinical trials. A study conducted with cancer patients, usually to evaluate a new treatment. Each study is designed to answer scientific questions and to find better ways to treat patients.

Computed tomography (tom-OG-rah-fee). An x-ray procedure that uses a computer to produce a detailed picture of a cross section of the body; also called CAT or CT scan.

Corpus. The body of the uterus.

Dilatation and curettage (dil-a-TAY-shun and KYOO-re-tahzh). A minor operation in which the cervix is expanded enough (dilatation) to permit the cervical canal and uterine lining to be scraped with a spoon-shaped instrument called a curette (curettage). This procedure also is called D and C.

Endometriosis (en-do-mee-tree-O-sis). A benign condition in which tissue that looks like endometrial tissue grows in abnormal places in the abdomen.

Endometrium (en-do-MEE-tree-um). The inner layer of the uterus.

Fallopian tubes (fa-LO-pee-in). Tubes (one on each side of the uterus) that transport the egg cells from the ovaries to the uterus.

Fetus (FEET-us). The unborn child developing in the uterus.

Fibroid (FY-broid). A benign uterine tumor.

Gynecologist (gy-na-KOL-o-jist). A doctor who specializes in treating diseases of the female reproductive organs.

Hormone therapy. Treatment of cancer by changing hormone levels in the body.

Hyperplasia (hy-per-PLAY-zha). A precancerous condition in which there is an increase in the number of normal cells lining the uterus.

Hysterectomy (hiss-ter-ECK-to-mee). An operation that removes the uterus and cervix.

Lymph (limf). The almost colorless fluid that bathes body cells and contains cells that help fight infection.

Lymph nodes. Small bean-shaped structures scattered throughout the body along the channels of the lymphatic system; also called the lymph glands. Nodes filter bacteria or cancer cells that may travel through the lymphatic system.

Lymphatic system (lim-FAT-ik). The lymph nodes, spleen, and thymus—which produce and store infection-fighting cells—and the network of channels that carry lymph.

Malignant (ma-LIG-nant). Cancerous (see Cancer).

Menopause. The time of a woman's life when menstrual periods permanently stop; also called "change of life."

Metastasis (me-TAS-ta-sis). The spread of a cancer from one part of the body to another. Cells in the metastatic tumor (the second tumor) are like those in the original tumor.

Myometrium (my-o-MEE-tree-um). The muscular outer layer of the uterus.

Oncologist (on-KOL-o-jist). A doctor who specializes in treating cancer.

Ovaries (O-var-eez). The pair of female reproductive glands in which the ova, or eggs, are formed. The ovaries are located in the lower abdomen, one on each side of the uterus.

Pap smear (Pap test). Microscopic examination of a sample of cells collected from the cervix.

Pathologist (path-OL-o-jist). A doctor who specializes in the diagnosis of disease by studying cells and tissues removed from the body.

Pelvis. The lower part of the abdomen, located between the hip bones. Organs in the female pelvis include the uterus, vagina, ovaries, fallopian tubes, bladder, and rectum.

Radiation therapy (ray-dee-AY-shun THER-a-pee). Treatment with high-energy radiation from x-rays or other sources.

Rectum. The last 5 to 6 inches of the colon leading to the outside of the body.

Salpingo-oophorectomy (sal-PING-o-OO-for-EK-to-mee). Surgical removal of the fallopian tubes and ovaries.

Speculum (SPEK-yoo-lum). An instrument used to widen the opening of the vagina so that the cervix is more easily visible.

Surgery. An operation.

Tumor. An abnormal mass of tissue.

Ultrasound. A diagnostic procedure that projects high-frequency sound waves into the body and changes the echoes into pictures.

Ureter (yu-REE-ter). The tube that carries urine from each kidney to the bladder.

Uterus (YOO-ter-us). Often called the womb, this is the organ in which a fetus develops. During pregnancy, the uterus expands. But when a woman is not pregnant, the uterus is small, hollow, and shaped like a flattened pear.

Vagina. The muscular canal extending from the uterus to the exterior of the body.

Resources

General information about cancer is widely available. Some helpful resources and publications are listed below. You also may wish to check your local library and to contact support groups in your community.

Cancer Information Service (CIS)
1-800-4-CANCER
The Cancer Information Service, a program of the National Cancer Institute, provides a nationwide telephone service for cancer patients and their families and friends, the public, and health care professionals. The staff can answer questions and can send booklets about cancer. They also know about local resources and services. One toll-free number, 1-800-4-CANCER (1-800-422-6237), connects callers all over the country to the office that serves their area. Spanish-speaking staff members are available.

American Cancer Society (ACS)
1599 Clifton Road, N.E.
Atlanta, GA 30329
1-800-ACS-2345
The American Cancer Society is a voluntary organization with a national office (at the above address) and local units all over the country. It supports research, conducts educational programs, and offers many services to patients and their families. It also provides free booklets on uterine cancer and on sexuality. To request booklets or to learn about services and activities in local areas, call the society's toll-free number, 1-800-ACS-2345 (1-800-227-2345), or the number listed under American Cancer Society in the white pages of the telephone book.

For Further Information

The booklets listed here may be helpful to cancer patients and their families. They are available free of charge from the National Cancer Institute. You may request them by calling 1-800-4-CANCER or writing:

Office of Cancer Communications
National Cancer Institute
Building 31, Room 10A24
Bethesda, MD 20892

Booklets About Cancer Treatment

♦ *Radiation Therapy and You: A Guide to Self-Help During Treatment*
♦ *Chemotherapy and You: A Guide to Self-Help During Treatment*
♦ *Eating Hints: Recipes and Tips for Better Nutrition During Cancer Treatment*
♦ *Questions and Answers About Pain Control* (also available from the American Cancer Society)
♦ *What Are Clinical Trials All About?*
♦ *What You Need to Know About Cancer of the Cervix*

Booklets About Living with Cancer

♦ *Taking Time: Support for People With Cancer and the People Who Care About Them*
♦ *Facing Forward: A Guide for Cancer Survivors*
♦ *When Cancer Recurs: Meeting the Challenge Again*
♦ *Advanced Cancer: Living Each Day*

■ **Document Source:**
U.S. Department of Health and Human Services, Public Health Service
National Institutes of Health
National Cancer Institute
NIH Publication No. 93-1562
Revised August 1991. Printed December 1992

See also: Chemotherapy and You: A Guide to Self-Help During Treatment (page 40); Endometrial Cancer (page 420); Radiation Therapy and You: A Guide to Self-Help During Treatment (page 56); What Are Clinical Trials All About? A Booklet for Patients with Cancer (page 68)

MISCELLANEOUS

■ ■ ■

ANABOLIC STEROIDS: LOSING AT WINNING

Learn About Steroids

Bear Bryant, the legendary University of Alabama football coach, used to say after his team would be unimpressive in winning: "Sometimes you lose when you win."

That pretty well sums up the use of anabolic steroids, too. You might win some muscle, but sooner or later you'll most likely be wearing a loser label.

Anabolic steroids may help put muscle on some people when they're used while lifting weights. However, the list of side effects or adverse reactions from steroids runs longer than the number of All-Americans that even Bear Bryant could produce in his many years of coaching.

Many people who use steroids are aware of the possible side effects, or adverse reactions, but they figure that most of the problems will be in the future and the future is a long way off. Not so. Acne, sexual function problems, rashes, and the infamous and uncontrollable "roid rages" are among the possible immediate consequences. Long-term side effects may include early heart disease and liver tumors.

The argument is made that anabolic steroids help a person recover from injuries. There is precious little evidence to support that claim. Actually, anabolic steroids aren't very popular as prescription drugs. They are used for certain types of cancer treatment and for some rare conditions, including a disease called hereditary angioedema, which is hardly a threat to those able to pump iron.

Anabolic steroids came to be used by athletes more than 30 years ago after the Russians and East European athletes dominated some international sports events. It was learned that their athletes had bolstered themselves with a male hormone called testosterone. Anabolic steroids are a synthetic version of testosterone, developed in the 1960s. Their American developer, Dr. John B. Ziegler, was later to tell *Sports Illustrated* that he wished he could have taken that chapter out of his life.

Those Communist athletes who won so many victories did so at great expense. They were taking so much of the male hormone that many of the male athletes had to be catheterized (a tube inserted in the penis) in order to urinate. The women were so masculine-appearing that chromosome tests had to be conducted to prove that they were females.

Testosterone has many jobs to do within the body. Among other things, it stimulates the development of bone, muscle, skin and hair growth as well as emotional responses. The body produces 2-1/2 to 10 milligrams of testosterone a day in an adult male. Of course, weight lifters are known to take many times that amount in a single day.

When the body gets too much testosterone, it reacts in many ways. One response may be to shut down skeletal growth mechanisms, resulting in stunted growth in children, or shriveled testicles, or lowered sperm counts, or balding.

Women produce very little of the hormone. So they take on masculine characteristics when they use steroids. Some of those traits never return to normal.

Long as it is, the list of side effects or adverse reactions from anabolic steroids may not be as long as it should be. That's because steroids haven't been studied in the amounts and combinations ("stacking") being taken today by many weight lifters. Nor does it take into account the adverse reactions that might result when steroids are taken with other drugs, such as those used to counteract unwanted steroid side effects.

Actually, steroids are not prescribed very often, so a black market has sprung up to supply athletes. However, buyers beware: Black-market steroids often come from underground laboratories or foreign countries and are of very questionable quality and purity. In fact, they may not even be steroids. The black market has problems of its own—in May 1987, for instance, 34 people were charged with conspiracy to make, smuggle and distribute counterfeit steroids after a federal investigation.

The National Football League has added anabolic steroids to its roster of test drugs. Players were tested in the training camps in August 1987 for the first time. Positive results bring suspensions and could lead to being thrown out of the league.

More musclemen, athletes and other sports officials are denouncing the drugs. Jesse Ventura, the TV wrestling commentator, movie star and muscleman in his own right, says he tried steroids, learned about them and realized "they have no place on my training table."

"Mr. Olympia"—Lee Haney—notes that muscle gain from steroids is only temporary and adds: "You'll ultimately make your best body-building gains if you avoid steroid usage and just concentrate on hard training and good nutrition."

In a letter to all NFL players, Commissioner Pete Rozelle said: "It is recommended that you educate yourself and your teammates about the hazards of anabolic steroids."

In other words, don't lose at winning. Pump iron, not trouble.

How You Can Lose with Steroids

Established Side Effects or Adverse Reactions from Anabolic Steroids Are:

acne
cancer
cholesterol increase
clitoris enlargement
death
edema (water retention in tissue)
fetal damage
frequent or continuing erections (mature males)
HDL (good cholesterol) decrease
heart disease
hirsutism (hairiness in women—irreversible)
increased frequency of erections (boys)
increased risk of coronary artery disease (heart attack, stroke)
jaundice
liver tumor
liver disease
male pattern baldness (in women—irreversible)
oily skin (females only)
peliosis hepatitis (a liver disease)
penis enlargement (young boys)
priapism (painful, prolonged erections)
prostate enlargement
shrunken testicles
sterility (reversible)
stunted growth
swelling of feet or lower legs
yellowing of the eyes or skin

Other Possible Side Effects or Adverse Reactions:

aggressive, combative behavior ("roid rage")
anaphylactic shock (from injections)
abdominal or stomach pains
black, tarry or light-colored stools
bone pain
breast development (sore or swelling—male)
chills
diarrhea
dark-colored urine
depression
fever
fatigue
feeling of discomfort (continuing)
frequent urge to urinate (mature males)
feeling of abdominal or stomach fullness
gallstones
hives
headache (continuing)
hypercalcemia (too much calcium)

high blood pressure
impotence
increased chance of injury to muscles tendons and ligaments plus longer recovery period from injuries
insomnia
kidney disease
kidney stones (from hypercalcemia)
listlessness
muscle cramps
menstrual irregularities
nausea or vomiting
purple or red-colored spots on body, inside of mouth, or nose
rash
septic shock (blood poisoning from injections)
sexual problems
sore tongue
unexplained darkening of skin
unexplained weight loss
unnatural hair growth
unpleasant breath odor (continuing)
unusual bleeding
unusual weight gain
urination problems
vomiting of blood

Sources: *Physicians Desk Reference*, 1987; *AMA Drug Evaluations*, 1986; *Death in the Locker Room* by Bob Goldman, D.O. with Patricia Bush, Ph.D. and Ronald Klatz D.O.; and *U.S. Pharmacopeia Drug Index*, Vol. 2, 1986.

■ **Document Source:**
U.S. Department of Health and Human Services, Public Health Service
Food and Drug Administration
DHHS Publication No. (FDA) 90-3171

DRUGS AND THE BRAIN

Introduction

We live in a world that sometimes seems saturated with drugs. If you have a headache, you take a pill. If you have a runny nose, you take another kind of pill. You cannot sleep very well? Well, there is a pill for that, too. Do you want to lose some weight or simply relax? You can take pills for all these things. Everywhere we turn, on the television and in the newspapers and magazines, we see advertisements that urge us to take some kind of drug for the myriad of problems, serious and superficial, which ail all of us.

So it should not be too surprising that, in addition to using legal drugs, people turn to illegal drugs or they abuse legal ones to try to solve their problems. People may be bored or anxious, or feel hopeless, and they turn to drugs to escape. Alcohol, tobacco, marijuana, cocaine, heroin, PCP, and a slew of other compounds do indeed change our moods and alter our perceptions. While some people are able to use some drugs in moderation, others cannot. They lose control of their drug-taking behavior and become addicted. Because drug abuse and addiction have become problems of significant consequence, it is important to understand why people abuse drugs and how drugs exert their addictive effects.

To begin with, we should bear in mind that drug abuse and drug addiction are entirely different phenomena. Drug abuse is a voluntary activity, but drug addiction is a compulsion. A drug abuser can choose whether or not to use a drug. People who are addicted, by contrast, have for all intents and purposes lost their free will to decide whether or not to use drugs. They feel they have no more choice about using drugs than they do about eating or breathing.

How can certain drugs produce such overpowering effects? The key lies in how these drugs affect the brain and some of its networks of nerve cells. To understand how drugs influence the brain, we need to examine some of the constituents of the brain and how they work.

The Brain and Its Nerve Cells

The brain can be divided into several large regions, each responsible for some of the activities vital for living. The brain's lowest portion, called the brain stem, controls basic functions such as heart rate, breathing, eating, and sleeping. When one of these basic needs must be fulfilled, the brain stem structures can direct the rest of the brain and body to work toward that end. While these structures may be simple, they can exert powerful effects on our behavior.

Above the brain stem and encompassing two-thirds of the human brain mass are the two hemispheres of the cerebral cortex. It is the cortex, the convoluted outer covering of nerve cells and fibers, that is the most recent part of the brain to evolve, developing completely only in mammals. Because they have a cortex, all mammals have more complex behavioral repertoires than creatures with simpler brains, like birds and reptiles. But, it is the large size and increased complexity of the human cerebral cortex that makes us different even from other mammals.

Though the cells throughout the entire extent of the cerebral cortex are remarkably similar, the cortex can be divided into dozens of specific areas, each with a highly specialized function. It is like a collection of small computers, each working on a different aspect of a large problem. Much of the cerebral cortex is devoted to our senses—enabling us to see, hear, smell, taste, and touch. Other areas give us the ability to generate complex movements; still other regions allow us to speak and understand words, and different regions altogether allow us to think, plan, and imagine.

On top of the brain stem and buried under the cortex, there is another set of more primitive brain structures called the limbic system. These limbic system structures are crucial for connecting the cortex, which deals mainly with the outside world, with our emotions and motivations, which reflect our internal environment and survival needs. These connections allow us to experience a wide range of feelings and to influence these feelings with our perceptions and actions. They also enable us to use our impressive cognitive abilities to help us do the things we need to do to survive. Two large limbic structures, called the hippocampus and the amygdala, are also critical for memory. Sensory information flows from the cortex to these primitive brain regions, which take into account what is going on inside the brain and body and then instruct the cortex to store what is important.

One of the reasons that drugs of abuse can exert such powerful control over our behavior is that they act directly on the more primitive brain stem and limbic structures, which can override the cortex in controlling our behavior. In effect, they eliminate the most human part of our brain from its role in controlling our behavior.

Surprisingly, the feeling of pleasure turns out to be one of the most important emotions for our survival. In fact, the feeling of pleasure is so important that there is a circuit of specialized nerve cells devoted to producing and regulating it. One important set of these nerve cells, which uses a special chemical messenger, a neurotransmitter called dopamine, sits at the very top of the brain stem. These dopamine-containing neurons relay messages about pleasure through their nerve fibers to nerve cells in a limbic structure called the nucleus accumbens. Still other fibers reach to a related part of the frontal region of the cerebral cortex. So, the pleasure circuit spans the survival-oriented brain stem, the emotional limbic system, and the complex information processor called the cerebral cortex.

The reason that pleasure, which scientists call reward, is a powerful biological force for our survival is that pleasure reinforces any behavior that elicits it. If you do something pleasurable, the brain is wired so that you tend to do that again. This is why a rat or a monkey so readily learns to press a lever for food. The animal does it because it is reinforcing—pressing the lever gets food and eating the food turns on the pleasure center, an action that helps ensure that the animal will do again what got him that food in the first place. And all of this happens unconsciously. We do not have to think about it or pay attention. It is an automatic brain function.

Thus, life's sustaining activities, such as eating a good meal or engaging in sex, activate this pleasure circuit. By doing so, they teach us to do these things again and again. But certain substances, including all the drugs that people abuse, also can potently activate the brain's pleasure circuit. Unfortunately, the more a person uses these drugs to get feelings of pleasure, the more the person learns to repeat the drug-taking behavior and the more the brain learns to depend on drugs to evoke pleasure.

So, that is the key reason why people repeatedly abuse drugs; drugs make them feel good by directly turning on the pleasure circuit. It also is a reason why drug addiction is so difficult to treat; addicts find that only drugs can give them pleasure. Drug addiction is a biologically based disease that alters the way the pleasure center, as well as other parts of the brain, function. By directly turning on our pleasure circuits, many addictive drugs make our brains behave as if these compounds were as important for survival as food, sex, and all the other natural rewards that also turn on the pleasure circuits. Thus, drugs pervert to a destructive end a strong emotion that helps to activate one of the brain's most powerful learning mechanisms.

This is a general description of how drugs influence our behavior by working on one important brain center. To really understand how drugs produce their effects, however, we need to understand how nerve cells and the molecules that make up these cells interact with the molecules that make up drugs.

To do this, we need to examine the fine structure of nerve cells, the communications network of the brain. Each nerve cell, or neuron, contains three important parts. The central cell body directs all the activities of the neuron. Messages from other nerve cells are relayed directly to the cell body through a set of branches called dendrites. Having examined the information relayed to it by its dendrites, the cell body then can send messages out to its neighbors through a cablelike fiber called an axon. But the axon does not make direct contact with the dendrites of other neurons. A tiny gap separates the terminal of the axon, sending the message from the dendrites of the cell with which it seeks to communicate. This gap is called a synapse.

The message is sent across the synaptic gap between the two nerve cells by a chemical called a neurotransmitter. The little packets of the neurotransmitter are released at the end of the axon and diffuse across the gap to bind to special molecules, called receptors, that sit on the surface of the dendrites of the adjacent nerve cell.

When the neurotransmitter couples to a receptor, it is like a key fitting into a lock that starts the process information flow in that neuron. First, this coupling allows the receptor molecules to link with other molecules that extend through the cell membrane to the inside of the cell. This is how the neurotransmitter that can only affect a receptor molecule sitting on the outside edge of the cell can change the way the cell behaves. Once the receptor activates these other molecules, its mission is complete. The neurotransmitter then is either destroyed or sucked back into the nerve cell that released it. This whole process is called chemical neurotransmission.

Almost all drugs that change the way the brain works do so by tinkering with chemical neurotransmission. Some drugs, like heroin, mimic the effects of a natural neurotransmitter. Others, like LSD, block receptors and thereby prevent neuronal messages from getting through. Still others, like cocaine, interfere with the process by which neurotransmitters are sucked up by the neurons that release them. Others, like caffeine and PCP, exert their effects by interfering with the way messages proceed from the surface receptors into the cell interior.

When drugs interfere with the delicate mechanisms through which nerve cells transmit, receive, and process the information critical for daily living, we lose some of our ability to control our own lives. The continued use of these drugs can actually change the way the brain works. This is the biological basis of addiction.

Observations of people and experiments with animals have taught us that addiction begins when a drug is inappropriately and repeatedly used to stimulate the nerve cells of the pleasure circuit of the brain. Rats hooked up to a drug pump will repeatedly press the lever for doses of illicit drugs that activate dopamine-containing nerve cells in the ventral tegmental area or the neurons that these cells end on in the nucleus accumbens and the frontal cortex. In fact, there is a remarkable similarity between the drugs humans like to abuse and the ones that laboratory monkeys will self administer. Given the opportunity, both monkeys and humans will use cocaine, amphetamines, heroin, alcohol, phenobarbital, nicotine, and virtually every opiate drug. Hallucinogens seem to be the only class of drugs that are preferred only by people.

Animal experiments have taught us that cocaine turns on the pleasure circuit by allowing dopamine to accumulate in the synapses where it is released. Because the amount of dopamine is allowed to build up, strong feelings of pleasure, even euphoria, are elicited. Heroin turns on the pleasure circuit by directly activating opiate receptors on other neurons in this circuit. Even drugs like marijuana, which animals do not like to self administer, can make it easier for other drugs or natural pleasures to turn on the pleasure circuit. This may be why people compulsively use even a relatively weak drug like marijuana.

So, people abuse drugs and animals self administer them because drugs turn on the pleasure center. They do this by altering the normal process of chemical neurotransmission. But, in order to understand why different people use different drugs and how repeated drug use can lead to addiction, it is useful to understand the specific effects of different classes of drugs and the particular brain areas they target.

Opiates

This drug class—which includes opium, codeine, morphine, and heroin—comes from the white, milky liquid exuded by the poppy flower. Opium, codeine, and morphine can be extracted directly from the fluid, while heroin is produced by chemically joining two molecules of morphine. Heroin injected into a vein reaches the brain in a mere 7 or 8 seconds and, because of its chemical structure, penetrates into the brain even faster than morphine, which is probably why most addicts in the United States choose heroin. Once heroin reaches the brain, it quickly binds to the opiate receptors that are found in many brain regions. Activation of the opiate receptors in the pleasure circuit causes intense euphoria, called a rush. This rush lasts only briefly, but is followed by a couple of hours of a relaxed, contented state.

By binding to opiate receptors in other parts of the brain and body, opiates also can stop diarrhea (an important medical use), depress breathing, and cause nausea and vomiting. People who try heroin for the first time often get nauseous or vomit, and some decide they will never use the drug again. But many get past this side effect.

Much more serious is heroin's ability, in large doses, to make breathing shallow or even stop altogether. It does this by binding to opiate receptors that are found on the neurons that control breathing. Activation of these opiate receptors by heroin actually causes the neurons to slow down or stop working altogether. Thousands of people have died because they stopped breathing after a heroin overdose. A number of years ago, however, scientists developed drugs that can block heroin from attaching to opiate receptors. These medications are called opiate antagonists. If someone who has overdosed on heroin is treated with one of these drugs in time, the heroin effects can be completely reversed.

In addition to their many other effects, opiates are the most potent painkillers available. Yet many people who may have had surgery or who are suffering from advanced cancer receive inadequate pain relief because they, their families, or their doctors worry they will become addicted to opiates. But the truth is, this rarely happens. Many studies have shown that pain patients can be treated effectively with strong opiates and either maintained indefinitely or, when their pain is gone, withdrawn from the drug with little problem.

One reason that opiates have so many effects is because opiate receptors are widely distributed throughout the brain and body. The brain also produces its own opiatelike neurotransmitters, called endorphins, that act just like but more weakly than morphine. Neurons that produce endorphins and neurons that contain opiate receptors are involved in many brain and body functions. The nucleus accumbens contains a large population of opiate receptors, which may be how opiates turn on the pleasure circuit, but regions of the brain involved in emotions and memory—the hippocampus—as well as the cerebral cortex also contain many receptors for opiates.

Cocaine

Cocaine comes from the leaves of the coca plant, which grows in the mountains of South America. One of the most highly addictive forms of cocaine is crack, a chemically altered form of cocaine that can be smoked. When a person smokes this drug, it enters the brain in seconds and produces a rush of euphoria and feelings of power and self-confidence.

Cocaine, like other stimulants, increases alertness, makes one feel more energetic, and suppresses hunger. In fact, a similar kind of stimulant—the amphetamines—for years were prescribed as appetite suppressants for dieters. One kind of amphetamine, methamphetamine, is now making its way back into illegal use in a smokeable form called ice. This, too, is a highly addictive drug.

Repeated exposure to stimulants can make a person feel anxious, hyperactive, and irritable. People can become psychotic, in a way that resembles paranoid schizophrenia, from taking too high a dose of these drugs. For many years, scientists have studied an animal model of psychosis induced by amphetamines to better understand the symptoms of schizophrenia. Finally, a cocaine or amphetamine overdose can cause tremors and lethal brain seizures.

By tracing the path of radioactive cocaine in the brain of human volunteers, researchers have tracked the drug's activity. For a period of up to about 6 minutes, when feelings of euphoria are most intense, cocaine can be found in the frontal cortex regions. After that time, the drug begins to dwindle in that area and is concentrated in another region densely packed with dopamine receptors and axons from dopamine-containing nerve cells.

Because cocaine acts to prevent reabsorption of the neurotransmitter dopamine after its release from nerve cells, cocaine addicts often have higher than normal levels of dopamine in their synapses. This may explain an important finding: the brains of chronic cocaine abusers appear to contain fewer dopamine receptors than normal brains. The excess dopamine causes the neurons that have dopamine receptors to decrease the number of dopamine receptors they make. This phenomenon is called down regulation and may explain the craving for cocaine that occurs during withdrawal from cocaine addiction.

When cocaine is no longer taken and dopamine levels return to their normal, lower concentration, the smaller number of dopamine receptors available for the neurotransmitter to bind to is insufficient to fully activate nerve cells. Because these nerve cells can no longer do their job, the end result may

be such common withdrawal symptoms as depression and a craving for the drug. The depression may reflect the brain's response to the lower level of dopamine action, and the craving is its way of telling the addict to get the dopamine level back up by taking cocaine. This is not unlike the way that hunger motivates us to eat.

Marijuana and Hallucinogens

Unlike opiates and stimulants, marijuana and hallucinogens (including LSD and mescaline) alter our perception of reality. These drugs distort the way our senses work and our sense of time, space, and self. In people who are particularly sensitive to them, hallucinogens can produce intense anxiety and even precipitate a psychotic episode.

It is not yet clear exactly how these effects are produced, but radioactive tracing shows that THC, the active ingredient in marijuana, binds to receptors that recognize it. There are many THC receptors in parts of the brain that coordinate movement. This may explain why animals given large doses of marijuana collapse and cannot move.

The hippocampus, a structure involved with the storage of memory, also contains many THC receptors. This may explain why people intoxicated with marijuana have poor short-term memory. Scientists already have shown that chronic administration of THC to rats actually can damage the hippocampus. They are trying to find out if this damage may lead to permanent memory impairment.

PCP

This drug has a variety of actions—it is a hallucinogen, a stimulant, and an anesthetic all in one. PCP blocks the way some receptors communicate their message to the inside of the cell and it also blocks certain kinds of receptors. It can produce euphoria, alleviate pain, and lead to disorganized thinking. Depending on the person, PCP can cause drowsiness or aggressiveness and passivity or hostility. A major concern about the drug is the unpredictability of its effects from one time to the next and from one person to the next.

Depressants

Alcohol may be the most familiar depressant, but this class of drugs also includes tranquilizers like valium and sleeping pills like phenobarbital. A major action of all of these drugs is to reduce anxiety. They may, however, first produce a brief period of excitement or euphoria before they produce calmness, sedation, and sleep.

In higher doses, these compounds can produce anesthesia and relax muscles, and some may serve as antiseizure medications. In fact, valium and phenobarbital are excellent antiepileptic medicines, but most people find them too sedating for regular use.

People who get drunk may feel alert at first, but then they start to feel depressed and lose their coordination. Most of us have seen the unpleasant and potentially dangerous behavior of drunks. An overdose of alcohol or other depressant can produce stupor and death. Another important effect of these drugs is to impair judgement. People who are drunk often think they are functioning well. This may help to explain why 23,000 people are killed by drunk drivers every year.

Designer Drugs

So-called "street or basement chemists" have designed a slew of compounds that differ only slightly from the chemical structure of other illegal drugs. Until a few years ago when the laws were changed, these compounds were technically legal, but still had the addictive effects of their chemical cousins. For example, people have modified the stimulant methamphetamine, developing a compound called MDMA, commonly known on the street as ecstacy. It has a combination of stimulant and hallucinogenic properties, but animal studies have shown that it causes a severe, possibly permanent loss of serotonin-containing nerve fibers of the cortex. The Drug Enforcement Administration has declared MDMA illegal.

In general, depending on the origin of the designer drug and how the source drug was modified, the new compound may have widely different properties ranging from stimulant to opiate to hallucinogenic.

Drugs and the Fetus

Many babies are now being born addicted to cocaine, PCP, or heroin. Normal development of the fetus is a highly complex and intricately timed process that is easily disrupted by drugs. The effects of drugs on the fetus can be absolutely devastating; there is no safe way for a pregnant woman to take drugs.

To understnad the effect of drugs on fetal development, consider the opiate receptors in the cortex of the adult and newborn monkey. An adult has three distinct, localized bands of opiate receptors while an infant has only one fairly uniform band.

Newborns actually have many more of these receptors than needed. In the normal course of development in animals, the extra receptors are gradually eliminated because no endorphin-containing nerve fibers contact them. Because they are never activated, they are eliminated. But if a mother is given opiates during her pregnancy, the fetus' opiate receptors all receive constant activation. As a consequence, the receptors do not disappear as they normally would and the normal functioning and continued development of the brain can be disrupted.

Addicted babies are irritable, sensitive, and unusually hard to handle. They appear to have developmental abnormalities as if their brains are trying to get back on track, attempting to develop properly even though they have been thrown off track by drugs. Because normal development is an exquisitely timed process that builds one event upon another, it is not surprising that drugs can disrupt it so easily.

The Steps to Addiction

No matter what kind of drug a person is using, nobody begins taking drugs thinking he or she will become addicted. The person says, "I can handle it. I'll just take this a few times and then I'll stop." The fact is, many people can do this. They can experiment with drugs and then stop. But many others cannot. And while we cannot predict who will and who will not get in trouble with drugs, we do know some of the steps along the path to addiction. Knowing the signposts along this route may help people recognize when they have gotten or are about to get into trouble.

Drugs make most people feel good; this is why they want to take drugs more than once or twice. In scientific terms, drug use is a "rewarding behavior" because the high or pleasure it induces tends to reinforce the drug-taking activity. For some people, this reinforcing experience in learning about the pleasures of drug use may lead from experimentation to more regular, social use of a drug. Many people start to use drugs at parties and with friends. Some people stay at this second level of use for many years and never get into trouble. There are, for example, many social drinkers who have never had a problem controlling their level of alcohol consumption.

But for other people, drug use does get out of hand. These people learn to take drugs for emotional support—one person had a tough day, another's boss yelled at her, still another has not done his homework and knows he will be in trouble at school. People get bored, lonely, or just do not like their world very much. Taking drugs to try to solve problems like these helps set the stage for addiction.

At first a person might say: "Well, I didn't do my homework tonight. I feel really guilty, so I'm going to get stoned, forget about it, and go to bed." Then it progresses—snorting cocaine in the stockroom, having a few drinks at lunch, or sneaking a drink or smoking dope in the bathroom to deal with stress. If this continues, physiological changes will begin to take place. Friends may even notice, "You know, he can drink anyone under the table. The guy has a hollow leg." What is happening is that the person has become tolerant to alcohol. If it used to take one or two drinks for that person to get high, after a period of drinking it takes three or four drinks, then five or six. Similarly, the dose needed to get high from marijuana, heroin, or crack also escalates. So the drug user is not only taking drugs more frequently, that person is exposing his or her body to higher doses.

Then, as regular drug use continues, a second related kind of change begins. The body of a habitual drug user begins to need the drug to work normally. The person cannot function without it; when the drug is not available, the person experiences symptoms of withdrawal. Deprived of the drug, the individual may feel anxious, generally lousy, or sick. Using the drug again alleviates these symptoms. Until a person goes into withdrawal, there may be little, if any, evidence that the user is physically dependent on a drug.

Most importantly, avoiding withdrawal is a powerful force motivating people to keep using drugs. The user now has entered a new stage in his or her relationship with drugs. The user not only needs drugs to produce pleasure, but the person must have them to avoid the pain and discomfort of withdrawal.

But physical dependence is not addiction. For example, people who take opiates to relieve chronic pain can become physically dependent on their painkilling medication. They would experience withdrawal if they suddenly stopped taking their narcotic. But the drug is not the focus of their existence. Indeed, they use their narcotic medication to live a normal life. Addicts, by contrast, have no life without their drugs. This difference may be why virtually all pain patients have no trouble giving up their opiates if their pain is relieved, while addicts tend to relapse into drug use even after they have been withdrawn and put in treatment for their addiction.

Addiction, then, is more than drug tolerance and physical dependence, though these may be necessary preconditions. Our experience with pain patients has taught us that the defining conditions for addiction also include psychological dependence on the drug. The addicts perceive themselves as chained to the drug and their behavior becomes characterized by compulsive drug-seeking and drug-taking behavior. The focus of life is obtaining drugs, taking drugs, getting high, and then getting more drugs. Everything else—family, friends, job—falls by the wayside. The addict may get fired because he or she cannot function while high; the addict's family may throw the person out because the individual has stolen their money to support a drug habit. At the same time, the addict now needs the drug not only for pleasure, but also to avoid the sick feeling associated with withdrawal. Thus, the addict's ability to choose whether or not to use a drug has been severely compromised because only drugs bring pleasure, the solution to most of life's problems has become drug use, and doing without drugs brings the anxiety and sickness of withdrawal.

Animal studies indicate that the destructive behavior associated with addiction is not unique to humans and thus confirms its biological basis. Rats given free access to cocaine will eventually kill themselves taking it, foregoing even food and drink. They just keep taking cocaine until they die. Some humans stop or seek help before their habit kills them, but others cannot. To make it worse, intravenous drug users run the risk of infecting themselves, their spouses, and their unborn children with AIDS. This fatal disease of the immune system is increasing most rapidly among intravenous drug users, including prostitutes who shoot up and then spread the disease among their customers.

Treatment

Addicts have a tremendous ability for self-delusion. Some believe and will tell others, "I can stop any time I want. I can handle it." These people are actively denying that their drug problem even exists. But eventually, such people can end up in the emergency room with an overdose, they can get busted selling or buying drugs, or they might even end up on the street rejected by friends and family. Many have to hit some kind of bottom that finally prompts them to seek treatment.

One of the first things to understand about treatment for drug addiction is that it is not a cure. There is no cure for addiction in the way that an ear infection or strep throat can be cured. Drug addiction is a chronic disease that has the potential for relapse. Successful treatment of drug addiction means that the addict significantly reduces use of the drug to which he or she is addicted and that the individual has learned new behaviors that help avoid drug use and other self-destructive activities.

From this perspective, drug addiction can be considered much like hypertension, atherosclerosis, or adult diabetes. These also are chronic diseases that are typically caused by voluntary activities, such as poor diet, poor stress management, and lack of exercise. These diseases cannot really be cured, but they can be controlled through appropriate changes in lifestyle and perhaps with the aid of some medications. Those who treat alcoholics have long recognized the chronic relapsing nature of alcohol addiction; even if an alcoholic has not taken a drink for years, that person is still referred to as "recovering," not "recovered." That is because they know that the potential for relapse always exists and that staying sober requires continuing effort. It is a life-long process. The same is true for any drug addict. The long-term goal in drug addiction treatment is to teach the addict how to live without drugs.

The first goal of any treatment program, however, must be to stop the use of illicit drugs. In order for any treatment program to work, a person's basic brain biochemistry has to be stabilized and allowed to return to normal so that both the problems that led to drug use in the first place as well as the problems caused by addiction can be addressed. The cessation of drug use often reduces the criminal or antisocial behaviors—including stealing, chronic lying, or the sharing of needles—associated with the drug habit. Often addicts must be taught new skills and habits to replace the destructive behaviors related to addiction.

Goals of Treatment

◆ Stop illicit drug use
◆ Stop criminal and antisocial activity
◆ Increase adaptive behavior
◆ Decrease spread of AIDS

There are essentially two different approaches that are now used to reach these goals. The first begins with detoxification, the process of removing the addictive substances from the addict's brain and body. This can be done slowly or quickly and often means undergoing withdrawal, though it is possible that the most extreme symptoms can be medically treated. After this process, a drug-free treatment can begin that emphasizes psychotherapy or counseling and group therapy sessions as ways to teach people to solve their problems without resorting to drugs. Many addicts also may have an underlying mental illness that must be treated before effective drug abuse treatment can begin. For otherwise healthy people with a stable family and a job, drug abuse treatments might be successfully undertaken on an outpatient basis.

For people without these social supports, or for those who have been deeply involved in criminal and antisocial activity, residing in a specially designed drug-free community for a year or two may be necessary. These communities typically feature strict control over behavior with rewards for appropriate behavior and punishments for failure to comply with the rules. Such communities not only protect the recovering addict from drugs and the environmental cues that often led to drug use in the past, but they also surround the addict with other people who are undergoing the same recovery process and who can act as role models and lend moral and psychological support.

Skills development, especially for the many adolescent addicts who never learned the social skills necessary to go to school or hold a job, is also critical for continued recovery. Many people have to learn new ways to cope with old problems. They may need remedial education to hold down a job or attend school; fear or shame about poor reading ability or other inadequate skills may have facilitated the turn to drugs in the first place. Without new skills to deal with the world, relapse into drug use becomes almost inevitable. Drug-free treatments aim to obliterate the old habits associated with drug use and replace those with new coping skills that are essential for a drug-free life.

The alternative to drug-free treatment is medication therapy. Currently, there are only two medications—methadone and naltrexone—that can be used for this type of therapy, and they are both useful only for opiate addicts. It is crucial to note, however, that medications by themselves are not effective treatments for addiction. They must be used as part of a comprehensive treatment program that includes many of the therapeutic activities described above.

Methadone, the best-known maintenance agent, replaces the heroin that addicts are taking. Like heroin, methadone is an opiate agonist, stimulating opiate receptors in the brain. But unlike heroin, which must be injected into a vein four to six times each day to avoid withdrawal, methadone can be taken by mouth and lasts for 24 hours. Instead of repeatedly disrupting brain chemistry, like those repeated shots of heroin do, it stabilizes the brain so an addict can participate in a recovery program. Given in a proper dose, methadone prevents withdrawal and blocks the effects of heroin if the addict should "shoot up" after taking the dose of methadone. It also helps to break the habit of repeatedly injecting drugs and it gets people off needles so their chance of contracting or spreading AIDS goes way down.

Methadone does not produce the intense euphoria associated with heroin and many people have been successfully maintained on methadone for years. These people are able to hold jobs, interact positively with their families, and contribute productively to society. There is little question that when it is properly used, methadone is an effective treatment for some heroin addicts.

Naltrexone is an opiate antagonist; it prevents heroin or other opiates from activating opiate receptors. A person taking naltrexone cannot get high from shooting up heroin. The problem with naltrexone is that most addicts do not want to take it and now it is used only by highly motivated addicts.

Drug-Free Treatment

◆ Detoxification
◆ Psychotherapy/counseling
◆ Psychosocial therapy
◆ Drug-free community
◆ Skills development

A new addition to some drug treatment programs is deconditioning procedures. Even months after they have stopped using drugs, people with a long history of drug use feel strong urges to use drugs again when they encounter places or situations in which they have used drugs in the past. They have been conditioned to expect to use drugs in those situations just like Pavlov's dogs were conditioned to salivate when they heard a bell that had previously been sounded whenever they received food. Although initially only the food caused salivation, after the food and bell are presented together often enough, the brain learns that the bell means food

and the bell itself causes the animal to salivate. This powerful learning mechanism, called pavlovian conditioning, takes place without us being aware of it and is very difficult to overcome. Deconditioning techniques were developed in animal experiments and are now being applied directly in some treatment programs.

Whether or not a person receives drug-free or maintenance treatment or there is deconditioning, a key component of successful recovery is some form of aftercare that usually includes regular attendance at group meetings with other recovering addicts. These groups, which are largely patterned after Alcoholics Anonymous, supply the support many people need to maintain their drug-free state. One reason they are productive is because addicts can effectively break through the psychological barriers of other addicts. They can best point out the lies that people tell themselves to rationalize their drug behavior, and they can offer poignant support because they are going through the same process of recovery. But whatever form of therapy or aftercare program an addict may use, it is important to understand that treatment can work.

Drugs, Genetics and Biology

Many people use drugs for years without getting addicted, while others report they felt like an addict the first time they smoked crack. Such observations beg the question: Is there a genetic component to drug addiction? Are some people simply born more vulnerable than others to the effects of drugs? Researchers have found evidence that at least some alcoholics are genetically predisposed to alcoholism. We do not know if people have a genetic predisposition to become addicted to other drugs, but some addicts report they do not use drugs to get high, but rather to feel normal. It may be they have an inborn chemical imbalance in brain chemistry that is corrected by drugs. Such people might have genetic predispositions to become addicted.

Other suggestive evidence has come from animal studies; rats can be bred either to work for cocaine or to avoid it, or to be dramatically affected by opiates or to have smaller than normal responses to the compounds. These different responses are due to the genetic makeup of the individual strains of animals.

But whether or not some people are genetically vulnerable to drug addiction, it seems clear that biology predisposes us to drug use. Drugs alter the way the brain works by acting directly on our nerve cells. Long-term drug use can lead to long-term changes in brain chemistry. We do not know whether these changes are permanent. Most alcoholics and other recovering addicts know that even one drink or snort of cocaine can lead to an uncontrollable binge of drug use. This suggests that addiction has caused permanent changes in the way the brain responds to drugs.

Because of all we have learned about how drugs affect the brain, scientists now are able to create new medications that may prevent the drugs from getting a foothold in the brain or that can reverse their effects. Currently, investigators at the National Institute on Drug Abuse and other research institutions are working hard to develop medications that may be used to treat addiction. A drug that can block cocaine's ability to stimulate nerve cells is an important priority. Other drugs that can block the drug hunger or craving, which is a common cause of relapse, also are being sought.

Because of what we have learned from studying both animals and people, it is now clear that addiction is a biologically based disorder of the brain that, like hypertension or diabetes, can be treated with medical and behavioral techniques. As our understanding of the addictive process and its consequences grows, we will continue to create new prevention and treatment techniques to improve our ability to deal with the devastation of addiction.

■ Document Source:
U.S. Department of Health and Human Services, Public Health Service
National Institutes of Health
Clinical Center Communications
NIH Publication No. 91-3172
June 1991

National Institute on Aging Age Page
FOOT CARE

Many common foot problems result from disease, years of wear and tear, ill-fitting or poorly designed shoes, poor circulation to the feet, or improperly trimmed toenails.

You can prevent foot problems by checking your feet regularly—or having them checked by a member of the family—and by practicing good foot hygiene. Podiatrists and primary care physicians (internists and family practitioners) are qualified to treat most foot problems; sometimes the special skills of an orthopaedic surgeon or dermatologist are needed.

Preventing Foot Trouble

Improving the circulation of blood to the feet can help prevent problems. Exposure to cold temperatures, wading or bathing in cold water, pressure from shoes on the feet, long periods of sitting or resting, or smoking can reduce blood flow to the feet. Even sitting with your legs crossed or wearing tight, elastic garters or socks (long elastic hose tend to be better) can affect circulation. On the other hand, elevating the feet, standing up and stretching, walking, and other forms of exercise promote good circulation. Gentle massage and warm foot baths (95°F) can also help increase circulation to the feet.

Wearing comfortable, well-fitting shoes can prevent many foot ailments. The upper part of the shoes should be made of a soft, flexible material to conform to the shape of the foot. Shoes made of leather allow the feet to "breathe" and can reduce the possibility of skin irritations. Soles should provide solid footing and not be slippery. Thick soles lessen pressure when walking on hard surfaces. Low-heeled shoes are safer and less damaging to the feet as well as more comfortable than high-heeled shoes, so limit the time you wear high heels.

Common Foot Problems

Fungal and bacterial conditions—including athlete's foot—occur because the feet are usually enclosed in a dark, damp, warm environment. This is an ideal growing place for fungi and bacteria. Such infections cause redness, blisters, peeling, and itching. If not treated promptly, an infection may become chronic and difficult to cure. To prevent infection, keep the feet—especially the area between the toes—clean and dry and expose the feet to sun and air whenever possible. If you are prone to fungal infections on your feet, you may want to dust your feet daily with a fungicidal powder.

Dry skin sometimes results in itching and burning feet. Dryness can be helped by applying a body lotion to the legs and feet every day and by using mild soaps. Since all soaps can dry the skin, use them sparingly. The best moisturizers are those containing petroleum jelly or lanolin. But be cautious about adding oils to bath water since it can make the feet and bathtub very slippery.

Corns and calluses are caused by the friction and pressure from bony areas rubbing against shoes. Layers of dead skin cells build up, and the pressure of this hard mass on sensitive nerves in the skin can be painful. A podiatrist or a physician can determine the cause of corns and calluses and can recommend treatment, which may include obtaining better-fitting shoes or special pads. Over-the-counter medicines, advertised as cures for corns, contain acids that destroy the tissue but do not treat the cause. Although not a cure, these medicines can sometimes reduce the need for surgery. Treating corns or calluses yourself may be harmful, especially if you have diabetes or poor circulation.

Warts are skin growths caused by viruses. They are sometimes painful and if left untreated, may spread. Since over-the-counter preparations rarely cure warts, professional care should be sought. A doctor can apply medicines, remove the wart surgically, or—while using an anesthetic pain killer—burn or freeze it off.

Bunions develop when big toe joints are out of line and become swollen and tender. Bunions may be caused by poor-fitting shoes that press on a deformity or an inherited weakness in the foot. If a bunion is not severe, wearing shoes cut wide at the instep and toes may provide relief. Protective pads can also cushion the painful area. Bunions can be treated by applying or injecting certain drugs, using whirlpool baths, or sometimes having surgery.

Ingrown toenails occur when a piece of the nail pierces the skin. This is usually caused by improperly trimmed nails. Ingrown toenails are especially common in the large toes. A podiatrist or doctor can remove the part of the nail that is cutting into the skin, which will allow the area to heal and control any infection. Ingrown toenails can usually be avoided by cutting the toenail straight across and level with the top of the toe.

Hammertoe results from a shortening of the tendons that control the movements of the toes. The knuckle of the toe is usually enlarged and the toe is drawn back. Over a period of time the joint enlarges and stiffens as it rubs against the shoe. This can cause a loss of balance since the affected toes provide less assistance in standing and walking. Hammertoe is treated by wearing shoes and stockings with plenty of toe room. In advanced cases, surgery is generally recommended.

Spurs are calcium growths that develop on bones of the feet. They are caused by strain on the muscles in the feet and are aggravated by prolonged standing, wearing badly fitting shoes, or being overweight. Sometimes they are completely painless, but at other times the pain can be severe. Treatments for spurs include using proper foot support, heel pads, heel cups, or other recommendations by a podiatrist or surgeon.

Resources

For more information on foot care, write to the American Podiatric Medical Association, 9312 Old Georgetown Road, Bethesda, MD 20814, or to the American Orthopaedic Foot and Ankle Society, 222 South Prospect, Park Ridge, IL 60068.

The National Institute on Aging offers a variety of information about health and aging. For a list of publications, write to the NIA Information Center, P.O. Box 8057, Gaithersburg, MD 20898-8057.

■ Document Source:
U.S. Department of Health and Human Services, Public Health Service
National Institutes of Health
National Institute on Aging
1992

A Reprint from FDA Consumer Magazine

GETTING THE LEAD OUT ... OF JUST ABOUT EVERYTHING

by Alexandra Greeley

A Puerto Rican family moved here from the Caribbean with high hopes for a better life. They set up housekeeping in low-income housing in eastern Massachusetts, and four of the six children developed lead poisoning, shattering family dreams.

When questioned, the 10-year-old son answers that he lives in the state of Boston and that George Washington is president of the United States. He cannot count to 30. His younger brother with severe lead poisoning is chronically restless. He is unable to sit still, and the doctor describes him as roaming around the doctor's office like "a caged animal."

In another case, the ninth of 10 children of a well-to-do Boston family had seizures and was in a coma as a child as a result of lead poisoning. She ultimately recovered and went to school and then to college. But her history shows she had tremendous emotional difficulties throughout her life and has managed to cope only because her family had the financial resources to help.

Not fictitious children, they represent but a few of the cases that John Graef, M.D., associate clinical professor at Harvard Medical School and chief of the lead and toxicology program at Children's Hospital in Boston, has encountered in his career. "I think we all get numbed by the numbers," he says. "These are real people. Statistics do not tell the whole

story. . . . One of the things that worries us is that no matter where we look, there are ways for lead to enter our bodies."

Despite successful cleanup efforts—such as the reduction in the numbers of lead-soldered food cans, which FDA has urged, and the removal of lead from gasoline—health problems caused by repeated exposure to lead continue to endanger Americans. And children are particularly vulnerable. According to the February 1991 *Strategic Plan for the Elimination of Childhood Lead Poisoning,* developed for the Department of Health and Human Services, "Lead poisoning remains the most common and societally devastating environmental disease of young children."

About Lead

Lead has no known functions or health benefits for humans. It is considered a metabolic poison (meaning it inhibits some of the basic enzyme functions) and has caused humanity untold ills.

"Once lead enters the body, it is treated like calcium because the body can't tell the difference between the two," says Joseph LaDou, M.D., chief of the division of occupational and environmental medicine, University of California in San Francisco. After several weeks, lead leaves the bloodstream and is absorbed by bone, where it can continue to accumulate over a lifetime.

Probably the first published link between lead ingestion or inhalation and illness or death was made in the second century B.C. by the Greek physician Nicander, who wrote graphically about the tortures of lead poisoning—foaming lips, bloated belly, drooping limbs, and an inflamed mouth. Without intervention, Nicander observed, "the sick man descends to the Stygian shades."

Since that time, scientists and physicians have catalogued a lengthy list of health effects that they attribute to lead: damage to the kidneys and liver, and to the nervous, reproductive, cardiovascular, immune, and gastrointestinal systems. In children, as scientists have recognized, lead has a particularly damaging effect on intellectual development. In addition, lead interferes with the manufacture of heme, the oxygen-carrying part of hemoglobin in red blood cells. Extremely high levels of lead in the body cause encephalopathy, or degenerative brain disease, which, if untreated, results in death. The most remarkable aspect about lead illnesses, notes HHS's study, is that they are completely preventable.

Children Most Vulnerable

As a poison, lead has its most profound effects on rapidly growing biological systems. For humans, explains Graef, that means on the fragile, developing fetus, infant and child.

But several other factors also account for why children are so vulnerable to lead poisoning. Children's behaviors and activities—putting their hands in their mouths, playing in dirt, and eating nonfood objects, for example—increase their exposure to lead, says Graef.

In addition, he continues, children absorb more nutrients than adults do. They sometimes are deficient in iron, particularly in infancy, which increases their tendency to absorb more lead, and their rate of mineral uptake in bone is "several times greater than that in adults," says Graef. "In every sense of the word, children and lead do not mix."

Because of their unique risks, John Rosen, M.D., professor of pediatrics at Montefiore Medical Center, New York City, points out that lead consumption in childhood can mean a lower IQ and impairment in reading, writing, math, visual and motor skills, language, abstract thinking, and concentration.

Children may also suffer irritability, insomnia, colic, and anemia, all of which are subtle indications of elevated blood lead levels. Lead can also impair children's growth.

Damage to the child's nervous system is permanent, says LaDou, and some experts are now suggesting that low doses of lead may be responsible for some behavioral problems that most people call hyperactivity, as with the Puerto Rican child who could not sit still in the doctor's office. Even the subtle effects may be permanent, says Sue Binder, M.D., chief of the Lead Poisoning Prevention Branch, the National Centers for Disease Control.

And, according to lead expert Herbert Needleman, M.D., professor of psychiatry and pediatrics at the University of Pittsburgh, "It is a reasonable assumption that 20 percent of delinquency is associated with lead intake."

A 1988 report issued by the Agency for Toxic Substances and Disease Registry (ATSDR) estimates that between 3 million and 4 million children suffer from exposure to lead at concentrations that place them at risk of adverse health effects. The same report says that about 200,000 children more are actually lead poisoned. Mike Bolger, Ph.D., toxicologist at FDA's Center for Food Safety and Applied Nutrition, says that now that most experts accept a lower standard for lead poisoning than was used in the ATSDR study, chances are that the number of children considered to be affected by lead will be higher. To date, Bolger adds, no estimates have been made of how many adults suffer from lead poisoning.

Fortunately, childhood deaths from severe lead poisoning have become very rare. The most recent case occurred at the Children's Hospital of Wisconsin in Milwaukee in September 1990, when Eric Rivera died of lead poisoning after consuming quantities of leaded paint chips, probably over a period of time.

Drug Approved

A new drug, recently approved by FDA, to chelate (or remove) lead from children may reduce illness and death from lead. Chelating agents work by binding to lead in the bloodstream and expediting its elimination from the body in urine. Before the development of Chemet (succimer), the only drug available to chelate lead was calcium disodium versenate (EDTA), which is administered intravenously in adults and by intramuscular injection in children. Chemet has been approved for use only in children who have lead levels above 45 micrograms per deciliter.

Chemet removes lead from the body while leaving essential trace elements. Although its use at present has been limited, its track record indicates that the new oral drug may prove to be invaluable: Chemet given every eight hours for five days to children with lead poisoning has produced a drop in blood lead levels up to 78 percent. The recommended treatment course lasts 19 days and does not require hospitali-

zation. Presently, therapeutic intervention is considered only when lead body burdens are high—that is, greater than 25 micrograms per deciliter. The proposed labeling for this new drug warns that Chemet is "not a substitute for preventing further exposure to lead."

Adults Also Benefit from Research

Although the scientific community has focused on helping children, adults have benefited from the efforts to reduce childhood lead poisoning, Bolger says. The health effects for adults may be almost as grim, although adults require larger quantities of lead to cause the same damaging effects.

Scientists know that lead attacks the adult's peripheral nervous system, but its effects on the central nervous system have not been adequately studied, says Bolger. Protecting pregnant women and women of childbearing age is particularly important—their bone lead stores may be released into the bloodstream, exposing not only them to lead, but also their fetuses.

Because lead accumulates over a lifetime, points out Kathryn Mahaffey, Ph.D., science advisor in the office of the director, National Institute of Environmental Sciences in North Carolina, people may be carrying around in their bones deposits of a toxic chemical. And lead may reenter the bloodstream at any time as a result of severe biologic stress—such as renal failure, pregnancy, and even menopause—and from prolonged immobilization and very severe disease, says Richard Wedeen, M.D., associate chief of staff, research and development, V.A. Medical Center, East Orange, N.J., and author of *Poison in the Pot: The Legacy of Lead.*

Adults' problems with lead may be difficult to recognize. "There's a delayed effect and it is difficult to prove," says Wedeen. "Lead may be linked to high blood pressure, strokes, and heart attacks as well as kidney disease." In addition, Wedeen says, it impairs reproduction. And lowered IQ in childhood may result in adults who do not perform well and who become disruptive members of society. He asserts that it is reasonable to believe that lead contaminates every biochemical function.

There may be racial implications as well, says Wedeen. For example, black males are six times overrepresented in end-stage renal disease programs in our society—and these figures, hypothesizes Wedeen, may well be related to lead exposure. (He adds that it is a well-known fact that black male children have the highest lead exposure and blood lead levels of any group in the United States.) Because lead exposure is certainly not the only cause of hypertension and kidney disease, diagnosis is complicated and obscured.

Symptoms of lead exposure may not be identified unless the doctor does specific kinds of testing, he says. Many adults with mental symptoms due to lead encephalopathy may be misdiagnosed as alcoholics. Conversely, believes Wedeen, adults who suffer from acute lead poisoning may become alcoholics and end up in mental institutions.

Body Levels

Measuring the level of lead in blood is the most common way to estimate how much lead is circulating in the body at that moment. Because lead migrates to the bone several weeks after entering the bloodstream, a number of scientists are in favor of using a more precise technique for measuring the actual extent of lead accumulation and poisoning as measured in bone and teeth.

Who's Doing What

The following list includes many of the agencies—and their areas of responsibility—involved with regulating lead exposure or researching the effects of lead.

FDA has responsibility for regulating lead in:

- bottled water
- calcium supplements
- ceramic and other foodware
- commercial coffee urns
- decorated glassware
- food, including ingredients and packaging
- lead crystal
- lead-soldered food cans

EPA (Environmental Protection Agency) researches and/or monitors lead content in air, water and soil, and has some involvement monitoring lead-based paints.

NIOSH (National Institute for Occupational Safety and Health) conducts research and surveillance on occupational lead exposure and offers health hazard evaluation programs on work sites when requested and industrial hygiene training.

OSHA (Occupational Safety and Health Administration) regulates lead exposure at the work site.

NIEHS (National Institute of Environmental Health Sciences) conducts basic biomedical research on human health effects of lead.

HUD (U.S. Department of Housing and Urban Development) funds public housing authorities to contain or remove lead-based paint in public housing units.

CPSC (Consumer Product Safety Commission) requires warning labels on lead solder for drinking water pipes; monitors lead paint on children's toys to ensure compliance with the federal standard limiting lead in paint to no more than 0.06 percent; regulates the labeling of artists' materials; and has issued safety warnings about hazards of use of lead-based paint in the home.

ATSDR (Agency for Toxic Substances and Disease Registry) is responsible for health assessment for areas near Superfund sites (toxic waste sites that pose an environmental threat); wrote case study on lead for health professionals; and authored 1988 congressional document about the nature and extent of lead poisoning of American children.

In the 1970s, scientists set the maximum safe blood lead level for adults at 45 micrograms per deciliter, and in 1985 for children at 25 micrograms per deciliter.

Since then, research has shown that adverse effects actually occur at far lower levels. Bolger says that for adults, lead toxicity is associated with blood lead levels as low as 30 micrograms per deciliter. For children, toxicity occurs at 10 micrograms per deciliter—a figure that CDC recognizes in a 1991 draft revision of an earlier statement in the booklet *Preventing Lead Poisoning in Young Children: A Statement by the Centers for Disease Control-January 1985*. He adds that researchers project that the average American carries about 5 to 6 micrograms per deciliter in the blood. "Because

lead serves no known function in the body, the amount of lead that is 'normal' is about zero," says Tom Matte, M.D., medical epidemiologist, Lead Poisoning Prevention Branch, CDC.

It's Almost Everywhere

Once extracted from its naturally occurring state as an ore, lead has had thousands of applications—in gasoline and solder, paint, water pipes, housewares decorations, pottery glazes and lead crystal ware, power plant scrubbers, and lead-acid batteries, to name a few. Lead's durability, malleability, mass, low melting point, and resistance to corrosion from many chemicals make it indispensable for many industries.

Jeffrey Zelms, chairman of the Lead Industries Association, Inc., says that the health impact of today's lead is not a significant nor unreasonable risk. But some experts would disagree. Although lead is naturally present in the earth's crust, its redistribution throughout the environment by industrial activities has become a global problem, says LaDou, adding, "Lead lasts forever in the environment," because it is dispersed into air, soil, dust, and water.

It's true that the most important environmental exposure today is coming from past uses of lead in solder, house paint, and car fuel, says Matte, and all those uses have been dramatically curtailed. But the legacy persists in the form of paint dust or chips in older homes where leaded paint still coats walls and as soil filled with lead particles emitted from leaded gasolines.

In 1991, concern arose over a possible lead hazard from the reuse by some people of plastic bread bags. In the June 1991 *American Journal of Public Health,* researchers from the University of Medicine and Dentistry of New Jersey-Robert Wood Johnson Medical School told about people turning bread bags inside out and reusing them to store food or pack lunches. The article noted with concern that lead-based ink was used on the labels of many bread bags. Right side out, the ink would not come in contact with the bread, but when the bags were turned inside out, the ink could have contaminated food stored in them.

However, since publication of the journal article, FDA has learned that lead-based inks are no longer used on bread bags. Neil Sass, Ph.D., of FDA's Center for Food Safety and Applied Nutrition, says it is now highly unlikely that consumers would come in contact with lead from this source.

But the risk of lead contamination was not the only problem with inverted bread wrappers. Who else handled the bag before it was turned inside out? There may have been dirty hands, insects, or microbial contaminants from other sources, none of which should be in contact with food.

Lead can leach from certain items that come in contact with food—such as improperly manufactured ceramic products (usually imported), lead crystal ware decanters used for storing wine and other liquids, lead crystal baby bottles, and some decorated drinking glasses and mugs.

FDA Sets Standards

Many agencies, such as FDA, the Environmental Protection Agency, and CDC, and numerous private groups have been

How to Avoid Lead Exposure

Lead may be almost everywhere, but consumers can take practical steps to limit their exposure to it. Several experts give the following advice:

Food and Food-Related Products

♦ Make sure children's hands are clean before they eat.

♦ If using leaded crystal ware for drinking, do not use it on a daily basis, do not store liquids in it, do not use it while pregnant, and do not let children use it. Lead crystal baby bottles should not be used for infant feeding.

♦ Some imported foods are still packed in lead-soldered cans. If your grocer cannot assure you that a particular product is not packed in a lead-soldered can, your best bet is to limit consumption of imported canned foods.

♦ If using older or imported ceramic products, avoid storing acidic foods in them or, better yet, have them tested. If they test high in lead, use only for decorative purposes or discontinue use or dispose of the item. There are at least four home lead test kits on the market:

  • *Test For Lead In Pottery* ($25) and *The FRANDON Lead Alert Kit* ($29.95), Frandon Enterprises Inc., P.O. Box 300321, Seattle, Wash. 98103, or (1-800) 359-9000.

  • *Lead Check Swabs* ($25) or Lead Check Swabs-Half Packs ($15), Hybri Vet Systems, Inc., P.O. Box 1210, Framingham, Mass. 01701, or (1-800) 262-LEAD.

  • *Lead Test* ($10), Verify, Inc., 1185 Chess Drive, Suite 202, Foster City, Calif. 94404-1109, or (1-415) 578-9401.

  • *LEAD CHECK II* ($25), distributed by Michigan Ceramic Supplies, 4048 Seventh St., P.O. Box 342, Wyandotte, Mich. 48192, or (1-313) 281-2300.

Household Paint

Although lead-based paints have been banned for use in residences, numerous older private homes and public housing units still contain these paints. As a precaution:

♦ Keep painted surfaces in good repair so that older layers of paint are not exposed, chipping or peeling.

♦ Do not allow children to eat paint chips.

♦ Hire only a professional contractor to remove lead-based paints from any surface. People can poison themselves by burning or scraping off layers of paint. Lead dust is generated and if not contained properly sticks to household surfaces and is dispersed into the air.

Water

In order for your water to contain lead, there must be a source, such as lead service lines to the house, brass faucets, and/or lead solder on water pipes. Jeff Cohen, chief of the Lead Task Force, at EPA's Office of Water, says that lead is not a hazard in everyone's home because, in general, lead levels in drinking water are low. But he says that concerned homeowners or apartment dwellers can take several steps to reduce lead content in water:

♦ Begin with a water analysis—usually available at a cost of $15—on your household water. Do not run the water for six to eight hours before testing—lead may leach from pipes into still water.

♦ If the analysis shows that lead levels are about 20 ppb or higher, let water run before first use in the morning for 30 seconds or until the water runs cool. This flushes the lines. Do not use hot water for drinking or cooking since lead leaches more easily into hot water.

♦ To take further action, call your local water supplier to find out if your home/apartment is connected to the water main by lead service connections. If so, and if the service lines belong to the water supplier, ask if they have plans to replace the lines. If you own the lines, the supplier can help locate the name of a contractor to change them.

♦ Never use lead solder to repair plumbing.

working for a long time to reduce lead levels in such primary sources as food, soil, water, dust, and air. Remarkable progress has been made in the past few years—most experts agree that blood lead levels in the general population have dropped dramatically since most leaded gasolines have been phased out, lead has been removed from interior house paints, and the number of foods packed in lead-soldered cans has been substantially reduced.

Replacement of lead solder in the manufacture of most food cans in the United States has had the most significant effect in reducing the amount of lead ingested by the average American, says Burke. As a result of ongoing dialogue with the American food canning industry, FDA has worked with food processors to change can design to eliminate use of lead solder. Since 1979, when about 90 percent of all American-produced food cans contained lead solder, the figure has dropped to a 1990 level of about 3.8 percent, and a spokesman

for the food processing industry expects that after mid-1991 no lead-soldered food cans will be produced domestically.

Reducing lead levels in food sources or products in contact with food surfaces has long been a major FDA effort. FDA initiated an enforcement program on lead-based pesticides in fruits and vegetables in 1930. Since then, FDA has monitored dietary intake of lead in its Total Diet Study and worked with the U.S. food processing industry, leading to the packing of baby foods and juices in glass containers, the elimination of lead solder from evaporated milk cans, and reduction in use of lead-soldered food cans.

Guidelines were established on allowable amounts of lead leachable from ceramic products—both domestic and imported—and silver-plated holloware. As concerns about lead exposure have grown, FDA has continued to monitor food for lower levels of lead and is further evaluating a variety of potential sources of dietary lead, such as ceramic ware, decorated glassware, calcium supplements, lead-containing wine bottle seals, some older commercial coffee urns, and food ingredients.

The lead glaze on most ceramic foodware sold in the United States is formulated, applied and fired in such a way that the final product is impervious to the effects of food and beverages. But if improperly formulated and fired, the lead from the glaze leaches into foods.

FDA set up requirements on how glazes test out on the final product and began setting limits for lead leaching from ceramic products in 1970 after a California family suffered acute lead poisoning from drinking orange juice stored in a pitcher bought in Mexico. Informal guidelines established by the agency in 1971 originally set leachable lead levels at 7 parts per million (ppm) for all ceramic ware products. These levels were tightened in 1979 and further reduced in 1991, because new information showed that lead can adversely affect the fetus, young children, and adults in amounts well below those previously believed to be harmful.

Current guidelines for lead leaching from ceramic ware are:

♦ 3 ppm for plates, saucers, and other flatware
♦ 2 ppm for small hollowware such as cereal bowls, but not cups and mugs
♦ 0.5 ppm for cups and mugs
♦ 1.0 ppm for large (greater than 1.1 liters) hollowware such as bowls, but not pitchers
♦ 0.5 ppm for pitchers

The amount of lead leaching from the pieces is measured in a standard test involving 24-hour contact of the piece with an acid solution.

Imported ceramic products have been a greater concern to FDA than those produced in the United States, because most violations of FDA standards have been from foreign sources. More than 60 percent of the ceramic foodware sold in the United States is imported from some 80 foreign countries.

FDA efforts are concentrated on testing ceramic products from countries with histories of violations of FDA standards. FDA also entered into an agreement in 1988 with the People's Republic of China. This agreement requires that the Chinese government certify that shipments to the United States have been tested and that they meet FDA requirements. FDA now is working toward similar agreements with other countries, including Italy, Spain, and Hong Kong.

Recent preliminary studies conducted by researchers at Columbia University and at FDA have suggested that alcoholic and some other beverages stored for prolonged periods in crystal ware decanters may leach lead from the crystal. Pending completion of more comprehensive studies conducted by FDA and the crystal ware industry, consumers may want to avoid storing foods or beverages in crystal glassware for extended periods. This advice is especially important for pregnant women and infants and children.

Road Map to the Future

In the ongoing battle against lead exposure and lead poisoning, HHS's 1991 *Strategic Plan* is intended as a road map to guide future programs. While elements of the plan are already in effect—reducing lead in paint, drinking water, and food, for example—authors of the plan convey a sense of urgency. As pointed out in the plan's preface, lead poisoning "has already affected millions of children, and it could affect millions more. Its impact on children is real, however silently it damages their brains and limits their abilities."

Two Agencies Look at Lead in Wine

A program to reduce consumers' exposure to lead from table wines was announced in September 1991 by FDA and the Bureau of Alcohol, Tobacco and Firearms. This is part of the U.S. government's overall efforts to reduce exposure to lead in the environment.

The agencies said their long-term plans include eliminating the use of lead foil capsules to cover the outside rim and cork of some wine bottles and setting a tolerance for lead residues in table wines produced in the future.

The announcement followed a review at ATF's request by FDA scientists of the potential risks of lead in table wine.

FDA intends to propose soon a regulation banning the future use of lead foil capsules. ATF test data show that the capsules can increase lead levels in wine by leaving lead salt deposits on a bottle's rim. These deposits dissolve when the wine is poured into a glass or container.

Wine consumers can reduce their lead exposure from foil-wrapped wines by removing the foil and cork and wiping the rim and exposed cork with a wet cloth or a cloth moistened with vinegar or lemon juice before drinking the wine.

"Pregnant and lactating women have long been advised to avoid alcoholic beverages, including wine," said FDA Commissioner David A. Kessler, M.D. "The recent findings provide another good reason to do this because even low levels of lead may pose a hazard to the fetus or nursing infant."

FDA has informed ATF that foreign and domestic table wines sold in the United States that contain lead levels above 300 parts per billion (ppb) could be harmful to consumers. FDA intends to propose a rule to establish a limit on lead in table wine. ATF has the authority to detain and seek recall of these products.

ATF issued a public report of test results on July 31. Its data showed that only 3 to 4 percent of table wines tested contained more than 300 ppb of lead.

Although ATF also analyzed a smaller number of other alcoholic beverages, FDA said that the data do not indicate that other classes of alcoholic beverages—including beer, sparkling or dessert wines, or spirits—warrant immediate concern.

As for its role, although it can count many successes, FDA is stepping up its lead efforts, says Burke. "We have recognized the increase in concern about lead exposure, and we are taking steps on a number of fronts that will reduce the potential for exposure," he says. FDA has set out a four-part approach that includes issuing regulations to reduce or eliminate certain lead sources; increasing cooperative and voluntary control activities with affected industries; developing information on effectiveness of existing controls and needs for new ones; and educating the public.

In the end, with a concerted national effort, lead poisoning can be eliminated within the next few decades.

Alexandra Greeley is a freelance writer in Reston, Va., who has written on food for Time-Life books, Newsday, *and the* South China Morning Post.

■ Document Source:
  U.S. Department of Health and Human Services, Public Health Service
  Food and Drug Administration, Office of Public Affairs, 5600 Fishers Lane, Rockville, Md. 20857
  DHHS Publication No. (FDA) 92-2249
  Reprinted and Revised from July-August 1991

HYPERTHERMIA: A HOT WEATHER HAZARD FOR OLDER PEOPLE

Warm weather and outdoor activity generally go hand in hand. However, it is important for older people to take action to avoid the severe health problems often caused by hot weather. "Hyperthermia" is the general name given to a variety of heat-related illnesses. The two most common forms of hyperthermia are heat exhaustion and heat stroke. Of the two, heat stroke is especially dangerous and requires immediate medical attention (see definition at conclusion of this brochure).

What causes hyperthermia?

Regardless of extreme weather conditions, the healthy human body keeps a steady temperature of 98.6° Fahrenheit (37° Centigrade). In hot weather, or during vigorous activity, the body perspires. As this perspiration evaporates from the skin, the body is cooled. If challenged by long periods of intense heat, the body may lose its ability to respond efficiently. When this occurs, a person can experience hyperthermia.

What can be done to prevent hyperthermia?

- Drink plenty of liquids, even if not thirsty.
- Dress in light-weight, light-colored, loose-fitting clothing.
- Avoid the midday heat and do not engage in vigorous activity during the hottest part of the day (noon–4 p.m.).
- Wear a hat or use an umbrella for shade.
- If possible, use air conditioners liberally or try to visit air-conditioned places such as libraries, shopping malls, and theaters. For an air conditioner to be beneficial it should be set below 80°F.
- If not used to the heat, get accustomed to it slowly by exposing yourself to it briefly at first and increasing the time little by little.
- Avoid hot, heavy meals. Do a minimum of cooking and use an oven only when absolutely necessary.
- Ask your physician whether you are at particular risk because of medication.

Who is at risk?

The temperature does not have to hit 100° for a person to be at risk. Both one's general health and/or lifestyle may increase a person's chance of suffering a heat-related illness.

Health factors which may increase risk include:

- poor circulation, inefficient sweat glands, and changes in the skin caused by the normal aging process.
- heart, lung, and kidney diseases, as well as any illness that causes general weakness or fever.
- high blood pressure or other conditions that require changes in diet. For example, people on salt restricted diets may increase their risk. However, salt pills should not be used without first asking a doctor.
- the inability to perspire, caused by medications including diuretics, sedatives and tranquilizers, and certain heart and blood pressure drugs.
- taking several drugs for various conditions. It is important, however, to continue to take prescribed medication and discuss possible problems with a physician.
- being substantially overweight or underweight.
- drinking alcoholic beverages.

Lifestyle factors that can increase risk include:

- unbearably hot living quarters. People who live in homes without fans or air conditioners should take the following steps to reduce heat discomfort: open windows at night; create cross-ventilation by opening windows on two sides of the building; cover windows when they are exposed to direct sunlight; and keep curtains, shades, or blinds drawn during the hottest part of the day.
- lack of transportation. People without fans or air conditioners often are unable to go to shopping malls, movie houses, and libraries because of illness and/or the lack of transportation. Friends or relatives might be asked to supply transportation on particularly hot days. Many communities, area agencies, religious groups, and senior citizen centers provide such services.
- overdressing. Because they may not feel the heat, older people may not dress appropriately in hot weather. Perhaps a friend or family member can help to select proper clothing. Natural fabrics such as cotton are best.
- visiting overcrowded places. Trips should be scheduled during non-rush-hour times and participation in special events should be carefully planned.
- not understanding weather conditions. Older people, particularly those at special risk (see health factors), should stay indoors on especially hot and humid days, particularly when there is an air pollution alert in effect.

How is hyperthermia treated?

If the victim is exhibiting signs of heat stroke, seek emergency assistance immediately. Without medical attention heat stroke is frequently deadly, especially for older people.

Heat exhaustion may be treated in several ways:

- ♦ Get the victim out of the sun and into a cool place—preferably one that is air-conditioned.
- ♦ Offer fluids but avoid alcohol and caffeine. Water and fruit and vegetable juices are best.
- ♦ Encourage the individual to shower or bathe, or sponge off with cool water.
- ♦ Urge the person to lie down and rest, preferably in a cool place.

How is hyperthermia detected?

A person with symptoms including headache, nausea, and fatigue after exposure to heat probably has some measure of a heat-related illness. It is important to recognize the difference between the very serious condition known as heat stroke and other heat-related illnesses. Persons experiencing any of these symptoms should consult a doctor.

Definitions

Heat stress. Occurs when a strain is placed on the body as a result of hot weather.

Heat fatigue. A feeling of weakness brought on by high outdoor temperature. Symptoms include cool, moist skin and a weakened pulse. The person may feel faint.

Heat syncope. A sudden dizziness experienced after exercising in the heat. The skin appears pale and sweaty but is generally moist and cool. The pulse may be weakened, and the heart rate is usually rapid. Body temperature is normal.

Heat cramps. Painful muscle spasms in the abdomen, arms, or legs following strenuous activity. The skin is usually moist and cool and the pulse is normal or slightly raised. Body temperature is mostly normal. Heat cramps often are caused by a lack of salt in the body, but salt replacement should not be considered without advice from a physician.

Heat exhaustion. A warning that the body is getting too hot. The person may be thirsty, giddy, weak, uncoordinated, nauseous, and sweating profusely. The body temperature is usually normal and the pulse is normal or raised. The skin is cold and clammy. Although heat exhaustion often is caused by the body's loss of water and salt, salt supplements should only be taken with advice from a doctor.

Heat stroke. Can be LIFE-THREATENING! Victims of heat stroke almost always die so immediate medical attention is essential when problems first begin. A person with heat stroke has a body temperature above 104°F. Other symptoms may include confusion, combativeness, bizarre behavior, faintness, staggering, strong rapid pulse, dry flushed skin, lack of sweating, possible delirium or coma.

Heat-related illnesses can become serious if preventive steps are not taken. It is important to realize that older people are at particular risk of hyperthermia. Many people die of heat stroke each year; most are over 50 years of age. With good, sound judgment and knowledge of preventive measures the summer can remain safe and enjoyable for everyone.

■ Document Source:
U.S. Department of Health and Human Services, Public Health Service
National Institutes of Health
National Institute on Aging
NIH Publication No. 89-2763
August 1989

A Reprint from FDA Consumer Magazine

NONSTEROIDAL ANTI-INFLAMMATORY DRUGS

by Dori Stehlin

How you take a drug makes a big difference in how well it will work and how safe it will be for you. Timing, what you eat and when you eat, proper dose, and many other factors can mean the difference between feeling better, staying the same, or even feeling worse. This drug information page is intended to help you make your treatment work as well as possible. It is important to note, however, that this is only a guideline. You should talk to your doctor or pharmacist about how and when to take any prescribed drugs.

This first installment of a series of articles on commonly prescribed drugs is about nonsteroidal anti-inflammatory drugs, often abbreviated NSAIDs.

Conditions These Drugs Treat

- ♦ symptoms such as redness, warmth, swelling, stiffness, and joint pain caused by rheumatoid arthritis, osteoarthritis, and other rheumatic conditions
- ♦ menstrual cramps
- ♦ pain, especially that associated with dental problems, gout, episiotomy (an incision made in a woman's perineum and vagina during childbirth to prevent tearing), tendinitis, bursitis, and injuries such as sprains and strains

NSAIDs are not a cure for arthritis or any other disease. These drugs temporarily relieve pain by blocking the body's production of chemicals known as prostaglandins, which are believed to be associated with the pain and inflammation of injuries and immune reactions.

How to Take NSAIDs

Indomethacin and phenylbutazone should always be taken with food. The food helps prevent an upset stomach, which NSAIDs can cause. Meclofenamate may be taken with meals. For other NSAIDs, however, your doctor may tell you to take the first several doses 30 minutes before or two hours after eating. This will help the medicine relieve the symptoms more quickly.

Generic Names	
diclofenac	meclofenamate
diflunisal	mefenamic acid
fenoprofen	naproxen
ibuprofen	phenylbutazone
indomethacin	piroxicam
ketoprofen	sulindac
ketorolac	tolmetin

Like food, antacids may prevent an upset stomach when you're taking NSAIDs. However, both food and some over-the-counter antacids may interfere with an NSAID's effectiveness. Ask your doctor for the best approach for a particular NSAID.

NSAID tablets and capsules should be washed down with eight ounces of water to help prevent the drugs from irritating the delicate lining of the esophagus and stomach. In addition, to let gravity help move the pills along—don't lie down for at least 15 to 30 minutes after each dose.

Be sure to take the right number of tablets or capsules for each dose. Liquid doses are best measured in special spoons available from your pharmacist. Teaspoons or tablespoons from the kitchen drawer are rarely the right dosage size.

Missed Doses

Ask your doctor what to do if you forget to take a dose. Some NSAIDs have a longer-lasting effect in the body than others, so you'll need your doctor's guidance on whether to make up a missed dose of the specific NSAID you are taking, or just wait until it's time for the next dose.

But never take a double dose.

Be sure to refill your prescriptions soon enough to avoid missing any doses.

Relief of Symptoms

Most NSAIDs start to relieve pain symptoms in about an hour. However, for long-term inflammation and for severe or continuing arthritis, relief may not come for a week to several weeks.

How long you will need to take the medicine depends on the condition being treated. Make sure you understand your doctor's instructions.

Side Effects and Risks

Common side effects include nausea, cramps, indigestion, and diarrhea or constipation. Other side effects can include increased sensitivity to sunlight, nervousness, confusion, headache, drowsiness, or dizziness. If you have any of these side effects, notify your doctor, but don't stop taking your medication on your own.

Occasionally, NSAIDs can cause ulcers or bleeding in the stomach or small intestine. Warning signs include severe cramps, pain or burning in the stomach or abdomen; diarrhea or black tarry stools, severe, continuing nausea, heartburn, or indigestion; or vomiting of blood or material that looks like coffee grounds. If any of these side effects occurs, stop taking the medicine and call your doctor immediately.

Other serious but rare reactions are:

♦ Anaphylaxis—Signs of this severe allergic reaction are very fast or difficult breathing, difficulty in swallowing, swollen tongue, gasping for breath, wheezing, dizziness, or fainting. A hive-like rash, puffy eyelids, change in face color, or very fast but irregular heartbeat or pulse may also occur. If any of these occurs, get emergency help at once.

♦ With phenylbutazone, sore throat or fever can be early signs that the drug has impaired the bone marrow's ability to produce blood cells. Call your doctor immediately. Because of the seriousness of this side effect, phenylbutazone is usually prescribed as a last resort and then for short periods only.

♦ Unusual swelling of the fingers, hands or feet, weight gain, or decreased or painful urination can indicate worsening of an underlying heart or kidney condition. If any of these symptoms occurs, call your doctor.

Don't store drugs in the bathroom medicine cabinet. Heat and humidity may cause the medicine to lose its effectiveness.

Keep all medicines, even those with child-resistant caps, out of the reach of children. Remember, the caps are child-resistant, not child-proof.

Discard medicines that have reached the expiration date shown on the label.

Precautions and Warnings

♦ NSAIDs should not usually be taken during pregnancy or while breast-feeding.

♦ People 65 and older are more likely to experience the side effects of NSAIDs and get sicker with those effects than younger adults.

♦ Alcoholic beverages should be avoided, as they increase the potential for stomach problems while taking NSAIDs.

♦ Don't take acetaminophen or aspirin or other salicylates with NSAIDs unless directed by your doctor. Taking these drugs along with NSAIDs may increase the risk of side effects.

♦ Tell your physician if you are taking any other medication—prescription or nonprescription.

♦ Before any surgery or dental work, tell the physician or dentist that you are taking NSAIDs.

♦ Don't drive or operate machines if the medicine makes you confused, drowsy, dizzy, or lightheaded. Learn how the medicine affects you first.

♦ NSAIDs can increase sensitivity to sunlight in some people. To avoid the risk of a serious sunburn, stay out of direct sunlight, especially between 10 a.m. and 3 p.m.; wear protective clothing; and apply a sunblock with a skin protection factor of 15.

■ Document Source:
U.S. Department of Health and Human Services, Public Health Service
Food and Drug Administration
Office of Public Affairs, 5600 Fishers Lane, Rockville, MD 20857
DHHS Publication No. (FDA) 90-3176
Reprinted June 1990

PAIN CONTROL AFTER SURGERY: A PATIENT'S GUIDE

Purpose of This Booklet

This booklet talks about pain relief after surgery. It explains the goals of pain control and the types of treatment you may receive. It also shows you how to work with your doctors and nurses to get the best pain control.

Reading the booklet should help you:

♦ Learn why pain control is important for your recovery as well as your comfort.
♦ Play an active role in choosing among options for treating your pain.

What Is Pain?

Pain is an uncomfortable feeling that tells you something may be wrong in your body. Pain is your body's way of sending a warning to your brain. Your spinal cord and nerves provide the pathway for messages to travel to and from your brain and the other parts of your body.

Receptor nerve cells in and beneath your skin sense heat, cold, light, touch, pressure, and pain. You have thousands of these receptor cells, most sense pain and the fewest sense cold. When there is an injury to your body—in this case surgery—these tiny cells send messages along nerves into your spinal cord and then up to your brain. Pain medicine blocks these messages or reduces their effect on your brain.

Sometimes pain may be just a nuisance, like a mild headache. At other times, such as after an operation, pain that doesn't go away—even after you take pain medicine—may be a signal that there is a problem. After your operation, your nurses and doctors will ask you about your pain because they want you to be comfortable, but also because they want to know if something is wrong. Be sure to tell your doctors and nurses when you have pain.

Treatment Goals

People used to think that severe pain after surgery was something they "just had to put up with." But with current treatments, that's no longer true. Today, you can work with your nurses and doctors before and after surgery to prevent or relieve pain.

Pain control can help you:

♦ Enjoy greater comfort while you heal.

♦ Get well faster. With less pain, you can start walking, do your breathing exercises, and get your strength back more quickly. You may even leave the hospital sooner.
♦ Improve your results. People whose pain is well-controlled seem to do better after surgery. They may avoid some problems (such as pneumonia and blood clots) that affect others.

Pain control: What are the options?

Both drug and non-drug treatments can be successful in helping to prevent and control pain. The most common methods of pain control are described below. You and your doctors and nurses will decide which ones are right for you. Many people combine two or more methods to get greater relief.

Don't worry about getting "hooked" on pain medicines. Studies show that this is very rare—unless you already have a problem with drug abuse.

Pain Control Methods You May Be Using

To get the best results, work with your doctors and nurses to choose the methods that will work best for you.

Your nurses and doctors want to make your surgery as pain free as they can. But you are the key to getting the best pain relief because pain is personal. The amount of type of pain you feel may not be the same as others feel—even those who have had the same operation.

Before surgery

Drug treatment: Take pain medicine.
Non-drug treatment: Understand what operation the doctor is doing, why it is being done, and how it will be done. Learn how to do deep breathing and relaxation exercises.

During surgery

Drug treatment: Receive general anesthesia, spinal anesthesia, or nerve blocks, or take a pain medicine through a small tube in your back (called an epidural).

After surgery

Drug treatment: Take a pain medicine as a pill, shot, or suppository, or through a tube in your vein or back.
Non-drug treatment: Use massage, hot or cold packs, relaxation, music or other pastimes to distract you, positive thinking, or nerve stimulation (TENS).

What Can You Do to Help Keep Your Pain Under Control?

These seven steps can help you help yourself.

Before surgery

1. Ask the doctor or nurse what to expect.

♦ Will there be much pain after surgery?
♦ Where will it occur?

♦ How long is it likely to last?

Being prepared helps put you in control. You may want to write down your questions before you meet with your doctor or nurse.

2. Discuss the pain control options with your doctors and nurses.

Be sure to:

♦ Talk with your nurses and doctors about pain control methods that have worked well or not so well for you before.
♦ Talk with your nurses and doctors about any concerns you may have about pain medicine.
♦ Tell your doctors and nurses about any allergies to medicines you may have.
♦ Ask about side effects that may occur with treatment.
♦ Talk with your doctors and nurses about the medicines you take for other health problems. The doctors and nurses need to know, because mixing some drugs with some pain medicines can cause problems.

3. Talk about the schedule for pain medicines in the hospital.

Some people get pain medicines in the hospital only when they call the nurse to ask for them. Sometimes there are delays, and the pain gets worse while they wait.

Today, two other ways to schedule pain medicines seem to give better results.

♦ Giving the pain pills or shots at set times. Instead of waiting until pain breaks through, you receive medicine at set times during the day to keep the pain under control.
♦ Patient controlled analgesia (PCA) may be available in your hospital. With PCA, you control when you get pain medicine. When you begin to feel pain, you press a button to inject the medicine through the intravenous (IV) tube in your vein.

For both ways, your nurses and doctors will ask you how the pain medicine is working and change the medicine, its dose, or its timing if you are still having pain.

4. Work with your doctors and nurses to make a pain control plan.

You should plan for pain control with your nurses and doctors. They need your help to design the best plan for you. When your pain control plan is complete, use the form to write down what will happen. Refer to it after your operation. Then keep it as a record if you need surgery in the future.

After surgery

5. Take (or ask for) pain relief drugs when pain first begins.

♦ Take action as soon as the pain starts.
♦ If you know your pain will worsen when you start working or doing breathing exercises, take pain medicine first. It's harder to ease pain once it has taken hold.

This is a key step in proper pain control.

6. Help the doctors and nurses "measure" your pain.

♦ They may ask you to rate your pain on a scale of 0 to 10. Or you may choose a word from a list that best describes the pain.
♦ You may also set a pain control goal (such as having no pain that's worse than 2 on the scale).
♦ Reporting your pain as a number helps the doctors and nurses know how well your treatment is working and whether to make any changes.
♦ They may ask you to use a "pain scale."

7. Tell the doctor or nurse about any pain that won't go away.

♦ Don't worry about being a "bother."
♦ Pain can be a sign of problems with your operation.
♦ The nurses and doctors want and need to know about it.

Stick with your pain control plan if it's working. Your doctors and nurses can change the plan if your pain is not under control. You need to tell the nurses and doctors about your pain and how the pain control plan is working.

Example—Slow Rhythmic Breathing for Relaxation*

1. Breathe in slowly and deeply.
2. As you breathe out slowly, feel yourself beginning to relax; feel the tension leaving your body.
3. Now breathe in and out slowly and regularly, at whatever rate is comfortable for you. You may wish to try abdominal breathing. If you do not know how to do abdominal breathing, ask your nurse to help.
4. To help you focus on your breathing and breathe slowly and rhythmically: Breathe in as you say silently to yourself, "in, two, three." Breathe out as you say silently to yourself, "out, two, three."

or

Each time you breathe out, say silently to yourself a word such as peace or relax.

5. You may imagine that you are doing this in a place that is very calming and relaxing for you, such as lying in the sun at the beach.

---

* From: McCaffery, M. and Beebe, A. (1989). *Pain: Clinical manual for nursing practice.* St. Louis: C.V. Mosby Company.

6. Do steps 1 through 4 only once or repeat steps 3 and 4 for up to 20 minutes.
7. End with a slow deep breath. As you breathe out say to yourself "I feel alert and relaxed."

Additional points: If you intend to do this for more than a few seconds, try to get in a comfortable position in a quiet place. You may close your eyes or focus on an object. This breathing exercise may be used for only a few seconds or for up to 20 minutes.

Benefits and Risks of Pain Treatment Methods

This information is provided to help you discuss your options with your doctors and nurses. Sometimes it is best to combine two or more of these treatments or change the treatments slightly to meet your individual needs. Your doctors and nurses will discuss this with you.

Pain Relief Medicines

Nonsteroidal anti-inflammatory drugs. Acetaminophen (for example, Tylenol), aspirin, ibuprofen (for example, Motrin), and other NSAIDs reduce swelling and soreness and relieve mild to moderate pain.

Benefits. There is no risk of addiction to these medicines. Depending on how much pain you have, these medicines can lessen or eliminate the need for stronger medicines (for example, morphine or another opioid).

Risks. Most NSAIDs interfere with blood clotting. They may cause nausea, stomach bleeding, or kidney problems. For severe pain, an opioid usually must be added.

Opioids. Morphine, codeine, and other opioids are most often used for acute pain, such as short-term pain after surgery.

Benefits. These medicines are effective for severe pain, and they do not cause bleeding in the stomach or elsewhere. It is rare for a patient to become addicted as a result of taking opioids for postoperative pain.

Risks. Opioids may cause drowsiness, nausea, constipation, itching, or interfere with breathing or urination.

Local anesthetics. These drugs (for example, bupivacaine) are given, either near the incision or through a small tube in your back, to block the nerves that transmit pain signals.

Benefits. Local anesthetics are effective for severe pain. Injections at the incision site block pain from that site. There is little or no risk of drowsiness, constipation, or breathing problems. Local anesthetics reduce the need for opioid use.

Risks. Repeated injections are needed to maintain pain relief. An overdose of local anesthetic can have serious consequences. Average doses may cause some patients to have weakness in their legs or dizziness.

Methods Used to Give Pain Relief Medicines

Tablet or liquid. Medicines given by mouth (for example, aspirin, ibuprofen, or opioid medications such as codeine).

Benefits. Tablets and liquids cause less discomfort than injections into muscle or skin, but they can work just as well. They are inexpensive, simple to give, and easy to use at home.

Risks. These medicines cannot be used if nothing can be taken by mouth or if you are nauseated or vomiting; sometimes these medicines can be given rectally (suppository form). There may be a delay in pain relief, since you must ask for the medicine and wait for it to be brought to you; also, these medicines take time to wear off.

Injections into skin or muscle.

Benefits. Medicine given by injection into skin or muscle is effective even if you are nauseated or vomiting; such injections are simple to give.

Risks. The injection site is usually painful for a short time. Medicines given by injection are more expensive than tablets or liquids and take time to wear off. Pain relief may be delayed while you ask the nurse for medicine and wait for the shot to be drawn up and given.

Injections into vein. Pain relief medicines are injected into a vein through a small tube, called an intravenous (IV) catheter. The tip of the tube stays in the vein.

Benefits. Medicines given by injection into a vein are fully absorbed and act quickly. This method is well suited for relief of brief episodes of pain. When a patient controlled analgesia (PCA) pump is used, you can control your own doses of pain medicine.

Risks. A small tube must be inserted in a vein. If PCA is used, there are extra costs for pumps, supplies, and staff training. You must want to use the pump and learn how and when to give yourself doses of medicine.

Injections into spine. Medicine is given through a small tube in your back (called an epidural or intrathecal catheter).

Benefits. This method works well when you have chest surgery or an operation on the lower parts of your body.

Risks. Staff must be specially trained to place a small tube in the back and to watch for problems that can appear hours after pain medicine is given. Extra cost is involved for staff time and training and to purchase pumps and supplies.

Non-Drug Pain Relief Methods

These methods can be effective for mild to moderate pain and to boost the pain-relief effects of drugs. There are no side effects. These techniques are best learned before surgery.

Patient teaching. **Learning about the operation and the pain expected afterwards (for example, when coughing or getting out of bed or a chair).**

Benefits. These techniques can reduce anxiety; they are simple to learn, and no equipment is needed.

Risks. There are no risks; however, patient attention and cooperation with staff are required.

Relaxation. Simple techniques, such as abdominal breathing and jaw relaxation, can help to increase your comfort after surgery.

Benefits. Relaxation techniques are easy to learn, and they can help to reduce anxiety. After instruction, you can use relaxation at any time. No equipment is needed.

Risks. There are no risks, but you will need instruction from your nurse or doctor.

Physical agents. Cold packs, massage, rest, and TENS therapy are some of the non-drug pain relief methods that might be used following surgery.

Benefits. In general, physical agents are safe and have no side effects. TENS, which stands for transcutaneous electrical nerve stimulation, is often helpful; it is quick to act and can be controlled by the patient.

Risks. There are no risks related to the use of physical techniques for managing pain. If TENS is used, there is some cost and staff time involved for purchasing the machine and instructing patients in its use. Also, there is only limited evidence to support the effectiveness of TENS for pain relief in certain situations.

Want to Know More?

The information in this booklet was taken from the *Clinical Practice Guideline for Acute Pain Management: Operative or Medical Procedures and Trauma.* The guideline was developed by a non-federal expert panel made up of doctors, nurses, other health care providers, an ethicist, and a consumer representative. The guideline development process was sponsored by the Agency for Health Care Policy and Research (AHCPR), an agency of the U.S. Public Health Service. Other guidelines on common health problems are being developed and will be released in the near future.

For more information about the guidelines or to receive additional copies of this booklet or other guideline materials, call 1-800-358-9295, or write to the AHCPR Publications Clearinghouse, P.O. Box 8547, Silver Spring, MD 20907.

■ Document Source:
U.S. Department of Health and Human Services, Public Health Service
Agency for Health Care Policy and Research
Executive Office Center, 2101 East Jefferson Street, Suite 501, Rockville, MD 20852
Publication No. AHCPR 92-0021

National Institute on Aging Age Page
WHEN YOU NEED A NURSING HOME

There are currently over 1.5 million residents of nursing homes in the United States, over two-thirds of whom are women. The nursing home population has been growing, and likely will continue to grow with the increase in numbers of older persons. While only 5 percent of the older population is in a nursing home at any one time, approximately 30 percent of all people can expect to spend some time in a nursing home setting.

Today's nursing homes are greatly improved and more accommodating to the needs of individuals than in the past. Still, most people prefer to remain in their own homes as long as possible. A number of choices are available in most communities that can help older people remain independent or to be cared for at home by their families. Community services may include homemaker/home health aide services, home-delivered meals, transportation and escort services, chore-workers, a friendly visitors program, adult day programs that provide social and health care services, respite care that provides temporary relief for caregivers, and emergency medical systems.

Long-Term Care Options

Although families often go to great lengths to keep older loved ones at home, they may not be able to provide the best physical and emotional care without experiencing undue stress. When home care and community services are no longer adequate, a person must decide on the best alternative arrangement for meeting personal and health care needs. The following options are available:

♦ **Residential care facilities** provide room and board and may offer social, recreational, and spiritual programs.
♦ **Continuing care communities,** a relatively new concept, ensure that all needs of the resident are met, including room and board, personal and health care, and social activities.
♦ **Assisted living facilities** include retirement homes and board and care homes. Services differ from location to location but usually include meals, recreation, security, and assistance with walking, bathing, and dressing.
♦ **Skilled nursing facilities** may be the best choice for those who require 24-hour medical care and supervision. Emphasis is on medical care with rehabilitative therapy to improve or maintain abilities.

Sometimes it is difficult to know when nursing home care is warranted. Ideally, a health care team will assess the level of care needed for the person and suggest the combination of services required. Health care teams are most likely to be found at university hospitals or community medical centers. The team should include the patient's doctor, a nurse, a social worker or psychiatric counselor, and a physical therapist.

Choosing a Nursing Home

Finding the right nursing home may also be difficult. It is wise to begin the search for a suitable nursing home well in advance of seeking admission. Often the best homes will have no vacancies and long waiting lists. You can obtain the names of nursing homes in the desired area(s) from the yellow pages of your telephone directory. Good homes may be known to other families in the community or your doctor. Your area agency on aging is also a good source for assistance in locating nursing homes in your area. Other sources include the social services department of a local hospital and your local or state health department.

Begin to eliminate from consideration those homes that do not meet your needs. Start with a telephone call to answer questions about vacancies, admission requirements, level of care provided, and participation in Medicare and Medicaid programs. (These Federal programs set certain minimum standards of care that must be met before a nursing home can be certified for participation. Nursing homes in some states can refuse to accept Medicaid patients, depending on the laws of the state.) You should also make sure that the nursing home has an up-to-date state license, and that the administrator's license is up-to-date as well. It is also a good idea to ask if the nursing home meets (or exceeds) the state fire regulations. This includes a sprinkler system, fire-resistant doors, and a plan for evacuating frail people.

Find out about access to medical and nursing services and about what arrangements exist for handling medical emergencies. You will also want to know what types of rehabilitation and social programs are offered to the residents, and you will want to evaluate the food service. Observing and talking to other residents and their families can provide you with useful information that you might not otherwise get from the staff. Look for evidence that staff members treat residents with respect and provide services tailored to the preferences and lifestyle of each individual. If you see residents restrained in any way, that nursing home will probably not be a satisfactory setting for your relative. You may want to drop in once or twice unannounced, perhaps in the evening, to get an idea of

---

Nursing Home Checklist

When you think a nursing home may be needed, plan and investigate before an emergency arises. These are some questions to guide you in making a decision:

Credentials

Does the home have a current state license?
Does the administrator have a current license?
Is the home certified for Medicare and Medicaid programs?

Residents

Do residents seem well cared for and generally content?
Are most residents out of their beds, dressed, and, when possible, occupied?
Are residents allowed to wear their own clothes and have some of their own furniture in their rooms?
Is a statement of patient's rights posted?
Is special care provided for Alzheimer's disease patients?

Facility

Is the atmosphere warm and pleasant?
Is the home accessible to family and friends?
Do rooms provide privacy?
Is there an activity room?
Is the nursing home clean, orderly, and reasonably free of unpleasant odors?
Are toilet and bathing facilities adequate and accessible to disabled persons?
Are grab bars, handrails, and emergency call buttons located in rooms and halls?
Does the building have smoke detectors, sprinkler systems, and emergency lighting?
Does the home have a security system to prevent confused residents from wandering out of the building?
What is the home's policy on the use of physical and chemical restraints?

Staff

Do employees show respect to residents?
Are enough nurses and aides on duty at all hours, including weekends?
Is the home sensitive to cultural and minority differences?
What is the average length of time staff have worked in the home?

Services

Is regular and emergency medical attention assured?
Does the home have arrangements with a hospital for transfer of patients in an emergency?
Are pharmaceutical services available and supervised by a qualified pharmacist?
Does the home offer physical therapy and rehabilitative services?
Are interesting activities scheduled, including trips outside the home?
Are arrangements made for residents to participate in religious practices?

Meals

Is a weekly menu available?
Are the dining room and kitchen clean?
Are meals nutritious, appetizing, and tasty? (Eat one.)
Does the staff assist residents who can't feed themselves?
Are special diets available for health needs, religious or ethnic preferences?

General

How do monthly costs compare with the cost of other homes?
Are financial and other policies specified in a contract?
Do the resident's assets remain in his or her control or that of the family?
Do you feel that this facility provides the best care for its residents?

General

How do monthly costs compare with the cost of other homes?
Are financial and other policies specified in a contract?
Do the resident's assets remain in his or her control or that of the family?
Do you feel that this facility provides the best care for its residents?

staffing levels and resident activities provided in the "off" hours.

Once a selection has been made, you will want to review and be sure you thoroughly understand the nursing home's contract or financial agreement. Since this is a legal contract, it is advisable to have a lawyer review the agreement before signing.

Other Personal Needs

Better nursing homes are designed with the needs of older people in mind. Aids such as handrails, low elevator buttons, easy-to-use furniture, call buttons in bedrooms and bathrooms, and wide doorways and ramps that are accessible to wheelchairs are all indications of an environment that encourages independence in residents. Color-coded hallways and directional signs are also useful, particularly for residents with mental impairments or those with poor vision. Such aids will help residents live more independently and exercise some control over their lives.

Opportunities for exercise and social activity should be available to nursing home residents as well. Nursing homes can provide safe, attractive places for residents to walk or push their wheelchairs. Nonglare windows with a view to the outdoors allow those who are immobile to view outside activities and seasonal changes. Staff can also help residents remain active and alert by including them in conversations and encouraging them to participate in social activities.

Furniture placed at the center of activity—such as in the lobby or at elevators—is more likely to attract people and encourage the development of friendly relationships in the nursing home. Small dining tables and lounge areas create a home-like atmosphere and help to motivate interaction between residents.

Personal privacy needs should be respected as much as possible. When rooms must be shared, screens or curtains can provide a measure of privacy. Places for individuals to have private conversations with friends or family members are desirable. It is also important to know that personal mail and documents are respected and that possessions are safe.

Making a Smooth Transition

Be prepared to ease the patient's transition to the nursing home. Such a change may affect the whole family and it will take some time to adjust to the new living arrangements. Some nursing homes have a social worker or nurse specialist who conducts preadmission group sessions for family members who can help the resident feel more comfortable by going with him or her on moving day and helping choose familiar items to bring along—family photos or favorite decorative items.

How often a family member visits the resident is an individual decision, but keep in mind that the presence of family members greatly helps to create a more personal atmosphere in the nursing home. Family visits offer reassurance to the resident that someone still cares. In fact, those residents whose families are involved in their care usually have higher morale and receive better care from the staff.

Resources

Persons who have problems with nursing homes may obtain assistance from the Nursing Home Ombudsman, a person in your state or local office on aging who investigates complaints and takes corrective action on behalf of nursing home residents.

Other sources of information include the following organizations:

The Nursing Home Information Service is an information and referral center for consumers of long-term care, their families, friends, and advocates. The service provides information on nursing homes and alternative community and health services, including a free guide on how to select a nursing home. For more information, write to the National Council of Senior Citizens, Nursing Home Information Service, National Senior Citizens Education and Research Center, Inc., 1331 F Street, NW, Washington, DC 20004.

The National Citizens Coalition for Nursing Home Reform helps local organizations work for nursing home reform and improvements in the long-term care system. To learn more about the coalition, write to the national office at 1224 M Street NW, Suite 301, Washington, DC 20005.

The American Association of Retired Persons can provide general information on long-term care for consumers. For a list of their publications, write to the AARP Health Advocacy Services, 601 E Street, NW., Washington, DC 20049. In addition, the AARP and the American Association of Homes for the Aging have information on continuing care communities. Write to the AARP/Housing Activities (at the address above) or to the AAHA at 901 E Street NW, Suite 500, Washington, DC 20004.

For a free list of NIA publications call 1-800-222-2225 or write to the National Institute on Aging Information Center, P.O. Box 8057, Gaithersburg, MD 20898-8057.

■ **Document Source:**
U.S. Department of Health and Human Services, Public Health Service
National Institutes of Health
National Institute on Aging
1992

A Reprint from FDA Consumer Magazine

WHO DONATES BETTER BLOOD FOR YOU THAN YOU?

The AIDS epidemic has had a great many consequences, few of them positive. But one favorable result has been increased use of a transfusion procedure by which persons facing elective surgery can donate their own blood to themselves before that surgery. Many people have become concerned about being exposed to AIDS through blood transfusions. Even though the risk of transfusion-transmitted AIDS appears to be very small, some people may feel any risk is too great.

Thus, the growing preference for a procedure called autologous (au-tol-o-gous) blood donation. (Autologous means "related to self.") It is based on the fact that donating before surgery, and receiving your own blood during and after surgery, is better and safer than receiving someone else's blood. (Blood intended for use by someone other than the donor is known as "homologous.")

All volunteer homologous blood donations in the United States are now tested for the presence of many infectious disease markers such as the antibody to the human immunodeficiency virus (the virus that causes AIDS), hepatitis B surface antigen, antibody to HCV (non-A, non-B), and syphilis. Homologous blood units testing positive for these markers must be discarded. This makes the risk of transmitting a virus through a homologous blood transfusion almost nonexistent.

Some advantages to donating one's own blood for later use are:

- reduced risk of infectious disease transmission
- reduced risk of transfusion reactions related to differences between donor and recipient, such as blood type
- more rapid replacement by your body of blood lost during surgery, since the bone marrow where blood cells form has already been activated by the process of donating blood
- less demand on the community blood supply.

Conditions that might prevent someone from donating blood to others do not necessarily prevent autologous donations. For example, people who would be ineligible to donate blood because they are on medication or because they have other medical conditions may be able to donate autologously. Age limits and other restrictions on blood donors also may vary for the autologous donor. An underlying principle of good surgical practice is to keep bleeding to a minimum, and transfusions are not needed for most planned operations. (Emergency surgery and some medical conditions account for the majority of transfusions. For this, a public blood supply must be maintained.) However, there are some procedures (generally orthopedic, cardiac, chest, gynecological, and blood vessel surgery) in which enough blood will be lost to require transfusing. Although blood transfusion is rarely needed during pregnancy and delivery, autologous donations may be appropriate in rare circumstances.

When autologous donation is suggested, the patient's physician and the local blood bank medical director determine if such a donation is indicated. The major consideration is simply the health of the patient.

Autologous donations can provide some or all of the blood components needed for surgery. However, autologous donations may not completely eliminate the possibility that the specific operation might need additional blood from other donors. Occasionally, some people may not be able to donate enough of their own blood to meet their needs. But even partial use of autologous blood will reduce the chance of an infection or adverse reaction from a transfusion of blood from other donors.

A study of 180 patients scheduled for elective surgery at a Boston hospital found that most could donate a unit of blood a week without becoming anemic. When the study was completed, it was found that a third of the patients had required no transfusions at all during or after their surgery, and another third had used only their already donated blood. Only one-third of the patients needed blood donated by other persons.

Advocates of autologous donation believe that wider use of the technique could help prevent shortages in the national blood supply, and the Boston hospital study seems to support that. But even if that is true, autologous donation is not encouraged solely because of any real or perceived shortage. Many physicians and blood bank medical directors endorse autologous blood donations and transfusions simply because autologous blood is the safest blood for people to receive.

Until a decade ago almost no patients used autologous transfusions. Few hospitals or blood banks even offered the service, which was generally reserved for persons with rare blood types or medical conditions. Despite all its attractions, autologous blood is still a very small part of all blood transfused in the United States. Blood bank officials estimate that perhaps 10 percent of transfusions in this country are autologous. Yet, figures compiled by the American Association of Blood Banks show that the practice of autologous transfusion increased enormously during the 1980s. There was a 17-fold increase in the number of autologous units donated before surgery between 1982 and 1988, and the use of autologous donations continues to increase.

Exploring available autologous blood donation options is important when transfusions are indicated. Scheduling autologous donations requires good planning by the attending physician with the local blood donor center and the patient, but the actual procedure of donating autologous blood is relatively simple. If transfusion is likely for a planned operation, there is sometimes more than one option for autologous transfusion:

- autologous donation before the surgery
- salvaging blood during surgery and "recycling" it
- salvaging blood after the operation from a surgical wound

Before Surgery

When autologous donation is suggested, the patient's physician will make arrangements with the local blood bank. How much and how often blood will be collected is decided by the physician. It's possible that iron supplements may be prescribed to build up the number of red blood cells to avoid anemia.

In autologous donation, a person can often give one unit of blood a week for up to six weeks, depending on the anticipated need. Each unit is just under a pint and is about 10 percent of the total blood supply of an average-size adult.

As the blood is taken, it is labeled for that patient's use and kept ready at the hospital for the operation. The last donation is usually made no closer than three days before the scheduled surgery. This allows the body time to replenish the fluid volume that has been removed.

As liquid blood, the donated units can be kept for up to 42 days, depending on the preservative used. If the red blood cells are appropriately frozen, the units may be kept for as long as 10 years.

Blood Salvage During Surgery

During an operation, lost blood can be collected from the bleeding site and returned to the patient. This may be done manually or using automated equipment. The blood cells may be washed prior to "recycling," or the blood may be returned without additional processing.

Some hospitals and medical centers have been using this approach to reducing the use of homologous blood for several years for some cardiac and orthopedic procedures and organ transplants. Many surgical patients facing procedures likely to require transfusions can benefit from intraoperative blood salvage, especially in cases where preoperative donation is impossible or inadequate. However, in some cases blood salvage is not recommended, such as in patients with infections. Just like any medical therapy, "recycled" blood has some risks, so patients should discuss this procedure with the physician, surgeon, and hospital to determine if it is right for them.

Blood Salvage After Surgery

Postoperative blood salvage is another technique of autologous transfusion in which blood is collected from the wound site following major surgery for reinfusion to that patient. This procedure is much less common, but its use is increasing for some selected orthopedic operations. Postoperative blood salvage may also be useful in heart surgery. Again, this procedure should be discussed with the physician.

What Does FDA Think About Autologous Blood?

Increased interest in autologous blood has prompted FDA's Center for Biologics Evaluation and Research to update recommendations and interpret existing regulations on collecting, handling, storing, shipping, and using autologous blood.

FDA recommends that all the tests required for homologous blood also be done for autologous blood. Many physicians and blood bank staff working with autologous blood also feel it should be tested for infectious agents at the time it is taken. If a unit fails one of the required tests, FDA recommends that it not be used. However, those units or blood components may be used for autologous transfusion if the patient's physician requests it in writing.

Unused autologous units may be destroyed or added to the homologous blood inventory if they have met all FDA requirements, including testing for infectious agents.

Blood banks and other facilities where blood is taken from donors follow these standards for procedures, equipment and staff. FDA is responsible for ensuring the safety of the nation's entire blood supply, which includes autologous blood and blood products. To that end, FDA routinely inspects blood donor centers to ensure that these strict standards are maintained.

If You Are Facing Surgery. . .

For most types of planned surgery, patients generally lose so little blood that they don't need blood transfusions. If you are going to have an operation, check with your doctor as soon as possible about your need for blood. Before determining that you should donate your own blood, your doctor must decide if the benefits outweigh any potential risks to you. However, when a transfusion is likely, use of autologous donations can decrease or eliminate exposure of patients to homologous blood. Although the risks of transfusion with homologous blood are very low, autologous transfusion remains the safest option for some patients. A "team approach" with your doctor, the blood collection facility, and you, the patient, is needed to determine what the safest autologous transfusion procedure may be.

A Blood-Chilling Experience

As public interest in blood donations has increased, a number of entrepreneurs have entered the market. These facilities will—at their locations around the country—collect, freeze and store your blood, and then deliver it to you—thawed and ready to use—when and if your physician calls for it.

Costs can be high, and shipping charges may be added. There is no guarantee the blood would be available when needed or that there would be time to thaw and ship it. (Under present FDA regulations, frozen blood may be kept for only 10 years and cannot be shipped between states.) In addition, frozen blood contains only red blood cells. If you need blood platelets or plasma, you may have to turn to the public blood supply.

The National Institutes of Health and several other health care centers endorse the use of autologous blood for elective surgery. But long-term storage or stock-piling with no indicated medical need is not routinely endorsed in this country. Many physicians feel there is no reason for healthy people to stockpile their own blood if they are not current candidates for surgery. It is recommended that you discuss any upcoming operation with your doctor to determine if you will need blood and, if so, what the safest procedure will be for you.

Seven Important Questions to Ask Your Doctor

1. Will I need blood for my operation?
2. Can I give blood in advance in case I need it?
3. Is there enough time before the operation to give the blood I will need?
4. Where should I go to give blood for my operation?
5. Can my blood be saved during the operation and given back to me if I need it?
6. What are the risks in giving or receiving my own blood?
7. Will I have to pay extra if I use my own blood?

■ Document Source:
U.S. Department of Health and Human Services, Public Health Service
Food and Drug Administration, HFI-40, Rockville, MD 20857.
DHHS Publication No. (FDA) 91-1148
Printed April 1993

APPENDIX A
PHYSICIAN DATA QUERY (PDQ)

■ ■ ■

Physician Data Query (PDQ)

Physician Data Query (PDQ) is a computer system that gives up-to-date information on cancer treatment. It is a service of the National Cancer Institute (NCI) for people with cancer and their families, and for doctors, nurses, and other health care professionals.

PDQ tells about the current treatments for most cancers. The information in PDQ is reviewed each month by cancer experts. It is updated when there is new information. The patient information in PDQ also tells about warning signs and how the cancer is found. PDQ also lists information about research on new treatments (clinical trials), doctors who treat cancer, and hospitals with cancer programs.

How to Use PDQ

You can use PDQ to learn more about current treatment for your kind of cancer. Bring the material from PDQ with you when you see your doctor. You can talk with your doctor, who knows you and has the facts about your disease, about which treatment would be best for you. Before you start your treatment, you might also want to seek a second opinion from a doctor who treats cancer.

Before you start treatment, you also may want to think about taking part in a clinical trial. A clinical trial is a study that uses new treatments to care for patients. Each study is based on past studies and what has been learned in the laboratory. Each trial answers certain scientific questions in order to find new and better ways to help cancer patients. During clinical trials, more and more information is collected about new treatments, their risks, and how well they do or do not work. If clinical trials show that the new treatment is better than the treatment currently being used, the new treatment may become the "standard" treatment. Listings of clinical trials are a part of PDQ. Many cancer doctors who take part in clinical trials are listed in PDQ.

If you want to know more about cancer and how it is treated, or if you wish to learn about clinical trials for your kind of cancer, you can call the National Cancer Institute's Cancer Information Service. The number is 1-800-4-CAN-CER (1-800-422-6237). The call is free and a trained counselor will talk with you and answer your questions.

PDQ may change when there is new information. Check with the Cancer Information Service to be sure that you have the most up-to-date information.

The Cancer Information Service can also send you free booklets. The following general booklets on questions related to cancer may be helpful:

- *What You Need to Know About Cancer*
- *Taking Time: Support for People With Cancer and the People Who Care About Them*
- *What Are Clinical Trials All About?*
- *Chemotherapy and You*
- *Radiation Therapy and You*
- *Eating Hints: Recipes and Tips for Better Nutrition During Cancer Treatment*
- *Advanced Cancer: Living Each Day*
- *When Cancer Recurs: Meeting the Challenge Again*

There are many other places you can get information about cancer treatment and services to help you. You can check the social service office at your hospital for local and national agencies that help with your finances, getting to and from treatment, care at home, and dealing with your problems. The American Cancer Society, for example, has many free services. Their local offices are listed in the white pages of the telephone book.

If you want to know more about cancer and how it is treated, or if you wish to learn about clinical trials for your kind of cancer, you can call the NCI's Cancer Information Service at 1-800-422-6237, toll free. A trained information specialist can talk with you and answer your questions.

APPENDIX B
HEALTH HOTLINES

■ ■ ■

Toll-Free Numbers from the National Library of Medicine's DIRLINE Database

Health Hotlines is a compilation of organizations with toll-free telephone numbers. It is derived from DIRLINE®, the National Library of Medicine's Directory of Information Resources Online. This database contains descriptions of over 15,000 organizations which serve as information resources and respond to inquiries in their subject areas.

Some of the subject areas included in **Health Hotlines** are AIDS, cancer, maternal and child health, aging, poison control centers, substance abuse, disabilities, and mental health. **Health Hotlines** also lists a variety of groups disseminating information on a number of specific diseases and disorders. Organizations fall into many categories including federal, state and local government agencies, information and referral centers, professional societies, support groups and voluntary associations.

Health Hotlines is provided as a community service to assist the public in locating health-related information. The toll-free telephone numbers in **Health Hotlines** were provided by the organizations and verified at the time of printing. The National Library of Medicine has not reviewed or evaluated the services of the organizations listed.

The inclusion of an organization in this publication does not constitute a recommendation or endorsement by the federal government of an organization's services or views.

ALM International
(American Leprosy Missions)
(800) 543-3131
1 ALM Way
Greenway, SC 29601

AMC Cancer Information and Counseling
(800) 525-3777
1600 Pierce St.
Denver, CO 80214

ABLEDATA
(800) 344-5405
(Product information for the handicapped and disabled)
Newington Children's Hospital
Adaptive Equipment Center
181 E. Cedar St.
Newington, CT 06111

Advocacy Center for the Elderly and Disabled
(800) 960-7705 (within Louisiana)
210 O'Keefe Ave., Ste. 700
New Orleans, LA 70112

Aeronational
(800) 245-9987
P.O. Box 538
Washington, PA 15301

AIDS Action Committee of Massachusetts
AIDS Education at Work
(800) 669-0696
131 Clarendon St.
Boston, MA 02116

AIDS Clinical Trials Information Service (ACTIS)
(800) TRIALS-A (874-2572)
(800) 243-7012 (TTY)
P.O. Box 6421
Rockville, MD 20859-6421

Air Ambulance America
(800) 262-8526
(800) 843-8418
9100 S. Dadeland Blvd.
Miami, FL 33156

Akron Regional Poison Control Center
Children's Hospital Medical Center of Akron
(800) 362-9922 (within Ohio)
281 Locust St.
Akron, OH 44308

Alabama AIDS Hotline
Alabama Department of Health
(800) 228-0469 (within Alabama)
State Office Bldg., Rm. 662
434 Monroe St.
Montgomery, AL 36130

Alabama Commission on Aging
(800) 243-5463 (within Alabama)
770 Washington Ave.
RSA Plaza, Ste. 470
Montgomery, AL 36130

Alabama Poison Center
(800) 462-0800 (within Alabama)
809 University Blvd., E
Tuscaloosa, AL 35401

Al-Anon, Alateen Family Group Hotline
(800) 344-2666
(800) 245-4656 (within New York)
(800) 443-4525 (within Canada)
P.O. Box 862, Midtown Station
New York, NY 10018-0862

Alaskan AIDS Assistance Association
(800) 478-AIDS (within Alaska)
417 W. 8th Ave.
Anchorage, AK 99501

Alcohol Rehab for the Elderly
(800) 354-7089
(800) 344-0824 (within Illinois)
P.O. Box 267
Hopedale, IL 61747

Alcoholism and Drug Addiction Treatment Center
(800) 382-4327 (within California)
McDonald Center
Scripps Memorial Hospital
9904 Genesee Ave.
La Jolla, Ca 92037

American Mental Health Counselors Association
    (AMHCA)
(800) 326-2642
5999 Stevenson Ave.
Alexandria, VA 22304

American Narcolepsy Association
(800) 222-6085
425 California Ave., Ste. 201
San Francisco, CA 94104

American Osteopathic Association
(800) 621-1773
142 E. Ontario St.
Chicago, IL 60611

American Paralysis Association
(800) 225-0292
500 Morris Ave.
Springfield, NJ 07081

American Parkinson Disease Association
(800) 223-2732
60 Bay St., Ste. 401
Staten Island, NY 10301

American Schizophrenia Association
(800) 847-3802
900 N. Federal Hwy.
Boca Raton, FL 33432
(See also: Huxley Institute for Biosocial Research)

American Self Help Clearinghouse
(800) 367-6274 (within New Jersey)
St. Clare's-Riverside Medical Center
Pocono Rd.
Denville, NJ 07834

American Social Health Association
(800) 227-8922 (National STD Hotline)
(800) 342-AIDS (National AIDS Hotline)
(800) 344-SIDA (Spanish)
(800) AIDS-TTY (Hearing Impaired)

P.O. Box 13827
Research Triangle Park, NC 27709

American Society for Dermatologic Surgery
(800) 441-2737
1567 Maple Ave., P.O. Box 3116
Evanston, IL 60204

American Society for Psychoprophylaxis in Obstetrics
    (ASPO/Lamaze)
(800) 368-4404
1101 Connecticut Ave., NW
Washington, DC 20036

American Society of Plastic and Reconstructive
    Surgeons
(800) 635-0635
4444 E. Algonquin Rd.
Arlington Heights, IL 60005

American Trauma Society
(800) 556-7890 (outside Maryland)
8903 Presidential Pkwy., Ste. 512
Upper Marlboro, MD 20772

Amyotrophic Lateral Sclerosis Association (ALSA)
(800) 782-4747
21021 Ventura Blvd., Ste. 321
Woodland Hills, CA 91364

Anchorage Poison Center
Providence Hospital
(800) 777-8189
P.O. Box 196604
Anchorage, AK 99519-0604

Ankylosing Spondylitis Association
(800) 777-8189
511 N. La Cienega, Ste. 216
Los Angeles, CA 90048

Arizona Department of Health Services
Office of HIV/AIDS Services
(800) 334-1540 (within Arizona)
3008 N. 3rd St.
Phoenix, AZ 85012

Arizona Poison and Drug Information Center
University of Arizona
(800) 362-0101 (within Arizona)
1501 N. Campbell Ave., Rm. 3204K
Tucson, AZ 85724

Arkansas Poison and Drug Information Center
(800) 482-8948 (within Arkansas)
University of Arkansas for Medical Sciences
4301 W. Markham St., Slot 522
Little Rock, AR 72205

Arthritis Consulting Services
(800) 327-3027
4620 N. State Rd. 7, Ste. 206
Ft. Lauderdale, FL 33319

Arthritis Foundation
(800) 283-7800
1314 Spring St., NW
Atlanta, GA 30309

Asthma and Allergy Foundation of America
(800) 7-ASTHMA (727-8462)
1717 Massachusetts Ave. NW, Ste. 305
Washington, DC 20036

Association of American Physicians and Surgeons
(800) 635-1196
1601 N. Tucson Blvd., Ste. 9
Tucson, AZ 85716

Association of Surgical Technologists
(800) 637-7433
8307 Shaffer Pkwy.
Littleton, CO 80127

Back Pain Hotline
(800) 247-BACK
Texas Back Institute
3801 W. 15th St.
Plano, TX 75075

Be Healthy, Inc.
Postitive Pregnancy and Parenting Fitness
(800) 433-5523
51 Saltrock Rd.
Baltic, CT 06330

Better Hearing Institute
Hearing Helpline
(800) 424-8576
5021-B Backlick Rd.
Annandale, VA 22003

Blind Children's Center
(800) 222-3566
(800) 222-3567 (within California)
4120 Marathon St.
P.O. Box 29159
Los Angeles, CA 90029-0159

Blinded Veterans Association
(800) 699-7079
477 H St. NW
Washington, DC 20001-2694

Blodgett Regional Poison Center
Blodgett Medical Center
(800) 632-2727 (within Michigan)
(800) 356-3232 (TTY)
1840 Wealthy St., SE
Grand Rapids, MI 49506

Blue Ridge Poison Center
Blue Ridge Hospital
(800) 451-1428
University of Virginia, P.O. Box 67
Charlottesville, VA 22901

Bowman Gray School of Medicine
Epilepsy Information Service
(800) 642-0500
(Comprehensive Epilepsy Program)
Medical Center Blvd.
Winston-Salem, NC 27157-1078

Bulemia Anorexia Self-Help (B.A.S.H.)
(800) BASH-STL (227-4785)
6125 Clayton Ave., Ste. 215
St. Louis, MO 63139-3295

California Department of Health
Office of AIDS
(800) 367-AIDS (within Northern California)
(800) 922-AIDS (within Southern California)
P.O. Box 942732
Sacramento, CA 94234-7320

California Self-Help Center
(800) 222-LINK (within California)
2349 Franz Hall
405 Hilgard Ave.
Los Angeles, CA 90024

California Teratogen Information Services and
    Clinical Research Program
University of California at San Diego
(800) 532-3749 (within California)
Department of Pediatrics
225 Dickinson St.
San Diego, CA 92103

Cancer Information Service
(800) 4-CANCER (in various states and regions)
Office of Cancer Communications, NCI/NIH
Bldg. 31, Rm. 10A24
9000 Rockville Pike
Bethesda, MD 20892

Candlelighters Childhood Cancer Foundation
(800) 366-CCCF (2223)
1312 18th St. NW
Washington, DC 20036

Cardinal Glennon Children's Hospital Regional Poison Center
(800) 366-8888
(800) 392-9111 (within Missouri)
1465 S. Grand Blvd.
St. Louis, MO 63104

Center for Self Help
Riverwood Center
(800) 336-0341 (within Michigan)
P.O. Box 547
Benton Harbor, MI 49022-0547

Central New York Poison Control Center
Upstate Medical Center
(800) 252-5655 (within central New York)
750 E. Adams St.
Syracuse, NY 13210

Central Ohio Poison Control Center
Children's Hospital
(800) 682-7625 (within Ohio)
700 Children's Dr.
Columbus, OH 43205

Central Pennsylvania Poison Center
University Hospital
(800) 521-6110
Milton S. Hershey Medical Center
Hershey, PA 17033

Central Washington Poison Center
Yakima Valley Memorial Hospital
(800) 572-9176 (within Washington)
2811 Tieton Dr.
Yakima, WA 98902

Chemical Referral Center
(800) 262-8200
2501 M St. NW
Washington, DC 20037

Chicago and Northeastern Illinois Regional Poison
    Control Center
Rush-Presbyterian-St. Luke's Medical Center
(800) 942-5969 (within Illinois)

1753 W. Congress Pkwy.
Chicago, IL 60612

Child Help USA
(800) 422-4453
6463 Independence Ave.
Woodland Hills, CA 91367

Children's Craniofacial Association
(800) 535-3643
10210 N. Central Expressway, LB 37
Dallas, TX 75231

Children's Hospice International
(800) 242-4453
901 N. Washington St., Ste. 700
Alexandria, VA 22314

Children's Hospital of Alabama
Regional Poison Control Center
(800) 292-6678 (within Alabama)
1600 Seventh Ave. S.
Birmingham, AL 35233

Children's Hospital of Michigan
Poison Control Center
(800) 462-6642 (within Michigan)
3901 Beaubien Blvd.
Detroit, MI 48201

Cleft Palate Foundation
(800) 242-5338
1218 Grandview Ave.
Pittsburgh, PA 15211

Clinical Genetic Services Center, Michigan
Henry Ford Hospital
Medical Genetics and Birth Defects Center
(800) 999-4340 (within Michigan)
2799 W. Grand Blvd.
Detroit, MI 48202

Clinical Genetic Services Center, Oregon
Emanuel Hospital
Department of Medical Genetics
(800) 237-7808
(800) 452-7032 Ext. 4726 (within Oregon)
2801 N. Gantenbein Ave.
Portland, OR 97227

Clinical Genetic Services Center, Pennsylvania
Pennsylvania Hospital
Division of Perinatology
(800) 336-5633
Spruce Bldg.
8th and Spruce Sts.
Philadelphia, PA 19107

Cocaine Anonymous
(800) 347-8998
3740 Overland Ave., Ste. G
Los Angeles, CA 90034

Colorado Department of Health
STD/AIDS Control
(800) 252-AIDS (within Colorado)
4210 E. 11th St.
Denver, CO 80220

Connecticut Department on Aging
(800) 443-9946 (within Connecticut)
175 Main St.
Hartford, CT 06106

Connecticut Poison Control Center
(800) 343-2722 (within Connecticut)
University of Connecticut Health Center
309 Farmington Ave.
Farmington, CT 06030

Consumer Product Safety Commission (CPSC)
(800) 638-2772 (Product Safety Line)
(800) 638-8270 (TTY National)
(800) 492-8104 (TTY Maryland)
Washington, DC 20207

Contact Lens Manufacturers Association
(800) 343-5367
421 King St., Ste. 224
Alexandria, VA 22314

Cooley's Anemia Foundation
(800) 221-3571
(800) 522-7222 (within New York)
105 E. 22nd St.
New York, NY 10010

Cornelia de Lange Syndrome Foundation
(800) 223-8355
(800) 735-2357 (Connecticut and Canada only)
(Birth defects information)
60 Dyer Ave.
Collinsville, CT 06022

Courage Stroke Network
(800) 553-6321
3915 Golden Valley Rd.
Golden Valley, MN 55422

Covenant House
(800) 999-9999
(Homeless youth—various locations in US and Canada)
460 W. 41st St.
New York, NY 10036

Crohn's and Colitis Foundation of America
(800) 343-3637
444 Park Ave. S., 11th Fl.
New York, NY 10018

Cystic Fibrosis Foundation
(800) 344-4823
6931 Arlington Rd.
Bethesda, MD 20814

Deafness Research Foundation
(800) 535-3323
9 E. 38th St., 7th Fl.
New York, NY 10016

Delaware AIDS Hotline
(800) 422-0429 (within Delaware)
P.O. Box 637
Dover, DE 19903

Delta Health Care
(800) 749-2255
711 E. Lamar, Ste. 211
Arlington, TX 76011

Department for Rights of Virginians with Disabilities
(800) 552-3962 (within Virginia)
101 N. 14th St., 17th Fl.
Richmond, VA 23219

Devereux Foundation
(800) 345-1292
(Treatment of emotionally, developmentally, and mentally handi-
    capped)
19 S. Waterloo Rd.
Devon, PA 19333

Device Experience Network
Division of Product Surveillance
Office of Compliance and Surveillance
Center for Devices and Radiological Health (FDA)
(800) 638-6725
FDA HFZ-343
8757 Georgia Ave.
Silver Spring, MD 20910

Duke Poison Control Center
North Carolina Regional Center
Duke University
(800) 672-1697 (within North Carolina)
P.O. Box 3007
Durham, NC 27710

Eating Disorders Helpline Unit
(800) 382-2832
Gracie Square Hospital
420 E. 76th St.
New York, NY 10021

Edna Gladney Center
(800) 433-2922
(800) GLADNEY (452-3639)
(800) 772-2740 (within Texas)
(Maternity home and infant placement agency)
2300 Hemphill
Fort Worth, TX 76110

Emergency Planning and Community Right-to-Know Hotline
Environmental Protection Agency
(800) 535-0202
401 M St. SW
Washington, DC 20460

Encore
Pennsylvania Department of Health
Office of Drug and Alcohol Programs
(800) 932-0912 (within Pennsylvania)
(Drug and alcohol information)
Health and Welfare Bldg.
6th and Commonwealth, P.O. Box 90
Harrisburg, PA 17120

Endometriosis Association
(800) 992-ENDO (3636)
P.O. Box 92187
Milwaukee, WI 53202

Epilepsy Foundation of America
(800) EFA-1000 (outside Maryland)
4351 Garden City Dr., Ste. 406
Landover, MD 20785

Facial Plastic Surgery Information Service
(800) 332-FACE (USA)
(800) 523-FACE (Canada)
1101 Vermont Ave. NW, Ste. 304
Washington, DC 20005

Familial Polyposis Registry
Cleveland Clinic Foundation
Department of Colorectal Surgery
(800) 321-5398, Ext. 6470

9500 Euclid Ave.
Cleveland, OH 44195

Family Survival Project for Care Givers of Brain
    Impaired Adults
(800) 445-8106 (within California)
425 Bush St., Ste. 500
San Francisco, CA 94108

Finger Lakes Regional Poison Center
University of Rochester Medical Center
(800) 333-0542 (within area codes 607, 315, 716)
Box 777
Rochester, NY 14642

Florida Department of Health-Rehabilitation
State AIDS Hotline
(800) FLA-AIDS (within Florida)
1317 Winewood Blvd.
Tallahassee, FL 32399

Florida Poison Information Center at the Tampa
    General Hospital
(800) 282-3171 (within Florida)
P.O. Box 1289
Tampa, FL 33601

Food Safety and Inspection Service
Meat and Poultry Hotline
(800) 535-4555
Department of Agriculture, Rm. 1165-S
Washington, DC 20250

Foundation Center
(800) 424-9836
79 5th Ave. at 16th St.
New York, NY 10003

French Foundation for Alzheimer's Research
(800) 477-2243
11620 Wilshire Blvd., Ste. 820
Los Angeles, CA 90025

Fresno Regional Poison Control Center
Fresno Community Hospital and Medical Center
(800) 346-5922 (within central California)
2823 N. Fresno St.
Fresno, CA 93712

Georgia Department of Human Resources
AID ATLANTA
(800) 551-2728 (AIDS Information Line)
1132 W. Peachtree St. NW
Atlanta, GA 30309-3624

Good Samaritan Project Teen
Teaching AIDS Prevention Program
(800) 234-8336 (4:00-8:00 pm Central time)
3030 Walnut St.
Kansas City, MO 64108

Guide Dog Foundation for the Blind
(800) 548-4337
371 E. Jericho Turnpike
Smithtown, NY 11787

Hawaii Poison Center
Kapiolani-Children's Medical Center
(800) 362-3585 (outer islands only)
1319 Punahou St.
Honolulu, HI 86826

Health Education Resource Organization (HERO)
Maryland AIDS Hotline
(800) 638-6252 (within Maryland)
(800) 553-3140 (TTD)
101 W. Read St., Ste. 825
Baltimore, MD 21201

Health Insurance Association of America
(800) 635-1271
1025 Connecticut Ave. NW
Washington, DC 20036-3998

Health Resources and Services Administration
Office of Health Facilities
(800) 492-0359 (English and Spanish, within Maryland)
(800) 638-0742 (English and Spanish, outside Maryland)
Department of Health and Human Services
Public Health Service
5600 Fishers Ln.
Rockville, MD 20857

Healthy Mothers, Healthy Babies Coalition
(800) 673-8444, Ext. 2458
409 12th St. SW
Washington, DC 20024-2188

Hearing Helpline
(800) 424-8576
P.O. Box 1840
Washington, DC 20013

HELPLINE
(800) 346-2211 (within New York)
(Human services and self-help clearinghouse)
22 W. Third St.
Corning, NY 14830

**Higher Education and Adult Training for People with Handi-
caps Resource Center**
(800) 544-3284
1 Dupont Circle
Washington, DC 20036-1193

Hill-Burton Free Hospital Care
(800) 638-0742
(800) 492-0359 (within Maryland)
Department of Health and Human Services
Public Health Service
Health Resources and Services Administration
Rockville, MD 20857

Histiocytosis Association of America
(800) 548-2758
609 New York Rd.
Glassboro, NJ 08028

Hospice Education Institute
(800) 331-1620
5 Essex Sq., Ste. 3-B
Essex, CT 06426-0713

Hudson Valley Poison Center
Nyack Hospital
(800) 336-6997 (within area codes 518, 914)
160 N. Midland Ave.
Nyack, NY 10960

Human Growth Foundation
(800) 451-6434
(Child growth abnormalities)
7777 Leesburg Pike, Ste. 2025
Falls Church, VA 22043

Huntington's Disease Society of America
(800) 345-4372
140 W. 22nd St., 6th Fl.
New York, NY 10011-2420

Huxley Institute for Biosocial Research
(800) 847-3802
900 N. Federal Hwy.
Boca Raton, FL 33432
(See also: American Schizophrenia Association)

Idaho Poison Control Center
St. Alphonsus Regional Medical Center
(800) 632-8000 (within Idaho)
1055 N. Curtis Rd.
Boise, ID 83704

Illinois Department of Public Health
AIDS Activity Section
State AIDS Hotline
(800) 243-AIDS (within Illinois)
525 W. Jefferson
Springfield, IL 62761

**IN *SOURCE (Indiana Resource Center for Families with
Special Needs)**
Indiana Parent Training Program (IPTP)
Education Surrogate Program of Indiana (ESPPI)
(800) 332-4433 (within Indiana)
833 Northside Blvd., Bldg. 1 Rear
South Bend, IN 46617

Indiana Department of Human Services
(800) 545-7763 (within Indiana)
402 W. Washington St.
P.O. Box 7083
Indianapolis, IN 46207-7083

Indiana Poison Center
Methodist Hospital of Indiana
(800) 382-9097 (within Indiana)
1701 N. Senate Blvd.
Indianapolis, IN 46206-1367

Information Center for Individuals with Disabilities
(800) 462-5015 (within Massachusetts)
Fort Point Pl., 1st Fl.
37-43 Wormwood St.
Boston, MA 02210-1606

Institute of Logopedics
(800) 835-1043
(Programs for multiply-handicapped children)
2400 Jardine Dr.
Wichita, KS 67219

Intermountain Regional Poison Control Center
(800) 456-7707 (within Utah)
50 N. Medical Dr., Bldg. 528
Salt Lake City, UT 84132

Iowa Self-Help Clearinghouse
Iowa Pilot Parents, Inc
(800) 383-4777
33 N. 12th St., P.O. Box 1151
Fort Dodge, IA 50501

Job Accommodation Network
(800) 526-7234
(800) 526-4698 (within West Virginia)
(for persons with disabilities seeking employment)
West Virginia University
809 Allen Hall

P.O. Box 6123
Morgantown, WV 26506-6123

Just Say No International
(800) 258-2766
1777 N. California Blvd., Ste. 210
Walnut Creek, CA 94596

Juvenile Diabetes Foundation (JDF)
(800) 223-1138
432 Park Ave. S, 16th Fl.
New York, NY 10016

Kansas Department of Health and Environment
AIDS Hotline
(800) 232-0040 (within Kansas)
Mills Bldg., Ste. 605
Topeka, KS 66612

Kansas Department on Aging
(800) 432-3535 (within Kansas)
Docking State Office Bldg., 122-S
Topeka, KS 66612-1500

Kentucky Department for Health Services
AIDS Health Education
(800) 564-AIDS (within Kentucky)
275 E. Main St.
Frankfort, KY 40621

Kentucky Regional Poison Center of Kosair Children's Hospital
(800) 722-5725 (within Kentucky)
P.O. Box 35070
Louisville, KY 40232-5070

Kevin Collins Foundation for Missing Children
(800) 272-0012
Box 590473
San Francisco, CA 94159

Kidsrights
(800) 892-5437
3700 Progress Blvd.
Mount Dora, FL 32757

La Leche League International
(800) 525-3243
P.O. Box 1209
Franklin Park, IL 60131-8209

Little People of America
(800) 243-9273
P.O. Box 9897
Washington, DC 20016

Living Bank
(800) 528-2971
(Organ donation)
P.O. Box 6725
Houston, TX 77625

Los Angeles County Medical Association Regional Poison Control Center
(800) 825-2722 (within California)
(800) 777-6476 (within California)
1925 Wilshire Blvd.
Los Angeles, CA 90057

Louisiana Department of Health and Hospitals
Office of Public Health
HIV/AIDS Services
(800) 992-4379 (within Louisiana)

325 Loyola Ave., Rm. 618
New Orleans, LA 70012

Lupus Foundation of America
(800) 558-0121
1717 Massachusetts Ave. NW, Ste. 203
Washington, DC 20036

Mahoning Valley Poison Center
St. Elizabeth Hospital Medical Center
(800) 426-2348
1044 Belmont St.
Youngstown, OH 44501

Maine AIDS Project
(800) 851-AIDS (within Maine)
22 Monument Sq.
Portland, ME 04101

Maine Poison Control Center at Maine Medical Center
(800) 442-6305 (within Maine)
22 Bramhall St.
Portland, ME 04102

Mary Bridge Poison Center
Multicare Medical Center
(800) 542-6319 (within Washington)
P.O. Box 5299
1317 S. K St.
Tacoma, WA 98405-0987

Maryland Poison Center
University of Maryland School of Pharmacy
(800) 492-2414 (within Maryland)
20 N. Pine St.
Baltimore, MA 21201

Massachusetts Department of Public Health
AIDS Health Education
(800) 235-2331 (within Massachusetts)
150 Tremont St.
Boston, MA 02111

Massachusetts Executive Office of Elder Affairs
(800) 882-2003 (within Massachusetts)
38 Chauncy St.
Boston, MA 02111

Massachusetts Nutrition Resource Center
(800) 322-7203 (within Massachusetts)
150 Tremont St.
Boston, MA 02111

Massachusetts Poison Control System
(800) 682-9211 (within Massachusetts)
300 Longwood Ave.
Boston, MA 02115

McKennan Hospital Poison Center
(800) 952-0123 (within South Dakota)
(800) 843-0505 (within Iowa, Minnesota, Nebraska)
P.O. Box 5045
800 E. 21st St.
Sioux Falls, SD 57117-5045

Medic Alert Foundation International
(800) ID-ALERT (432-5378)
(800) 344-3226 (within California)
2323 Colorado
Turlock, CA 95381-1009

Medical and Chirurgical Faculty of the State of Maryland Library
(800) 492-1056 (within Maryland)
1211 Cathedral St.
Baltimore, MD 21201

Medical College of Ohio
Poison and Drug Information Center
(800) 321-8383 (within Ohio)
300 Arlington Ave.
Toledo, OH 49614

Meniere's Network
(800) 545-4327
2000 Church St., Box 111
Nashville, TN 37236

Mercy Hospital Poison Control Center
(800) 848-6946 (regional)
2001 Vail Ave.
Charlotte, NC 28207

Metro-Help
National Runaway Switchboard
(800) 621-4000
(800) 621-3230 (within Illinois)
3080 N. Lincoln Ave.
Chicago, IL 60657
(See also: Runaway Hotline)

Michigan Department of Health
Office on AIDS Prevention
(800) 872-AIDS (within Michigan)
3423 N. Logan
Lansing, MI 48906

Michigan Self-Help Clearinghouse
(800) 752-5858 (within Michigan)
109 W. Michigan Ave., Ste. 900
Lansing, MI 48933

Mid-America Poison Control Center
University of Kansas Medical Center
(800) 332-6633 (within Kansas)
3900 Rainbow Blvd.
Kansas City, KS 66103

Mid-Atlantic AIDS Regional Education and Training Center
(800) 332-UMAB, Ext. 2382
University of Maryland at Baltimore
520 W. Lombard St.
Baltimore, MD 21201

Middle Tennessee Regional Poison and Clinical Toxicology Center
(800) 288-9999 (regional)
1161 21st Ave. S.
501 Oxford House
Nashville, TN 37232-4632

Minnesota Regional Poison Center
St. Paul-Ramsey Medical Center
(800) 222-1222 (within Minnesota)
640 Jackson St.
St. Paul, MN 55101

Missing Children Help Center
(800) USA-KIDS (872-5437)
410 Ware Blvd., Ste. 400
Tampa, FL 33619

Mississippi Department of Health
HIV/AIDS Prevention Program

(800) 826-2961 (within Mississippi)
P.O. Box 1700
Jackson, MS 39215

Mothers Against Drunk Drivers
(800) 438-6233 (Victim hotline)
P.O. Box 541688
Dallas, TX 75354-1688

Myasthenia Gravis Foundation
(800) 541-5454
53 W. Jackson Blvd., Ste. 660
Chicago, IL 60604

National AIDS Hotline
Centers for Disease Control
(800) 342-AIDS
(800) 344-SIDA (Spanish)
(800) AIDS-TTY (Hearing Impaired)
Atlanta, GA 30033

National AIDS Information Clearinghouse
(800) 458-5231
P.O. Box 6003
Rockville, MD 20850

National Alliance of Blind Students
(800) 424-8666
1155 15th St. NW, Ste. 720
Washington, DC 20005

National Association for Parents of Visually Impaired
(800) 562-6265
2180 Linway Dr.
Beloit, WI 53511

National Association for Sickle Cell Disease, Inc.
(800) 421-8453
3345 Wilshire Blvd., Ste. 1106
Los Angeles, CA 90010-1880

National Association for the Education of Young Children
(800) 424-2460
1834 Connecticut Ave. NW
Washington, DC 20009-5786

National Association of People with AIDS (NAPWA)
(800) 673-8538
P.O. Box 18345
Washington, DC 20036

National Center for Missing and Exploited Children
(800) 843-5678
2101 Wilson Blvd., Ste. 550
Arlington, VA 22201

National Center for Stuttering
(800) 221-2483
200 E. 33rd St.
New York, NY 10016

National Center for Vision and Aging
The Lighthouse
(800) 334-5497
800 2nd Ave.
New York, NY 10017

National Center for Youth with Disabilities (NCYD)
(800) 333-5497
University of Minnesota
Box 721-YMHC

Harvard St. at E. River Rd.
Minneapolis, MN 55455

National Child Abuse Hotline
(800) 422-4453
Box 630
Hollywood, CA 90028

National Child Safety Council
Childwatch
(800) 222-1464
P.O. Box 1368
Jackson, MI 49204

National Clearinghouse for Alcohol and Drug
Information
(800) SAY-NOTO (729-6686)
P.O. Box 2345
Rockville, MD 20852

National Cocaine Hotline
(800) 262-2463
P.O. Box 100
Summit, NJ 07902-0100

National Council on Alcoholism and Drug Dependent Hope-
line
(800) NCA-CALL (622-2255)
12 W. 21st St., Ste. 700
New York, NY 10010

National Council on Child Abuse and Family Violence
(800) 222-2000
1155 Connecticut Ave. NW, Ste. 300
Washington, DC 20036

National Council on the Aging
(800) 424-9046
409 3rd St. SW, 2nd Fl.
Washington, DC 20024

National Domestic Violence Hotline
Michigan Coalition Against Domestic Violence
(800) 333-SAFE (7233)
P.O. Box 463100
Mt. Clemens, MI 48043

National Down Syndrome Congress
(800) 232-NDSC (6372)
1800 Dempster St.
Park Ridge, IL 60068-1146

National Down Syndrome Society
(800) 221-4602
666 Broadway
New York, NY 10012

National Drug Information and Referral Line
National Institute on Drug Abuse
(800) 662-HELP (4357)
4635 Fishers Ln.
Rockville, MD 20852

National Easter Seal Society
(800) 221-6827
70 E. Lake St.
Chicago, IL 60601

National Eye Care Project
(800) 222-EYES (3937)
(Medical and surgical care for the elderly at no out-of-pocket ex-
pense)
P.O. Box 9688
San Francisco, CA 94101-9688

National Eye Research Foundation
(800) 621-2258
910 Skokie Blvd., #207A
Northbrook, IL 60062

National Fire Protection Association
(800) 344-3555
Battermarch Park
Quincy, MA 02269

National Foundation for Depressive Illness
(800) 248-4344
P.O. Box 2257
New York, NY 10116

National Head Injury Foundation
(800) 444-6443
1140 Connecticut Ave. NW, Ste. 812
Washington, DC 20036

National Headache Foundation
(800) 843-2256
5252 N. Western Ave.
Chicago, IL 60625

National Health Information Center
(800) 336-4797
P.O. Box 1133
Washington, DC 20013-1133

National Hearing Aid Society
Hearing Aid Helpline
(800) 521-5247
20361 Middlebelt Rd.
Livonia, MI 48152

National Highway Traffic Safety Administration
Auto Safety Hotline
(800) 424-9393
400 7th St. SW, Rm. 5319
Washington, DC 20590

National Hospice Organization
(800) 658-8898
1901 N. Moore St., Ste. 901
Arlington, VA 22209

National Information Center for Children and Youth with
Handicaps
(800) 999-5599
P.O. Box 1492
Washington, DC 20013

National Information Center for Orphan Drugs and Rare Dis-
eases
(800) 456-3505
P.O. Box 1133
Washington, DC 20013-1133

National Information Clearinghouse for Infants with Disabili-
ties and Life-Threatening Conditions
Center for Developmental Disabilities
(800) 922-9234
University of South Carolina
Benson Bldg., 1st Fl.
Columbia, SC 29208

National Information System for Health Related
Services
(800) 922-9234
(800) 922-1107 (within South Carolina)
University of South Carolina

Benson Bldg., 1st Fl.
Columbia, SC 29208

National Institute for Occupational Safety and Health (NIOSH)
(800) 356-4674
4676 Columbia Pkwy.
Cincinnati, OH 45226

National Jewish Center for Immunology and Respiratory Medicine
LUNGLINE
(800) 222-LUNG (5864)
1400 Jackson St.
Denver, CO 80206

National Kidney Foundation
(800) 622-9010
30 E. 33rd St.
New York, NY 10016

National Library Services for the Blind and Physically Handicapped
Library of Congress
(800) 424-8567
1291 Taylor St. NW
Washington, DC 20542

National Lymphedema Network
(800) 541-3259
2211 Post St., Ste. 404
San Francisco, CA 94115

National Mental Health Association
(800) 969-6642
1021 Prince St.
Alexandria, VA 22314-2971

National Multiple Sclerosis Society (NMSS)
(800) 642-8236
733 3rd Ave., 6th Fl.
New York, NY 10017

National Native American AIDS Prevention Center
Indian AIDS Hotline
(800) 283-AIDS
3515 Grand Ave., Ste. 100
Oakland, CA 94610

National Neurofibromatosis Foundation
(800) 323-7938
141 Fifth Ave., Ste. 7-S
New York, NY 10010

National Organization for Rare Disorders
(800) 999-6673
P.O. Box 8923
New Fairfield, CT 06812

National Organization on Disability (NOD)
(800) 248-ABLE (2253)
910 16th St. NW, Ste. 600
Washington, DC 20006

National Osteopathic Foundation (NOF)
(800) 621-1773
142 E. Ontario St.
Chicago, IL 60611

National Parents' Resource Institute for Drug Education (PRIDE)
(800) 677-7433
Hurt Bldg., #210

50 Hurt Plaza
Atlanta, GA 30303

National Parkinson Foundation
(800) 327-4545
(800) 433-7022 (within Florida)
1501 NW 9th Ave.
Miami, FL 33136

National Pesticide Telecommunications Network
(800) 858-7378
Texas Tech University
Thompson Hall, Rm. S129
Lubbock, TX 79430

National Reference Center for Bioethics Literature
Joseph and Rose Kennedy Institute of Ethics
(800) MED-ETHX (633-3849)
Georgetown University
Washington, DC 20057

National Rehabilitation Information Center
(800) 34-NARIC (346-2742)
8455 Colesville Rd., Ste. 935
Silver Spring, MD 20910

National Resource Center on Homelessness and Mental Illness
(800) 444-7415
262 Delaware Ave.
Delmar, NY 12054

National Retinitis Pigmentosa Foundation
(800) 638-2300
1401 Mount Royal Ave., 4th Fl.
Baltimore, MD 21217
(See also: R P Foundation Fighting Blindness)

National Reye's Syndrome Foundation, Inc
(800) 233-7393
(800) 231-7393 (within Ohio)
P.O. Box 829
Bryan, OH 43506

National Runaway Switchboard
(800) 621-4000
3080 N. Lincoln
Chicago, IL 60657
(See also: Metro-Help)

National STD Hotline
(800) 227-8922
(Sexually transmitted diseases)
Centers for Disease Control
Atlanta, GA 30333

National Safety Council
(800) 621-7619
444 N. Michigan Ave.
Chicago, IL 60611

National Second Surgical Opinion Program
(800) 638-6833
200 Independence Ave. SW
Washington, DC 20201

National Sheriffs' Association Aids Project
(800) 424-7827
1450 Duke St.
Alexandria, VA 22314

National Society to Prevent Blindness
(800) 221-3004
500 E. Remington Rd.
Schaumburg, IL 60173

National Spinal Cord Injury Association
(800) 962-9629
600 W. Cummings Park, Ste. 2000
Woburn, MA 01801

National Stroke Association
(800) 787-6537
300 E. Hampden Ave., Ste. 240
Englewood, CO 80110

National Sudden Infant Death Syndrome Foundation
(800) 221-SIDS (outside Maryland)
10500 Little Patuxent Pkwy., Ste. 420
Columbia, MD 21044

National Support Center for Persons with Disabilities
(800) 426-2133
P.O. Box 2150
Atlanta, GA 30301-2150

National Tuberous Sclerosis Association
(800) 225-6872
8000 Corporate Dr., Ste. 120
Landover, MD 20785

Nebraska Department of Health
AIDS Project Hotline
(800) 782-AIDS (within Nebraska)
3624 Leavenworth
Omaha, NE 68105

Nevada AIDS Hotline
Department of Human Resources
STD/HIV Program
(800) 842-AIDS (within Nevada)
505 E. King St., Rm. 104
Carson City, NV 89710

New England Headache Treatment Program
(800) 245-0088
778 Longridge Rd.
Stamford, CT 06902

New Hampshire Division of Public Health Services
Bureau of Disease Control, AIDS Program
(800) 752-AIDS (within New Hampshire)
6 Hazen Dr.
Concord, NH 03301-6527

New Hampshire Poison Information Center
(800) 562-8236 (within New Hampshire)
2 Maynard St.
Hanover, NH 03756

New Jersey Department of Health
AIDS Division
(800) 624-2377 (within New Jersey)
C.N. 360, 363 W. State St.
Trenton, NJ 08625

New Jersey Poison Information and Education System
(800) 962-1253 (within New Jersey)
201 Lyons Ave.
Newark, NJ 07112

New Mexico Agency on Aging
(800) 432-2080 (within New Mexico)
224 E. Palace Ave., 4th Fl.
Santa Fe, NM 87503

New Mexico Poison and Drug Information Center
(800) 432-6866 (within New Mexico)
University of New Mexico
2400 Marble St.
Albuquerque, NM 87131

New York State Department of Health
AIDS Institute
(800) 541-AIDS (within New York) (General Information)
(800) 872-2777 (HIV Counseling)
(800) 962-5065 (Confidentiality Law)
(800) 542-AIDS (Drug Assistance Program)
Corning Tower Bldg., Rm. 359
Empire State Plaza
Albany, NY 12237

New York State Office for the Aging
Senior Citizens' Hot Line
(800) 342-9871 (within New York)
Empire State Plaza
Agency Bldg. 2
Albany, NY 12223

North Carolina Department of Human Resources
CARELINE
(800) 662-7030 (within North Carolina)
325 N. Salisbury St.
Raleigh, NC 27611

North Dakota State Department of Health and
**   Consolidated Laboratories**
AIDS Program
(800) 472-2180 (within North Dakota)
State Capitol Bldg., 600 East Blvd.
Bismarck, ND 58505

North Texas Poison Center
Saint Vincent Health Center
(800) 822-3232 (within Pennsylvania, New York, Ohio)
232 W. 25th St.
Erie, PA 16544

Occupational Hearing Service
Dial A Hearing Screen Test
(800) 222-3277
(800) 345-3277 (within Pennsylvania)
P.O. Box 1880
Media, PA 19063

Office of Minority Health Resource Center
(800) 444-6472
P.O. Box 37337
Washington, DC 20013-7337

Ohio Department of Health
Ohio AIDS Hotline
(800) 332-AIDS (within Ohio)
1500 W. 3rd Ave., Ste. 329
Columbus, OH 43266-0588

Oklahoma Poison Control Center
Children's Hospital of Oklahoma
(800) 522-4611 (within Oklahoma)
940 NE 13th
Oklahoma City, OK 73126

Oklahoma State Health Department
Oklahoma AIDS Information Line
(800) 535-AIDS (within Oklahoma)
P.O. Box 53551
Oklahoma City, OK 73126

Open Quest Institute
(800) 444-9999
(Crisis intervention and substance abuse counseling)
309 S. Raymond
Pasadena, CA 91105

Oregon AIDS Hotline
(800) 777-AIDS (within Oregon)
408 SW 2nd, Ste. 412
Portland, OR 97204

Oregon Department of Human Services
Senior Citizens Division
(800) 232-3020 (within Oregon)
313 Public Service Bldg.
Portland, OR 97227

Oregon Drug and Alcohol Information Center
(800) 237-7808, Ext. 3673
(800) 452-7032 (within Oregon)
100 N. Cook
Portland, OR 97227

Oregon Poison Center
Oregon Health Sciences University
(800) 452-7165 (within Oregon)
3181 SW Sam Jackson Park Rd.
Portland, OR 97201

Orton Dyslexia Society
(800) ABCD-123 (outside Maryland)
724 York Rd.
Baltimore, MD 21204

PMS Access
(800) 22-4PMS
(Information on premenstrual syndrome)
P.O. Box 9326
Madison, WI 53715

Palmetto Poison Center
University of South Carolina College of Pharmacy
(800) 922-1117 (within South Carolina)
Columbia, SC 29208

Parents Anonymous (PA)
(800) 421-0353
(800) 352-0386 (within California)
6733 S. Sepulveda Blvd., Ste. 270
Los Angeles, CA 90045

Parkinson's Education Program USA
(800) 344-7872
3900 Birch St., Ste. 105
Newport Beach, CA 92660

Pennsylvania Department of Health
Bureau of HIV/AIDS Factline
AIDS Factline
(800) 662-6080 (within Pennsylvania)
P.O. Box 90
Harrisburg, PA 17108

Pennsylvania Department of Health
(800) 932-0912 (within Pennsylvania)
Health & Welfare Bldg., Rm. 929
6th and Commonwealth
Harrisburg, PA 17120
(See also: Encore)

People's Medical Society
(800) 624-8773
462 Walnut St.
Allentown, PA 18102

Plan International, USA
(800) 556-7918
(Foster Parents)
155 Plan Way
Warwick, RI 02886

Planned Parenthood Federation of America
(800) 829-7732
810 7th Ave.
New York, NY 10019

The Poison Center
Chidren's Memorial Hospital
(800) 955-9119 (within Nebraska)
(800) 228-9515 (surrounding states)
8301 Dodge St.
Omaha, NE 68114

Practitioner Reporter System
(800) 638-6725 (Defect reporting)
(Reporting of product defects)
12601 Twinbrook Pkwy.
Rockville, MD 20852

Pride Institute
(800) 54-PRIDE
(Addiction treatment center for gay and lesbian population)
14400 Martin Dr.
Eden Prairie, MN 55344

Project Inform
(800) 334-7422 (within California)
(800) 822-7422 (outside California)
(Information on experimental drugs for AIDS, ARC, and HIV infection)
1965 Market St., Ste. 220
San Francisco, CA 94103

R P Foundation Fighting Blindness
(800) 683-5555
1401 Mt. Royal Ave., 4th Fl.
Baltimore, MD 21217
(See also: National Retinitis Pigmentosa Foundation)

Recovery of Male Potency
(800) 835-7667
27211 Lahser Rd., Ste. 208
Southfield, MI 48034

Regional Poison Control System and Cincinnati Drug and Poison Information Center
University of Cincinnati Medical Center
(800) 872-5111 (within Ohio)
231 Bethesda Ave., M.L. 144
Cincinnati, OH 45267-0144

Rocky Mountain Poison and Drug Center
(800) 332-3073 (within Colorado)
(800) 525-5042 (within Montana)
(800) 442-2702 (within Wyoming)
645 Bannock St.
Denver, CO 80204-4507

Runaway Hotline
(800) 231-6946
(800) 392-3552 (within Texas)
P.O. Box 12428

Austin, TX 78711
(See also: Metro-Help, National Runaway Switchboard)

Saginaw Regional Poison Center
(800) 451-4585 (within Michigan)
Saginaw General Hospital
1447 N. Harrison St.
Saginaw, MI 48602

St. John's Hospital Regional Poison Resource Center for Central and Southern Illinois
(800) 252-2022 (within Illinois)
800 E. Carpenter St.
Springfield, IL 62769

St. Luke's Poison Center
St. Luke's Regional Medical Center
(800) 352-2222 (within Iowa, Nebraska, South Dakota)
2720 Stone Park Blvd.
Sioux City, IA 51104

San Diego Regional Poison Center
(800) 876-4766 (regional)
UC San Diego Medical Center
225 Dickinson St., H-925
San Diego, CA 92103-1990

San Francisco AIDS Foundation
(800) 367-2437 (within Northern California)
P.O. Box 6182
25 Van Ness Ave., Ste. 660
San Francisco, CA 94102-6182

San Francisco Bay Area Regional Poison Control Center
San Francisco General Hospital
(800) 523-2222 (regional)
1001 Potrero Ave., Rm. 1E86
San Francisco, CA 94110

Santa Clara Valley Medical Center Regional Poison Center
(800) 662-9886 (within California)
751 S. Bascom Ave.
San Jose, CA 95128

Schuy/Line
Schuyler Self-Help Clearinghouse
(800) 348-0448 (within New York)
425 Pennsylvania Ave.
Elmira, NY 14904

Seattle Poison Center
Children's Hospital and Medical Center
(800) 732-6985 (within Washington)
4800 Sand Point Way NE
P.O. Box C5371
Seattle, WA 98105-0371

Shriners Hospital Referral Line
(800) 237-5055
(Free orthopedic or burn care for children)
2900 Rocky Point Dr.
Tampa, FL 33607

Simon Foundation
(800) 237-4666
(Incontinence information)
P.O. Box 815
Wilmette, IL 60091

South Carolina Department of Health
AIDS Project
(800) 322-AIDS (within South Carolina)

2600 Bull St.
Columbia, SC 29201

South Dakota Department of Health
AIDS Hotline
(800) 592-1861 (within South Dakota)
523 E. Capital
Pierre, SD 57501

Spina Bifida Association of America
(800) 621-3141
1700 Rockville Pike, Ste. 250
Rockville, MD 20852

Spinal Cord Injury Hotline
(800) 526-3456
2201 Argonne Dr.
Baltimore, MD 21218

Spokane Poison Center
(800) 572-5842 (within Washington and N. Idaho)
711 S. Cowley
Spokane, WA 99202

Stark County Poison Control Center
Timken Mercy Medical Center
(800) 722-8662 (within Ohio)
1320 Timken Mercy Dr.
Canton, OH 44708

Sturge-Weber Foundation
(800) 627-5482
P.O. Box 460931
Aurora, CO 80046

Susquehanna Poison Center
Geisinger Medical Center
(800) 352-7001 (within Pennsylvania)
N. Academy Ave.
Danville, PA 17822-2005

Tennessee Department of Health and Environment
(800) 342-3145 (within Tennessee)
(Medicaid information)
344 Cordell Hull Bldg.
Nashville, TN 37247-0101

Tennessee Department of Health and Environment
State AIDS Hotline
(800) 525-AIDS (within Tennessee)
C2-221 Cordell Hull Bldg.
Nashville, TN 37247-4947

Terri Gotthelf Lupus Research Institute
(800) 82-LUPUS (825-8787)
3 Duke Pl.
South Norwalk, CT 06854

Texas State Poison Center
(800) 392-8548
University of Texas Medical Branch
Clinical Science Bldg., Rm. 1202
Galveston, TX 77550-2780

Tourette Syndrome Association (TSA)
(800) 237-0717
42-40 Bell Blvd.
Bayside, NY 11361

Triad Poison Center
Moses H. Cone Memorial Hospital
(800) 722-2222 (within North Carolina)
1200 N. Elm St.
Greensboro, NC 27401-1020

Tripod Grapevine
(800) 352-8888
(800) 287-4763 (within California)
(Hearing-impaired children)
2901 N. Keystone St.
Burbank, CA 91504

UC Davis Medical Center
Regional Poison Control Center
(800) 342-9293 (within Northern California)
2315 Stockton Blvd., Rm. 1151
Sacramento, CA 95817

UC Irvine Regional Poison Center
(800) 544-4404 (within Southern California)
UC Irvine Medical Center
101 The City Dr., Rte. 78
Orange, CA 92668-3298

U.S. Department of Health and Human Services
Social Security Administration
(800) 234-5SSA (5772)
6401 Security Blvd.
Baltimore, MD 21235

United Cerebral Palsy Association, Inc.
(800) USA-1UCP (872-1827)
7 Penn Plaza, Ste. 804
New York, NY 10001

United Network for Organ Sharing (UNOS)
(800) 24-DONOR (243-6667)
P.O. Box 13770
Richmond, VA 23225

United Scleroderma Foundation
(800) 722-4673
P.O. Box 399
Watsonville, CA 95077-0399

Utah Department of Health
AIDS Information and Referral Line
(800) 537-1046 (within Utah)
288 North 1460 West
P.O. Box 16660
Salt Lake City, UT 84116

Variety Club Poison and Drug Information Center
Iowa Methodist Medical Center
(800) 362-2327 (within Iowa)
1200 Pleasant St.
Des Moines, IA 50309

Vermont Department of Health
(800) 464-4343 (within Vermont)
60 Main St.
P.O. Box 70
Burlington, VT 05402

Vermont Department of Health
AIDS Education
(800) 882-AIDS (within Vermont)
60 Main St.
P.O. Box 70
Burlington, VT 05402

Virginia Department for the Aging
(800) 552-4464 (within Virginia)
700 E. Franklin St., 10th Fl.
Richmond, VA 23219-2327

Virginia Department of Health
Bureau of STD/AIDS

(800) 533-4148 (within Virginia)
P.O. Box 2448
Richmond, VA 23218

Virginia Poison Center
Virginia Commonwealth University
(800) 552-6337 (within Virginia and TDD)
Box 522 MCV Station
Richmond, VA 23298-0522

Vision Foundation, Inc.
(800) 852-3029 (within Massachusetts)
818 Mt. Auburn St.
Watertown, MA 02172

Visiting Nurse Association of America
(800) 426-2547
3801 E. Florida Ave., Ste. 206
Denver, CO 80210

Washington State Department of Health
Health Promotion and Chronic Disease Prevention
Office of Prevention and Education Services
(800) 272-AIDS (within Washington)
Airdustrial Park, Bldg. 9
Olympia, WA 98504

West Virginia Department of Health
State AIDS Hotline
(800) 642-8244 (within West Virginia)
1422 Washington St. E
Charleston, WV 25301

West Virginia Poison Center
West Virginia University School of Pharmacy
(800) 642-3625 (within West Virginia)
3110 MacCorkle Ave., SE
Charleston, WV 25304

West Virginia University
West Virginia Rehabilitation Research Training Center
(800) 624-8284
1 Dunbar Plaza, Ste. E
Dunbar, WV 25064

West Virginia University School of Pharmacy
Drug Information Center
(800) 352-2501 (within West Virginia)
Morgantown, WV 26506

Western New York Regional Poison Control Center
Children's Hospital of Buffalo
(800) 888-7655 (within New York and western Pennsylvania)
219 Bryant St.
Buffalo, NY 14222

Western Ohio Regional Poison and Drug Information Center
Children's Medical Center
(800) 762-0727 (within Ohio)
1 Children's Plaza
Dayton, OH 45404

Wisconsin Clearinghouse
(Drug and alcohol prevention materials)
(800) 322-1468
University of Wisconsin
P.O. Box 1468
Madison, WI 57301-1468

Wisconsin Department of Health and Social Services
AIDS Program
(800) 334-AIDS (within Wisconsin)
1 W. Wilson St.

P.O. Box 309
Madison, WI 53701

Women's Sports Foundation
Information and Referral Service
(800) 227-3988
342 Madison Ave., Ste. 728
New York, NY 10173

Wyoming Department of Health
Division on Aging
(800) 442-2766 (within Wyoming)
Hathaway Bldg.
Cheyenne, WY 82002

Wyoming HIV/AIDS Prevention Program
(800) 327-3577 (within Wyoming)
Hathaway Bldg.
Cheyenne, WY 82002

YMCA of the USA
(800) USA-YMCA (872-9622)
101 N. Wacker
Chicago, IL 60606

Y-Me Breast Cancer Support Program
(800) 221-2141 (9-5 Central Time)
18220 Harwood Ave.
Homewood, IL 60430

■ Document Source:
   U.S. Department of Health and Human Services, Public Health
   Service
   National Institutes of Health
   National Library of Medicine
   NIH Publication No. 92-2780
   January 1992

APPENDIX C
STATE AGENCIES ON AGING

■ ■ ■

Alabama
Executive Director
Alabama Commission on Aging
770 Washington Avenue, Suite 470
RSA Plaza
Montgomery, Alabama 36130
(205) 242-5743

Alaska
Executive Director
Older Alaskans Commission
P.O. Box C, MS 0209
Juneau, Alaska
(907) 465-3250

American Samoa
Director
Territorial Administration on Aging
Government of American Samoa
Pago Pago, American Samoa 96799
(684) 633-1251

Arizona
Administrator
Aging and Adult Administration
Department of Economic Security
1789 West Jefferson—950A
Phoenix, Arizona 85007
(602) 542-4446
*1-(800) 352-3792

Arkansas
Deputy Director
Division of Aging and Adult Services
Arkansas Department of Human Services
Main & 7th Streets
Donaghey Building, Suite 1428
Little Rock, Arkansas 72301
(501) 682-2441

California
Director
California Department of Aging
1600 K Street
Sacramento, California 95814
(916) 322-5290

Colorado
Director
Aging and Adult Services
Department of Social Services

1575 Sherman Street, 10th Floor
Denver, CO 80203-1714
(303) 866-5905

Commonwealth of the Northern Mariana Islands
Administrator
Office on Aging
Department of Community and Cultural Affairs
Civic Center
Saipan, Mariana Islands 96950
(670) 234-6011

Connecticut
Commissioner
Connecticut Department on Aging
175 Main Street
Hartford, Connecticut 06106
(203) 566-3238
*1-(800) 443-9946

Delaware
Director
Delaware Division on Aging
Department of Health and Human Services
1901 North Dupont Highway—Second Floor
New Castle, Delaware 19720
(302) 577-4791
*1-(800) 223-9074

District of Columbia
Executive Director
District of Columbia Office on Aging
Executive Office of the Mayor
1424 K Street, N.W., Second Floor
Washington, D.C. 20005
(202) 724-5622

Florida
Secretary
Florida Department of Elder Affairs
Building 1—Room 317
1317 Winewood Boulevard
Tallahassee, Florida 32399-0700
(904) 922-5297
1-(800) 342-0825

Georgia
Director
Office of Aging
Department of Human Resources
Sixth Floor

*In-State Toll-Free Number

878 Peachtree Street, N.E.
Atlanta, Georgia 30309
(404) 894-5333

Guam
Administrator
Division of Senior Citizens
Department of Public Health and Social Services
P.O. Box 2816
Government of Guam
Agana, Guam 96910
(671) 734-2942

Hawaii
Executive Director
Hawaii Executive Office on Aging
335 Merchant Street, Room 241
Honolulu, Hawaii 96813
(808) 548-0100

Idaho
Director
Idaho Office on Aging
Statehouse, Room 108
Boise, Idaho 83720
(208) 334-3833

Illinois
Director
Illinois Department of Aging
421 East Capitol Avenue
Springfield, Illinois 62701
(217) 785-2870
1-(800) 252-8966

Indiana
Commissioner
Indiana Department of Human Services
251 North Illinois Street
P.O. Box 7083
Indianapolis, Indiana 46207-7083
(317) 232-1139
1-(800) 545-7763

Iowa
Executive Director
Department of Elder Affairs
Jewett Building, Suite 236
914 Grand Avenue
Des Moines, Iowa 50319
(515) 281-5187
1-(800) 532-3213

Kansas
Secretary
Kansas Department of Aging
Docking State Office Building, 122-S
915 S.W. Harrison
Topeka, Kansas 66612-1500
(913) 296-4986
1-(800) 432-3535

Kentucky
Director
Division for Aging Services
Cabinet for Human Resources
Department for Social Services
275 East Main Street
Frankfort, Kentucky 40621
(502) 564-6930

Louisiana
Director
Governor's Office of Elderly Affairs
P.O. Box 80374
Baton Rouge, Louisiana 70898-0374
(504) 925-1700

Maine
Director
Bureau of Maine's Elderly
Department of Human Services
State House—Station 11
Augusta, Maine 04333
(207) 626-5335

Maryland
Director
Maryland Office on Aging
301 West Preston Street
Baltimore, Maryland 21201
(301) 225-1102
*1-(800) 338-0153

Massachusetts
Secretary
Massachusetts Executive Office of Elder Affairs
38 Chauncy Street
Boston, Massachusetts 02111
(617) 727-7750
*1-(800) 882-2003

Michigan
Director
Office of Services to the Aging
P.O. Box 30026
Lansing, Michigan 48909
(517) 373-8230

Minnesota
Executive Secretary
Minnesota Board on Aging
444 Lafayette Road, 4th Floor
St. Paul, Minnesota 55155-3843
(612) 296-2770
*1-(800) 652-9747

Mississippi
Director
Council on Aging
Division of Aging and Adult Services
421 West Pascagoula Street
Jackson, Mississippi 39203
(601) 949-2070
*1-(800) 222-7622

Missouri
Director
Division of Aging
Department of Social Services
2701 W. Main Street, P.O. Box 1337
Jefferson City, Missouri 65102
(314) 751-3082
*1-(800) 235-5503

Montana
Coordinator
Governor's Office of Aging
Capitol Station, Room 219
Helena, Montana 59620
(406) 444-3111
*1-(800) 332-2272

*In-State Toll-Free Number

Nebraska
Director
Department on Aging
301 Centennial Mall South
P.O. Box 95044
Lincoln, Nebraska 68509
(402) 471-2306

Nevada
Administrator
Division for Aging Services
State Mail Room
Las Vegas, Nevada 89158
(702) 486-3545

New Hampshire
Director
Division of Elderly and Adult Services
New Hampshire Department of Health and Human
    Services
6 Hazen Drive
Concord, New Hampshire 03301
(603) 271-4390
*1-(800) 852-3311

New Jersey
Director
New Jersey Division on Aging
Department of Community Affairs
101 South Broad Street—CN 807
Trenton, New Jersey 08625-0807
(609) 292-0920
*1-(800) 792-8820

New Mexico
Director
New Mexico State Agency on Aging
La Villa Rivera Building, 4th Floor
224 East Palace Avenue
Santa Fe, New Mexico 87501
(505) 827-7640
*1-(800) 432-2080

New York
Director
New York State Office for the Aging
Agency Building #2, Empire State Plaza
Albany, New York 12223-0001
(518) 474-5731
*1-(800) 342-9871

North Carolina
Director
North Carolina Division on Aging
Department of Human Resources
Kirby Building
1985 Umstead Drive
Raleigh, North Carolina 27603
(919) 733-3983
*1-(800) 722-7030

North Dakota
Director
Aging Services Division
North Dakota Department of Human Services
State Capitol Building
Bismarck, North Dakota 58505
(701) 224-2577
*1-(800) 472-2622

Ohio
Director

Ohio Department of Aging
50 West Broad Street—9th Floor
Columbus, Ohio 43215
(614) 466-5500

Oklahoma
Division Administrator
Aging Services Division
Department of Human Services
P.O. Box 25352
Oklahoma City, Oklahoma 73125
(405) 521-2327

Oregon
Administrator
Senior and Disabled Services Division
Department of Human Resources
313 Public Service Building
Salem, Oregon 97310
(503) 378-4728

Pennsylvania
Secretary
Pennsylvania Department of Aging
231 State Street (Barto Building)
Harrisburg, Pennsylvania 17101
(717) 783-1550

Puerto Rico
Executive Director
Puerto Rico Office of Elderly Affairs
Call Box 50063
Old San Juan Station, Puerto Rico 00902
(809) 721-0753

Republic of Palau
Director
State Agency on Aging
Department of Social Services
Republic of Palau
Koror, Palau 96940

Rhode Island
Director
Department of Elderly Affairs
160 Pine Street
Providence, Rhode Island 02903
(401) 277-2858
*1-(800) 752-8088

South Carolina
Executive Director
South Carolina Commission on Aging
400 Arbor Lake Drive, Suite B-500
Columbia, South Carolina 29223
(803) 735-0210
*1-(800) 922-1107

South Dakota
Administrator
Office of Adult Services and Aging
Richard F. Kneip Building
700 Governors Drive
Pierre, South Dakota 57501-2291
(605) 773-3656

Tennessee
Executive Director
Tennessee Commission on Aging
706 Church Street, Suite 201
Nashville, Tennessee 37219-5573
(615) 741-2056

*In-State Toll-Free Number

Texas
Executive Director
Texas Department on Aging
P.O. Box 12786
Capitol Station
Austin, Texas 78711
(512) 444-2727
*1-(800) 252-9240

Utah
Director
Utah Division of Aging & Adult Services
120 North 200 West, Room 4A
P.O. Box 45500
Salt Lake City, Utah 84145-0500
(801) 538-3910

Vermont
Commissioner
Department of Rehabilitation and Aging
103 S. Main Street
Waterbury, Vermont 05676
(802) 241-2400
*1-(800) 642-5119

Virgin Islands
Commissioner
Virgin Islands Department of Human Services
Barbel Plaza South
Charlotte Amalie
St. Thomas, Virgin Islands 00802
(809) 774-0930

Virginia
Commissioner
Virginia Department for the Aging
700 East Franklin Street—10th Floor
Richmond, Virginia 23219-2327

(804) 225-2271
*1-(800) 552-4464

Washington
Assistant Secretary
Aging and Adult Services Administration
Department of Social and Health Services
Mail Stop OB-44-A
Olympia, Washington 98504
(206) 586-3768
*1-(800) 422-3263

West Virginia
Executive Director
West Virginia Commission on Aging
State Capitol Complex—Holly Grove
1900 Kanawha Boulevard East
Charleston, West Virginia 25305-0160
(304) 558-3317
*1-(800) 642-3671

Wisconsin
Director
Bureau on Aging
Department of Health and Social Services
Room 480
1 West Wilson Street
P.O. Box 7851
Madison, Wisconsin 53707
(608) 266-2536

Wyoming
Administrator
Commission on Aging
Hathaway Building, 1st Floor
Cheyenne, Wyoming 82002
(307) 777-7986

*In-State Toll-Free Number

TITLE INDEX

■ ■ ■

SUBJECT INDEX

■ ■ ■

by Kay Banning